Medical Language
For Modern Health Care

Fifth Edition

Rachel C. Basco, MS, RRT
Bossier Parish Community College

Rhonna Krouse-Adams, MS
College of Western Idaho

David M. Allan, MA, MD

Mc
Graw
Hill

MEDICAL LANGUAGE FOR MODERN HEALTH CARE, FIFTH EDITION

1 2 3 4 5 6 7 8 9 LMN 27 26 25 24 23 22

ISBN 978-1-260-01794-6 (bound edition)
MHID 1-260-01794-X (bound edition)
ISBN 978-1-264-11115-2 (loose-leaf edition)
MHID 1-264-11115-0 (loose-leaf edition)

Portfolio Manager: *Marah Bellegarde*
Product Developers: *Erin DeHeck, Joan Weber*
Marketing Manager: *Jim Connely*
Content Project Managers: *Jeni McAtee, Brent dela Cruz*
Buyer: *Susan K. Culbertson*
Designer: *David Hash*
Content Licensing Specialist: *Beth Cray*
Cover Image: *Shutterstock/Liya Graphics*
Compositor: *Straive*

Library of Congress Cataloging-in-Publication Data
Names: Basco, Rachel C., author. | Krouse-Adams, Rhonna, author.
Title: Medical language for modern health care / Rachel C. Basco, MS, RRT,
    Bossier Parish Community College, Rhonna Krouse-Adams, MS, College of
    Western Idaho.
Description: Fifth edition. | New York, NY : McGraw-Hill Education, [2023]
    | Revised edition of: Medical language for modern health care / David M.
    Allan, MA, MD, Rachel C. Basco, MS, RRT, Bossier Parish Community
    College. 2019. Fourth edition. | Audience: Ages 18+
Identifiers: LCCN 2021045788 (print) | LCCN 2021045789 (ebook) | ISBN
    9781260017946 (paperback) | ISBN 9781264111190 (ebook)
Subjects: LCSH: Medicine—Terminology—Programmed instruction.
Classification: LCC R123 .A43 2023 (print) | LCC R123 (ebook) | DDC
    610.1/4—dc23/eng/20211001
LC record available at https://lccn.loc.gov/2021045788
LC ebook record available at https://lccn.loc.gov/2021045789

Rachel Curran Basco

Rachel Basco earned her BS in Cardiopulmonary Science and MS in Health Sciences from Louisiana State University Health Science Center, School of Allied Health Professions. She worked as a registered respiratory therapist for 10 years and then began her career in college instruction in respiratory therapy at LSU-SAHP in Shreveport, LA. She is an Assistant Professor at Bossier Parish Community College in Bossier City, LA . She instructs medical terminology and anatomy & physiology courses.

Rachel resides in Shreveport with her husband and always finds time to visit her relatives in Colorado, Texas, and her home state of Wisconsin.

Rhonna Krouse-Adams

Rhonna Krouse-Adams is an Associate Professor in the department of Health Sciences at the College of Western Idaho. She received a MS from Boise State University. In 2009. Rhonna was provided the unique opportunity to be a founding member of a brand-new community college that opened in 2010. There she was able to build the Health Science Department and a nationally recognized Public Health degree. Presently, Rhonna serves as the curriculum developer for both the health science and public health programs and developing educational content for her school and others. Her present project is with the League of Innovation, CDC, AHA developing CEC modules for health care workers on infectious disease.

David Allan

David Allan received his medical training at Cambridge University and Guy's Hospital in England. He was Chief Resident in Pediatrics at Bellevue Hospital in New York City before moving to San Diego, California.

Dr. Allan has worked as a family physician in England, a pediatrician in San Diego, and Associate Dean at the University of California, San Diego School of Medicine. He has designed, written, and produced more than 100 award-winning multimedia programs with virtual reality as their conceptual base. Dr. Allan resides happily in San Diego and enjoys the warmth of the people, the weather, and the beaches.

BRIEF CONTENTS

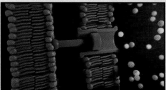
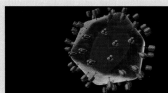
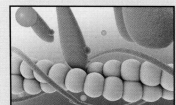
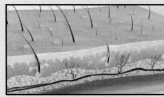

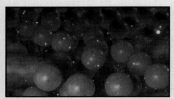
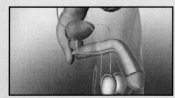
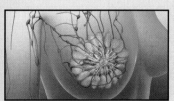
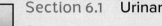

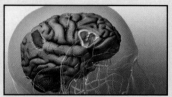
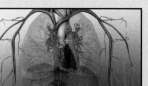
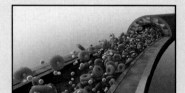
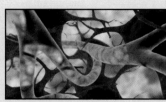

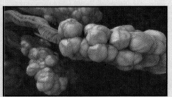
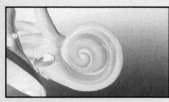

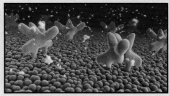
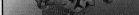
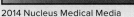
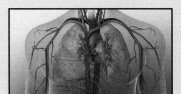

CHAPTER 22 Pharmacology: *The Language of Pharmacology* 698

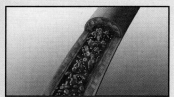

2014 Nucleus Medical Media

We wish to acknowledge with great appreciation the most valuable contributions that Karen Lockyer, BA, RHIT, CPC, made to the first three editions of this book. Karen's expertise and knowledge were intrinsic to the foundation of the book's approach. The text wouldn't be what it has become without her involvement. We would also like to thank Michele Kaufman, PharmD, BCGP for her contributions and assistance with Chapter 22: Pharmacology.

Thank you as well to the extraordinary efforts of a talented group of individuals at McGraw Hill Education who made this textbook and its ancillaries come together: Portfolio Director, Michelle Vogler; Portfolio Manager, Marah Bellegarde; Product Developer, Erin DeHeck; Marketing Manager, Jim Connely; SmartBook Product Developer, Joan Weber; Project Managers, Jeni McAtee and Brent dela Cruz; Designer, David Hash; and Content Licensing Specialist, Beth Cray.

We would like to recognize the valuable contributions of those who helped guide our developmental decisions with their insightful reviews and suggestions:

Fifth Edition Reviewers

Hiren Darji
Ancora Education

Tim Gilmore
Louisiana State University

Barbara Goldman
Palm Beach State College

Michael D. Gruich
Stark State Colllege

Dr. Shahin Kanani
Seminole State College of Florida

Dr. Kristine N. Kraft
University of Akron

Kren McManus
North Hennepin Community College

Sean F. Peck
Arizona Western College

Shari Smith
McCann School of Business and Technology

Cheryl Travelstead
Tidewater Community College

Danette Vercher
Ancora Education

Medical terminology is not just another subject for which you memorize the facts and then forget them when you move on to your next course. Medical language will be used throughout your studies, as well as every day on your job. Health care professionals use specific terms to describe and talk about objects and situations they encounter each day.

Like every language, medical terminology changes constantly as new knowledge is discovered. Modern medical terminology is a language constructed over centuries, using words and elements from Greek and Latin origins as its building blocks. Some 15,000 or more words are formed from 1,200 Greek and Latin roots. It serves as an international language, enabling medical scientists from different countries and in different medical fields to communicate with a common understanding.

In your world as a health care professional, medical terminology enables you to communicate with your team leader, with other health care professionals on your team, and with other professionals in different disciplines outside your team. Understanding medical terminology also enables you to translate the medical terms into language your patients can understand, thus improving the quality of their care and demonstrating your professionalism. Your understanding of medical terminology will make you a successful student and health professional.

ORGANIZATION OF CONTENT

In this new edition, chapters have been organized for consistency and continuity to enhance student retention. For all major organ systems, the chapters will be placed in sections and will begin with an overview of the anatomy and physiology of the system. The following section will cover the common pathology associated with that organ system. The final sections will cover diagnostic and therapeutic procedures along with pharmacology. Each chapter is structured around a consistent and unique framework of learning devices including illustrations, Word Analysis and Definition (WAD) tables, and end-of-section Checkpoints. Regardless of the organ system being covered, the structure enables you to develop a consistent learning strategy, making the fifth edition of Medical Language For Modern Health Care a superior learning tool.

Word Analysis and Definition Boxes and Case Reports

The medical terms covered in each lesson are introduced in context and then to facilitate easy reference and review, the terms also are listed in boxes as a group. The **Word Analysis and Definition (WAD) boxes** list the term and its pronunciation, elements, and definition in a concise, color-coded, at-a-glance format. **Case Reports** can be found within Checkpoints and Chapter-End exercises providing the students opportunities to apply and reinforce their knowledge of medical terms.

Section and Chapter-End Exercises

Each section ends with exercises designed to allow you to check your basic understanding of the terms you just learned. These checkpoints can be used by instructors as assignments or in-class activities or by students for self-evaluation.

At the end of each chapter, you will find chapter review of exercises that ask you to apply what you learned in all the lessons of a chapter. These exercises reinforce learning of each chapter's terms and help you go beyond mere memorization to think critically about the medical language you use. In addition to reviewing and recalling the definitions of terms learned in the chapter, you will be asked to use medical terms in new and different ways.

Additional Learning Tools

Did you know? boxes appear throughout each chapter and provide additional interesting pieces of information that related to the chapter content. Each chapter also includes an abbreviation table and a Disorder or Disease table.

NEW TO THE FIFTH EDITION:

- Learning outcomes have been streamlined for each chapter for easy organization and assessment.
- Every chapter has been reorganized into sections that are consistent across all chapters.
- Chapters have been updated with the latest trends in medicine, including COVID-19.
- The case studies have been enhanced to support practical application of the terms learned.
- Pronunciation questions have been added to each chapter to develop effective communication.
- Multiple new activities have been added to the instructor manual to enhance in-person and online learning.

NEW TO CONNECT WITH THE FIFTH EDITION:

- All Connect questions are now tagged to CAAHEP and ABHES requirements for easy assessment and reporting for accreditation.
- All new activities were added to support medical terminology fundamentals for each organ system.
- New Application-Based Activities bring pathology to life for your students.

INSTRUCTOR RESOURCES

The following materials are available to help you and your students work through the material in the book; all are available in the Instructor Resources under the Library tab in Connect (available only to instructors who are logged in to Connect).

- Instructor's Manual
- PowerPoint Presentation
- Answer Keys
- Test Bank

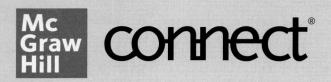

Instructors: Student Success Starts with You

Tools to enhance your unique voice

Want to build your own course? No problem. Prefer to use an OLC-aligned, prebuilt course? Easy. Want to make changes throughout the semester? Sure. And you'll save time with Connect's auto-grading too.

65%
Less Time Grading

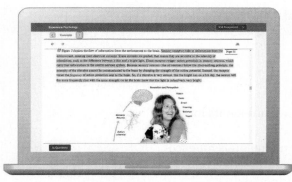

Laptop: McGraw Hill; Woman/dog: George Doyle/Getty Images

Study made personal

Incorporate adaptive study resources like SmartBook® 2.0 into your course and help your students be better prepared in less time. Learn more about the powerful personalized learning experience available in SmartBook 2.0 at **www.mheducation.com/highered/connect/smartbook**

Affordable solutions, added value

Make technology work for you with LMS integration for single sign-on access, mobile access to the digital textbook, and reports to quickly show you how each of your students is doing. And with our Inclusive Access program you can provide all these tools at a discount to your students. Ask your McGraw Hill representative for more information.

Padlock: Jobalou/Getty Images

Solutions for your challenges

A product isn't a solution. Real solutions are affordable, reliable, and come with training and ongoing support when you need it and how you want it. Visit **www.supportateverystep.com** for videos and resources both you and your students can use throughout the semester.

Checkmark: Jobalou/Getty Images

Students: Get Learning that Fits You

Effective tools for efficient studying

Connect is designed to help you be more productive with simple, flexible, intuitive tools that maximize your study time and meet your individual learning needs. Get learning that works for you with Connect.

Study anytime, anywhere

Download the free ReadAnywhere app and access your online eBook, SmartBook 2.0, or Adaptive Learning Assignments when it's convenient, even if you're offline. And since the app automatically syncs with your Connect account, all of your work is available every time you open it. Find out more at **www.mheducation.com/readanywhere**

> *"I really liked this app—it made it easy to study when you don't have your textbook in front of you."*
>
> - Jordan Cunningham, Eastern Washington University

Calendar: owattaphotos/Getty Images

Everything you need in one place

Your Connect course has everything you need—whether reading on your digital eBook or completing assignments for class, Connect makes it easy to get your work done.

Learning for everyone

McGraw Hill works directly with Accessibility Services Departments and faculty to meet the learning needs of all students. Please contact your Accessibility Services Office and ask them to email accessibility@mheducation.com, or visit **www.mheducation.com/about/accessibility** for more information.

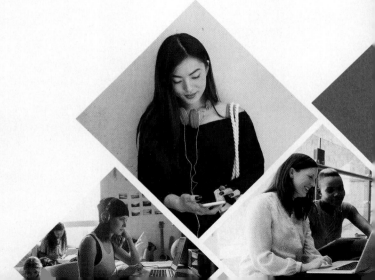

Top: Jenner Images/Getty Images, Left: Hero Images/Getty Images, Right: Hero Images/Getty Images

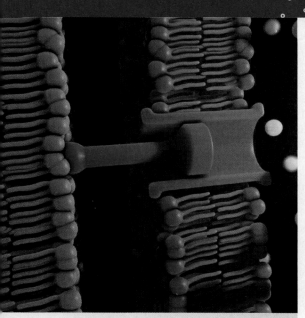

Nucleus Medical Media

1

The Anatomy of Medical Terms
The Foundation of Medical Language

Chapter Learning Outcomes

LO 1.1 Identify and utilize the roots and combining forms to form medical terms.

LO 1.2 Identify and utilize suffixes and prefixes to build medical terms.

LO 1.3 Recognize medical terms taken directly from Greek, Latin, or Old English words.

LO 1.4 Differentiate between medical terms that are spelled and/or pronounced similarly.

The technical language of medicine has been developed logically from Latin and Greek roots because it is in Latin and Greek cultures that the concept of treating patients began. This medical language provides all the health professionals involved in the care of a patient with the ability to communicate with each other by using medical terms with precise meanings. To be a qualified health professional it is necessary to be able to speak the language of medicine.

Medical terms are built from individual parts, or elements, that form the anatomy of the word. Upon completion of this chapter, you will be able to.

The Logic of Medical Terminology

Understanding and being comfortable with the technical language of medicine are keys to a successful career as a health professional. Your ability to use and understand the technical language to communicate verbally and in writing are essential for patient safety, high-quality patient care, precise interaction with other health professionals, and your own self-esteem as a health professional.

Your confidence in using medical terms will increase as you understand the logic of how each term is built from its individual parts, or elements. In addition, understanding the logic of this process will help you analyze or deconstruct an unknown medical term and break it down into its elements so that its meaning can be understood.

The **elements** of a medical term are its **roots**, **suffixes**, and **prefixes**, and the vast majority of these elements are derived from Latin and Greek origins. Throughout this book, when words are broken down, the elements will be color coded.

Throughout this book, look for the following patterns:

- **Roots**, **combining forms**, and **combining vowels** will be colored **pink**.
- **Prefixes** will be colored **green** and come before the root.
- **Suffixes** will be colored **blue** and come after the root.

This will be discussed in greater length.

Roots

Every medical term has a **root**—the element that provides the core meaning of the word. A **root** is the constant foundation and core of a medical term.

- **Roots** are usually of Greek or Latin origin.
- All medical terms have one or more **roots**.
- A **root** can appear anywhere in the term.
- More than one **root** can have the same meaning.
- A **root** plus a **combining vowel** creates a **combining form**.
- The word *pneumonia* has the **root** *pneumon-*, taken from the Greek word meaning *lung* or *air*. The Greek **root** *pneum-* also means lung or air. *Pneumonia* is an infection of the lung tissue.
- The **root** *pulmon-* is taken from the Latin word meaning *lung*. A *pulmonologist* is a specialist who treats lung diseases.

Combining Forms

Roots are often joined to other elements in a medical term by adding a **combining vowel**, such as the letter "o," to the end of the **root**, like *pneum-*, to form pneum/o-.

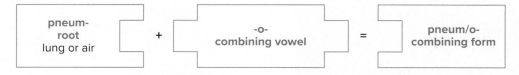

Throughout this book, whenever a term is presented, a **slash** (/) will be used to separate the combining vowel from the **root**. Other examples of this approach are as follows:

- Adding the **combining vowel** "o" to the Latin **root** *pulmon-* makes the **combining form** *pulmon/o-*.

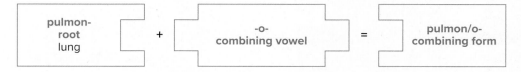

Any vowel, "a," "e," "i," "o," or "u," can be used as a **combining vowel**.

- The root *respir-* means *to breathe*. Adding the combining vowel "a" makes the combining form *respir/a-*.

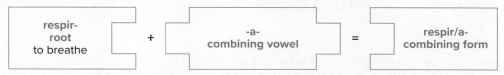

- The root *bronch-* is derived from the Greek word for *windpipe* and is one of the two subdivisions of the trachea that carry air to and from the lungs. Adding the combining vowel "o" to the root *bronch-* makes the combining form *bronch/o-*.

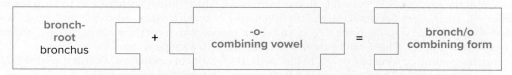

Many medical terms contain more than one root; when two roots occur together, they are always joined by a combining vowel, as in the following example:

- The word **hemopneumothorax** has the root *hem-*, from the Greek word meaning *blood*; the root *pneum-*, from the Greek word meaning *air* or *lung*; and the suffix -thorax, from the Greek word meaning *chest*. The combining vowel "o" is added to these two roots to make the combining forms *hem/o* and *pneum/o-*. A combining vowel is used to join a root (*pneum-*) to a suffix that begins with a consonant (-thorax). A **hemopneumothorax** is the presence of air and blood in the space that surrounds the lungs in the chest. As blood and air fill the pleural cavity, the lungs cannot expand and respiration is not possible, thus forcing the affected lung to collapse.

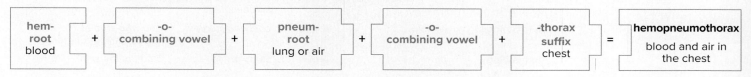

- Different roots can have the same meaning. *Pulmon-* and *pneumon-* both mean *lung, air.*

Check Point Section 1.1

A. Review what you have just learned about roots and combining forms. *Select the correct answer to the statement.* **LO 1.1, 1.2**

root   combining form   combining vowel   suffix   prefix

1. Roots and combining forms can go before a _____.

2. This element does not have a meaning; it serves to make the word easier to pronounce: _____.

3. A _____ can go before a root.

4. The _____ is the root plus a combining vowel.

B. Identify the word parts of a medical term. *Use the provided medical term to correctly answer the questions.* **LO 1.1**

1. In the word **pneumonia,** the root is:
   - **a.** *pneum-*
   - **b.** *pneumon-*
   - **c.** *-ia*
   - **d.** *-nia*

2. In the medical term **pulmonologist,** the root is:
   - **a.** *pulm-*
   - **b.** *pulmon-*
   - **c.** *-logist*
   - **d.** *-gist*

3. The combining vowel in the medical term **respiratory** is:
   - **a.** *-a-*
   - **b.** *-o-*
   - **c.** *-i-*
   - **d.** *-e-*

Section 1.2 Suffixes

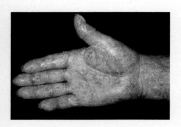

▲ Figure 1.1 Dermatitis due to a latex glove.

Dr. P. Marazzi/Science Source

A **suffix** is a group of letters positioned at the end of a medical term. It attaches to the end of a **root** or **combining form**. **Suffixes** can have more than one meaning. If a **suffix** begins with a consonant, add a **combining vowel** to the **root**. If a **suffix** starts with a vowel, no **combining vowel** is needed. An occasional medical term can have two **suffixes**. For example, the **root gene-**, meaning origin or gene, is teamed with the **suffix -tic**, which means pertaining to, to form the word genetic, *pertaining to a gene*. Again, the **root gene-** is teamed with the **suffix -tics**, which means *knowledge of,* to form the word genetics, *the knowledge of or the science of the inheritance of characteristics*. Also, the **root gene-** can be teamed with two **suffixes**, **-tic**, *pertaining to,* and *-ist, a specialist,* to form the word geneticist, *pertaining to a specialist in genetics*. There can be more than one **suffix** in a single word.

Using the combining form of **cardi/o**, in the medical specialty of cardiology, a cardiologist will often diagnose a cardiopathy. The **suffix -logy**, which means *study of;* the **suffix -logist**, which means *one who studies* or *a specialist;* and the suffix **-pathy**, which means *disease,* all give different meanings in the sentence "in the specialty of cardiology, a cardiologist will often diagnose a cardiopathy."

Another example of the use of **suffixes** is in the medical specialty of dermatology, when a dermatologist will often diagnose a case of dermatitis *(Table 1.1, Figure 1.1)*.

Table 1.1 Use of Suffixes

Complete Word	Root **or** Combining Form	Suffix	Meaning of Suffix	Meaning of Word
dermatitis	dermat-	-itis	*inflammation*	*inflammation of the skin*
dermatologist	dermat/o-	-logist	*one who studies*	*one who studies the skin, specialist in dermatology*
dermatology	dermat/o-	-logy	*study of*	*study of the skin*

In *dermatitis,* the **suffix -itis** starts with a vowel, so there is no need for a **combining vowel**, and the **suffix** is attached directly to the **root**.

In a different example of the use of **suffixes**, an orthopedic surgeon operating on a joint can perform an arthroscopy, an arthrodesis, or an arthroplasty, all different operations with different outcomes, as shown in *Table 1.2*.

Table 1.2 Different Meanings of Suffixes

Complete Word	Combining Form	Suffix	Meaning of Suffix	Meaning of Word
arthroscopy	arthr/o-	-scopy	*visual examination*	*visual examination of a joint*
arthrodesis	arthr/o-	-desis	*fixation*	*fixation of a joint*
arthroplasty	arthr/o-	-plasty	*surgical repair*	*repair of a joint*

You always need a **combining vowel** before a **suffix** that begins with a consonant (e.g., dermatology, arthroplasty).

Classification of Suffixes

One strategy to help you understand medical terms is to divide suffixes into different types, such as diagnostic, surgical, pathologic, and descriptive or adjectival.

Diagnostic Suffixes

This group of suffixes, when added to a root or combining form, produces a medical term that is a diagnosis or a procedure or test to identify the nature of an illness.

The roots/combining forms hem/o and hemat/o both mean *blood*. Adding diagnostic suffixes can produce a variety of diagnostic medical terms throughout the body systems *(Table 1.3)*.

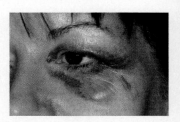

▲ **Figure 1.2** Hematoma (black eye) following a fall.
Dr. P. Marazzi/Science Source

Table 1.3 Diagnostic Suffixes

Diagnostic Suffix	Meaning of Suffix	Word Example	Meaning of Word Example
-chezia	pass a stool	hemat/ochezia	passage of a bloody stool
-crit	to separate	hemat/ocrit	percentage of red blood cells in the blood
-gram	record	cardi/ogram	record derived from the heart
-graph	instrument for recording	cardi/ograph	instrument for recording the heart
-lysis	destruction	hem/olysis	destruction of red blood cells
-oma	tumor, mass	hematoma *(Figure 1.2)*	collection of blood in a tissue
-philia	attraction	hem/ophilia	an inherited blood disease
-ptysis	spit	hem/optysis	to cough up bloody sputum
-rrhage	to flow profusely	hem/orrhage	to bleed profusely
-rrhoid	to flow	hem/orrhoid	painful anal swelling of venous blood
-uria	urine	hematuria	blood in the urine

As you go through each body system in the book, there will be additional diagnostic suffixes you will learn in relation to the actual diagnoses made at that point in the book.

Surgical Suffixes

When added to a root or combining form, surgical suffixes produce medical terms that describe the invasive surgical procedure performed on the body *(Table 1.4)*.

Table 1.4 Surgical Suffixes

Surgical Suffix	Meaning of Suffix	Word Example	Meaning of Surgical Procedure
-centesis	surgical puncture	arthr/ocentesis	surgical puncture of a joint space with a needle
-desis	fixation	arthr/odesis	surgical fixation of the bones of a joint
-ectomy	surgical removal	appendectomy	surgical removal of the appendix
-plasty	surgical repair	rhin/oplasty	surgical repair of the nose
-rrhaphy	surgical suture	herni/orrhaphy	surgical suture of a hernia
-stomy	surgical formation of an opening	trache/ostomy	surgical formation of an artificial opening into the trachea into which a tube is inserted
-tomy	surgical incision	trache/otomy	surgical incision into the trachea
-tripsy	crushing	lith/otripsy	crushing of a stone (calculus), for example, in the ureters

Pathologic Suffixes

When added to a **root** or **combining form**, this type of **suffix** produces a medical term that describes a symptom or sign of a disease process *(Table 1.5)*.

Table 1.5 Pathologic Suffixes

Pathologic Suffix	Meaning of Suffix	Word Example	Meaning of Pathologic Term
-algia	*pain*	**arthr**algia	*pain in a joint(s)*
-ectasis	*dilation*	**bronchi**ectasis	*chronic dilation of bronchi*
-edema	*accumulation of fluid in tissues*	**lymph**edema	*swelling in tissues as a result of obstruction of lymphatic vessels*
-emesis	*vomiting*	**hemat**emesis	*vomiting of blood*
-genesis	*form, produce*	**oste/o**genesis	*formation of new bone*
-itis	*inflammation*	**cyst**itis	*inflammation of the urinary bladder*
-oma	*tumor, mass*	**hemat**oma	*mass of blood leaked outside blood vessels into tissues*
-osis	*abnormal condition*	**cyan**osis	*dark blue coloration of blood due to lack of oxygen*
-pathy	*disease*	**neur/o**pathy	*any disease of the nervous system*
-penia	*deficiency, lack of*	**erythr/o**penia	*decrease in red blood cells*
-phobia	*fear of*	**agora**phobia	*an unfounded fear of public places that arouses a state of panic*
-stenosis	*narrowing*	**arteri/o**stenosis	*abnormal narrowing of an artery*

Adjectival Suffixes

As you learn new medical terms in each body system chapter in this book, you will see that there are 28 **suffixes** that mean *pertaining to.* These **suffixes** are used as adjectives to describe the root. Examples of adjectival **suffixes** are:

- **-ac cardiac** pertaining to the heart
- **-ary pulmonary** pertaining to the lungs
- **-ior posterior** pertaining to the back of the body

   Those 28 suffixes are -ac, -al, -ale, -alis, -ar, -aris, -ary, -atic, -ative, -eal, -ent, -etic, -ial, -ic, -ica, -ical, -ine, -ior, -iosum, -ious, -istic, -ius, -nic, -ous, -tic, -tiz, -tous, -us.

Noun Suffixes

Several **suffixes** do not fall under any of the earlier classifications but maintain the root or combining form as a noun *(Table 1.6)*.

Table 1.6 Noun Suffixes

Noun Suffix	Meaning of Suffix	Word Example	Meaning of Word Example
-iatry	*treatment, medical specialty*	**psychiatry**	*diagnosis and treatment of mental disorders*
-ician	*expert, specialist*	**pediatrician**	*medical specialist in children's development and disorders*
-icle	*small, minute*	**ossicle** (Figure 1.3)	*small bone, relating to the three small bones in the middle ear*
-ist	*expert, specialist*	**dentist**	*specialist in disorders of the orofacial complex*
-istry	*medical specialty*	**dentistry**	*specialty in disorders of the orofacial complex*
-ole	*small, minute*	**arteriole**	*small artery*
-ule	*small, minute*	**venule**	*small vein*

Ossicles

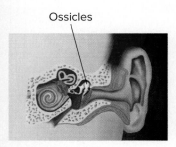

▲ **Figure 1.3** Ossicles of the middle ear. BSIP SA/ Alamy Stock Photo

   Note that in *Table 1.6,* three **suffixes** mean "small," two **suffixes** mean "specialist," and two **suffixes** mean "medical specialty."

A. Building onto the elements of roots, combining vowels, and combining forms are the prefixes and suffixes of medical terminology. *Prefixes and suffixes are additional word elements that give further meaning to a root or combining form. Develop your knowledge of more word elements with the following exercise. Choose T if the statement is true. Choose F if the statement is false.* **LO 1.1, 1.2**

1. In a medical term, the suffix will always appear at the end.   T   F

2. In the terms **arthroscopy** and **arthrodesis,** the combining form is the same, but the suffix is different.   T   F

3. If a suffix begins with a consonant, you will need a combining vowel before it.   T   F

B. Identify the meaning of the word by the suffix. *The medical terms below are commonly used by people who are not necessarily in the medical field. Using what you may already know, identify the meaning of the suffix of medical terms. Match the definition on the left with the correct term it is describing on the right.* **LO 1.2**

1. _____ a specialist   **a.** agoraphobia

2. _____ afraid of   **b.** pneumonectomy

3. _____ study of   **c.** dentist

4. _____ removal of   **d.** dermatitis

5. _____ inflammation of   **e.** biology

Section 1.3 Prefixes

Prefixes can be one letter or a group of letters. **Prefixes** are added directly to the beginning of the term, to the **root** or **combining form** and do not require **combining vowels**. An occasional medical term can have two **prefixes**. **Prefixes** can have more than one meaning. That being said, every medical term will not have a prefix.

For example, you can add the different prefixes **peri-** and **endo-** to the same root, cardi-, to produce the different words **peri**cardium and **endo**cardium, which have very different meanings, as shown in *Table 1.7*.

Table 1.7 Use of Prefixes

Complete Word	Prefix	Meaning of Prefix	Meaning of Word
pericardium	peri-	*around*	*structure around the heart*
endocardium	endo-	*inside*	*structure inside the heart*

Note that **-um** is a **suffix** meaning *structure*.

Similarly, **epi**gastric, **hypo**gastric, and **endo**gastric all have the same root, gastr-, but because of the different prefixes, **epi-, hypo-,** and **endo-,** have very different meanings, as shown in *Table 1.8*.

Table 1.8 Different Meanings of Prefixes

Complete Word	Prefix	Meaning of Prefix	Meaning of Word
epigastric	epi-	*above*	*pertaining to above the stomach*
hypogastric	hypo-	*below*	*pertaining to below the stomach*
endogastric	endo-	*inside*	*pertaining to inside the stomach*

Note that **-ic** is a **suffix** meaning *pertaining to.*

Classification of Prefixes

Many **prefixes** can be classified into **prefixes** of position, **prefixes** of number or measurement, and **prefixes** of direction (*Tables 1.9, 1.10, 1.11*).

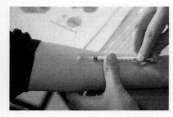

▲ **Figure 1.4** **Intradermal injection.** Andrew Aitchison/Contributor/Getty Images

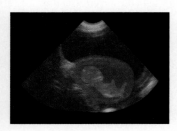

▲ **Figure 1.5** **Obstetric ultrasonography of a 22-year-old woman.** The 12-week-old fetus is *in brown.* The placenta is *in green.* Warrick G./Science Source

Table 1.9 Prefixes of Position

Position Prefix	Meaning of Prefix	Word Example	Meaning of Medical Term
ante-	before, forward	antevert	to tilt forward, as a uterus can
anti-	against	antibiotic	an agent that can destroy bacteria and other microorganisms
circum-	around	circumcision	to cut around the penis to remove the foreskin
endo-	inside, inner	endocrine	a gland that secretes directly into the blood
epi-	above, over, upon	epidermis	the top layer of the skin
exo-	outside, outward	exocrine	a gland that excretes outwardly through ducts
hyper-	above, excessive	hypertrophy	increase in size
hypo-	below	hypodermis	tissue layer below the top layer of the skin
inter-	between	intercostal	the space between two ribs
intra-	inside, within	intradermal (Figure 1.4)	within the skin
para-	adjacent, alongside	paranoid	having delusions of persecution
peri-	around	perinatal	around the time of birth
post-	after	postnatal	after the time of birth
pre-	before	prenatal	before the time of birth
retro-	backward	retrovert	to tilt backward, as a uterus can
supra-	above, excessive	suprapubic	above the pubic bone
trans-	across, through	transdermal	going across or through the skin
ultra-	higher, beyond	ultrasound (Figure 1.5)	very high-frequency sound waves

Table 1.10 Prefixes of Number and Measurement

Measurement Prefix	Meaning of Prefix	Word Example	Meaning of Medical Term
bi-	two, twice, double	bilateral	pertaining to or related to two sides of the body
brady-	slow	bradycardia	slow heart rate
di-	two	diplegia	paralysis of corresponding parts on both sides of the body
eu-	normal	eupnea	normal breathing
hemi-	half	hemiparesis	weakness of one side (half) of the body
macro-	large	macrocyte	large red blood cell
micro-	small	microcyte	small red blood cell
mono-	single, one	monocyte	white blood cell with a single nucleus
multi-	many	multipara	woman who has given birth at least twice
pan-	all	pancytopenia	deficiency of all types of blood cells
poly-	excessive	polyuria	excessive production of urine
primi-	first	primipara	woman who has given birth for the first time
quadri-	four	quadriplegia	paralysis of all four limbs
tachy-	rapid	tachycardia	rapid heart rate
tri-	three	tricuspid	having three points—a tricuspid heart valve has three flaps
uni-	single, one	unipolar	pertaining to one pole; neuron having a single process

Table 1.11 Prefixes of Direction and Location

Directional Prefix	Meaning of Prefix	Medical Term Example	Meaning of Medical Term
ab-	*away from*	abduction	*action of moving away from the midline*
ad-	*toward*	adduction	*action of moving toward the midline*
ante-	*coming before, in front of*	antevert	*to tilt forward*
post-	*coming after, behind*	postnatal	*occurring after birth*
sub-	*under, beneath*	subdural	*in the space under the dura mater*
syn-	*coming together*	synapse	*junction between two nerve cells*

Check Point Section 1.3

A. Review the prefixes and terms in Table 1.9. *Select the correct answer to complete each statement.* **LO 1.2**

1. The location of the tumor was *above the pubic bone.* The tumor is located _____.

   a. hypogastric   **b.** transdermal   **c.** suprapubic   **d.** ultrasonic

2. The *transdermal* route of drug administration goes:

   a. through the skin.   **b.** in an IV.   **c.** through the mouth.   **d.** in the rectum.

3. *Postpartum* occurs

   a. before delivery.   **b.** during delivery.   **c.** after delivery.

4. *Retroverted* means

   a. tilted sideways.   **b.** tilted forward.   **c.** tilted backward.

B. Answer the following questions regarding the proper use of prefixes. *Choose T if the statement is True. Choose F if the statement is False.* **LO 1.2**

1. They usually appear in the beginning of a term.		T	F
2. They can attach to a root or combining form.		T	F
3. Every term must have a prefix.		T	F
4. Some terms can have more than one prefix.		T	F
5. Prefixes can be classified into prefixes of position, number or measurement, or direction.		T	F

Section 1.4   Unique Medical Words

Greek, Latin, and Old English Words

Some medical terms are solid and cannot be broken down into elements. Examples are virus, a Latin word meaning poison, and toxin, a Greek word meaning poison. Though they have the same meaning in their original language, when they are converted to modern medical language, they have very different meanings. These solid words have to be recognized and their meanings memorized.

- **medical,** from a Latin term meaning *to heal;* it means *pertaining to the practice of medicine.*
- **care,** an Old English word meaning *to worry;* when you care for your patients, you look after them and are concerned about them.
- **breath,** an Old English word meaning *a single cycle of inhaling and exhaling.*
- **cough,** an Old English word meaning *to expel breath from the lungs.*
- **mucus,** a Latin word for *a clear, sticky secretion.*
- **record,** a Latin word meaning *to remember;* a medical *record* is a written account of a patient's medical history.

- **patient,** an Old English term meaning *to suffer* or *undergo;* the term refers to a person who is under medical or surgical treatment.
- **knee,** an Old English word meaning *an angular shape;* today it refers to the **joint** (a Latin word for junction) between the upper and lower leg.
- **apex,** a Latin word meaning *tip* or *summit* (as in Mount Everest); the apex of the heart is the downward-pointing tip of the cone-shaped heart.
- **patent,** a Latin word meaning *open* or *exposed; a patent* blood vessel is open to the circulation of freely flowing blood (Note the difference in the word **patient**).
- **quadrant,** a Latin word meaning *a quarter;* the abdomen is divided into four *quadrants* by horizontal and vertical planes that intersect at the umbilicus.
- **umbilicus,** which is a Latin word for the *navel or belly button.*
- **toxin,** a Greek word meaning *poison; a toxin* is a poisonous substance formed by a cell, such as a bacterium.
- **lymph,** a Latin word meaning *clear spring water; lymph* is a clear, shimmering fluid collected from the body tissues.
- **breech,** an Old English word meaning *buttocks;* in obstetrics, a fetus is in a *breech* presentation when the buttocks, rather than the head, are the presenting part at delivery.
- **specialist,** a Latin word meaning *of a given species; a specialist* devotes professional attention to a particular subject area.

Terms That Are Alike

Precision in both written and verbal communication is essential for a health professional, with great attention given to detail. There are many words in the medical language that are very similar to each other in both their spelling and pronunciation. Examples are:
- **ilium,** pronounced **ill-ee-um,** a bone in the pelvis
- **ileum,** pronounced the same way, **ill-ee-um,** a segment of the small intestine
- **ureter,** the tube from the kidney to the bladder
- **urethra,** the tube from the bladder to the outside
- **trapezius,** a muscle in the back
- **trapezium,** a bone in the wrist
- **malleus,** a small bone in the middle ear
- **malleolus,** a bony protuberance at the ankle
- **neurology,** the study of diseases of the nervous system
- **urology,** the study of diseases of the kidney and bladder

Check Point Section 1.4

A. The following medical terms are all of Greek or Latin origin. *Match the definition on the left with the correct term it is describing on the right.* **LO 1.3**

_____ 1. tip or summit		**a.** patent
_____ 2. buttocks		**b.** mucus
_____ 3. poison		**c.** apex
_____ 4. clear, sticky secretion		**d.** breech
_____ 5. open		**e.** toxin

B. Choose the correct spelling of medical terms taken directly from Greek, Latin, or Old English words. LO 1.3, 1.4

1. A tube from the bladder to the outside.
   a. ureethra
   b. urethra
   c. ureter
   d. ureetere

2. The study of the diseases of the nervous system.
   a. urology
   b. ureology
   c. neurlogy
   d. neurology

3. A muscle in the back.
   a. ilium
   b. ileum
   c. trapezius
   d. trapezium

4. A small bone in the middle ear.
   a. ileum
   b. ilium
   c. malleolus
   d. malleus

The Anatomy of Medical Terms

Challenge Your Knowledge

A. Identify the statements below as either true or false. Choose T if the statement is true. Choose F if the statement is false. **LO 1.1**

1. A term never has more than one root.   T   F

2. Some terms will have no combining vowel.   T   F

3. A combining vowel changes the meaning of the word.   T   F

4. A vowel must always be present in a combining form. T   F

B. The root/combining form is the core meaning of the word. Choose the correct definition for the root/combining form for each term. **LO 1.1**

1. The term *hypogastric* relates to under or below the

   a. chest.   **c.** stomach.

   b. skin.   **d.** lungs.

2. The term *neuralgia* means pain in a

   a. nerve.   **c.** heart.

   b. joint.   **d.** cell.

3. The term *subdermal* means pertaining to below the

   a. chest.   **c.** stomach.

   b. skin.   **d.** lungs.

4. The term *cardiac* means pertaining to the

   a. lungs.   **c.** kidneys.

   b. joints.   **d.** heart.

5. The term *arthritis* means inflammation of the

   a. lungs.   **c.** kidneys.

   b. joints.   **d.** heart.

6. The term *erythrocyte* means cell that is

   a. large.   **c.** red.

   b. round.   **d.** swollen.

7. The term *bronchitis* means inflammation of a

   a. kidney.   **c.** bronchus.

   b. eye.   **d.** joint.

8. The term *hematology* means the study of

   a. blood.   **c.** the heart.

   b. skin.   **d.** the mind.

C. Match the Greek/Latin elements in the first column with their meanings in the second column. LO 1.1, 1.4

_____ **1.** pneum

_____ **2.** hemat

_____ **3.** lymph

_____ **4.** thorax

_____ **5.** arthr

_____ **6.** respir

_____ **7.** mucus

_____ **8.** patent

a. to breathe

b. open

c. clear, sticky secretion

d. tip or summit

e. buttocks

f. chest

g. skin

h. joint

_____ 9. toxin

_____ 10. apex

_____ 11. dermat

_____ 12. breech

i. blood

j. air, lung

k. clear spring water

l. poison

D. **Spelling is most important in medical terminology.** For example, **ilium** and **ileum** may be similar in appearance and sound, but the difference of one letter makes each a different body part. Select the correct spelling for the following terms. **LO 1.3, 1.4**

1. The _____ of the small intestine was infected.

    a. ileum   **b.** ilium   **c.** illium

2. The _____ system keeps you breathing.

    a. respieratory   **b.** respiratory   **c.** resspiratory

3. Inflammation of the heart is _____.

    a. carditus   **b.** carditis   **c.** cardiitis

4. A muscle in the back is the _____.

    a. trapeze   **b.** trapezium   **c.** trapezius

5. A bony protuberance in your ankle is the _____.

    a. maleus   **b.** malius   **c.** malleolus

E. **Use your newly acquired knowledge of medical language to correctly answer the following questions.** Let the roots and combining forms be your guide. Choose the correct answer to complete each statement. **LO 1.1**

1. This term means one who studies the skin.

    a. dermatologist

    b. urologist

    c. neurologist

2. This term relates to the intestines and the stomach.

    a. gastroenterology

    b. cardiology

    c. dermatology

3. This term relates to the process of breathing.

    a. apex

    b. toxic

    c. respiratory

4. This term relates to the stomach.

    a. gastritis

    b. gynecology

    c. dermatitis

5. This term relates to a joint.

    a. urethritis

    b. arthritis

    c. neuralgia

F. Use the correct medical term to complete the sentence. Use the words to complete each sentence below. Fill in the blanks.
LO 1.1, 1.2, 1.3

bladder   breech   cardiologist   ileum   ilium   kidney   lymph   malleolus   trapezium   ureter   urethra

1. A _____ is a specialist in the care of the heart.

2. The _____ is a tube from the kidney to the bladder.

3. Urology is the study of diseases of the _____ and _____.

4. A segment of the small intestine is the _____.

5. _____ means the buttocks, not the head, present first at delivery.

6. _____ is the tube from the bladder to the outside.

7. _____ is a fluid collected from body tissues.

8. A bone in the wrist is the _____.

9. The bony protuberance at the ankle is the _____.

10. The _____ is a bone in the pelvis.

G. Because much of clinical documentation centers on surgeries, knowledge of surgical suffixes is most important—especially for coders. LO 1.2

Matching
Match the definition in the first column with the correct term it is describing in the second column.

Term	Meaning
_____ 1. scopy	A. surgical repair
_____ 2. desis	B. visual examination
_____ 3. plasty	C. surgical fixation

Combine these suffixes with the combining form arthr/o and fill in the blanks with the correct medical term.

4. The surgeon wants a closer look inside Mr. Parker's knee so he is scheduled for an _____ tomorrow morning.

5. Mary Collins has torn her knee ligaments playing high school basketball. Her treatment plan includes scheduling an _____ to reattach them. (fixation)

6. June Larkin had a bad skiing accident while on vacation. Her tendons and ligaments in her knee will require extensive surgery to get her walking again without crutches. She needs an _____. (repair)

Case Reports

A. Case Reports demonstrate how medical terminology is used in context. Using the skills of identifying the meaning of the prefix, root/combining form, and suffix will help you learn the meaning of each term. Correctly answer the following questions. **LO 1.1, 1.2**

 Case Report (CR) 1.1

You are

. . . a **respiratory therapist** working with Tavis Senko, MD, a **pulmonologist** at Fulwood Medical Center.

You are communicating with

. . . Mrs. Sandra Schwartz, a 43-year-old woman referred to Dr. Senko by her primary care physician, Dr. Andrew McDonald, an **internist.** Mrs. Schwartz has a persistent abnormality on her chest x-ray. You have been asked to determine her **pulmonary** function prior to a scheduled **bronchoscopy.**

This summary of a Case Report

. . . illustrates for you the use of some simple medical terms. Modern health care and medicine have their own language. The medical terms all have precise meanings, which enable you, as a health professional, to communicate clearly and accurately with other health professionals involved in the care of a patient. This communication is critical for patient safety and the delivery of high-quality patient care.

From her medical records, you can see that 2 months ago Mrs. Schwartz developed a right upper lobe (RUL) **pneumonia.** After treatment with an **antibiotic,** a follow-up chest x-ray (CXR) showed some residual collapse in the right upper lobe and a small right **pneumothorax.** Mrs. Schwartz has smoked a pack a day since she was a teenager. Dr. Senko is concerned that she has lung cancer and has scheduled her for a **bronchoscopy.**

1. Dr. Senko is a specialist in the treatment of the:

    a. heart.   **b.** kidneys.   **c.** lungs.   **d.** ear, nose, and throat.

2. The _____ of the term *bronchoscopy* means windpipe.

    a. combining form   **b.** root   **c.** prefix   **d.** suffix

3. In the medical term *antibiotic,* the prefix is:

    a. an-   **b.** ant-   **c.** anti-

4. The word element *respir* is a:

    a. combining form.   **b.** root.   **c.** prefix.   **d.** suffix.

5. Identify the terms that have word elements that mean *lung.* (Choose all that apply)

    a. Pneumonia   **b.** Bronchoscopy   **c.** Internist   **d.** Pulmonologist   **e.** Therapist

B. This Case Report has several terms using the same root element but with different suffixes. Correctly answer the following questions. **LO 1.1, 1.2**

 Case Report (CR) 1.2

You are

. . . a **genetic** nurse working with **geneticist** Ingrid Hughes, MD, PhD, in the **Genetics** Department at Fulwood Medical Center.

Your patient is

. . . Mrs. Geraldine Long, a 37-year-old administrative assistant who has been referred by primary care **physician** Susan Lee, MD. Mrs. Long has twin girls who are 12 years old. She is an award-winning ballroom dancer who does not smoke, drinks alcohol occasionally, and rehearses her dance routines four or five days each week. Her mother, aged 62, is being treated for ovarian cancer. Her mother's sister is being treated for breast cancer and has been found to carry a **gene mutation** associated with breast cancer. Mrs. Long's **mammogram** is normal. She has requested **genetic screening.**

1. Identify the suffixes that mean specialist. (Choose all that apply)

   a. -ist   **b.** -ics   **c.** -ician   **d.** -tic

2. Provide the medical term that has two suffixes: _____

3. The root of the term *geneticist* means:

   a. pertaining to.   **b.** specialist.   **c.** origin.   **d.** cancer.

C. This Case Report focuses on medical terms that are based in Greek, Latin, and Old English. Correctly answer the following questions. **LO 1.1, 1.3**

 Case Report (CR) 1.3

You are

. . . a **medical** assistant working for Russell Gordon, MD, a primary **care** physician at Fulwood Medical Center.

Your patient is

. . . Mr. William Doyle, a 72-year-old retired long-distance truck driver and a lifetime pack-a-day smoker. He is complaining of shortness of **breath,** increased **cough,** and production of sticky yellow **mucus.** In his medical **record,** you see that he has had stones in both ureters and is frequently a **patient** in the urology department, and that he has had both **knees** replaced. You begin to examine him.

1. Provide the medical term that refers to a *joint:* _____

2. Provide the medical term that means *to suffer:* _____

3. Mr. Williams has a problem inhaling and exhaling air. He has a problem with his:

   a. breath.   **b.** cough.   **c.** kidneys.   **d.** mucus.   **e.** knees.

D. Read Case Report 1.4 and correctly answer the questions that follow. **LO 1.3**

 Case Report (CR) 1.4

You are

. . . a medical assistant employed by Russell Gordon, MD, a primary care physician at Fulwood Medical Center.

Your patient is

. . . Mrs. Connie Bishop, a 55-year-old woman who presents with a swelling in her lower abdomen and shortness of breath. She has no gynecologic or gastroenterologic symptoms. Her previous medical history shows recurrent dermatitis of her hands since a teenager and an arthroscopy for a knee injury at age 40. Physical examination reveals a circular mass 6 inches in diameter in the left lower quadrant of her abdomen. There is no abnormality in her respiratory or cardiovascular system.

Your role is to maintain her medical record and document her care, assist Dr. Gordon during his examinations, explain the examination and treatment procedures to Mrs. Bishop, and facilitate her referral for specialist care.

1. What type of skin problem has Mrs. Bishop had since she was a teenager? _____

2. Which term in the case study means pertaining to the stomach and small intestines? _____

3. Her knee injury required what type of procedure? _____

4. Does she have any issues with her lungs or heart? (yes or no) _____

5. Do her symptoms indicate a possible problem with her ileum? (yes or no) _____

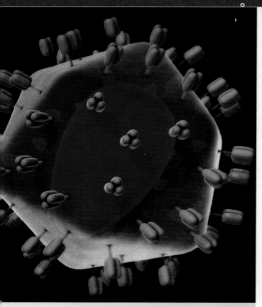

CHAPTER
2

Word Analysis and Communication
The Language of Health Care

Chapter Sections

Chapter Learning Outcomes

LO 2.1   Deconstruct a medical term into its basic elements.

LO 2.2   Use word elements to identify or construct a medical term.

LO 2.3   Connect the singular and plural components of medical terms.

LO 2.4   Employ the phonetic system used to pronounce medical terms.

LO 2.5   Communicate with precision in both written and verbal forms.

Section 2.1 Word Analysis and Definition

Word Analysis and Definition

When you see a medical term you do not understand, the first step you can take to analyze, decipher, or deconstruct the term is to break it down into its component elements, or parts.

For words you need to define, first identify the suffix. Then, go to the front of the word and define the elements, moving from the front of the word to the suffix.

For example, in the term **endocarditis,** the suffix at the end of the word is -itis, which means *inflammation.*

That leaves **endocard-**. The first word element is **endo-**, a prefix meaning *inside.* The next element is **-card-**, a root meaning *heart.* Now you can assemble the pieces together to form the word meaning *inflammation of the heart.*

That leaves **endo-**, a prefix meaning *inside.* Now you can assemble the pieces together to form the word meaning *inflammation of the inside of the heart:*

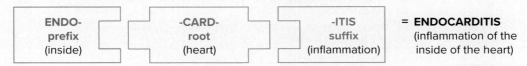

| ENDO- prefix (inside) | -CARD- root (heart) | -ITIS suffix (inflammation) | = ENDOCARDITIS (inflammation of the inside of the heart) |

You also have learned that the suffix **-um** means *a structure.* So changing the word to **endocardium** would be the structure that lines the inside of the heart.

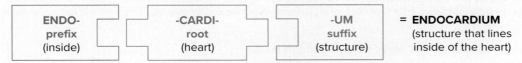

| ENDO- prefix (inside) | -CARDI- root (heart) | -UM suffix (structure) | = ENDOCARDIUM (structure that lines inside of the heart) |

Therefore, you can understand that **endocarditis** is used to mean that the endocardium lining the heart has become inflamed or infected. Both **-card-** and **-cardi-** are roots meaning *heart.*

Another example is the word **hemorrhage.** The suffix **-rrhage** following the combining vowel "o" is borrowed from the Greek word meaning *to flow profusely.* The combining form **hem/o-** is from the Greek word for *blood.* The elements of the medical term **hemorrhage** are assembled together and used to mean *profuse bleeding.*

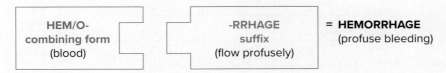

| HEM/O- combining form (blood) | -RRHAGE suffix (flow profusely) | = HEMORRHAGE (profuse bleeding) |

In this book, when the medical terms are broken down into their elements, a hyphen is used to isolate each major element and to identify its position in the whole word.

When a combining form is used, the combining vowel is separated from the root by a slash (/).

WORD	PRONUNCIATION	ELEMENTS		DEFINITION
diagnosis (noun)	die-ag-**NO**-sis	P/	**dia-** *complete*	The determination of the cause of a disease, injury or congenital defect
		R/	**-gnosis** *knowledge*	
diagnoses (pl)	die-ag-**NO**-seez			
diagnostic (adj)	die-ag-**NOS**-tik	S/	**-tic** *pertaining to*	Pertaining to or a diagnosis
(**Note:** The "is" in gnosis is deleted to allow the word to flow.)				
diagnose (verb)	die-ag-**NOSE**	R/	**-gnose** *recognize an abnormal condition*	To make a diagnosis
endocarditis	**EN**-doh-kar-**DIE**-tis	S/	**-itis** *inflammation, infection*	Inflammation of the lining of the heart
(**Note:** The root "-card-" is the root used when the heart condition is **cardi-tis** or a type of **carditis**.)		P/	**endo-** *within, inner, inside*	
		R/	**-card-** *heart*	
endocardium	**EN**-doh-**KAR**-dee-um	S/	**-um** *structure*	The inside lining of the heart
		P/	**endo-** *within, inner*	
		R/	**-cardi-** *heart*	
hemorrhage	**HEM**-oh-raj	S/	**-rrhage** *to flow profusely*	To bleed profusely
		R/CF	**hem/o-** *blood*	

Check Point Section 2.1

A. To analyze a medical term, simply break the elements down (deconstruct them) into their basic forms. *To construct a new term, take the appropriate elements, put them in the correct position in the term, and build your term.* **Note:** *Remember that not every term will have all elements present at the same time.* **LO 2.1, 2.2**

1. To deconstruct: Take the medical term **endocarditis** and break it down into elements.

The prefix _____ means _____.

The root _____ means _____.

The suffix _____ means _____.

2. To deconstruct: Take the medical term **hemorrhage** and break it down into elements.

The prefix _____ means _____.

The root _____ means _____.

The suffix _____ means _____.

3. To deconstruct: Take the medical term **endocardium** and break it down into elements.

The prefix _____ means _____.

The root _____ means _____.

The suffix _____ means _____.

Section 2.2 Plurals and Pronunciation

Plurals

When you change a medical term from singular to plural, it is not as simple as adding an *s*, as you often can in the English language. Unfortunately, in medical terms, the end of the word changes in ways that were logical in Latin and Greek but have to be learned by memory in English. This is shown in *Table 2.1.*

Table 2.1 Singular and Plural Forms

Singular Ending	Plural Ending	Examples	Singular Ending	Plural Ending	Examples
-a		axilla	-on		ganglion
	-ae	axillae		-a	ganglia
-ax		thorax	-um		septum
	-aces	thoraces		-a	septa
-en		lumen	-us**		viscus
	-ina	lumina		-era	viscera
-ex		cortex	-us**		villus
	-ices	cortices		-i	villi
-is*		diagnosis	-us**		corpus
	-es	diagnoses		-ora	corpora
-is*		epididymis	-x		phalanx
	-ides	epididymides		-ges	phalanges
-ix		appendix	-y		ovary
	-ices	appendices		-ies	ovaries
-ma		carcinoma	-yx		calyx
	-mata	carcinomata		-yces	calyces

*Note: Both singular terms can end in -is. You have to know on a case-by-case basis which singular terms change to -es and which ones change to -ides.
**The same applies to the singular terms ending in -us—some will form plurals with -era, -i, or -ora.

Pronunciation

In your role as a health professional, pronouncing medical terms correctly and precisely is not only about understanding conversations with your peers or a physician. It is also a matter of ensuring patient safety and providing high-quality patient care.

Correct pronunciation is essential so that other health professionals with whom you are working can understand what you are saying. Throughout this textbook, the pronunciation of each medical term will be written out phonetically using modern English forms. The part(s) of the word to which you give the strongest, or primary, emphasis is (are) written in bold, uppercase letters.

For example, the term **gastroenterology** will be phonetically written **GAS**-troh-en-ter-**OL**-oh-jee, whereas the term **gastritis,** which means *inflammation of the stomach,* will be phonetically written as gas-**TRY**-tis. **Hemorrhage** will be written as **HEM**-oh-raj, whereas the term **hemostasis,** which means *the stopping of bleeding,* will be written he-moh-**STAY**-sis.

The only way you can learn how to pronounce medical terms is to say them repeatedly and have your pronunciation checked against a standard, which is found in McGraw-Hill Connect.

Check Point Section 2.2

A. Forming plurals of medical terms will be less difficult if you follow the rules and apply them correctly. *The rules are given to you in the following chart—practice changing the medical terms from singular to plural. Fill in the chart.* **LO 2.3**

Singular	Plural	Singular Term	Plural Term
-a	-ae	axilla	1.
-um	-a	septum	2.
-ax	-aces	thorax	3.
-en	-ina	lumen	4.
-ex	-ices	cortex	5.
-is	-es	diagnosis	6.
-on	-a	ganglion	7.
-us	-i	villus	8.
-ix	-ices	appendix	9.
-x	-ges	phalanx	10.

Precision in Communication

This year in the United States, more than 400,000 people will die because of drug reactions and medical errors. Many of these deaths are due to inaccurate or imprecise written or verbal communications between the different members of the health care team.

Being a health professional requires the utmost attention to detail and precision, both in written documentation and in verbal communication. A patient's life could be in your hands. In addition, the medical record in which you document a patient's care and your actions is a legal document. It can be used in court as evidence in professional medical liability cases.

When you understand the individual word elements that make up a medical term, you are better able to clearly understand the medical terms you are using. For example, if **hypotension** (low blood pressure) is confused with **hypertension** (high blood pressure), incorrect treatments could be prescribed. Confusing the terms **ureter** (the tube from the kidney to the bladder) with **urethra** (the tube from the bladder to the outside) could lead to disastrous consequences.

Each chapter will end with a Case Report for you to practice precision in written and verbal communication. Your review may require you to interpret medical terms, identify word elements within them, and their meanings. Correct interpretation of medical terms is important when communicating with patients and their families.

Use of Word Analysis

Ureter (you-REET-er) and **urethra** (you-REE-thra) are both simple words with no **prefix**, **combining vowel**, or **suffix**. They are derived from the Greek word for *urine*. They are similar words but have very different anatomic locations (*Chapter 6*).

To deconstruct the word **hypotension** (HIGH-poh-TEN-shun), start with the **suffix -ion**, which means *a condition*. Next, the **prefix hypo-** means *below* or *less than normal*. The **root -tens-** is from the Latin word for *pressure*. Place the pieces together to form a word meaning *condition of below-normal pressure*, or low blood pressure.

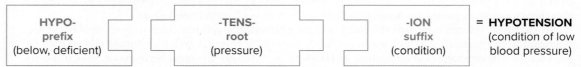

To deconstruct the term **costovertebral** (kos-toe-VER-teh-bral), start with the **suffix -al**, which means *pertaining to*. Separated by the **combining vowel "o"** are two **roots**, **cost-** and **-vertebr-**. The **combining form cost/o-** is from the Latin word for *a rib*. **-Vertebr-** is from the Latin word for *backbone or spine*. So you have *pertaining to the rib and the spine*.

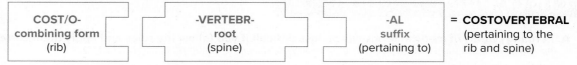

It is common that Greek and Latin terms have suffixes attached to them. These suffixes often mean *pertaining to*. For example, abdominal has the suffix -al changing the meaning of abdomen to *pertaining to the abdomen*. In proper documentation, a physician would order an abdominal x-ray rather than an abdomen x-ray.

Learning the meaning of word elements guides you to the meaning of medical terms. Instead of memorizing the meaning of each word, look for the word element you are familiar with. You might be familiar with the term insomnia which means *the inability to sleep*. The suffix -ia means *condition of*. Learning the meaning of the suffix can help you learn the meaning of other terms with the same suffix. For example, the term pyrexia. Because you know the suffix -ia means *condition of*, all you will need to learn is the meaning of the root element. The root element is pyrex-, which means *fever, heat*. Putting the elements together, pyrexia means *condition of fever or heat*. A condition of fever or heat is abnormal; therefore, the definition of pyrexia is *an abnormally high body temperature or fever*.

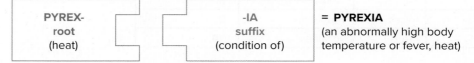

Word Introduction
Word Analysis and Definition

S = Suffix   P = Prefix   R = Root   R/CF = Combining Form

WORD	PRONUNCIATION		ELEMENTS	DEFINITION
abdomen	**AB**-doh-men		Latin *abdomen*	The part of the trunk that lies between the thorax and the pelvis
abdominal	ab-**DOM**-in-al	S/ R/	**-al** *pertaining to* **abdomin-** *abdomen*	Pertaining to the abdomen
costovertebral	kos-toe-**VER**-teh-bral	S/ R/CF R/	**-al** *pertaining to* **cost/o-** *rib* **-vertebr-** *vertebra*	Pertaining to the rib and spine
hypertension	**HIGH**-per-**TEN**-shun	S/ P/ R/	**-ion** *action, condition* **hyper-** *excessive* **-tens-** *pressure*	Persistent high arterial blood pressure
hypotension	**HIGH**-poh-**TEN**-shun	P/	**hypo-** *low, below*	Persistent low arterial blood pressure
pyrexia	pie-**REK**-see-ah	S/ R/	**-ia** *condition* **pyrex-** *fever, heat*	An abnormally high body temperature or fever
ureter (**Note:** Two "e" s = two tubes.)	you-**REET**-er		Greek *urinary canal*	Tube that connects the kidney to the urinary bladder
urethra	you-**REE**-thra		Greek *urethra*	Canal leading from the urinary bladder to the outside

Check Point Section 2.3

A. Precision in communication. *Verbal and written communication must always be precise and accurate for patient safety and legal requirements. Develop your eyes' and ears' ability to distinguish correct pronunciations, word choice, and spelling to ensure documentation and communication accuracy. Fill in the following blanks:* **LO 2.2, 2.5**

1. If the doctor tells you a patient's blood pressure readings are elevated, does the patient have **hypertension** or **hypotension?**

   _____

2. When describing a person's pain, would you say that a person has **abdomen** pain or **abdominal** pain?

   _____

3. Does urine travel from a kidney to the bladder through a **ureter** or **urethra?**

   _____

4. In the term **costovertebral,** the word element cost/o refers to which body part?

   _____

SECTION 2.3 Precision in Communication   23

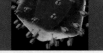

Chapter 2 Review

2014 Nucleus Medical Media

Word Analysis and Communication

Challenge Your Knowledge

A. **Select the correct answer to the following statement.** **LO 2.3, 2.5**

1. *Costovertebral* pertains to the

   a. rib and colon.   **d.** lung and rib.

   b. heart and rib cage.   **e.** rib and kidney.

   c. rib and spine.

B. **Recall your pronunciation.** Select the correct answer that completes each statement. **LO 2.4, 2.5**

1. What is the correct pronunciation of *pyrexia?*

   a. pie-**RECK**-si-a   **d.** pie-**REK**-see-ah

   b. **PIE-RECK**-ci-a   **e.** py-rek-**SEE**-ah

   c. **PY**-rek-sia

2. What is the correct pronunciation of *costovertebral?*

   a. **KOSTO**-ver-**TREE**-bral   **d.** **COSTO**-ver-tree-bral

   b. cost-o-**VER**-tre-bal   **e.** kosto-ver-tree-**BAL**

   c. kos-toe-**VER**-teh-bral

3. What is the correct pronunciation of abdominal?

   a. ab-**DOM**-in-al   **d.** ab-**DOH**-min-el

   b. ab-**DOME**-i-nal   **e.** **AB**-dom-**IN**-el

   c. **AB**-doh-men

C. **To help you master plurals, practice changing singular endings to plural and plural endings to singular in the following exercise.** If you are given a singular word, change it to plural. If you are given a plural word, change it to singular. The first one is done for you. **LO 2.3**

Word	Singular	Plural
1. carcinomata	carcinoma	
2. ovaries		
3. ganglia		
4. lumen		
5. villi		
6. cortices		
7. calyx		

24 CHAPTER 2 REVIEW Word Analysis and Communication

8. epididymis _____   _____

9. axilla _____   _____

10. viscus _____   _____

11. appendices _____   _____

12. corpora _____   _____

13. diagnoses _____   _____

14. thoraces _____   _____

D. Precision in documentation means using the correct form of the term, as well as the correct term. Medical terms can take the forms of noun (thing), verb (action), or adjective (description). Fill in the blank with the correct term. **LO 2.5**

diagnosis   diagnose   diagnostic   diagnoses

1. After performing several _____ tests, the physician has confirmed his _____.

2. In addition to her diabetes, the patient has several other _____.

3. The physician was unable to _____ the patient's condition because the patient refused the prescribed tests.

E. Use the appropriate medical language to answer the questions. Select the correct answer that completes each statement or answers each question. **LO 2.1, 2.2**

1. Which one of the following terms would describe the condition of a person with an increased body temperature?

   a. pyrexia   **d.** villus

   b. fainting   **e.** endocardium

   c. hemorrhage

2. Inflammation of the lining of the heart is

   a. cardiology.   **d.** cardiologist.

   b. cardiac.   **e.** endocardium.

   c. endocarditis.

3. Which term might be used to describe an area of the ribcage?

   a. hypertensive   **d.** costovertebral

   b. urethra   **e.** ureter

   c. hypotensive

4. Which one of the following terms would a heart specialist use to describe a heart condition?

   a. cortices   **d.** abdominal

   b. urethra   **e.** dermatitis

   c. endocarditis

F. Use the word elements to identify the correct medical term. Select the correct answer to answer each question. **LO 2.2**

1. Which medical term has an element meaning *to flow profusely?*

    a. corpora   **d.** pyrexia

    b. endocardium   **e.** diagnosis

    c. hemorrhage

2. Which medical term has an element meaning *a structure?*

    a. endocarditis   **d.** appendix

    b. cardiologist   **e.** cardiology

    c. endocardium

3. Which medical term has an element meaning *condition?*

    a. pyrexia   **d.** hemostasis

    b. carcinoma   **e.** gastroenterology

    c. diagnoses

4. Which medical term has an element meaning *inflammation?*

    a. gastroenterologist   **d.** gastric

    b. gastritis   **e.** gastrology

    c. gastrologist

5. Which medical term has an element meaning *knowledge of an abnormal condition?*

    a. cortices   **d.** seizure

    b. diagnosis   **e.** pyrexia

    c. convulsion

G. Speak and spell with precision in medical communication. All terms presented are spelled phonetically to make them easier for you to learn to pronounce. Be sure you can speak them correctly as well as spell them correctly! Practice, practice, practice. Choose the best answer, and then fill in the blanks. **LO 2.4, 2.5**

1. The correct pronunciation for an inflammation of the heart is

    a. EN-do-kar-di-tis

    b. en-**DO**-kard-itis

    c. EN-doh-kar-**DIE**-tis

The correct spelling of this term is _____.

2. An abnormally high body temperature is

    a. pie-**REK**-see-ah

    b. **PIE**-rek-seeah

    c. pie-**REK**-see-**AH**

    The correct spelling of this term is _____.

3. Profuse bleeding is termed a

    a. **HEM**-oh-raj

    b. hem-**OH**-raj

    c. **HEM**-oh-**RAJ**

    The correct spelling of this term is _____.

H. **Spelling comprehension.** Select the correct spelling of the term. **LO 2.5**

1. a. pyrexcia	**b.** pyrexia	**c.** pirixia	**d.** pyrixea	**e.** pirexia
2. a. endocardites	**b.** endocarditis	**c.** endocaritis	**d.** endoarites	**e.** endacardites
3. a. hemorrhege	**b.** hemorrage	**c.** hemmorrhage	**d.** hemmorage	**e.** hemorrhage
4. a. diagnosis	**b.** deagnossis	**c.** diagnnosis	**d.** diaggnosis	**e.** diagnosiss
5. a. hypotenssion	**b.** hopotension	**c.** hypotension	**d.** hypotennsion	**e.** hipotension
6. a. costovertebrral	**b.** costovertebral	**c.** costoverrtibral	**d.** castovertebal	**e.** costovertebal
7. a. hemostassis	**b.** hemostasis	**c.** hematsasis	**d.** hemmostassis	**e.** hemastasis
8. a. urethrra	**b.** ureathra	**c.** urettra	**d.** ureathrra	**e.** urethra

I. **Provide the correct term based on the meaning provided below.** Fill in the blank with the correct term. **LO 2.2**

Meaning	Term
1. abnormally high fever	_____
2. pertaining to the ribs and spine	_____
3. stopping bleeding	_____
4. more than one carcinoma	_____
5. low blood pressure	_____
6. canal leading from the urinary bladder to the outside	_____
7. determination of the cause of a disease	_____
8. to bleed profusely	_____
9. inflammation of the inside of the heart	_____
10. more than one appendix	_____

Case Reports

A. **After reading the following Case Report, correctly answer the following questions.** The answers to the questions may not be in the Case Report itself but can be found in the chapter content. **LO 2.1, 2.2, 2.3**

 Case Report (CR) 2.1

You are

. . . an EMT employed in the Emergency Department at Fulwood Medical Center.

Your patient is

. . . Barbara Rotelli, a 17-year-old woman, who presents with **pyrexia** and shaking chills. On her medical record, you read that her physical examination reveals splinter **hemorrhages** under her fingernails and a heart murmur. There is blood in her urine. She had dental surgery four days ago. A provisional **diagnosis** is made of acute **endocarditis.** You are to prepare her for admission to intensive care.

1. *Pyrexia* has an element that means *fever* or *heat.* What is that element? _____

2. If Ms. Rotelli had more than one diagnosis, how would you document that term? _____

3. *Endocarditis* has a prefix that means _____.

B. **After reading the following Case Report, correctly answer the following questions.** The answers to the questions may not be in the Case Report itself but can be found in the chapter content. **LO 2.2**

 Case Report (CR) 2.2

You are

. . . a radiology technician working in the Radiology Department of Fulwood Medical Center.

Your patient is

. . . Mrs. Matilda Morones, a 38-year-old woman who presents with sudden onset of severe, colicky right-flank pain and pain in her **urethra** as she passes urine.

The physical examination revealed that Mrs. Morones is in severe distress, with marked tenderness in the right **costovertebral** angle and in the right lower quadrant of her **abdomen.** Microscopy of her urine showed numerous red blood cells. The **stat abdominal** x-ray you have taken reveals a radiopaque stone in the right **ureter.** She has now become faint and is in **hypotension.**

How are you going to communicate Mrs. Morones's condition as you ask for help and then document her condition and your response?

1. The location of Mrs. Morones's stone is _____ her urinary bladder.

   a. above

   b. below

2. The x-ray was ordered to be taken:

   a. in the order it was received.

   b. tomorrow in the early morning.

   c. before midnight.

   d. immediately.

3. Identify the phrase that best describes her condition.

   a. The position of the stat x-ray caused Mrs. Morones to vomit.

   b. Mrs. Morones's has intense pain in her chest and she fainted.

   c. The red blood cells in her urine caused high blood pressure.

   d. There is a stone in her kidney causing blood in her urine.

   e. Mrs. Morones has low blood pressure and she has lost consciousness.

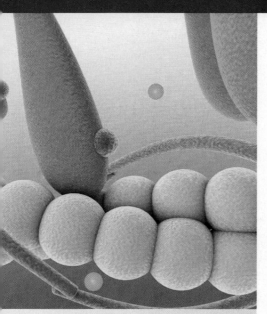

CHAPTER
3

The Body as a Whole
The Language of Anatomy

Chapter Sections

Chapter Learning Outcomes

Upon completion of this chapter, you will be able to:

LO 3.1 Use roots, combining forms, suffixes, and prefixes to construct and analyze medical terms related to the anatomy and physiology of the body as a whole.

LO 3.2 Spell and pronounce medical terms related to the body as a whole.

LO 3.3 Identify the elements that compose the body and discuss the structure and functions of cells.

LO 3.4 Describe the four primary tissue groups found in the body.

LO 3.5 Distinguish between the different organ systems and their major organs.

LO 3.6 Discuss the roles of DNA, genes, and medical genetics and its applications in modern medicine.

LO 3.7 Describe the different anatomical positions, planes, and directions of the body.

LO 3.8 Map the body cavities and describe the abdominal quadrants and the nine regions of the abdomen.

LO 3.9 Apply knowledge of medical terms relating to the body as a whole in documentation, medical records, and communication.

LO 3.10 Identify and correctly use abbreviations of terms used in anatomy and physiology related to the body as a whole.

Human life starts with a single zygote, which as it grows divides into new cells. As the cells continue dividing, they specialize into all the different organs and tissues of the body. Effective medical diagnosis and treatment recognizes that a cell in our body should function in harmony with every other cell. Understanding all the systems of the body is critical for accurate diagnosis of pathology and identifying an effective treatment.

Section 3.1 Organization of the Body

The Body's Levels of Organization

All the elements of your body interact with one another to enable your body to be in constant change as it reacts to the environment, to the nourishment you give it, and to the thoughts and emotions that you express to it.

- The whole body or organism is composed of **organ** systems.
    - Organ systems are composed of **organs.**
        - Organs are composed of **tissues.**
            - Tissues are composed of **cells.**
                - Cells are composed in part of **organelles.**
                    - Organelles are composed of **molecules.**
                        - Molecules are composed of **atoms.**
                            - The **nucleus** of a cell directs all the activities of a cell.

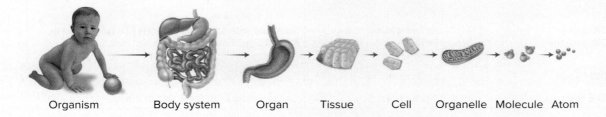

Organism   Body system   Organ   Tissue   Cell   Organelle   Molecule   Atom

The Cell

This single fertilized cell, the **zygote,** is the result of the **fertilization** of an egg **(oocyte)** by a sperm and is the origin of every cell in your body *(Figure 3.1)*. The oocyte divides and multiplies into millions of cells that are the basic unit of every tissue and organ. The structure and all of the functions of your tissues and organs are due to their cells. The **cell** is the basic unit of life. **Cytology** is the study of this cell structure and function. Your understanding of the cell will form the basis for your knowledge of the anatomy and physiology of every tissue and organ.

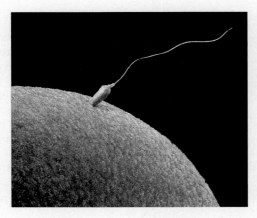

▲ **Figure 3.1** Fertilization of egg by single **sperm.** Francis Leroy, Biocosmos/Science Source

---

Did you know...

- Estimates of the total number of cells in the human body vary from 50 trillion to 70 trillion cells.

- The number of cells in your own body is constantly changing, as cells die and new cells take their place.

- In addition to your own cells, there are 10 times as many microorganisms (bacterial and fungal cells) residing on the skin, in saliva, in the conjunctiva, in the vagina, and in the gastrointestinal tract.

- These microorganisms (normal flora) participate in maintaining normal health, and under normal circumstances do not cause disease.

WORD	PRONUNCIATION		ELEMENTS	DEFINITION
atom	**AT**-om		Greek *indivisible*	A small unit of matter
cell	SELL		Latin *a storeroom*	The smallest unit capable of independent existence
cellular (adj)	**SELL**-you-lar	S/	-ar *pertaining to*	Pertaining to a cell
		R/	**cellul-** *small cell*	
cytology	sigh-**TOL**-oh-jee	S/	**-logy** *study of*	Study of the cell
		R/CF	**cyt/o-** *cell*	
cytologist	sigh-**TOL**-oh-jist	S/	**-logist** *one who studies*	Specialist in the study of cells
fertilization	**FER**-til-eye-**ZAY**-shun	S/	**-ation** *process*	Union of a male sperm and a female egg
fertilize (verb)	**FER**-til-ize	R/	**fertiliz-** *to bear*	
molecule	**MOLL**-eh-kyul	S/	**-ule** *small*	Very small particle consisting of two or more atoms held tightly together
molecular (adj)	mo-**LEK**-you-lar	R/	**molec-** *mass*	
(***Note:*** The two suffixes are joined by two vowels, therefore the *e* in *ule* is not used.)		S/	**-ar** *pertaining to*	
oocyte	**OH**-oh-site	S/	**-cyte** *cell*	Female egg cell
		R/CF	**o/o-** *egg*	
organ	**OR**-gan		Latin *instrument, tool*	Structure with specific functions in a body system
organelle	**OR**-gah-nell	S/	**-elle** *small*	Part of a cell having a specialized function(s)
		R/	**organ-** *organ*	
tissue	**TISH**-you		Latin *to weave*	Collection of similar cells
zygote	**ZYE**-goht		Greek *yoked*	Cell resulting from the union of the sperm and egg

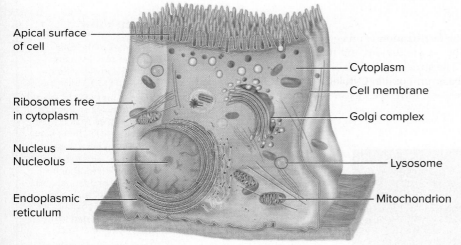

Apical surface of cell

Ribosomes free in cytoplasm

Nucleus
Nucleolus

Endoplasmic reticulum

Cytoplasm

Cell membrane

Golgi complex

Lysosome

Mitochondrion

▲ **Figure 3.2** Structure of a representative cell.

Structure and Functions of Cells

As the zygote divides, every cell derived from it becomes a small, complex factory that carries out these **basic functions of life:**

- Manufacture of proteins and lipids
- Production and use of energy
- Communication with other cells
- Replication of **deoxyribonucleic acid (DNA)**
- Reproduction

All your cells contain a fluid called **cytosol (intracellular** fluid) surrounded by a **cell membrane** *(Figure 3.2).* A single cell may have 10 billion protein molecules inside it.

The cell membrane is made of proteins and lipids and allows water, oxygen, glucose, **electrolytes, steroids,** and alcohol to pass through it. On the outside of the cell membrane are receptors that bind to chemical messengers, such as **hormones** sent by other cells. These are the chemical signals by which your cells communicate with each other. The **cytoplasm** is a clear, gelatinous substance containing cytosol and crowded with different organelles. **Organelles** are small structures that carry out special **metabolic** tasks, the chemical processes that occur in the cell. Examples of organelles are:

- **Nucleus**
- Endoplasmic reticulum
- Golgi complex or apparatus
- **Mitochondria**
- **Nucleolus**
- Ribosomes
- Lysosomes

Organelles

The **nucleus** is the largest organelle and located between the cell membrane and the cytoplasm *(Figure 3.2)*. It directs all the activities of the cell. Most of your cells have one nucleus; red blood cells have none, and some liver cells and muscle cells contain many nuclei. The nucleus is surrounded by its own membrane, which has small openings called *pores*. Every minute, hundreds of molecules pass through the pores. These molecules include the raw materials for the DNA and ribonucleic (RNA) synthesis that is ongoing inside the nucleus. Forty-six molecules of DNA and their associated **proteins** are packed into each nucleus as thin strands called **chromatin.** When cells divide, the chromatin condenses to form 46 more densely coiled bodies called **chromosomes.**

Word Analysis and Definition: The Cell

S = Suffix   P = Prefix   R = Root   R/CF = Combining Form

WORD	PRONUNCIATION		ELEMENTS	DEFINITION
chromatin	**KROH**-ma-tin	S/ R/	**-in** *substance, chemical compound* **chromat-** *color*	Substance composed of DNA that forms chromosomes during cell division
chromosome	**KROH**-moh-sohm	S/ R/CF	**-some** *body* **chrom/o-** *color*	Body in the nucleus that contains DNA and genes
cytoplasm	**SIGH**-toh-plazm	S/ R/CF	**-plasm** *something formed* **cyt/o-** *cell*	Clear, gelatinous substance that forms the substance of a cell except for the nucleus
cytosol	**SIGH**-toh-sawl	S/ R/CF	**-sol** *solution* **cyt/o-** *cell*	Liquid portion of the cell
deoxyribonucleic acid (DNA)	dee-**OCK**-see-**RYE**-boh-noo-**KLEE**-ik **ASS**-id		**deoxyribose** *sugar* **nucleic acid** *protein*	Source of hereditary characteristics found in chromosomes
electrolyte	ee-**LEK**-troh-lite	S/ R/CF	**-lyte** *soluble* **electr/o-** *electric*	Substance that, when dissolved in a suitable medium, forms electrically charged particles
hormone hormonal (adj)	**HOR**-mohn hor-**MOHN**-al	 S/	Greek *set in motion* **-al** *pertaining to*	Chemical formed in one tissue or organ and carried by the blood to stimulate or inhibit a function of another tissue or organ Pertaining to a hormone
intracellular	in-trah-**SELL**-you-lar	S/ P/ R/	**-ar** *pertaining to* **intra-** *within* **-cellul-** *small cell*	Within the cell
membrane membranous (adj)	**MEM**-brain **MEM**-brah-nus	 S/	Latin *parchment* **-ous** *pertaining to*	Thin layer of tissue covering a structure or cavity Pertaining to a membrane
metabolism metabolic (adj)	meh-**TAB**-oh-lizm met-ah-**BOL**-ik	S/ R/ S/	**-ism** *condition* **metabol-** *change* **-ic** *pertaining to*	The constantly changing physical and chemical processes occurring in the cell Pertaining to metabolism
nucleolus	nyu-**KLEE**-oh-lus	S/ R/CF	**-lus** *small* **nucle/o-** *nucleus*	Small mass within the nucleus
nucleus nuclei (pl) nuclear (adj)	**NYU**-klee-us **NYU**-klee-eye **NYU**-klee-ar	 S/ R/	Latin *kernel* **-ar** *pertaining to* **nucle-** *nucleus*	Functional center of a cell or structure Pertaining to the nucleus
steroid steroidal (adj)	**STER**-oyd **STER**-oy-dal	S/ R/	**-oid** *resemble* **ster-** *solid*	Large family of chemical substances found in many drugs, hormones, and body components
synthesis	**SIN**-the-sis	P/ R/	**syn-** *together* **-thesis** *to arrange*	The process of building a compound from different elements

Ribosomes are organelles involved in the manufacture of **protein** from simple materials. This process is called **anabolism.**

Each nucleus (*Figure 3.3*) contains a **nucleolus,** a small dense body composed of RNA and protein. It manufactures ribosomes that migrate through the nuclear membrane pores into the cytoplasm.

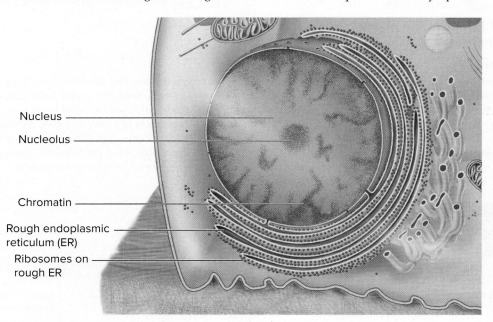

Nucleus

Nucleolus

Chromatin

Rough endoplasmic reticulum (ER)

Ribosomes on rough ER

▲ **Figure 3.3** **The nucleus.**

The **endoplasmic reticulum** is an organelle that manufactures steroids, cholesterol and other lipids, and proteins. It also detoxifies alcohol and other drugs.

Lysosomes are organelles that are the garbage disposal units of the cell. They digest and dispose of worn-out organelles as part of the process of cell death. They also digest foreign particles and bacteria.

Mitochondria (mitochondrion, singular**)** are the powerhouses of the cells. They extract energy by breaking down compounds such as glucose and fat. This process is called **catabolism.** The energy is used to do the work of the cell: for example, to make a muscle contract.

Tissues

The knee contains examples of all the different major groups of tissue and will be used to illustrate the relation of structure to function in the different tissues. Tissues hold your body together. The many tissues of your body have different structures for specialized functions. The different tissues are made of similar cells with unique materials around them that are manufactured by the cells. **Histology** is the study of the structure and function of tissues. The four primary tissue groups are outlined in *Table 3.1.*

Table 3.1 The Four Primary Tissue Groups

Type	Function	Location
Connective	Bind, support, protect, fill spaces, store fat	Widely distributed throughout the body; for example, in blood, bone, cartilage, and fat
Epithelial	Protect, **secrete,** absorb, **excrete**	Cover body surface, cover and line internal organs, compose glands
Muscle	Movement	Attached to bones, in the walls of hollow internal organs, and in the heart
Nervous	Transmit impulses for coordination, sensory reception, motor actions	Brain, spinal cord, nerves

WORD	PRONUNCIATION	ELEMENTS		DEFINITION
anabolism	an-**AB**-oh-lizm	S/ R/	-ism *condition* anabol- *build up*	The buildup of complex substances in the cell from simpler ones as a part of metabolism
catabolism	kah-**TAB**-oh-lizm	S/ R/	-ism *condition* catabol- *break down*	Breakdown of complex substances into simpler ones as a part of metabolism
epithelium	ep-ih-**THEE**-lee-um	S/ P/ R/CF	-um *structure* epi- *upon* -thel/i- *nipple*	Tissue that covers surfaces or lines cavities
epithelial (adj)	ep-ih-**THEE**-lee-al	S/	-al *pertaining to*	Pertaining to epithelium
excrete	eks-**KREET**		Latin *separate*	To pass waste products of metabolism out of the body
excretion (noun)	eks-**KREE**-shun			Removal of waste products of metabolism out of the body
histology	his-**TOL**-oh-jee	S/ R/CF	-logy *study of* hist/o- *tissue*	Structure and function of cells, tissues, and organs
histologist	his-**TOL**-oh-jist	S/	-logist *one who studies*	Specialist in the structure and function of cells, tissues, and organs
lysosome	**LIE**-soh-sohm	S/ R/CF	-some *body* lys/o- *decompose*	Enzyme that digests foreign material and worn-out cell components
mitochondrion	my-toe-**KON**-dree-on	S/ R/CF R	-ion *action, condition* mit/o- *thread* -chondr- *cartilage, rib, granule*	Organelle that generates, stores, and releases energy for cell activities
mitochondria (pl)	my-toe-**KON**-dree-ah			
protein	**PRO**-teen	S/ R/CF	-in *substance, chemical compound* prot/e- *first*	Class of food substances based on amino acids
ribosome	**RYE**-bo-sohm	S/ R/CF	-some *body* rib/o- *like a rib*	Structure in the cell that assembles amino acids into protein
secrete secretion (noun)	se-**KREET** se-**KREE**-shun		Latin *release*	To produce a chemical substance in a cell and release it from the cell

Connective Tissues in the Knee Joint

The knee joint provides an excellent example of how different types of tissues form the knee joint to allow for the functions of walking, bending, and running. These tissues and roles are listed below:

- **Bone** is the hardest connective tissue due to the presence of calcium mineral salts, mostly calcium phosphate. Cells that make up bone tissue are
  - **Osteoblasts** deposit bone **matrix** (*Figure 3.4*) in concentric patterns around a central canal containing a blood vessel. As a result, every osteoblast is close to a supply of **nutrients** from the blood.
  - **Osteocytes** are former osteoblasts that maintain the bone matrix.
  - **Osteoclasts** dissolve the bone matrix to release calcium and phosphate into the blood when these chemicals are needed elsewhere.
- **Cartilage** has a flexible, rubbery matrix that allows it, as a meniscus, to function as a shock absorber and as a gliding surface where two bones meet to form a joint. Cartilage also forms the shape of your ear, the tip of your nose, and your larynx. Cartilage has very few blood vessels and heals poorly or not at all. Cells of cartilage include
  - Chrondroblasts, which deposit the cartilage matrix.
  - Chrondrocytes, which are former chondroblasts that maintain the cartilage matrix.
  - Fibers, which give the cartilage strength and flexibility.

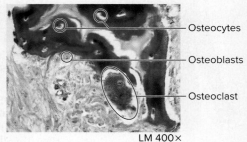

Osteocytes

Osteoblasts

Osteoclast

LM 400×

▲ **Figure 3.4** **Bone tissue.**
Al Telser/McGraw Hill

- **Ligaments** are strips or bands of fibrous connective tissue *(Figure 3.5)*. Cells called **fibroblasts** form a gelatinous (jellylike) matrix and closely packed, parallel **collagen** fibers. These fibers provide the strength the ligament needs. Their blood supply is poor, so they do not heal well without surgery.
- **Tendons** are thick, strong ligaments that attach muscles to bone.
- The **joint capsule** of the knee joint is attached to the tibia and femur, encloses the joint cavity, and is made of thin, collagenous fibrous connective tissue. It is strengthened by fibers that extend over it from the ligaments and muscles surrounding the knee joint. These features are common to most joints.
- The inner surface of many joint capsules is lined with **synovial membrane,** which secretes **synovial fluid.** This fluid is a slippery lubricant retained in the joint cavity by the capsule. It has a texture similar to raw egg white. It makes joint movement almost friction-free and distributes nutrients to the cartilage on the joint surfaces of bone.
- **Muscle** tissue stabilizes the knee joint. Extensions of the tendons of the *quadriceps femoris,* the large muscle in front of the thigh, and of the *semimembranosus muscle* on the rear of the thigh, are major stabilizers. The muscles themselves respectively extend and flex the joint. The structure and functions of these and other skeletal muscles are described in *Chapter 14.*
- **Nervous** tissue extensively supplies all the knee structures, which is why a knee injury is excruciatingly painful. The structure and functions of nervous tissue are described in *Chapter 9.*

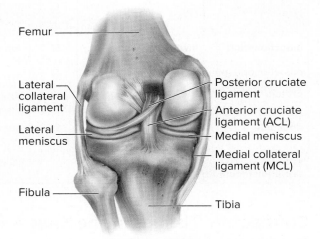

Femur

Lateral collateral ligament

Lateral meniscus

Fibula

Posterior cruciate ligament

Anterior cruciate ligament (ACL)

Medial meniscus

Medial collateral ligament (MCL)

Tibia

Posterior view

▲ **Figure 3.5** Ligaments of the knee joint.

Organs and Organ Systems

Organs

An **organ** is a structure composed of several tissues that work together to carry out specific functions. For example, the skin is an organ that has different tissues in it such as epithelial cells, hair, nails, and glands.

Each organ has well-defined anatomic boundaries separating it from adjacent structures and performs a particular function. The different organs in an organ system are usually interconnected. For example, in the urinary organ system, the organs are the kidneys, ureters, bladder, and urethra, and they are all connected *(Figure 3.6)* as they work to eliminate fluid waste from the body. See *Table 3.2* to review the organs of each body system.

Organ Systems

An **organ system** is a group of organs with a specific collective function, such as digestion, circulation, or respiration. For example, the nose, pharynx, larynx, trachea, and bronchi work together to achieve the total function of respiration.

The body has 11 organ systems, shown in *Table 3.2.* The muscle and skeleton can be considered one organ system, the musculoskeletal system.

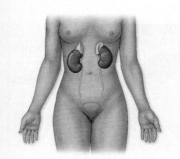

▲ **Figure 3.6** Organs of the urinary system.
©McGraw-Hill Education

WORD	PRONUNCIATION		ELEMENTS	DEFINITION
capsule capsular (adj)	KAP-syul KAP-syu-lar	S/ R/ S/	-ule *little* caps- *box* -ar *pertaining to*	Fibrous tissue layer surrounding a joint or some other structure Pertaining to a capsule
cartilage	KAR-tih-lij		Latin *gristle*	Nonvascular firm, connective tissue found mostly in joints
chondroblast chondrocyte	KON-droh-blast KON-droh-site	S/ R/CF S/	-blast *germ cell* chondr/o- *cartilage* -cyte *cell*	Cartilage-forming cell Cartilage cell
collagen	KOL-ah-jen	S/ R/CF	-gen *produce, form* coll/a- *glue*	Major protein of connective tissue, cartilage, and bone
fibroblast	FIE-bro-blast	S/ R/CF	-blast *germ cell* fibr/o- *fiber*	Cell that forms collagen fibers
matrix	MAY-triks		Latin "mater" *mother*	Substance that surrounds cells, is manufactured by the cells, and holds them together
nutrient	NYU-tree-ent	S/ R/	-ent *end result* nutri- *nourish*	A substance in food required for normal physiologic function
osteoblast osteoclast osteocyte	OS-tee-oh-blast OS-tee-oh-klast OS-tee-oh-site	S/ R/CF S/ S/	-blast *germ cell* oste/o- *bone* -clast *break* -cyte *cell*	Bone-forming cell Bone-removing cell Bone-maintaining cell
synovia (**Note:** The fluid resembles the white of an egg) synovial (adj)	so-**NOH**-vee-uh sih-**NOH**-vee-al	S/ P/ R/ S/ R/CF	-ia *pertaining to* syn- *together* -ov- *egg* -al *pertaining to* synov/i- *synovial membrane*	Pertaining to the fluid in a joint. Pertaining to synovial fluid and synovial membrane
tendon	TEN-dun		Latin *sinew*	Fibrous band that connects muscle to bone

All your organ systems work together to ensure that your body's internal environment remains relatively constant. This process is called **homeostasis.** For example, your digestive, respiratory, and circulatory organ systems work together so that (a) every cell in your body receives adequate nutrients and oxygen and (b) waste products from the breakdown of these nutrients during cell metabolism are removed. Your cells can then function normally. Disease affecting an organ or organ system disrupts this game plan of homeostasis.

Table 3.2 Organ Systems

Organ System	Major Organs	Major Functions
Integumentary	Skin, hair, nails, sweat glands, sebaceous glands	Protect tissues, regulate body temperature, support sensory receptors
Skeletal	Bones, ligaments, cartilages, tendons	Provide framework, protect soft tissues, provide attachments for muscles, produce blood cells, store inorganic salts
Muscular	Muscles	Cause movements, maintain posture, produce body heat
Nervous	Brain, spinal cord, nerves, sense organs	Detect changes, receive and interpret sensory information, stimulate muscles and glands
Endocrine	Glands that secrete hormones: pituitary, thyroid, parathyroid, adrenal, pancreas, ovaries, testes, pineal, thymus	Control metabolic activities of organs and structures
Cardiovascular	Heart, blood vessels	Move blood and transport substances throughout body
Lymphatic	Lymph vessels and nodes, thymus, spleen	Return tissue fluid to the blood, carry certain absorbed food molecules, defend body against infection
Digestive	Mouth, tongue, teeth, salivary glands, pharynx, esophagus, stomach, liver, gallbladder, pancreas, small and large intestines	Receive, break down, and absorb food; eliminate unabsorbed material
Respiratory	Nasal cavity, pharynx, larynx, trachea, bronchi, lungs	Control Intake and output of air, exchange gases between air and blood
Urinary	Kidneys, ureters, urinary bladder, urethra	Remove wastes from blood, maintain water and electrolyte balance, store and transport urine
Reproductive	*Male:* scrotum, testes, epididymides, vas deferens, seminal vesicles, prostate, bulbourethral glands, urethra, penis	Produce and maintain sperm cells, transfer sperm cells into female reproductive tract, secrete male hormones
	Female: ovaries, uterine (fallopian) tubes, uterus, vagina, vulva	Produce and maintain egg cells, receive sperm cells, support development of an embryo, function in birth process, secrete female hormones

WORD	PRONUNCIATION	ELEMENTS		DEFINITION
cardiovascular	KAR-dee-oh-VAS-kyu-lar	S/ R/CF R/	-ar *pertaining to* cardi/o- *heart* -vascul- *blood vessel*	Pertaining to the heart and blood vessels
digestive	die-JEST-iv	S/ R/	-ive *nature of* digest- *to break down*	Pertaining to the breakdown of food into elements suitable for cell metabolism
endocrine	EN-doh-krin	P/ R/CF	endo- *within* -crin/e *secrete*	Pertaining to a gland that produces an internal or hormonal secretion
homeostasis (**Note:** *Hemo*stasis is very different.)	ho-mee-oh-STAY-sis	S/ R/CF	-stasis *stand still, control* home/o- *the same*	Stability or equilibrium of a system or the body's internal environment
integumentary	in-TEG-you-MEN-tah-ree	S/ R/	-ary *pertaining to* integument- *covering of the body*	Pertaining to the covering of the body (the skin)
lymphatic	lim-FAT-ik	S/ R/	-atic *pertaining to* lymph- *lymph*	Pertaining to lymph or the lymphatic system
muscular	MUSS-kyu-lar	S/ R/	-ar *pertaining to* muscul- *muscle*	Pertaining to muscle or muscles
nervous	NER-vus		Latin *nerve*	Pertaining to a nerve
organ	OR-gan		Greek *instrument*	Structure with specific functions in a body system
reproductive	ree-pro-DUC-tiv	S/ P/ R/	-ive *nature of, pertaining to* re- *again* -product- *lead forth*	Relating to the process by which organisms produce offspring
respiratory	RES-pir-ah-TOR-ee		Latin *breathing*	Relating to the process of exchanging oxygen and carbon dioxide
skeletal	SKEL-eh-tal	S/ R/	-al *pertaining to* -skelet- *skeleton*	Pertaining to the bony skeleton
urinary	YUR-in-air-ee	S/ R/	-ary *pertaining to* urin- *urine*	Pertaining to urine

Check Point Section 3.1

A. As you begin your study of *medical language, it is important to realize the logic of how terms are formed.* Elements are building blocks. There is always a root, but you may not see the root in the same position in every term. Not every term requires a prefix and/or a suffix. Fill in the blanks. LO 3.1, 3.3

1. The female egg cell is known as an _____ / _____

2. This term does not start with a prefix; it starts with a combining form and ends with a suffix.

    Study of the cell: _____ / _____

3. This term also begins with a combining form, which is a root plus a combining vowel. The term ends with a suffix. Pertaining to the cell: _____ / _____

B. Continue building your knowledge of elements. *Add the elements that will complete this medical term. Fill in the blanks.* **LO 3.1, 3.3**

1. Within the cell   _____/cellul/ _____

2. Substance of a cell except for the nucleus   _____/plasm

3. Chemical substance found in drugs   _____/oid

C. Seek and find the medical terms that are defined as follows. *Fill in the blank with the correct term.* **LO 3.3, 3.9**

1. small organ _____

2. thin layer of tissue covering a structure or cavity _____

3. electrically charged particles _____

4. functional center of a cell or structure _____

D. Continue analyzing the logic of medical language. *Fill in the blanks.* **LO 3.1, 3.3**

1. Which term refers to an enzyme? _____

2. Find a term that contains an element that means *water* _____

3. Which term refers to breaking substances down? _____

E. Define word elements. *Given the word element, identify its meaning.* **LO 3.1**

1. The meaning of the word element -*logy:*
   a. pertaining to   b. composed of   c. one who studies   d. study of

2. The meaning of the word element -*al:*
   a. pertaining to   b. composed of   c. structure   d. study of

3. The meaning of the word element -*logist:*
   a. one who studies   b. tissue   c. upon   d. structure

F. Understanding elements is the key to a large medical vocabulary. *Work with the following exercise to increase your knowledge of medical language. Fill in the blanks.* **LO 3.4**

osteoblast osteoclast osteocyte

1. The three terms list above all refer to (select one)   a. cartilage   b. bone   c. collagen   The element they have in common is: _____

2. The element that changes in every term is the (select one):   P   R   CF   S

3. The suffix that means germ cell is: _____

4. The suffix that means break is: _____

5. The suffix that means cell is: _____

G. Match the appropriate medical term in the first column to the descriptions given in the *second column.* **LO 3.4**

_____   1. synovial   a. bone forming cell

_____   2. meniscus   b. connects muscle to bone

_____   3. tendon   c. slippery lubricant

_____   4. osteoblast   d. shock absorber

H. Use your knowledge of the building blocks of terms, and deconstruct the following terms into their basic elements. *This will give you a better picture of how the words were formed. Fill in the blanks. The first one is done for you.* **LO 3.1**

1. homeostasis   home/o/stasis

2. urinary   _____/_____

3. cardiovascular   _____/_____/_____

4. respiratory   _____/_____/_____

Section 3.2 Basic Genetics and Genetic Medicine

DNA and Genes

Inside the cell nucleus are packed 46 molecules of **deoxyribonucleic acid (DNA)** as thin strands called **chromatin.** When cells divide, the chromatin condenses with **histone** proteins to form 23 pairs (46 total) of densely coiled bodies called **chromosomes.** Twenty-two of these pairs look the same in both males and females. In the 23rd pair, females have two copies of the X chromosome; males have one X and one Y. The picture of the human chromosomes lined up in pairs is called a **karyotype** *(Figure 3.7).*

The information in DNA is stored as a code of four chemical bases: adenine (A), guanine (G), cytosine (C), and thymine (T). The total human DNA contains about 3 billion bases, and more than 99% of those bases are the same in all people. The sequence of these bases determines the building and maintaining of the organism's cells, similar to the way in which letters of the alphabet appear in order to form words and sentences.

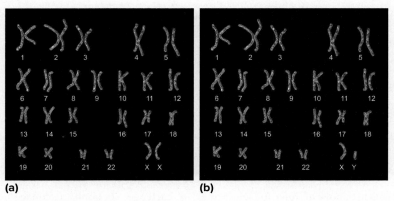

(a) (b)

▲ **Figure 3.7** **Human karyotype.** (a) Kateryna Kon/Shutterstock (b) Kateryna Kon/Shutterstock

The **chromosomal** DNA bases pair with each other—A with T and C with G—and are attached to a sugar molecule and a phosphate molecule. A base, sugar, and phosphate form a **nucleotide.** Nucleotides are arranged in two long strands to form a spiral called a double **helix.**

The nuclear DNA in the chromosomes is the **hereditary** material, each unit of which is called a **gene.** The genes act as instructions to make molecules of different proteins. Each person has two copies of each gene, one inherited from each parent. Most genes are the same in all people; only less than one percent is slightly different between people. These small differences contribute to each person's unique physical features. Humans are thought to have between 20,000 and 25,000 genes. This total is called the **genome.**

Mitosis

The critical property of DNA is that it can **replicate,** make copies of itself, so that when cells divide, each new cell has an exact copy of the DNA present in the old cell. This cell division is called **mitosis,** in which a cell duplicates all of its contents, including its chromosomes, to form two identical daughter cells. When mitosis is not performed correctly, abnormal cells, such as cancer cells, can result.

Mutations and Epigenetic Changes

A permanent alteration of the nucleotide sequence of the genome of an organism is called a **mutation.** Mutations may or may not produce visible changes in the observable characteristics (**phenotype**) of an organism. Mutations play a part in both normal and abnormal biological processes including evolution, cancer, and the development of the immune system.

Chemical compounds that become added to single genes can regulate their activity to produce modifications known as **epigenetic** changes. These changes can remain as cells divide and can be inherited through generations. Environmental influences from pollution, drugs, pharmaceuticals, aging, and diets can also produce epigenetic modifications, such as cancers, mental disorders, and degenerative and metabolic disorders.

Word Analysis and Definition: DNA

WORD	PRONUNCIATION		ELEMENTS	DEFINITION
epigenetics	EP-ih-jeh-NET-iks	S/ P/ R/	-tics *pertaining to* epi- *above, over* -gene *to create*	The study of disorders produced by the effects of chemical compounds (e.g., pollutants) or environmental influences (such as diet) on genes
gene genetic (adj)	JEEN jeh-NET-ik	S/ R/	Greek *birth* -tic *pertaining to* gene- *to create*	The functional unit of heredity on a chromosome Pertaining to genetics
genome (*Note:* The vowel "e" at the end of gene- is dropped to make the composite word flow more easily.)	JEE-nome	R/ S/	gene- *to create* -ome *a mass of something*	A complete set of chromosomes
helix	HEE-liks		Greek *a coil*	A spiral of nucleotides in the structure of DNA
heredity	heh-RED-ih-tee		Latin *an heir*	The transmission of characteristics from parent to offspring
hereditary	heh-RED-ih-ter-ee	S/ R/	-ary *pertaining to* heredit- *inherited through genes*	Transmissible from parent to offspring
histone	HIS-tone	S/ R/	-one *chemical* hist- *tissue*	A simple protein found in the cell nucleus
karyotype	KAIR-ee-oh-type	S/ R/CF	-type *model* kary/o- *nucleus*	The chromosome characteristics of an individual cell
mitosis	my-TOH-sis		Greek *thread*	Cell division to create two identical cells, each with 46 chromosomes
mutation	myu-TAY-shun		Latin *to change*	A permanent alteration in the nucleotide sequence of the genome
nucleotide (*Note:* The "t" at the end of nucleo- is added to make the composite word flow more easily.)	NYU-klee-oh-tide	R/CF S/	nucle/o- *nucleus* -ide *having a particular quality*	Combination of a DNA base, a sugar molecule, and a phosphate molecule
phenotype	FEE-noh-type	S/ R/CF	-type *model* phen/o- *appearance*	Manifestation of a genome
replicate	REP-lih-kate		Latin *a reply*	To produce an exact copy

Genetic Medicine

Medical genetics is the application of genetics to medical care. Genetic medicine is the newer term for medical genetics and incorporates areas such as gene therapy, personalized (precise) medicine, and predictive medicine.

Every person has a unique variation of the human genome and an individual's health stems from this genetic variation interacting with behaviors (drinking, smoking, etc.) and influences from the environment (chemical pollution in some form). Knowing the genetic makeup will enable more accurate diagnoses to be made, the source of the disease to be understood, and earlier, more accurate treatments or the prevention of progression of the disease provided. This concept is called *personalized medicine.*

One way that the biological variant is seen is responsiveness to drugs. Attention deficit hyperactivity disorder (ADHD) medications only work for one out of ten preschoolers, cancer drugs are effective for only one out of four patients, and depression drugs work for six out of ten patients. The drug Tamoxifen used to be prescribed to women with a form of breast cancer (BRCA), but 65% developed resistance to it. These women were found to have a mutation in their CYP2D6 gene that made Tamoxifen an ineffective treatment.

Personalized medicine can assist with preventive care. Women are already being genotyped for mutations in the BRCA1 (BReast CAncer gene 1) and BRCA2 (BReast CAncer gene 2) genes if they have a family history of breast or ovarian cancer. Women that test positive for both mutations can consider preventative and treatment that are specific to genetic mutations.

Cytogenetics is the study of chromosome abnormalities to determine a cause for developmental delay, mental retardation, birth defects, and **dysmorphic** features, and chromosomal abnormalities are often detected in cancer cells.

Gene therapy is an experimental technique to replace a mutated gene that causes disease with a healthy copy, inactivate a mutated gene that is functioning improperly, or introduce a new gene into the body to prevent or help cure a disease. The **therapeutic** genes are introduced into body cells, and some 600 clinical trials utilizing this form of therapy are underway in the United States.

Predictive medicine looks at the probability of a disease and allows preventive measures to be taken. Examples are newborn screening to identify genetic disorders that can be treated early in life, and **prenatal** testing to look for diseases and conditions in an **embryo** or **fetus** whose parents have an increased risk of having a baby with a genetic or chromosomal disorder.

Word Analysis and Definition: Genetics

S = Suffix   P = Prefix   R = Root   R/CF = Combining Form

WORD	PRONUNCIATION		ELEMENTS	DEFINITION
cytogenetics	SIGH-toh-jeh-NET-iks	S/ R/CF R/	-tics *pertaining to* cyto- *cell* -gene- *create*	Study of chromosomal abnormalities in a cell
dysmorphology	dis-mor-FOLL-oh-jee	S/ P/ R/CF	-logy *study of* dys- *difficult, bad* -morph/o- *shape*	The study of developmental structural defects
dysmorphic	dis-MOR-fik	S/	-ic *pertaining to*	Possessing a developmental structural defect
embryo	EM-bree-oh		Greek *a young one*	Developing organism from conception until the end of the eighth week
fetus	FEE-tus		Latin *offspring*	Human organism from the end of the eighth week to birth
personalized	PER-son-al-ized	S/ R/	-ized *affected in a specific way* personal- *an individual*	Designed to meet someone's individual needs
predictive	pree-DIK-tiv	S/ P/ R/	-ive *quality of* pre- *before* -dict- *consent*	The likelihood of a disease or disorder being present or occurring in the future
prenatal	pree-NAY-tal	S/ P/ R/	-al *pertaining to* pre- *before* -nat- *born*	Before birth
therapy therapeutic	THAIR-ah-pee THAIR-ah-PYU-tik		Greek *medical treatment* Greek *curing of a disorder or disease*	Systematic treatment of a disease, dysfunction, or disorder Curing or capable of curing a disorder or disease

Check Point Section 3.2

A. Use your knowledge of medical terminology related to genetics. *Insert the correct term in the appropriate statement.* **LO 3.6**

gene   genome   mitosis   chromosome   chromatin

1. When the cell is maintaining normal function, DNA and proteins are contained within thin strands of _____
_____.

2. When the cell is dividing, DNA wraps around the proteins and is contained within densely coiled bodies called _____
_____.

3. The unit of nuclear DNA in the chromosomes is called a _____.

4. A _____ is a complete set of chromosomes.

5. The process of _____ occurs when a cell creates an exact copy of itself and divides into two identical cells.

B. Discuss the applications of medical genetics. *Choose the correct answer to complete the following statements.* **LO 3.6**

1. The replacement of a mutated gene with a healthy copy is termed:

   a. predictive medicine.   b. cytogenetics.   c. gene therapy.   d. personalized medicine.

2. The study of chromosome abnormalities in a cell is:

   a. cytogenetics.   b. dysmorphology.   c. prenatal therapy.   d. precise medicine.

3. _____ medicine uses genetics to determine accurate treatments for an existing condition.

   a. Personalized   b. Preventative   c. Cytogenetic   d. Predictive

C. Not all terms can be deconstructed. *It is sometimes necessary to memorize the medical terms of Greek and Latin origin. Given the definition, provide the term that is being described. Fill in the blanks.* **LO 3.6, 3.9**

1. Systematic treatment of a disease, dysfunction, or disorder. _____

2. Human organism from conception to the end of the eighth week. _____

3. Human organism from the end of the eighth week to birth. _____

4. Curing or capable of curing a disorder or disease. _____

Section 3.3 Anatomic Position, Planes, and Directions

Anatomic Position

Terms have been developed over the past several thousand years to enable you to describe clearly where different anatomic structures and lesions are in relation to each other. To communicate effectively with other health professionals, it is critical that you are able to use the terminology to describe these positions and relative positions. When all **anatomic** descriptions are used, it is assumed that the body is in the anatomic position. The body is standing erect with feet flat on the floor, face and eyes facing forward, and arms at the sides with the palms facing forward *(Figure 3.8)*.

When your palms face forward, the forearm is **supine.** When you lie down flat on your back, you are supine. When your palms face backward, the forearm is **prone.** When you lie down flat on your abdomen, you are prone.

Directional Terms

Directional terms describe the position of one structure or part of the body relative to another; for example, **cephalic** vs. **caudal, ventral** vs. **dorsal,** and **proximal** vs. **distal.** These directional terms are shown in *Figures 3.8* and *3.9.*

Anatomic Planes

Different views of the body are based on imaginary "slices" producing flat surfaces that pass through the body *(Figure 3.10)*. The three major anatomic planes are

- **Transverse** or **horizontal**—a plane passing across the body parallel to the floor and perpendicular to the body's long axis. It divides the body into an upper (**superior**) portion and a lower (**inferior**) portion.
- **Sagittal**—a vertical plane that divides the body into right and left portions.
- **Frontal** or **coronal**—a vertical plane that divides the body into front (**anterior**) and back (**posterior**) portions.

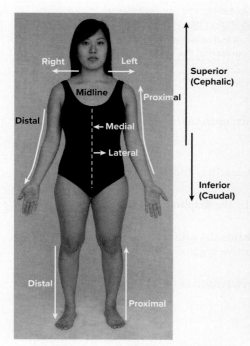

▲ **Figure 3.8** Anatomic position with directional terms. Aaron Roeth Photography

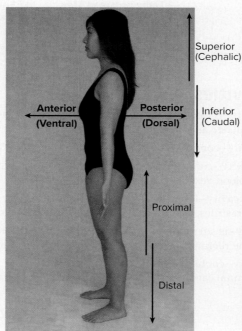

▲ **Figure 3.9** Directional terms. Aaron Roeth Photography

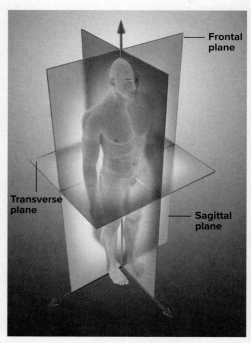

▲ **Figure 3.10** Anatomic planes. Springer Medizin/Science Source

S = Suffix   P = Prefix   R = Root   R/CF = Combining Form

WORD	PRONUNCIATION	ELEMENTS		DEFINITION
anatomy	ah-**NAT**-oh-mee	P/ R/ S/	ana- *away from* -tomy- *section* -ic *pertaining to*	Study of the structures of the human body
anatomic (adj)	an-ah-**TOM**-ik			Pertaining to anatomy
anterior (opposite of posterior)	an-**TER**-ee-or	S/ R/	-ior *pertaining to* anter- *before, front part*	Front surface of body; situated in front
caudal (opposite of cephalic)	**KAW**-dal	S/ R/	-al *pertaining to* caud- *tail*	Pertaining to or nearer to the tail
cephalic (opposite of caudal)	se-**FAL**-ik	S/ R/	-ic *pertaining to* cephal- *head*	Pertaining to or nearer to the head
coronal (equivalent to frontal)	**KOR**-oh-nal	S/ R/	-al *pertaining to* coron- *crown*	Pertaining to the vertical plane dividing the body into anterior and posterior portions
distal (opposite of proximal)	**DISS**-tal	S/ R/	-al *pertaining to* dist- *away from the center*	Situated away from the center of the body
dorsal (equivalent to posterior)	**DOR**-sal	S/ R/	-al *pertaining to* dors- *back*	Pertaining to the back or situated behind
frontal (equivalent to coronal)	**FRON**-tal	S/ R/	-al *pertaining to* front- *front*	In front; relating to the anterior part of the body
inferior (opposite of superior)	in-**FEE**-ree-or	S/ R/	-ior *pertaining to* infer- *below*	Situated below
posterior (opposite of anterior)	pos-**TER**-ee-or	S/ R/	-ior *pertaining to* poster- *coming behind*	Pertaining to the back surface of the body; situated behind
prone (opposite of supine)	PRONE		Latin *bending forward*	Lying face-down, flat on your abdomen
proximal (opposite of distal)	**PROK**-sih-mal	S/ R/	-al *pertaining to* proxim- *nearest*	Situated nearest the center of the body
sagittal	**SAJ**-ih-tal	S/ R/	-al *pertaining to* sagitt- *arrow*	Pertaining to the vertical plane through the body, dividing it into right and left portions
superior (opposite of inferior)	soo-**PEE**-ree-or	S/ R/	-ior *pertaining to* super- *above*	Situated above
supine (opposite of prone)	soo-**PINE**		Latin *bend backward*	Lying face-up, flat on your spine
transverse	trans-**VERS**		Latin *crosswise*	Pertaining to the horizontal plane dividing the body into upper and lower portions
ventral (equivalent to anterior)	**VEN**-tral	S/ R/	-al *pertaining to* ventr- *belly*	Pertaining to the abdomen or situated nearer the surface of the abdomen

Body Cavities

The body contains many **cavities.** Some, like the nasal cavity, open to the outside. Five cavities do not open to the outside and are shown in *Figure 3.11.*

- **Cranial** cavity—contains the brain within the skull.
- **Thoracic** cavity—contains the heart, lungs, thymus gland, trachea, and esophagus, as well as numerous blood vessels and nerves.
- **Abdominal** cavity—is separated from the thoracic cavity by the **diaphragm** and contains the stomach, intestines, liver, spleen, pancreas, and kidneys.
- **Pelvic** cavity—is surrounded by the pelvic bones and contains the urinary bladder, part of the large intestine, the rectum, the anus, and the internal reproductive organs.
- **Spinal** cavity—contains the spinal cord.
    The abdominal cavity and pelvic cavity are collectively referred to as the **abdominopelvic** cavity.

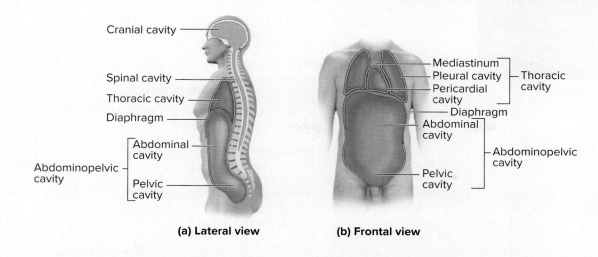

Figure 3.11 Body cavities. (a) lateral view; (b) frontal view.

Cranial cavity

Spinal cavity

Thoracic cavity

Diaphragm

Abdominal cavity

Abdominopelvic cavity

Pelvic cavity

(a) Lateral view

Mediastinum

Pleural cavity

Pericardial cavity

Thoracic cavity

Diaphragm

Abdominal cavity

Abdominopelvic cavity

Pelvic cavity

(b) Frontal view

Abdominal Quadrants and Regions

One way of referring to the locations of abdominal structures and to the site of abdominal pain and other abnormalities is to divide the abdominal region into **quadrants,** as shown in *Figure 3.12a.* The locations are **right upper quadrant (RUQ), left upper quadrant (LUQ), right lower quadrant (RLQ),** and **left lower quadrant (LLQ).** Each quadrant has a three-letter abbreviation as shown—for example, RUQ.

The **abdomen** can also be divided into nine **regions** *(Figure 3.12b).* The central region is called the **umbilical** region, as it is located around the **umbilicus.** The areas above and below that region are named relative to the stomach—**epigastric,** above the stomach, and **hypogastric,** below the stomach.

The six remaining regions are on the right and left sides of these three central regions. The upper regions on either side of the epigastric region, which sit below the ribs, are named the right and left **hypochondriac** regions. The regions on either side of the umbilical region are named the right and left **lumbar** regions (according to the area of the spine nearby). The regions on either side of the hypogastric region are named the right and left **inguinal** (groin) regions.

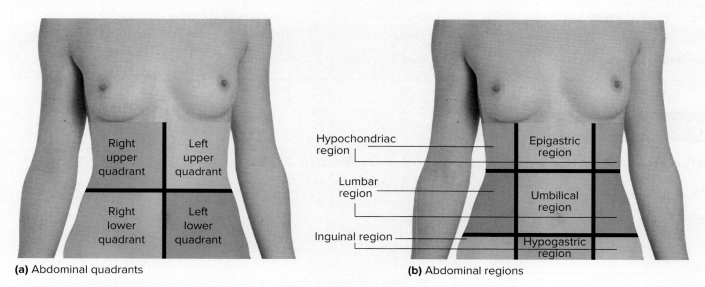

Right upper quadrant

Left upper quadrant

Right lower quadrant

Left lower quadrant

(a) Abdominal quadrants

Hypochondriac region

Lumbar region

Inguinal region

Epigastric region

Umbilical region

Hypogastric region

(b) Abdominal regions

▲ **Figure 3.12** **Regional anatomy.** (a) JW Ramsey/McGraw Hill (b) JW Ramsey/McGraw Hill

Word Analysis and Definition: Body Cavities, Abdominal Quadrants, and Regions

S = Suffix   P = Prefix   R = Root   R/CF = Combining Form

WORD	PRONUNCIATION		ELEMENTS	DEFINITION
abdomen abdominal (adj) abdominopelvic	AB-doh-men ab-DOM-in-al ab-DOM-ih-noh-PEL-vik	 S/ R/ S/ R/CF R/	Latin *abdomen* -al *pertaining to* abdomin- *abdomen* -ic *pertaining to* abdomin/o- *abdomen* -pelv- *pelvis*	Part of the trunk between the thorax and the pelvis Pertaining to the abdomen Pertaining to the abdomen and pelvis
cavity cavities (pl)	KAV-ih-tee KAV-ih-tees		Latin *hollow place*	Hollow space or body compartment
cranial	KRAY-nee-al	S/ R/CF	-al *pertaining to* crani- *skull*	Pertaining to the skull
diaphragm	DIE-ah-fram		Greek *diaphragm, fence*	The musculomembranous partition separating the abdominal and thoracic cavities
epigastric epigastrium (noun)	ep-ih-GAS-trik ep-ih-GAS-tree-um	S/ P/ R/ S/	-ic *pertaining to* epi- *above* gastr- *stomach* -ium *structure*	Pertaining to the abdominal region above the stomach The upper central region of the abdomen located between the costal margins and the subcostal plane
hypochondriac	high-poh-KON-dree-ack	S/ P/ R/CF	-iac *pertaining to* hypo- *below* -chondr *cartilage*	Pertaining to below the cartilage below the ribs
hypogastric	high-poh-GAS-trik	S/ P/ R/	-ic *pertaining to* hypo- *below* -gastr- *stomach*	Pertaining to the abdominal region below the stomach
inguinal	ING-gwi-nal	S/ R/	-al *pertaining to* inguin- *groin*	Pertaining to the groin
lumbar	LUM-bar	S/ R/	-ar *pertaining to* lumb- *lower back, loin*	Pertaining to the region in the back and sides between the ribs and pelvis
pelvic	PEL-vic	S/ R/	-ic *pertaining to* pelv- *pelvis*	Pertaining to the pubic bone
quadrant	KWAD-rant		Latin *one quarter*	One-quarter of a circle
umbilical umbilicus (noun)	um-BIL-ih-kal um-BIL-ih-kus	S/ R/	-al *pertaining to* umbilic- *belly button (navel)*	Pertaining to or around the umbilicus or the center of the abdomen Pit in the abdomen where the umbilical cord entered the fetus

Check Point Section 3.3

A. Identify directional terms. *Identify the term that has the opposite meaning. Fill in the blank.* **LO 3.1, 3.7**

1. ventral _____

2. caudal _____

3. distal _____

4. posterior _____

5. superior _____

B. Identify the planes of the body. *Identify the plane that is being described. Fill in the blank.* **LO 3.7**

1. This plane divides the body into right and left sides: _____

2. This plane is also known as the frontal plane: _____

3. This plane is also known as the horizontal plane: _____

C. Take a closer look at the breakdown of medical terms. *The medical term is given to you. Break it down into elements with a slash (/). See how the combination of elements will give you the meaning of the entire term. <u>The first one is done for you.</u> Fill in the blanks.* **LO 3.1, 3.7**

1. *epigastrium* $\dfrac{epi}{above}$ / $\dfrac{gastr}{stomach}$ / $\dfrac{ium}{structure}$

2. *hypogastric* _____ / _____ / _____

3. *abdominopelvic* _____ / _____ / _____

D. Create medical terms related to the body cavities. *Fill in the blank with the missing word elements.* **LO 3.1, 3.8**

1. The quadrants mark the areas of the _____ /al cavity.

2. The center of the abdominal regions is the _____ /al region.

The Body as a Whole
Challenge Your Knowledge

A. **Demonstrate your knowledge of directional terms and abbreviations by identifying the correct choice.** Select the correct answer that completes each statement. **LO 3.7, 3.8, 3.10**

1. The epigastric region is _____ the stomach.

   a. above

   b. below

2. Therefore, the epigastric region is _____ to the stomach.

   a. superior

   b. inferior

3. The umbilical region is so named because it is in the _____ of the abdomen.

   a. center

   b. back

4. The umbilical region is _____ to the epigastric region.

   a. inferior

   b. superior

5. In the abbreviation LLQ, the first "L" means _____.

   a. lower

   b. left

6. The spine is _____ to the heart.

   a. anterior

   b. posterior

7. The nose is _____ to the chin.

   a. superior

   b. inferior

8. The umbilicus is _____ to the spine.

   a. dorsal

   b. ventral

9. The toes are _____ to the knee.

   a. distal

   b. proximal

B. **Latin and Greek terms.** There is no easy way to remember these—you just have to know them so that you can relate to their meanings. Match the terms in 1–10 to the meanings in a-j. **LO 3.3, 3.4, 3.6, 3.9**

_____ 1. secrete	**a.**	a storeroom
_____ 2. helix	**b.**	to change
_____ 3. hormone	**c.**	gristle
_____ 4. ligament	**d.**	release
_____ 5. cell	**e.**	band
_____ 6. matrix	**f.**	coil
_____ 7. mutation	**g.**	mother
_____ 8. membrane	**h.**	to set in motion
_____ 9. cartilage	**i.**	sinew
_____ 10. tendon	**j.**	parchment

C. **Knowledge of anatomic locations on the body will make your communications with other health professionals precise.** Challenge yourself with the following questions. Choose T if the statement is true. Choose F if the statement is false. **LO 3.7, 3.8**

1. Standing erect with feet flat on the floor, face and eyes facing forward, and arms at the side with palms facing forward is the anatomical position.   T   F

2. A transverse plane is a horizontal plane.   T   F

3. Frontal and sagittal planes are both vertical planes.   T   F

4. Inferior is situated above another part of the body.   T   F

5. *Dorsal* means the same as *anterior*.   T   F

6. The abdominal cavity contains the urinary bladder.   T   F

7. The thoracic cavity is superior to the pelvic cavity, and the pelvic cavity is inferior to the abdominal cavity.   T   F

8. The diaphragm divides the pelvic cavity and the abdominal cavity.   T   F

9. In RUQ, "Q" means *quadrant*.   T   F

10. The RUQ and the LUQ are divided by a sagittal plane.   T   F

D. **What am I? Fill in the blanks with the correct answers. LO 3.3, 3.5**

1. Anabolism + catabolism = _____.

2. The largest organelle that directs all the activities of the cell is the _____.

3. This forms the tip of your nose, the shape of your ear, and the larynx: _____.

4. The relatively constant internal environment in the body is _____.

5. Standing erect, with feet flat on the floor, face and eyes facing forward, and arms at the side, palms facing forward is _____.

E. **Use the language of anatomy to answer the questions.** Select the correct answer to each question. **LO 3.7**

1. Which of the following medical terms is NOT an anatomic plane?

   a. transverse   **d.** supine

   b. frontal   **e.** coronal

   c. sagittal

2. Which of the following medical terms is NOT a correct pair of opposites?

   a. anterior   posterior

   b. inferior   superior

   c. dorsal   proximal

   d. prone   supine

   e. caudal   cephalic

3. Which of the following medical terms has an element meaning *nearest*?

   a. ventral
   b. proximal
   c. supine
   d. sagittal
   e. superior

4. Which of the following terms means the same thing as *coronal*?

   a. frontal
   b. superior
   c. ventral
   d. dorsal
   e. cephalic

5. If dorsal is *equivalent to* posterior, it means they are

   a. nouns.
   b. verbs.
   c. adjectives.
   d. the same.
   e. the opposite.

F. **Anatomic positions and planes.** You must know anatomic positions to prepare a patient for any type of procedure or surgery. Anatomic planes can help define radiologic studies. Using this knowledge, fill in each blank with the correct term that completes each statement. **LO 3.7**

   1. The surgeon needs his patient in the _____ position to remove a lesion on his back.

   2. To prepare for a knee arthroscopy, the patient will be in the _____ position.

   3. When the palms of the hands are faced up, the forearms are in the _____ position.

   4. A plane that divides the body into an upper, or superior, portion and a lower, or inferior, portion is called a _____ plane.

   5. A frontal plane can also be called a _____ plane.

G. **Use the language of anatomy to answer the following questions about the cell.** Select the correct answer that completes each statement or answers each question. **LO 3.3**

   1. Which one of the following medical terms is *not* an organelle?

      a. lysosomes
      b. nucleolus
      c. endoplasmic reticulum
      d. sulcus
      e. mitochondria

   2. The fluid contained inside the cell is termed

      a. cytoplasm.
      b. endoplasm.
      c. ectoplasm.
      d. synovial fluid.
      e. plasma.

   3. What surrounds and protects the cell?

      a. Golgi complex
      b. endoplasmic reticulum
      c. lysosomes
      d. ribosomes
      e. cell membrane

   4. What are the chemical messenger cells called?

      a. lymphocytes
      b. erythrocytes
      c. electrolytes
      d. hormones
      e. minerals

   5. What type of tasks do organelles carry out?

      a. excretory
      b. sensory
      c. metabolic
      d. communicative
      e. reproductive

H. Build medical terms using your knowledge of elements and their proper position in a medical term. Fill in the blanks. **LO 3.1, 3.3, 3.8**

1. Small mass   molec/_____

2. Pertaining to below the stomach   _____ /_____ /ic

3. Manifestation of a genome   _____ /o/type

4. Pertaining to urine   urin/_____

5. A change in condition (when the elements are taken literally)   _____ /ism

6. Small organ   organ/_____

7. Small nucleus   nucle/o/_____

8. Enzyme that digests foreign material   lys/o/_____

I. Body cavities. The organ is given to you in the following chart. Fill in the chart. Organize the terms in the correct body cavity, and then place the organ in the correct body system. Note: There are two answers to every question. **LO 3.5, 3.8, 3.9**

Organ	Body Cavity	Body System
brain	1.	2.
gallbladder	3.	4.
heart	5.	6.
kidneys	7.	8.
lungs	9.	10.
pituitary	11.	12.
prostate	13.	14.
spleen	15.	16.
uterus	17.	18.

J. Multiple choice is the format used for most national certification examinations. Choose the correct answer to the statement or question. **LO 3.2, 3.3, 3.4, 3.5, 3.6**

1. The single, fertilized cell is called the
   a. mitochondria.   d. zygote.
   b. ribosome.   e. blastocyst.
   c. organelle.

2. The word *membrane* means
   a. small organ.
   b. fluid inside a cell.
   c. thin layer of tissue.
   d. chemical substance.
   e. molecule with electrical charge.

3. Possessing a developmental structural defect is
   a. mutation.   d. metabolic.
   b. anatomic.   e. phenotype.
   c. dysmorphic.

4. Which of the following functions as a shock absorber?
   a. cartilage   d. ligament
   b. muscle   e. blood vessel
   c. tendon

5. The prefix *endo-* means

  a. outside.
  b. within.
  c. around.
  d. behind.
  e. across.

6. The study of the function of tissues is called

  a. cytology.
  b. cardiology.
  c. dermatology.
  d. histology.
  e. gastroenterology.

7. The type of cell that forms cartilage is a

  a. chondroblast.
  b. chondrocyte.
  c. osteocyte.
  d. osteoclast.
  d. osteoblast.

8. How many quadrants are in the abdominal region?

  a. one
  b. two
  c. three
  d. four
  e. five

9. *Hypogastric* refers to a

  a. body region.
  b. body opening.
  c. body quadrant.
  d. body cavity.
  e. body plane.

10. What forms the gliding surface where two bones meet to form a joint?

  a. cartilage
  b. blood vessels
  c. collage
  d. ligaments
  e. lymph

K. **Spelling comprehension.** Select the correct spelling of the term. **LO 3.2**

1. a. organale   **b.** orgenele   **c.** organelle   **d.** orgenelle   **e.** organel

2. a. sinovial   **b.** sinnovial   **c.** synoveal   **d.** synevial   **e.** synovial

3. a. rybosome   **b.** ribosonme   **c.** rhibosome   **d.** ribosome   **e.** rhybosone

4. a. diaphram   **b.** diaphrame   **c.** diaphragm   **d.** deaphragm   **e.** diafragm

5. a. feneotyp   **b.** feenotipe   **c.** pheneotype   **d.** pheenotype   **e.** phenotype

6. a. nucklii   **b.** nucleei   **c.** nuclei   **d.** neuclei   **e.** nucklie

7. a. zygoat   **b.** zigote   **c.** zygote   **d.** zigotte   **e.** zygoate

8. a. endockrine   **b.** endocrine   **c.** endoccrine   **d.** endockryne   **e.** endocrin

9. a. osteocyte   **b.** osteoscyte   **c.** osteyosite   **d.** osteeoscite   **e.** osteasyte

10. a. histology   **b.** historyology   **c.** hystology   **d.** hestology   **e.** historology

L. **Discuss the body cavities.** Place each organ in the correct body cavity. Fill in the blanks. **LO 3.5, 3.8**

  1. stomach   cavity: _____

  2. spinal cord   cavity: _____

  3. bladder   cavity: _____

  4. pancreas   cavity: _____

  5. thymus gland   cavity: _____

M. **Comprehend, spell, and write medical terms pertaining to the body as a whole so that you communicate and document accurately and precisely in any health care setting.** You are given the meaning of the term. Spell it correctly and write it on the line. **LO 3.2, 3.6, 3.7, 3.8, 3.9**

1. muscle separating the thoracic and abdominal cavities   _____

2. abdominal region above the stomach   _____

3. in the body system building path, what organelles are composed of   _____

4. a group of organic food compounds that includes sugar and starch   _____

5. pertaining to, or nearer, the head   _____

6. the chromosome characteristics of an individual cell   _____

7. the manifestation of a genome   _____

8. study of disorders produced by the effects of pollutants or diet on genes   _____

N. **Describe the medical terms for the different anatomic positions, planes, and directions of the body.** Identify which of the following terms apply to anatomic position, planes, or directions of the body. Select the correct choice. **LO 3.7**

1. caudal

  a. anatomic position

  b. planes

  c. directions

2. transverse

  a. anatomic position

  b. planes

  c. directions

3. superior

  a. anatomic position

  b. planes

  c. directions

4. prone

  a. anatomic position

  b. planes

  c. directions

5. distal

  a. anatomic position

  b. planes

  c. directions

O. **Apply correct medical terms to the anatomy and physiology of the body as a whole.** Choose T if the answer is True. Choose F if the answer is False. **LO 3.5**

1. Muscles are in the immune system.   T   F

2. The reproductive system vocabulary is divided into male and female terms.   T   F

3. Teeth are considered part of the digestive system.   T   F

4. One of the functions of the urinary system is to remove wastes from the blood.   T   F

Case Reports

A. **Members of a health care team requires correct reading and comprehending medical content.** Use Case Report 3.1 to correctly answer the following questions. Not all answers are found in the Case Report but can be found in the Chapter 3 text. **LO 3.9, 3.10**

Case Report (CR) 3.1

You are

. . . a certified medical assistant (CMA) employed as an in vitro fertilization coordinator in the Assisted Reproduction Clinic at Fulwood Medical Center.

Your patient is

. . . Mrs. Mary Arnold, a 35-year-old woman who has been unable to conceive. **In vitro fertilization** was recommended. After **hormone** therapy, several healthy and mature eggs were recovered from her **ovary.** The eggs were combined with her husband's **sperm** in a laboratory dish where **fertilization** occurred to form a single cell, called a **zygote.** The cells were allowed to divide for 5 days to become **blastocysts,** and then four blastocysts were implanted in her **uterus.**

Your role is to guide, counsel, and support Mrs. Arnold and her husband through the implementation and follow-up for the process.

---

1. The procedure *in vitro fertilization* can be abbreviated. Provide the abbreviation here: _____

2. There is a term in Case Report 3.1 that can be replaced with oocytes. Insert the term here: (make sure it in its plural form):

   _____

3. Which test would indicate that successful implantation has taken place?

   a. Genome

   b. Pregnancy test

   c. Phenotype

   d. Prenatal therapy

B. Members of a health care team require correct interpretation and translation of medical content. Use Case Report 3.2 to correctly answer the following questions. Not all answers are found in the Case Report but can be found in the Chapter 3 text. **LO 3.4, 3.9 and 3.10**

 Case Report (CR) 3.2

You are

. . . a physical therapy assistant employed in the Rehabilitation Unit in Fulwood Medical Center.

Your patient is

. . . Mr. Richard Josen, a 22-year-old man who injured tissues in his left knee playing football *(Figure 3.13)*.

Using arthroscopy, the orthopedic surgeon removed Mr. Josen's torn **anterior cruciate ligament** (ACL) and replaced it with a graft from his patellar ligament. The torn medial collateral ligament was sutured together. The tear in his medial meniscus was repaired. His rehabilitation, in which you play a key role, focuses on strengthening the **muscles** around his knee joint and helping him regain joint mobility.

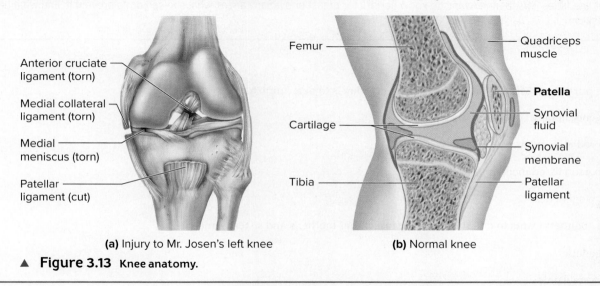

(a) Injury to Mr. Josen's left knee   **(b)** Normal knee

▲ **Figure 3.13 Knee anatomy.**

1. In this Case Report there is a knee structure that can be abbreviated. Provide the abbreviation here: _____.

2. The injured structures are on the _____ and _____ of the knee. Choose the two answers that correctly fill in the blanks.

   a. middle   **b.** outside   **c.** front   **d.** back

3. The patellar ligament gets its name from the:

   a. muscle to muscle attachment.   **c.** length of the tissue.

   b. organ it originates from.   **d.** bone it attaches to.

4. Which level of structural organization do ligaments fit into?

   a. organ system   **b.** organ   **c.** tissue   **d.** cell

5. Your job would be to focus on two areas. Select these two areas:

   a. joint mobility.   **b.** cartilage healing.   **c.** bone density.   **d.** muscle strength.

C. Case Reports contain information that combine content from different chapter sections. Use Case Report 3.3 to correctly answer the following questions. Not all answers are found in the Case Report but can be found in the Chapter 3 text. **LO 3.5 and 3.9**

Case Report (CR) 3.3

You are
. . . a physician's assistant (PA) in the Genetic Counseling Clinic at Fulwood Medical Center.

Your patient is
. . . Mrs. Patricia Bennet, a 52-year-old office manager with two daughters, aged 30 and 25. Mrs.

Bennett's sister, aged 55, recently had a mastectomy for breast cancer and is now receiving chemotherapy. Their mother died of ovarian cancer in her late fifties. Mrs. Bennet wants to know her risk for breast or ovarian cancer, what she can do to prevent it, and what her daughters' risks are.

1. The purpose of Mrs. Bennett's visit with you today is to determine her:

   a. gene therapy.

   b. predictive medicine.

   c. personalized medicine.

   d. cytogenetics.

2. Mrs. Bennett wants to determine if the cause of her mother's and sister's cancer is:

   a. genetic.

   b. dysmorphic.

   c. causative.

   d. therapeutic.

3. The types of cancer that affected Mrs. Bennett's sister and mother were of the _____ system.

   a. digestive

   b. urinary

   c. endocrine

   d. reproductive

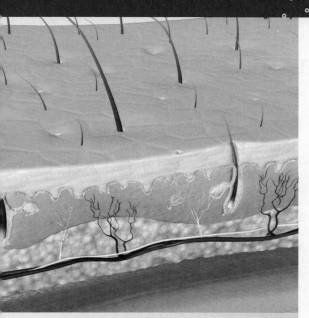

2014 Nucleus Medical Media

Integumentary System
The Language of Dermatology

Chapter Sections

Chapter Learning Outcomes

Upon completion of this chapter, you will be able to:

LO 4.1 Identify and describe the anatomy and physiology of the integumentary system.

LO 4.2 Use roots, combining forms, suffixes, and prefixes to construct and analyze medical terms related to the integumentary system.

LO 4.3 Spell medical terms related to the integumentary system.

LO 4.4 Pronounce medical terms related to the integumentary system.

LO 4.5 Describe diagnostic procedures utilized in dermatology.

LO 4.6 Identify and describe burns, lesions, and pathological conditions related to the integumentary system.

LO 4.7 Describe the therapeutic procedures and pharmacologic agents used in dermatology.

LO 4.8 Apply knowledge of medical terms relating to dermatology to documentation, medical records, and communication.

LO 4.9 Identify and correctly use abbreviations used in dermatology.

LO 4.10 Identify health professionals involved in the care of dermatology patients.

Health professionals involved in the care of patients with dermatological diseases include

- **Dermatologists,** who are medical specialists in diseases of the skin.
- **Dermatopathologists,** who are medical specialists in dermatology and surgical pathology and who focus on the study of cutaneous diseases at a microscopic level.
- **Cosmetic surgeons,** who are board certified by the American Board of Cosmetic Surgery to enhance appearance through elective surgical and medical procedures.
- **Plastic surgeons,** who are board certified by the American Board of Plastic Surgery to reconstruct facial and body defects due to birth disorders, trauma, burns, and disease.
- **Nurse practitioners** and **physician assistants,** who with extensive training and experience in dermatology work under the supervision of dermatologists.
- **Estheticians,** also called *skin care therapists,* who perform various cosmetic procedures for the treatment of the skin. They do not diagnose, prescribe medications, or suggest treatments.

Section 4.1 Functions and Structure of the Skin

Functions of the Skin

The **integumentary system** consists of the skin and its associated organs. The skin is also known as the **cutaneous** membrane. The cutaneous membrane is made up the **epidermis, dermis,** and **hypodermis** *(Figure 4.1).* The study and treatment of the integumentary system is called **dermatology.** This organ system receives more medical and personal attention than any other organ system. Your understanding of its structure and functions will be used every day in your professional and personal life.

The skin is the largest organ in your body and accounts for 7% to 8% of body weight. The skin is the most vulnerable of all your organs because it is continually exposed to chemicals, trauma, infection, radiation, temperature change, humidity variation, and all the pollution of modern life. The skin is an important part of a person's self-image and an important part of total patient care.

The skin is a barrier that is not easily broken. Few infectious organisms can penetrate the skin on their own. Those that do use accidental breaks in the skin or rely on animals such as mosquitoes, fleas, or ticks to puncture the skin to allow access for the infectious organisms. The skin is also a barrier to solar radiation, including ultraviolet (UV) rays.

A summary of the functions of the skin:

- **Protection.** The skin is a physical barrier against injury, chemicals, ultraviolet rays, microbes, and toxins.

- **Water resistance.** You don't swell up every time you take a bath because your skin is water resistant. It also prevents water from leaking out from the body tissues.

- **Temperature regulation.** A network of capillaries in the skin opens up or dilates (vasodilation) when your body is too hot so that the blood flow increases and the heat from the blood dissipates through your skin. When your body is cold, the capillary network narrows (vasoconstriction), blood flow decreases, and heat is retained in your body.

- **Vitamin D synthesis.** As little as 15 to 30 minutes of sunlight daily allows your skin cells to initiate the metabolism of vitamin D, which is essential for bone growth and maintenance.

- **Sensation.** Nerve endings that detect touch, pressure, heat, cold, pain, vibration, and tissue injury are particularly numerous on your face, fingers, palms, soles, nipples, and genitals.

- **Excretion and secretion.** Water and small amounts of waste products from cell metabolism are lost through the skin by excretion (the process of removal of waste products from the body) and by secretion (the process of producing and releasing a substance by a tissue or organ of the body) from your sweat glands.

- **Social functions.** The skin reflects your emotions, blushing when you are self-conscious, going pale when you are frightened, wrinkling when you dislike something.

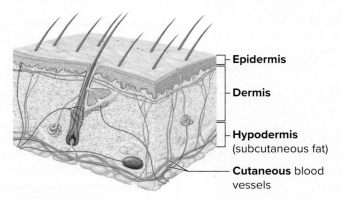

▲ **Figure 4.1** Structure of the cutaneous membrane.

WORD	PRONUNCIATION	ELEMENTS		DEFINITION
cutaneous	kyu-**TAY**-nee-us	S/ R/CF	**-us** *pertaining to* **cutane/o-** *skin*	Pertaining to the skin
dermis dermal (adj)	**DER**-miss **DER**-mal		Greek *skin*	Connective tissue layer of the skin beneath the epidermis
dermatology	der-mah-**TOL**-oh-jee	S/ R/CF	**-logy** *study of* **dermat/o-** *skin*	Medical specialty concerned with disorders of the skin
dermatologist	der-mah-**TOL**-oh-jist	S/	**-logist** *one who studies*	Medical specialist in diseases of the skin
epidermis	ep-ih-**DER**-miss	P/ R/	**epi-** *upon* **-dermis** *skin*	Top layer of the skin
esthetics esthetician	es-**THET**-iks es-the-**TI**-shun	S/ R/	Greek *sensation* **-ician** *specialist* **esthet-** *beauty*	Concerned with beauty A therapist who enhances the beauty of the skin
integument	in-**TEG**-you-ment		Latin *a covering*	Organ system that covers the body, the skin being the main organ within the system
integumentary (adj)	in-**TEG**-you-**MEN**-tah-ree	S/ R/	**-ary** *pertaining to* **integument-** *covering of the body*	Pertaining to the covering of the body
squamous cell	**SKWAY**-mus **SELL**		Latin *scaly*	Flat scalelike epithelial cell

Structure of the Skin

Epidermis

The most superficial layer of the skin is the epidermis. This layer

- Protects underlying structures.
- Withstands the toxic pollution of modern life.
- Sheds its superficial cells and renews them continually throughout life.
- Provides a waterproof barrier.

The epidermis is an **epithelial** tissue, which consists of four to five layers of cells, most of which are **keratinocytes.** Keratinocytes are formed in the bottommost layer of the epidermis, **stratum basale,** and then pushed up (migrate) to the topmost layer of the epidermis, the **stratum corneum** *(Figure 4.2).* The palms of the hands and the soles of the feet have five layers; all other areas of the body have four. From superficial to deep, these layers are:

- **Stratum corneum:** a layer of compact, dead cells packed with **keratin.** These dead cells have no nuclei and are continually shed. Keratin is a tough, scaly protein that is also the basis for hair and nails.
- **Stratum lucidum:** only found in the palm of the hands and the soles of the feet, it is a thin translucent layer of cells. These cells, **keratinocytes,** are filled with a protein that becomes keratin.
- **Stratum granulosum:** these keratinocytes produce a fatty mixture that covers the surface of the cells and waterproofs them. This waterproof barrier not only stops water from getting in and out but also cuts off the supply of nutrients to the keratinocytes above it and they die.
- **Stratum spinosum:** the keratinocytes contain nuclei and are firmly attached to each other by numerous spines (hence "spinosum"). This enables the epidermis to be firm and strong.
- **Stratum basale:** a single layer of cells that form the keratinocytes. This layer also contains **melanocytes,** which produce the dark pigment **melanin,** and the **tactile** (touch) cells attached to sensory nerve fibers. The process by which keratinocytes migrate from this layer to the skin's surface, where they are shed as dead cells, takes about a month.

Did you know...

- The skin provides protection, contains sensory organs, and helps control body temperature.
- The stratum granulosum waterproofs the skin.
- The stratum spinosum holds the epidermis together.

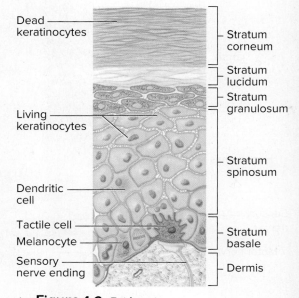

▲ **Figure 4.2** Epidermis.

WORD	PRONUNCIATION	ELEMENTS		DEFINITION
epithelial (adj)	ep-ih-**THEE**-lee-al	S/ P/ R/CF	-al *pertaining to* epi- *upon* -thel/i- *nipple*	Relating to or consisting of epithelium
epithelium	ep-ih-**THEE**-lee-um	S/	-um *tissue*	Tissue that covers surfaces or lines cavities
keratin keratinocyte	**KER**-ah-tin ke-**RAT**-in-oh-site	S/ R/CF	**Greek** *keratin* -cyte *cell* keratin/o- *keratin*	Protein found in the dead outer layer of skin and in nails and hair Cell producing a tough, horny protein (keratin) in the process of differentiating into the dead cells of the stratum corneum
melanin melanocyte	**MEL**-ah-nin **MEL**-an-oh-cyte	S/ R/CF	Greek *black* -cyte *cell* melan/o- *black*	Black pigment found in skin, hair, retina Cell that synthesizes (produces) melanin
stratum strata (pl) stratum basale	**STRAH**-tum **STRAH**-tah **STRAH**-tum ba-**SAL**-eh	S/ R/ R/	-um *structure* strat- *layer* basal/e *deepest part*	A layer of tissue Deepest layer of the epidermis, from which the other cells originate and migrate
stratum corneum	**STRAH**-tum **COR**-nee-um	R/	corne- *having a horn*	Outermost layer of the epidermis that has cells containing keratin; the layer is tough and thick, like a horn
stratum granulosum	**STRAH**-tum gran-you-**LOH**-sum	S/ R/	-sum *pick up* granul/o- *small grain*	Layer of the epidermis where the cells contain granules of lipids
stratum lucidum	**STRAH**-tum **LOO**-si-dum	R/	lucid- *clear*	Layer of the epidermis only found on the palms of the hands and the soles of the feet
stratum spinosum	**STRAH**-tum spy-**NOH**-sum	S/	Latin *spiny*	Layer of the epidermis where the cells appear to have spines
tactile	**TAK**-tile		Latin *to touch*	Relating to touch

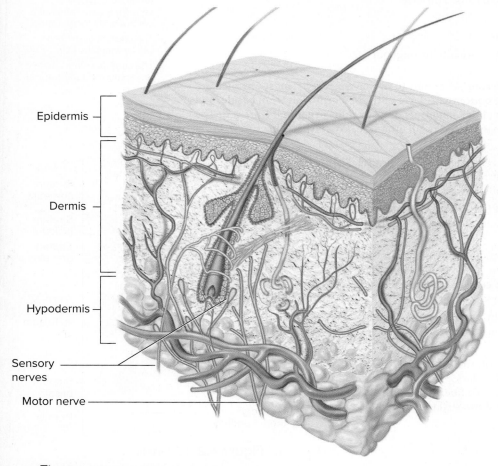

Epidermis

Dermis

Hypodermis

Sensory nerves

Motor nerve

▲ **Figure 4.3** Dermis and its organs.

Dermis

Figure 4.3 shows that the **dermis** is a much thicker tissue layer than the epidermis. The dermis is a type of connective tissue consisting mainly of **collagen,** a type of protein fiber produced by **fibroblasts.** Collagen provides strength and flexibility to the cutaneous membrane. The dermis is well supplied with blood vessels and nerves and contains the accessory skin organs: sweat glands, sebaceous glands, hair follicles, and nail roots. The accessory skin organs will be discussed later in this chapter. The boundary between the dermis and the epidermis is distinct: irregular and wavy.

Hypodermis

The **hypodermis,** the layer beneath the dermis, is the site of **subcutaneous** fat (**adipose** tissue). It is also called the **subcutaneous tissue layer** and is often referred to as **SC** in clinical documentation.

Word Analysis and Definition: Structures of the Skin

S = Suffix   P = Prefix   R = Root   R/CF = Combining Form

WORD	PRONUNCIATION	ELEMENTS		DEFINITION
adipose	**ADD**-i-pose	S/ R/	**-ose** *condition* **adip-** *fat*	Containing fat
collagen	**KOL**-ah-jen	S/ R/	**-gen** *producing* **coll/a-** *glue*	Major protein of connective tissue, cartilage, and bone
fibroblast	**FIE**-bro-blast	S/ R/CF	**-blast** *germ cell* **fibr/o-** *fiber*	Cell that forms collagen fibers
hypodermis	high-poh-**DER**-miss	P/ R/	**hypo-** *below* **-dermis** *skin*	Tissue layer below the dermis
hypodermic (adj)	high-poh-**DER**-mik	S/ R/	**-ic** *pertaining to* **-derm-** *skin*	Beneath the skin
subcutaneous hypodermic (syn)	sub-kew-**TAY**-nee-us	S/ P/ R/CF	**-ous** *pertaining to* **sub-** *below* **-cutane/o** *skin*	Below the skin

Check Point Section 4.1

A. Build your knowledge of the elements in the language of dermatology. *Choose the best answer.* **LO 4.1**

1. Choose the term that has a word element meaning *study of:*

   a. dermatology   **b.** dermatologist   **c.** dermatitist

2. The term **cutaneous** means *pertaining to*

   a. skin   **b.** mass   **c.** tumor

B. Apply the correct rule for plurals and form the plural of the term. **LO 4.3**

1. There are many (strata/stratum) of the epidermis.

2. The most superficial layer of the epidermis, (strata/stratum) corneum, contains only dead keratinocytes.

C. Number the layers of the epidermis in the correct order, from superficial to deep. The most superficial layer is "1"; the deepest layer is "5." LO 4.1

_____ stratum lucidum

_____ stratum basale

_____ stratum granulosum

_____ stratum corneum

_____ stratum spinosum

D. Deconstruct medical terms to determine their meaning. *Identify the meaning of the word elements in each term.* **LO 4.1**

1. The root in the term **melanocyte** means:

   a. layer   **b.** black   **c.** spiny   **d.** cell   **e.** touch

2. The root in the term **lucidum** means:

   a. layer   **b.** pertaining to   **c.** structure   **d.** protein   **e.** clear

3. The suffix *-cyte* means:

   a. structure   **b.** pertaining to   **c.** small   **d.** state of   **e.** cell

E. Find the missing elements and build the terms. *Fill in the blanks.* **LO 4.2, 4.3**

1. pertaining to below the skin: _____ /derm/_____

2. containing fat: adip/_____

3. pertaining to below the skin: _____ /cutane/_____

F. Answer the following questions regarding terms relating to the structure of the skin. LO 4.1

1. The type of cells that produce fibers is called a:

  a. melanocyte   **b.** keratinocyte   **c.** fibroblast   **d.** adipose   **e.** stratum

2. The type of connective tissue found in the hypodermis:

  a. epithelium   **b.** collagen   **c.** adipose   **d.** keratin

Section 4.2 Accessory Skin Organs

Hair Follicles and Sebaceous Glands

Hair follicles and their associated sebaceous glands, sweat glands, and nails are organs located in your skin. They each have specific anatomical and physiologic characteristics. You must understand their roles in the different functions of the skin and in diseases that affect the skin. Each hair follicle has a **sebaceous gland** opening into it *(Figure 4.4).* The gland secretes into the follicle a mixture of oily, acidic **sebum** and broken-down cells from the base of the gland.

Hair

Each hair, no matter where it is on your body or scalp, originates from epidermal cells at the base (matrix) of a hair follicle. As these cells divide and grow, they push older cells upward away from the source of nutrition in the hair papilla. The cells become keratinized and die. They rest for a while; and when a new hair is formed, the old, dead hair is pushed out and drops off.

In cross-section, each hair has three layers *(Figure 4.5).* Its core, the **medulla,** is composed of loosely arranged cells containing a flexible keratin. The **cortex** is composed of densely packed cells with a harder keratin that gives hair its stiffness. These cells also contain pigment. The outer **cuticle** is a single layer of scaly, dead keratin cells.

Straight hair is round in cross-section *(Figure 4.5a and b).* Curly hair is oval *(Figure 4.5c and d).* Two pigments derived from **melanin (eumelanin** and **pheomelanin)** give hair its natural color. Black and dark brown hair have a lot of a dark form of the pigment eumelanin in the cells of the cortex *(Figure 4.5b).* Blonde hair has little of this dark pigment but a lighter form of pheomelanin *(Figure 4.5a).* Red hair has a lot of the lighter pigment *(Figure 4.5c).* White or gray hair has little pigment *(Figure 4.5d).*

A problem with the scalp hair follicle occurs in men when a combination of genetic influence and excess testosterone produces "top of the head" baldness. In most people, aging causes **alopecia,** thinning of the hair and baldness as the follicles shrink and produce thin, wispy hairs.

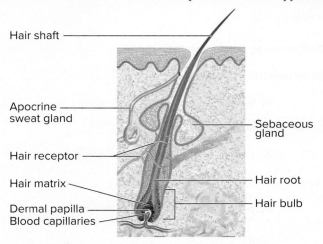

Hair shaft

Apocrine sweat gland

Hair receptor

Hair matrix

Dermal papilla

Blood capillaries

Sebaceous gland

Hair root

Hair bulb

▲ **Figure 4.4** Hair follicle and sebaceous gland.

Scalp hair is thick enough to retain heat. Body hair has no specific function in our present evolution because, in most people, it is too thin to retain heat. Beard, pubic, and **axillary** (armpit) hair reflect sexual maturity. Stronger hairs guard the nostrils and ears to prevent foreign particles from entering. Similarly, eyelashes protect the eyes, and eyebrows help keep perspiration from running into the eyes.

Melanin is in the black skin melanocytes of dark-skinned people and is the pigment generated by sunbathing and tanning. The absence of melanin produces **albinism.**

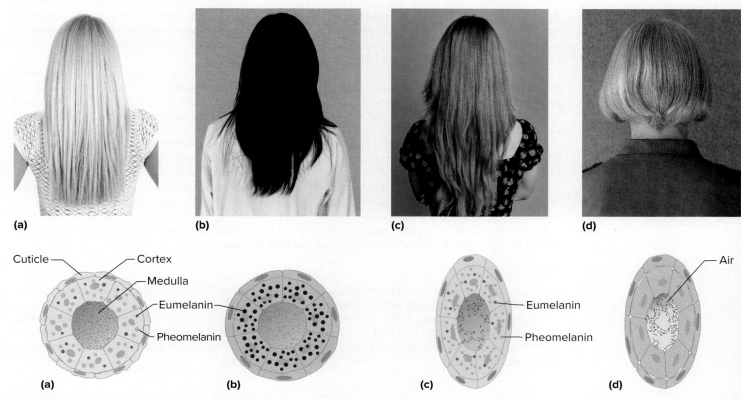

▲ **Figure 4.5** **Basis of hair color and texture.** (a) vgajic/E+/Getty Images (b) Rawpixel.com/Shutterstock (c) Krakenimages.com/Shutterstock.com (d) Studio Light and Shade/Shutterstock

Word Analysis and Definition: Skin and Hair

S = Suffix   P = Prefix   R = Root   R/CF = Combining Form

WORD	PRONUNCIATION		ELEMENTS	DEFINITION
albinism	**AL**-bih-nizm	S/	-ism *condition*	Genetic disorder with lack of melanin
albino	al-**BY**-no	R/CF	albin/o- *white*	Person with albinism
alopecia	al-oh-**PEE**-shah		Greek *mange*	Partial or complete loss of hair, naturally or from medication
axilla	ak-**SIL**-ah		Greek *region under a bird's wing*	Medical name for the armpit
axillae (pl)	ak-**SIL**-ee			
axillary (adj)	**AK**-sill-air-ee			Pertaining to the axilla
cortex	**KOR**-teks		Latin *outer covering*	Outer portion of an organ, such as bone
cortical (adj)	**KOR**-tih-kal			Gray covering of cerebral hemispheres
cortices (pl)	**KOR**-tih-sees			
cuticle	**KEW**-tih-cul		Diminutive of cutis *skin*	Nonliving epidermis at the base of the fingernails and toenails, and the outer layer of hair
medulla	meh-**DULL**-ah		French *middle*	Central portion of a structure surrounded by cortex
medullary (adj)	**MED**-ul-ah-ree			
melanin	**MEL**-ah-nin		Greek *black*	Black pigment found in skin, hair, and retina
eumelanin	**YOU**-mel-ah-nin	P/	eu- *good, normal*	The dark form of the pigment melanin
		R/	-melanin *black*	
pheomelanin	**FEE**-oh-mel-ah-nin	P/	pheo- *gray*	The lighter form of melanin

Sweat Glands

You have 3 million to 4 million **eccrine** (**merocrine**) sweat glands *(Figure 4.6)* scattered all over your skin, with higher concentrations on your palms, soles, and forehead.

Their main function is to produce the watery perspiration (sweat) that cools your body. Your sweat is 99% water; the rest is made up of electrolytes such as sodium chloride, which gives the sweat its salty taste. Some waste products of cell metabolism are also secreted.

In the dermis, the sweat gland is a coiled tube lined with epithelial cells that secrete the sweat. Around the tube, muscle cells contract to squeeze the sweat up the tube directly to the surface of the skin. Perspiration is a normal process to cool the body and remove waste products. An excessive amount of sweating, as seen with very stressful situations or medical conditions, such as a myocardial infarction (heart attack), is termed **diaphoresis.**

In your armpits (axillae), around your nipples, in your groin, and around your anus, **apocrine** sweat glands produce a thick, cloudy secretion that interacts with normal skin bacteria to produce a distinct, noticeable smell. The ducts of these glands lead directly into hair follicles *(see Figure 4.6).* They respond to sexual stimulation and stress and secrete chemicals called **pheromones,** which have an effect on the sexual behavior of other people.

Ceruminous glands are found in the external ear canal, where their secretions combine with sebum and dead epidermal cells to form earwax (**cerumen**). This wax waterproofs the external ear canal and kills bacteria.

Sweat gland functions are severely affected in a group of diseases termed *ectodermal dysplasia,* manifested in the reduction or absence of sweat. They can be involved in the infections that engulf the nearby hair follicles and sebaceous glands.

Mammary glands, a type of modified sweat gland, serve a distinct purpose in reproduction and are therefore discussed in *Chapter 8* under the female reproductive system.

Nails

Nails are formed from the stratum corneum of the epidermis. They consist of closely packed, thin, dead cells that are filled with parallel fibers of hard keratin.

Fingernails grow about 1 mm per week. New cells are added by cell division in the nail **matrix,** which is protected by the nail fold of skin and the cuticle at the base of the nail *(Figure 4.7).* The nail rests on the nail bed, which consists of the living layers of the epidermis and the strata basale, spinosum, and granulosum.

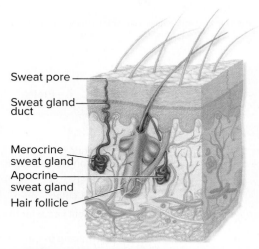

▲ **Figure 4.6** Sweat glands.

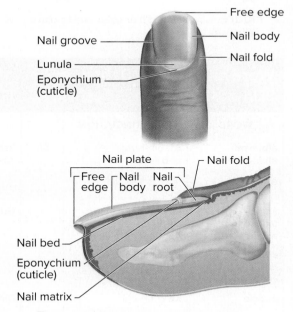

▲ **Figure 4.7** Anatomy of a fingernail.

WORD	PRONUNCIATION		ELEMENTS	DEFINITION
apocrine	AP-oh-krin	P/ R/	apo- *different from* -crine *secrete*	Apocrine sweat glands open into the hair follicle
cerumen ceruminous (adj)	seh-ROO-men seh-ROO-mih-nus		Latin *wax*	Waxy secretion of the ceruminous glands of the external ear
eccrine	EK-rin		Greek *to secrete*	Coiled sweat gland that occurs in skin all over the body
matrix matrices (pl)	MAY-triks		Latin *womb*	Substance that surrounds cells, is manufactured by the cells, and holds them together
merocrine	MARE-oh-krin	P/ R/	mero- *partial* -crine *secrete*	Another name for eccrine
pheromone (*Note:* The *horin hormone* is dropped to ease pronunciation)	FAIR-oh-moan	P/ R/	pher- *carrying* -hormone *excite, stimulate*	Substance that carries and generates a physical attraction for other people

Check Point Section 4.2

A. Match the definition to the term

1. eccrine
2. pheromone
3. diaphoresis
4. apocrine
5. albinism

6. sebaceous gland
7. body hair
8. cerumen
9. ectodermal dysplasia

10. nails

a. reduction or absence of sweat
b. excessive sweating
c. absence of melanin
d. has no specific function
e. secretes into the follicle a mixture of oily, acidic sebum and broken-down cells
f. sweat gland
g. effect sexual behavior
h. ear wax
i. formed from the stratum corneum of the epidermis
j. sweat glands that open into the hair follicle

B. Answering the following questions about the language of dermatology. *Fill in the blanks regarding statements about the hair.*
   LO 4.1, 4.2, 4.3

1. The root melanin denotes the color _____.

2. The medical term for *armpit* is _____.

3. The plural form of *cortex* is _____.

4. The central portion of a structure is the _____, which means _____.

5. The outer portion of an organ is the _____.

6. The medical term for baldness is _____.

7. *Alopecia* can result from natural causes or from _____.

C. The following nouns all have an adjectival form. *Fill in the blanks.* **LO 4.3**

1. Noun: axilla   Adjective: _____

2. Noun: cortex   Adjective: _____

3. Noun: medulla   Adjective: _____

Section 4.3 Disorders and Diseases of the Skin and Accessory Organs

Disorders of the Skin

Carcinomas

Squamous cell carcinoma *(Figure 4.8)* arises from keratinocytes in the stratum spinosum. It appears as a flattened reddish or brownish plaque and can have a rough, scaly or crusted surface. It responds well to surgical removal but can **metastasize** (spread) to lymph glands if neglected.

   Basal cell carcinoma *(Figure 4.9)* begins in the cells of the stratum basale and invades the dermis and epidermis. It is the most common skin cancer and is also the least dangerous because it does not metastasize.

   Sunlight can also be an irritant to the skin, not only by burning it but by leading to cancer when there is excessive exposure. Any congenital lesion of the skin, including various types of birthmarks and all **moles,** is referred to as a **nevus.**

   Malignant melanoma *(Figure 4.10)* is the least common skin cancer but is the most deadly. It arises from the melanocytes in the stratum basale. It metastasizes quickly and is fatal if neglected.

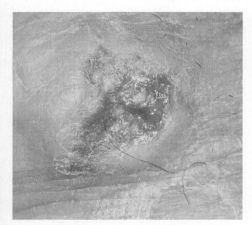

▲ **Figure 4.8** Squamous cell carcinoma.
Biophoto Associates/Science Source

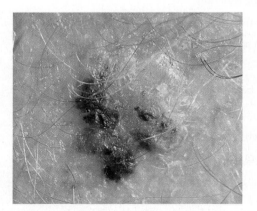

▲ **Figure 4.9** Basal cell carcinoma.
Biophoto Associates/Science Source

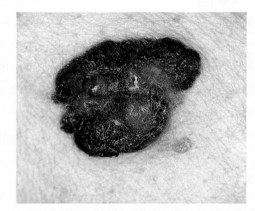

▲ **Figure 4.10** Malignant melanoma.
James Stevenson/Science Source

Pressure Sores

When a patient lies in one position for a long period, the pressure between the bed and bony body projections, like the lower spine or heel, cuts off the blood supply to the skin and **decubitus (pressure) ulcers** can appear *(Figure 4.11)*. The protective function of the skin is broken, and germs can enter the body. Pressure sores begin as a reddened area of the skin. With continued pressure on the skin overlying the bony structure, the epidermis may form blisters and erode (wear away). If the pressure continues, the dermis wears away, and then the hypodermis. If it continues, the muscles and bones can be affected.

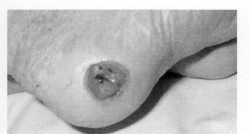

▲ **Figure 4.11** Decubitus ulcer on heel.
Mediscan/Alamy Stock Photo

WORD	PRONUNCIATION		ELEMENTS	DEFINITION
basal	**BAY**-sal	S/ R/	**-al** *pertaining to* **bas-** *lower part*	Pertaining to the lower part of a structure
carcinoma	kar-sih-**NOH**-mah	S/ R/	**-oma** *tumor, mass* **carcin-** *cancer*	A malignant epithelial tumor
decubitus ulcer	de-**KYU**-bit-us **UL**-ser	P/ R/ R/	**de-** *from* **-cubitus** *lying down* **ulcer** *sore*	Sore caused by lying down for long periods of time
lesion	**LEE**-zhun		Latin *injury*	Pathological change or injury in a tissue
malignant	mah-**LIG**-nant	S/ R/	**-ant** *pertaining to* **malign-** *harmful*	Having the properties of being locally invasive and able to spread to distant parts of the body
melanoma	**MEL**-ah-**NOH**-mah	S/ R/	**-oma** *tumor, mass* **melan-** *black*	Malignant tumor formed from cells that produce the pigment melanin
metastasis	meh-**TAS**-tah-sis	P/ R/	**meta-** *beyond* **-stasis** *stay in one place*	Spread of a disease from one part of the body to another
metastasize	meh-**TAS**-tah-size	S/ R/	**-ize** *affect in a specific way* **-stat-** *stand still*	To spread to distant parts
mole	MOLE		Latin *spot*	Benign localized area of melanin-producing cells
nevus nevi (pl)	**NEE**-vus **NEE**-vie		Latin *mole, birthmark*	Congenital or acquired lesion of the skin
pathology	pa-**THOL**-oh-jee	S/ R/CF R/	**-logy** *study of* **path/o-** *disease* **-log-** *to study*	Medical specialty dealing with the structural and functional changes of a disease process or the cause, development, and structural changes in disease
pathologic (adj)	path-oh-**LOJ**-ik	S/	**-ic** *pertaining to*	Pertaining to the changes in the body induced by disease

Dermatitis

Dermatitis *(Figure 4.12)* results from direct exposure to an irritating agent. **Atopic (allergic) dermatitis** develops when the body becomes sensitive to an **allergen. Allergenic** agents include latex, nickel in jewelry, or poison ivy. This whole-body involvement is seen by systemic symptoms of pruritus distant from the local irritant site.

    Eczema is a general term used for inflamed, itchy skin conditions. When the itchy skin is scratched, it becomes **excoriated** and produces the dry, red, scaly patches characteristic of eczema. **Vesicles** containing serous fluid may form. Continued scratching can cause the rash to "weep" **serous** fluid that can lead to crusting of the area. There are numerous types of eczema, the most common type being **atopic** dermatitis, which is caused by an allergic reaction, such as when a person develops an **allergy** to nickel.

    Ichthyosis is a condition of dry, scaly skin. The skin is flaky and resembles the skin of a fish. This condition is usually inherited, but it also can be acquired.

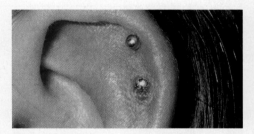

▲ **Figure 4.12** **Dermatitis of ear due to nickel sensitivity.** Dr P. Marazzi/Science Source

Skin Infections

The skin is also susceptible to many different types of infections. The following are examples.

Viral Infections

Warts (verrucas) are caused by the human papillomavirus invading the epidermis and causing the outer epidermal cells to produce a roughened projection from the skin surface. Human papillomavirus is discussed extensively in *Chapter 8.*

    Varicella-zoster virus causes **chickenpox** in unvaccinated people, forming macules, papules, and vesicles. The virus can then remain dormant in the peripheral nerves for decades before erupting as the painful vesicles of **herpes zoster (shingles)** *(Figure 4.13).*

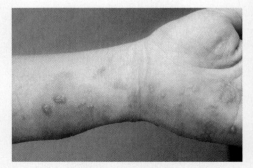

▲ **Figure 4.13** **Shingles, Zoster, or Herpes Zoster symptoms on arm.** Akhararat Wathanasing/Alamy Stock Photo

WORD	PRONUNCIATION	ELEMENTS		DEFINITION
allergen (*Note:* The duplicate letter "g" is deleted to better form the word.)	**AL**-er-jen	S/ R/ R/	**-gen** *to produce* **all-** *different, strange* **-erg-** *work*	Substance producing a hypersensitivity (allergic) reaction
allergic allergy	ah-**LER**-jic **AL**-er-jee	S/ S/	**-ic** *pertaining to* **-ergy** *process of working*	Pertaining to or suffering from an allergy Hypersensitivity to a particular allergen
atopy atopic	**AY**-toh-pee ay-**TOP**-ik		Greek *strangeness*	State of hypersensitivity to an allergen; allergic
dermatitis	der-mah-**TYE**-tis	S/ R/	**-itis** *inflammation* **dermat-** *skin*	Inflammation of the skin
eczema eczematous (adj)	**EK**-zeh-mah ek-**ZEM**-ah-tus	S/ R/	Greek *to boil or ferment* **-tous** *pertaining to* **eczema-** *eczema*	Inflammatory skin disease often with a serous discharge Pertaining to or resembling eczema
excoriate	eks-**KOR**-ee-ate	S/ P/ R/	**-ate** *composed of, pertaining to* **ex-** *away from, out of* **-cori-** *skin*	To scratch
excoriation (noun)	eks-**KOR**-ee-**AY**-shun	S/	**-ation** *process*	Scratch mark
ichthyosis	ik-thee-**OH**-sis	S/ R/	**-osis** *condition* **ichthy-** *fish*	Scaling and dryness of the skin
latex	**LAY**-tecks		Latin *liquid*	Manufactured from the milky liquid in rubber plants; used for gloves in patient care
pruritus pruritic (adj)	proo-**RYE**-tus proo-**RIT**-ik		Latin *to itch*	Itching Itchy
serous	**SEER**-us		Latin *serum*	Thicker and less transparent than water
vesicle	**VES**-ih-kull		Latin *small sac*	Small sac containing liquid; for example, a blister

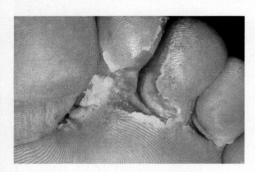

▲ **Figure 4.14** **Tinea pedis between toes.** SPL/Science Source

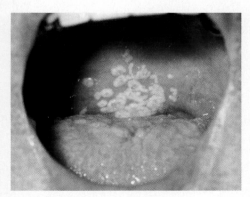

▲ **Figure 4.15** **Oral thrush.** Dr. P. Marazzi/ Science Source

Fungal Infections

Tinea is a general term for a group of related skin infections caused by different species of fungi. The fungi live on, and are strictly confined to, the nonliving stratum corneum and its derivatives, hair and nails, where keratin provides their food. The different types of tinea take their name from the location of the infection.

Tinea pedis, athlete's foot, causes itching, redness, and peeling of the foot, particularly between the toes *(Figure 4.14)*. **Tinea capitis** describes infection of the scalp (ringworm); **tinea corporis** is the name for infections of the body. **Tinea cruris** ("jock itch") is the name for infections of the groin. The fungus spreads from animals, from the soil, and by direct contact with infected individuals. **Tinea versicolor** is characterized by brown and white patches on the trunk.

The yeastlike fungus **Candida** can produce recurrent infections of the skin, nails, and mucous membranes. The first sign can be a recurrent diaper rash or **thrush** in infants. Older children can show recurrent or persistent lesions on the scalp. In adults, chronic **candidiasis** can affect the mouth (**thrush**) *(Figure 4.15)* and vagina, as well as the skin. It can also be associated with diseases of the immune system *(see Chapter 12)*.

Parasitic Infestations

A **parasite** is an organism that lives in contact with and feeds off another organism (host). This process is called an **infestation.** It is different from an **infection.**

Lice are small, wingless, blood-sucking parasites that produce the disease **pediculosis** by attaching their eggs (nits) to hair and clothing *(Table 4.1)*.

Scabies ("itch mites") produce an intense, itching rash, often in the genital area, waist, breast, and armpits. The mites live and lay eggs under the skin.

The skin normally sheds its cells. These tiny specks form some of the dust on our furniture, floors, and carpets. The house dust mite *(Figure 4.16)* thrives on the keratin of these cells and lives well on carpets, upholstery, pillows, and mattresses. Many people are allergic to the inhaled feces of these parasites.

Table 4.1 Pediculosis

Louse (lice, pl)	Attachment of Eggs	Disease
Pediculus capitis	Hair of scalp	Pediculosis capitis
Phthirus pubis (crab-shaped)	Pubic hair	Pediculosis cruris (crabs)
Pediculus humanus	Clothing, body hair	Pediculosis corporis

Bacterial Infections

Staphylococcus aureus (commonly called *staph*) is the most common bacterium to invade the skin and is the cause of pimples, boils, **carbuncles,** and **impetigo.** It can infect hair follicles and the surrounding tissues to produce **furuncles** and carbuncles. Staph can cause a **cellulitis** of the epidermis and dermis.

Necrotizing fasciitis is caused when some strains of staph and strep produce enzymes that are very toxic and digest the connective tissues and spread into muscle layers.

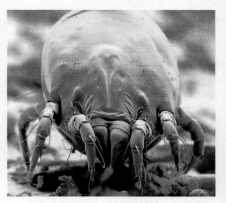
▲ **Figure 4.16** House dust mite.
Eye of Science/Science Source

Word Analysis and Definition: Disorders of the Skin

S = Suffix   P = Prefix   R = Root   R/CF = Combining Form

WORD	PRONUNCIATION		ELEMENTS	DEFINITION
Candida candidiasis thrush	**KAN**-did-ah can-dih-**DIE**-ah-sis THRUSH	 S/ R/	Latin *dazzling white* -iasis *condition, state of* candid- *Candida*	A yeastlike fungus Infection with the yeastlike fungus *Candida* Infection with *Candida albicans*
carbuncle	**KAR**-bunk-ul		Latin *carbuncle*	Infection composed of many furuncles in a small area, often on the back of the neck
cellulitis	sell-you-**LIE**-tis	S/ R/	-itis *inflammation* cellul- *small cell*	Infection of subcutaneous connective tissue
furuncle	**FU**-rung-kel		Latin *a boil*	An infected hair follicle that spreads into the tissues around the follicle
herpes zoster shingles (syn)	**HER**-pees **ZOS**-ter		**herpes** *to creep or spread* **zoster** *belt, girdle*	Painful eruption of vesicles that follows a dermatome or nerve root on one side of the body
impetigo	im-peh-**TIE**-go		Latin *scabby eruption*	Infection of the skin that produces thick, yellow crusts
infection	in-**FEK**-shun	S/ R/	-ion *process* infect- *tainted, internal invasion*	Invasion of the body by disease-producing microorganisms
infestation	in-fes-**TAY**-shun	S/ R/	-ation *process* infest- *invade*	Act of being invaded on the skin by a troublesome other species, such as a parasite
louse lice (pl)	LOWSE LICE		Old English *louse*	Parasitic insect
necrotizing fasciitis	neh-kroh-**TIZE**-ing fash-eh-**EYE**-tis	S/ R/CF S/ S/ R/CF	-ing *quality of* necr/o- *death* -tiz- *pertaining to* -itis *inflammation* fasc/i – *fascia*	Inflammation of fascia, producing death of the tissue
parasite	**PAR**-ah-site		Greek *guest*	An organism that attaches itself to, lives on or in, and derives its nutrition from another species
pediculosis	peh-dick-you-**LOH**-sis	S/ R/	-osis *condition* pedicul- *louse*	An infestation with lice
scabies	**SKAY**-bees		Latin *to scratch*	Skin disease produced by mites
tinea	**TIN**-ee-ah		Latin *worm*	General term for a group of related skin infections caused by different species of fungi
tinea capitis	**TIN**-ee-ah **CAP**-it-us	S/ R/	-is *pertaining to* capit- *head*	Fungal infection of the scalp
tinea corporis	**TIN**-ee-ah **KOR**-por-is	S/ R/	-is *pertaining to* corpor- *body*	Fungal infection of the body
tinea cruris	**TIN**-ee-ah **KROO**-ris	S/ R/	-is *pertaining to* crur- *leg*	Fungal infection of the groin
tinea pedis tinea versicolor	**TIN**-ee-ah **PED**-is **TIN**-ee-ah **VERSE**-ih-col-or	R/ R/CF R/	ped- *child* vers/i- *to turn* -color *color*	Fungal infection of the foot Fungal infection of the trunk in which the skin loses pigmentation
verruca	ver-**ROO**-cah		Latin *wart*	Wart caused by a virus

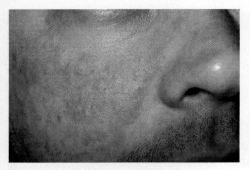

▲ **Figure 4.17** Systemic lupus erythematosus. Dr P. Marazzi/Science Source

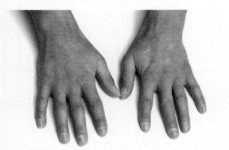

▲ **Figure 4.18** Scleroderma. SPL/Science Source

Diseases of the Skin

Collagen Diseases

Collagen, a fibrous protein, accounts for 30% of total body protein. Therefore, collagen diseases can have a dramatic effect all over the body. Collagen diseases, **autoimmune** or otherwise, attack collagen or other components of connective tissue.

Systemic lupus erythematosus (SLE), an autoimmune disease, occurs most commonly in women and produces characteristic skin lesions. A butterfly-shaped red rash on both cheeks joined across the bridge of the nose is commonly seen *(Figure 4.17).* It is associated with fever, fatigue, joint pains, and multiple internal organ involvement.

Rosacea produces a facial rash similar to that of SLE, and the underlying capillaries become enlarged and show through the skin. It is thought to be worsened by alcohol and spicy food. Its etiology is unknown. It has no **systemic** complications.

Scleroderma is a chronic, persistent autoimmune disease, occurring more often in women and characterized by hardening and shrinking of the skin that makes it feel leathery *(Figure 4.18).* Joints show swelling, pain, and stiffness. Internal organs such as the heart, lungs, kidneys, and digestive tract can be involved in a similar process. The etiology is unknown, and there is no effective treatment.

Other Skin Diseases

Psoriasis *(Figure 4.19)* is marked by itchy, flaky, red patches of skin of various sizes covered with white or silvery scales. It appears most commonly on the scalp, elbows, and knees. Its cause is unknown.

Vitiligo produces pale, irregular patches of skin. It is thought to have an autoimmune etiology.

Skin Manifestations of Internal Disease

Signs of the presence of cancer inside the body are often shown by skin lesions, even before the cancer has produced **symptoms** or been diagnosed.

Dermatomyositis *(Figure 4.20)* is often associated with ovarian cancer, which can appear within 4 to 5 years after the skin disease is diagnosed. It is an inflammatory condition causing symptoms of muscle weakness and a characteristic skin rash found around the eyes.

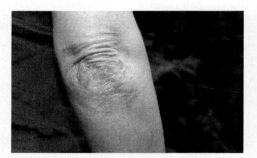

▲ **Figure 4.19** Psoriasis. Dave Bolton/Getty Images

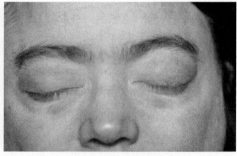

▲ **Figure 4.20** Periorbital rash of dermatomyositis. Medical-on-line/Alamy Stock Photo

WORD	PRONUNCIATION	ELEMENTS		DEFINITION
autoimmune	aw-toh-im-YUNE	P/ R/CF	auto- *self, same* -immune *immune response*	Immune reaction directed against a person's own tissue.
dermatomyositis	**DER**-mah-toh-**MY**-oh-site-is	S/ R/CF R/	-itis *inflammation* dermat/o- *skin* -myos- *muscle*	Inflammation of the skin and muscles
psoriasis	so-**RYE**-ah-sis		Greek *the itch*	Rash characterized by reddish, silver-scaled patches
rosacea	roh-**ZAY**-she-ah		Latin *rosy*	Persistent erythematous rash of the central face
scleroderma	sklair-oh-**DERM**-ah	R/ R/CF	-derma *skin* scler/o- *hard*	Thickening and hardening of the skin due to new collagen formation
sign (objective) symptom (subjective) symptomatic (adj)	SINE **SIMP**-tum simp-toh-**MAT**-ik	 S/ R/	Latin *mark* Greek *sign* -ic *pertaining to* symptomat- *symptoms*	Physical evidence of a disease process Departure from normal health experienced by the patient Pertaining to the symptoms of a disease
systemic lupus erythematosus	sis-**TEM**-ik **LOO**-pus er-ih-**THEE**-mah-toh-sus	S/ R/ S/ R/	-ic *pertaining to* system- *body system* lupus *wolf* -osus *condition* erythemat- *redness*	Inflammatory connective tissue disease affecting the whole body
vitiligo	vit-ill-**EYE**-go		Latin *skin blemish*	Nonpigmented white patches on otherwise normal skin

Acne

Around puberty, **androgens** are thought to trigger excessive production of sebum from the glands, which then brings excessive numbers of broken-down cells toward the skin surface. This blocks the follicle, forming a **comedo** (whitehead or blackhead). Comedones can stay closed, leading to **papules,** or can **rupture,** allowing bacteria to get in and produce **pustules.** These are the classic signs of **acne,** which is said to affect, in different degrees, about 85% of people between 12 and 25 years *(Figure 4.21).* For many acne patients, treatment is difficult during puberty and the face can be scarred.

A different skin problem involving the sebaceous glands is **seborrheic dermatitis.** The glands are thought to be inflamed and to produce a different sebum. The skin around the face and scalp is reddened and covered with yellow, greasy scales. In infants, this condition is called cradle cap. Seborrheic dermatitis of the scalp produces dandruff. **Dandruff** is clumps of these keratinocytes stuck together with **sebum,** oil from **sebaceous** glands.

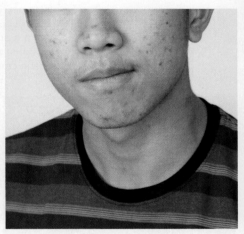

▲ **Figure 4.21** **Acne.** ©Teim/Shutterstock.com RF

WORD	PRONUNCIATION		ELEMENTS	DEFINITION
acne	**AK**-nee		Greek *point*	Inflammatory disease of sebaceous glands and hair follicles
androgen	**AN**-droh-jen	S/ R/CF	**-gen** *to produce* **andr/o-** *male*	Hormone that promotes masculine characteristics
comedo comedones (pl)	**KOM**-ee-doh		Latin *eat up*	A whitehead or blackhead caused by too much sebum and too many keratin cells blocking the hair follicle
cyst cystic (adj)	SIST **SIS**-tik	S/ R/	Greek *sac, bladder* **-ic** *pertaining to* **cyst-** *cyst, bladder*	An abnormal, fluid-containing sac Relating to a cyst
dandruff	**DAN**-druff		Old English *scurf*	Seborrheic scales from the scalp
papule	**PAP**-yul		Latin *pimple*	Small, circumscribed elevation on the skin
pustule	**PUS**-tyul		Latin *pustule*	Small protuberance on the skin that contains pus
rupture	**RUP**-tyur		Latin *break*	Break or tear of any organ or body part
sebaceous glands sebum	se-**BAY**-shus GLANDZ **SEE**-bum	S/ R	**-ous** *pertaining to* **sebace-** *sebum* Latin *wax*	Glands in the dermis that open into hair follicles and secrete an oily fluid called sebum Waxy secretion of the sebaceous glands
seborrhea seborrheic (adj)	seb-oh-**REE**-ah seb-oh-**REE**-ik	S/ R/CF S/	**-rrhea** *flow* **seb/o-** *sebum* **-ic** *pertaining to*	Excessive amount of sebum Pertaining to seborrhea

Diseases of Nails

Fifty percent of all nail disorders are caused by fungal infections and are labeled **onychomycosis** *(Figure 4.22)*. They begin in nails constantly exposed to moisture and warmth; for example, in warm shoes when associated with poor foot hygiene, in the hands of a restaurant dishwasher, under artificial fingernails, and in pedicure bowls if they are not sanitized. The fungus grows under the nail and leads to brittle cracked nails that separate from the underlying nail bed.

Paronychia *(Figure 4.23)* is a bacterial infection, usually staphylococcal, of the base of the nail. The nail fold and cuticle become swollen, red, and painful, and pus forms under the nail and can escape at the side of the nail.

The nail of the big toe can grow into the skin at the side of the nail, particularly if pressured by tight, narrow shoes. Infection can then get underneath this ingrown toenail.

The nails can reflect systemic illness. In anemia, the nail bed is pale, and the nails can become spoon-shaped. In conditions producing chronic **hypoxia,** the fingers, toes, and nails become clubbed. **Malnutrition** or severe illness can produce horizontal white lines in the nails.

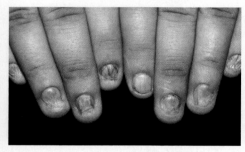

▲ **Figure 4.22** Onychomycosis (fungal infection). ©Dr. Harout Taniellian/ Photo Researchers, Inc.

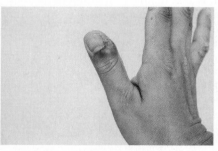

▲ **Figure 4.23** Paronychia, with pus at the corner of the nail bed. kckate16/ Shutterstock

Word Analysis and Definition: Disorders of the Glands and Nails

S = Suffix   P = Prefix   R = Root   R/CF = Combining Form

WORD	PRONUNCIATION	ELEMENTS		DEFINITION
diaphoretic	DIE-ah-foh-RET-ic	S/ R/	-etic *pertaining to* diaphor- *sweat*	Pertaining to sweat or perspiration
diaphoresis	DIE-ah-foh-REE-sis	S/	-esis *abnormal*	Abnormal amount of sweat or perspiration
hypoxia	high-POK-see-ah	S/ P/ R/	-ia *condition* hyp- *below* -ox- *oxygen*	Decrease below normal levels of oxygen in tissues, gases, or blood
hypoxic (adj)	high-POK-sik	S/	-ic *pertaining to*	Deficient in oxygen
malnutrition	mal-nyu-TRISH-un	S/ P/ R/	-ion *process* mal- *bad, inadequate* -nutrit- *nourishment*	Inadequate nutrition from poor diet or inadequate absorption of nutrients
onychomycosis	oh-ni-koh-my-KOH-sis	S/ R/CF R/	-osis *condition* onych/o- *nail* -myc- *fungus*	Condition of a fungus infection in a nail
paironychia (*Note:* The vowel "a" at the end of para- is dropped to make the composite word flow more easily.)	pair-oh-NICK-ee-ah	S/ P/ R/	-ia *condition* para- *alongside* -onych- *nail*	Infection alongside the nail

Check Point Section 4.3

A. Demonstrate that you are able to spell medical terms related to disorders of the skin. *Fill in the blank.* **LO 4.3, 4.6**

1. The medical term that means the same as *mole* is _____.

2. A cancerous tumor originating in the deepest layer of the epidermis is termed a _____ cell carcinoma.

3. The plural form of the term *nevus* is _____.

4. A _____ is a malignant tumor of cells that produce melanin.

B. Medical terms can have small differences that make them entirely new words. *Fill in the blanks with the correct terms.* **LO 4.6**

allergens   **allergenic**   **allergy**   **allergic**

1. After many _____ tests, it was determined that she was _____ to mold.

2. There were too many _____ substances in the carpet, therefore it was removed from the room.

3. Dust mites, peanuts, and pollen can be _____ to some people.

C. One of the following terms is a noun (person, place, or thing), and the other term is a verb (action). *Identify the noun and verb.* **LO 4.2**

1. Excori<u>ate</u>   Noun or verb: _____

2. Excori<u>ation</u>   Noun or verb: _____

D. Demonstrate that you are able to spell medical terms related to disorders of the skin. *Fill in the blanks.* **LO 4.3, 4.6**

1. A condition caused by lice infestation: _____

2. Inflammation of a small cell: _____

E. The terms for skin conditions are similar. *It is important to know the specific differences in skin conditions. Fill in the blanks.* **LO 4.3, 4.6**

1. One infected hair follicle that spreads to surrounding tissues: _____

2. A small area of many infected hair follicles: _____

3. Skin infection characterized by thick, yellow crusts: _____

4. Skin infection caused by mites: _____

5. Skin infection caused by fungus (nonspecific): _____

6. Infection caused by the fungus *Candida* (two terms mean the same thing): _____ and _____

F. Building medical terms and taking them apart force you to focus on the elements they contain. *Understanding elements is the key to increasing your medical vocabulary. Deconstruct the following terms to increase your knowledge of their elements.* **LO 4.2**

1. In the term **erythematosus,** the root means:

    a. condition of   b. blemish   c. red   d. inflammation

2. In the term **symptomatic,** the suffix means:

    a. pertaining to   b. inflammation   c. painful   d. condition of

3. In the term **dermatomyositis,** the word element that means *skin* is a:

    a. root/combining form   b. prefix   c. suffix

4. In the term **autoimmune,** the word element that means *self* is a:

    a. root/combining form   b. prefix   c. suffix

G. Indicate if the statement is true or false. **LO 4.6**

1. A *pustule* is filled with pus.   True   False

2. *Acne* is a degenerative disease of the skin.   True   False

3. A *cystic lesion* is filled with hard, packed cells.   True   False

4. A *comedo* can be either a whitehead or a blackhead.   True   False

H. Work on understanding the meanings of the elements. *From the given definition, construct medical terms relating to the definition. Fill in the blanks.* **LO 4.1, 4.2, 4.6**

1. Fungal infection of the nail: onych/o/_____ /osis

2. Coiled sweat gland that occurs all over the body: mer/o/_____

3. Substance that carries and generates attraction for other people: _____ /omone

4. Infection alongside the nail: par/_____ /ia

I. Answer the following questions about the medical terms relating to diseases of the nail. *Fill in the blanks.* **LO 4.3, 4.6**

paronychia   onychomycosis   hypoxia   malnutrition

1. Clubbing of the nails can occur with chronic _____.

2. An infection alongside the nail is termed _____.

3. A fungal infection of the nails is termed _____.

4. A person suffering from _____ may have visible white lines in the nail bed.

Section 4.4 Burns and Injuries to the Skin

Burns

Burns are the leading cause of *accidental* death. The immediate threats to life are from fluid loss, infection, and the systemic effects of burned dead tissue. **Shock** can develop when a large amount of skin surface area is burned.

Burns are classified according to the depth of tissue involved *(Figure 4.24):*

- **First-degree (superficial) burns** involve only the epidermis and produce inflammation with redness, pain, and slight **edema.** Healing occurs in 3 to 5 days without scarring.
- **Second-degree (partial-thickness) burns** involve the epidermis and dermis but leave some of the dermis intact. They produce redness, blisters, and more severe pain. Healing occurs in 2 to 3 weeks with minimal scarring.
- **Third-degree (full-thickness) burns** involve the epidermis, dermis, and subcutaneous tissues, which are often completely destroyed. **Eschar** *(Figure 4.24c)* develops and is treated with **debridement**. Healing takes a long time and involves using skin grafts.
- **Fourth-degree burns** destroy all layers of the skin and involve tendons, muscles, and sometimes bones.

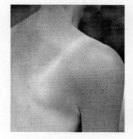 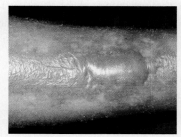 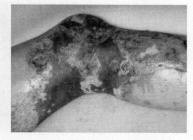

(a) First degree (superficial) **(b)** Second degree (partial thickness) **(c)** Third degree (full thickness)

▲ **Figure 4.24** **Degrees of burns.** (a) Sheila Terry/Science Source (b) Dr. P. Marazzi/Science Source (c) John Radcliffe Hospital/Science Source

Word Analysis and Definition: Related to Burns

S = Suffix   P = Prefix   R = Root   R/CF = Combining Form

WORD	PRONUNCIATION	ELEMENTS		DEFINITION
debridement	day-**BREED**-mon	S/ P/ R/	-ment *resulting state* de- *take away* -bride- *rubbish*	The removal of injured or necrotic tissue
edema edematous (adj)	ee-**DEE**-mah ee-**DEM**-ah-tus	S/ R/	Greek *swelling* -tous *pertaining to* edema- *swelling*	Excessive collection of fluid in cells and tissues Marked by edema
eschar	**ESS**-kar		Greek *scab of a burn*	The burned, dead tissue lying on top of third-degree burns
shock	SHOCK		German *to clash*	Sudden physical or mental collapse or circulatory collapse

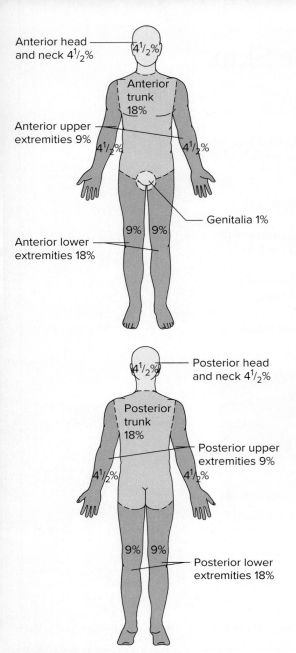

Anterior head and neck 4½%

4½%

Anterior trunk 18%

Anterior upper extremities 9%

4½% 4½%

Genitalia 1%

Anterior lower extremities 18%

9% 9%

Posterior head and neck 4½%

4½%

Posterior trunk 18%

Posterior upper extremities 9%

4½% 4½%

Posterior lower extremities 18%

9% 9%

▲ **Figure 4.25** Rule of Nines.

Burns (continued)

Burn injury to the lungs through damage from heat or smoke inhalation is responsible for 60% or more of fatalities from burns.

In partial-thickness burns, **regeneration** of the skin can occur from remaining cells in the stratum basale, from residual hair follicles and sweat glands, and from the edges of the burned area. In full-thickness burns, there is no dermal tissue left for regeneration, and skin grafts are needed. The ideal graft is an **autograft** taken from another location on the patient. It is not rejected by the immune system.

If the patient's burns are too extensive, **allografts** from another person are needed. These are provided by skin banks and are taken from deceased people (cadavers). A **homograft** is another name for an allograft. A **xenograft,** or **heterograft,** is a graft from another species, for example, pigs.

Artificial skin is being developed commercially and can stimulate the growth of connective tissues from the patient's underlying tissue.

Regions of Skin Surface Area

The skin's surface area can be divided into six regions, each one of which is a fraction or multiple of 9% of the total surface area. This is called the Rule of Nines (*Figure 4.25*).

The treatment and prognosis for a burn patient depend, in part, on the extent of the body surface that is affected. This is estimated by applying the Rule of Nines to determine the percentage of the skin's surface affected by burns:

- Head and neck are assigned 9% (4½% anterior and 4½% posterior).
- Each arm is 9% (4½% anterior and 4½% posterior).
- Each leg is 18% (9% anterior and 9% posterior).
- The anterior trunk is 18%.
- The posterior trunk is 18%.
- The genitalia are 1%.

Word Analysis and Definition: Burn Treatment

S = Suffix P = Prefix R = Root R/CF = Combining Form

WORD	PRONUNCIATION		ELEMENTS	DEFINITION
allograft	**AL**-oh-graft	P/	allo- *other*	Skin graft from another person or cadaver
		R/	-graft *transplant*	
homograft (syn)	**HOH**-moh-graft	P/	homo- *same, alike*	
autograft	**AWE**-toh-graft	P/	auto- *self*	A graft using tissue taken from the individual who is receiving the graft
		R/	-graft *transplant*	
regenerate	ree-**JEN**-eh-rate	S/	-ate *composed of*	To reconstitute a lost part
		P/	re- *again*	
		R/	-gener- *produce*	
regeneration (noun)	ree-**JEN**-eh-**RAY**-shun	S/	-ation *process*	Reconstitution of a lost part
xenograft	**ZEN**-oh-graft	P/	xeno- *foreign*	A graft from another species
		R/	-graft *transplant*	
heterograft (syn)	**HET**-er-oh-graft	P/	hetero- *different*	

Wounds and Tissue Repair

If you cut yourself with paper and produce a shallow **laceration** primarily in the epidermis, the epithelial cells along its edges will divide rapidly and fill in the gap. An adhesive bandage helps the process by pulling the edges together.

If you cut yourself more deeply, extending the **wound** into the dermis or hypodermis, or if a surgeon makes an **incision,** then blood vessels in the dermis break and blood escapes into the wound *(Figure 4.26a).*

This escaped blood forms a **clot** in the wound. The clot consists of protein (**fibrin**) together with **platelets** (also called **thrombocytes**), blood cells, and dried tissue fluids trapped in the fibers. **Macrophages** come into the wound with the escaped blood. They digest and clean up the tissue debris. The surface of the clot dries and hardens in the air to form a **scab.** The scab seals and protects the wound from becoming infected *(Figure 4.26b).*

The clot begins to be invaded by new capillaries from the surrounding dermis. Three or four days after the injury, fibroblasts migrate into the wound and form new collagen fibers that pull the wound together. This soft tissue in the wound is called **granulation tissue** and in unsutured wounds takes a couple of weeks to completely form *(Figure 4.27).*

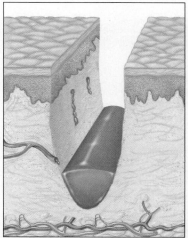

(a) Bleeding into the wound

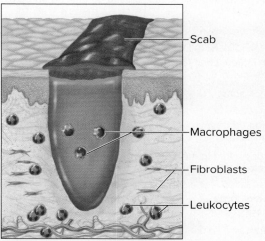

(b) Scab formation and macrophage activity

— Scab

— Macrophages

— Fibroblasts

— Leukocytes

▲ **Figure 4.26** Wound healing.

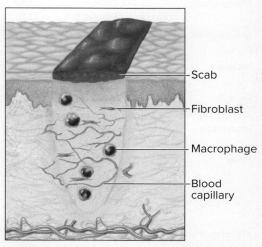

— Scab

— Fibroblast

— Macrophage

— Blood capillary

▲ **Figure 4.27** Formation of granulation tissue.

As healing continues, surface epithelial cells from the edges of the wound migrate into the area underneath the scab. As this new epithelium thickens, the scab loosens and falls off. Inside the wound, new collagen fibers formed by the fibroblasts form a **scar** to replace the granulation tissue *(Figure 4.28).* In unsutured wounds, this takes up to a month to complete.

Suturing brings together the edges of the wound to enhance tissue healing. It also reduces the risk of infection and the amount of scarring. A liquid skin adhesive can sometimes be used in place of **sutures.** Some sutures eventually dissolve, avoiding the need for suture removal. The scar formation and remodeling process may go on for more than a year.

In some people, there is excessive fibrosis and scar tissue formation, producing raised, irregular, lumpy, shiny scars called **keloids** *(Figure 4.29).* They can extend beyond the edges of the original wound and often return if they are surgically removed. They are most common on the upper body and earlobes.

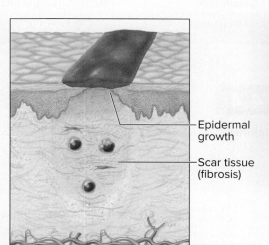

— Epidermal growth

— Scar tissue (fibrosis)

▲ **Figure 4.28** Scar formation.

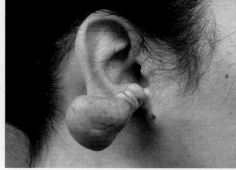

▲ **Figure 4.29** A keloid of the earlobe. **This scar resulted from piercing the ear for earrings.** BSIP/Contributor/Getty Images

Surgery on the skin is now being performed using light beams called **lasers.** These beams of light can be focused precisely to vaporize specific lesions on the superficial layers of the skin. The beams remove lesions and create a fresh surface over which new skin can grow. Healing takes 10 to 15 days and goes through the process described above, with clotting and scabbing.

A superficial scraping of the skin, a mucous membrane, or the cornea *(see Chapter 16)* is called an **abrasion.**

Word Analysis and Definition: Tissue Damage and Repair

S = Suffix   P = Prefix   R = Root   R/CF = Combining Form

WORD	PRONUNCIATION		ELEMENTS	DEFINITION
abrasion	ah-**BRAY**-shun		Latin *to scrape*	Area of skin or mucous membrane that has been scraped off
clot	KLOT		German *to block*	The mass of fibrin and cells that is produced in a wound
fibrin fibrous (adj)	**FIE**-brin **FIE**-brus	 S/ R/	Latin *fiber* -ous *pertaining to* fibr- *fiber*	Stringy protein fiber that is a component of a blood clot Tissue containing fibroblasts and fibers
granulation	gran-you-**LAY**-shun	S/ R/	-ation *process* granul- *small grain*	New fibrous tissue formed during wound healing
incision	in-**SIZH**-un	S/ R/	-ion *action, condition* incis- *cut into*	A cut or surgical wound
keloid	**KEY**-loyd		Greek *stain*	Raised, irregular, lumpy, shiny scar due to excess collagen fiber production during healing of a wound
laceration	lass-eh-**RAY**-shun	S/ R/	-ation *process* lacer- *to tear*	A tear of the skin
laser	**LAY**-zer		acronym for **L**ight **A**mplification by **S**timulated **E**mission of **R**adiation	Intense, narrow beam of monochromatic light
macrophage	**MAK**-roh-fayj	P/ R/	macro- *large* -phage *to eat*	Large white blood cell that removes bacteria, foreign particles, and dead cells
platelet (also called thrombocyte)	**PLAYT**-let		Greek *small plate*	Cell fragment involved in clotting process
scab	SKAB		Old English *crust*	Crust that forms over a wound or sore during healing
scar	SKAR		Greek *scab*	Fibrotic seam that forms when a wound heals
suture	**SOO**-chur		Latin *seam*	Stitch to hold the edges of a wound together
wound	WOOND		Old English *wound*	Any injury that interrupts the continuity of skin or a mucous membrane

Check Point Section 4.4

A. Define the terms associated with burn injuries. *Match the terms in the first column with their correct definition in the second column.* **LO 4.6**

_____ 1. regenerate

_____ 2. eschar

_____ 3. debridement

_____ 4. shock

_____ 5. edema

a. sudden physical collapse

b. burned, dead tissue

c. excessive collection of fluid in cells and tissues

d. to reconstitute a lost part

e. removal of injured or necrotic tissue

B. Compare and contrast the meanings of word elements that describe the types of skin grafts. *Fill in the blank with the correct term.* **LO 4.6, 4.7**

1. A graft from another species is a **xenograft** and a _____.

2. A graft from another person is an **allograft** and a _____.

3. A graft taken from one part a person's body and placed elsewhere on the same body: _____

C. Remembering the meaning of the word element can help you easily identify the type of skin grafts. *Match the prefix to its meaning.* **LO 4.2, 4.7**

_____ 1. *hetero-*   **a.** other

_____ 2. *allo-*   **b.** same, alike

_____ 3. *xeno-*   **c.** self

_____ 4. *homo-*   **d.** different

_____ 5. *auto-*   **e.** foreign

D. Reviewing the elements and definitions will help you work out the answers. *Put on your thinking cap. Fill in the blanks.* **LO 4.6**

1. Reorder these terms into the order of their occurrence. Place a 1 for the process that occurs first, ending with 4 for the process that occurs last.

   _____scab   _____scar   _____clot   _____wound

2. An excess amount of scar tissue is termed a _____.

3. What is the soft tissue in the wound-healing process called? _____

4. The type of cell that produces collagen is a _____.

5. A scraping of the skin is termed an _____.

6. A tear in the skin is termed a _____.

7. What is another name for a stitch used to close a wound? _____

Section 4.5 Procedures and Pharmacology

Diagnostic Procedures

The most important procedures in making a diagnosis of a skin lesion are a careful history of the etiology and progression of the lesion and a careful visual examination to define the clinical appearance of the lesion.

Diascopy, in which a finger or a microscope slide is pressed against a lesion to see if it blanches, helps define a vascular (inflammatory) lesion, which blanches, from a hemorrhagic lesion (petechia or purpura) which does not blanch.

Microscopic examination of skin scrapings helps diagnose fungal infections and scabies. Tzank testing by scraping the base of vesicles and staining them with a Giemsa stain shows multinucleated giant cells of herpes simplex or zoster under microscopy.

Cultures using swabs taken from lesions and implanted in the appropriate growth medium are utilized to diagnose some viruses (e.g., herpes simplex) and certain bacteria.

Biopsy (Bx) of a skin lesion using a punch biopsy, excision of a whole lesion, or shaving of the lesion for microscopic examination is valuable in diagnosing malignancies, fungal diseases, and immune diseases.

Wood's light (black light) is used to define the borders of pigmented lesions before excision, show the presence of *Pseudomonas* infection (**fluoresces** green), and distinguish the **hypopigmentation** of vitiligo, which fluoresces a deep ivory white.

Therapeutic Procedures

Photodynamic therapy in a series of sessions exposes the skin in acne to a high-intensity blue light and creates a toxic environment in which bacteria in the sebaceous glands cannot live. In addition to treating acne, photodynamic therapy can be used to treat precancerous lesions called **actinic keratoses,** which have the potential to develop into squamous cell carcinomas.

Laser therapy is used for the management of birthmarks, vascular lesions, warts, and skin disorders like vitiligo.

Chemical peels are **cosmetic** procedures performed on the face, neck, or hands. An acid solution such as glycolic acid, salicylic acid, or carbolic acid (phenol) is applied to small areas of skin to reduce fine facial lines and wrinkles, treat sun damage, and reduce age spots and dark patches (**melasma**).

Cryotherapy is used frequently to treat acne, scars, sebaceous plaques, and some skin cancers. Liquid nitrogen is sprayed onto the affected area of skin to cause peeling or scabbing.

Botox is a prescription medicine that blocks signals from nerves to muscles. When injected into superficial muscles, the injected muscle can no longer contract, causing facial wrinkles and lines to temporarily relax and soften.

Dermal fillers such as Restylane and Juvederm help to diminish facial lines and wrinkles by restoring subcutaneous volume and fullness to the face as subcutaneous fat is lost in the natural aging process.

Word Analysis and Definition: Diagnostic and Therapeutic Procedures

S = Suffix   P = Prefix   R = Root   R/CF = Combining Form

WORD	PRONUNCIATION		ELEMENTS	DEFINITION
actinic	ak-**TIN**-ik	S/ R/	-ic *pertaining to* actin- *ray*	Pertaining to the sun
biopsy biopsy removal	**BIE**-op-see **BIE**-op-see re-**MUV**-al	S/ R/CF	-opsy *to view* bi/o- *life*	Removing tissue from a living person for laboratory examination Used for small tumors when complete removal provides tissue for a biopsy and cures the lesion
cosmetic	koz-**MET**-ik		Greek *an adornment*	A concern for appearance
cryosurgery	cry-oh-**SUR**-jer-ee	S/ R/CF R/	-ery *process of* cry/o- *icy cold* -surg- *operate*	Use of liquid nitrogen or argon gas in a probe to freeze
cryotherapy	**CRY**-oh-**THAIR**-ah pee	R/CF R/	cry/o- *icy cold* -therapy *medical treatment*	The use of cold in the treatment of disease
culture	**KUL**-chur		Latin *tillage*	The growth of microorganisms on or in media
diascopy	di-**AS**-koh-pee	P/ S/	dia- *through* -scopy *to examine, to view*	Examination of superficial skin lesions with pressure
fluoresce	flor-**ESS**		Greek *bright color*	Emit a bright-colored light when irradiated with ultraviolet or violet-blue rays
keratosis keratoses (pl)	ker-ah-**TOH**-sis ker-ah-**TOH**-seez	S/ R/	-osis *condition* kerat- *horny*	Epidermal lesion of circumscribed overgrowth of the horny layer
melasma	meh-**LAZ**-mah		Greek *black spot*	Patchy pigmentation of the skin
microscope microscopic (adj)	**MY**-kroh-skope **MY**-kroh-**SKOP**-ik	P/ R/ S/	micro- *small* -scope *instrument for viewing* -ic *pertaining to*	Instrument for viewing something small that cannot be seen in detail by the naked eye Visible only with the aid of a microscope
pigment hypopigmentation	**PIG**-ment **HIGH**-poh-pig-men-**TAY**-shun	 S/ P/ R/	Latin *paint* -ation *process* hypo- *below normal* -pigment- *color*	A coloring matter or stain Below normal melanin relative to the surrounding skin

Dermatologic Pharmacology

A wide range of **topical pharmacologic** agents of different types can be used in the treatment of skin lesions either to relieve symptoms or to cure the disease.

- **Anesthetics:** topical agents that relieve pain or itching on the skin's surface. Benzocaine is used for this purpose as a numbing **cream.** It is used prior to injections, for oral ulcers, for hemorrhoids, and for infant teething.
- **Antibacterials:** topical agents that eliminate bacteria that cause skin lesions. Neomycin **ointment** is commonly used.
- **Antifungals:** topical agents that eliminate or inhibit the growth of fungi. Nystatin (*Mycostatin, Nilstat*) is used as a cream or ointment. Terbinafine (*Lamisil*) is used as a cream or ointment. Clotrimazole (*Canesten, Clomazol*) and ketaconazole (*Ketopine, Daktagold*) are *imadazoles* available in creams, sprays, **lotions,** and **shampoos.** Amphotericin B (*Fungizone*) is used locally to treat oral candidiasis (thrush), and in intravenous (IV) therapy for systemic fungal infections.
- **Antipruritics:** topical lotions, ointments, creams, or sprays that relieve itching. **Corticosteroids** such as hydrocortisone are most frequently used.
- **Biologics:** administered as an injection or intravenously, these agents block immune system reactions that cause psoriasis. Examples of biologics adalimumab (*Humira*), dupilumab (*Dupixent*), infliximab (*Remicade*), risankizumab (*Skyrizi*), and secukinumab (*Cosentyx*).
- **Keratolytics:** topical agents that peel away the skin's stratum corneum from the other epidermal layers. Salicylic acid is used for this purpose in the treatment of acne, psoriasis, ichthyoses, and dandruff. It is available in the form of wipes, creams, **lotions, gels,** ointments, and **shampoos** in strengths varying from 3% to 20%.
- **Parasiticides:** topical agents that kill parasites living on the skin. Hexachlorocyclohexane (*Lindane 1%*) is used in lotion or shampoo form to kill lice if other methods have failed.
- **Retinoids:** derivatives of retinoic acid (vitamin A) used under the strict supervision of a physician in the treatment of acne, sun spots, and psoriasis. Tretinoin (*Retin-A*) is used topically for acne; isoretinoin (*Accutane*) is taken orally for severe acne; etretinate (*Tegison*) is taken orally to treat severe psoriasis; and adapalene (*Differin*) is used topically for psoriasis and acne.

Classes of Topical Medications
Solutions are usually a powder dissolved in water or alcohol.
Lotions are usually a powder mixed with oil and water to be thicker than a solution.
Gels are a semisolid **emulsion** in an alcohol base.
Creams are an emulsion of oil and water that is thicker than a lotion and holds its shape when removed from its container. They penetrate the outer stratum corneum layer of skin.
Ointments are a homogenous semisolid preparation, 80% a thick oil and 20% water, that lies on the skin. They can also be used on the mucous membranes of the eye, vulva, anus, and nose, and are emulsifiable with the mucous membrane secretions.
Transdermal patches are a very precise time-released method to deliver a drug. Release of the drug can be controlled by **diffusion** through the adhesive that covers the whole patch or through a membrane with adhesive only on the patch rim.

WORD	PRONUNCIATION	ELEMENTS		DEFINITION
anesthetic	an-es-**THET**-ik	S/ P/ R/	-ic *pertaining to* an- *without* -esthet- *sensation,* *perception*	Substance that takes away feeling and pain
antibacterial	**AN**-tee-bak-**TEER**-ee-al	S/ P/ R/CF	-al *pertaining to* anti- *against* -bacter/i-	Destroying or preventing the growth of bacteria
antifungal antipruritic	**AN**-tee-**FUN**-gul **AN**-tee-pru-**RIT**-ik	R/ S/ P/ R/	fung- *fungus* -ic *pertaining to* anti- *against* -prurit- *itch*	Destroying or preventing the growth of a fungus Medication against itching
cream	KREEM		Latin *thick juice*	A semisolid emulsion
diffusion	dih-**FYU**-zhun	S/ R/	-ion *process* diffus- *movement*	The process by which small particles move between tissues
emulsion	ee-**MUL**-shun	S/ R/	-ion *process* emuls- *suspension in a* *liquid*	Very small particles suspended in a solution
keratolytic	**KER**-ah-toh-**LIT**-ik	S/ R/CF R/	-ic *pertaining to* kerat/o- *horn* -lyt- *loosening*	Causing separation or loosening of the horny layer (stratum corneum) of the skin
parasiticide	par-ah-**SIT**-ih-side	S/ R/CF	-cide *to kill* parasit/i *parasite*	Agent that destroys parasites
retinoid	**RET**-ih-noyd		Derived from retinoic acid	A cream that is a derivative of vitamin A used to treat acne and wrinkles
topical	**TOP**-ih-kal	S/ R/	-al *pertaining to* topic- *local*	Medication applied to the skin to obtain a local effect

Check Point Section 4.5

A. Identify the proper diagnostic procedure or treatment for each condition. *Use the words from the provided word bank to complete the sentences. Fill in the blank.* **LO 4.5**

diascopy   Juvederm   cryotherapy   Botox   fluoresce

1. Injecting _____ into the skin will fill areas to reduce the appearance of aging.

2. Acne can be treated with _____ to freeze the cells of the affected area.

3. Pigmented or hypopigmented areas can be better seen when they _____ with Wood's light.

4. Pressing on an area of skin to see if it blanches is termed _____.

5. The injection of _____ can reduce the appearance of wrinkles by paralyzing the affected muscles.

B. Defining the meaning of word elements can help you to quickly decipher the meaning of medical terms. *Choose the correct answer to each question.* **LO 4.2, 4.5**

1. The word element that means *cold:*

   a. *dia-*   **b.** *-therapy*   **c.** *cry/o-*   **d.** *hypo-*

2. The word element *dia-* means:

   a. to view   **b.** through   **c.** light   **d.** two

3. The word element *-scopy* means:

    a. to view   **b.** scrape   **c.** suture   **d.** inject

4. The suffix that means *condition of* is:

    a. *-osis*   **b.** *-ic*   **c.** *-itis*   **d.** *-al*

C. Practice your *language of pharmacology* by correctly filling in the blanks of patient documentation. LO 4.7, 4.8

Mrs. Robison brought in her 8-year-old daughter to the doctor because the child had a red ring–like rash on her abdomen. Dr. Palmer examined the child and diagnosed her with tinea corporis. She prescribed terbinafine cream to be applied to the site twice daily for 6 weeks.

1. Dr. Palmer prescribed an _____ cream to cure the patient's tinea corporis.

2. She prefers to provide _____ application of the medication because it stays local to the site of the infection.

D. Define the classes of topical medications. *Topical medications come in a variety of forms to best deliver medication to the skin. Match the description of the form of the medication to its term.* **LO 4.7**

Term		Meaning
_____	**1.** gel	**a.** adhesive membrane attached to the surface of the skin
_____	**2.** lotion	**b.** semisolid emulsion in an alcohol base
_____	**3.** ointment	**c.** powder dissolved in alcohol or water
_____	**4.** transdermal patch	**d.** powder mixed with oil and water; thicker than a solution
_____	**5.** solution	**e.** semisolid preparation of oil and water

Table 4.2 Chapter 4 Abbreviations

Abbreviation	Meaning
Bx	biopsy
PDT	Photodynamic therapy

Table 4.3 Comparison of Selected Skin Disorders—Signs, Symptoms, and Treatments

Skin Disorder or Disease	Sign	Symptom	Treatment
Eczema	Red rash, may have vesicles	Itchy skin	Anesthetic Corticosteroid
Psoriasis	Flakey, red patches covered by silvery scales	Itchy skin	Keratolytic (salicylic acid) Retinoids Biologics
Dandruff	White flakes or clumps in scalp		Keratolytic (salicylic acid)
Ichthyoses	Dry, scaly skin		Keratolytic (salicylic acid)
Acne	Pustules		Keratolytic (salicylic acid) Retinoids
Pediculosis	Nits attached to hair	Itchy area surrounding hair (hair of scalp, hair of pubis, body hair)	Parasiticide

2014 Nucleus Medical Media

Integumentary System

Challenge Your Knowledge

A. **Match the type of skin graft with its correct definition.** The definitions can be used more than once. **LO 4.7**

_____ **1.** homograft

_____ **2.** autograft

_____ **3.** allograft

_____ **4.** xenograft

_____ **5.** heterograft

a. skin graft taken from the individual who is receiving the graft

b. skin graft from another person or cadaver

c. a graft from another species

B. **Plurals.** Follow the rules and form the plurals for the following terms. **LO 4.1, 4.3**

1. papilla   Plural: _____

2. matrix   Plural: _____

3. cortex   Plural: _____

4. axilla   Plural: _____

C. **Abbreviations appear in written documentation and must be used correctly.** From the sentences, give the abbreviation of the description in italics. **LO 4.8, 4.9**

1. Please inject the medication *into the hypodermis.*

_____

2. The pathologist performed a(n) *examination of the* nail matrix shaving to determine the presence of nail melanoma.

_____

D. **Skin diseases can affect any and all parts of the body.** Some skin diseases are an early manifestation of a more serious internal problem. Match the symptom or association in the left column with the correct medical term in the right column. You have more answer choices than you need. **LO 4.6**

_____ **1.** cause unknown; silvery scales

_____ **2.** butterfly rash

_____ **3.** associated with ovarian cancer

_____ **4.** enlarged capillaries show through skin

_____ **5.** pale patches of skin

_____ **6.** shrinking of skin; hardening

a. pemphigus vulgaris

b. vitiligo

c. rosacea

d. psoriasis

e. seborrheic lesions

f. scleroderma

g. systemic lupus erythematosus

h. herpes zoster

i. dermatomyositis

E. **Use your knowledge of the language of dermatology to make the connection with the following medical terms.** Match the medical terms in the left column with the descriptions in the right column. **LO 4.5, 4.6**

_____ 1. pruritus

_____ 2. edema

_____ 3. malignancy

_____ 4. systematic

_____ 5. excoriate

a. can infiltrate or metastasize

b. body as a whole

c. swelling

d. to scratch

e. itching

F. **Identify the correct dermatologic condition or procedure.** Choose the correct answer. **LO 4.1–4.9**

1. Use of liquid nitrogen to freeze or kill abnormal tissue is called:

a. biopsy

b. patch test

c. cryosurgery

d. hypodermic injection

e. infestation

2. A laceration that is _superficial_ is not very:

a. swollen

b. edematous

c. deep

d. purulent

e. infected

3. Keratinized stratified squamous epithelium is:

a. stratum corneum

b. dandruff

c. hair follicle

d. sweat

e. dermatitis

4. An ointment, cream, or spray prescribed to relieve itching is called:

a. antifungal

b. keratolytic

c. antipruritic

d. retinoid

e. antibacterial

5. Subcutaneous fat is another name for:

a. epidermis

b. hypodermis

c. dermis

d. adipose tissue

e. follicles

6. A congenital lesion of the skin, including birthmarks and moles, is called a:

a. macule

b. papule

c. vesicle

d. nevus

e. melanoma

7. Another name for a pressure ulcer is:

a. eczema

b. excoriation

c. decubitus

d. edematous

e. serous

8. Strep enzymes digest connective tissue and spread into muscle layers in:

a. lesions

b. atopic dermatitis

c. cellulitis

d. ulcers

e. necrotizing fasciitis

9. The medical term for shingles is:

a. eczema

b. herpes zoster

c. impetigo

d. candidiasis

e. pediculosis

10. A facial butterfly rash is associated with which autoimmune disease?

a. SC

b. HIV

c. SLE

d. TB

e. MRSA

G. **Medical terms that are nouns can also have an adjectival form that must be used in some cases.** Test your knowledge of the correct form of the term to use in the following sentences. **LO 4.3**

    1. This puncture wound has completely penetrated the _____.

    a. dermis   **b.** dermal

    2. This burn wound has completely penetrated the _____ layer of skin.

    a. dermis   **b.** dermal

    3. Please take this specimen to the _____ department.

    a. pathological   **b.** pathology

    4. The _____ diagnosis has not yet been determined.

    a. pathological   **b.** pathology

    5. The _____ properties of the aloe lotion reduced the pain in the sunburn.

    a. anesthesia   **b.** anesthetic

H. **Build your medical language of dermatology.** Complete the medical terms by filling in the blanks. The first one has been done for you. **LO 4.1, 4.2, 4.5, 4.6, 4.7**

    1. Study of disorders of the skin   dermato/*logy*

    2. To scratch the skin   ex/_____/ate

    3. Sore caused by lying in bed   _____/cubitus

    4. Infestation with lice   _____/osis

    5. Takes away feeling and pain   an/_____/ia

    6. Medication against itching   anti/_____/ic

I. **Terminology challenge.** Use the following medical terms to complete the sentences. **LO 4.3, 4.6**

    metastasis   metastasize   metastatic

    1. The surgeon predicted that the lesion would _____ to the liver.

    2. The _____ lesion received radiation therapy, while the primary lesion was surgically removed.

    3. The pathology report confirmed that there was no _____ of the lesion.

J. **Identify the type of secretions from each gland of the integumentary system.** Match the secretion with the gland type. **LO 4.1**

    _____ **1.** cerumen   **a.** sweat at groin and armpits

    _____ **2.** milk   **b.** ear wax

    _____ **3.** apocrine   **c.** typical sweat

    _____ **4.** eccrine   **d.** mammary

K. Write the term for the condition that is being described. Interpret each statement that may be given to you from a patient to the correct medical term. Fill in the blank. **LO 4.6, 4.8**

1. "My child fell off his skateboard and scraped off a lot of skin from her leg." She has a large _____.

2. "I was cutting up vegetables and accidentally gave myself a deep cut to my hand." He has a _____.

3. "After my cut on my arm, I developed a large, thickened, shiny scar." He has developed a _____.

4. "My daughter has several patches of skin that do not have any pigment." She may have a condition called _____.

L. Identify the correct topical skin treatment for each condition. Choose the best answer for each question. **LO 4.7**

1. A treatment to kill lice:

   a. antipruritic   **b.** keralytic   **c.** retinoid   **d.** parasiticide

2. A cream that would relieve itching due to allergies:

   a. retinoid   **b.** corticosteroid   **c.** antifungal   **d.** antibacterial

3. A topical treatment for tinea pedis is a(n) _____ cream:

   a. parasiticide   **b.** antibacterial   **c.** antifungal   **d.** anesthetic

4. A topical treatment for acne is a(n) _____ cream:

   a. retinoid   **b.** corticosteroid   **c.** antifungal   **d.** antibacterial

M. Identify the health professionals involved in the care of dermatological patients. From the given description, choose the medical professional that would be involved in the care of the patient. Fill in the blank. **LO 4.10**

dermatologist   nurse practitioner   dermatopathologist   plastic surgeon   esthetician

1. Uses a microscope to examine a skin sample: _____

2. Medical specialist in the care and diagnosis of skin disorders: _____

3. Utilizes corrective surgery to correct deformities due to injury or birth defects: _____

4. Professional who uses cosmetic procedures to beautify the skin: _____

5. Works under the direction of a physician to treat skin disorders: _____

N. Pronunciation is important whether you are saying the word or listening to a word from a coworker. Identify the proper pronunciation of the following medical terms. **LO 4.4, 4.8, 4.10**

1. The correct pronunciation for a benign localized area of melanin is

   a. kar-sih-**NOH**-mah

   b. **KAH**-sin-oh-**MAH**

   c. mel-ahn-**OM**-ah

   d. **MEL**-ah-**NO**-mah

   Correctly spell the term: _____

2. The correct pronunciation for the protein found in the dead outer layer of skin is

    a. KER-ah-tin

    b. KE-rah-**TEN**

    c. MEL-ah-nin

    d. MEL-a-nine

Correctly spell the term: _____

3. The correct pronunciation for seborrheic scales from the scalp is

    a. DA-nd-ryuf

    b. DAN-druff

    c. SEE-bum

    d. SAY-byum

Correctly spell the term: _____

4. The correct pronunciation for deficient in oxygen

    a. DAY-ah-for-**EE**-**SIS**

    b. DIE-ah-foh-**REE**-sis

    c. high-**POCK**-sik

    d. HIGH-pox-sike

Correctly spell the term: _____

5. The correct pronunciation for a therapist who enhances the beauty of the skin

    a. EES-thee-**TISH**-on

    b. es-the-**TI**-shun

    c. DEER-mah-**TOLL**-oh-jist

    d. der-mah-**TOL**-oh-jist

Correctly spell the term: _____

Case Reports

A. **Apply your knowledge of the language of dermatology to the following Case Report.** Use Case Report 4.1 to correctly answer each question or complete each statement below. Not all answers are found in the Case Report but can be found in the *Chapter 4* text. **LO 4.9, 4.10**

 Case Report (CR) 4.1

You are

. . . a clinical medical assistant working in the office of **dermatologist** Dr. Lenore Echols, a member of the Fulwood Medical Group.

Your patient is

. . . Mr. Rod Andrews, a 60-year-old man, who shows you three skin lesions—two on his left forearm and one on the back of his left hand. On questioning him, you learn that he has been living for the past 10 years in Arizona and has returned to the area to be near his daughter and young grandchildren. You find no other skin lesions on his body.

When Dr. Echols examined Mr. Andrews, she determined clinically that two of his lesions were basal cell **carcinomas** and she treated them with **cryosurgery.** She believed that the third lesion was a **squamous cell** carcinoma, and she performed a **biopsy removal** of that **lesion.** You sent it to the laboratory with a request for **pathological** diagnosis and determination of whether the lesion had been completely removed. This is done by ensuring that a normal skin margin completely surrounds the lesion when it is examined under the microscope.

1. Provide the abbreviation for biopsy: _____

2. Which medical specialist would likely examine the biopsied skin?

   a. Esthetician   **b.** Dermatologist   **c.** Dermatopathologist   **d.** Cosmetic surgeon

3. Is it possible for cryosurgery to remove normal tissue?

   a. Yes   **b.** No

4. Based on the information provided in the Case Report, how could Mr. Andrews decrease his chances of developing these types skin carcinomas?

   a. Reduce his exposure to air pollution.   **c.** Wear long sleeves to cover his arms.

   b. Apply keratolytic skin lotions.   **d.** Stop smoking tobacco products.

5. The pathology reports that the biopsy lacks a normal skin margin. What does this mean?

   a. The lesion is a squamous cell carcinoma.   **c.** The biopsy sample removed all the cancerous tissue.

   b. The lesion is not a squamous cell carcinoma.   **d.** The biopsy sample did not remove all the cancerous tissue.

B. **Apply your knowledge of the language of dermatology to the following Case Report.** Use Case Report 4.2 to correctly answer each question or complete each statement below. Not all answers are found in the Case Report but are related to the *Chapter 4* text. **LO 4.9, 4.10**

 Case Report (CR) 4.2

Fulwood Medical Center

Mrs. Rose McGinnis, a 72-year-old widow, was in a nursing home for the past 6 months. She was unable to get out of bed since surgery to repair a broken hip. She was depressed and difficult to feed and nurse. Two months ago, she developed **decubitus ulcers** over her buttocks and left heel. The ulcer over her buttocks became infected with a methicillin-resistant *Staphylococcus aureus* (MRSA). Staphylococcal septicemia ensued, and she died.

1. Which of Mrs. McGinnis's conditions caused her decubitus ulcers to form?

    a. Surgical hip repair   **b.** Depression   **c.** MRSA Septicemia   **d.** Lack of movement

2. Do decubitus ulcers only form on people that are lying down?

    a. Yes   **b.** No

C. **Apply your knowledge of the language of dermatology to the following Case Report.** Use Case Report 4.3 to correctly answer each question or complete each statement below. **LO 4.5–4.8**

 Case Report (CR) 4.3

Ms. Cheryl Fox is a 37-year-old nursing assistant working in a surgical unit in Fulwood Medical Center. Recently her fingers have become red and itchy, with occasional vesicles. She has also noticed irritation and swelling of her earlobes and a generalized pruritus. Over the weekend, both the itching and the rash on her hands worsened. A patch test by her dermatologist showed her to be allergic to nickel in rings that she wears on both hands and in her earrings. She wore these on weekends and not during her workdays.

1. What diagnostic test did Ms. Fox have to determine the cause of her condition?

    a. itching   **b.** patch test   **c.** nickel   **d.** blood serum

2. Identify her symptoms. Choose all that apply.

    a. vesicle   **b.** pruritus   **c.** allergies   **d.** swelling

3. What part of her body was edematous?

    a. fingers   **b.** earlobes   **c.** abdomen   **d.** toes

4. Write the term in the above Case Report that means *itching:* _____

5. What is the *allergen* that Ms. Fox is allergic to? _____

6. A likely diagnosis for Ms. Fox would be:

    a. melanoma   **b.** dermatitis   **c.** vitiligo   **d.** candidiasis

D. **Case report questions.** Read Case Report 4.4. You should feel more comfortable with the medical terminology now and will be able to answer the questions that follow. **LO 4.2, 4.7**

 Case Report (CR) 4.4

You are

. . . a burn technologist employed in the Burn Unit at Fulwood Medical Center.

Your patient is

. . . Mr. Steven Hapgood, a 52-year-old man, admitted to the Fulwood Burn Unit with severe burns over his face, chest, and abdomen.

After an evening of drinking, Mr. Hapgood was smoking in bed and fell asleep. His next-door neighbors in the apartment building smelled smoke and called 911. In the Burn Unit, his initial treatment included large volumes of intravenous fluids to prevent shock.

Your role will be to participate in Mr. Hapgood's care as a member of the Burn Unit team and to document the care and his response to it. Mr. Hapgood's burns were mostly third-degree. The protective ability of the skin to prevent water loss had been removed, as had the skin barrier against infection. The burned, dead tissue forms an eschar that can have toxic effects on the digestive, respiratory, and cardiovascular systems. The eschar was surgically removed by debridement.

1. Based on the Rule of Nines, approximately what percent of Mr. Hapgood's body was burned?

    a. 16%   **b.** 18%   **c.** 20%   **d.** 22%

2. The first treatment that Mr. Hapgood received was:

    a. CPR   **b.** removal of the eschar

    c. IV fluids   **d.** skin grafts

    e. wound therapy

3. _____ is the medical term for burned, dead tissue lying on top of third-degree burns.

    a. Eschar   **b.** Wheal   **c.** Vesicle   **d.** Eczema   **e.** Vitiligo

4. His burns involved only the:

    a. epidermis   **c.** epidermis, dermis, and hypodermis

    b. epidermis and dermis   **d.** epidermis, dermis, hypodermis, and muscles

5. Mr. Hapgood's loss of skin makes him at increased risk of:

    a. ulcers   **b.** infection   **c.** furuncles   **d.** wheals

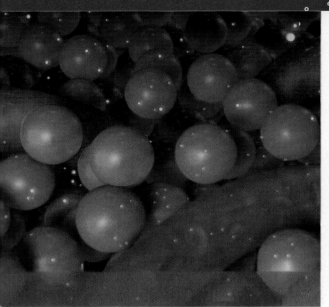

2014 Nucleus Medical Media

CHAPTER
5

Digestive System
The Language of Gastroenterology

Chapter Sections

5.1 The Digestive System

5.2 Mouth, Pharynx, and Esophagus

5.3 Digestion—Stomach, Small, and Large Intestine

5.4 Digestion—Liver, Gallbladder, and Pancreas

5.5 Disorders of the Digestive System

5.6 Procedures and Pharmacology of the Digestive System

Chapter Learning Outcomes

Upon completion of this chapter, you will be able to:

LO 5.1 Identify and describe the anatomy and physiology of the digestive system.

LO 5.2 Use roots, combining forms, suffixes, and prefixes to construct and analyze medical terms related to the digestive system.

LO 5.3 Spell medical terms related to the digestive system.

LO 5.4 Pronounce medical terms related to the digestive system.

LO 5.5 Describe diagnostic procedures utilized in gastroenterology.

LO 5.6 Identify and describe disorders and pathological conditions related to the digestive system.

LO 5.7 Describe the therapeutic procedures and pharmacologic agents used in gastroenterology.

LO 5.8 Apply knowledge of medical terms relating to gastroenterology to documentation, medical records, and communication.

LO 5.9 Identify and correctly use abbreviations of terms used in gastroenterology.

LO 5.10 Identify health professionals involved in the care of gastroenterology patients.

In your future career as a health professional, you may work directly or indirectly with one or more of the health professionals involved in **gastroenterology:**

- **Gastroenterologists** are medical specialists in the field of gastroenterology.
- **Proctologists** are surgical specialists in diseases of the anus and rectum.
- **Dentists** are licensed practitioners in the anatomy, physiology, and pathology of the oral-facial complex.
- **Periodontists** are specialists in diseases of the tissues surrounding the teeth.
- **Nutritionists** are professionals who prevent and treat illness by promoting healthy eating habits.
- **Dieticians** manage food services systems and promote sound eating habits.

Section 5.1 The Digestive System

Digestive Tract and Accessory Organs

There are basic elements of anatomy, physiology, and medical terminology that apply throughout the different parts of the digestive system. Every cell in your body requires a constant supply of nourishment. The cells cannot travel, so the nourishment has to be brought to them in a form that can be absorbed across their cell membrane. The foods that you ingest cannot be used in their existing form by the cells. The digestive system, through its alimentary canal, breaks down the nutrients in the food into elements that can be transported to the cells via the blood and **lymphatics**. This physical breakdown of food into smaller sizes and the chemical change of food into the basic elements of lipids, amino acids, and sugars is termed **digestion.** These elements can then be transported across the cell membrane into the cell.

The **digestive system** consists of the digestive tract (**alimentary canal**), which is a hollow tube that extends from the **mouth** to the anus, and accessory organs connected to the digestive tract to assist in digestion. The accessory organs project into or secrete liquids into the digestive tract.

The term **gastrointestinal (GI)** technically refers to the stomach and **intestines** but is often used to mean the whole digestive system. **Gastroenterology** is the study of the digestive system. A **gastroenterologist** is a physician who specializes in the digestive system.

The alimentary canal (*Figure 5.1*) includes the

- **Mouth**
- **Esophagus**
- Small **intestine**
- Pharynx
- Stomach
- Large **intestine**

The **accessory organs** of digestion include the

- Teeth
- Salivary glands
- Gallbladder
- Tongue
- Liver
- Pancreas

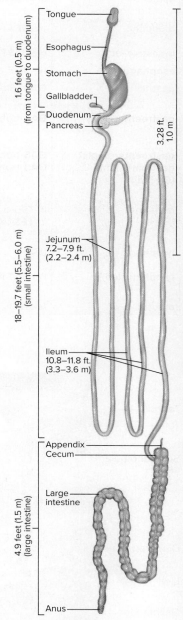

▲ **Figure 5.1** Digestive tract.

WORD	PRONUNCIATION	ELEMENTS		DEFINITION
alimentary	al-ih-**MEN**-tar-ee	S/ R/	-ary *pertaining to* aliment- *nourishment*	Pertaining to the digestive tract
digestion	die-**JEST**-shun	S/ R/	-ion *action* digest- *to break down*	Breakdown of food into elements suitable for cell metabolism
digestive (adj)	die-**JEST**-iv	S/	-ive *nature of*	Pertaining to digestion
esophagus	ee-**SOF**-ah-gus		Greek *gullet*	Tube linking the pharynx and the stomach
gastric	**GAS**-trik	S/ R/	-ic *pertaining to* gastr- *stomach*	Pertaining to the stomach
gastroenterology	**GAS**-troh-en-ter-**OL**-oh-jee	S/ R/CF R/CF	-logy *study of* gastr/o- *stomach* -enter/o- *intestine*	Medical specialty of the stomach and intestines
gastroenterologist	**GAS**-troh-en-ter-**OL**-oh-jist	S/	-logist *one who studies*	Medical specialist in gastroenterology
gastrointestinal (GI) (adj)	**GAS**-troh-in-**TESS**-tin-al	S/ R/CF R/	-al *pertaining to* gastr/o- *stomach* -intestin- *gut, intestine*	Pertaining to the stomach and intestines
intestine	in-**TES**-tin		Latin *intestine, gut*	The digestive tube from stomach to anus
intestinal (adj)	in-**TES**-tin-al	S/ R/	-al *pertaining to* intestin- *intestine, gut*	
lymph	LIMF		Latin *spring water*	A clear fluid collected from tissues and transported by vessels to venous circulation
lymphatic (adj)	lim-**FAT**-ik	S/ R/	-atic *pertaining to* lymph- *lymph*	Pertaining to lymph
mouth	MOWTH		Old English *mouth*	External opening of a cavity or canal

Functions of the Digestive System

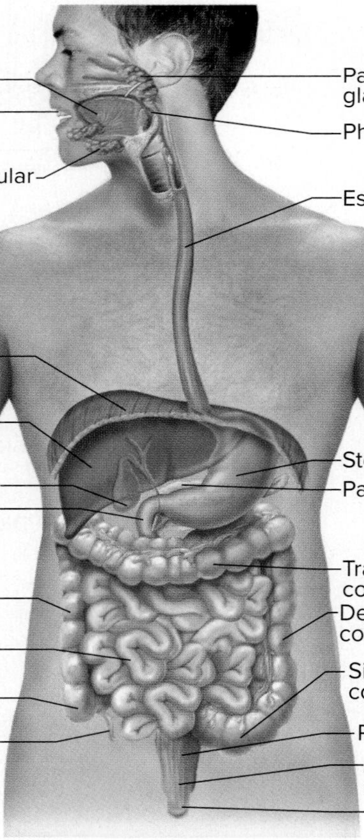

Tongue
Teeth
Submandibular gland
Diaphragm
Liver
Gallbladder
Duodenum
Ascending colon
Small intestine
Cecum
Appendix

Parotid gland
Pharynx
Esophagus
Stomach
Pancreas
Transverse colon
Descending colon
Sigmoid colon
Rectum
Anal canal
Anus

▲ **Figure 5.2** The digestive system.

1. **Ingestion**—the selective intake of food into the mouth.
2. **Propulsion**—the movement of food from the mouth to the anus *(Figure 5.2)*. Normally, this takes 24 to 36 hours. **Deglutition,** or swallowing, moves the **bolus** of food from the mouth into the esophagus. **Peristalsis,** or waves of contraction and relaxation, moves material through most of the alimentary canal. **Segmental contractions** in the small intestine move food back and forth to mix it with digestive secretions.
3. **Digestion**—the breakdown of foods into forms that can be transported to and absorbed into cells. This process has two components:
   a. **Mechanical digestion** breaks larger pieces of food into smaller ones without altering their chemical composition. This process exposes a larger surface area of the food to the action of digestive enzymes with which to interact.
   b. **Chemical digestion** breaks down large molecules of food into smaller and simpler chemicals. This process is carried out by digestive enzymes produced by the salivary glands, stomach, small intestine, and pancreas.

   The digestive **enzymes** have three main groups:
   - **Amylases** that digest carbohydrates into sugars
   - **Lipases** that digest fats into fatty acids
   - **Proteases** that digest proteins into amino acids
4. **Secretion**—the addition throughout the digestive tract of secretions that lubricate, liquefy, and digest the food. Mucus lubricates the food and the lining of the tract. Water liquefies the food to make it easier to digest and absorb. Enzymes digest the food.
5. **Absorption**—the movement of nutrient molecules out of the digestive tract and through the epithelial cells lining the tract into the blood or lymph for transportation to body cells.
6. **Elimination**—the process by which the unabsorbed residue of food is removed from the body.

Word Analysis and Definition: Functions of the Digestive System

S = Suffix   P = Prefix   R = Root   R/CF = Combining Form

WORD	PRONUNCIATION		ELEMENTS	DEFINITION
absorption absorb (verb)	ab-**SORP**-shun ab-**SORB**		Latin *to swallow*	Uptake of nutrients and water by cells in the GI tract
amylase	**AM**-il-aze	S/ R/	-ase *enzyme* amyl- *starch*	Enzyme that breaks down starch
bolus	**BOH**-lus		Greek *lump*	Single mass of a substance
contraction contract	kon-**TRAKT**-shun kon-**TRAKT**	S/ R/	-ion *action* contract- *to shorten* Latin *draw together*	A shortening of a muscle, which increases tension To shorten
deglutition	dee-glue-**TISH**-un	S/ R/	-ion *action* deglutit- *to swallow*	The act of swallowing
elimination	e-lim-ih-**NAY**-shun	S/ R/	-ation *process* elimin- *throw away*	Removal of waste material from the digestive tract
enzyme	**EN**-zime	P/ R/	en- *in* -zyme *fermenting, enzyme*	Protein that induces changes in other substances
ingestion	in-**JEST**-shun	S/ R/	-ion *action* ingest- *carry in*	Intake of food or drink into the digestive tract
lipase	**LIE**-paze	S/ R/	-ase *enzyme* lip- *fat*	Enzyme that breaks down fat
peristalsis	per-ih-**STAL**-sis	P/ R/	peri- *around* -stalsis *constrict*	Waves of alternate contraction and relaxation of alimentary canal wall to move food through the digestive tract
protease	**PROH**-tee-aze	S/ R/CF	-ase *enzyme* prot/e- *protein*	Enzyme that breaks down protein
secrete secretion (noun)	se-**KREET** se-**KREE**-shun		Latin *to separate*	To release or give off, as substances produced by cells Production by a cell or gland
segment segmental (adj)	**SEG**-ment seg-**MENT**-al	S/ R/	Latin *to cut* -al *pertaining to* segment- *section*	A section of an organ or structure Pertaining to a segment

Check Point Section 5.1

A. Analyzing the elements can tell you a lot about a medical term. *Fill in the blanks.* **LO 5.1, 5.2**

1. Analyzing the two combining forms shows that the term **gastroenterology** relates to the _____ and the _____.

2. In the term **gastric,** the root _____ has the same meaning as the combining form _____ in the term **gastroenterology.**

3. The _____ is the tube that connects the stomach to the anus. The _____ is the tube that connects the pharynx to stomach. The beginning the alimentary canal is the _____.

B. The body process or action has been described for you. *Match the definition in the left column to the correct medical term in the right column.* **LO 5.1**

_____ **1.** Swallowing

_____ **2.** Helps lubricate, liquefy, and digest food

_____ **3.** Increased muscular tension

_____ **4.** Removal of waste material

a. contraction

b. elimination

c. deglutition

d. secretion

C. Build the medical terms by filling in their missing elements. LO 5.1, 5.2

1. Enzyme that breaks down protein: _____/ase

2. Removal of waste material from the digestive tract: _____/ation

3. Enzyme that breaks down fat: lip/_____

4. Enzyme that breaks down starch: _____/ase

5. Pertaining to a section of an organ or structure: _____/al

6. Waves that move food in intestines: peri/_____.

Section 5.2 Mouth, Pharynx, and Esophagus

The Mouth and Mastication

When you pop a piece of chicken and some vegetables into your mouth, you start a cascade of digestive tract events that occur during the following 24 to 36 hours. In this chapter, you will follow a meal of chicken and vegetables as it goes through the digestive tract. The mouth, or **oral** cavity *(Figure 5.3)*, is the entrance to your digestive tract and is the first site of mechanical digestion (through **mastication,** chewing) and of chemical digestion (through an enzyme in saliva).

The cheeks contain the buccinator muscles. These muscles hold the chicken and vegetables in place while you chew and your teeth crush and tear them.

The roof of the mouth is called the **palate.** The anterior two-thirds is the bony hard palate. The posterior one-third is the muscular soft palate. The hard palate is covered with folds of epithelium called **rugae,** which assist the tongue to manipulate food for mechanical and chemical digestion prior to swallowing. The soft palate has a projection called the **uvula** that closes off the nasopharynx during swallowing.

The **tongue** *(Figure 5.4)* moves food around your mouth and helps the cheeks, lips, and gums hold the food in place while you chew it. Small, rough, raised areas on the tongue, called **papillae,** contain some 4,000 taste buds that react to the chemical nature of the food to give you the different sensations of **taste.** A taste bud cell lives for 7 to 10 days and is then replaced.

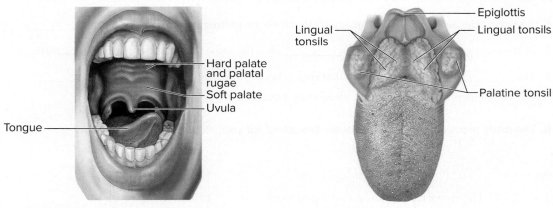

▲ **Figure 5.3** Mouth (oral cavity).

▲ **Figure 5.4** Tongue.

Word Analysis and Definition: The Mouth

S = Suffix   P = Prefix   R = Root   R/CF = Combining Form

WORD	PRONUNCIATION	ELEMENTS		DEFINITION
masticate (verb)	**MAS**-tih-kate	S/ R/	**-ate** *pertaining to, composed of* **mastic-** *chew*	To chew
mastication (noun)	mas-tih-**KAY**-shun	S/	**-ation** *process*	The process of chewing
oral	**OR**-al	S/ R/	**-al** *pertaining to* **or-** *mouth*	Pertaining to the mouth
palate	**PAL**-uht		Latin *palate*	Roof of the mouth
papilla papillae (pl)	pah-**PILL**-ah pah-**PILL**-ee		Latin *small pimple*	Any small projection
ruga rugae (pl)	**ROO**-gah **ROO**-jee		Latin *wrinkle*	A fold, ridge, or crease
taste	TAYST		Latin *to taste*	Sensation from chemicals on the taste buds
tongue	TUNG		Latin *tongue*	Mobile muscle mass in mouth; bears the taste buds
uvula	**YOU**-vyu-lah		Latin *grape*	Fleshy projection of the soft palate

Adult Teeth

The normal adult has 32 teeth, 16 rooted in the upper jaw (maxilla) and 16 in the lower jaw (mandible). The teeth are the hardest structures in your body, and different teeth *(Figure 5.5)* are designed to handle food in different ways. The eight **incisors** are shaped like a chisel to slice and cut into food. The four **cuspids** have a pointed tip for puncturing and tearing. The eight **bicuspids** and twelve **molars** have flattened surfaces for grinding and crushing food. Your wisdom teeth are molars.

Each tooth has two main parts:

- The **crown,** which projects above the gum and is covered in **enamel,** the hardest substance in the body.

- The **root,** which anchors the tooth to the jaw.

The bulk of the tooth is composed of **dentin,** a substance like bone but harder *(Figure 5.6)*. The dentin surrounds a central **pulp cavity** that contains blood vessels, nerves, and connective tissue. The blood vessels and nerves reach this cavity from the jaw through tubular **root canals.** The **gingiva** is a soft pink tissue that surrounds and attaches to teeth and the jaw bones. The area around the tooth is referred to as the **periodontal region.**

Salivary Glands

Salivary glands secrete saliva. The two **parotid** glands, the two **submandibular** glands, the two **sublingual glands** *(Figure 5.7)*, and numerous minor salivary glands scattered in the mucosa of the tongue and cheeks secrete more than a quart of saliva each day.

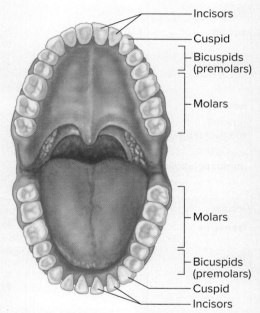

▲ **Figure 5.5** Adult teeth.

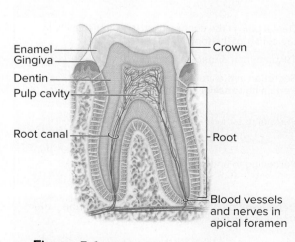

▲ **Figure 5.6** Anatomy of a molar.

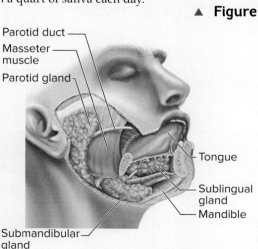

▲ **Figure 5.7** Salivary glands.

Saliva is 95% water, and its functions are to

- Begin starch digestion with the enzyme amylase.
- Begin fat digestion with the enzyme lipase.
- Prevent the growth of bacteria in the mouth with the enzyme **lysozyme** and the protective **immunoglobulin A (IgA)** *(see Chapter 12)*.
- Produce mucus to lubricate food to make it easier to swallow.

   Imagine that you are eating a piece of chicken with some vegetables. By the end of the mastication process, the chicken has been torn and ground into small pieces by your teeth, and its fat has begun to be digested by the lipase in your saliva. The vegetables have been ground into small pieces as well, and the starch in them has begun to be digested by the amylase in your saliva. The food has been lubricated, mixed together, and formed into a bolus ready to be swallowed.

Word Analysis and Definition: The Mouth and Mastication

S = Suffix   P = Prefix   R = Root   R/CF = Combining Form

WORD	PRONUNCIATION		ELEMENTS	DEFINITION
bicuspid (also called **premolar**)	by-**KUSS**-pid	S/ P/ R/	**-id** *having a particular quality* **bi-** *two* **-cusp-** *point*	Having two points; a bicuspid (premolar) tooth has two points
crown	KROWN		Latin *crown*	Part of the tooth above the gum
cuspid	**KUSS**-pid	S/ R/	**-id** *having a particular quality* **cusp-** *point*	Tooth with one point
dentin (also spelled **dentine**)	**DEN**-tin	S/ R/	**-in** *substance, chemical compound* **dent-** *tooth*	Dense, ivory-like substance located under the enamel in a tooth
enamel	ee-**NAM**-el		French *enamel*	Hard substance covering a tooth
gingiva **gingival** (adj)	**JIN**-jih-vah **JIN**-jih-vul	S/ R/	Latin *gum* **-al** *pertaining to* **gingiv-** *gums*	Tissue surrounding teeth and covering the jaw Pertaining to the gums
immunoglobulin	**IM**-you-noh-**GLOB**-you-lin	S/ R/CF R/	**-in** *chemical compound* **immun/o-** *immune response* **-globul-** *protein*	Specific protein evoked by an antigen; all antibodies are immunoglobulins
incisor	in-**SIGH**-zor		Latin *to cut into*	Chisel-shaped tooth
lysozyme	**LIE**-soh-zime	S/ R/CF	**-zyme** *enzyme* **lys/o-** *dissolve*	Enzyme that dissolves the cell walls of bacteria
molar	**MOH**-lar		Latin *millstone*	One of six teeth in each jaw that grind food
parotid	pah-**ROT**-id	S/ P/ R/	**-id** *having a particular quality* **par-** *beside* **-ot-** *ear*	Parotid gland is the salivary gland beside the ear
periodontal	**PER**-ee-oh-**DON**-tal	S/ P/ R/	**-al** *pertaining to* **peri-** *around* **-odont-** *tooth*	Around a tooth
pulp	PULP		Latin *flesh*	Dental pulp is the connective tissue in the cavity in the center of the tooth
root	ROOT		Old English *beginning*	Fundamental or beginning part of a structure
saliva **salivary** (adj)	sa-**LIE**-vah **SAL**-ih-var-ee	S/ R/	Latin *spit* **-ary** *pertaining to* **saliv-** *saliva*	Secretion in the mouth from salivary glands Pertaining to saliva
sublingual	sub-**LING**-wal	S/ P/ R/	**-al** *pertaining to* **sub-** *underneath* **-lingu-** *tongue*	Pertaining to underneath the tongue
submandibular	sub-man-**DIB**-you-lar	S/ P/ R/	**-ar** *pertaining to* **sub-** *underneath* **-mandibul-** *the jaw*	Pertaining to underneath the mandible
symptom **symptomatic** **asymptomatic**	**SIMP**-tum simp-toe-**MAT**-ik	S/ R/ P/	Greek *sign* **-ic** *pertaining to* **symptomat-** *symptom* **a-** *without*	Departure from the normal experienced by the patient Pertaining to the symptoms of a disease Absence of symptoms

Deglutition (Swallowing)—Pharynx and Esophagus

The pieces of chicken and vegetables that you ingested have now been sliced and ground into small particles by the teeth, partially digested and lubricated by saliva, and rolled into a bolus between the tongue and the hard palate, the bony roof of the mouth (*Figure 5.8*). The bolus is now ready to be swallowed **(deglutition).**

- **Phase One.** As you swallow, the bolus of food is pushed backward by your tongue into the **oropharynx.** Once the bolus is in your oropharynx, the tongue contracts against the hard palate and pushes up the soft palate and uvula to close off the **nasopharynx** at the back of the nose. This prevents food from going up into your nasopharynx and nose (*see Figure 5.8*).

- **Phase Two.** Surrounding the oropharynx are circular muscles called **constrictors.** These muscles contract, forcing the bolus down through the laryngopharynx toward the **esophagus** and pushing the **epiglottis** closed so that food cannot enter the airways to the lungs, the larynx, and trachea (*Figure 5.9*).

- **Phase Three.** When the bolus reaches the lower end of the **pharynx,** the upper **esophageal sphincter** relaxes and the bolus enters the esophagus, where contractions of the muscles in the wall move the bolus toward the stomach (*Figure 5.10*).

- **Phase Four.** The esophageal sphincter at the lower end of the esophagus **(cardiac sphincter)** relaxes to allow the bolus to enter the stomach (*Figure 5.11*).

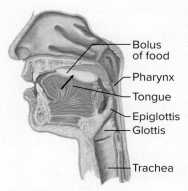

- Bolus of food
- Pharynx
- Tongue
- Epiglottis
- Glottis
- Trachea

▲ **Figure 5.8** Deglutition (swallowing): phase one.

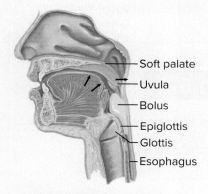

- Soft palate
- Uvula
- Bolus
- Epiglottis
- Glottis
- Esophagus

▲ **Figure 5.9** Deglutition (swallowing): phase two.

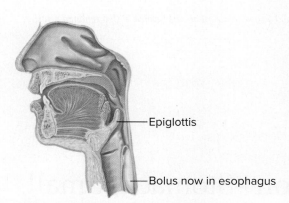

- Epiglottis
- Bolus now in esophagus

▲ **Figure 5.10** Deglutition (swallowing): phase three.

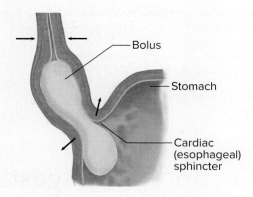

- Bolus
- Stomach
- Cardiac (esophageal) sphincter

▲ **Figure 5.11** Deglutition (swallowing): phase four.

WORD	PRONUNCIATION		ELEMENTS	DEFINITION
cardiac	KAR-dee-ak	S/ R/	-ac *pertaining to* cardi- *heart*	Pertaining to the heart
constrictor	kon-STRIK-tore	S/ R/	-or *a doer, one who does, that which does something* constrict- *narrow, to narrow*	Muscle that contracts or compresses an organ
deglutition	dee-glue-TISH-un		Latin *to swallow*	The act of swallowing
epiglottis	ep-ih-GLOT-is	P/ R/	epi- *above* -glottis *windpipe*	Leaf-shaped plate of cartilage that shuts off larynx during swallowing
esophagus esophageal (adj)	ee-SOF-ah-gus ee-SOF-ah-JEE-al	 S/ R/	Greek *gullet* -eal *pertaining to* esophag- *esophagus*	Tube linking the pharynx and stomach Pertaining to the esophagus
nasopharynx	NAY-zoh-FAIR-inks	R/CF R/	nas/o- *nose* -pharynx *throat*	Region of the pharynx at the back of the nose and above the soft palate
oropharynx	OR-oh-FAIR-inks	R/CF R/	or/o- *mouth* -pharynx *throat*	Region at the back of the mouth between the soft palate and the tip of the epiglottis
pharynx	FAIR-inks		Greek *throat*	Air tube from the back of the nose to the larynx
sphincter	SFINK-ter		Greek *band, lace, or anything that binds tight*	Bank of muscle that encircles an opening; when it contracts, the opening squeezes closed

Check Point Section 5.2

A. Many medical terms have Latin origins and cannot be deconstructed. *Fill in the blank.* **LO 5.1**

1. The roof of the mouth is termed the _____.

2. During swallowing, the _____ covers the entrance to the nose from the back of the throat.

3. Taste buds are located on the sides of the tongue's _____.

4. The _____ that covers the hard palate aid in mechanical digestion of food.

B. Study the terms and elements. *Notice that some terms are formed with only a prefix and a root, while others are formed with a root and a suffix. Write the correct element on each blank that needs an element.* **LO 5.1, 5.2**

1 submandibular _____/_____/_____
               P   R   S

2. sublingual _____/_____/_____
              P   R   S

Section 5.3 Digestion—Stomach, Small, and Large Intestine

Digestion in the Stomach

The bolus of food that you swallowed has passed down the esophagus. It now enters the stomach, and the process of digestion begins in earnest. The stomach continues the mechanical breakdown of the food particles and begins the chemical digestion of protein and fats. It is in the small intestine that the greatest amount of digestion and absorption occurs. The stomach's peristaltic contractions mix different boluses of food together and also push the more liquid contents toward the **pylorus** (*Figure 5.12*). These contractions and the digestive process work on the boluses of food to produce a mixture of semidigested food called **chyme.**

The cells of the lining of the stomach secrete the following:

- **Mucin**—continues to lubricate food and protects the stomach lining. Mucin combines with the other secretions to become **mucus.**

- **Hydrochloric acid (HCl)**—breaks up the connective tissue of the chicken and the cell walls of the vegetables that you ingested a few seconds ago. It also destroys any pathogens that enter your stomach along with the food you eat.

- **Pepsinogen**—is converted by hydrochloric acid to **pepsin,** an active enzyme that starts to digest the protein in the chicken and vegetables.

- **Intrinsic factor**—is essential for the absorption of vitamin B_{12} in the small intestine. Neither chicken nor vegetables contain this factor.

- **Chemical messengers**—stimulate other cells in the gastric mucosa. One of these messengers, **gastrin,** stimulates both the production of HCl and pepsinogen by the stomach cells and the peristaltic contractions of the stomach.

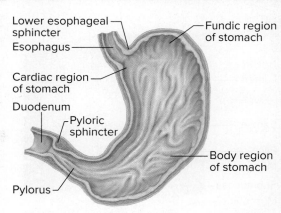

▲ **Figure 5.12** Stomach.

Liquids exit the stomach within 1½ to 2 hours after ingestion. A typical meal like your chicken and vegetables takes 3 to 4 hours to exit. The resulting chyme is held in the pylorus. Peristaltic waves squirt 2 to 3 mL of the chyme at a time through the **pyloric sphincter** into the **duodenum.**

Anywhere from 40 minutes to 2 hours after consuming that chicken and vegetable dinner mentioned earlier, your food is partially digested by the salivary and stomach enzymes described previously.

Word Analysis and Definition: Stomach Digestion

S = Suffix   P = Prefix   R = Root   R/CF = Combining Form

WORD	PRONUNCIATION		ELEMENTS	DEFINITION
chyme	KIME		Greek *juice*	Semifluid, partially digested food passed from the stomach into the duodenum
duodenum	du-oh-**DEE**-num	S/	-um *structure*	The first part of the small intestine; approximately 12 finger-breadths (9 to 10 inches) in length
		R/	**duoden-** *Latin for twelve*	
duodenal (adj)	du-oh-**DEE**-nal	S/	-al *pertaining to*	Pertaining to the duodenum
gastrin	**GAS**-trin	S/	-in *substance*	Hormone secreted in the stomach that stimulates secretion of HCl and increases gastric motility
		R/	**gastr-** *stomach*	
hydrochloric acid (HCl)	high-droh-**KLOR**-ic **ASS**-id	S/	-ic *pertaining to*	The acid of gastric juice
		R/CF	**hydr/o-** *water*	
		R/	-chlor- *green*	
intrinsic factor	in-**TRIN**-sik **FAK**-tor	S/	-ic *pertaining to*	Substance secreted by the stomach that is necessary for the absorption of vitamin B_{12}
		R/	**intrins-** *on the inside*	
		R/	**factor** *maker*	
malabsorption (**Note:** The last *b* in *absorb* changes to a *p* to ease pronunciation.)	mal-ab-**SORP**-shun	S/	-tion *process*	To bring in inadequate gastrointestinal absorption of nutrients
		P/	**mal-** *back*	
		R/	-absorb- *swallow*	
mucus	**MYU**-kus		Latin *slime*	Sticky secretion of cells in mucous membranes
mucous (adj)	**MYU**-kus	S/	-ous *pertaining to*	Relating to mucus or the mucosa
		R/	**muc-** *mucus*	
mucin	**MYU**-sin	S/	-in *chemical compound*	Protein element of mucus
pepsin	**PEP**-sin		Greek *to digest*	Enzyme produced by the stomach that breaks down protein
pepsinogen	pep-**SIN**-oh-jen	S/	-gen *produce*	Enzyme converted by HCl in stomach to pepsin
		R/CF	**pepsin/o-** *pepsin*	
pylorus	pie-**LOR**-us	S/	-us *pertaining to*	Exit area of the stomach proximal to the duodenum
		R/	**pylor-** *gate*	
pyloric (adj)	pie-**LOR**-ik	S/	-ic *pertaining to*	Pertaining to the pylorus

Small Intestine

The small intestine, called "small" because of its diameter, finishes the process of chemical digestion and is responsible for the absorption of most of the nutrients.

Four major layers are present in the wall of the small intestine and in all areas of the digestive tract (*Figure 5.13*):

1. **Mucosa,** or mucous membrane—the layer containing the epithelial cells that line the tract, intestinal glands that secrete the digestive enzymes, and supportive connective tissue. Fingerlike shapes of mucosa called **villi** project into the lumen of the intestine.

2. **Submucosa**—a thick connective tissue layer containing blood vessels, lymphatic vessels, and nerves.

3. **Muscularis**—an inner, circular layer of smooth muscle and an outer longitudinal layer of smooth muscle. When the inner circular layer contracts, it decreases the diameter of the tract. When the outer longitudinal layer contracts, it shortens the tract. These two movements create peristalsis and segmental contractions.

4. **Serosa**—an outermost layer of thin connective tissue and a single layer of epithelial cells.

Most of the digestive organs lie within the abdominal cavity (*see Chapter 3*), which is lined by a moist serous membrane called the **peritoneum. Parietal** peritoneum lines the wall of the abdominal cavity. **Visceral** peritoneum (a serosa) covers the external surface of the digestive organs.

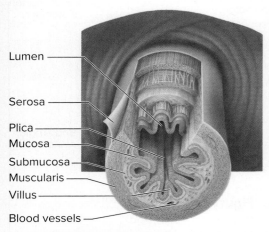

▲ **Figure 5.13** **Tissue layers of digestive tract.** An example of the most typical histologic structure of the tract.

The intestines are suspended from the back wall of the abdominal cavity by a translucent membrane called the **mesentery,** a continuation of the peritoneum. A fatty portion of the mesentery, called the **greater omentum** (*Figure 5.14*), hangs like an apron in front of all the intestines.

The small intestine (*Figure 5.15*) occupies much of the abdominal cavity, extends from the pylorus of the stomach to the beginning of the large intestine, and has three segments:

1. The **duodenum** is the first 9 to 10 inches of the small intestine. It receives chyme from the stomach, together with pancreatic juices and bile. Here, stomach acid is neutralized, fats are broken up by the bile acids, and pancreatic enzymes take over chemical digestion.

2. The **jejunum** makes up about 40% of the small intestine's length. It is the primary region for chemical digestion and nutrient absorption.

3. The **ileum** makes up about 55% of the small intestine's length. It ends at the **ileocecal** valve, a sphincter that controls entry into the large intestine.

From the duodenum to the middle of the ileum, the lining of the small intestine is folded into circular folds called **plicae.** Along their surface, the plicae have tiny fingerlike villi. The plicae and villi increase the surface area over which secretions can act on the food and through which nutrients can be absorbed. The folds also act as "speed bumps" to slow down the movement of chyme through the small intestine. The cells at the tip of the villi are shed and renewed every 3 or 4 days.

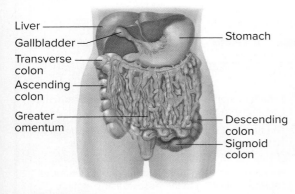

▲ **Figure 5.14** **Greater omentum.**

Digestion in the Small Intestine

After leaving the stomach as chyme, the food spends 3 to 5 hours in the small intestine, from which most of the nutrients are absorbed.

Secretion from the small intestine cells is mostly water, mucus, and enzymes. Peristaltic movements of the small intestine have three functions:

1. To mix chyme with intestinal and pancreatic juices and with bile.

2. To churn chyme to make contact with the mucosa for digestion and absorption.

3. To move the residue toward the large intestine.

Anywhere from four to six hours after consuming that chicken and vegetable dinner mentioned earlier, your food has passed through the small intestine and is ready to be moved into the large intestine. Most of the protein, carbohydrate, and fat of your meal has been broken down by enzymes into basic nutrients and absorbed into your bloodstream.

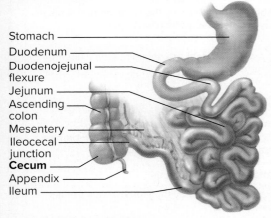

▲ **Figure 5.15** **Small intestine.**

WORD	PRONUNCIATION	ELEMENTS		DEFINITION
duodenum	du-oh-**DEE**-num	S/ R/	-um *structure* **duoden-** Latin for *twelve*	The first part of the small intestine; approximately 12 finger-breadths (9 to 10 inches) in length
ileum ileocecal (adj)	**ILL**-ee-um **ILL**-ee-oh-**SEE**-cal	 S/ R/CF R/	Latin *to roll up* -al *pertaining to* **ile/o-** *ileum* **-cec-** *cecum*	Third portion of the small intestine Pertaining to the junction of the ileum and cecum (the first part of the large intestine)
jejunum jejunal (adj)	je-**JEW**-num je-**JEW**-nal	 R/ S/	jejun Latin *empty* **jejun-** *empty* -al *pertaining to*	Segment of small intestine between the duodenum and the ileum where most of the nutrients are absorbed Pertaining to the jejunum
mesentery mesenteric (adj)	**MESS**-en-ter-ree **MESS**-en-ter-ik	P/ R/ S/	**mes-** *middle* **-entery** *intestine* -ic *pertaining to*	A double layer of peritoneum enclosing the abdominal viscera Pertaining to the mesentery
mucosa (another name for **mucous membrane**) mucosal (adj) submucosa	myu-**KOH**-sah myu-**KOH**-sal sub-mew-**KOH**-sa	 S/ P/ R/	Latin *mucus* -al *pertaining to* **sub-** *under* **-mucosa** *lining of a cavity*	Lining of a tubular structure Pertaining to the mucosa Tissue layer underneath the mucosa
muscularis	muss-kyu-**LAR**-is	S/ R/	-aris *pertaining to* **muscul-** *muscle*	The muscular layer of a hollow organ or tube
omentum omental (adj)	oh-**MEN**-tum oh-**MEN**-tal	 S/	Latin *membrane that drapes over the intestines* -al *pertaining to*	Membrane that drapes over the intestines Pertaining to the omentum
parietal	pah-**RYE**-eh-tal	S/ R/	-al *pertaining to* **pariet-** *wall*	Pertaining to the wall of an organ or a body cavity
peritoneum peritoneal (adj)	per-ih-toh-**NEE**-um per-ih-toh-**NEE**-al	 S/ R/	Latin *to stretch over, peritoneum* -al *pertaining to* **peritone-** *peritoneum*	Membrane that lines the abdominal cavity Pertaining to the peritoneum
plica plicae (pl)	**PLEE**-cah **PLEE**-key		Latin *fold*	Fold in a mucous membrane
serosa serosal (adj)	seh-**ROH**-sa seh-**ROH**-sal	 S/ R/	Latin *serous, watery* -al *pertaining to* **seros-** *watery consistency*	Outermost covering of the alimentary tract Pertaining to serosa
villus villi (pl)	**VILL**-us **VILL**-eye		Latin *shaggy hair*	Thin, hairlike projection, particularly of a mucous membrane lining a cavity
viscus (**Note: Viscous** is pronounced the same but means something *sticky.*) viscera (pl) visceral (adj)	**VISS**-kus **VISS**-er-ah **VISS**-er-al	 R/ S/	Latin *internal organ* **viscer-** *soft parts* -al *pertaining to*	Hollow, walled, internal organ Internal organs, particularly in the abdomen Pertaining to the internal organs

Chemical Digestion, Absorption, and Transport

When the remains of the chicken and vegetable arrive in your duodenum, they have been reduced to very small particles by mastication and gastric peristalsis, and they have been mixed with other food to form boluses. Thus far, 10% of their carbohydrates has been partially digested by salivary amylase, operating mostly in the mouth; 10% to 15% of their protein has been partially digested by proteases in the stomach; and 10% of their fats has been digested by the salivary lipase operating in the stomach.

Carbohydrates are ingested in three forms:

1. Polysaccharides, such as starches.

2. Disaccharides, such as sucrose (table sugar) and lactose (milk sugar).

3. Monosaccharides, such as glucose (the basic sugar), fructose (found in fruits), and galactose (found in milk).

Did you know...

- Proteins are broken down into amino acids.
- Minerals are electrolytes.

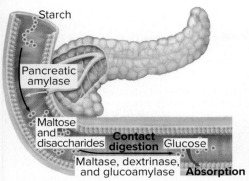

▲ **Figure 5.16** Starch digestion in the small intestine.

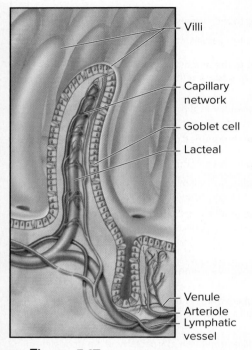

Villi

Capillary network

Goblet cell

Lacteal

Venule
Arteriole
Lymphatic vessel

▲ **Figure 5.17** Intestinal villi.

In the small intestine, polysaccharides are broken down by pancreatic amylase into disaccharides (*Figure 5.16*). Disaccharides are broken down to monosaccharides by maltase and dextrinase, enzymes secreted by the cells lining the villi of the small intestine.

The monosaccharides are taken up by the lining cells and transferred to the capillaries of the villi. They are then carried by the portal vein to the liver, where the nonglucose sugars are converted to glucose.

Proteins arrive in the duodenum and small intestine only 10% to 20% digested by gastric pepsin. Enzymes attached to the villi of the small intestine, together with the pancreatic enzyme trypsin, break down the remaining proteins to **amino acids.**

The amino acids are taken in by the epithelial cells of the small intestine, released into the capillaries of the villi, and carried away in the hepatic portal circulation. They are transported into cells all over the body, to be used as building blocks for new tissue formation.

Lipids (including fats) enter the duodenum and small intestine as large globules that have to be emulsified by bile salts into smaller droplets so that pancreatic lipase can digest the fats into very small droplets of free fatty acids and monoglycerides. There is enough pancreatic lipase in the duodenum to digest average amounts of fat within 1 or 2 minutes.

The very small droplets are absorbed by the intestinal cells and then taken into the lymphatic system by the **lacteals** inside the villi. The white, fatty lymphatic **chyle** eventually reaches the thoracic duct and is transferred into the left subclavian vein of the bloodstream. The chyle is carried by the blood and stored in adipose tissue.

The fat-soluble vitamins (A, D, E, and K) are absorbed with the lipids.

Water that is ingested is 92% absorbed by the small intestine and taken into the bloodstream through the capillaries in the villi (*Figure 5.17*). Water-soluble vitamins (C and the B-complex) are absorbed with water with the exception of vitamin B_{12}. This is a large molecule that has to bind with intrinsic factor from the stomach so that cells in the distant ileum can receive it and pass it through to the bloodstream.

Minerals are absorbed along the whole length of the small intestine. Iron and calcium are absorbed according to the body's needs. The other minerals are absorbed regardless of need, and the kidneys excrete the surplus.

Word Analysis and Definition: Absorption and Macro-nutrients

S = Suffix   P = Prefix   R = Root   R/CF = Combining Form

WORD	PRONUNCIATION	ELEMENTS		DEFINITION
amino acid	ah-**MEE**-noh **ASS**-id	R/CF	**amin/o** *nitrogen compound* **acid** Latin *sour*	The basic building block of protein
carbohydrate	kar-boh-**HIGH**-drate	S/ R/CF R/	**-ate** *composed of* **carb/o-** *carbon* **-hydr-** *water*	Group of organic food compounds that includes sugars, starch, glycogen, and cellulose
chyle	KILE		Greek *juice*	A milky fluid that results from the digestion and absorption of fats in the small intestine
lacteal	**LAK**-tee-al	S/ R/CF	**-al** *pertaining to* **lact/e-** *milk*	A lymphatic vessel carrying chyle away from the intestine
lipid	**LIP**-id		Greek *fat*	General term for all types of fatty compounds; for example, cholesterol, triglycerides, and fatty acids
mineral	**MIN**-er-al	S/ R/	**-al** *pertaining to* **miner-** *mines*	Inorganic compound usually found in earth's crust
protein	**PRO**-teen		Greek *first, primary*	Class of food substances based on amino acids

Structure and Functions of the Large Intestine

Structure of the Large Intestine

After the nutrients have been digested and absorbed in the small intestine, the residual materials have to be prepared in the large intestine for elimination from the body. The large intestine is so named because its diameter is much greater than that of the small intestine. It forms a **perimeter** in the abdominal cavity around the central mass of the small intestine (*Figure 5.18*).

At the junction between the small and large intestines, a ring of smooth muscle called the **ileocecal sphincter** forms a one-way valve. This allows chyme to pass into the large intestine and prevents the contents of the large intestine from backing up into the ileum.

At the beginning of the large intestine, the **cecum** is a pouch in the lower right quadrant of the abdomen (*Figure 5.18*). A narrow tube with a closed end, the **vermiform appendix,** projects downward from the cecum. The function of the appendix is not known.

The ascending **colon** begins at the cecum and extends upward until, just underneath the liver, it makes a sharp left turn at the hepatic **flexure** and becomes the transverse colon. At the left side of the abdomen, near the spleen at the splenic flexure, the transverse colon turns downward to form the descending colon. At the pelvic brim, the descending colon makes an S-shaped curve, the **sigmoid** colon, which descends in the pelvis to become the **rectum** and then the **anal canal.**

The rectum has three transverse folds, rectal valves that enable it to retain feces while passing gas (**flatus**). Intestinal gas is 90% nitrogen and oxygen, ingested while breathing and eating, together with methane, hydrogen, sulfites, and carbon dioxide contributed from bacterial fermentation of undigested food. This yields pungent ammonia and foul-smelling hydrogen sulfide to give gas and feces their characteristic odor.

The anal canal is the last 1 to 2 inches of the large intestine, opening to the outside as the **anus.** The mucous membrane is folded into six to eight longitudinal anal columns. **Feces** pressing against the columns causes them to produce more mucus to lubricate the canal during **defecation.** Two **sphincter** muscles guard the anus (*Figure 5.19):* an internal sphincter, composed of smooth muscle from the intestinal wall, and an external sphincter, composed of skeletal muscle that you can control voluntarily.

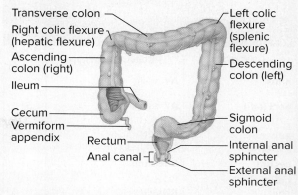

▲ **Figure 5.18 Large intestine.** Anatomy of the large intestine.

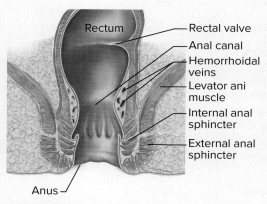

▲ **Figure 5.19** Anal canal.

Functions of the Large Intestine

- **Absorption** of water and electrolytes. The large intestine receives more than 1 L (1.05 quarts) of chyme each day from the small intestine and reabsorbs water and electrolytes to reduce the volume to 100 to 150 mL of feces to be eliminated by **defecation.**

- **Secretion** of mucus that protects the intestinal wall and holds particles of **fecal** matter together.

- **Digestion** by the bacteria that inhabit the large intestine of any food remnants that have escaped the digestive enzymes of the small intestine.

- **Peristalsis,** which, in the large intestine, happens only a few times a day to produce mass movements toward the rectum. Often when you ingest food into your stomach, your **gastrocolic reflex** will generate a mass movement of feces.

- **Elimination** of materials that were not digested or absorbed.

Word Analysis and Definition: The Large Intestine

WORD	PRONUNCIATION		ELEMENTS	DEFINITION
anus	AY-nuss		Latin *ring*	Terminal opening of the digestive tract through which feces are discharged
anal (adj)	AY-nal	S/ R/CF	-al *pertaining to* an/o- *anus*	Pertaining to the anus
appendix	ah-PEN-dicks		Latin *appendage*	Small blind projection from the pouch of the cecum
vermiform	VER-mih-form		Latin *wormlike*	Worm shaped; used as a descriptor for the appendix
cecum	SEE-kum		Latin *blind*	Blind pouch that is the first part of the large intestine
colon	KOH-lon		Greek *colon*	The large intestine, extending from the cecum to the rectum
colic	KOL-ik	S/ R/	-ic *pertaining to* col- *colon*	Spasmodic, crampy pains in the abdomen
feces	FEE-sees		Latin *dregs*	Undigested, waste material discharged from the bowel
fecal (adj)	FEE-kal	S/ R/	-al *pertaining to* fec- *feces*	Pertaining to feces
defecation	def-eh-KAY-shun	S/ P/	-ation *process* de- *from, out of*	Evacuation of feces from the rectum and anus
defecate (verb)	DEF-eh-kate	S/	-ate *process*	Process of defecation
flatus	FLAY-tus		Latin *blowing*	Gas or air expelled through the anus
flatulence	FLAT-you-lents	S/	-ence *forming*	Excessive amount of gas in the stomach and intestines
flatulent (adj)	FLAT-you-lent	R/	flatul- *excessive gas*	
flexure	FLECK-shur		Latin *bend*	A bend in a structure
gastrocolic reflex	gas-troh-KOL-ik REE-fleks	S/ R/CF R/ R/	-ic *pertaining to* gastr/o- *stomach* -col- *colon* reflex *bend back*	Mass movement of feces in the colon and the desire to defecate caused by taking food into stomach
ileocecal sphincter	ILL-ee-oh-SEE-cal SFINK-ter	S/ R/CF R/	-al *pertaining to* ile/o- *ileum* -cec- *cecum* sphincter Greek *band*	Band of muscle that encircles the junction of the ileum and cecum
perimeter	peh-RIM-eh-ter	P/ R/	peri- *around* -meter *measure*	An edge or border
rectum	RECK-tum		Latin *straight*	Terminal part of the colon from the sigmoid to the anal canal
rectal (adj)	RECK-tal	S/ R/	-al *pertaining to* rect- *rectum*	Pertaining to the rectum
sigmoid	SIG-moyd	S/ R/	-oid *resembling* sigm- Greek *letter "S"*	Sigmoid colon is shaped like an "S"

Check Point Section 5.3

A. Define the actions of the secretions of the stomach. *Match the secretion in the first column with its function listed in the second column.* **LO 5.1**

_____ 1. intrinsic factor

_____ 2. pepsin

_____ 3. mucus

_____ 4. hydrochloric acid

a. protects the lining of the stomach

b. destroys pathogens

c. allows for absorption of vitamin B_{12}

d. enzyme that breaks down protein

B. Greek and Latin terms do not deconstruct into basic elements, so you must know them for what they are. *Build your knowledge of these terms by matching the phrase in the left column to the correct medical term in the right column.* **LO 5.1**

_____ 1. To roll up   **a.** viscus

_____ 2. Membrane that drapes over the intestines   **b.** peritoneum

_____ 3. Watery   **c.** mucosa

_____ 4. Shaggy hair   **d.** plica

_____ 5. Internal organ   **e.** omentum

_____ 6. Fold   **f.** ileum

_____ 7. Empty   **g.** serosa

_____ 8. To stretch over   **h.** villus

_____ 9. Lining of a tubular structure   **i.** jejunum

C. Apply your medical vocabulary to answer the following questions about digestion. *Select the correct answer that completes each statement.* **LO 5.1, 5.2**

1. The suffix that is used to form the names of enzymes is

   a. *-ic*   **b.** *-al*   **c.** *-ase*   **d.** *-ous*   **e.** *-ion*

2. Which of the following terms means *a milky fluid resulting from the digestion and absorption of fats in the small intestine?*

   a. lipid   **b.** chyme   **c.** protease   **d.** chyle   **e.** lacteal

3. The group of organic food compounds that includes sugars, starch, glycogen, and cellulose is

   a. proteins   **b.** fats   **c.** lipids   **d.** carbohydrates   **e.** calories

4. The root *hydr-* means

   a. blood   **b.** juice   **c.** water   **d.** milk   **e.** bile

D. Apply your medical vocabulary to answer the following questions about digestion. *Select the correct answer that completes each statement.* **LO 5.1**

1. The general term for all fatty compounds is

   a. bile   **b.** protein   **c.** carbohydrate   **d.** lipid   **e.** protease

2. What is another name for a mineral?

   a. enzyme   **b.** electrolyte   **c.** lipid   **d.** hormone   **e.** fatty acid

3. The majority of water is absorbed in the:

   a. pancreas   **b.** stomach   **c.** small intestine   **d.** large intestine

E. Memorizing the meaning of word elements will help you to understand the meaning of many medical terms. *Match the word element in the first column with its correct meaning in the second column.* **LO 5.1, 5.2**

_____ 1. *sigm-*   **a.** forming

_____ 2. *peri-*   **b.** colon

_____ 3. *col-*   **c.** measure

_____ 4. *-ence*   **d.** Greek letter "S"

_____ 5. *meter-*   **e.** around

F. Some words cannot be deconstructed. *Correctly complete each sentence. Use the italicized word as a clue to the correct term. Fill in the blank.*
   LO 5.1, 5.3

1. The *blind* pouch of the large intestine is the _____.

2. The structure of the large intestine that is shaped like a *ring* is the _____.

3. The appendix has a *wormlike* appearance, and therefore is often termed as the _____ appendix.

4. The large intestine has several *bends* that are each termed as a _____.

Section 5.4 Digestion—Liver, Gallbladder, and Pancreas

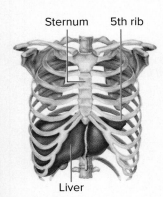

Sternum   5th rib

Liver

▲ **Figure 5.20**
Location of liver.

Liver

The liver and pancreas secrete enzymes that are responsible for most of the digestion that occurs in the small intestine. You must understand the function of these enzymes as they relate to digestion. The **liver,** the body's largest *internal* organ, is a complex structure located under the right ribs and below the diaphragm *(Figure 5.20).*

   The liver has multiple functions, including to:

- **Manufacture** and **excrete bile.** Although it contains no digestive enzymes, bile plays key roles in digestion. It neutralizes the acidic chyme so that pancreatic enzymes can function. Bile salts **emulsify** fat. **Bile acids** are synthesized from **cholesterol,** and bile also contains cholesterol and fat-soluble vitamins.
- **Remove** the pigment **bilirubin** from the bloodstream and excrete it in bile. Bilirubin is produced as a breakdown product of hemoglobin during phagocytosis by macrophages in the spleen and liver. It is dark yellow and is responsible for the brown color of feces and for the yellow color of skin in **jaundice.**
- **Remove** excess glucose (sugar) from the blood and store it as **glycogen** and release glucose when needed by the body.
- **Convert** proteins and fats into glucose, a process called **gluconeogenesis.**
- **Store** fat and the fat-soluble vitamins A, D, E, and K.
- **Manufacture** blood proteins, including those necessary for clotting *(see Chapter 11).*
- **Remove** toxins from the blood.

   A major reason that the liver can perform all these functions is that venous blood is returned from all the small intestines to join into the **portal vein** that takes the blood directly to the liver.

   The liver cells **secrete** bile into narrow channels that converge on the underside of the liver to form the common **hepatic duct.**

   Several hours after consuming that chicken and vegetable dinner mentioned earlier, the bile manufactured by the liver neutralizes the acidic chyme and emulsifies the fat.

Word Analysis and Definition: The Liver

S = Suffix   P = Prefix   R = Root   R/CF = Combining Form

WORD	PRONUNCIATION	ELEMENTS		DEFINITION
bile	BILE		Latin *bile*	Fluid secreted by the liver into the duodenum
bile acids	BILE **ASS**-ids	S/	-ary *pertaining to*	Steroids synthesized from cholesterol
biliary (adj)	**BILL**-ee-air-ee	R/CF	bil/i- *bile*	Pertaining to bile or the biliary tract
bilirubin	bill-ee-**RU**-bin	S/ R/CF	-rubin *rust colored* bil/i- *bile*	Bile pigment formed in the liver from hemoglobin
cholesterol	koh-**LESS**-ter-ol	S/ R/CF	-sterol *steroid* chol/e- *bile*	Steroid formed in liver cells; the most abundant steroid in tissues, which circulates in the plasma attached to proteins of different densities
duct	DUKT		Latin *to lead*	Tube or channel that carries a substance
emulsify	ee-**MUL**-sih-fie	S/ R/	-ify *to become* emuls- *suspend in a liquid*	Break up into very small droplets to suspend in a solution (emulsion)
emulsion (noun)	ee-**MUL**-shun	S/	-sion *state, condition*	System containing two liquids, one of which is in the form of small globules that are dispersed throughout the other
excrete	eks-**KREET**		Latin *separate*	To pass waste products of metabolism out of the body
excretion (noun)	eks-**KREE**-shun	S/ R/	-ion *action* excret- *separate*	Removal of waste products of metabolism out of the body
gluconeogenesis	**GLU**-koh-nee-oh-**JEN**-eh-sis	S/ R/CF R/CF	-genesis *creation* gluc/o- *sugar* -neo- *new*	Formation of glucose from noncarbohydrate sources
glycogen	**GLIE**-koh-jen	S/ R/CF	-gen *produce, create* glyc/o- *sugar*	The body's principal carbohydrate reserve, stored in the liver and skeletal muscle
hepatic	hep-**AT**-ik	S/ R/	-ic *pertaining to* hepat- *liver*	Pertaining to the liver
hepatitis	hep-ah-**TIE**-tis	S/	-itis *inflammation*	Inflammation of the liver
liver	**LIV**-er		Old English *liver*	Body's largest internal organ, located in right upper quadrant of abdomen
pancreas	**PAN**-kree-as		Greek *sweetbread*	Lobulated gland, the head of which is tucked into the curve of the duodenum
portal vein	**POR**-tal VANE		Latin *gate*	The vein that carries blood from the intestines to the liver

Gallbladder and Biliary Tract

On the underside of the liver is the **gallbladder** *(Figure 5.21a),* which stores and concentrates the bile that the liver produces. The cystic duct from the gallbladder joins with the hepatic duct to form the common bile duct. The system of ducts to get the bile from the liver to the duodenum is called the biliary tract *(Figure 5.21b).*

When acid and fat arrive in the duodenum, cells in the lining of the duodenum secrete a hormone, **cholecystokinin,** which causes the gallbladder to contract and force bile into the bile duct and, from there, into the duodenum. Cholecystokinin also stimulates the production of pancreatic enzymes.

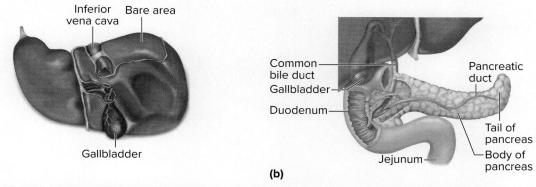

(a)   (b)

▲ **Figure 5.21 Gallbladder and biliary tract.** (a) Underside of liver. (b) Anatomy of gallbladder, pancreas, and biliary tract.

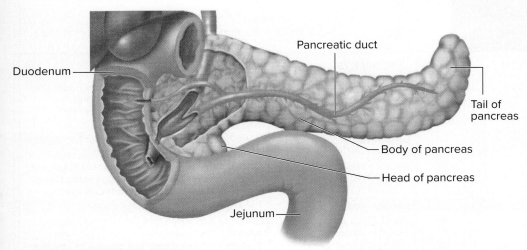

Duodenum

Pancreatic duct

Tail of pancreas

Body of pancreas

Head of pancreas

Jejunum

▲ **Figure 5.22** The pancreas.

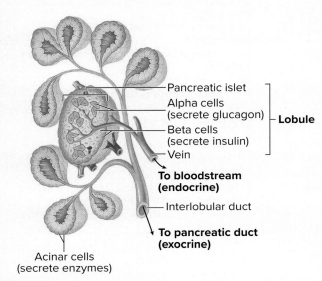

Pancreatic islet

Alpha cells (secrete glucagon)

Beta cells (secrete insulin)

Vein

Lobule

To bloodstream (endocrine)

Interlobular duct

To pancreatic duct (exocrine)

Acinar cells (secrete enzymes)

▲ **Figure 5.23** Exocrine and endocrine aspects of pancreas.

Pancreas

The **pancreas** (*Figure 5.22*) is a spongy gland, the head of which is encircled by the duodenum. Most of the pancreas secretes digestive juices; this is a part of the pancreas called an **exocrine gland** (*Figure 5.23*), and the **pancreatic** digestive juices formed in the **acinar cells of the exocrine part of the pancreas** are excreted through the pancreatic duct. The pancreatic duct joins the common bile duct shortly before it opens into the duodenum (*Figure 5.22*). Pancreatic and bile juices then enter the duodenum.

In the same parts of the pancreas as those in which pancreatic enzymes are produced, pancreatic **islet cells** secrete the hormones insulin and glucagon (*see Chapter 17*), which go directly into the bloodstream. This part of the pancreas is an **endocrine gland** (*Figure 5.23*). Thus, the pancreas is both an exocrine and endocrine gland.

The exocrine pancreatic juices contain:

1. **Electrolytes,** including the alkaline sodium bicarbonate, that make the pancreatic juice alkaline and help neutralize the acid chyme as it comes from the stomach.

2. **Enzymes:**

   • **Amylase** breaks down the **polysaccharide** starch into **disaccharides** and **monosaccharides.**

   • **Lipase** breaks down **triglyceride** fat molecules into **fatty acids** and **monoglycerides.**

   • **Trypsin, chymotrypsin,** and **carboxypeptidase** split proteins into their amino acids.

Pancreatic exocrine secretions are regulated by both the nervous and endocrine systems. While food is being digested in the stomach, nervous impulses stimulate the pancreas to produce its juices. When chyme enters the duodenum, the hormone **secretin,** produced in the duodenal mucosa, stimulates the pancreas to produce large volumes of watery fluid. Another hormone, cholecystokinin, is produced in the intestinal mucosa to stimulate production of pancreatic enzymes. Both hormones travel from the intestine via the bloodstream to the pancreas.

WORD	PRONUNCIATION	ELEMENTS		DEFINITION
acinar cells	**ASS**-in-ar SELLS	S/ R/	-ar *pertaining to* acin- *grape*	Enzyme-secreting cells of the pancreas
carboxypeptidase	kar-box-ee-**PEP**-tid-ase	S/ R/ R/	-ase *enzyme* carboxy- *group of organic compounds* -peptid- *digestion*	Enzyme that breaks down protein
cholecystokinin	**KOH**-leh-sis-toh-**KIE**-nin	S/ R/CF R/CF	-kinin *move in* chol/e- *bile* -cyst/o- *bladder*	Hormone secreted by the lining of the intestine that stimulates secretion of pancreatic enzymes and contraction of the gallbladder
electrolytes	ee-**LEK**-troh-lites	S/ R/CF	-lyte *soluble* electr/o *electric*	Substances, that when dissolved in a suitable medium, forms electrically charged particles
endocrine gland	**EN**-doh-krin GLAND	P/ R/CF	endo- *within* -crin/e *secrete*	A gland that produces an internal or hormonal secretion and secretes it into the bloodstream
exocrine gland	**EK**-soh-krin GLAND	P/ R/CF	exo- *outward* -crin/e *secrete*	A gland that secretes outwardly through excretory ducts
fatty acid	**FAT**-ee **ASS**-id		Old English *fat* Latin *sour*	An acid obtained from the hydrolysis of fats
gallbladder	**GAWL**-blad-er	R/	gall- *bile* Old English *bladder*	Receptacle on inferior surface of the liver for storing bile
islet cells	**EYE**-let SELLS		islet *small island*	Hormone-secreting cells of the pancreas
monoglyceride	mon-oh-**GLISS**-eh-ride	S/ P/ R/	-ide *having a particular quality* mono- *one* -glycer- *glycerol*	A fatty substance with a single fatty acid
triglyceride	trie-**GLISS**-eh-ride	P/	tri- *three*	Substance with three fatty acids
monosaccharide	**MON**-oh-**SACK**-ah-ride	S/ P/ R/	-ide *having a particular quality* mono- *one* -sacchar- *sugar*	Simplest form of sugar; for example, glucose A combination of two monosaccharides; for example, table sugar
disaccharide	die-**SACK**-ah-ride	P/	di- *two*	A combination of many saccharides; for example, starch
polysaccharide	pol-ee-**SACK**-ah-ride	P/	poly- *many*	
pancreas	**PAN**-kree-as		Greek *sweetbread*	Lobulated gland, the head of which is tucked into the curve of the duodenum
pancreatic (adj)	pan-kree-**AT**-ik	S/ R/	-ic *pertaining to* pancreat- *pancreas*	Pertaining to the pancreas
secretin	se-**KREE**-tin	S/ R/	-in *substance, chemical compound* secret- *separate*	Hormone produced by duodenum to stimulate pancreatic juice
trypsin	**TRIP**-sin	S/	-in *substance, chemical compound*	Enzyme that breaks down protein
chymotrypsin	kie-moh-**TRIP**-sin	R/ R/CF	tryps- *friction* chym/o-*chyme*	Trypsin found in chyme

Checkpoint Section 5.4

A. Use this exercise as a quick review of the elements related to the liver. *Select the correct answer that completes each statement.*
   LO 5.1, 5.2

1. In the term **hepatic,** the root means

   a. pancreas   **b.** stomach   **c.** liver

2. The term **gallstone** is composed of

   a. root + combining form   **b.** root + root   **c.** root + suffix

3. The term **biliary** is composed of a

   a. prefix + root   **b.** root + suffix   **c.** combining form + suffix

4. In the term **gluconeogenesis,** *neo* means

   a. never   **b.** new   **c.** negative

B. Work on recognizing the elements. *Fill in the chart.* **LO 5.1, 5.2, 5.3, 5.6**

Element	Meaning of Element	Type of Element (Prefix, Root, Combining Form, Suffix)	Medical Term Containing This Element
osis	1.	2.	3.
hemo	4.	5.	6.
asc	7.	8.	9.
cirrh	10.	11.	12.
chole	13.	14.	15.
stat	16.	17.	18.

C. Describe the anatomy and function of the pancreas. *Choose the correct answer to the following questions.* **LO 5.1**

1. The exocrine function of the pancreas is the secretion of:

   a. bile   **b.** insulin   **c.** glucagon   **d.** pancreatic juice

2. On the pH scale, pancreatic juice is:

   a. alkaline   **b.** acidic

3. The pancreas is:

   a. in the left lower quadrant   **b.** superior to the diaphragm   **c.** surrounded by the curve of the duodenum   **d.** lateral to the stomach

Section 5.5 Disorders of the Digestive System

Overall Digestive System Disorders

A large number of disorders produce symptoms from the gastrointestinal tract but have no specific lesions discoverable in any part of the tract. These disorders include:

- **Food intolerance** has gastrointestinal symptoms such as bloating, cramps, gas, heartburn, diarrhea, and general nonspecific symptoms such as irritability and headache. It is usually diagnosed by keeping a food diary to identify which foods are triggering the symptoms so that they can be avoided.
- **Food allergies** are estimated by the Centers for Disease Control and Prevention (CDC) to affect 8% of children and 4% of adults. An **allergic** reaction to food occurs when the immune system (*see Chapter 12*) overreacts to a food antigen, identifying it as a danger, and triggering a protective response. A food that triggers only mild symptoms on one occasion can cause severe symptoms on another occasion. Gastrointestinal symptoms involve vomiting, stomach cramps, and difficulty swallowing. Eight types of food account for 90% of all allergic food reactions: eggs, milk, peanuts, tree nuts, fish, shellfish, wheat, and soy. Skin-prick tests and blood tests can indicate whether food-specific **immunoglobulin** E (IgE) **antibodies** are present in the body. Management of the allergy is to avoid consuming the food.
- **Irritable bowel syndrome** (IBS) is a symptom-based diagnosis with chronic abdominal pain, abdominal discomfort, bloating, and either diarrhea or **constipation.** There is no known organic cause and routine testing shows no abnormality. Dietary adjustments involving fiber intake and psychological interventions can help.
- **Inflammatory bowel disease** (IBD) involves chronic inflammation of all or part of the digestive tract, but primarily includes ulcerative colitis and Crohn's disease.
- **Aging** has less effect on the digestive system than on other organ systems. In the small intestine, **lactase** levels decrease, leading to intolerance of dairy products (**lactose** intolerance). In the large intestine, there is a slight slowing of the movement of contents, leading to constipation.

Gastrointestinal Bleeding

Bleeding can occur anywhere in the gastrointestinal (GI) tract from a variety of causes, as described in the preceding sections. The bleeding can be internal and painless. It can present in different ways to provide a clue to the site of bleeding:

- **Hematemesis**—the vomiting of bright red blood, which indicates an upper GI source of ongoing bleeding (esophagus, stomach, duodenum).
- **Vomiting of "coffee grounds" (coffee ground emesis)**—occurs when bleeding from an upper GI source has slowed or stopped; red hemoglobin has been converted to brown hematin by gastric acids.
- **Hematochezia**—the passage of bright red bloody stools, which usually indicates lower GI bowel bleeding from the sigmoid colon, rectum, or anus.
- **Melena**—the passage of black tarry stools, which usually indicates upper GI bleeding. The blood is digested and hemoglobin is oxidized as it passes through the intestine to produce the black color. Melena can continue for several days after a severe hemorrhage.
- **Occult blood**—blood is present in the stool but its amount is too small to be seen. The chronic source of the bleeding can be anywhere in the GI tract.

Consuming black licorice, Pepto-Bismol, or blueberries can produce black stools.

Word Analysis and Definition: Overall Digestive System Disorders

S = Suffix   P = Prefix   R = Root   R/CF = Combining Form

WORD	PRONUNCIATION		ELEMENTS	DEFINITION
aging	AY-jing		Latin *old*	The process of growing old
allergy	AL-er-jee	P/ R/ R/	all- *other* -ergy *process of working* -erg *work*	An acquired sensitivity to certain proteins
allergen allergic (adj)	AL-er-jen ah-LER-jic	R/ S/	-gen *to produce* -ic *pertaining to*	The substance that incites an allergic reaction Relating to any response to an allergen
antibody antibodies (pl)	AN-tih-body AN-tih-bod-ees	P/ R/	anti- *against* -body *substance*	Protein produced in response to an antigen
antigen	AN-tih-jen	P/ R/	anti- *against* -gen *to produce*	Substance capable of triggering an immune response
constipation	kon-stih-PAY-shun	S/ R/	-ation *process* constip- *press together*	Hard, infrequent bowel movements
emesis hematemesis	EM-eh-sis he-mah-TEM-eh-sis	R/ S/	Greek *vomiting* hemat- *blood* -emesis *vomiting*	Condition of vomiting Vomiting of red blood
hematochezia	he-mat-oh-KEY-zee-ah	S/ R/CF	-chezia *pass a stool* hemat/o- *blood*	The passage of red, bloody stools
immunoglobulin	IM-you-noh-GLOB-you-lin	S/ R/CF R/	-in *chemical compound* immun/o- *immune response* -globul- *protein*	Specific protein evoked by an antigen; all antibodies are immunoglobulins
intolerance intolerant (adj)	in-TOL-er-ance in-TOL-er-ant		Latin *unable to cope with*	Inability of the small intestine to metabolize a particular dietary constituent Possessing intolerance
lactose lactase	LAK-toes LAK-tase	S/ R/ S/	-ose *condition* lact- *milk* -ase *enzyme*	The disaccharide in cow's milk Enzyme that breaks down lactose to glucose and galactose
melena	mel-EN-ah		Greek *black*	The passage of black, tarry stools
occult	oh-KULT		Latin *to hide*	Not visible on the surface
vomit (verb) vomit (noun)	VAH-mit		Latin *to spew forth, discharge*	Expel contents from the stomach, though the esophagus, and out the mouth Matter vomited from the stomach

Disorders of the Mouth

An accumulation of dental **plaque** (a collection of oral microorganisms and their products) or **dental calculus (tartar),** calcified deposits at the gingival margin of the teeth, is a precursor to dental disease.

Dental **caries,** tooth decay and cavity formation, is an erosion of the tooth surface caused by bacteria *(Figure 5.24)*. If untreated, it can lead to an **abscess** at the root of the tooth. **Gingivitis** is an infection of the gums. **Periodontal disease** occurs when the gums and the jawbone are involved in a disease process. In **periodontitis,** infection causes the gums to pull away from the teeth, forming pockets that become infected. The infection can spread to the underlying bone. Infection of the gums with a purulent discharge is called **pyorrhea.**

The term **stomatitis** is used for any infection of the mouth. The most common infections are

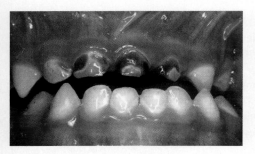

▲ **Figure 5.24 Dental caries.** Child with dental caries. Ted Croll/Science Source

- **Mouth ulcers,** also called **canker** sores, which are erosions of the mucous membrane lining the mouth. The most common type are **aphthous ulcers,** which occur in clusters of small ulcers and last for 3 or 4 days. They are usually related to stress or illness. Ulcers can also be caused by trauma.

- **Cold sores,** also known as fever blisters *(Figure 5.25)*, which are recurrent ulcers of the lips, lining of the mouth, and gums due to infection with the virus **herpes simplex type 1 (HSV-1).**

- **Thrush** *(Figure 5.26)*, an infection occurring anywhere in the mouth and caused by the fungus *Candida albicans*. This fungus typically is found in the mouth, but it can multiply out of control as a result of prolonged antibiotic or steroid treatment, cancer chemotherapy, or diabetes. A newborn baby can acquire oral thrush from the mother's vaginal yeast infection during the birth process.

- **Leukoplakia,** a white plaque seen anywhere in the mouth. It is more common in the elderly, it is often associated with smoking or chewing tobacco, and approximately 3% turn into oral cancer. Patients whose immune systems are compromised, for example, with **human immunodeficiency virus (HIV),** are susceptible to leukoplakia.

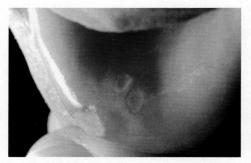

▲ **Figure 5.25 Cold sores.** Ulcer inside lower lip. defun/Getty Images

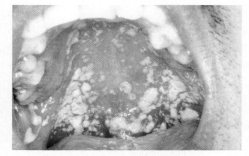

▲ **Figure 5.26 Oral thrush.** Mediscan/ Alamy Stock Photo

- **Oral cancer** *(Figure 5.27)*, which is mostly squamous cell **carcinoma,** occurring often on the lip. Eighty percent of oral cancers are associated with smoking or chewing tobacco. Metastasis occurs to lymph nodes, bone, lung, and liver. The 5-year survival rate is only 51%.

- **Halitosis,** the medical term for bad breath, which can be found in association with any of the above mouth disorders.

- **Glossodynia,** a painful burning sensation of the tongue. It occurs in postmenopausal women. Its etiology is unknown, and there is no successful treatment.

- **Cleft palate,** a congenital fissure in the median line of the palate. It is often associated with a cleft lip.

- **Sjögren syndrome,** an autoimmune disease that attacks the glands that produce saliva and tears. Symptoms include dry mouth and eyes. It is associated with other autoimmune diseases, such as rheumatoid arthritis.

WORD	PRONUNCIATION	ELEMENTS		DEFINITION
abscess	**AB**-sess		Latin *a going away*	A collection of pus
aphthous ulcer	**AF**-thus **UL**-ser		Greek *ulcer*	Painful small oral ulcer (canker sore)
canker; canker sore (also called **mouth ulcer**)	**KANG**-ker SOAR		Latin *crab*	Nonmedical term for aphthous ulcer
carcinoma	kar-sih-**NOH**-mah	S/ R/	-oma *tumor, mass* carcin- *cancer*	A cancerous (malignant) and invasive epithelial tumor
caries	**KARE**-eez		Latin *dry rot*	Bacterial destruction of teeth
gingivitis	jin-jih-**VIE**-tis	S/ R/	-itis *inflammation* gingiv- *gums*	Inflammation of the gums
gingivectomy	jin-jih-**VEC**-toe-mee	S/	-ectomy *surgical excision*	Surgical removal of diseased gum tissue
glossodynia	gloss-oh-**DIN**-ee-ah	S/ R/CF	-dynia *pain* gloss/o- *tongue*	Painful, burning tongue
halitosis	hal-ih-**TOE**-sis	S/ R/	-osis *condition* halit- *breath*	Bad odor of the breath
leukoplakia	loo-koh-**PLAY**-kee-ah	S/ R/CF R/	-ia *condition* leuk/o- *white* -plak- *plate, plaque*	White patch on oral mucous membrane, often precancerous
periodontics	**PER**-ee-oh-**DON**-tiks	S/ P/ R/	-ics *knowledge of* peri- *around* -odont- *tooth*	Branch of dentistry specializing in disorders of tissues around the teeth
periodontist periodontitis	**PER**-ee-oh-**DON**-tist **PER**-ee-oh-don-**TIE**-tis	S/ S/	-ist *specialist* -itis *inflammation*	Specialist in periodontics Inflammation of tissues around a tooth
plaque	PLAK		French *plate*	Patch of abnormal tissue
pyorrhea	pie-oh-**REE**-ah	S/ R/CF	-rrhea *flow* py/o- *pus*	Purulent discharge
Sjögren syndrome	**SHOW**-gren **SIN**-drome		Henrik Sjögren, 1889–1986, Swedish ophthalmologist	Autoimmune disease that attacks the glands that produce saliva and tears
stomatitis	**STOW**-ma-**TIE**-tis	S/ R/	-itis *inflammation* stomat- *mouth*	A general term given to any infection of the mouth
syndrome	**SIN**-drome	P/ R/	syn- *together* -drome *course*	A collection of signs and symptoms that typify a disease
tartar (also called **dental calculus**)	**TAR**-tar		Latin *crust on wine casks*	Calcified deposit at the gingival margin of the teeth
thrush	THRUSH		Root unknown	Infection with *Candida albicans*
ulcer ulceration	**ULL**-cer ull-cer-**A**-shun	S/ R/	Latin *sore* -ation *a process* ulcer- *a sore*	Erosion of an area of skin or mucosa Formation of an ulcer

Disorders of the Esophagus

- **Esophagitis** is inflammation of the lining of the esophagus that produces a **postprandial** burning chest pain **(heartburn),** pain on swallowing, and occasional hematemesis.

- **Gastroesophageal reflux disease (GERD)** is the **regurgitation** of stomach contents back into the esophagus, often when a person is lying down at night. The patient experiences burning sensations in the chest and mouth from the acidity of the regurgitation. The acidity can also irritate and ulcerate the lining of the esophagus, causing it to bleed. Scar tissue can form and cause an esophageal **stricture,** with difficulty in swallowing **(dysphagia).**

- **Hiatal hernia** occurs when a portion of the stomach protrudes **(herniates)** through the diaphragm alongside the esophagus at the esophageal **hiatus** *(Figure 5.28).* Reflux of acid stomach contents into the esophagus causes an **esophagitis.** Surgical repair sometimes is necessary and is called a **herniorrhaphy.**

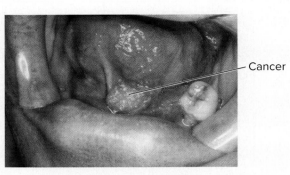

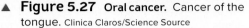

▲ **Figure 5.27** **Oral cancer.** Cancer of the tongue. Clinica Claros/Science Source

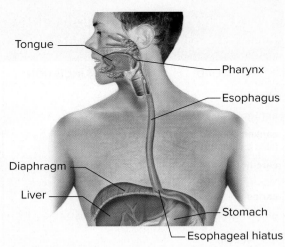

▲ **Figure 5.28** **Esophageal hiatus.**

- **Esophageal varices** are **varicose** veins of the esophagus. They are **asymptomatic** until they rupture, causing massive bleeding and hematemesis. They are a complication of cirrhosis of the liver *(see Section 5.5)*.
- **Cancer of the esophagus** arises from the lining of the tube. **Symptoms** are difficulty in swallowing **(dysphagia),** a burning sensation in the chest, and weight loss. Risk factors include cigarettes, alcohol, betel nut chewing, and esophageal reflux.

Word Analysis and Definition: Disorders of the Esophagus

S = Suffix   P = Prefix   R = Root   R/CF = Combining Form

WORD	PRONUNCIATION		ELEMENTS	DEFINITION
dysphagia	dis-**FAY**-jee-ah	P/ R/	**dys-** *difficult* **-phagia** *swallowing*	Difficulty in swallowing
esophagitis	ee-**SOF**-ah-**JIE**-tis	S/ R/	**-itis** *inflammation* **esophag-** *esophagus*	Inflammation of the lining of the esophagus
gastroesophageal	**GAS**-troh-ee-sof-ah-**JEE**-al	S/ R/CF R/CF	**-al** *pertaining to* **gastr/o-** *stomach* **-esophag/e** *esophagus*	Pertaining to the stomach and esophagus
hernia herniorrhaphy herniate (verb)	**HER**-nee-ah **HER**-nee-**OR**-ah-fee **HER**-nee-ate	S/ R/CF S/	*Latin rupture* **-rrhaphy** *suture* **herni/o-** *hernia* **-ate** *pertaining to*	Protrusion of a structure through the tissue that normally
hiatus hiatal (adj)	high-**AY**-tus high-**AY**-tal	S/ R/	*Latin an aperture* **-al** *pertaining to* **hiat-** *aperture*	An opening through a structure Pertaining to an opening through a structure
postprandial (adj)	post-**PRAN**-dee-al	S/ P/ R/	**-ial** *pertaining to* **post-** *after* **-prand-** *meal*	Following a meal
reflux	**REE**-fluks	P/ R/	**re-** *back* **-flux** *flow*	Backward flow
regurgitation	ree-gur-jih-**TAY**-shun	S/ P/ R/	**-ation** *process* **re-** *back* **-gurgit-** *flood*	Expelling contents of the stomach into the mouth, short of vomiting
symptom symptomatic asymptomatic	**SIMP**-tum simp-toe-**MAT**-ik	S/ R/ P/	*Greek sign* **-ic** *pertaining to* **symptomat-** *symptom* **a-** *without*	Departure from the normal experienced by the patient Pertaining to the symptoms of a disease Absence of symptoms
varix varices (pl) varicose (adj)	**VAIR**-iks **VAIR**-ih-seez **VAIR**-ih-kos		*Latin dilated vein*	Dilated, tortuous vein Characterized by or affected with varices
stricture	**STRICK**-shur		*Latin to draw tight*	Narrowing of a tube

Disorders of the Stomach

Distention or irritation of any part of the digestive tract can lead to vomiting. A message is sent via the **vagus** nerve to the vomiting center in the brain, which, in turn, stimulates the muscles of the diaphragm and abdominal wall to forcefully contract and expel the stomach contents upward into the esophagus and out the mouth.

- **Gastritis** is an inflammation of the lining of the stomach, producing symptoms of epigastric pain, a feeling of fullness, nausea, and occasional bleeding. Gastritis can be caused by common medications such as aspirin and nonsteroidal anti-inflammatory drugs (NSAIDs), by radiotherapy and chemotherapy, and by alcohol and smoking. Treatment is directed at removing the factors causing the gastritis by acid neutralization and suppression of gastric acid

- **Peptic ulcers** occur in the stomach and duodenum when the balance between the acid gastric juices and the protection of the mucosal lining breaks down, causing an **erosion** of the lining by the acid *(Figure 5.29)*. Most peptic ulcers are caused by the bacterium *Helicobacter pylori (H. pylori)*, which produces enzymes that weaken the protective mucus. These ulcers respond to an antibiotic. Use of NSAIDs increases the incidence of peptic ulcers, particularly in the elderly. **Dyspepsia,** epigastric pain with bloating and nausea, is the most common symptom.

- **Gastric ulcers** are peptic ulcers occurring in the stomach. Symptoms are epigastric burning pain after food, nausea, vomiting, and belching. Bleeding can occur from **erosion** of a blood vessel. If untreated, the ulcer can erode through the entire wall, causing a **perforation.**

- **Gastric cancer** can be asymptomatic for a long period and then cause **indigestion, anorexia,** abdominal pain, and weight loss. It affects men twice as often as women. It metastasizes to lymph nodes, liver, peritoneum, chest, and brain.

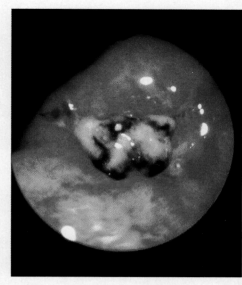

▲ **Figure 5.29 Bleeding peptic ulcer.** The yellow floor of the ulcer shows black blood clots. Fresh blood is around the ulcer margin. CNRI/Science Source

Word Analysis and Definition: Disorders of the Stomach

S = Suffix   P = Prefix   R = Root   R/CF = Combining Form

WORD	PRONUNCIATION	ELEMENTS		DEFINITION
anorexia	an-oh-**RECK**-see-ah	S/ P/ R/	**-ia** *condition* **an-** *without* **-orex-** *appetite*	Severe lack of appetite; or an aversion to food
distend distention	dis-**TEND** dis-**TEN**-shun	 S/ P/ R/	Latin *stretch apart* **-tion** *process, being* **dis-** *apart, away* **-ten-** *pressure*	To swell, stretch Being stretched by pressure from the inside
dyspepsia	dis-**PEP**-see-ah	S/ P/ R/	**-ia** *condition* **dys-** *difficult, bad* **-peps-** *digestion*	"Upset stomach," epigastric pain, nausea, and gas
erosion	ee-**ROH**-shun		Latin *to gnaw away*	A shallow ulcer in the lining of a structure
gastritis	gas-**TRY**-tis	S/ R/	**-itis** *inflammation* **gastr-** *stomach*	Inflammation of the lining of the stomach
peptic	**PEP**-tik	S/ R/	**-ic** *pertaining to* **pept-** *digest*	Relating to the stomach and duodenum
perforation	per-foh-**RAY**-shun	S/ R/	**-ion** *action* **perforat-** *bore through*	Erosion that progresses to become a hole through the wall of a structure
vagus	**VAY**-gus		Latin *wandering*	Tenth (X) cranial nerve; supplies many different organs throughout the body

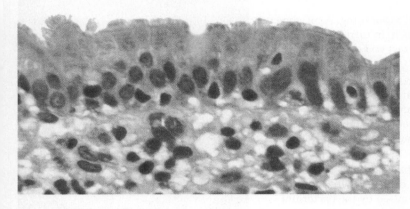

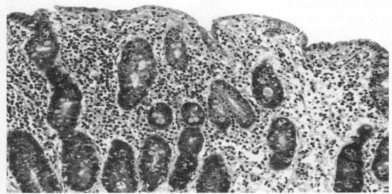

▲ **Figure 5.30** Photomicrograph of celiac disease showing atrophy of duodenal villi. Biophoto Associates/Science Source

Disorders of the Small Intestine

Disorders of the small intestine are due to inflammation, bleeding, allergies, intestinal motility, or cancer.

Common disorders of the small intestine are:

- **Gastroenteritis,** or inflammation of the stomach and small intestine, can result in acute vomiting and diarrhea. It can be caused by a variety of viruses and bacteria (including, occasionally, the parasite *Giardia lamblia*) and is initiated by contact with contaminated food (food poisoning) and water.
- Bleeding from the small intestine is usually caused by a duodenal ulcer.
- **Celiac disease** is an autoimmune disease where the ingestion of gluten damages the small intestine *(Figure 5.20)*. Gluten is a protein found in wheat, rye, and barley. Symptoms can include abdominal swelling, gas, pain, weight loss, fatigue, and weakness. Treatment is a strict gluten-free diet.
- An **intussusception** occurs when a part of the small intestine slides into a neighboring portion of the small intestine—much like the way that parts of a collapsible telescope slide into each other. Eighty percent of intussusceptions can be cured with an enema; the remaining 20% require surgical intervention.
- **Ileus (paralytic ileus)** is a disruption of the normal peristaltic ability of the small intestine. It can be caused by a bowel obstruction or by intestinal paralysis. Risk factors for paralytic ileus include GI surgery, diabetic ketoacidosis *(see Chapter 17),* peritonitis, and medications, such as opiates.
- **Cancer** of the small intestine occurs infrequently compared with tumors in other parts of the GI tract. An **adenocarcinoma** is the most common malignant tumor of the small bowel.

Disorders of Absorption

- **Malabsorption syndromes** refer to a group of diseases in which intestinal absorption of nutrients is impaired.
- **Malnutrition** can arise from malabsorption or from insufficient food intake as a result of famine, poverty, loss of appetite due to cancer, or terminal illness. Many of the poor and elderly in this country suffer from malnutrition.
- **Lactose intolerance** occurs when the small intestine is not producing sufficient **lactase** to break down the milk sugar lactose. The result is **diarrhea** and cramps. Lactase can be taken in pill form before eating dairy products, and/or lactose can be avoided by using soy products rather than milk products.
- **Crohn's disease** (or **regional enteritis**) is an inflammation of the small intestine (frequently in the ileum) and occasionally also in the large intestine. The symptoms are abdominal pain, diarrhea, fatigue, and weight loss. Malabsorption is common, and children with Crohn's disease may have delayed development and stunted growth.
- **Constipation** occurs when fecal movement through the large intestine is slow, causing too much water to be reabsorbed by the large intestine. The feces become hardened. Factors causing constipation are lack of dietary fiber, lack of exercise, and emotional upset.
- **Gastroenteritis (stomach "flu")** is an infection of the stomach and intestine that can be caused by a large variety of bacteria and viruses. It causes vomiting, diarrhea, and fever. An outbreak of gastroenteritis can sometimes be traced to contaminated food or water. The Norwalk virus and rotaviruses are major causes of diarrhea in infants and children.
- **Dysentery** is a severe form of bacterial gastroenteritis with blood and mucus in frequent, watery stools. It can lead to **dehydration.**

WORD	PRONUNCIATION	ELEMENTS		DEFINITION
celiac	**SEE**-lee-ack	S/ R/	-ac *pertaining to* celi- *abdomen*	Relating to the abdominal cavity
celiac disease	**SEE**-lee-ack diz-**EEZ**	P/ R/	dis- *apart* -ease *normal function*	Disease caused by sensitivity to gluten
constipation	kon-stih-**PAY**-shun	S/ R/	-ation *process* constip- *press together*	Hard, infrequent bowel movements
Crohn's disease (also called **regional enteritis**)	KRONES diz-**EEZ** **REE**-jun-al en-ter-**EYE**-tis		Burrill Crohn, 1884–1993, New York gastroenterologist	Inflammatory bowel disease with narrowing and thickening of the terminal small bowel
dehydration	dee-high-**DRAY**-shun	S/ P/ R/	-ation *a process* de- *without* -hydr- *water*	Process of losing body water
diarrhea	die-ah-**REE**-ah	P/ S/	dia- *complete, through* -rrhea *flow, discharge*	Abnormally frequent and loose stools
dysentery	**DIS**-en-tare-ee	P/ R/	dys- *bad, difficult* -entery *intestine*	Disease with diarrhea, bowel spasms, fever, and dehydration
gastroenteritis	**GAS**-troh-en-ter-**EYE**-tis	S/ R/CF R/	-itis *inflammation* gastr/o- *stomach* -enter- *intestine*	Inflammation of the stomach and intestines
intolerance	in-**TOL**-er-ance		Latin *unable to cope with*	Inability of the small intestine to digest and dispose of a particular dietary constituent
lactose lactase	**LAK**-toes **LAK**-tase	S/ R/	Latin *milk sugar* -ase *enzyme* lact- *milk*	The disaccharide found in cow's milk Enzyme that breaks down lactose to glucose and galactose
malabsorption	mal-ab-**SORP**-shun	S/ P/ R/	-ion *action, condition* mal- *bad* -absorpt- *to swallow*	Inadequate gastrointestinal absorption of nutrients
malnutrition	mal-nyu-**TRISH**-un	S/ P/ R/	-ion *action, condition* mal- *bad* nutri- *nourish*	Inadequate nutrition from poor diet or inadequate absorption of nutrients

Disorders of the Large Intestine and Anal Canal

Disorders of the Large Intestine

Appendicitis is the most common cause of acute abdominal pain in the right lower quadrant. On palpation, tenderness over the **McBurney point,** one-third the distance from the anterior superior iliac crest to the umbilicus *(see Chapter 3)*, suggests appendicitis. If neglected, the inflamed appendix can rupture, leading to **peritonitis.** This is strongly suggested by the presence of *rebound tenderness,* in which a stab of severe pain is produced when the abdominal wall, which has been pressed in slowly, is released rapidly.

Diverticulosis is the presence of small pouches (**diverticula**) bulging outward through weak spots in the lining of the large intestine *(Figure 5.31)*. They are asymptomatic until the pouches become infected and inflamed, a condition called **diverticulitis.** This condition causes abdominal pain, vomiting, constipation, and fever. Complications, such as perforation and abscess formation, can occur. The most likely cause of diverticular disease (diverticulosis and diverticulitis) is a low-fiber diet.

Ulcerative colitis is an extensive inflammation and ulceration of the lining of the large intestine. It produces bouts of bloody diarrhea, crampy pain, and often weight loss and electrolyte imbalance.

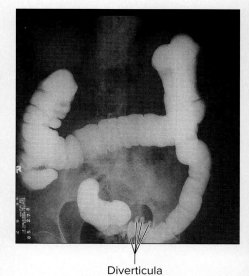

Diverticula

▲ **Figure 5.31** **Barium enema showing diverticulosis.** Susan Leavine/Science Source

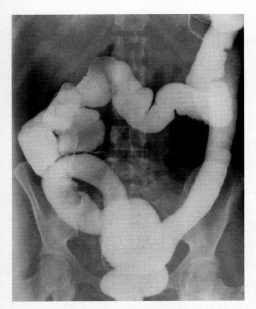

▲ **Figure 5.32** Barium enema showing cancer of the colon (orange area). SPL/ Science Source

Irritable bowel syndrome (IBS) is an increasingly common large-**bowel** disorder, presenting with crampy pains, gas, and changes in bowel habits to either constipation or diarrhea. There are no anatomic changes seen in the bowel, and the cause is unknown.

Polyposis is a condition of multiple polyps. **Polyps** are masses of tissue arising from the wall of the large intestine and other tube-like structures that protrude into the bowel **lumen.** They vary in size and shape. Most are benign. Endoscopic biopsy can determine if they are **precancerous** or cancerous.

Colon and **rectal cancers** *(Figure 5.32)* are the second leading cause of cancer deaths after lung cancer. The majority occur in the rectum and sigmoid colon. These cancers spread by:

1. Direct extension through the bowel wall.
2. **Metastasis** to regional lymph nodes.
3. Moving down the lumen of the bowel.
4. Bloodborne **metastases** to liver, lung, bone, and brain.

Obstruction of the large bowel can be caused by cancers, large polyps, or diverticulitis.

Intussusception is a form of obstruction whereby a tumor in the lumen of the bowel, together with its segment of bowel, is telescoped into the immediately distal segment of bowel.

Proctitis is inflammation of the lining of the rectum, often associated with ulcerative colitis, Crohn's disease, or radiation therapy. Symptoms are **anorectal** pain, rectal bleeding, and excess mucus in the **stool.**

Disorders of the Anal Canal

Hemorrhoids are dilated veins in the submucosa of the anal canal, often associated with pregnancy, chronic constipation, diarrhea, or aging. They protrude into the anal canal (internal hemorrhoid) or bulge out along the edge of the anus (external hemorrhoid) producing pain and bright red blood from the anus. A thrombosed hemorrhoid, in which blood has clotted, is very painful.

Anal fissures are tears in the lining of the anal canal, such as may occur with difficult **bowel** movements (**BM**s).

Anal fistulas occur following abscesses in the anal glands. The anal canal has six or seven glands in the posterior canal that secrete mucus to lubricate the canal. If the glands become infected, abscesses form that, when they heal, can form a passage (fistula) between the anal canal and the skin outside the anus.

WORD	PRONUNCIATION	ELEMENTS		DEFINITION
appendicitis	ah-pen-dih-**SIGH**-tis	S/ S/ R/	**-ic-** *pertaining to* **-itis** *inflammation* **append-** *appendix*	Inflammation of the appendix
bowel	**BOUGH**-el		Latin *sausage*	Another name for intestine
colitis	koh-**LIE**-tis	S/ R/	**-itis** *inflammation* **col-** *colon*	Inflammation of the colon
diverticulum diverticula (pl) diverticulosis	die-ver-**TICK**-you-lum die-ver-**TICK**-you-lah **DIE**-ver-tick-you-**LOH**-sis	S/ R/ S/	**-um** *tissue* **diverticul-** *by-road* **-osis** *condition*	A pouchlike opening or sac from a tubular structure (e.g., gut) Presence of a number of small pouches in the wall of the large intestine
diverticulitis	**DIE**-ver-tick-you-**LIE**-tis	S/	**-itis** *inflammation*	Inflammation of the diverticula
fissure	**FISH**-ur		Latin *slit*	Deep furrow or cleft
fistula	**FIS**-tyu-lah		Latin *pipe, tube*	Abnormal passage
hemorrhoid hemorrhoids (pl) hemorrhoidectomy	**HEM**-oh-royd **HEM**-oh-roy-**DEK**-toh-me	S/ R/CF S/	**-rrhoid** *flow* **hem/o-** *blood* **-ectomy** *excision*	Dilated rectal vein producing painful anal swelling Surgical removal of hemorrhoids
intussusception	**IN**-tuss-sus-**SEP**-shun	S/ P/ R/	**-ion** *action* **intus-** *within* **-suscept-** *to take up*	The slipping of one part of bowel inside another to cause obstruction
lumen	**LOO**-men		Latin *light, window*	The interior space of a tubelike structure
McBurney point	mack-**BUR**-nee POYNT		Charles McBurney, 1845–1913, New York surgeon	One-third the distance from the anterior superior iliac spine to the umbilicus
metastasis metastases (pl)	meh-**TAS**-tah-sis meh-**TAS**-tah-seez	P/ R/	**meta-** *beyond* **-stasis** *placement*	Spread of a disease from one part of the body to another
peritoneum peritoneal (adj) peritonitis	per-ih-toh-**NEE**-um **PER**-ih-toh-**NEE**-al **PER**-ih-toh-**NIE**-tis	S/ R/CF S/ S/	**-um** *tissue* **periton/e-** *stretch over* **-al** *pertaining to* **-itis** *inflammation*	Membrane that lines the abdominal cavity Pertaining to the peritoneum Inflammation of the peritoneum
polyp polyposis polypectomy	**POL**-ip pol-ih-**POH**-sis pol-ip-**ECK**-toh-mee	S/ R/ S/	Latin *foot, stalk* **-osis** *condition* **polyp-** *polyp* **-ectomy** *excision*	Mass of tissue that projects into the lumen of a hollow organ Presence of several polyps Excision or removal of a polyp
precancerous	pree-**KAN**-sir-us	S/ P/ R/	**-ous** *pertaining to* **pre-** *before* **-cancer-** *cancer*	Lesion from which a cancer can develop
proctitis	prok-**TIE**-tis	S/ R/	**-itis** *inflammation* **proct-** *anus and rectum*	Inflammation of the lining of the rectum
stool	STOOL		Old English *chair, seat*	Matter expelled from a bowel movement
ulcerative	**UL**-sir-ah-tiv	S/ R/	**-ative** *quality of* **ulcer-** *a sore*	Marked by an ulcer or ulcers

Disorders of the Liver

Hepatitis is an inflammation of the liver causing jaundice. Viral hepatitis is the most common cause of hepatitis and is related to three major types of virus:

1. **Hepatitis A virus (HAV)** is highly contagious and causes a mild to severe infection. It is transmitted by the **fecal-oral route** through contaminated food. It frequently occurs in schools, camps, and institutions.

2. **Hepatitis B virus (HBV)** is transmitted through contact with blood, semen, vaginal secretions, saliva, or a needle prick and through sharing contaminated needles. Some people become chronic carriers of the virus in their blood.

3. **Hepatitis C virus (HCV)** is transmitted by blood-to-blood contact; it is often asymptomatic. It can be cured in 51% of patients with antiviral treatment but can progress to chronic hepatitis and cirrhosis.

4. **Hepatitis D virus (HDV)** can occur only in the presence of HBV. In 2017 outbreaks of HDV infection have been seen in homeless populations.

5. **Hepatitis E** is similar to hepatitis A and occurs mostly in underdeveloped countries.

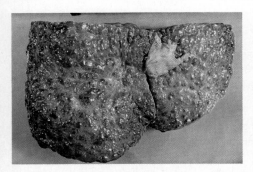

▲ **Figure 5.33** Cirrhosis of liver. Biophoto
Associates/Science Source

Other causes of hepatitis include abuse of alcohol; autoimmune hepatitis; metabolic disorders such as **Wilson disease** and diabetes mellitus; other viruses, such as mononucleosis and cytomegalovirus; and drugs such as acetaminophen.

Symptoms include nausea, vomiting and loss of appetite, joint pain, and sore muscles. Signs include jaundice, fever, and tenderness in the right upper quadrant of the abdomen.

Chronic hepatitis occurs when the acute hepatitis is not healed after 6 months. It progresses slowly, can last for years, and is difficult to treat.

Cirrhosis of the liver is a chronic, irreversible disease, replacing normal liver cells with hard, fibrous scar tissue *(Figure 5.33)*. It is the seventh leading cause of death in the United States. The most common cause of **cirrhosis** is alcoholism. In cirrhosis, the damage sustained to the liver is irreversible, and there is no known cure. Treatment is symptomatic. When cirrhosis blocks the flow of blood in the portal vein, the back-pressure produces **ascites,** an accumulation of fluid in the abdominal cavity.

Cancer of the liver as a primary cancer typically arises in patients with chronic liver disease, usually from HBV infection. A more common form of liver cancer is secondary deposits of metastases from a primary cancer in the colon, lung, breast, or prostate.

Hemochromatosis is caused by the absorption of too much iron, which is stored throughout the body, mostly in the liver, and can lead to liver failure.

Hyperbilirubinemia, too much bilirubin in the blood, is caused when red cells break down, producing the yellow pigment bilirubin. Newborn babies cannot get rid of the bilirubin easily and it can build up in the blood and other tissues, producing a yellow discoloration of the skin and eyes called **jaundice.** About 60% of term newborns and 80% of premature babies develop hyperbilirubinemia. There are several causes of this condition:

- **Physiologic jaundice,** a "normal" response in the first few days of life.

- **Breast milk jaundice,** which occurs in about 2% of breastfed babies, peaking around 2 weeks of age and persisting up to 3 to 12 weeks. No treatment is necessary.

- **Breast feeding failure jaundice,** when there is difficulty establishing breast feeding, resulting in dehydration, decreased urine production, and build up of bilirubin in the blood and tissues. It goes away once breast feeding is established.

- **Hemolytic disease of the newborn (Rh disease)** *(see Chapter 11)* produces jaundice as too many red blood cells (**RBCs**) break down and release bilirubin to cause jaundice.

- **Inadequate liver function** due to infection or other rare problems, which can also produce jaundice.

Wilson disease is the retention of too much copper in the liver and also can lead to liver failure.

Disorders of the Gallbladder

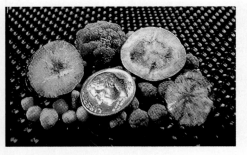

▲ **Figure 5.34** Gallstones. Southern Illinois
University/Science Source

Gallstones (cholelithiasis) can form in the gallbladder from excess cholesterol, bile salts, and bile pigment *(Figure 5.34)*. The stones can vary in size and number. Risk factors are **obesity,** high-cholesterol diets, multiple pregnancies, and rapid weight loss. Mrs. Jacobs presented in the Emergency Department with the classic gallstone symptoms of severe waves of right upper quadrant pain (**biliary colic**), nausea, and vomiting. **Cholelithotomy** is the operative removal of one or more gallstones. If small stones become impacted in the common bile duct, this is called **choledocholithiasis.** This can cause biliary colic and jaundice (see the following).

Cholecystitis is an acute or chronic inflammation of the gallbladder usually associated with cholelithiasis and obstruction of the cystic duct with a stone. Acute colicky pain in the right upper quadrant with nausea and vomiting are followed by jaundice, dark urine (because bilirubin backs up into the blood and is excreted by the kidneys), and pale-colored stools (because bilirubin cannot get into the duodenum).

Icterus (jaundice) is a symptom of many different diseases in the biliary tract and liver. It is a yellow discoloration of the skin and sclera of the eyes *(see Chapter 16)* caused by deposits of bilirubin just below the outer layers of the skin. Bilirubin is a breakdown product of hemoglobin that occurs as old **red blood cells (RBCs)** are destroyed. Bilirubin is removed from the bloodstream by the liver and excreted in bile.

Jaundice occurs when there is an increased concentration of bilirubin circulating in the bloodstream. There are three categories of disease that cause jaundice:

1. **Obstructive jaundice** is a result of the blockage of bile between the liver and the duodenum, usually due to gallstones in the common bile duct or to a carcinoma of the head of the pancreas imping ing on the common duct.

2. **Hemolytic jaundice** results from an accelerated destruction of RBCs such that the liver cannot remove the excess bilirubin fast enough. This is most often seen in newborn infants with hemolytic jaundice due to blood group incompatibility between mother and infant.

3. **Hepatocellular jaundice** occurs when an infection or poison injures the liver cells, preventing the removal of bilirubin from the blood. This occurs in viral hepatitis.

Disorders of the Pancreas

Pancreatitis is inflammation of the pancreas. The acute disease ranges from a mild, self-limiting episode to an acute life-threatening emergency with severe abdominal pain, nausea, vomiting, and a rapid fall in blood pressure. In the **chronic** form, there is a progressive destruction of pancreatic tissue leading to **malabsorption** and **diabetes.** Factors in the development of pancreatitis are biliary tract disease, gallstones, and alcoholism. The pancreatic enzyme trypsin builds up and digests parts of the pancreas, causing the intense pain.

Pancreatic cancer is the fourth-leading cause of cancer-related death. It occurs twice as often in males as in females. Incidence peaks in the 40- to 60-year-old range. The cancer can be asymptomatic in its early stages and is difficult to detect. The 5-year survival rate after diagnosis is 5–10%. The treatment is surgical resection of the pancreas.

Diabetes, in which endocrine insulin production is shut down or severely reduced or its effects are resisted by body cells, is discussed in *Chapter 17.*

Cystic fibrosis (CF) is an inherited disease that becomes apparent in infancy or childhood. It affects exocrine glands in multiple body systems, including the respiratory and digestive systems.

Word Analysis and Definition: Disorders of the Liver, Gallbladder, and Pancreas

S = Suffix   P = Prefix   R = Root   R/CF = Combining Form

WORD	PRONUNCIATION		ELEMENTS	DEFINITION
ascites	ah-**SIGH**-teez	S/ R/	-ites *associated with* asc- *belly*	Accumulation of fluid in the abdominal cavity
biliary colic	**BILL**-ee-air-ee**KOL**-ik	S/ R/CF S/ R/	-ary *pertaining to* bil/i- *bile* -ic *pertaining to* col- *colon*	Severe waves of pain in the right upper quadrant due to a gallstone blocking the bile duct
cholecystitis	**KOH**-leh-sis-**TIE**-tis	S/ R/CF R/	-itis *inflammation* chol/e *bile* -cyst- *bladder*	Inflammation of the gallbladder
choledocholithiasis	koh-leh-**DOH**-koh-lih-**THIGH**-ah-sis	S/ R/CF R/	-iasis *condition* choledoch/o- *common bile duct* -lith- *stone*	Presence of a gallstone(s) in the common bile duct
cholelithiasis	**KOH**-leh-lih-**THIGH**-ah-sis	S/ R/CF	-iasis *condition* chol/e- *bile*	Condition of having bile stones (gallstones)
cirrhosis	sir-**ROH**-sis	S/ R/	-osis *condition* cirrh- *yellow*	Extensive fibrotic liver disease
hemochromatosis	**HEE**-moh-kroh-mah-**TOH**-sis	S/ R/CF R/	-osis *condition* hem/o- *blood* -chromat- *color*	Dangerously high levels of iron in the body with deposition of iron pigments in tissues
hepatitis	hep-ah-**TIE**-tis	S/ R/	-itis *inflammation* hepat- *liver*	Inflammation of the liver
hyperbilirubinemia	**HIGH**-per-**BILL**-ee-**RU**-bin-**EE**-mee-ah	S/ P/ R/	-emia *blood condition* hyper- *above* -bilirubin- *bilirubin*	High level of bilirubin in the blood
jaundice	**JAWN**-dis		French *yellow*	Yellow staining of tissues with bile pigments, including bilirubin
Wilson disease			Samuel Alexander Kinnier Wilson, 1878–1937, British neurologist	Genetic disorder in which copper accumulates in the body, which can lead to liver failure

A. Abbreviations used in general disorders of the gastrointestinal system. *Healthcare providers often use abbreviations when communicating verbally and in writing. Fill in the blank with the correct abbreviation from the provided word bank.* **LO 5.6, 5.9**

IBD   IBS   GI

1. The patient has been diagnosed with ulcerative colitis, and therefore has a form of _____.

2. A problem of the digestive tract would be considered to be a _____ disorder.

3. A patient complaining of unpredictable bouts of diarrhea that had no known cause was diagnosed with _____.

B. Describe disorders of the gastrointestinal system. *Determine if the statements are accurate. Choose T if the statement is true, choose F if the statement is false.* **LO 5.6**

1. A food allergy involves the immune system.	T	F
2. A lack of a digestive enzyme causes a food allergy.	T	F
3. Melena is a sign of active bleeding.	T	F
4. Aging has the least effect on the digestive system compared to the other body systems.	T	F
5. Hematochezia is a sign of active bleeding.	T	F

C. Enter the correct suffix to complete the medical terms. *Fill in the blanks.* **LO 5.2, 5.6**

1. Inflammation of the gums   gingiv/_____

2. Specialized branch of dentistry   periodont/_____

3. Painful, burning tongue   glosso/_____

4. Inflammation around a tooth   periodont/_____

5. Bad breath   halit/_____

6. Purulent discharge   pyo/_____

7. Precancerous white patches   leukoplak/_____

D. Some of the terms in this chapter are particularly hard to spell and pronounce. *Select the correct spelling for the medical term(s) that complete each sentence.* **LO 5.1, 5.6, 5.7**

1. (Hyatus/Hiatus) is the Latin word for *opening* and is the opening through the diaphragm for the (esophagis/esophagus).

2. The (eppiglotis/epiglottis) is a leaf-shaped plate of cartilage that acts to cover the opening of the (larynix/larynx) during deglutition.

3. The uvula covers the (nasopharynx/nasopharnyx) during (deglutition/degluition).

4. The cardiac (sphinter/sphincter) is a circular muscle that opens to allow the bolus into the (stomech/stomach).

E. Deconstruct the following medical terms into basic elements. *The definitions of the elements will help you understand the meaning of the term. Select the correct answer that completes each statement.* **LO 5.2, 5.6**

1. The meaning of the prefix in the medical term **dyspepsia** is:

   a. digestion   c. difficult

   b. condition   d. stomach

2. The meaning of the root in the medical term **peptic** is:

   a. pump   c. ulcer

   b. digestion   d. digest

3. The meaning of the suffix in the medical term **perforation** is:

   a. action   c. pertaining to

   b. condition   d. inflammation

4. The meaning of the root in the medical term **anorexia** is:

   a. digestion   c. without

   b. stomach   d. appetite

F. Given the description of a disorder of the stomach, give the condition. *Fill in the blank.* **LO 5.2, 5.3, 5.9**

1. This condition can be caused by *Helicobacter pylori*: _____ ulcer

2. Inflammation of the lining of the stomach: _____

3. Regurgitation of the stomach contents back into the esophagus (write the abbreviation): _____

G. Match the disorder of the small intestine in column one with the statement describing it in column two. **LO 5.6**

_____ 1. ileus

_____ 2. constipation

_____ 3. celiac disease

_____ 4. *Giardia lamblia*

_____ 5. intussusception

a. Parasite that causes gastroenteritis

b. Part of the small intestine slides into a neighboring part

c. Disruption of the normal peristalsis of the small intestine

d. Hard, infrequent bowel movements

e. Allergy to gluten

H. Use your knowledge of the small intestine and answer the questions. *Choose T if the statement is true. Choose F if the statement is false.* **LO 5.6**

1. People with constipation complain of frequent trips to the bathroom to pass soft stools.　　　　T　　　F

2. Gastroenteritis can result in acute vomiting and diarrhea.　　　　T　　　F

3. Bleeding from the small intestine is usually from an infection.　　　　T　　　F

4. Cancer of the small intestine is a common occurrence.　　　　T　　　F

5. Risk factors for paralytic ileus include GI surgery, diabetic ketoacidosis, and medicines such as opiates.　　　　T　　　F

I. In this exercise, the root or combining form remains the same, but the addition of other elements will construct entirely different medical terms. *Use this group of elements, in addition to* **chol/e,** *to form the medical terms that are defined. Some elements you will use more than once; some elements you will not use at all. Fill in the blanks.* **LO 5.1, 5.2, 5.3, 5.6**

1. The element *chol/e* means _____.

2. The element *choledoch/o* means _____.

Add these elements to **chol/e** *or* **choledoch/o** *to form the medical terms defined as follows:*

lith	lysis	iasis	graphy	osis	cyst
kinin	nephr/o	cyst/o	hemat/o	itis	

3. Condition of gallstones in the common bile duct　_____

4. Condition of having bile stones (gallstones)　_____

5. Inflammation of the gallbladder　_____

J. Define the disorders of the pancreas. *Match the disorder of the pancreas with its correct description.* **LO 5.6**

_____ 1. cystic fibrosis

_____ 2. pancreatitis

_____ 3. diabetes

a. lack of insulin production

b. genetic condition affecting the pancreas

c. can be caused by biliary disease, gallstones, or alcholism

K. The suffix is your first clue to the meaning of a word. *Match the word element in the first column with its correct meaning in the second column. Some answers you will use twice because more than one suffix can have the same meaning. One answer will not be used at all.* **LO 5.2**

_____ **1.** -um

_____ **2.** -ous

_____ **3.** -osis

_____ **4.** -ion

_____ **5.** -itis

_____ **6.** -rrhoid

_____ **7.** -ative

_____ **8.** -al

_____ **9.** -ectomy

a. flow

b. action

c. inflammation

d. tissue

e. pertaining to

f. condition

g. excision

h. quality of

i. study of

Section 5.6 Procedures and Pharmacology of the Digestive System

Diagnostic Procedures

Nasogastric aspiration and lavage are used to detect upper GI bleeding. The presence of bright red blood in the lavage material indicates active upper GI bleeding; "coffee grounds" indicate the bleeding has slowed or stopped.

Enteroscopy uses an oral, flexible **endoscope** containing light-transmitting fibers or a video transmitter to visualize and biopsy tumors and ulcers and to control bleeding from the esophagus, stomach, and duodenum. Visualization of the stomach is called **gastroscopy;** visualization of the esophagus, stomach, and duodenum is called **panendoscopy.**

Capsule endoscopy enables examination of the entire small intestine by ingesting a pill-sized video capsule with its own camera and light source that sends images to a data recorder worn on the patient's belt.

Double balloon endoscopy uses two balloons at the tip of the endoscope that are inflated sequentially to move the endoscope further into the small intestine than with a usual endoscope.

Angiography uses injected dye to highlight blood vessels and is used to detect the site of bleeding in the GI tract.

In a **digital rectal examination (DRE)** the physician palpates the rectum and prostate gland with a gloved, lubricated index finger to determine the presence of lesions.

Proctoscopy is procedure performed with a proctoscope that allows for the visual examination of the anus, rectum and sigmoid colon to look for diseases, causes of rectal bleeding or check on abnormal results seen during a barium enema.

Anoscopy is an examination of the anus and lower rectum using a rigid instrument. Flexible **sigmoidoscopy** examines the rectum and sigmoid colon and **flexible colonoscopy** examines the whole length of the colon.

In a **barium swallow,** the patient ingests barium sulfate, a contrast material, to show details of the pharynx and esophagus on x-ray.

In a **barium meal,** barium sulfate is used to study the stomach and duodenum on x-ray (*Figure 5.35*). They are less accurate than enteroscopy at identifying bleeding lesions.

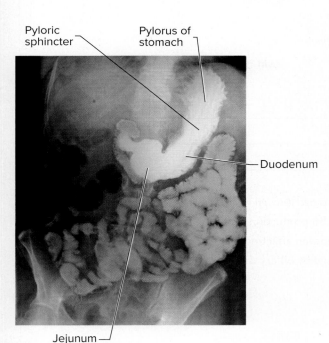

Pyloric sphincter

Pylorus of stomach

Duodenum

Jejunum

▲ **Figure 5.35** **Barium meal showing pylorus and duodenum.** Scott Camazine/Science Source

Barium enema uses the contrast material barium sulfate, which is injected into the large intestine as an enema and x-ray films are taken (*Figure 5.36*).

Fecal occult blood test (Hemoccult) is used to detect the presence in the stool of blood not visible to the naked eye. It is a good first screening test for cancer of the large intestine.

Pancreas endoscopic ultrasound (EUS) is a type of endoscopic examination that enables detailed imaging and analysis of the pancreas. A thin tube tipped with an ultrasound probe is inserted through the mouth down into the stomach and the first part of the small intestine. The probe emits sound waves that bounce off surrounding structures, and these sound waves are recaptured by the probe and converted to black and white images that can be interpreted by the physician. EUS is of great value in assessing pancreatic tumors and cysts and acute and chronic pancreatitis.

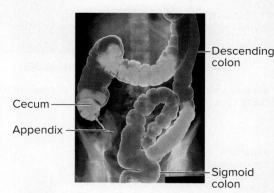

Descending colon

Cecum

Appendix

Sigmoid colon

▲ **Figure 5.36** **Barium enema of the large intestine.** CNRI/Science Source

Liver Function Tests

Liver function tests (LFTs) are a group of tests to show how well your liver is functioning. They are divided into four categories:

1. **Measuring liver proteins in blood serum**

   - Measuring proteins, albumin, and globulin *(see Chapter 7)*, which are low when there is liver damage.

2. **Measuring liver enzymes in blood serum**

   - Measuring enzymes made in the liver, known as **transaminases**, including **alanine aminotransferase (ALT**; also known as **serum glutamic-pyruvic transaminase,** or SGPT) and **aspartate aminotransferase (AST**; also known as **serum glutamic oxaloacetic acid transaminase,** or SGOT). Elevated levels of these enzymes in the blood indicate liver damage.

3. **Measuring cholestatic liver enzymes in the blood serum**

   - Measuring **alkaline phosphatase (ALP)**, which metabolizes phosphorus and makes energy available for the body. Elevated blood levels are found in liver and biliary tract disorders.

   - Measuring **gamma-glutamyl transpeptidase (GGT)**, which is elevated in liver disease.

4. **Measuring bilirubin in the bloodstream**

   - **Bilirubin** is formed in the liver from hemoglobin and secreted into the biliary system. If the liver is damaged, bilirubin can leak out into the bloodstream, producing elevated levels and jaundice.

S = Suffix   P = Prefix   R = Root   R/CF = Combining Form

WORD	PRONUNCIATION	ELEMENTS		DEFINITION
alanine aminotransfer (ALT)	AL-ah-neen ah-MEE-noh-TRANS-fer-aze	S/ R/CF R/ R/	alanine *an amino acid* -ase *enzyme* amin/o- *nitrogen compound* -transfer- *carry*	Enzymes that are found in liver cells and leak out into the bloodstream when the cells are damaged, enabling liver damage to be diagnosed
aspartate aminotransferase (AST)	as-PAR-tate	R/	aspartate *an amino acid*	A salt of aspartic acid
angiography	an-jee-OG-rah-fee	S/ R/CF	-graphy *process of recording* angio- *blood vessel*	Process of recording the image of blood vessels after injection of contrast material
anoscopy	A-nos-koh-pee	S/ R/CF	-scopy *to examine* an/o- *anus*	Endoscopic examination of the anus
aspiration	AS-pih-RAY-shun	S/ R/CF	-ion *process* aspirat- *to breathe on*	Removal by suction of fluid or gas from a body cavity
cholangiography	KOH-lan-jee-OG-rah-fee	S/ R/ R/CF	-graphy *process of recording* chol- *bile* -angi/o- *blood vessel, lymph vessel*	X-ray of the bile ducts after injection or ingestion of a contrast medium
colonoscopy	koh-lon-OSS-koh-pee	S/ R/CF	-scopy *to examine* colon/o- *colon*	Endoscopic examination of the colon
digital	DIJ-ih-tal	S/ R/	-al *pertaining to* digit- *finger or toe*	Pertaining to a finger or toe
endoscope	EN-doh-skope	P/ S/	endo- *within, inside* -scope *instrument for viewing*	Instrument to examine the inside of a tubular or hollow organ
endoscopic (adj) endoscopy	EN-doh-SKOP-ik en-DOS-koh-pee	S/ S/	-ic *pertaining to* -scopy *to examine*	Pertaining to the use of an endoscope The use of an endoscope
enema	EN-eh-mah		Greek *injection*	An injection of fluid into the rectum
enteroscopy	en-ter-OSS-koh-pee	S/ R/CF	-scopy *to examine, to view* enter/o- *intestine*	The examination of the lining of the digestive tract
gastroscope	GAS-troh-skope	S/	-scope *instrument for viewing*	Instrument to view the inside of the stomach
gastroscopy	gas-TROS-koh-pee	R/CF S/	gastr/o- *stomach* -scopy *to examine*	Endoscopic examination of the stomach
ileoscopy	ill-ee-OS-koh-pee	S/ R/CF	-scopy *to examine* ile/o- *ileum*	Endoscopic examination of the ileum
lavage	lah-VAHZH		Latin *to wash*	Washing out of a hollow cavity, tube, or organ
pancreatography	PAN-kree-ah-TOG-raff-ee	S/ R/CF	-graphy *process of recording* pancreat/o- *pancreas*	Process of recording the structure of the pancreas
panendoscopy	pan-en-DOS-koh-pee	S/ P/ P/	-scopy *to examine* pan- *all* -endo- *within, inside*	Endoscopic examination of the esophagus, stomach and duodenum
phosphatase	FOS-fah-tase	S/ R/	-ase *enzyme* phosphat- *phosphorus*	Enzyme that liberates phosphorus
proctoscopy	prok-TOSS-koh-pee	S/ R/CF	-scopy *to examine* proct/o- *anus and rectum*	Examination of the inside of the anus and the rectum by proctoscope or rectoscope
sigmoidoscopy	sig-moi-DOS-koh-pee	S/ R/CF	-scopy *to examine* sigmoid/o- *sigmoid colon*	Endoscopic examination of the sigmoid colon
ultrasound	UL-trah-sownd	P/ R/	ultra- *higher* -sound *noise*	Very-high-frequency sound waves

Therapeutic Procedures

Many of the diagnostic procedures in the previous section can also be used as therapeutic procedures. For example, endoscopy can be used to remove polyps, biopsy suspicious lesions, stop bleeding, and be used as screening procedures for cancer.

Laparoscopy uses a thin, lighted tube inserted through an **incision** in the abdominal wall to examine abdominal and pelvic organs. Biopsy samples can be taken through the **laparoscope,** and in many cases, surgery can be performed instead of using a much larger incision. Laparoscopy is done to check for and remove abnormal tumors; fix **hiatal** and **inguinal hernias;** and perform several procedures on the organs of the digestive system.

An **appendectomy** completely removes the appendix. This procedure is performed on patients with acute appendicitis.

Organs that can be fully or partially resected are the liver (**lobectomy**), esophagus (**esophagectomy**), stomach (**gastrectomy**), duodenum (**duodenectomy**), and colon (**colectomy**).

Intestinal resections are used to surgically remove diseased portions of the intestine. The remaining portions of the intestine can be joined back together through an **anastomosis** *(Figure 5.37a)*. If there is insufficient bowel remaining for an anastomosis, an **ostomy** *(Figure 5.37b)* can be performed, where the end of the bowel opens onto the skin at a **stoma. Ileostomy** and **colostomy** are two such procedures.

Bariatric surgeries are used to help patients lose weight by surgically separating the stomach into smaller section which decreases the amount of food it takes for a patient to fill full. The gastric bypass procedure, also called **Roux-en-Y,** separates the stomach in to a small and a large section. The smaller section is connected a distal section of intestine, bypassing most of the stomach and a section of the small intestine while bile flows down another section of intestine *(Figure 5.38)*. The **sleeve gastrectomy** procedure removes the larger lower section of the stomach leaving a smaller-sized stomach.

A **cholelithotomy** is the operative removal of one or more gallstones. A **cholecystectomy** completely removes the gall bladder to treat complications of the gallbladder such as cholelithiasis and choledocholithiasis.

Endoscopic retrograde cholangiopancreatography (ERCP) is used to diagnose and treat problems in the biliary ductal system. Through an endoscope, the physician can see the inside of the duodenum and inject radiographic contrast dye into the biliary tract ducts. Gallstones and cancer can be treated with this technique.

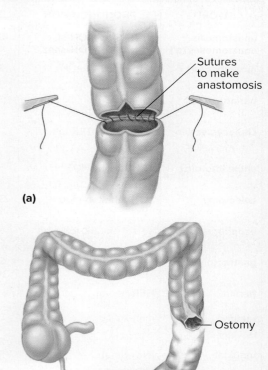

(a)

Sutures to make anastomosis

Ostomy

(b)

▲ **Figure 5.37** Intestinal resections.

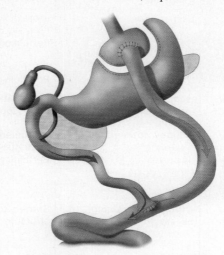

▲ **Figure 5.38** Roux-en-Y Surgery.
Monica Schroeder/Science Source

WORD	PRONUNCIATION	ELEMENTS		DEFINITION
anastomosis anastomoses (pl)	ah-**NAS**-to-**MOH**-sis ah-**NAS**-to-**MOH**-seez	S/ R/	-osis *condition* anastom- *join together*	A surgically made union between two tubular structures
appendectomy	ah-pen-**DEK**-toh-mee	S/ R/	-ectomy *surgical excision* append- *appendix*	Surgical removal of the appendix
bariatric	bar-ee-**AT**-rik	S/ R/	-atric *treatment* bari- *weight*	Treatment of obesity
cholecystectomy	**KOH**-leh-sis-**TEK**-toh-mee	S/ R/CF R/	-ectomy *surgical excision* chol/e- *bile* -cyst- *bladder*	Surgical removal of the gallbladder
cholelithotomy	**KOH**-leh-lih-**THOT**-oh-mee	S/ R/	-otomy *surgical incision* -lith- *stone*	Surgical incision to remove a gallstone(s)
colectomy	**KOH**-lehk-toh-mee	S/ R/	-ectomy *surgical excision* col- *colon*	Surgical removal of all or part of the colon
esophagectomy	ee-sof-ah-**JEK**-toh-mee	S/ R/	-ectomy *surgical excision* esophag- *esophagus*	Surgical removal of all or part of the esophagus
gastrectomy	gas-**TREK**-toh-mee	S/ R/	-ectomy *surgical excision* gastr- *stomach*	Surgical removal of all or part of the stomach
hernia	**HER**-nee-ah		Latin *rupture*	Protrusion of a structure through the tissue that normally contains it
hiatal	high-**AY**-tal	S/ R/	-al *pertaining to* hiat- *aperture*	Pertaining to an opening through a structure
inguinal	**IN**-gwin-al	S/ R/	-al *pertaining to* inguin- *groin*	Pertaining to the groin
laparoscopy	lap-ah-**ROS**-koh-pee	S/ R/CF	-scopy *to view* lapar/o- *abdomen in general*	Examination of the contents of the abdomen using an endoscope
laparoscope	**LAP**-ah-roh-skope	S/	-scope *instrument for viewing*	Instrument (endoscope) used for viewing the abdominal contents
laparoscopic (adj)	**LAP**-ah-rah-**SKOP**-ik	S/	-ic *pertaining to*	Pertaining to laparoscopy
lobectomy	low-**BEK**-toh-mee	S/ R/	-ectomy *removal* lob- *lobe*	Surgical removal of a lobe
ostomy (*Note:* an "s" is removed for the purpose of spelling)	**OS**-toh-mee	S/ R/	-stomy *new opening* os- *mouth*	Surgery to create an artificial opening into a tubular structure
colostomy	ko-**LOS**-toh-mee	R/	col- *colon*	Artificial opening from the colon to the outside of the body
ileostomy	ill-ee-**OS**-toh-mee	R/	ile- *ileum*	Artificial opening from the ileum to the outside of the body
resection	ree-**SEK**-shun	S/ P/	-ion *action, condition* re- *back*	Removal of a specific part of an organ or structure
resect (verb)		R/	-sect- *cut off*	
retrograde	**RET**-roh-grade	P/ R/	retro- *backward* -grade *going*	Reversal of a normal flow
Roux-en-Y	**ROO**-on-**Y**		César Roux, a Swiss surgeon, 1857–1934	Surgical procedure to reduce the size of the stomach
stoma	**STOH**-mah		Greek *mouth*	Artificial opening

Gastrointestinal Drugs
Drugs to Treat Excess Gastric Acid

Antacids, which are taken orally, neutralize gastric acid and relieve heartburn and acid indigestion. Examples of antacids include:

- aluminum hydroxide and magnesium hydroxide (*Maalox, Mylanta*)
- magnesium hydroxide (*Milk of Magnesia*)
- calcium carbonate (*Tums, Rolaids*)

Histamine-2 receptor antagonists (H$_2$-blockers) block signals that tell the stomach cells to produce acid. They are used to treat gastroesophageal reflux (GERD) and esophagitis. Examples include:

- cimetidine (*Tagamet*)
- famotidine (*Pepcid*)
- ranitidine (*Zantac*)
- nizatidine

Proton pump inhibitors (PPIs) suppress gastric acid secretion in the lining of the stomach by blocking the secretion of gastric acid from the cells into the lumen of the stomach. Examples include:

- omeprazole (*Prilosec*)
- lansoprazole (*Prevacid*)
- esomeprazole (*Nexium*)

A new form of PPI called imidazopyridine (*Tenatoprazole*) appears to be extremely effective in reducing gastric acid.

Misoprostol (*Cytotec*) inhibits the secretion of gastric acid and is approved for the prevention of nonsteroidal anti-inflammatory drug (NSAID)–induced gastric acid.

Sucralfate (*Carafate*) reacts with gastric acid (hydrogen chloride **[HCl]**) to form a paste that binds to stomach mucosal cells and inhibits the diffusion of acid into the stomach lumen. It also forms a protective barrier on the surface of an ulcer. Its main use is in the **prophylaxis** of stress ulcers.

Anti–*H. pylori* therapy for the treatment of peptic ulcer and chronic gastritis is given with a combination of two antibiotics (e.g., amoxicillin [generic] and clarithromycin [generic]) and a proton pump inhibitor.

Drugs to Treat Nausea and Vomiting

Antiemetics, drugs that are effective against vomiting and nausea, are used to treat motion sickness and the side effects of opioid analgesics, general anesthetics, and chemotherapy. The types of antiemetics include:

- **Serotonin antagonists,** which block serotonin receptors in the central nervous system and GI tract. They are used to treat postoperative and chemotherapy nausea and vomiting. Examples include dolasetron (*Anzemet*), granisetron, and ondansetron (*Zofran*).
- **Dopamine antagonists,** which act in the brain. They are inexpensive but have an extensive side-effect profile and have been replaced by serotonin antagonists. Examples include chlorpromazine and prochlorperazine.
- **Antihistamines,** which are used to treat motion sickness, morning sickness in pregnancy, and opioid nausea. Examples include diphenhydramine (*Benadryl*) and promethazine (*Phenergan*).
- **Cannabinoids,** which are used in patients with **cachexia** or who are unresponsive to other antiemetics. Examples include cannabis (medical marijuana) and dronabinol (*Marinol*).

Drugs to Treat Constipation

Laxative drugs are used to treat chronic constipation:

- If increased water and fiber are unsuccessful, OTC forms of magnesium hydroxide are the first-line agents to be used.
- Linaclotide (*Linzess*) and lubiprostone (*Amitiza*) are indicated for the treatment of constipation due to irritable bowel syndrome (IBS-C). It acts on the epithelial cells of the GI tract to produce a chloride-rich fluid that softens the stool and increases bowel **motility.**

Drugs to Treat Diarrhea

Antidiarrheal drugs are widely available OTC. Examples include loperamide (*Imodium A-D, Maalox*), which reduces bowel motility; bismuth subsalicylate (*Pepto-Bismol*), which decreases the secretion of fluid into the intestine; and attapulgite (*Kaopectate*), which pulls diarrhea-causing substances away from the GI tract; as well as enzymes and nutrients. A combination of diphenyloxylate and atropine (*Lomotil*), a Schedule V drug, reduces bowel motility. Eluxadoline (*Viberzi*) slows is indicated in the treatment of diarrhea associated with IBS (IBS-D). Rifaximin (*Xifaxan*) is an antibiotic to treat traveler's diarrhea and IBS-D.

Word Analysis and Definition: Gastrointestinal Drugs

WORD	PRONUNCIATION	ELEMENTS		DEFINITION
antacid (*Note:* anti is shortened to ant-)	ant-**ASS**-id	P/ R/	ant- *against* -acid acid	Agent that neutralizes acidity
antidiarrheal	**AN**-tee-die-ah-**REE**-al	S/ P/ P/ S/	-al *pertaining to* anti- *against* -dia- *complete, through* -rrhea *flow, discharge*	Drug that prevents abnormally frequent and loose stools
antiemetic	**AN**-tee-eh-**MEH**-tik	P/ R/	anti- *against* -emetic *causing vomiting*	Agent that prevents vomiting
antihistamine	an-tee-**HISS**-tah-meen	P/ R/ R/CF	anti- *against* -hist- *tissue* -amine *nitrogen compound*	Drug that can be used to treat allergic symptoms or prevent vomiting
cachexia	kah-**KEK**-see-ah	P/ R/	cach- *bad* -exia *condition of body*	A general weight loss and wasting of the body
cannabinoid	can-**AH**-bi-noyd	S/ R/	-oid *resembling* cannabin- *hemp*	A group of chemical compounds, some of which increase appetite and others treat nausea and vomiting
laxative	**LAK**-sah-tiv	S/ R/CF	-tive *pertaining to* lax/a- *looseness*	An oral agent that promotes the expulsion of feces
motility	moh-**TILL**-ih-tee	S/ R/	-ility *condition, state of* mot- *to move*	The ability for spontaneous movement
prophylaxis	pro-fih-**LAX**-is		Greek *to guard before*	Prevention of a disease
proton pump inhibitor (PPI)	**PROH**-ton PUMP in-**HIB**-ih-tor	R/ R/ S/ R/	proton *first* pump *pump* -or *a doer* inhibit- *repress*	Agent that blocks production of gastric acid

Check Point Section 5.6

A. Notice that some terms are formed with only a prefix and a root, while others are formed with a root and a suffix. *The only element that needs to be present in every term is a root or combining form.* *The definitions for the terms are given, as well as the element placement in the term. Write the correct element on each blank.* **LO 5.2, 5.6**

1. Abnormally frequent and loose stools _____ /_____

2. Infrequent bowel movements _____ /_____

3. Enzyme that breaks down lactose _____ /_____

4. Relating to the abdominal cavity _____ /_____

5. Disease with fever, diarrhea, and bowel spasms _____ /_____

B. Utilize the correct terms for patient documentation. *When communicating verbally and in writing, it is crucial to use correct medical terminology. Using the terms provided below, fill in the blanks with the correct term. Not all terms will be used.* **LO 5.5, 5.8**

endoscopy   proctoscopy   colonoscopy   enema   gastroenterologist   sigmoidoscopy   barium   angiography

A patient was complaining of blood in his stool. The physician requested that you schedule a **(1)**_____ **(2)**_____ with the radiology department. One week later, the test results came back and were inconclusive. The physician decided that further tests were needed, and therefore wished to view the inside of the intestines. Because the physician believed the source of the bleeding was in the large intestine, she ordered a **(3)**_____. The medical assistant called the hospital's **(4)**_____ department.

C. Use word elements to build medical terms. Many therapeutic procedures differ by one word element. *Given the definition of the procedure, provide the correct word element to create the medical term. Fill in the blank.* **LO 5.2, 5.3, 5.7**

1. Surgical incision to remove a gallstone: cholelitho/_____

2. Surgical removal of the appendix: _____/ectomy

3. Surgery to create an opening from a tubular structure to the outside: _____/tomy

4. Surgical removal of the gallbladder: chole/_____/ectomy

5. Artificial opening from the ileum to the outside of the body: ile/_____/tomy

D. Deconstruct medical terms to determine their meanings. *By knowing the meaning of word elements, you can decipher the meaning of the medical term. Choose the correct answer for each question.* **LO 5.7, 5.9**

1. In the procedure ERCP, the "E" stands for

   a. enteric   **b.** echo   **c.** endoscopic   **d.** electrical

2. In the procedure of inserting a nasogastric tube, the practitioner inserts the tube through the

   a. nose   **b.** mouth   **c.** stomach   **d.** rectum

3. In the procedure ERCP, the "C" tells you that the organ being treated is the

   a. stomach   **b.** pancreas   **c.** biliary ducts   **d.** duodenum

4. In an anastomosis, the root means

   a. removal   **b.** creation of an opening   **c.** join together   **d.** incision

E. Read the statements carefully and match them with the right drugs. *Match the definition in the first column with the correct medication it is describing in the second column.* **LO 5.7**

_____	1. used to suppress gastric acid secretions	**a.** Maalox
_____	2. used to treat opioid nausea	**b.** Imodium
_____	3. neutralizes gastric acid and relieves heartburn	**c.** Tagamet
_____	4. used for treatment of postoperative nausea	**d.** Nexium
_____	5. antidiarrheal drug	**e.** Benadryl
_____	6. blocks production of stomach acid	**f.** Zofran

Table 5.2 Chapter 5 Abbreviations

Abbreviation	Meaning	Abbreviation	Meaning
ALP	alkaline phosphatase	HCV	hepatitis C virus
ALT	alanine aminotransferase (also known as SGPT)	HDV	hepatitis D virus
AST	aspartate aminotransferase (also known as SGOT)	HIV	human immunodeficiency virus
BM	bowel movement	HSV-1	herpes simplex virus, type 1
CDC	Centers for Disease Control and Prevention	IBD	inflammatory bowel disease
CF	cystic fibrosis	IBS	irritable bowel syndrome
CMA	Certified Medical Assistant	IgE	immunoglobulin E
ERCP	endoscopic retrograde cholangiopancreatography	LFT	liver function test
ESR	erythrocyte sedimentation rate	NSAIDs	nonsteroidal anti-inflammatory drugs
EUS	endoscopic ultrasound	PPI	proton pump inhibitor
GERD	gastroesophageal reflux disease	RBC	red blood cell
GGT	gamma-glutamyl transpeptidase	SGOT	serum glutamic oxaloacetic acid transaminase (also known as AST)
GI	gastrointestinal	SGPT	serum glutamic-pyruvic transaminase (also known as ALT)
H2-blocker	histamine-2 receptor antagonist	SSA	Sjögren syndrome antibody A
HAV	hepatitis A virus	SSB	Sjögren syndrome antibody B
HBV	hepatitis B virus	WBC	white blood cell
HCl	hydrochloric acid		

Table 5.3 Comparison of Selected Gastrointestinal Disorders—Signs, Symptoms, and Treatments

Disorder or Disease	Signs and Symptoms	Diagnostic Tests	Treatment
Appendicitis	Pain in right lower quadrant, vomiting	Rebound tenderness, ultrasonography	Laparoscopic or open surgery, antibiotics
Crohn's disease	abdominal pain, diarrhea, fatigue, weight loss	Capsule endoscopy	Corticosteroids, biologics
Dental caries	Tooth decay, tooth pain	X-ray	Dental filling or tooth removal by dentist
Dysphagia	Swallowing difficulty	Barium swallow, endoscopy	Treat the cause which may be an obstruction or muscular weakness, for example
Gingivitis	Bleeding gums, swollen, red gums with pockets		Tooth brushing, mouth wash, cleaning by dentist or periodontist
Irritable bowel syndrome	Chronic abdominal pain and discomfort, chronic diarrhea, and constipation	Rule out other disorders such as lactose intolerance, celiac disease, or Crohn' disease	Dietary adjustments. Pharmacologic treatment for symptoms. Antidiarrheal or laxative

Digestive System

Challenge Your Knowledge

A. **A dental assistant, or anyone working in an Oral Surgery Department, needs to have a thorough knowledge of the mouth and the mastication process.** Your knowledge of medical terms will help you communicate with the dentist or oral surgeon and the patients. Match the definition in the first column with the correct structure it is describing in the second column. **LO 5.1, 5.6**

_____ 1. Grind and crush food	**a.** mouth
_____ 2. Projects above the gum/covered with enamel	**b.** pulp cavity
_____ 3. Wrinkle	**c.** root canal
_____ 4. Destroys tooth enamel and dentin	**d.** caries
_____ 5. Contains blood vessels, nerves, tissue	**e.** root
_____ 6. Harder than bone	**f.** gingivitis
_____ 7. Oral cavity	**g.** papillae
_____ 8. Dental decay	**h.** crown
_____ 9. Anchors tooth to jaw	**i.** tartar
_____ 10. Inflammation of the gum	**j.** rugae
_____ 11. Nerves reach the tooth through this	**k.** bicuspids and molars
_____ 12. Contain the taste buds	**l.** dentin

B. **A medical term that is a noun can also have an adjective form.** Each statement has the noun form in parentheses; you must fill in the correct form of the adjective on the blank. Fill in the blanks. **LO 5.3**

1. The patient's (digestion) _____ symptoms were resolved with the new medication.

2. Due to an obstruction, the (pylorus) _____ sphincter was necrotic.

3. The (feces) _____ sample showed the presence of blood.

4. The patient is suffering from (pancreas) _____ cancer.

5. The (saliva) _____ gland was removed and sent to pathology.

6. Due to infection, the patient's (intestine) _____ surgery has been postponed until next week.

7. (Hemolysis) _____ jaundice results from RBC destruction and excess bilirubin.

8. The patient's (esophagus) _____ varices were bleeding.

9. The (laparoscope) _____ surgery poses less risk to the patient.

10. The (segment) _____ resection of the intestine is scheduled for later today.

C. **Abbreviations.** Choose the abbreviation that is best described in the statement, and fill it in on the blank provided. There are more answers than questions. Fill in the blanks. **LO 5.1, 5.6, 5.9**

| GI | SSA | GERD | BMI | HAV | SGOT | CF | BM |

1. Final act of elimination   Abbreviation: _____

2. Backing up into the esophagus   Abbreviation: _____

3. Digestive system component   Abbreviation: _____

4. Liver disease indicator   Abbreviation:_____

5. Inherited disease that affects exocrine glands   Abbreviation: _____

D. **Be aware of singular and plural terms.** Insert the correct medical terms in the blanks; watch for spelling. You will not use all the terms. **LO 5.3**

| diverticulitis | diverticulum | diverticulosis | diverticula |

1. What starts out as a single _____ can be followed by many other _____.

   The condition of having a number of these small pouches in the wall of the intestine is known as _____.

   Should these pouches become inflamed, _____ will result.

| metastasses | metastases | metastize | metastasis |

2. What was originally thought to be a single _____ to the patient's lung was proved to be multiple

   _____ to lung, kidney, and bone.

| polypectomy | polyposis | polyp (singular) |

3. The first polyp was found on sigmoidoscopy. A follow-up colonoscopy 6 months later found several more (plural)

   _____ in the large intestine. Diagnosis is _____. Proposed

   treatment is _____.

| peritoneum | peritonitis | peritoneal |

4. The _____ laceration sliced completely through the _____. Because of an

   infection in the wound, the patient developed _____.

E. Word elements are the keys to unlocking medical terms. Assess your knowledge of elements with this exercise. **LO 5.1–5.8**

1. Where is the inflammation in **hepatitis?**

   a. belly   d. mouth

   b. liver   e. intestine

   c. pancreas

2. In the term **submucosa,** the prefix means

   a. over   d. inside

   b. under   e. across

   c. around

3. The color denoted in the term **leukoplakia** is

   a. green   d. yellow

   b. black   e. red

   c. white

4. The element **os** means

   a. stomach   d. liver

   b. mouth   e. ear

   c. eye

5. If the root **cyst** means *bladder,* what is a **cystectomy?**

   a. bladder irrigation   d. bladder laceration

   b. bladder removal   e. bladder hemorrhage

   c. bladder examination

6. If a medication is given **postprandially,** you will take it after

   a. exercise   d. a vitamin

   b. drinking water   e. waking up

   c. a meal

7. **Gingivitis** has a root that means

   a. opening   d. decay

   b. teeth   e. enzyme

   c. gum

8. A **cholecystectomy** is

   a. a procedure   d. a discharge

   b. a diagnosis   e. an instrument

   c. an inflammation

9. What is the adjective used to describe a dilated, tortuous vein?

   a. adipose   d. pyloric

   b. varicose   e. segmental

   c. edematous

10. On the basis of the suffix, you know that the **peritoneum** will be

    a. an opening   d. a tumor

    b. an incision   e. a matrix

    c. a structure

F. Deconstruct. Deconstruct the following medical terms related to the digestive system. Write each element in the appropriate area of the chart. If a term does not have a particular element, write n/a. Fill in the blanks. The first one has been done for you. **LO 5.1, 5.2, 5.5, 5.6**

Medical Term	Prefix	Meaning of Prefix	Root	Meaning of Root	Suffix	Meaning of Suffix	Meaning of Term
stomatitis	1. n/a	2. n/a	3. stom	4. mouth	5. itis	6. inflammation	7. Inflammation of the mucous membrane of the mouth
sublingual	8.	9.	10.	11.	12.	13.	14.
dyspepsia	15.	16.	17.	18.	19.	20.	21.
intussusception	22.	23.	24.	25.	26.	27.	28.
flatulence	29.	30.	31.	32.	33.	34.	35.

G. Check the accuracy of your chart documentation. The following patients have presented to the gastroenterology clinic today. Can you correctly complete their documentation? Fill in the blanks. **LO 5.3, 5.5, 5.8**

1. Caroline Mason presents today with severe _____ (vomiting of blood), which has been getting progressively worse. _____ (looking within by a scope) reveals _____-atous (swollen) _____ (pertaining to the esophagus) _____ (dilated veins).

2. Andrew Baker reported to the Fulwood Emergency Room yesterday with symptoms of _____ (following a meal) burning chest pain and _____ (vomiting of blood). Dr. Lee admitted him to the GI service for further diagnostic tests and possible surgery.

H. Medical abbreviations must be interpreted correctly to ensure precision in communication and patient safety. Match the correct abbreviation in the first column to the defined meanings in the second column. **LO 5.9**

_____ 1. CF   a. use increases incidence of peptic ulcers

_____ 2. IBS   b. blocks production of gastric acid

_____ 3. GI   c. an intestinal diagnosis

_____ 4. PPI   d. an inherited disease

_____ 5. NSAIDs   e. refers to two specific organs

I. Can you interpret the following colonoscopy report for this patient? If you need to, consult a dictionary or your glossary for additional help. Fill in the blanks. **LO 5.2, 5.3, 5.5, 5.6, 5.8**

Preoperative Diagnosis: History of (H/O) multiple colonic polyps.

Postoperative Diagnosis: Normal colon.

In the left lateral position, the colonoscope was advanced into the rectum without difficulty. Examination of the rectum was normal. The sigmoid and descending colon revealed extensive diverticular disease but no evidence of colonic polyp disease. The transverse colon was examined to the hepatic flexure. There were no abnormalities of the transverse colon. The ascending colon was examined to the ileocecal valve. There were no abnormalities of the ascending colon. The patient tolerated the procedure well and was discharged from the endoscopy suite in good condition. In view of his age and a clean colonoscopy, I have recommended no further surveillance.

1. Analyze the prefixes. What is the difference between the pre- and postoperative diagnoses?

pre- = _____ post- = _____

2. Describe the left lateral position:

    a. side

    b. belly

    c. back

3. What instrument was used for this procedure? _____

4. Deconstruct **diverticulosis.** Suffix:_____; Root/Combining Form: _____

5. Define **polyp.**

    a. mass of tissue projecting into hollow organ

    b. erosion of tissue causing bleeding

    c. bulging of veins

    d. death of tissue wall

J. **Precision in documentation.** Get the stone in the right place: **cholelithiasis** or **choledocholithiasis?** Make the correct choice of medical terminology for the digestive system. Fill in the blanks. **LO 5.3**

    1. The patient's films revealed a stone in the common bile duct.

    Diagnosis:

    _____

    2. The presence of a stone in the patient's gallbladder was confirmed by the radiologist.

    Diagnosis:

    _____

K. **Supply the missing element that will complete the medical term.** Fill in the blanks. The first one is done for you. **LO 5.1, 5.5, 5.6**

    1. Inflammation of the appendix   appendic / __itis_____

    2. Part of the colon shaped like an "S"   sigm / _____

    3. Pertaining to the anus   an / _____

    4. Excessive amount of gas   flatul / _____

    5. Inflammation of the anus and rectum   _____ / itis

    6. Presence of polyps   polyp / _____

    7. Examination of the contents of the abdomen using an endoscope   /o / scopy / _____

    8. Evacuation of feces from the rectum and anus   de / fec / _____

    9. An edge or a border   peri / _____

    10. Inflammation of the colon   / itis / _____

L. **Many medical terms that are nouns also have an adjectival form.** Correctly apply these six medical terms to the following sentences. Fill in the blanks. **LO 5.3**

    mucous   **mucin**   **mucus**   **mucosal**   **mucosa**   **submucosa**

    1. The lining of a tubular structure is referred to as the _____.

    2. A sticky film containing mucin is _____.

    3. The term for *pertaining to* the mucosa is _____.

    4. The tissue layer beneath the mucosa is the _____.

    5. _____ is a secretion from the mucosal glands.

    6. _____ means *relating to mucus or the mucosa.*

M. Medications used to treat disorders of the gastrointestinal tract. Select the correct answer that will complete each statement.
LO 5.7

1. Antihistamines treat

    a. diarrhea   **c.** nausea and vomiting

    b. constipation   **d.** excess gastric acid

2. Imodium A-D® treats

    a. diarrhea   **c.** nausea and vomiting

    b. constipation   **d.** excess gastric acid

3. Histamine-2 blockers treat

    a. diarrhea   **c.** nausea and vomiting

    b. constipation   **d.** excess gastric acid

4. Proton pump inhibitors treat

    a. diarrhea   **c.** nausea and vomiting

    b. constipation   **d.** excess gastric acid

5. Laxative drugs treat

    a. diarrhea   **c.** nausea and vomiting

    b. constipation   **d.** excess gastric acid

N. Correct pronunciation is key when communicating to other health care providers, patients, and their families. Choose the correct pronunciation for each medical term. **LO 5.4, 5.5**

1. The last syllable of the term rugae rhymes with:

    a. bee.

    b. bay.

    c. bye.

2. The first syllable in the term sphincter rhymes with:

    a. rank   **c.** rink

    b. bike   **d.** beak

3. The suffix in the term leukoplakia sounds like:

    a. ee-ah   **c.** ee-ay

    b. i-ah   **d.** i-ay

4. Identify the proper pronunciation of dysentery:

    a. DIS-en-tare-ee   **c.** dice-en-tar-EE

    b. DIS-en-tar-eh   **d.** di-**YICE**-en-**TARE**-ee

5. The correct pronunciation for the term that means an examination of the inside of the anus and rectum:

    a. pan-en-**DOS**-koh-pee

    b. EN-te-oss-**KOH**-pee

    c. prok-**TOSS**-koh-pee

    d. koh-**LON**-oss-**KOH**-pee

Case Reports

O. **After reading Case Report 5.1, answer the following questions.** Select the correct answer to complete each statement or answer each question. **LO 5.6, 5.8**

 ## Case Report (CR) 5.1

You are
. . . a Certified Medical Assistant working with Susan Lee, MD, a primary care physician at Fulwood Medical Center.

Your patient is
. . . Mrs. Sandra Jacobs, a 46-year-old mother of four. Your task is to document her care.

Documentation

Mrs. Sandra Jacobs, a 46-year-old mother of four, presents in Dr. Susan Lee's primary care clinic with episodes of crampy pain in her right upper quadrant associated with nausea and vomiting. The pain often occurs after eating fast food. She has not noticed fever or jaundice. Physical examination reveals an obese white woman with a positive **Murphy sign.** Her BP is 170/90. A provisional diagnosis of **gallstones** has been made. She has been referred for an ultrasound examination, and an appointment has been made to see Dr. Stewart Walsh in the Surgery Department.

I explained to her the etiology of her gallstones and the need for surgical removal of the stones, and I discussed with her a low-fat, 1500-calorie diet sheet.

Luisa Guitterez, CMA. 10/12/12, 1430 hrs.

---

1. In which quadrant is Mrs. Jacobs having pain?

   a. LUQ   **c.** RUQ

   b. LLQ   **d.** RLQ

2. The fact that she does not have jaundice rules out a disorder of the:

   a. stomach   **c.** gallbladder

   b. liver   **d.** pancreas

3. What is a *positive Murphy sign?*

   a. pain in the right upper quadrant

   b. accumulation of fluid in the peritoneum

   c. blood in the stool

   d. vomit that appears as coffee grounds

4. What additional diagnostic procedure is she scheduled for?

   a. sigmoidoscopy   **c.**   barium enema

   b. cholecystectomy   **d.**   ultrasound

C. **Read the letter below.** After reading the letter, answer the following questions. The answers to the questions may not be in the letter itself but can be found in the chapter content. **LO 5.5, 5.8, 5.10**

Fulwood Medical Center
3333 Medical Parkway, Fulwood, MI 01234
555-247-6100

Department of: **Bariatric** Surgery

To: Charles Leavenworth, MD
Medical Director
Lombard Insurance Company

From: Stewart Walsh, MD, FACS
Chief of Surgery
Center for Bariatric Surgery
Fulwood Medical Center

10/06/20

Dear Doctor Leavenworth,

Request for authorization of surgery

Re: Mrs. Martha Jones
Subscriber ID 056437

Mrs. Jones is a 52-year-old former waitress, recently divorced. She is 5 feet 4 inches tall and weighs 275 pounds. She has type 2 diabetes with frequent episodes of hypoglycemia and also ketoacidosis, requiring three different hospitalizations. She now has diabetic retinopathy and peripheral vasculitis. Complicating this is hypertension (185/110), coronary artery disease, and pulmonary edema. Exercise is out of the question because she has marked osteoarthritis of her knees and hips. Mrs. Jones is now housebound, dependent on transportation to our medical center. In spite of monthly meetings with our nutritionist, she has gained 25 pounds in the past 6 months.

At a case conference earlier today, we all recognized that unless we were able to reduce and control her weight, we had no hope of controlling any of her other multiple problems.

Therefore, I am proposing to perform a **Roux-en-Y gastric** bypass using a laparoscopic approach. We will need to admit her 2 days prior to surgery to control her blood sugar and cardiovascular problems and anticipate that she will remain in the hospital for 2 days after surgery, barring any complications. My surgical technologist and I have spent time with Mrs. Jones explaining the procedure and its risks, and she is aware and accepting of these. She is also very aware of the necessary follow-up to the procedure and the counseling required for a new lifestyle.

We believe not only that this is an essential procedure medically but that it will reduce in the long term the financial burden of her multiple therapies and improve the quality of the patient's life. Enclosed is supportive documentation of her current history and medical problems.

Your company has designated our hospital as a Center of Excellence for weight-loss surgery, and I look forward to your prompt agreement with this approach for this patient.

Sincerely,

Stewart Walsh, MD, FACS
Chief of Surgery
Fulwood Medical Center

---

1. The device used to perform the procedure will be inserted into the:

   a. peritoneal space   **b.** thorax   **c.** abdomen   **d.** mouth

2. The surgical department specializes in the treatment of:

   a. obesity   **b.** gastric disorders   **c.** diabetes   **d.** malnutrition

3. The surgical procedure will reduce the size of the:

   a. gallbladder   **c.** large intestine

   b. stomach   **d.** small intestine

D. After reading the following Case Report, correctly answer the following questions. The answers to the questions may not be in the Case Report itself but can be found in the chapter content. **LO 5.5, 5.9, 5.10**

 Case Report (CR) 5.2

You are

. . . a Certified Medical Assistant working with Susan Lee, MD, a primary care physician at Fulwood Medical Center.

Your patient is

. . . Mrs. Helen Schreiber, a 45-year-old high school principal. Your task is to document her care.

Documentation

Mrs. Helen Schreiber, a 45-year-old high school principal, presents with a 6-month history of dry mouth, bleeding gums, and difficulty in chewing and swallowing food. She complains of having canker sores that don't seem to go away.

Questioning by Dr. Susan Lee, her primary care physician, reveals that she also has dry eyes, is having pain in some joints of both hands, and has felt fatigued. Her previous medical history is uneventful. Physical examination shows a dry mouth, mild red, swollen gums, and an **ulcer** on the back of the lower lip. Her salivary glands are not swollen. Her eyes show no ulceration or conjunctivitis. The metacarpophalangeal joints of both index fingers are swollen, stiff, and tender. All other systems show no abnormality.

Initial laboratory reports show anemia, decreased **WBC** count, and an elevated **ESR.** Dr. Lee made a provisional diagnosis of **Sjogren syndrome.** The results of studies for **SSA** and **SSB** antibodies and for rheumatoid factor titers are pending, as are x-rays of her hands.

Mrs. Schreiber was given advice about symptomatic treatment for her dry mouth and will be seen again in 1 week.

Luisa Guitterez, **(5)**_____ 06/12/12,1530 hrs.

---

1. The medical term that means "red, swollen gums" is:

   a. difficulty chewing   **b.** gingivitis   **c.** dry mouth   **d.** headache

2. Which medical term correctly documents a "canker sore?"

   a. Ileus   **b.** Glossodynia   **c.** Aphthous ulcer   **d.** Halitosis

3. The results of her "tests" came from a sample of her:

   a. saliva   **b.** blood   **c.** urine

4. The letter "E" in the abbreviation ESR stands for _____.

5. Provide the abbreviation that correctly documents your profession for (5) _____

E. **After reading the following Case Report, correctly answer the following questions.** The answers to the questions may not be in the Case Report itself but can be found in the chapter content. **LO 5.6, 5.8, 5.10**

Case Report (CR) 5.3

You are
. . . an **EMR** working in the Emergency Department at Fulwood Medical Center.

Your patient is
. . . Mrs. Jan Stark, a 36-year-old pottery maker. Your task is to document her visit.

Documentation
Mrs. Jan Stark, a 36-year-old pottery maker, was admitted to the Emergency Department at 2015 hrs.

She stated that she had passed between 20 and 30 watery, gray stools in the previous 24 hours. She had not passed urine for more than 12 hours. She was markedly **dehydrated** and responded well to infusion of lactated Ringer solution and then D5NS (5% dextrose in normal 0.9% saline).

Mrs. Stark describes that

Questioning revealed that, for the past 10 years, after meals she had severe abdominal cramping followed by diarrhea and feeling very bloated and gassy. These symptoms were associated with severe headaches and fatigue. During those episodes, her stools were greasy and pale. In the past 3 or 4 months, she has had some difficulties with fine movements as she works on her pottery wheel and has had tingling in her fingers and toes.

Dr. Homer Hilinski, emergency physician, believes her dehydration is a result of a **malabsorption syndrome.** An appointment has been made for her to see Dr. Cameron Grabowski, gastroenterologist, tomorrow. She was discharged to her husband's care at midnight. She has been advised to stay on fluids only and to return to the Emergency Room **(ER)** if the diarrhea returns.

Sunil Patel, EMT-1.10/21/12, 0100 hrs.

1. Mrs. Stark's dehydration was due to:

   a. excessive urination

   b. not drinking enough fluids

   c. her intestines not absorbing water

   d. inflammation of her stomach

2. How was Mrs. Stark's infusion administered?

   a. Through her veins

   b. Via a tube to her stomach

   c. She drank the fluid

   d. Through her rectum

3. The medical term that correctly replaces her symptom of "feeling bloated and gassy" is:

   a. flatulence   **b.** flatulent   **c.** flatus

4. Dr. Grabowski is a specialist in the treatment of disorders of the:

   a. mouth

   b. stomach and intestines

   c. stomach only

   d. liver

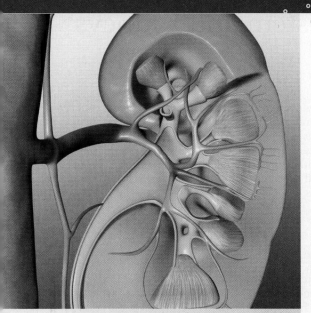

2014 Nucleus Medical Media

Urinary System
The Language of Urology

Chapter Sections

6.1 Urinary System and Kidneys

6.2 Ureters, Urinary Bladder, and Urethra

6.3 Disorders of the Urinary System

6.4 Procedures and Pharmacology

Chapter Learning Outcomes

Upon completion of this chapter, you will be able to:

LO 6.1 Identify and describe the anatomy and physiology of the urinary system.

LO 6.2 Use roots, combining forms, suffixes, and prefixes to construct and analyze medical terms related to the urinary system.

LO 6.3 Spell medical terms related to the urinary system.

LO 6.4 Pronounce medical terms related to the urinary system.

LO 6.5 Describe diagnostic procedures utilized in urology.

LO 6.6 Identify and describe disorders and pathological conditions related to the urinary system.

LO 6.7 Describe the therapeutic procedures and pharmacologic agents used in urology.

LO 6.8 Apply knowledge of medical terms relating to urology to documentation, medical records, and communication.

LO 6.9 Identify and correctly use abbreviations of terms used in urology.

LO 6.10 Identify health professionals involved in the care of urological patients.

Health professionals involved in the diagnosis and treatment of patients with problems with the urinary system include

- **Urologists,** who are specialists in the diagnosis and treatment of patients with diseases of the urinary system.
- **Nephrologists,** who are specialists in the diagnosis and treatment of diseases of the kidney.
- **Urologic nurses and nurse practitioners,** who are registered nurses with advanced academic and clinical experience in urology.

Urinary System

Although the respiratory system *(see Chapter 13)* excretes carbon dioxide and water; the integumentary system *(see Chapter 4)* excretes water, inorganic salts, and lactic acid in sweat; and the digestive tract *(see Chapter 5)* excretes water, salts, lipids, bile pigments, and other wastes, the urinary system carries the major burden of excretion. Within the urinary system, the kidneys are the agents that eliminate the waste products. If the kidneys fail to function, the other three systems of excretion are not able to replace them. Therefore, the kidney is a vital organ, and it brings with it a whole new set of terminology. The urinary system *(Figure 6.1)* consists of six organs:

- Two **kidneys (2)**
- A single **urinary bladder (1)**
- Two **ureters (2)**
- A single **urethra (1)**

The process of removing metabolic waste is called **excretion.** It is an essential process in maintaining homeostasis *(see Chapter 3)*. The metabolic wastes include carbon dioxide from cellular respiration, excess water and electrolytes, **nitrogenous** compounds from the breakdown of proteins, and **urea.** If these wastes are not eliminated, they poison the whole body.

In the body's cells, protein is broken down *(see Chapter 3)* into **amino acids.** When an amino acid is broken down, **ammonia** is produced. Ammonia is extremely toxic to cells. The liver quickly converts it to the less toxic urea, which is **excreted** by the kidneys in the form of **urine.**

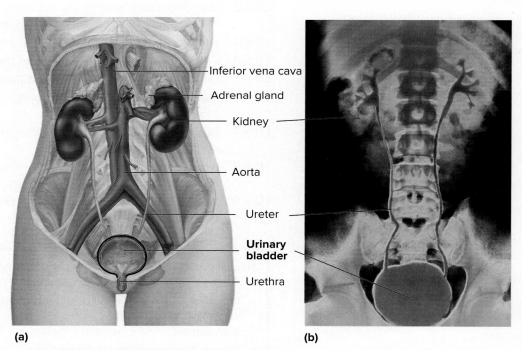

Did you know...

- **Urology** is the medical specialty of the diagnosis and treatment of diseases of the urinary system.
- The **kidney** is the major organ that eliminates the waste products of cellular metabolism.

(a) (b)

▲ **Figure 6.1 The urinary system.** (a) Major organs. (b) Structures of the urinary system are visible in this colored **intravenous pyelogram** (IVP). (b) CNRI/SPL/Science Source

WORD	PRONUNCIATION	ELEMENTS		DEFINITION
amino acid	ah-**MEE**-noh **ASS**-id	R/CF	**amin/o** nitrogen containing **acid** Latin sour	The basic building block for protein
ammonia	ah-**MOHN**-ih-ah	S/ R/	-ia condition **ammon-** ammonia	Toxic breakdown product of amino acids
bladder	**BLAD**-er		Old English bladder	Hollow sac that holds fluid; for example, urine or bile
excretion excrete (verb)	eks-**KREE**-shun eks-**KREET**		Latin remove	Removal of waste products of metabolism out of the body To pass out of the body the waste products of metabolism
kidney	**KID**-nee		Greek kidney	Organ of excretion
nephrology	neh-**FROL**-oh-jee	S/ R/CF	-logy study of **nephr/o** kidney	Medical specialty of diseases of the kidney
nephrologist	neh-**FROL**-oh-jist	S/	-logist one who studies, specialist	Medical specialist in diseases of the kidney
nitrogenous	ni-**TROJ**-en-us	S/ R/CF R/	-ous pertaining to **nitr/o-** nitrogen -gen- create	Containing or generating nitrogen
renal	**REE**-nal	S/ R/	-al pertaining to **ren-** kidney	Pertaining to the kidney
urea	you-**REE**-ah		Greek urine	End product of nitrogen metabolism expelled in urine
ureter (**Note:** Two "e's" = two tubes.) ureteral (adj)	you-**REET**-er you-**REE**-ter-al	 S/ R/	Greek urinary canal -al pertaining to **ureter-** ureter	Tube that connects the kidney to the urinary bladder (**Note:** The roots for **urethra** and **ureter** are different.) Pertaining to the ureter
urethra (**Note:** One "e" = one tube.) urethral (adj)	you-**REE**-thra you-**REE**-thral	 S/ R/	Greek urethra -al pertaining to **urethr-** urethra	Canal leading from the bladder to outside (**Note:** The roots for **urethra** and **ureter** are different.) Pertaining to the urethra
urine urinary (adj)	**YUR**-in **YUR**-in-air-ee	 S/ R/	Latin urine -ary pertaining to **urin-** urine	Fluid and dissolved substances excreted by kidney Pertaining to urine
urinate (verb)	**YUR**-in-ate	S/	-ate composed of, pertaining to	To pass urine
urination	yur-ih-**NAY**-shun	S/	-ation process	The act of passing urine
urology	you-**ROL**-oh-jee	S/ R/CF	-logy study of **ur/o-** urinary system	Medical specialty of disorders of the urinary system
urologist urologic (adj)	you-**ROL**-oh-jist yur-roh-**LOJ**-ik	S/ S/	-logist one who studies -ic pertaining to	Medical specialist in disorders of the urinary system Pertaining to urology

Kidneys

Each kidney is a bean-shaped organ about the size of a clenched fist. It is located on either side of the vertebral column behind the peritoneum and lies against the deep muscles of the back. The left kidney is behind the spleen, and the right kidney is behind and below the liver (*Figure 6.2a*).

The functions of the kidneys are to:

- **Filter** blood to eliminate wastes.
- **Regulate** blood volume and pressure by eliminating or conserving water as necessary.
- **Maintain homeostasis** by controlling the quantities of water and electrolytes that are eliminated.
- **Secrete** the enzyme **renin,** which raises arterial blood pressure.
- **Secrete** the hormone **erythropoietin,** which acts on the bone to release red blood cells.
- **Synthesize vitamin D** to contribute to maintaining normal blood calcium levels.

Waste-laden blood enters the kidney at its **hilum** (*Figure 6.2b*) through the renal artery. Excess water, urea, and other waste products are **filtered** from the blood by the kidney, collected in the ureter, and carried off to the bladder through the renal pelvis at the hilum. The filtered blood exits through the renal vein at the hilum.

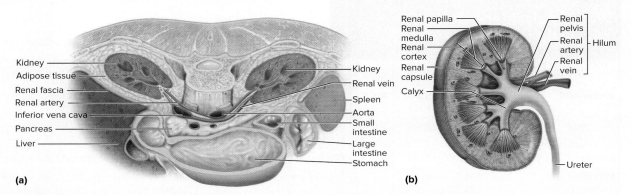

(a)

Kidney
Adipose tissue
Renal fascia
Renal artery
Inferior vena cava
Pancreas
Liver

Kidney
Renal vein
Spleen
Aorta
Small intestine
Large intestine
Stomach

(b)

Renal papilla
Renal medulla
Renal cortex
Renal capsule
Calyx

Renal pelvis
Renal artery
Renal vein

Hilum

Ureter

▲ **Figure 6.2** **Kidney.** (a) Transverse section of abdomen showing position of kidneys. (b) Longitudinal section of a kidney.

Each kidney has three regions *(see Figure 6.2b):*

- An outer renal **cortex**—containing about 1 million **nephrons,** the basic filtration unit of the kidney.

- An inner renal **medulla**—containing the collecting ducts, which merge together to form about 30 papillary ducts, that enter into a **calyx.**

- A central renal **pelvis**—a funnel-shaped structure into which the calyces open, and which forms the ureter.

In the cortex, the renal artery divides into smaller and smaller arterioles, each of which enters a nephron and divides into a network of approximately 50 capillaries, known as a **glomerulus.** Each glomerulus is encased in the **glomerular capsule.** Because the blood is under pressure and the capillaries and glomerular capsule are **permeable,** much of the fluid from the blood filters through the capillary wall and glomerular capsule into the renal tubule, which includes the **nephron loop,** sometimes called the **loop of Henle** *(Figure 6.3).*

This **filtrate** entering the renal tubule contains water, urea, glucose, electrolytes, amino acids, and vitamins. Red blood cells, platelets, and plasma proteins are too large to pass through the capillary membrane, and they remain in the blood.

Approximately 180 liters (45 gallons) of filtrate are formed each day. As the filtrate passes down the renal tubule, over 90% of the water is returned to the blood by **reabsorption.** Glucose and minerals are also returned to the blood. Some residual wastes in the blood are secreted from the blood into the tubule. These interchanges between the filtrate in the tubule and the blood are made possible by a mesh of capillaries that surrounds the renal tubule *(Figure 6.3).* The material that remains in the tubule is urine. It consists of excess water, electrolytes, and urea.

The renal tubules merge to form collecting ducts *(Figure 6.3)* that merge into the calyces and then form the **renal pelvis** and become the **ureter.**

Purified blood is returned from the **peritubular** mesh of capillaries to the circulatory system through the renal vein.

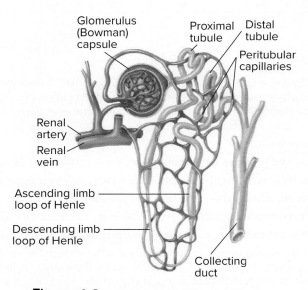

Glomerulus (Bowman) capsule
Proximal tubule
Distal tubule
Peritubular capillaries
Renal artery
Renal vein
Ascending limb loop of Henle
Descending limb loop of Henle
Collecting duct

▲ **Figure 6.3** **Glomerulus and renal tubule.**

WORD	PRONUNCIATION		ELEMENTS	DEFINITION
calyx calyces (pl)	**KAY**-licks **KAY**-lih-sees		Greek *cup of a flower*	Funnel-shaped structure
cortex cortices (pl) cortical (adj)	**KOR**-teks **KOR**-tih-sees **KOR**-tih-kal	 S/ R/	Latin *tree bark* -ical *pertaining to* cort- *cortex*	Outer portion of an organ Pertaining to the cortex
erythropoietin	eh-**RITH**-roh-**POY**-ee-tin	S/ R/CF	-poietin *the maker* erythr/o- *red*	Protein secreted by the kidney that stimulates red blood cell production
filter	**FIL**-ter		Latin *to filter through the material felt*	A porous substance through which a liquid or gas is passed to separate out contained particles; or to use a filter
filtrate	**FIL**-trate	S/ R/	-ate *composed of, pertaining to* filtr- *strain through*	That which has passed through a filter
filtration	fil-**TRAY**-shun	S/	-ation *process*	Process of passing liquid through a filter
glomerulus glomeruli (pl) glomerular (adj)	glo-**MAIR**-you-lus glo-**MAIR**-you-lee glo-**MAIR**-you-lar	 R/ S/	Latin *small ball of yarn* glomerul- *glomerulus* -ar *pertaining to*	Plexus of capillaries; part of a nephron Pertaining to or affecting a glomerulus or glomeruli
hilum hila (pl)	**HIGH**-lum **HIGH**-lah		Latin *small bit*	The part where the nerves and blood vessels enter and leave an organ
medulla	meh-**DULL**-ah		French *middle*	Central portion of a structure surrounded by cortex
nephron nephron loop (loop of Henle)	**NEF**-ron **NEF**-ron LOOP LOOP of **HEN**-lee		Greek *kidney* Friedrich Henle, 1809–1885, German anatomist, pathologist, and histologist	Filtration unit of the kidney; glomerulus + renal tubule Part of the renal tubule where reabsorption occurs
pelvis	**PEL**-vis		Latin *basin*	A cup-shaped cavity, as in the pelvis of the kidney
peritubular	**PER**-ih-**TOO**-byu-lar	S/ P/ R/	-ar *pertaining to* peri- *around* -tubul- *small tube*	Surrounding the small renal tubules
permeable	**PER**-mee-ah-bull	S/ R/CF	-able *capable of* perm/e- *pass through*	Allowing passage of substances through a membrane
semipermeable impermeable	sem-ee-**PER**-me-ah-bull im-**PER**-me-ah-bull	P/ P/	semi- *half* im- *not, in*	Freely permeable to water but not to solutes When nothing is allowed passage
absorb reabsorption (**Note:** The last *b* in *absorb* changes to a *p* to ease pronunciation.)	ab-**SORB** ree-ab-**SORP**-shun	 S/ P/ R/	Latin *swallow* -tion *process* re- *back* -absorb- *swallow*	To bring in The taking back into the blood of substances that had previously been filtered out from it
renin	**REE**-nin	S/ R/	-in *substance* ren- *kidney*	Enzyme secreted by the kidney that causes vasoconstriction

Check Point Section 6.1

A. The same but different. *More than one word element can have the same meaning. In this body system,* **nephr/o** *and* **ren-** *both mean kidney. The elements are not interchangeable—one particular element will be used for a specific term. You need to know them individually. Fill in the blanks. Read carefully!* **LO 6.1, 6.2, 6.10**

1. Medical specialist in kidney treatment   _____/ _____/ _____

2. Medical specialty in kidney diseases   _____/ _____/ _____

3. Pertaining to the kidney   _____/ _____

B. Employ the *language of urology* to correctly match the medical term to the brief description. LO 6.1

_____ 1. hollow sac that holds fluids

_____ 2. organ of excretion

_____ 3. connects kidney to bladder

_____ 4. canal leading from bladder to outside the body

a. kidney

b. ureter

c. urethra

d. bladder

C. Deconstruct the following medical terms into their basic elements. *Fill in the blanks.* **LO 6.1, 6.2**

1. Passage of a substance through a filter   _____/_____

2. Enzyme that causes vasoconstriction   _____/_____

3. Surrounding the small renal tubules   _____/_____/_____

4. Blood that reclaims previously filtered substances   _____/_____/_____/_____

D. Three of these terms refer to the regions of the kidney. *Choose the correct three terms and match them to the region.* **LO 6.1**
peritubular   cortex   glomerular capsule   pelvis   nephron loop   medulla

1. outer region   _____

2. inner region   _____

3. central region   _____

Section 6.2 Ureters, Urinary Bladder, and Urethra

Ureters

Each **ureter** is a muscular tube, about 10 inches long (25.5 cm) and ¼ inch (0.6 cm) wide, that lies on the posterior abdominal wall. The ureters function is to carry urine from the renal pelvis to the urinary bladder.

Each ureter passes obliquely through the muscle wall of the bladder. As pressure builds in a filling bladder, the muscle wall compresses the ureter and prevents urine from being forced back up the ureter to the kidneys.

In addition to gravity pulling the urine from the renal pelvis to the bladder, **intermittent** waves in the muscular wall **(peristalsis)** of the ureter, beginning at the renal pelvis, squeeze urine down the ureter and squirt the urine into the bladder.

Urinary Bladder and Urethra

Urethra

The final passageway for the urine to escape to the outside is the **urethra,** a thin-walled tube that takes urine from the floor of the bladder to the outside. At the base of the bladder, the muscular wall is thickened to form the **internal urethral sphincter.** As the urethra passes through the skeletal muscles of the pelvic floor, the **external urethral sphincter** provides voluntary control of **micturition.**

In the female *(see Figure 6.5)*, the urethra is only about 1.5 inches long, and it opens to the outside anterior to the vagina *(see Figure 6.7)*. In the male *(Figure 6.4)*, the urethra is 7 to 8 inches in length and passes through the penis. In both the male and the female, the opening of the urethra to the outside is called the **external urinary meatus.**

Micturition

The **urinary bladder** is a hollow, muscular organ on the floor of the pelvic cavity, posterior to the pubic symphysis *(Figure 6.5)*. When the bladder is distended, it rises upward and can be palpated above the symphysis pubis.

When the bladder contains about 200 mL of urine, stretch receptors in its wall trigger the **micturition reflex.** However, voluntary control of the external sphincter can keep that sphincter contracted and can hold urine in the bladder until you decide to urinate. The passage of urine can be described as **urination, micturition,** or **voiding.**

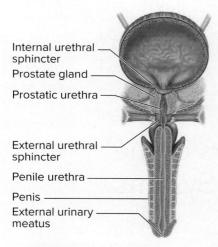

▲ **Figure 6.4** Male urinary bladder and urethra.

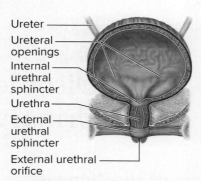

▲ **Figure 6.5** Female urinary bladder and urethra.

Word Analysis and Definition: Ureters, Urinary Bladder, and Urethra

S = Suffix   P = Prefix   R = Root   R/CF = Combining Form

WORD	PRONUNCIATION		ELEMENTS	DEFINITION
external	ek-**STURN**-al	S/	Latin *on the outside* -al *pertaining to*	Outside a structure or organ
intermittent	**IN**-ter-**MIT**-ent	S/ P/ R/	-ent *end result* inter- *between* -mitt- *send*	Alternately ceasing and beginning again
internal	**IN**-tur-nl	S/	Latin *on the inside* -al *pertaining to*	Inside a structure or organ
meatus	mee-**AY**-tus		Latin *a passage*	The external opening of a passage
micturition	mik-choo-**RISH**-un	S/ R/	-ition *process* mictur- *pass urine*	Act of passing urine
micturate	**MIK**-choo-rate	S/	-ate *composed of, pertaining to*	Pass urine
oblique obliquely	ob-**LEEK** ob-**LEEK**-lee	S/	Latin *slanted* -ly *going toward*	Slanting; projection that is neither frontal nor lateral Going toward a slanting direction
peristalsis	pair-ih-**STAL**-sis	P/ R/	peri- *around* -stalsis *constrict*	Waves of alternate contraction and relaxation along a tube to move its contents onward
peristaltic (adj)	pair-ih-**STAL**-tik	S/	-tic *pertaining to*	Pertaining to peristalsis
reflex	**REE**-fleks		Latin *to bend back*	An involuntary response to a stimulus
reflux	**REE**-fluks	P/ R/	re- *back* -flux *flow*	Backward flow
sphincter	**SFINK**-ter		Greek *band*	Band of muscle that encircles an opening; when the muscle contracts, the opening squeezes closed
urination	yur-ih-**NAY**-shun	S/ R/CF	-ation *process* urin/a- *urine*	The passing of urine Latin urine
void	VOYD		Latin *to empty*	To evacuate urine or feces

A. Describe the structures of the bladder and urethra. *Indicate if the following statements are accurate. If the statement is true, choose T. If the statement is false, choose F.* **LO 6.1**

1. The length of the urethra is the same for males and females.   T   F

2. Micturition, voiding, and urination are synonyms.   T   F

3. Humans have control over the micturition reflex.   T   F

4. In both males and females, urine exits the urinary meatus.   T   F

5. There are two urethral sphincters.   T   F

6. The presence of 100 mL of urine in the bladder triggers the urge to void.   T   F

Section 6.3 Disorders of the Urinary System

Disorders of the Kidneys

Renal cell carcinoma is the most common form of kidney cancer and occurs twice as often in men as in women. The cancer develops in the lining cells of the renal tubules.

Nephroblastoma, or **Wilms tumor,** is a malignant kidney tumor of childhood, usually appearing between ages 3 and 8 years.

Benign kidney tumors, such as **renal adenoma,** are usually asymptomatic, are discovered incidentally, and are not life-threatening.

Acute glomerulonephritis is an inflammation of the glomerulus. It damages the glomerular capillaries, allows protein and red blood cells to leak into the urine, and interferes with the clearance of waste products. In its acute form, it can develop rapidly after an episode of strep throat infection, most often in children. The *Streptococcus* bacteria do not invade the kidney but stimulate the immune system to overproduce antibodies that damage the glomeruli.

Chronic glomerulonephritis can occur with no history of kidney disease and present as kidney failure. It also occurs in **diabetic nephropathy** and can be associated with autoimmune diseases such as lupus erythematosus; human immunodeficiency virus (HIV) can cause glomerular disease even before developing into acquired immunodeficiency syndrome (AIDS).

Nephrotic syndrome involves large amounts of protein leaking out into the urine so that the level of protein in the blood falls. The types of nephrotic syndrome are described in *Table 6.1.* The most obvious symptom is fluid retention with edema of the ankles and legs.

Interstitial nephritis is an inflammation of the spaces between the renal tubules. Most often it is acute and temporary. It can be an allergic reaction to or a side effect of drugs such as penicillin or ampicillin, NSAIDs, and diuretics.

Pyelitis is inflammation of the renal pelvis due to bacterial infection. If pyelitis is not effectively treated, it often progresses to **pyelonephritis,** an infection of the renal pelvis and kidney tissue. Most often it occurs as part of a total urinary tract infection (UTI), commencing in the urinary bladder. It has a high mortality rate in the elderly and in people with a compromised immune system *(see Chapter 4).* It requires aggressive antibiotic therapy.

Did you know...

- Of all renal cancers, 25% to 30% relate directly to smoking.
- As little as 1 mL of blood will turn the urine red.
- Hematuria can be caused by a lesion anywhere in the urinary system.
- The acute form of glomerulonephritis has a 100% recovery rate.
- Acute interstitial nephritis causes 15% of cases of acute renal failure.

Table 6.1 Types of Nephrotic Syndrome

Disease (as Seen on Biopsy)	Description
Minimal change disease	Most common in children; responds to steroids
Focal segmental glomerulosclerosis (FSGS)	Cause unknown; little response to treatment
Membranous nephropathy	Cause unknown; may respond to immunosuppressive treatment
Diabetes	Occurs if blood sugar has been poorly controlled

WORD	PRONUNCIATION		ELEMENTS	DEFINITION
adenoma	AD-eh-NOH-mah	S/ R/	-oma *tumor* aden- *gland*	Benign tumor that originates from glandular tissue
benign (adj)	bee-NINE		Latin *kind*	Denoting the nonmalignant character of a neoplasm or illness
carcinoma	kar-sih-NOH-mah	S/ R/	-oma *tumor* carcin- *cancer*	A cancerous (malignant) and invasive epithelial tumor
glomerulonephritis	glo-MAIR-you-loh-nef-RIE-tis	S/ R/CF R/	-itis *inflammation* glomerul/o- *glomerulus* -nephr- *kidney*	Infection of the glomeruli of the kidney
interstitial	in-ter-STISH-al	S/ P/ R/	-ial *pertaining to* inter- *between* -stit- *space*	Pertaining to the spaces between cells in a tissue or organ
nephritis	neh-FRIE-tis	S/ R/	-itis *inflammation* nephr- *kidney*	Inflammation of the kidney
nephroblastoma	NEF-roh-blas-TOH-mah	S/ R/CF R/	-oma *tumor, mass* nephr/o- *kidney* -blast- *embryonic, immature cell*	Cancerous kidney tumor of childhood
Wilms tumor (syn)	WILMZ TOO-mor		Max Vilms, 1867–1918, German surgeon	
nephropathy	neh-FROP-ah-thee	S/ R/CF	-pathy *disease* nephr/o- *kidney*	Any disease of the kidney
nephrotic syndrome	neh-FROT-ik SIN-drome	S/ R/CF	-tic *pertaining to* nephr/o- *kidney*	Glomerular disease with marked loss of protein
nephrosis (syn)	neh-FRO-sis	S/	-osis *condition*	
pyelitis	pie-eh-LIE-tis	S/ R/	-itis *inflammation* pyel- *renal pelvis*	Inflammation of renal pelvis
pyelonephritis	PIE-eh-loh-neh-FRIE-tis	R/CF R/	pyel/o- *renal pelvis* -nephr- *kidney*	Inflammation of the kidney and renal pelvis

Hypertension, with its high blood pressure, can damage the renal arterioles and glomeruli, causing them to thicken and narrow. This reduces their capability to remove wastes and excess water, which can cause the blood pressure (BP) to rise even more.

Polycystic kidney disease (PKD) is an inherited disease. Large, fluid-filled cysts grow within the kidneys and press against the kidney tissue. Finally, the kidneys cannot function effectively.

Acute renal failure (ARF) makes the kidneys suddenly stop filtering waste products from the blood. The causes of acute renal failure include:

- **Severe burns, trauma,** or **complicated surgery**—with a drastic drop in blood pressure and the release of myoglobin from injured muscles *(see Chapter 14).* Myoglobin lodges in the renal tubules and blocks the flow of urine.

- **Drugs**—including pain medications such as aspirin and ibuprofen, antibiotics such as streptomycin and gentamicin, and contrast dyes used in angiography.

- **Toxins**—such as heavy metals (mercury is one) and excessive alcohol.

- **Systemic infections**—septicemia.

- **Blood disorders**—such as idiopathic thrombocytopenic purpura or disseminated intravascular coagulation *(see Chapter 11).*

Chronic renal failure (CRF), or **chronic kidney disease (CKD),** is a gradual loss of renal function. Symptoms and signs may not appear until kidney function is less than 25% of normal.

The causes of chronic renal failure include diabetes—type 1 and type 2 *(see Chapter 17);* hypertension; kidney diseases; and lead poisoning.

End-stage renal disease (ESRD) means the kidneys are functioning at less than 10% of their normal capacity. At this point, life cannot be sustained, and either dialysis or kidney transplant is needed.

The signs and symptoms of kidney failure can include **oliguria** (reduction of urine output), **anuria** (cessation of urine output), confusion, seizures, and coma due to the buildup of toxins.

Did you know...

- Acute renal failure is usually reversible.
- Chronic renal failure has no cure.

Hematuria (blood in the urine) can be caused by lesions anywhere in the urinary system; this includes trauma (including long-distance running), infections, medications (such as quinine and phenytoin), and congenital diseases (such as sickle cell anemia). In **microscopic hematuria,** the urine is not red, and red blood cells can be seen only under a microscope or identified by a urine dipstick. Normal urine contains no blood. Excessive consumption of beets, rhubarb, and red food coloring can cause urine to be colored red. This is not hematuria. Also, in the collection of urine from a woman during menstruation, the urine can be contaminated with blood, giving the impression of hematuria.

Polyuria (excessive urine production) has multiple causes ranging from increased fluid intake, diuretic medication, diabetes insipidus, and uncontrolled diabetes mellitus (*see Chapter 8*).

Nocturia can be due to drinking too much fluid before bedtime or due to diuretics. It can occur when there is an obstruction to urethra, such as an enlarged prostate, because the bladder is unable to fully empty.

Azotemia is the buildup of urea (nitrogenous waste products) in the blood. **Uremia** is the complex of symptoms resulting from excess nitrogenous waste products in the blood, as seen in renal failure.

Protein is not detected normally in urine. Its presence (**proteinuria**) indicates infection or urinary tract disease.

Glucose in the urine (**glycosuria**) is a spillover into the urine when the nephrons are damaged or diseased or blood sugar is high in uncontrolled diabetes.

Word Analysis and Definition: Disorders of the Kidney

S = Suffix   P = Prefix   R = Root   R/CF = Combining Form

WORD	PRONUNCIATION		ELEMENTS	DEFINITION
anuria	an-**YOU**-ree-ah	S/ P/ R/	**-ia** *condition* **an-** *lack of, without* **-ur-** *urine*	Absence of urine production
azotemia	az-oh-**TEE**-mee-ah	S/ R/	**-emia** *blood condition* **azot-** *nitrogen*	Excess nitrogenous waste products (urea) in the blood
glycosuria (*Note:* The "s" is added to make the word flow.)	**GLIE**-koh-**SYU**-ree-ah	S/ R/CF R/	**-ia** *condition* **glyc/o-** *glucose* **-ur-** *urine*	Presence of glucose in urine
hematuria	hee-mah-**TYU**-ree-ah	S/ R/ R/	**-ia** *condition* **hemat-** *blood* **-ur-** *urine*	Blood in the urine
hypertension	**HIGH**-per-**TEN**-shun	S/ P/ R/	**-ion** *action, condition* **hyper-** *excessive* **-tens-** *pressure*	Persistent high arterial blood pressure
microscopic	**MY**-kroh-**SKOP**-ik	P/ R/ S/	**micro-** *small* **-scope** *instrument for viewing* **-ic** *pertaining to*	Visible only with the aid of a microscope
nocturia	nok-**TYU**-ree-ah	S/ P/ R/	**-ia** *condition* **noct-** *night* **-ur-** *urine*	Excessive urination at night
oliguria	ol-ih-**GYUR**-ee-ah	S/ P/ R/	**-ia** *condition* **olig-** *scanty* **-ur-** *urine*	Scanty production of urine
polycystic	pol-ee-**SIS**-tik	S/ P/ R/	**-ic** *pertaining to* **poly-** *many* **-cyst-** *bladder, cyst*	Composed of many cysts
polyuria	pol-ee-**YOU**-ree-ah	S/ P/ R/	**-ia** *condition* **poly-** *excessive* **-ur-** *urine*	Excessive production of urine
proteinuria	pro-tee-**NYU**-ree-ah	S/ R/ R/	**-ia** *condition* **protein-** *protein* **-ur-** *urine*	Presence of protein in urine
uremia	you-**REE**-mee-ah	S/ R/	**-emia** *blood condition* **ur-** *urine*	A condition caused by excess urea and other nitrogenous wastes in the blood

Nephrolithiasis

Stones **(calculi)** begin in the pelvis of the kidney as a tiny grain of undissolved material, usually a mineral called calcium oxalate *(Figure 6.6)*. When the urine flows out of the kidney, the grain of material is left behind. Over time, more material is deposited and a stone is formed. The presence of stones is called **nephrolithiasis.**

Most stones enter the ureter while they are still small enough to pass down the ureter into the bladder and out of the body in urine. **Hydronephrosis** occurs when a calculus lodges in the ureter, blocks the flow of urine, and, because of the back-flow pressure, causes the renal pelvis to dilate. **Spasmodic** pain can be felt in the ureter.

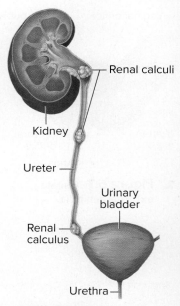

▲ **Figure 6.6 Renal calculi.** Calculi can become lodged at different sites in the ureters.

Word Analysis and Definition: Nephrolithiasis

S = Suffix   P = Prefix   R = Root   R/CF = Combining Form

WORD	PRONUNCIATION	ELEMENTS		DEFINITION
calculus calculi (pl)	**KAL**-kyu-lus **KAL**-kyu-lie		Latin *pebble*	Small stone
hydronephrosis	**HIGH**-droh-neh-**FROH**-sis	S/ P/ R/CF	**-osis** *condition* **hydro-** *water* **-nephr/o-** *kidney*	Dilation of pelvis and calyces of a kidney
hydronephrotic (adj)	**HIGH**-droh-neh-**FROT**-ik	S/	**-tic** *pertaining to*	Pertaining to or suffering from the dilation of the pelvis and calyces of the kidney
nephrolithiasis	**NEF**-roh-lih-**THIGH**-ah-sis	S/ R/CF R/	**-iasis** *condition* **nephr/o-** *kidney* **-lith-** *stone*	Presence of a kidney stone
spasmodic (**Note:** One "m" is taken out.)	spaz-**MOD**-ik	S/ R/ R/	**-ic** *pertaining to* **spasm-** *spasm* **-mod-** *nature, form*	Having intermittent spasms or contractions

Disorders of the Urinary Bladder and Urethra

Urinary Tract Infection

A **urinary tract infection (UTI)** occurs when bacteria invade and multiply in the urinary tract. The portal of entry for the bacteria is through the urethra. Because the female urethra is shorter than the male urethra and opens to the surface near the anus *(Figure 6.7)*, bacteria from the gastrointestinal tract can more easily invade the female urethra. This is why women are more prone than men to UTIs. Once UTIs have occurred, they often recur.

Infection of the urethra is called **urethritis;** infection of the urinary bladder is **cystitis.** If cystitis is untreated, infection can spread up the ureters to the renal pelvis, causing pyelitis, and carry on to reach the renal cortex and nephrons, causing pyelonephritis.

Urinary Incontinence

Loss of control of your bladder is called **urinary incontinence.** The result is wet clothes. About 12 million adults in America have urinary incontinence. It is most common in women over the age of 50 years.

Did you know...

- Ten million doctor visits each year in the United States are for UTIs.
- Aging itself is not a cause of urinary incontinence.
- Incontinence is not a way of life. It can be helped.
- Cigarette smoking contributes to more than 50% of bladder cancers.
- Bladder cancer is more common in men than women. It is the fourth most common cancer in men and the eighth in women *(see Chapter 20)*.

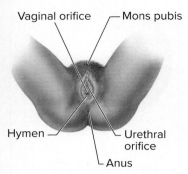

Vaginal orifice — Mons pubis

Hymen —

Urethral orifice

Anus

▲ **Figure 6.7** Female external genitalia.

There are four types of urinary incontinence:

- **Stress incontinence.** Urine leaks because of sudden pressure on the lower stomach muscles when you cough, laugh, sneeze, lift something heavy, or exercise. It is most common in women, with previous pregnancy and childbirth being risk factors.
- **Urge incontinence.** The need to urinate comes on too fast for you to get to the toilet. It is often **idiopathic** but can be associated with UTI, diabetes, stroke, Alzheimer and Parkinson disease, or bladder cancer.
- **Overflow incontinence.** Small amounts of urine leak from a bladder that is always full because you cannot empty it. This occurs when an enlarged prostate gland or tumor blocks the outflow of urine from the bladder. It also occurs in spinal cord injuries and as a side effect of some medications.
- **Functional incontinence.** You cannot get to the toilet in time because of arthritis or any other disease that makes moving quickly difficult.

Urinary retention is the abnormal, involuntary holding of urine in the bladder. **Acute retention** can be caused by an obstruction in the urinary system; for example, an enlarged prostate in the male *(see Chapter 7)* or neurologic problems such as multiple sclerosis. It can be a side effect of anticholinergic drugs that include tricyclic antidepressants *(see Chapter 18).* **Chronic retention** can be caused by untreated obstructions in the urinary tract such as an enlarged prostate.

Transitional cell carcinoma is the most common type of bladder cancer, arising in the transitional cells of the lining of the bladder. A primary symptom of bladder cancer is hematuria.

Word Analysis and Definition: Disorders of the Urinary Bladder and Urethra

S = Suffix   P = Prefix   R = Root   R/CF = Combining Form

WORD	PRONUNCIATION	ELEMENTS		DEFINITION
cystitis	sis-**TIE**-tis	S/ R/	-itis *inflammation* cyst- *bladder*	Inflammation of the urinary bladder
dysuria	dis-**YOU**-ree-ah	S/ P/ R/	-ia *condition* dys- *bad, difficult* -ur- *urine*	Difficulty or pain with urination
frequency	**FREE**-kwen-see	S/ R/	-ency *state of, quality of* frequ- *repeated, often*	The number of times something happens in a given time (e.g., passing urine)
idiopathic	**ID**-ih-oh-**PATH**-ik	S/ R/CF R/	-ic *pertaining to* idi/o- *personal, distinct* -path- *disease*	Pertaining to a disease of unknown etiology (cause)
incontinence	in-**KON**-tin-ens	S/ P/ R/	-ence *state of, quality of* in- *in, not* -contin- *hold together*	Inability to prevent discharge of urine or feces
incontinent (adj)	in-**KON**-tin-ent	S/	-ent *pertaining to, end result*	Denoting incontinence
retention	ree-**TEN**-shun		Latin *hold back*	A holding in of what should normally be discharged (e.g., urine)
urethritis	you-ree-**THRIE**-tis	S/ R/	-itis *inflammation* urethr- *urethra*	Inflammation of the urethra

Check Point Section 6.3

A. Differentiate the types of kidney disorders. *Match the kidney disorder in the first column with its correct description in the second column.* **LO 6.6**

Term	Meaning
_____ 1. renal adenoma	**a.** condition only diagnosed in children
_____ 2. nephroblastoma	**b.** malignant condition of the kidney; develops in the cells of the renal tubules
_____ 3. nephrotic syndrome	**c.** can develop as a result of strep throat infection
_____ 4. renal cell carcinoma	**d.** benign and usually asymptomatic
_____ 5. acute glomerulonephritis	**e.** condition that causes leakage of proteins into the urine; edema of the ankles and legs is a common sign

B. Abbreviations are commonly used in written and verbal communication. *Demonstrate your understanding of kidney disorders by selecting the correct kidney disorder abbreviation that completes each sentence.* **LO 6.6, 6.9**

CRF   ARF   PKD   ESRD

1. An athlete has sprained her knee. She self-treats it with very large doses of ibuprofen, which can lead to _____.

2. Diabetes that is not well managed can lead to _____.

3. An inherited disease in which fluid-filled sacs are present within the kidney is known as _____.

C. Identify the meanings of the word elements in each term. *Recalling the meanings of word elements aids in determining the definition of medical terms.* **LO 6.2, 6.6**

1. The meaning of the prefix in the term *hypertension* is:

   a. pressure   b. condition   c. excessive   d. low

2. The meaning of the prefix in the term *oliguria* is:

   a. urine   b. scanty   c. condition   d. blood

3. The meaning of the suffix in the term *hematuria* is:

   a. urine   b. condition   c. blood   d. inflammation

4. The root *azot-* means:

   a. nitrogen   b. protein   c. sugar   d. without

5. The prefix *poly-* means:

   a. sac   b. fluid   c. scanty   d. many

D. Define the different types of disorders related to the urinary bladder and urethra. *Choose the correct answer that completes each statement.* **LO 6.1, 6.6**

1. The portal of entry for bacteria to infect the urinary bladder is the:

   a. urethra   b. ureter   c. blood   d. kidney

2. The medical term that defines *infection of the bladder* is:

   a. pyelitis   b. cystitis   c. incontinence   d. retention

3. The urologist was unable to determine the cause of the Juan's urethritis. This means that:

   a. The urologist will refer Juan to a nephrologist.

   b. The cause of the inflamed urethra is due to a bacterial infection.

   c. The urologist does not know why Juan's urethra is inflamed.

   d. Juan is unable to urinate due an enlarged prostate.

4. The medical term *incontinence* is defined as a(n)

   a. inability to empty the bladder   b. loss of the micturition reflex

   c. loss of bladder control   d. infection of the bladder and urethra

5. A primary symptom of bladder cancer is

   a. urea in the blood   b. inability to empty the bladder

   c. blood in the urine   d. pain with urination

E. Describe the different types of urinary incontinence. *Match the type of incontinence in column one with its correct definition in the second column.* **LO 6.6**

Term		Meaning
_____	**1.** overflow incontinence	**a.** urine leaks because the need to urinate comes on too fast to make it to the toilet in time to void
_____	**2.** stress incontinence	**b.** urine leaks because the bladder is always full
_____	**3.** functional incontinence	**c.** urine leaks because another condition prevents the person from reaching the toilet in time to void
_____	**4.** urge incontinence	**d.** urine leaks due to sudden pressure, like a cough

Section 6.4 Procedures and Pharmacology

Diagnostic Procedures

Urinalysis

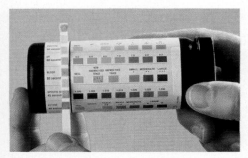

▲ **Figure 6.8** Urinalysis dipstick being compared against color chart on container. Saturn Stills/Science Source

A **dipstick** (a plastic strip bearing paper squares of reagent) is the most cost-effective method of screening urine *(Figure 6.8)*. After the stick is dipped in the urine specimen, the color change in each segment of the dipstick is compared to a color chart on the container. Dipsticks can screen for pH, specific gravity, protein, blood, glucose, ketones, bilirubin, **nitrite,** and leukocyte esterase (see the following).

Routine **urinalysis (UA)** in the laboratory can include the following tests:

- **Visual observation** examines **color** and **clarity.** Normal urine is pale yellow or amber in color and clear. Cloudiness indicates excess cells or cellular material. Red and cloudy indicates red blood cells.

- **Odor** of normal urine has a slight "nutty" scent. Infected urine has a foul odor. **Ketosis** gives urine a fruity odor.

- **pH** measures how acidic or alkaline urine is *(see Chapter 3)*.

- **Specific gravity (SG)** measures how dilute or concentrated the urine is.

- **Protein** is often found in urine. Detection of protein in urine may be benign or a sign of other disorders such as nephrotic syndrome.

- **Glucose** is normally present in the urine in very small amounts and is not detected by urinalysis. When a urinalysis detects glucose, further tests are conducted to determine its cause.

- **Ketones** are present in the urine in **diabetic ketoacidosis** *(see Chapter 17)* or in starvation.

- **Leukocyte esterase** indicates the presence of white blood cells (WBCs) in the urine, which in turn can indicate a UTI.

- **Urine culture** from a clean-catch specimen is the definitive test for a UTI. Culture of the organism and testing of its sensitivity to different antibiotics enables appropriate antibiotic therapy to be prescribed.

Microscopic urinalysis is performed on the solids deposited by centrifuging a specimen of urine. It can reveal red blood cells (RBC's), WBC's, renal tubular epithelial cells stuck together to form **casts,** WBCs stuck together to form casts, and bacteria.

Other Diagnostic Procedures

- **KUB.** An x-ray of the abdomen that shows the kidneys, ureters, and bladder.
- **IVP.** A contrast material containing iodine is injected intravenously, and its progress through the urinary tract is then recorded on a series of rapid x-ray images.
- **Retrograde pyelogram.** Contrast material is injected through a urinary catheter into the ureters to locate stones and other obstructions.
- **Voiding cystourethrogram (VCUG).** Contrast material is inserted into the bladder through a catheter and x-rays are taken as the patient urinates.
- **Computed tomography (CT) scan.** X-ray images show cross-sectional views of the kidneys and bladder.
- **Magnetic resonance imaging (MRI).** Magnetic fields are used to generate cross-sectional images of the urinary tract.
- **Ultrasound imaging (US).** High-frequency sound waves and computer generated noninvasive images of the kidneys.
- **Renal angiogram.** X-rays with contrast material are used to assess blood flow to the kidneys.
- **Cystoscopy.** A pencil-thin, flexible, tubelike optical instrument (**cystoscope**) is inserted through the urethra into the bladder to examine directly the lining of the bladder to determine the causes of hematuria, urinary frequency, urgency, incontinence or urinary retention, and to take a biopsy if needed. Cystoscopy with biopsy is the definitive test for bladder cancer.

Methods of Urine Collection

- **Random collection** is taken with no precautions regarding contamination. It is often used for collecting samples for drug testing.
- **Early morning collection** is used to determine the ability of the kidneys to concentrate urine following overnight dehydration.
- **Clean-catch, midstream specimen** is collected after the external urethral meatus is cleaned. The first part of the urine is passed, and a sterile collecting vessel is introduced into the urinary stream to collect the last part.
- **Twenty-four-hour collection** is used to determine the amount of protein being excreted and to estimate the kidneys' filtration ability.
- **Suprapubic transabdominal needle aspiration** of the bladder is used in newborns and small infants to obtain a pure sample of urine.
- **Catheterization of the bladder** can be used as a last resort to obtain a urine specimen. A soft plastic or rubber tube (catheter) is inserted through the urethra into the bladder to drain and collect urine.

WORD	PRONUNCIATION	ELEMENTS		DEFINITION
cast	KAST		Latin *pure*	A cylindrical mold formed by materials in kidney tubules
cystoscope	**SIS**-toh-skope	S/	-scope *instrument for viewing*	An endoscope to view the inside of the bladder
		R/CF	cyst/o- *bladder*	
cystoscopy	sis-**TOS**-koh-pee	S/	-scopy *to examine*	The process of using a cystoscope
cystourethrogram	sis-toh-you-**REETH**-roh-gram	S/	-gram *a record*	X-ray image during voiding to show structure and function of bladder and urethra
		R/CF	cyst/o- *bladder*	
		R/CF	-urethr/o- *urethra*	
ketone	**KEY**-tone		Greek *acetone*	Chemical formed in uncontrolled diabetes or in starvation
ketosis	key-**TOH**-sis	S/	-sis *condition*	Excess production of ketones
		R/CF	ket/o- *ketones*	
ketoacidosis	**KEY**-toh-ass-ih-**DOH**-sis	R/CF	-acid/o- *acid, low pH*	Excessive production of ketones, making the blood acidic
nitrite	**NIE**-trite		Greek *niter, saltpeter*	Chemical formed in urine by *Escherichia coli (E. coli)* and other microorganisms
pyelogram	**PIE**-el-oh-gram	S/	-gram *recording*	X-ray image of renal pelvis and ureters
		R/CF	pyel/o- *renal pelvis*	
retrograde	**RET**-roh-grade	P/	retro- *backward*	Reversal of a normal flow; for example, back from the bladder into the ureters
		R/	-grade *going*	
stage	STAYJ		Latin *status, to stand*	A description of the distribution and extent of dissemination of a cancer disease process
suprapubic	**SOO**-prah-**PYU**-bik	S/	-ic *pertaining to*	Above the symphysis pubis
		P/	supra- *above*	
		R/	-pub- *pubis*	
urinalysis	you-rih-**NAL**-ih-sis	S/	-lysis *to separate*	Examination of urine to separate it into its elements and define their kind and/or quantity
		R/CF	urin/a- *urine*	

Therapeutic Procedures

Renal Stones

For renal stones that do not pass down the ureter into the bladder and out of the body in urine, there are several treatment options:

- **Watchful waiting.** With pain medication to relieve symptoms, the hope is that the stone can be passed.
- **Extracorporeal shock wave lithotripsy (ESWL).** With ESWL, a machine called a **lithotripter** from outside the body generates sound waves that crumble the stone into small pieces that can pass down the ureter into the bladder and be voided.
- **Ureteroscopy.** A small, flexible **ureteroscope** is passed through the urethra and bladder into the ureter. Devices can be passed through the endoscope to remove or fragment the stone.
- **Percutaneous nephrolithotomy.** A **nephroscope** is inserted through the skin and into the kidney to locate and remove the stone.
- **Open surgery.** A surgical incision is made to expose the ureter and remove the stone; this is rarely done.

Nephrectomy

A **nephrectomy** is the removal of a kidney, entirely or partially. Nephrectomies are typically performed to treat renal carcinomas. Surgical methods to perform nephrectomies are open, laparoscopic, or via a robotic system.

Radical nephrectomy is the removal of the entire kidney and surrounding tissues to treat renal carcinoma.

A **donor nephrectomy** is the removal of a healthy kidney from a person so that it can be given to a person needing a healthy kidney.

Partial nephrectomy is the removal of the diseased tissue of the kidney while leaving the healthy kidney tissue.

Kidney Failure

Dialysis is an artificial method of removing waste materials and excess fluid from the blood in end-stage renal disease. It is not a cure, but can prolong life. There are several types of kidney dialysis: in treatment of acute renal failure (ARF), the goal is to treat the underlying disease. Dialysis may be necessary while the kidneys are healing.

- **Hemodialysis** *(Figure 6.9)* filters the blood through an artificial kidney machine (**dialyzer**). Most patients require 12 hours of dialysis weekly, usually in three sessions.

- **Peritoneal dialysis** uses a solution that is infused into and drained out of the patient's abdominal cavity through a small flexible catheter implanted into the patient's abdominal cavity. The dialysis solution extracts wastes and excess fluid from the blood through the network of capillaries in the peritoneal lining of the abdominal cavity.

- **Continuous ambulatory peritoneal dialysis (CAPD)** *(Figure 6.10)* is performed by the patient at home usually four times each day, seven days a week.

- **Continuous cycling peritoneal dialysis (CCPD)** uses a machine to automatically infuse dialysis solution into and out of the abdominal cavity during sleep.

A **kidney transplant** provides a better quality of life than dialysis, provided a suitable donor can be found *(see Chapter 12)*. A **sibling** or blood relative can often qualify as a donor. If not, tissue banks across the country can search for a kidney from an accident victim or a donor who has died.

Urinary Bladder

Cystoscopy can be used therapeutically to remove stones, polyps, and some types of tumors. It can also be used to perform a transurethral resection of the prostate (**TURP**) to remove tissue from the inner portion of the prostate gland in men with benign prostatic hyperplasia (**BPH**).

For acute or chronic lower urinary tract obstruction in which the urethra is blocked, a flexible urethral catheter (**Foley catheter**) is passed into the bladder. The catheter can be left indwelling, or the patient can perform clean intermittent catheterization. If a Foley catheter cannot be passed, a suprapubic tube can be placed through the lower anterior abdominal wall into the bladder.

Treatment for urinary incontinence depends on the cause. If a medical or surgical problem is present, then the incontinence can go away when the problem is treated. **Bladder training** and **biofeedback** lengthen the time between the urges to go to the toilet. **Kegel exercises** strengthen the muscles of the pelvic floor. Medications, for example, oxybutynin, are used for urge incontinence. Surgery can pull up the bladder and secure it if pelvic floor muscles are weak (**cystopexy**). Absorbent underclothing is available.

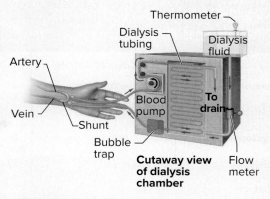

▲ **Figure 6.9** Hemodialysis.

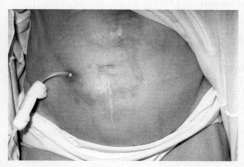

▲ **Figure 6.10** Continuous ambulatory peritoneal dialysis. Mediscan/Alamy Stock Photo

WORD	PRONUNCIATION		ELEMENTS	DEFINITION
ambulatory (adj)	**AM**-byu-lah-tor-ee	S/ R/	**-ory** *relating to* **ambulat-** *walk*	Relating to walking
catheter	**KATH**-eh-ter		Greek *to send down*	Hollow tube that allows passage of fluid into or out of a body cavity, organ, or vessel
cystopexy	**SIS**-toh-pek-see	S/ R/CF	**-pexy** *surgical fixation* **cyst/o-** *bladder*	Surgical procedure to support the urinary bladder
dialysis	die-**AL**-ih-sis	P/ R/	**dia-** *complete* **-lysis** *to separate*	An artificial method of filtration to remove excess waste materials and water from the body
dialyzer	die-**A**-lie-zer	S/	**-lyzer** *separator*	Machine that performs dialysis
hemodialysis	**HEE**-moh-die-**AL**-ih-sis	R/CF	**hem/o-** *blood*	An artificial machine-based method to remove wastes from the blood
extracorporeal	**EKS**-trah-kor-**POH**-ree-al	S/ P/ R/	**-eal** *pertaining to* **extra-** *outside* **-corpor-** *body*	Outside the body
Kegel exercises	**KEE**-gal **EKS**-er-size-ez		Arnold Kegel, 1894–1981, American gynecologist	Contraction and relaxation of the pelvic floor muscles to improve urethral and rectal sphincter function
lithotripsy	**LITH**-oh-trip-see	S/ R/CF	**-tripsy** *to crush* **lith/o-** *stone*	Crushing stones by sound waves
lithotripter	**LITH**-oh–trip-ter	S/	**-tripter** *crusher*	Instrument that generates the sound waves
nephrectomy	neh-**FREK**-toh-mee	S/ R/	**-ectomy** *removal of* **nephr-** *kidney*	Surgical removal of a kidney
nephrolithotomy	**NEF**-roh-lih-**THOT**-oh-mee	S/ R/CF R/CF	**-tomy** *surgical incision* **nephr/o-** *kidney* **lith/o-** *stone*	Incision to remove a renal stone
nephroscope	**NEF**-roh-skope	S/ R/CF	**-scope** *instrument for viewing* **nephr/o-** *kidney*	Endoscope to view the inside of the kidney
nephroscopy	neh-**FROS**-koh-pee	S/	**-scopy** *to examine*	Visual examination of the kidney
percutaneous	**PER**-kyu-**TAY**-nee-us	S/ P/ R/CF	**-us** *pertaining to* **per-** *through* **cutane/o-** *skin*	Pertaining to through the skin
transplant	**TRANZ**-plant	P/ R/	**trans-** *across* **-plant** *insert, plant*	The act of transferring tissue from one person to another
ureteroscope	you-**REE**-ter-oh-skope	S/ R/CF	**-scope** *instrument for viewing* **ureter/o-** *ureter*	Endoscope to view the inside of the ureter
ureteroscopy	you-**REE**-ter-**OS**-koh-pee	S/	**-scopy** *to examine*	Endoscopic examination of the inside of the ureter

Pharmacology of the Urinary System

There are several distinct classes of drugs with different effects on the urinary system.

Diuretics

Diuretic drugs increase urine output by the kidney—they promote this **diuresis** by altering how the kidney handles sodium. If the kidney excretes more sodium, then water excretion will also increase. **Loop diuretics** such as furosemide (*Lasix*) are more powerful than **thiazide** diuretics such as hydrochlorothiazide. The most frequent problem with both forms of diuretics is **hypokalemia,** and potassium supplements are usually prescribed with them. Acetazolamide (*Diamox*) is a weak diuretic that also lowers the intraocular pressure in glaucoma (*see Chapter 16*).

Renal Drugs

Pyelonephritis, which is inflammation of the pelvis of the kidney usually spreading from a **urinary tract infection (UTI),** is treated aggressively with antibiotics, such as an aminoglycoside (*Gentamycin*) together with ampicillin or ceftriaxone (*Rocephin*).

Nephrotic syndrome is treated initially with corticosteroids (*Prednisolone*) and cytostatic drugs, such as cyclophosphamide (*Cytoxan*) and cyclosporine (*Cyclosporin A*), are used for relapses.

Renal cell carcinoma is resistant to both radiation and chemotherapy, metastases are treated with targeted therapies using drugs such as temsirolimus (*Torisel*) and bevacizumab (*Avastin*).

Renal transplant patients receive a regimen of drugs to prevent rejection. The most common regimen is a cocktail of tacrolimus (*Prograf*), mycophenolate (*Cellcept*), and prednisone (generic).

Nonrenal Urinary Tract Drugs

Antibiotics are the usual treatment for UTIs no matter in which part of the urinary system the infection is located. The specific antibiotic to be used is determined by the **sensitivity** of the organism obtained by **culture** of the urine specimen. UTIs, including **cystitis,** are treated with antibiotics, such as trimethoprim (*Trimpex, Primsol*), nitrofurantoin (*Furadantin, Macrobid*), or one of the many cephalosporins. Infections that spread from the urinary tract to the epididymis (epididymitis) and the testes (orchitis) are treated with cefalexin or ciprofloxacin.

Cranberry juice may make the inside wall of the bladder slippery, preventing bacteria from sticking to it. Studies on its effectiveness to treat or prevent UTIs show mixed results.

In patients with chronic renal disease and diminished renal function, dosing of renally excreted drugs should be adjusted by reducing the dose, increasing the dosing interval, or both. Drugs that have to be adjusted include antihypertensive agents, hypoglycemic agents, antimicrobials, analgesics, NSAIDs, and many herbal products.

A **urinary analgesic** phenazopyridine (*Pyridium*), a dye, is used to provide symptomatic relief in acute cystitis and is often prescribed after the use of an indwelling Foley catheter, cystoscopy, or urinary bladder surgery. It produces a vivid dark orange to red color in the urine.

Alpha-blocking agents (**alpha-blockers**) relax smooth muscle in the body. They can be used to relax the smooth muscle in the ureters and make them wider to help a kidney stone pass more easily.

There are no reliable medications that can prevent renal stones from forming, though alkalinization of the urine with acetazolamide (*Diamox*) can help.

Drugs for Sexually Transmitted Diseases

Sexually transmitted diseases (STDs) are caused by a variety of organisms in both men and women and primarily affect the **genitalia.** They require different drug treatments, depending on the organism.

- **Chlamydia** is treated with a single dose of azithromycin (*Zithromax* and others) or a week of doxycycline (*Vibramycin* and others) in both sexes.

- **Trichomoniasis** is treated with metronidazole (*Flagyl*) or tinidazole (*Tindamax*).

- **Gonorrhea** has become resistant to most classes of antibiotics except cephalosporins, such as ceftriaxone (*Rocephin*) and cefixime (*Suprax*).

- **Bacterial vaginosis** is treated with metronidazole (*Flagyl*) or clindamycin (*Cleocin*).

- **Pelvic inflammatory disease (PID),** which is usually a complication of *Chlamydia* or gonorrhea, is treated with antibiotic combinations of two drugs—for example, cefotetan (*Cefotan*) and doxycycline (*Vibramycin*); clindamycin (*Cleocin*) and gentamicin (*Garamycin*); or cefoxitin (*Cefotan*) and doxycycline (*Vibramycin*).

- **Genital herpes infections** have no cure, but antiviral medications, such as acyclovir (*Zovirax*), famaciclovir (*Famvir*), and valacyclovir (*Valtrex*), can prevent or cut short outbreaks.

- **Syphilis** in its early stages requires a single dose of IM penicillin. If the infection has been present for more than a year, additional doses are required.

- **Human papilloma virus (HPV)** has 40 different types that infect the genital area. HPV can cause cervical cancer. There is no known treatment, but two vaccines are approved by the FDA. *Cervarix* protects against HPV types 16 and 18. *Gardasil* protects against types 6, 11, 16, and 18. Both protect against HPV types that cause 70% of cervical cancers, and *Gardasil* protects against HPV types that cause 90% of genital warts.

- **Human immunodeficiency virus (HIV) infections** have no cure. The aim of treatment is to maintain a good quality of life and prevent the development of **acquired immunodeficiency syndrome (AIDS).** Highly active antiretroviral therapy (**HAART**) is a combination of at least three drugs belonging to at least two types of **antiretroviral** agents. Without HAART, HIV infection progresses to AIDS in approximately 9 to 10 years.

The sexually transmitted diseases—chlamydia, trichomoniasis, gonorrhea, syphilis—are detailed in *Chapter 8.*

Prostate Drugs

Prostatitis is usually an extension of an *E. coli* UTI. In the acute phase, antibiotics such as trimethoprim-sulfamethoxazole (*Bactrim, Septa*), fluoroquinolones (*Floxin, Cipro*), or doxycycline (*Vibramycin*) are given for 14 days. If the disease is chronic, the regimen is continued for 4 to 12 weeks.

Benign prostatic hypertrophy (BPH) is commonly treated with medications. **Alpha blockers,** such as doxazosin (*Cardura*), tamsulosin (*Flomax*), or alfuzosin (*Uroxatral*), relax smooth muscle at the bladder neck to allow a freer flow of urine. **5-alpha-reductase inhibitors,** such as finasteride (*Proscar, Propecia*) and dutasteride (*Avodart*), inhibit the production of dihydrotestosterone, which is believed to stimulate the prostate cells to grow. **Tadalafil** (*Cialis*) show promise for treating this condition.

Prostate cancer is treated primarily with surgery or radiation therapy. Other treatments such as hormonal or chemotherapy are not approved by the Federal Drug Administration (FDA).

Other Nonrenal Urinary Tract Drugs

Erectile dysfunction (ED) can be treated with drugs designed to improve the flow of blood to the penis. Examples include sildenafil (*Viagra*), tadalafil (*Cialis*), vardenafil (*Levitra*), and alprostadil (*Edex, Caverject*), which is injected into one of the corpus cavernosa of the penis. The latter drug is sometimes used for the treatment of **impotence.**

Urinary incontinence, which is any involuntary leakage of urine, almost always results from an underlying treatable medical condition. In an **overactive bladder,** which causes incontinence, drugs that relax the bladder muscle wall can alleviate the symptoms. They include tolterodine (*Detrol*), oxybutynin (*Ditropan*), trospium (*Sanctura*), solifenacin (*Vesicare*), darifenacin (*Enablex*), and an oxybutynin skin patch (*Oxytrol*).

Word Analysis and Definition: Pharmacology of the Urinary System

S = Suffix   P = Prefix   R = Root   R/CF = Combining Form

WORD	PRONUNCIATION		ELEMENTS	DEFINITION
alpha-blocking agent	**AL**-fah **BLOK**-ing **A**-jent		**alpha-** Greek *first letter*	Drugs that relax smooth muscle
alpha-blockers			**block** French *inhibit*	
analgesia	an-al-**JEE**-zee-ah	S/ P/ R/	**-ia** *condition* **an-** *without* **-alges-** *sensation of pain*	State in which pain is reduced
analgesic (adj)	an-al-**JEE**-zik	S/	**-ic** *pertaining to*	Substance that produces analgesia
antiretroviral (adj)	**AN**-tee-**REH**-troh-**VIE**-rul	S/ P/	**-al** *pertaining to* **anti-** *against*	An agent that inhibits or kills any virus of the family
retrovirus	**RET**-roh-vi-rus	P/ R/	**-retro-** *back, backward* **-vir-** *virus*	A virus with RNA core genetic material
culture	**KUL**-chur		Latin *to till*	The reproduction of microorganisms (e.g., bacteria) on or in various media
diuresis (*Note:* The *a* is dropped)	die-you-**REE**-sis	S/ P/ R/	**-esis** *abnormal condition* **dia-** *complete* **-ur-** *urinary system*	Excretion of large volumes of urine
diuretic (adj)	die-you-**REH**-tik	S/	**-etic** *pertaining to*	Agent that increases urine output
dysfunction	dis-**FUNK**-shun	P/ R/	**dys-** *difficult, painful* **-function-** *perform*	Difficulty in performing
dysfunctional (adj)	dis-**FUNK**-shun-al	S/	**-al** *pertaining to*	Having difficulty in performing
genital	**JEN**-it-al	S/ R/	**-al** *pertaining to* **genit-** *primary male or female sex organs*	Relating to the male or female sex organs
genitalia	**JEN**-ih-**TAY**-lee-ah	S/	**-ia** *condition*	External and internal organs of reproduction
hypokalemia	**HIGH**-poh-kah-**LEE**-mee-ah	S/ P/ R/	**-emia** *blood condition* **hypo-** *below, low* **-kal-** *potassium*	Low concentration of potassium in the blood
impotence	**IM**-poh-tence		Latin *inability*	Inability to achieve an erection
overactive	**OH**-ver-**AK**-tiv	S/ P/ R/	**-ive** *function, connection* **over-** *above* **-act-** *process of doing*	An exaggerated response
sensitivity	sen-si-**TIV**-ih-tee	S/ R/	**-ity** *condition, state* **sensitiv-** *feeling*	Denoting the susceptibility of a microorganism to inhibition or destruction by a given antibiotic
vaginosis	vah-jih-**NOH**-sis	S/ R/	**-osis** *condition* **vagin-** *vagina*	Any disease of the vagina
vaginitis	vah-jih-**NIE**-tis	S/	**-itis** *inflammation*	Inflammation of the vagina

Check Point Section 6.4

A. Apply your knowledge of medical language to this exercise. *All the questions can be answered using terms from this spread. Select the best answer.* **LO 6.5**

1. An x-ray image taken during voiding:

    a. retrograde   **b.** pyelogram   **c.** KUB   **d.** cystourethrogram

2. Reversal of normal flow:

    a. reflex   **b.** retrograde   **c.** regenerate   **d.** retention

3. Excessive ketones in the blood, making it acidic:

    a. ketosis   **b.** ketoacidosis   **c.** ketone

4. Separating urine into its elements:

    a. urinalysis   **b.** cystourethrogram   **c.** retrograde   **d.** pyelogram

B. Abbreviations are used in written and verbal communication. *Complete each sentence with the correct abbreviations. Use the provided abbreviations to fill in the blanks.* **LO 6.7, 6.9**

| BPH | CAPD | CCPD | ESWL | TURP |

1. The nephrologist recommended that the patient have _____ to assist in the passing of his kidney stones.

2. Because of his _____, Mr. Plaza suffered from overflow incontinence.

3. Mrs. Doskos prefers to receive her dialysis while she sleeps, and therefore the nephrologist recommended _____ to dialyze her blood.

4. _____ is used to remove sections of an enlarged prostate.

5. _____ allows the patient to walk around while receiving dialysis.

C. Construct terms using word elements. *Given the definition, complete each medical term with the correct missing element. Fill in the blank. The first one has been done for you.* **LO 6.1, 6.2, 6.9**

1. Relating to walking   <u>ambulat</u>/ory
2. Surgical procedure to support the urinary bladder.   cysto/ _____
3. Visual examination of the kidney.   _____ /scopy
4. Pertaining to through the skin.   _____ /cutaneo/us
5. Incision to remove a stone.   nephro/litho/ _____
6. Artificial method to remove wastes from the blood.   _____ /dia/lysis

D. Demonstrate the proper use of medical terms. *Suffixes change the meanings of words and how they are to be used in verbal and written communication. Complete each sentence with the proper term provided in parentheses. Fill in the blank.* **LO 6.2, 6.3, 6.7, 6.8**

1. The _____ (**diuretic/diuresis**) medication was given to increase Mrs. Bienvenue's urinary output.

2. The patient needed _____ (**analgesia/analgesic**) to relieve the moderate pain caused by the cystitis.

3. Morphine relieves pain and therefore is an _____ (**analgesia/analgesic**).

4. The nephrologist recommend that _____ (**diuretic/diuresis**) be utilized to quickly relieve the excess fluid in the patient's interstitial tissues.

SECTION 6.4 Procedures and Pharmacology 165

E. Identify the purpose and effects of medications used to treat urinary system conditions. *Select the term that correctly answers each question.* **LO 6.7**

1. In order to choose the correct antibiotic, the physician must order a urine:

    a. blocker   **b.** culture   **c.** analgesic   **d.** chemotherapeutic

2. A side effect of some diuretics is:

    a. hypokalemia   **b.** carcinoma   **c.** bacterial infection   **d.** analgesia

3. The usual treatment for an UTI is:

    a. radiation   **b.** diuresis   **c.** surgery   **d.** antibiotics

4. A dye that produces an analgesic effect in the urinary system is:

    a. ibuprofen   **b.** aspirin   **c.** phenazopyridine   **d.** cyclophosphamide

F. Review what you learned in the earlier chapters about word elements. *Choose the correct answer for each question.* **LO 6.1, 6.2, 6.7**

1. What is most unusual about the term *antiretroviral?*

    a. it has two prefixes

    b. it does not have a root

    c. it has only one suffix

    d. it lacks a combining vowel

2. Vaginosis would be found in which body system?

    a. male

    b. female

3. Which of the following medications will not cure vaginal infections?

    a. *Cipro*

    b. *Flagyl*

    c. *Valtrex*

    d. *Tindamax*

G. Match the condition with the drug(s) used to treat it. *Choose the correct term in the second column.* **LO 6.6, 6.7, 6.9**

_____ **1.** syphilis	**a.**	antibiotic combination of two drugs
_____ **2.** HP	**b.**	HAART
_____ **3.** PID	**c.**	IM penicillin
_____ **4.** bacterial vaginosis	**d.**	no known treatment
_____ **5.** HIV	**e.**	*Flagyl*

H. Match the condition with the drug(s) or other treatment types used to treat it. *Choose the correct term in the second column.* **LO 6.7**

_____ 1. Prostate cancer	**a.** solifenacin
_____ 2. Erectile dysfunction	**b.** Bactrim, Cipro
_____ 3. Prostatitis	**c.** alpha blockers or alfuzosin
_____ 4. Benign prostatic hypertrophy	**d.** radiation therapy
_____ 5. Overactive bladder	**e.** sildenafil, tadalafil

I. Precision in communication involves correct spelling. *Select the pair of terms that is spelled incorrectly. Rewrite them as correct on the following lines.* **LO 6.6, 6.7**

1. **a.** dysfunction   overactive

   b. inhibbitors   impotance

   c. erectile   cavernosa

   d. prostatitise   genital

   e. genitalia   pelvic

2. Corrected first terms: _____

3. Corrected second terms: _____

Table 6.2 Chapter 6 Abbreviations

Abbreviation	Meaning	Abbreviation	Meaning
AIDS	acquired immunodeficiency syndrome	HPV	human papilloma virus
ARF	acute renal failure	IV	intravenous
BP	blood pressure	IVP	intravenous pyelogram
BPH	benign prostatic hyperplasia	KUB	x-ray of abdomen to show **k**idneys, **u**reters, and **b**ladder
CAPD	continuous ambulatory peritoneal dialysis	MRI	magnetic resonance imaging
CCPD	continuous cycling peritoneal dialysis	PID	pelvic inflammatory disease
CKD	chronic kidney disease; also known as chronic renal failure	PKD	polycystic kidney disease
CRF	chronic renal failure; also known as chronic kidney disease	SG	specific gravity
CT	computed tomography	STD	sexually transmitted disease
ED	erectile dysfunction	TNM	tumor, nodes, and metastases (tumor staging method)
EMT-P	emergency medical technician–paramedic	TURP	transurethral resection of the prostate
ESRD	end-stage renal disease	UA	urinalysis
ESWL	extracorporeal shock wave lithotripsy	US	ultrasound
HAART	highly active antiretroviral therapy	UTI	urinary tract infection
HIV	human immunodeficiency virus	VCUG	voiding cystourethrogram
HPI	history of present illness	VS	vital signs

Table 6.3 Comparison of Common Urinary Disorders

Disorder or Disease	Signs and Symptoms	Diagnostic Tests	Treatment
Prostatitis	Dysuria, hematuria, flu-like symptoms	Urinalysis, blood tests, CT	Antibiotics, alpha-blockers if condition is not due to infection, NSAIDs for pain
Benign prostatic hypertrophy	Problems with urinating such as difficulty in starting urination or not completely emptying the bladder	Urinalysis to rule out infection, cystoscopy	Medication—alpha-blockers or 5-alpha-reductase inhibitors and tadalafil (*Cialis*) or TURP via cystoscopy
Prostate cancer			Surgery or radiation
Renal stones	Hematuria, proteinuria, swelling in face, hands, feet, and abdomen	Urinalysis, KUB, ultrasound, CT	ESWL, ureteroscopy, percutaneous nephrolithotomy, open surgery
Urinary incontinence due to overactive bladder	Sudden urge to urinate, frequent urination	Urinalysis, measurements of bladder function	Kegel exercises, incontinence medications
Kidney failure	Decreased amount or urine production, swelling in legs, fatigue	Measure urine production, urinalysis, blood test, ultrasound, CT	Dialysis or transplant
UTI	Abdominal pain, dysuria	Urinalysis, culture to identify bacteria causing infection	Antibiotics

2014 Nucleus Medical Media

Urinary System

Challenge Your Knowledge

A. System review. Understanding the structure and function of the urinary system will give you a better grasp of the terminology. Choose the correct answers to the following questions. **LO 6.1, 6.2, 6.6**

1. Where does waste-laden blood enter the kidney?

a. the fascia   d. the renal vein

b. the glomerulus   e. the portal vein

c. the hilum

2. The medical term to describe urine being forced back up the ureter to the kidneys is

a. reflux   d. absorption

b. filtration   e. micturition

c. excretion

3. What results if the kidney produces too much renin?

a. hematuria   c. hypertension

b. oliguria   d. anuria

4. What is the end product of amino acid metabolism?

a. ammonia   d. nitrates

b. glycogen   e. renin

c. lipid

5. What do urethritis, cystitis, pyelitis, and pyelonephritis all have in common?

a. infection   d. fever

b. skin rash   e. kidney

c. bladder

6. Each kidney is the size of a(n)

a. orange   d. bean

b. golf ball   e. ping-pong ball

c. clenched fist

7. All of the nephrons are located in the kidney's

a. medulla   d. cortex

b. calyces   e. hilum

c. pelvis

8. The external opening of a passage is called a

a. meatus   d. bladder

b. urethra   e. hilum

c. ureter

9. The glomerulus is encased in

a. a blood vessel   d. the glomerular capsule

b. a muscle   e. the urethra

c. renal fascia

10. Nephrotic syndrome involves large amounts of _____ leaking out into the urine.

a. protein   d. blood

b. sugar   e. white blood cells

c. red blood cells

11. Muscular tube, about 10 inches long, that carries urine to the bladder. This describes the

a. ureter   c. renal vein

b. urethra   d. nephron

12. Another name for a kidney stone is

a. UTI   d. hematuria

b. calculus   e. lithotripsy

c. tumor

13. Water is returned to the blood by

a. excretion   d. elimination

b. filtration   e. respiration

c. reabsorption

2014 Nucleus Medical Media

B. **Abbreviations are not helpful if you do not understand their meaning and cannot use them to communicate safely and effectively.** Demonstrate that you can put the appropriate abbreviation in the correct context. You will not use every abbreviation listed to fill in the blanks. **LO 6.5, 6.6, 6.9**

ARF	ESWL	KUB	SPA
BUN	GRF	MRI	TNM
CRF	IV	PKD	UA
ESRD	IVP	SG	UTI

1. Dr. Lee ordered the _____ medication stat.

2. The patient informed me that there is a history of _____ in his family.

3. The patient with the kidney stone is scheduled for _____ early tomorrow morning.

4. The patient's renal carcinoma was staged using the _____ method.

5. The patient returns with her second _____ this month. Medication is prescribed.

C. **Review.** One or more roots or combining forms can have the same meaning. Demonstrate that you can use these elements correctly. *Remember: They are not interchangeable.* One particular root or combining form goes with a specific suffix. Fill in the blanks. **LO 6.2, 6.6, 6.9**

-al	-in	-ic	-logist	-ectomy	-itis	-logist	-logy

1. Having intermittent spasms or contractions   spasmod/ _____

2. Expert in the study of the kidney   nephro/ _____

3. Pertaining to the kidney   ren/ _____

4. Removal of the kidney   nephr/ _____

5. Kidney enzyme that causes vasoconstriction   ren/ _____

6. Inflammation of the kidney   nephr/ _____

7. Study of the kidney   nephro/ _____

8. Specialist in kidney diseases   nephro/ _____

D. Matching. Confirm that your knowledge of the language of the urinary system and its functions is accurate. Match the statements in the first column to the correct answers in the second column. **LO 6.6, 6.7**

_____ 1. Outside the body   **a.** uremia

_____ 2. Pertaining to a disease of unknown cause   **b.** idiopathic

_____ 3. Donor organ to recipient   **c.** catheter

_____ 4. Reversal of normal flow   **d.** extracorporeal

_____ 5. Hollow tube   **e.** retrograde

_____ 6. Loss of bladder control   **f.** dialyzer

_____ 7. Disease state resulting from renal failure   **g.** transplant

_____ 8. Artificial kidney machine   **h.** incontinence

E. Each of these diagnoses relates to a specific organ in the urinary system. Fill in the chart. **LO 6.6, 6.7**

Diagnosis	Organ in the Urinary System
1. urethritis	
2. cystitis	
3. nephritis	
4. ureteritis	

F. Tests and procedures. Patients with urinary problems will be sent for various renal function tests and diagnostic procedures that may result in a surgical procedure. Any of the following procedures might be ordered for your patient. Do you know their purpose? Be prepared to discuss which terms are tests and which are procedures. **LO 6.5, 6.7**

_____ 1. Contrast material injected to locate stones   **a.** dialysis

_____ 2. Collection of bladder sample in newborns   **b.** transplant

_____ 3. Incision for removal of kidney stone   **c.** KUB

_____ 4. Crushing renal stone by sound waves   **d.** retrograde pyelogram

_____ 5. Assess blood flow to the kidneys   **e.** cystoscopy

_____ 6. Tissue bank matching of donor to recipient   **f.** nephrolithotomy

_____ 7. Treatment for renal cell carcinoma   **g.** nephrectomy

_____ 8. X-ray of the abdominal urinary organs   **h.** needle aspiration

_____ 9. Viewing the bladder through a scope   **i.** renal angiogram

_____ 10. Filtering blood through an artificial kidney machine   **j.** lithotripsy

G. **Patient documentation.** Answer the questions as they relate to the example of documentation presented below. Choose the correct answer for each question. **LO 6.6, 6.7, 6.8**

Documentation

A 68-year-old female presents with hematuria, dysuria, and left-flank pain. I ordered a KUB and an IVP to ascertain the possibility or extent of obstruction. Test results indicate one large and several small calculi impacted in her left ureter just below the renal hilum. Patient would prefer ESWL, but surgical laparoscopy, I think, will offer better and quicker results to alleviate her pain. Patient will proceed with surgery tomorrow.

1. What are the patient's symptoms? (Choose all that apply.)

    a. KUB   **b.** calculi   **c.** hematuria   **d.** pain

2. What diagnostic tests were performed? (Choose all that apply.)

    a. KUB   **b.** calculi   **c.** ESWL   **d.** laparoscopy   **e.** hilum

3. What organs were checked in these tests? (Choose all that apply.)

    a. kidneys   **b.** ureters   **c.** bladder   **d.** urethra

4. What is a *laparoscopy*?

    a. removal of calculi   **c.** procedure to view the inside of the abdomen

    b. procedure to crush stones   **d.** surgical fixation of the urinary bladder

5. What is a preoperative diagnosis for this patient?

    a. urinary tract infection   **c.** renal calculi

    b. bladder cancer   **d.** acute renal failure

H. Roots and combining forms are the foundation of a medical term. Differentiate their meanings by analyzing the rest of the term. If the term does not have a particular word element, write n/a. Fill in the blanks. **LO 6.2, 6.6**

Medical Term	Meaning of Prefix	Meaning or Root/ Combining Form	Meaning of Suffix	Meaning of Term
anuria	1.	2.	3.	4.
dysuria	5.	6.	7.	8.
micturition	9.	10.	11.	12.
uremia	13.	14.	15.	16.
oliguria	17.	18.	19.	20.
interstitial	21.	22.	23.	24.

I. Correct pronunciation of medical terms is necessary when communicating to health care professional and to the patient and their friends and family members. Choose the correct answer to the following questions.

1. In the term *urethra,* the letter "e" is pronounced like the letter "e" in:

   a. bet   **b.** new   **c.** break   **d.** me

2. The bolded letter "o" in the following term *nephrology* is pronounced like the "o" in:

   a. throat   **b.** rot   **c.** goose   **d.** boy

3. Identify the correct pronunciation for each term:

   a. meatus—**MEET**-us

   b. adenoma—**AID**-ehno-may

   c. nephritis—neh-**FRIE**-tis

   d. pyelogram—**PEE**-el-oh-gram

4. The bolded letters in the term "**anal**gesic" are correctly pronounced:

   a. an-al   **b.** ane-al   **c.** uh-null   **d.** een-el

5. In the term *renin,* the "e" is pronounced like the "e" in:

   a. bet   **b.** new   **c.** break   **d.** me

Case Reports

A. After reading the following Case Report, correctly answer the following questions. The answers to the Case Report may not be in the Case Report itself but can be found in the chapter content. **LO 6.2, 6.5, 6.8, 6.9, 6.10**

Case Report (CR) 6.1

You are

. . . a surgical physician assistant working with Phillip Johnson, a medical doctor specializing in the study of the urinary tract at Fulwood Medical Center.

Your patient is

. . . Mr. Nelson Hughes, a 58-year-old school principal. Mr. Nelson Hughes had been well until a few months before his surgery, when he noticed a vague, aching pain in his left loin. One week before surgery, he suddenly passed bright red urine. **Urinalysis** showed (1)_____. Physical examination revealed an enlarged left kidney. IVP and other imaging tests showed a tumor 3 inches in diameter in the center of the left kidney. Bone scan was normal, indicating no **metastases** to bone.

Earlier today you assisted at Mr. Hughes's surgery. A **laparoscopic radical nephrectomy** for a **tumor- nodes-metastases (TNM) stage II renal cell carcinoma** (2)_____ with no evidence of local invasion or lymph node involvement (3)_____ was performed.

You are making your afternoon hospital visits to Dr. Johnson's patients. Your job is to assess Mr. Hughes's postoperative state and determine whether postoperative complications exist.

2014 Nucleus Medical Media

1. Based on the color of his urine, what condition did the urinalysis show? _____

2. When communicating with Mr. Hughes and his family, rather than use the term *carcinoma*, you what word might you use so they understood his condition? _____

3. When documenting, *no evidence of local invasion or lymph node involvement*, which one word would replace this status? _____

4. The diagnostic test that showed that presence of a tumor evaluated which of the following organs? (Choose all that apply)

    a. Kidney   **b.** Bladder   **c.** Urethra   **d.** Ureters

5. Which of the following conditions indicate the status of the "N" of the abbreviation TNM?

    a. No metastases to the lymph node   **c.** Radical nephrectomy

    b. Lack of tumor to the kidney   **d.** Lack of metastases to the bone

6. Which term correctly describes Dr. Johnson's specialty?

    a. Enterologist   **b.** Urologist   **c.** Gynecologist   **d.** Nephrologist

7. Which two letters abbreviate Dr. Johnson's doctoral degree? (Do not add periods to the abbreviation) _____

B. After reading the following Case Report, correctly answer the following questions. The answers to the Case Report may not be in the Case Report itself but can be found in the chapter content. **LO 6.1, 6.3, 6.5, 6.8, 6.9, 6.10**

 ## Case Report (CR) 6.2

You are

. . . an **EMT-P** working in the Emergency Department of Fulwood Medical Center.

Your patient is

. . . Mr. Justin Leandro, a 37-year-old construction worker who is complaining of a sudden onset of excruciating pain in his right abdomen and back an hour previously while at work. The pain is **spasmodic** and radiates down into his groin. He has vomited once and keeps having the urge to urinate but cannot. He has no previous medical history of significance.

Vital signs (VS) T 99.4°F, P 92, R 20, BP 130/86. Abdomen slightly distended, with tenderness in the right upper and lower quadrants and flank. A dipstick test showed blood in his urine.

Provisional diagnosis: stone in right ureter. An **IV** line was inserted, and 2 mg morphine sulfate given by IV push at 1540.

An x-ray of Mr. Leandro's kidneys, ureters, and bladder showed a suspicious lesion halfway down his right ureter, and the **pyelogram** confirmed that this was a renal stone blocking the ureter.

---

1. If Mr. Leandro's pain had a "sudden onset," is it acute or chronic? _____

2. Provide the abbreviation for *intravenous pyelogram*: _____

3. Provide the three letters that abbreviate the specific type of X-ray Mr. Leandro had: _____

4. What does the "P" stand for in your job as an EMT-P? (Do not capitalize the term) _____

5. The one word that describes the results of his dipstick urinalysis is: _____

6. Mr. Leandro does not know what the term ureter means. Which of the following phrases would you use to explain it to him?

    a. "It is the tube from your bladder through your penis."

    b. "It is the part of the kidney that filters blood."

    c. "It is the tube from your kidney to the bladder."

    d. "It is the inside lining of your bladder."

C. **After reading the following Case Report, correctly answer the following questions.** The answers to the Case Report may not be in the Case Report itself but can be found in the chapter content. **LO 6.1, 6.5, 6.6, 6.7, 6.8, 6.9**

 ### Case Report (CR) 6.3

You are

. . . a medical assistant working in the office of Dr. Susan Lee, a primary care physician at Fulwood Medical Center.

Your patient is

. . . Mrs. Caroline Dobson, a 32-year-old housewife. You have asked her to describe the reason for her visit to the office today.

Patient Interview

Mrs. Dobson:

"Since yesterday afternoon I've had a lot of pain low down in my belly and in my lower back. I keep having to go to the bathroom every hour or so to pee. It's often difficult to start, and it burns as it comes out. I've had this problem twice before when I was pregnant with my two kids, so I've started drinking cranberry juice. I've been shivering since I woke up this morning, and the last urine I passed was pink. Was that due to the cranberry juice?"

Mrs. Dobson described many of the symptoms of cystitis. She had suprapubic and low-back pain. She had increased frequency of micturition with dysuria and had difficulty in and burning on micturition. Her pink urine is probably hematuria.

2014 Nucleus Medical Media

1. The pain that Mrs. Dobson describes being "low down in my belly" can be documented as being:

a. Suprapubic   **b.** Flank   **c.** Groin   **d.** Perineum

2. Which diagnostic test would quickly determine the cause of her pink urine?

a. Ureteroscopy

b. Dipstick urinalysis

c. Voiding cystourethrogram

d. Hemodialysis

3. Using the term dysuria in your documentation would describe Mrs. Dobson's:

a. pain in her back and lower belly.

b. increased frequency in using the bathroom.

c. difficulty in starting to micturate.

d. shivering and pink urine.

4. Drinking cranberry juice is thought to

a. dissolve kidney stones.

b. treat urinary tract infections.

c. decrease urethral pain.

d. relax the urinary bladder walls.

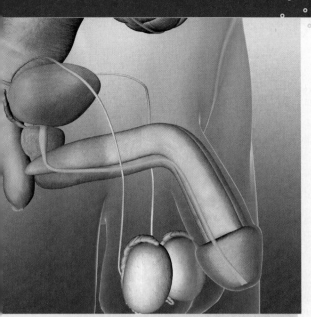

2014 Nucleus Medical Media

CHAPTER

7

Male Reproductive System

The Language of Reproduction

Chapter Sections

Chapter Learning Outcomes

LO 7.1 Identify and describe the anatomy and physiology of the male reproductive system and its accessory glands.

LO 7.2 Use roots, combining forms, suffixes, and prefixes to construct and analyze medical terms related to the male reproductive system.

LO 7.3 Spell medical terms related to the male reproductive system.

LO 7.4 Pronounce medical terms related to the male reproductive system.

LO 7.5 Describe diagnostic procedures utilized in urology.

LO 7.6 Identify and describe disorders and pathological conditions related to the male reproductive system.

LO 7.7 Describe the therapeutic procedures and pharmacologic agents used in the male reproductive system.

LO 7.8 Apply knowledge of medical terms relating to male reproductive system to documentation, medical records, and communication.

LO 7.9 Identify and correctly use abbreviations of terms used in male reproductive system.

LO 7.10 Identify health professionals involved in the care of male reproduction patients.

The health professionals involved in the diagnosis and treatment of problems with the male reproductive system include:

- **Urologists,** who are specialists in the diagnosis and treatment of diseases of the urinary system.
- Health care professionals with training and expertise in providing urologic patient care, including **nurse practitioners, physicians' assistants,** and **technologists.**

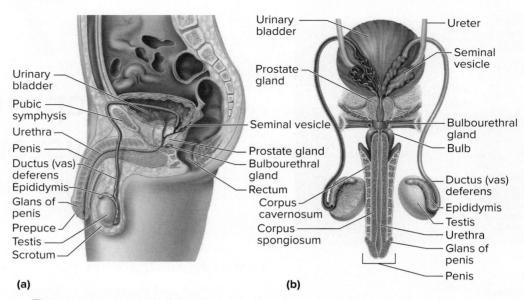

▲ **Figure 7.1** **Male reproductive system.** (a) Male pelvic cavity: midsagittal section. (b) Male reproductive organs.

Male Reproductive System

Unlike every other organ system, the reproductive system is not essential for an individual human to survive. However, without the reproductive system, the human species could not survive. The male reproductive system ensures the sexual maturation of each male; influences male behavior; and produces, maintains, and transports the male sex cells (sperm cells) to the female reproductive tract. The male reproductive organ system *(Figure 7.1)* consists of:

1. **Primary sex organs** or **gonads:** the **testes**

2. **Secondary sex organs:**

   a. **Penis**

   b. **Scrotum**

   c. **System of ducts,** including the **epididymis, ductus (vas) deferens,** and **urethra**

3. **Accessory glands:**

   a. **Prostate**

   b. **Seminal vesicles**

   c. **Bulbourethral (Cowper) glands**

Perineum

The **external genitalia** (the penis, scrotum, and testes) occupy the **perineum,** a diamond-shaped region between the thighs. Its border is at the pubic symphysis anteriorly and the coccyx posteriorly *(Figure 7.2)*. The anus is also in the perineum.

Scrotum

The **scrotum** is a skin-covered sac between the thighs. Its midline shows a distinct ridge called the **raphe.** It marks the position of the internal **median septum** that divides the scrotum into two compartments. Each compartment contains a testis.

The scrotum's function is to provide a cooler environment for the testes than that inside the body. This is because sperm are best produced and stored at a few degrees cooler than the internal body temperature.

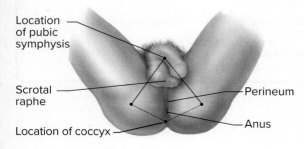

▲ **Figure 7.2** **Male perineum.**

WORD	PRONUNCIATION	ELEMENTS		DEFINITION
bulbourethral	**BUL**-boh-you-**REE**-thral	S/ R/CF R/	**-al** *pertaining to* **bulb/o-** *bulb* **-urethr-** *urethra*	Pertaining to the bulbous penis and urethra
ductus deferens	**DUK**-tus **DEH**-fuh-renz		**ductus** Latin *to lead* **deferens** Latin *carry away*	Tube that receives sperm from the epididymis
vas deferens (syn)	VAS **DEH**-fuh-renz		**vas** Latin *blood vessel, duct*	
epididymis	EP-ih-**DID**-ih-miss	S/ P/ R/	**-is** *belonging to* **epi-** *above* **-didym-** *testis*	Coiled tube attached to the testis
genitalia	JEN-ih-**TAY**-lee-ah	S/ R/	**-ia** *condition* **genit-** *primary male or female sex organs*	External and internal organs of reproduction
genital (adj)	JEN-ih-tal	S/	**-al** *pertaining to*	Relating to reproduction or to the male or female sex organs
gonad gonads (pl)	**GOH**-nad **GOH**-nads		Greek *seed*	Testis or ovary
penis penile (adj)	**PEE**-nis **PEE**-nile	S/ R/	Latin *tail* **-ile** *pertaining to* **pen-** *penis*	Conveys urine and semen to the outside Pertaining to the penis
perineum	PER-ih-**NEE**-um		Greek *perineum*	Area between thighs, extending from the coccyx to the pubis
perineal (adj)	PER-ih-**NEE**-al	S/ R/CF	**-al** *pertaining to* **perin/e-** *perineum*	Pertaining to the perineum
raphe	**RAY**-fee		Greek *seam*	Line separating two symmetrical structures
scrotum scrotal (adj)	**SKROH**-tum **SKROH**-tal	S/ R/	Latin *scrotum* **-al** *pertaining to* **scrot-** *scrotum*	Sac containing the testes Pertaining to the scrotum
semen seminal vesicle	**SEE**-men **SEM**-in-al **VES**-ih-kull	S/ R/ S/ R/	Latin *seed* **-al** *pertaining to* **semin-** *semen* **-le** *small* **vesic-** *sac containing fluid*	Penile ejaculate containing sperm and seminal fluid Sac of ductus deferens that produces seminal fluid
seminiferous	sem-ih-**NIF**-er-us	S/ R/CF R/	**-ous** *pertaining to* **semin/i-** *semen* **-fer-** *to bear*	Pertaining to carrying semen
testicle (also called **testis**)	**TES**-tih-kul		Latin *small testis*	One of the male reproductive glands
testicular (adj)	tes-**TICK**-you-lar	S/ R/	**-ar** *pertaining to* **testicul-** *testicle*	Pertaining to the testicle
testis testes (pl)	**TES**-tis **TES**-teez		Latin *testis*	A synonym for testicle

Testes, Testosterone, and Spermatic Cords

In the adult male, each testis is a small, oval organ about 2 inches (5 cm) long and ¾ inch (2 cm) wide *(Figure 7.3)*. Each testis is covered by a serous membrane, the **tunica vaginalis,** which has an outer parietal layer and an inner visceral layer separated by serous fluid.

Inside the testis, thin septa subdivide the testis into some 250 lobules *(Figure 7.3)*. Each lobule contains three or four **seminiferous tubules** in which several layers of germ cells are in the process of becoming sperm.

Between the seminiferous tubules are the interstitial cells. They produce hormones called **androgens.**

Testosterone

Testosterone is the major androgen produced by the interstitial cells of the testes. It has the following effects:

- **Sustains** the male reproductive tract throughout adulthood.
- **Stimulates spermatogenesis;** testosterone levels peak at age 20, and then decline steadily to one-third of that level at age 65.

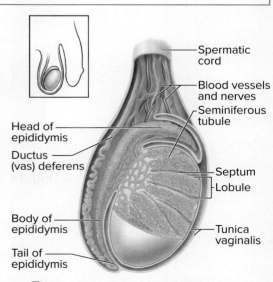

▲ **Figure 7.3** **The testis and associated structures.**

- **Inhibits** the secretion of female hormones at age 65, and continues declining after that age.
- **Stimulates** the development of male secondary sex characteristics at **puberty.**
- **Enlarges** the **spermatic** ducts and accessory glands of the male reproductive system.
- **Stimulates** a burst of growth at puberty—including increased muscle mass, higher **basal metabolic rate (BMR),** and larger larynx (this effect deepens the voice).
- **Stimulates** erythropoiesis, giving men a higher red blood cell (RBC) count than women.
- **Stimulates** the brain to increase **libido** (sex drive) in the male.

Did you know...

The mature, adult male testes produce up to 100,000,000 sperm per day.

Spermatic Cord

The blood vessels and nerves to the testis arise in the abdominal cavity. They pass through the inguinal canal, where they join with connective tissue to form a spermatic cord that suspends each testis in the scrotum *(see Figure 7.3)*. The left testis is suspended lower than the right. Within the cord are an artery, a plexus of veins, nerves, a thin muscle, and the ductus (vas) deferens (the passage into which sperm go when they leave the testis).

Spermatogenesis

Spermatogenesis is the process in which the germ cells of the seminiferous tubules mature and divide **(mitosis)** and then undergo two divisions called **meiosis.** The four daughter cells differentiate into **spermatids** and then **spermatozoa (sperm)** *(Figure 7.4)*. The germ cells have 23 pairs of chromosomes (a total of 46). Because of meiosis, each sperm has only 23 chromosomes that can combine at fertilization with the 23 chromosomes in a female oocyte (egg).

The mature sperm has a pear-shaped head and a long tail *(Figure 7.5)*. The nucleus of the head contains 23 chromosomes.

The tail **(flagellum)** provides the movement as the sperm swims up the female reproductive tract.

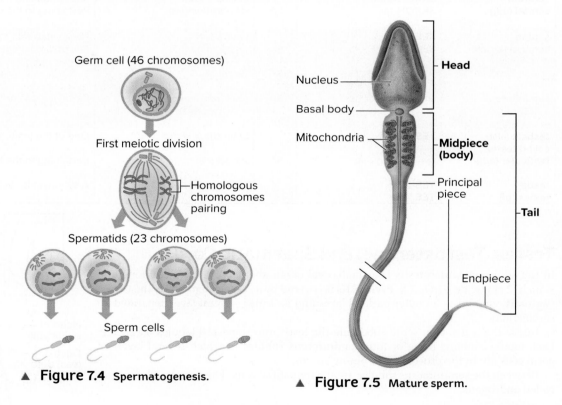

▲ **Figure 7.4** **Spermatogenesis.**

▲ **Figure 7.5** **Mature sperm.**

Word Analysis and Definition Testes, Testosterone, and Spermatic Cords

S = Suffix   P = Prefix   R = Root   R/CF = Combining Form

WORD	PRONUNCIATION		ELEMENTS	DEFINITION
androgen	**AN**-droh-jen	S/ R/CF	**-gen** *form, create* **andr/o-** *masculine*	Hormone that promotes masculine characteristics
flagellum flagella (pl)	fla-**JELL**-um fla-**JELL**-ah		Latin *small whip*	Tail of a sperm
libido	li-**BEE**-doh		Latin *lust*	Sexual desire
meiosis	my-**OH**-sis	S/ R/	**-osis** *condition* **mei-** *lessening*	Two rapid cell divisions, resulting in half the number of chromosomes
mitosis	my-**TOH**-sis	S/ R/	**-osis** *condition* **mit-** *threadlike structure*	Cell division to create two identical cells, each with 46 chromosomes
puberty	**PYU**-ber-tee		Latin *grown up*	Process of maturing from child to young adult
seminiferous tubule	sem-ih-**NIF**-er-us **TU**-byul	S/ R/CF R/	**-ous** *pertaining to* **semin/i-** *semen* **-fer-** *to bear*	Coiled tubes in the testes that produce sperm
sperm (also called spermatozoon) spermatozoa (pl) spermatic (adj)	SPERM **SPER**-mat-oh-**ZOH**-ah **SPER**-mat-ik	 S/ R/CF S/	Greek *seed* **-zoa** *animals* **spermat/o-** *sperm* **-ic** *pertaining to*	Mature male sex cell Sperm (plural of spermatozoon) Pertaining to sperm
spermatid spermatogenesis	**SPER**-mah-tid **SPER**-mat-oh-**JEN**-eh-sis	S/ R/ R/CF S/	**-id** *having a particular quality* **spermat-** *sperm* **spermat/o-** *sperm* **genesis** *origin, creation*	A cell late in the development process of sperm The process by which male germ cells differentiate into sperm
testosterone	tes-**TOSS**-ter-ohn	S/ R/CF	**-sterone** *steroid* **test/o-** *testis*	Powerful androgen produced by the testes
tunica vaginalis	**TYU**-nih-kah vaj-ih-**NAHL**-iss	 S/ R/	**tunica** Latin *coat* **-alis** *pertaining to* **vagin-** *sheath, vagina*	Covering, particularly of a tubular structure. The tunica vaginalis is the sheath of the testis and epididymis

Check Point Section 7.1

Case Report (CR) 7.1

You are

. . . an EMT-P working in the Emergency Department at Fulwood Medical Center.

Your patient is

. . . Joseph Davis, a 17-year-old high school senior. He is brought in by his mother at 0400 hrs. He complains of sudden onset of pain in his left **testicle** 3 hours earlier that woke him up. The pain is intense and has made him vomit. VS: T 99.2°F, P 88, R 15, BP 130/70. Examination reveals his left testicle to be enlarged, warm, and tender. His abdomen is normal to palpation.

At your request, Dr. Helinski, the emergency physician on duty, examines him immediately. He diagnoses a **torsion** of the patient's left testicle.

His diagnosis is a torsion of the patient's left testicle. Joseph Davis presented with typical symptoms and signs of testicular torsion. The affected testis rapidly became painful, tender, swollen, and inflamed.

Emergency surgery was performed, and the testis and cord were manually untwisted through an incision in the scrotum. The testis was stitched to surrounding tissues to prevent a recurrence.

A. In your own words. *You could be working in the Emergency Department when this patient comes in. Using the information presented in Case Report (CR) 7.1, document the case in the patient's record. Use the following terms to fill in the blanks. One term will be used more than once.* **LO 7.1, 7.6, 7.8**

testicular   **testes**   **testicle**

This patient presented to the ED because of pain in his left **1.** _____. Both **2.** _____ were examined, but the left **3.** _____ was enlarged, warm, and tender. The emergency physician on duty diagnosed **4.** _____ torsion. Patient will be scheduled for surgery immediately.

B. Deconstruction of medical terms is a tool for analyzing the meaning. *In the following chart, you are given a medical term. Deconstruct the term into its root (or combining form) and suffix. Note that none of these terms have prefixes, and not all of the terms have a suffix. Write the element in the appropriate column. The first one is done for you.* **LO 7.1, 7.2**

Term	Root/Combining Form	Suffix
androgen	*andro*	*-gen*
testosterone	**1.**	**2.**
meiosis	**3.**	**4.**
vaginalis	**5.**	**6.**

C. Define medical terms related to the male reproductive system. *Write the term the definition is describing. Fill in the blanks.* **LO 7.1, 7.3**

1. A type of androgen: _____

2. Pertaining to a sheath: _____

3. Two rapid cell divisions, resulting in half the number of chromosomes: _____

4. Hormone that promotes masculine characteristics: _____

Section 7.2 The Penis, Spermatic Ducts, and Accessory Glands

Penis

The structure of the penis is specifically designed to meet its two main functions:

· Deposit semen in the female vagina around the cervix.

· Enable urine to flow to the outside.

It is essential that the anatomy, physiology, and terminology of the penis as related to performing these two functions be understood.

The external, visible part of the penis comprises the **shaft** and the **glans** *(Figure 7.6a)*, at the tip of which the external urethral meatus is located. The skin of the penis is very loosely attached to the shaft to permit expansion during erection. The skin continues over the glans as the **prepuce** (foreskin). A ventral fold of tissue, the **frenulum,** attaches the skin to the glans. The glans and facing prepuce contain sebaceous glands that produce a waxy secretion called **smegma.**

The shaft of the penis contains three erectile vascular bodies *(Figure 7.6b)*:

- Paired **corpora cavernosa** are located dorsolaterally.
- A single **corpus spongiosum** is located inferiorly. It contains the urethra and goes on to form the glans.

The corpora cavernosa are composed of a network of venous sinuses surrounding a central artery. **Erection** occurs when the sinuses fill with blood, causing the erectile bodies to distend and become rigid. It is a parasympathetic nervous system response to stimulation.

Ejaculation occurs when the sympathetic nervous system stimulates the smooth muscle of the ductus deferens, ejaculatory ducts, and the prostate gland to contract. The seminal vesicles contract so that their fluids join to form semen. The internal urethral sphincter also contracts so that urine cannot enter the urethra and semen cannot enter the bladder.

Prepuce (Foreskin)

The functions of the prepuce (foreskin) *(see Figure 7.7)* are to cover and protect the glans and produce smegma, a lubricant containing lipids, cell debris, and some natural antibiotics.

Penile Urethra

The penile urethra passes through the single erectile body, the corpus spongiosum, to the external urethral meatus.

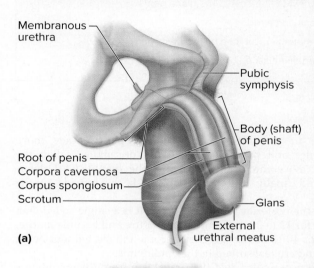

Membranous urethra
Pubic symphysis
Body (shaft) of penis
Root of penis
Corpora cavernosa
Corpus spongiosum
Scrotum
Glans
External urethral meatus

(a)

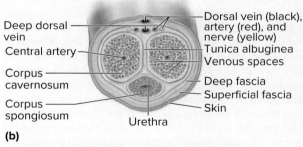

Deep dorsal vein
Central artery
Corpus cavernosum
Corpus spongiosum
Urethra
Dorsal vein (black), artery (red), and nerve (yellow)
Tunica albuginea
Venous spaces
Deep fascia
Superficial fascia
Skin

(b)

▲ **Figure 7.6** **Anatomy of penis.** (a) External anatomy. (b) Cross-sectional view.

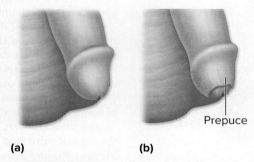

Prepuce

(a)   **(b)**

▲ **Figure 7.7** **Prepuce.** (a) Circumcised penis. (b) Uncircumcised penis. Electronic Publishing Services, Inc., NY/McGraw Hill

WORD	PRONUNCIATION	ELEMENTS		DEFINITION
cavernosa	kav-er-**NOH**-sah	S/ R/	-osa *like* cavern- *cave*	Resembling a cave
corpus corpora (pl)	**KOR**-pus **KOR**-por-ah		Latin *body*	Major part of a structure
erection	ee-**REK**-shun	S/ R/	-ion *process, condition* erect- *straight, to set up*	Distended and rigid state of an organ
erectile (adj)	ee-**REK**-tile	S/	-ile *capable of*	Capable of erection or being distended with blood
frenulum	**FREN**-you-lum		Latin *small bridle*	Fold of mucous membrane between the glans and prepuce
glans	GLANZ		Latin *acorn*	Head of the penis or clitoris
prepuce	**PREE**-puce		Latin *foreskin*	Fold of skin that covers the glans penis
shaft	SHAFT		Old English *sceaft*	Resembling a rod
smegma	**SMEG**-mah		Greek *ointment*	Oily material produced by the glans and prepuce
spongiosum	spun-jee-**OH**-sum	S/ R/	-um *structure* spongios- *sponge*	Spongelike tissue

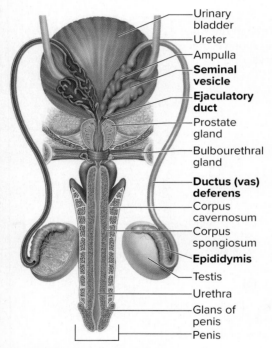

Urinary bladder
Ureter
Ampulla
Seminal vesicle
Ejaculatory duct
Prostate gland
Bulbourethral gland
Ductus (vas) deferens
Corpus cavernosum
Corpus spongiosum
Epididymis
Testis
Urethra
Glans of penis
Penis

▲ **Figure 7.8** Components of male reproductive ducts.

Spermatic Ducts

As the sperm cells mature in the testes over a 60-day period, they move down the seminiferous tubules and pass into a network of tubules called the **rete testis.** From here, they move into the epididymis, the ductus (vas) deferens, the ejaculatory duct, and finally the urethra to reach the outside of the body *(Figure 7.8).*

The epididymis adheres to the posterior side of the testis. It is a single coiled duct in which the sperm are stored for 12 to 20 days until they mature and become **motile.** Stored sperm remain fertile for 40 to 60 days. If they become too old without being **ejaculated,** they disintegrate and are reabsorbed in the epididymis.

The ductus (vas) deferens is a muscular duct that travels up from the epididymis in the scrotum and through the inguinal canal *(see Chapter 5)* into the pelvic cavity *(see Figure 7.8).* Here the ductus turns medially and passes behind the urinary bladder and widens into a terminal **ampulla,** which joins with the duct of the seminal **vesicle.**

The **ejaculatory duct,** formed by the ductus deferens and seminal vesicle, is a short (¾-inch or 2-cm) duct that passes through the prostate gland and empties its contents of sperm and seminal fluid (semen) into the urethra.

The male prostate and urethra have both **urologic** and **reproductive** functions, as the flow of urine and semen goes through both organs. Disorders of the prostate and urethra produce symptoms and signs that arise in both areas. This makes it essential to have knowledge of their anatomy, physiology, and terminology to be able to understand both functions.

WORD	PRONUNCIATION	ELEMENTS		DEFINITION
ampulla	am-**PULL**-ah		Latin *two-handled bottle*	Dilated portion of a canal or duct
ejaculate (**Note:** This term can be a verb or noun.)	ee-**JACK**-you-late	S/ R/	-ate *composed of, pertaining to* ejacul- *shoot out*	To expel suddenly, or the semen expelled in ejaculation
ejaculation	ee-**JACK**-you-**LAY**-shun	S/	-ation *process*	Process of expelling semen
motile	**MOH**-til	S/ R/	-ile *capable* mot- *to move*	Capable of spontaneous movement
motility (noun)	moh-**TILL**-ih-tee	S/	-ility *condition, state of*	The ability for spontaneous movement
reproductive	ree-pro-**DUC**-tiv	S/ P/ R/	-ive *nature of, pertaining to* re- *again* -product- *lead forth*	Relating to the process by which organisms produce offspring
reproduction (noun)	ree-pro-**DUC**-shun	S/	-ion *action, process*	The process by which organisms produce offspring
rete testis	**REE**-teh **TES**-tis		**rete** Latin *net* **testis** Latin *testis*	Network of tubules between the seminiferous tubules and the epididymis
vesicle	**VES**-ih-kull		Latin *a blister*	Small sac containing liquid; for example, a blister or, in this case, semen

Accessory Glands

Seminal fluid contains components produced by all three accessory glands (*Figure 7.9*). The functions of seminal fluid are to:

- **Provide nutrients** to the sperm as they are in the urethra and female reproductive tract.
- **Neutralize acid secretions** of the vagina (in which sperm cannot survive).
- **Provide hormones** (**prostaglandins**) that widen the opening of the cervix to enable sperm to enter more easily.
- **Provide the fluid vehicle** in which sperm can swim.

The two seminal vesicles are located on the posterior surface of the urinary bladder. The wall of each vesicle contains mucosal folds. They produce a viscous, yellowish, alkaline fluid that contains fructose and prostaglandins. Fructose is a sugar that provides energy for the sperm.

Did you know...

- Combined with sperm, the seminal fluid becomes semen.
- The male testes produce up to 100 million sperm per day.
- A normal sperm count is in the range of 75 to 150 million sperm per mL of semen.
- A normal ejaculation consists of 2 to 5 mL of semen.

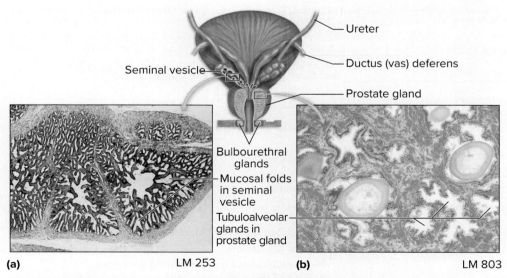

(a) LM 253   **(b)** LM 803

▲ **Figure 7.9** **Accessory glands of the male reproductive system.** (a) Seminal vesicle. (b) Prostate gland. (a) Biophoto Associates/Science Source (b) Alvin Telser/McGraw Hill

The single **prostate gland** is located immediately below the bladder and anterior to the rectum and surrounds the urethra and the **ejaculatory** duct. It is composed of 30 to 50 glands that open directly into the urethra. The glands secrete a slightly milky fluid that contains:

- **Citric acid,** a nutrient for sperm.
- **An antibiotic** that combats **urinary tract infections (UTIs)** in males.
- **Clotting factors** that hold the sperm together in a sticky mass until **ejaculation.**
- **Prostate-specific antigen (PSA),** an enzyme that helps liquefy the sticky mass following ejaculation.

The two bulbourethral glands are located one on each side of the membranous urethra. Each gland has a short duct leading into the spongy (penile) urethra. The glands secrete a clear, slippery, alkaline mucus that protects the sperm as they pass through the urethra by neutralizing any residual acid urine. It also acts as a lubricant during sexual intercourse.

Semen is derived from the secretions of several glands:

- 5% comes from the testicles and epididymis.
- 50% to 80% comes from the seminal vesicles.
- 15% to 33% comes from the prostate gland.
- 2% to 5% comes from the bulbourethral glands.

Word Analysis and Definition: Accessory Glands

S = Suffix   P = Prefix   R = Root   R/CF = Combining Form

WORD	PRONUNCIATION		ELEMENTS	DEFINITION
prostate	PROS-tate (**Note:** *not* PROS-trate.)		Greek *one standing before*	Organ surrounding the beginning of the urethra
prostatic (adj)	pros-**TAT**-ik	S/ R/	-tic *pertaining to* prosta- *prostate*	Pertaining to the prostate
prostaglandin	PROS-tah-**GLAN**-din	S/ R/ R/	-in *chemical* prosta- *prostate* -gland- *gland*	Hormone present in many tissues, but first isolated from the prostate gland
semen	**SEE**-men		Latin *seed*	Penile ejaculate containing sperm and seminal fluid

Check Point Section 7.2

A. Recall and review. *Become familiar with the terms relating to the spermatic ducts and accessory gland and how they relate clinical conditions related to the male reproductive system.* **LO 7.1, 7.3, 7.9, 7.10**

1. After leaving the testis, sperm are stored in the _____.

2. The ductus deferens widens at the _____ and then joins the ejaculatory duct.

3. The specialist treating the male reproductive system is a(n) _____.

4. What is the abbreviation for the procedure in which a finger is inserted into the rectum to evaluate the prostate gland? _____.

5. In the term *rete testis,* the word *rete* is Latin for the word _____.

B. Test your knowledge of the language of male reproduction. *Choose the best answer.* **LO 7.1, 7.2, 7.9**

1. PSA is
   a. an enzyme that liquefies semen
   b. an antibiotic that coats the urethra
   c. a diagnostic test for testicular torsion
   d. a hormone that dilates the cervix

2. The two bulbourethral glands are located
   a. near the ureters
   b. on each side of the membranous urethra
   c. behind the seminal vesicles
   d. on top of the prostate gland
   e. under the vas deferens

3. The suffix in the term **prostaglandin** tells you it is a
a. hormone
b. enzyme
c. protein
d. chemical
e. blood cell

4. **Semen** is derived from the secretions of several glands:
a. testicles, epididymis
b. accessory glands
c. thymus gland
d. a, b, and c
e. a and b only

5. The **prostate gland** is located
a. below the bladder and posterior to the rectum
b. beside the bladder and anterior to the rectum
c. below the bladder and anterior to the rectum
d. beside the bladder and posterior to the rectum
e. between the bladder and the kidney

6. The root for **prostatic** is
a. *adeno-*
b. *prosta-*
c. *gland-*
d. *ren-*
e. *nephro-*

7. What provides energy for sperm?
a. citric acid
b. prostaglandins
c. fructose
d. a and c
e. none of these

8. What is a nutrient for sperm?
a. alkaline mucus
b. acid urine
c. citric acid
d. normal flora
e. acid secretions of the vagina

9. In the abbreviation **PSA,** the "A" stands for
a. antidiuretic
b. antibiotic
c. antigen
d. antibody
e. allergen

10. What is the fluid vehicle for sperm?
a. bloodstream
b. lymph system
c. plasma
d. aqueous humor
e. seminal fluid

C. Many medical terms have Greek and Latin origins and cannot be deconstructed. *Match the term in the first column with its meaning in the second column.* **LO 7.1**

Term	Meaning
_____ 1. glans	a. acorn
_____ 2. corpora	b. small bridle
_____ 3. prepuce	c. body
_____ 4. smegma	d. foreskin
_____ 5. frenulum	e. ointment

Section 7.3 Disorders of the Male Reproductive System

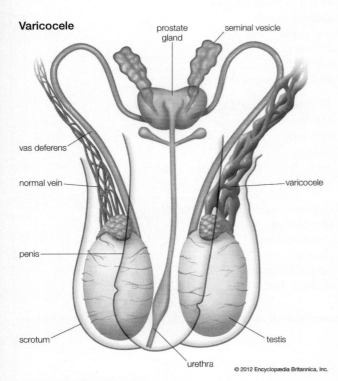

Varicocele

prostate gland
seminal vesicle
vas deferens
normal vein
penis
scrotum
varicocele
testis
urethra

© 2012 Encyclopædia Britannica, Inc.

▲ **Figure 7.10** Illustration of varicocele, showing varicose dilated veins of the spermatic cord in the scrotum. Universal Images Group North America LLC/Alamy Stock Photo

Did you know...

- The testis in testicular torsion will die in some 6 hours unless the blood supply is restored.
- **Self-examination of the testes (SET)** for swelling or tenderness should be performed monthly by all men.

Disorders of the Testes

Cryptorchism occurs when a testis fails to descend from the abdomen into the scrotum before the boy is 12 months old. In the embryo, the testes develop inside the abdomen at the level of the kidney. They must then migrate down the abdomen into the scrotum.

Testicular torsion is the twisting of a testis on its spermatic cord. As the testis twists, the spermatic cord has to twist because it is fixed in the abdomen. The testicular artery in the twisted cord becomes blocked, and the blood supply to the testis is cut off. The condition occurs in men between puberty and age 25. In half the cases, it starts in bed at night.

Varicocele *(Figure 7.10)* is a condition in which the veins in the spermatic cord become dilated and tortuous as varicose veins.

Hydrocele is a collection of excess fluid in the space between the visceral and parietal layers of the tunica vaginalis of the testis. It is most common after age 40. The diagnosis can be confirmed by transillumination, shining a bright light on the swelling to see the shape of the testis through the translucent excess fluid *(Figure 7.11)*. Surgical removal is performed for large hydroceles.

Spermatocele is a collection of sperm in a sac formed in the epididymis. It occurs in about 30% of men, is benign, and rarely causes symptoms. It does not require treatment unless it becomes bothersome.

Epididymitis and **epididymoorchitis (orchitis)** are both inflammatory diseases. Epididymitis is inflammation of the epididymis; epididymoorchitis is inflammation of the epididymis and testis. Orchitis is usually a consequence of epididymitis. They are most commonly caused by a bacterial infection spreading from a urinary tract infection or infection of the prostate. They also can be caused by sexually transmitted diseases (STDs), such as gonorrhea or chlamydia *(see Chapter 6)*.

A viral cause of orchitis is mumps. In males past puberty who develop mumps, 30% will develop orchitis, and 30% of those will develop resulting testicular atrophy. If the testicular infection is bilateral, **infertility** can result. Mumps is avoidable by immunization during childhood.

Testicular cancer usually develops in men younger than 40.

Forty percent of testicular cancers are **seminomas,** made up of immature germ cells. Nonseminomas occur in different combinations of **choriocarcinoma,** embryonal cell, and **teratoma.**

Disorders of the Prostate Gland

By the age of 20, the prostate weighs about 20 grams. It remains at that weight until age 45 to 50, when it begins to grow again. By age 80, some 90% of men have **benign prostatic hyperplasia (BPH)** *(Figure 7.12)*. This is a noncancerous enlargement that compresses the prostatic urethra to produce symptoms of:

- Difficulty starting and stopping the urine stream.
- **Nocturia, polyuria,** and **dysuria.**

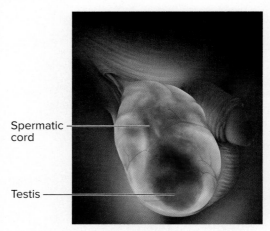

Spermatic cord

Testis

▲ **Figure 7.11** Transillumination of hydrocele showing testis and spermatic cord. Brian Evans/Science Source

WORD	PRONUNCIATION	ELEMENTS		DEFINITION
choriocarcinoma	KOH-ree-oh-kar-sih-NOH-mah	S/ R/CF R/	-oma *tumor* chori/o- *membrane, chorion* -carcin- *cancer*	Highly malignant cancer in a testis or ovary
cryptorchism (syn: cryptorchidism)	krip-TOR-kizm	S/ P/ R/	-ism *condition* crypt- *hidden* -orch- *testicle*	Failure of one or both testes to descend into the scrotum
epididymitis	EP-ih-did-ih-MY-tis	S/ P/ R/	-itis *inflammation* epi- *above* -didym- *testis*	Inflammation of the epididymis
epididymoorchitis (syn: orchitis)	ep-ih-DID-ih-moh-or-KIE-tis	S/ P/ R/CF R/	-itis *inflammation* epi-*above* didym/o- *testis* -orch- *testicle*	Inflammation of the epididymis and testicle
hydrocele	HIGH-droh-seal	S/ R/CF	-cele *cave* hydr/o- *water*	Collection of fluid in the space of the tunica vaginalis
infertility	in-fer-TIL-ih-tee	S/ P/ R/	-ity *condition* in- *not* -fertil- *able to conceive*	Failure to conceive
orchitis epididymoorchitis (syn)	or-KIE-tis	S/ R/	-itis *inflammation* orch- *testicle*	Inflammation of the testis
seminoma	sem-ih-NOH-mah	S/ R/	-oma *tumor, mass* semin- *scatter seed*	Neoplasm of germ cells of a testis
spermatocele	SPER-mat-oh-seal	S/ R/CF	-cele *cave, swelling* spermat/o- *sperm*	Cyst of the epididymis that contains sperm
teratoma	ter-ah-TOH-mah	S/ R/	-oma *tumor, mass* terat- *monster, malformed fetus*	Neoplasm of a testis or ovary containing multiple tissues from other sites in the body
torsion	TOR-shun		Latin *to twist*	The act or result of twisting
varicocele	VAIR-ih-koh-seal	S/ R/CF	-cele *cave, swelling* varic/o- *varicosity*	Varicose veins of the spermatic cord

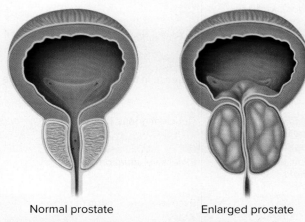

Normal prostate   Enlarged prostate

▲ **Figure 7.12** Normal prostate and prostate with BPH.

Did you know...

- Survival from prostate cancer is up to 80% if it is detected before it spreads outside the gland.
- Male infertility is involved in 40% of the 2.6 million infertile married couples in the United States (data from the **National Institutes of Health [NIH]**).

Prostatic cancer affects more than 10% of men over the age of 50, and its incidence is increasing. It forms hard nodules in the periphery of the gland and is often asymptomatic in its early stages because it does not compress the urethra.

Several treatment options involving radiotherapy are available *(see Chapter 20)*. Sometimes, a **radical prostatectomy,** with complete surgical removal of the prostate and surrounding tissues, is performed.

Prostatitis is inflammation of the prostate gland. It occurs in three main types:

Type I—an acute bacterial infection with fever, chills, frequency, dysuria, and hematuria.

Type II—a chronic bacterial infection with less severe symptoms.

Type III—a chronic nonbacterial prostatitis in which the urinary symptoms are present, but no bacteria can be detected. This is the most common type. Its etiology is unknown, and treatment is difficult.

Male Infertility

Male infertility is the inability to conceive after at least one year of unprotected intercourse. The primary causes of infertility are:

1. Impaired sperm production:
   a. Cryptorchism
   b. **Anorchism** (absence of one or both testes)
   c. Testicular trauma
   d. Testicular cancer
   e. Orchitis after puberty
2. Impaired sperm delivery:
   a. Infections and blockage of spermatic ducts.
3. Testosterone deficiency **(hypogonadism):**
   a. Medications to treat hypertension and/or high cholesterol.
   b. Environmental endocrine disrupters that adversely affect the endocrine system; examples are phthalates in plastics and dioxins in paper production.

In the United States each year, 500,000 men choose to be made infertile **(sterile)** by having a vasectomy.

Word Analysis and Definition: Disorders of the Prostate Gland and Male Infertility

S = Suffix   P = Prefix   R = Root   R/CF = Combining Form

WORD	PRONUNCIATION	ELEMENTS		DEFINITION
anorchism	an-**OR**-kizm	S/ P/ R/	-ism *condition* an- *without, lack of* -orch- *testicle*	Absence of testes
dysuria	dis-**YOU**-ree-ah	S/ P/ R/	-ia *condition* dys- *difficult, painful* -ur- *urine*	Pain or difficulty when urinating
hyperplasia	high-per-**PLAY**-zee-ah	S/ P/ R/	-ia *condition* hyper- *excessive* -plas- *molding, formation*	Increase in the number of the cells in a tissue or organ
hypogonadism	**HIGH**-poh-**GOH**-nad-izm	S/ P/ R/	-ism *condition* hypo- *deficient* -gonad- *testes or ovaries*	Deficient gonad production of sperm, eggs, or hormones
nocturia	nok-**TYU**-ree-ah	S/ P/ R/	-ia *condition* noct- *night* -ur- *urine*	Excessive urination at night
polyuria	pol-ee-**YOU**-ree-ah	S/ P/ R/	-ia *condition* poly- *excessive* -ur- *urine*	Excessive production of urine
prostatitis	pross-tah-**TIE**-tis	S/ R/	-itis *inflammation* prostat- *prostate*	Inflammation of the prostate
sterile sterility	**STER**-ill steh-**RIL**-ih-tee	 S/ R/	Latin *barren* -ity *state, condition* steril- *barren*	Unable to fertilize or reproduce Inability to reproduce

Disorders of the Penis

Disorders of the Penis

Trauma to the penis can vary from being caught in a pants zipper to a fracture of an erect penis during vigorous sexual intercourse.

Peyronie disease is a marked curvature of the erect penis caused by fibrous tissue. Its etiology is unknown.

Priapism is a persistent, painful **erection** when blood cannot escape from the erectile tissue. It can be caused by drugs (such as epinephrine), blood clots, or spinal cord injury.

Cancer of the penis occurs most commonly on the glans and is rare in circumcised men. Circumcision also offers some protection against HIV infection.

Syphilis can cause flat pink or gray growths called **condylomata** or a sore called a **chancre**.

Other sexually transmitted diseases (STDs) can produce small, firm genital warts called **condylomata acuminata** or firm, dimpled growths called **molluscum contagiosum.** The STDs are discussed in detail in *Chapter 6*.

Erectile dysfunction (impotence) is the inability to develop or maintain an erection of the penis during sexual activity. The problem can be caused by cardiovascular disease, diabetes, trauma from prostatectomy surgery, drug side effects, potassium deficiency, and psychological reasons.

Premature ejaculation occurs when a man ejaculates so quickly during intercourse that it causes embarrassment.

Disorders of the Prepuce

Disorders of the prepuce include:

- **Balanitis**—infection of the glans and foreskin with bacteria or yeast.

- **Balanoposthitis**—is an inflammation of the glans penis and the prepuce.

- **Phimosis**—a condition in which the foreskin is tight because of a small opening and cannot be retracted over the glans for cleaning *(Figure 7.13)*. It can lead to balanitis.

- **Paraphimosis**—a condition in which the retracted foreskin cannot be pulled forward to cover the glans.

In all of these conditions, particularly if they are recurrent, circumcision as an adult may be necessary.

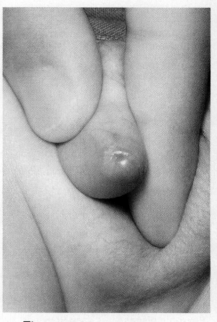

▲ **Figure 7.13** **Phimosis.** Cardiff and Vale NHS Trust/Wellcome Images

Disorders of the Penile Urethra

Urethritis is an inflammation of the urethra. It can be caused by:

- The same bacteria that cause UTIs *(see Chapter 6)*.

- STDs such as chlamydia and gonorrhea *(see Chapter 8)*.

- Herpes simplex virus and cytomegalovirus *(see Chapter 8)*.

- Chemical irritants such as spermicides and contraceptive gels.

Urethritis presents with dysuria, increased frequency of urination, and discharge from the penis. After urine culture to identify the organism, antibiotics will clear a bacterial infection, usually without complications.

Urethral stricture is scarring that narrows the urethra. It results from infection or injury. It produces a less forceful stream of urine and can be a cause of UTI.

Hypospadias is a congenital defect in which the opening of the urethra is on the undersurface of the penis instead of at the head of the glans *(Figure 7.14)*. It can be corrected surgically.

Epispadias is a congenital defect in which the opening of the urethra is on the **dorsum** of the penis. It can be corrected surgically.

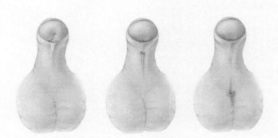

▲ **Figure 7.14** **Hypospadias.**
Centers for Disease Control.

Word Analysis and Definition: Disorders of the Penis

S = Suffix   P = Prefix   R = Root   R/CF = Combining Form

WORD	PRONUNCIATION		ELEMENTS	DEFINITION
acuminata	a-**KYU**-min-**AH**-ta	S/ R/	**-ata** *action, place* **acumin-** *to sharpen*	Tapering to a point
balanitis	**BAL**-a-**NIE**-tis	S/ R/	**-itis** *inflammation* **balan-** *glans penis*	Inflammation of the glans penis
balanoposthitis	**BAL**-a-no-pos-**THI**-tis	S/ R/CF R/	**-itis** *inflammation* **balan/o-** *glans penis* **-posth-** *prepuce*	Inflammation of the glans and prepuce of the penis
chancre	**SHAN**-ker		Latin *cancer*	Primary lesion of syphilis
condyloma condylomata (pl)	kon-dih-**LOH**-ma kon-dih-**LOH**-ma-tah		Greek *a knob*	Warty growth on external genitalia
contagiosum contagious (adj)	kon-**TAY**-jee-oh-sum kon-**TAY**-jus		Latin *to touch closely*	Infection spread from one person to another by direct contact Able to be transmitted, as infections transmitted from person to person or from person to air or surface to person
dorsum	**DOR**-sum		Latin *back*	Upper, posterior, or back surface
epispadias	ep-ih-**SPAY**-dee-as	S/ P/ R/	**-ias** *condition* **epi-** *above* **-spad-** *tear or cut*	Condition in which the urethral opening is on the dorsum of the penis
hypospadias	high-poh-**SPAY**-dee-as	S/ P/ R/	**-ias** *condition* **hypo-** *below* **-spad-** *tear or cut*	Urethral opening more proximal than normal on the ventral surface of the penis
impotence	**IM**-poh-tence		Latin *inability*	Inability to achieve an erection
molluscum contagiosum	moh-**LUS**-kum kon-**TAY**-jee-oh-sum	S/ R/	**-um** *structure* **mollusc-** *soft* Latin *to touch closely*	A soft, round tumor of skin caused by a virus; it is sexually transmitted when these tumors are located on or near the genitals
paraphimosis phimosis	**PAR**-ah-fi-**MOH**-sis fi-**MOH**-sis	S/ P/ R/	**-osis** *condition* **para-** *abnormal* **-phim-** *muzzle*	Condition in which a retracted prepuce cannot be pulled forward to cover the glans Condition in which the prepuce cannot be retracted
Peyronie disease	pay-**ROH**-nee diz-**EEZ**		François de la Peyronie, 1678–1747, French surgeon	Penile bending and pain on erection
priapism	**PRY**-ah-pizm		Priapus, mythical Roman god of procreation	Persistent erection of the penis
stricture	**STRICK**-shur		Latin *to draw tight*	Narrowing of a tube
syphilis	**SIF**-ih-lis		Possibly from the Latin poem "Syphilis sive Morbus Gallicus" by Fracastorius	Sexually transmitted disease caused by a spirochete
urethritis	you-ree-**THRIE**-tis	S/ R/	**-itis** *inflammation* **urethr-** *urethra*	Inflammation of the urethra

Check Point Section 7.3

A. Recognition. *As you become more familiar with elements (especially suffixes), you will be able to recognize medical terms that are procedures and diagnoses. Choose the correct answer.* **LO 7.1, 7.2, 7.6**

1. The root in the term **anorchism** means:

   a. hidden   b. testicle   c. reproductive   d. condition

2. In the term **hypogonadism,** the prefix means:

   a. below   b. above   c. deficient   d. excessive

3. The root in the term **hyperplasia** is:

   a. hyper   b. plas   c. ia

4. The meaning of the root in the term **hyperplasia** is:

   a. excessive   b. formation   c. condition   d. below

B. Matching. *Match the type of prostatitis with its correct description.* **LO 7.6**

	Term		Meaning
_____	1. Type I	a.	an acute bacterial infection with fever, chills, frequency, dysuria, and hematuria
_____	2. Type II	b.	a chronic bacterial infection with less severe symptoms
_____	3. Type III	c.	chronic nonbacterial prostatitis with urinary symptoms, but no bacteria can be detected

C. Latin and Greek terms stand alone and do not deconstruct into several elements the way other terms do. *Match the medical term in the first column to its definition in the second column.* **LO 7.6**

_____	1. chancre	a.	warty growth on external genitalia
_____	2. contagiosum	b.	transmitted, as an infection spread from one person to another by direct contact
_____	3. condyloma	c.	inability to achieve an erection
_____	4. impotence	d.	primary lesion of syphilis
_____	5. contagious	e.	to touch closely

D. Construct medical terms using word elements. *Complete the medical terms being described. Fill in the blanks.* **LO 7.2, 7.6**

1. Inflammation of the epididymis: epi/ _____ /itis

2. Highly malignant cancer in the testis or ovary: chorio/ _____ /oma

3. Swelling containing water: _____ /cele

4. Neoplasm of the germ cells of the testis: semin/ _____

5. Inflammation of the testis: orch/ _____

6. Varicose veins of the spermatic cord: varico/ _____

Diagnostic Procedures

A **digital rectal examination (DRE),** in which a lubricated, gloved finger is inserted into the rectum, is part of a routine physical examination in men and women. In men it is used to check for enlargement or other abnormalities of the prostate gland.

Prostate-specific antigen (PSA) is a protein produced by cells of the prostate gland, and the PSA test measures the level of PSA in a man's blood. The level is increased in cancer of the prostate, benign prostatic hyperplasia (BPH), and acute prostatitis.

Prostate biopsy is commonly performed under ultrasound guidance to remove samples of tissue for pathologic analysis. MRI-guided biopsies or a hybrid of MRI images with ultrasound also can be used.

Therapeutic Procedures

Circumcision, the removal of the foreskin, can be indicated in an adult for pathological phimosis, **refractory** balanoposthitis, and chronic urinary tract infections. In many religions, circumcision is a ritual in the neonatal period or at varying ages before puberty. In the United States, 85% of all males are circumcised in the neonatal period. In Europe, less than 20% are circumcised.

Orchiopexy is a **surgical** procedure to move an undescended testicle (**cryptorchid**) from the abdomen into the scrotum and permanently fix it there.

Orchiectomy (orchidectomy) is the removal of one or both testicles and is the initial treatment for testicular cancer, followed by chemotherapy and sometimes radiation therapy. It is also a procedure for gender affirmation surgery for transgender women, and advanced prostate cancer to stop the production of testosterone.

Urethrotomy is incision of the urethra to relieve stricture caused by injury or infection.

Benign prostatic hypertrophy (BPH) can be treated surgically by **transurethral resection of the prostate (TURP),** in which a **resectoscope** is inserted through the penile urethra to remove prostate tissue obstructing the urethra; **transurethral incision of the prostate (TUIP),** in which the urethra is widened by incision in the neck of the bladder and in the prostate gland; laser surgery, which removes prostate tissue by **ablation** (melting) or **enucleation** (cutting) through insertion of a scope through the penile urethra; or open simple **prostatectomy,** in which the portion of the prostate gland blocking urine flow is removed through incisions or **laparoscopy** in the abdomen.

Cancer of the prostate can be treated by closely watching (active surveillance) it for early-stage, asymptomatic, slow-growing lesions; external beam **radiation therapy** or **brachytherapy,** in which many rice-sized radioactive seeds are implanted in the prostate; **cryosurgery,** in which small needles containing a very cold gas are inserted in the cancer using ultrasound images as guidance; **radical prostatectomy,** to remove the prostate gland, surrounding tissue, and lymph nodes surgically; and **chemotherapy.**

Proton beam radiation therapy delivers beams of protons to the prostate tumor. This therapy is under investigation to compare its effectiveness to traditional radiation therapy.

In a **vasectomy,** performed under local anesthesia, the ductus deferens is pulled through a small incision in the scrotum and cut in two places, a 1-centimeter segment is removed, and the ends are cauterized and tied (*Figure 7.15*). The procedure to reverse (repair) a vasectomy is called a **vasovasotomy.**

Pharmacology

BPH can be treated with medication to make urination easier and medication to prevent the growth of the prostate gland.

Alpha-blockers make urination easier by relaxing muscle fibers in the prostate and the urinary bladder neck muscles These medications include alfuzosin (*Uroxatral*), doxazosin (*Cardura*), tamsulosin (*Flomax*), and silodosin (*Rapaflo*).

5-alpha reductase inhibitors block hormones that spur the growth of the gland. These medications include finasteride (*Proscar*) and dutasteride (*Avodart*).

Prostate cancer can be treated with hormone therapy using medications that stop the body from producing testosterone, which prostate cancer cells need to grow, or **anti-androgens** that block testosterone from reaching the cancer cells.

Prostatitis is usually a bacterial infection and requires treatment with appropriate **antibiotics.**

Treatment of the underlying cause of erectile dysfunction can relieve the difficulty of maintaining an erection, and phosphodiesterase type 5 inhibitors (PDE5) such as avanafil (*Stendra*), sildenafil citrate (*Viagra*), tadalafil (*Cialis*), and vardenafil HCl (*Levitra*) are now in common use. Less common treatments are a penile prosthesis or a penile pump.

Did you know...

- **Vasectomy** is almost 100% successful in producing male sterility.
- **Vasovasostomy** is a microsurgical procedure to suture back together (**anastomosis**) the cut ends of the ductus deferens if requested sometime after vasectomy.

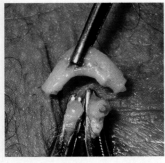

▲ **Figure 7.15** Vasectomy being performed. SPL/Science Source

WORD	PRONUNCIATION		ELEMENTS	DEFINITION
ablation	ab-**LAY**-shun	S/ P/ R/	-ion *action* ab- *away from* -lat- *to take*	Removal of tissue to destroy its function
alpha-blocking agent alpha-blockers	**AL**-fah **BLOK**-ing **A**-jent		**alpha-** Greek *first letter* **block** French *inhibit*	Drugs that relax smooth muscle
biopsy	**BI**-op-see	S/ R/CF	-opsy *to view* bi/o- *life*	Removing tissue from a living person for laboratory examination
brachytherapy	brah-kee-**THAIR**-ah-pee	P/ R	brachy- *short* -therapy *treatment*	Radiation therapy in which the source of irradiation is implanted in the tissue to be treated
circumcision	ser-kum-**SIZH**-un	S/ P/ R/	-ion *process, action* circum- *around* -cis- *to cut*	To remove part or all of the prepuce
cryosurgery	cry-oh-**SUR**-jer-ee	S/ R/CF R/	-ery *process of* cry/o- *icy cold* -surg- *operate*	Use of liquid nitrogen or argon gas to freeze and kill abnormal tissue
digital	**DIJ**-ih-tal	S/ R/	-al *pertaining to* digit- *finger or toe*	Pertaining to a finger or toe
enucleation	ee-nu-klee-**A**-shun	S/ P/ R/	-ation *process* e- *out of, from* -nucle- *kernel*	Removal of an entire structure without rupture
orchiectomy (orchidectomy)	or-kee-**ECK**-toh-mee	S/ R/CF	-ectomy *surgical excision* orch/i- *testicle*	Removal of one testis or both testes
orchiopexy	**OR**-kee-oh-**PEK**-see	S/ R/CF	-pexy *surgical fixation* orchi/o- *testicle*	Surgical fixation of a testis in the scrotum
prostatectomy	pross-tah-**TEK**-toh-mee	S/ R/	-ectomy *surgical excision* prostat- *prostate*	Surgical removal of the prostate
radiation	ray-dee-**AY**-shun	S/ R/	-ation *process* radi- *radiation*	The sending forth of x-rays or other rays for treatment or diagnosis
radical surgery	**RAD**-ih-kal **SUR**-jeh-ree	 S/ R/	radical Latin *root* -ery *condition, process of* surg- *operate*	Surgical procedure in which the affected organ is removed along with the blood and lymph supply to that organ
refractory	ree-**FRACK**-tor-ee		Latin *to oppose*	Resistant to treatment
resection	ree-**SEK**-shun	S/ P/ R/	-ion *action* re- *back* -sect- *cut off*	Removal of a specific part of an organ or structure
resectoscope	ree-**SEK**-toe-skope	S/ R/CF	-scope *instrument for viewing* resect/o- *cut off*	Endoscope for the transurethral removal of lesions
surgical	**SUR**-jih-kal	S/ R/	-ical *pertaining to* surg- *operate*	Relating to surgery
transurethral	**TRANS**-you-**REE**-thral	S/ P/ R/	-al *pertaining to* trans- *across, through* -urethr- *urethra*	Procedure performed through the urethra
urethrotomy	you-ree-**THROT**-oh-mee	S/ R/CF	-tomy *surgical incision* urethr/o- *urethra*	Incision of a stricture of the urethra
vasectomy	vah-**SEK**-toh-mee	S/ R/	-ectomy *surgical excision* vas- *duct*	Excision of a segment of the ductus (vas) deferens
vasovasostomy (also called **vasectomy reversal**)	**VAY**-soh-vay-**SOS**-toh-mee	S/ R/CF	-stomy *new opening* vas/o- *duct*	Reanastomosis of the ductus deferens to restore the flow of sperm

Check Point Section 7.4

A. Construct medical terms. *Recalling the meanings of word elements assists you in determining the meaning of a medical term. From the given definition, provide the missing word element. Fill in the blanks.* **LO 7.2, 7.5, 7.7**

1. Use of liquid nitrogen to freeze abnormal tissue.   _____/surgery

2. Removal of a specific part of an organ or tissue.   re/_____/ion

3. Excision of a section of the ductus deferens.   vas/_____

4. Surgical fixation of a testis in the scrotum   _____/pexy

5. Pertaining to a finger or toe   _____/al

6. Removal of tissue to destroy its function.   _____/lat/ion

7. Removal of entire structure without rupture   e/_____/ation

8. Radiation therapy for which the source of radiation is implanted into the tissue to be treated   _____/therapy

Table 7.1 Chapter 7 Abbreviations

Abbreviation	Meaning	Abbreviation	Meaning
BMR	basal metabolic rate	PSA	prostate-specific antigen
BPH	benign prostatic hyperplasia	SET	self-examination of the testes
c/o	complains of	STD	sexually transmitted disease
DRE	digital rectal examination	TUIP	transurethral incision of the prostate
ED	erectile dysfunction	TURP	transurethral resection of the prostate
LCC-ST	Liaison Council on Certification for the Surgical Technologist	VS	vital signs, which include T (temperature), P (pulse rate), R (respiration rate), and BP (blood pressure)
PDE5	phosphodiesterase type 5 inhibitor		

Table 7.2 Comparison of Common Male Reproduction Disorders

Disorder	Signs and Symptoms	Diagnostic Tests	Treatment
Balanitis	Pain and irritation on the glans Redness on penis Itching under the foreskin Foul smell Dysuria	Physical examination	Antifungal creams Antibiotics Improved personal hygiene
Urethritis	Pain or burning during urination Increased urge to urinate	Physical examination	Antibiotics
Urethral stricture	Incomplete bladder emptying Increased urge to urinate Decreased urine stream	Retrograde urethrogram Cystoscopy	Surgical treatment to widen the urethra
Priapism	Erection lasting 4 hours or longer	Physical examination	Ice packs Methods to reduce the amount of blood in the penis
Epididymitis	Pain in scrotum Testicular swelling Fever and chills Dysuria	Physical exam Urinalysis Ultrasound	Antibiotics Ice packs NSAIDs

Male Reproductive System

Challenge Your Knowledge

A. **Language of male reproductive system.** Every day on the job in the Urology Clinic, you will be asked to apply the language of urology to the anatomy and physiology of the male reproductive system. Select the correct choice. **LO 7.1**

1. The prostate, seminal vesicles, and bulbourethral glands are

   a. gonads   **d.** secondary sex organs

   b. primary sex organs   **e.** accessory vessels

   c. accessory glands

2. The tube that carries the sperm from the epididymis:

   a. glans   **d.** raphe

   b. urethra   **e.** vesicle

   c. vas (ductus) deferens

3. A male secondary sex organ:

   a. prostate   **d.** bulbourethral glands

   b. testis   **e.** penis

   c. seminal vesicle

4. The final portion of the tubular system of the male reproductive system is the:

   a. testes   **d.** penis

   b. urethra   **e.** scrotum

   c. prostate

5. The skin-covered sac between the thighs of males:

   a. rete testis   **d.** ductus deferens

   b. perineum   **e.** scrotum

   c. median septum

B. **Apply the language of urology to the anatomy and physiology of the male reproductive system.** Select the correct choice. **LO 7.1**

1. Androgens are

   a. enzymes   **d.** special nerve cells

   b. vitamins   **e.** flagella

   c. hormones

2. The penis, scrotum, and testes collectively are known as

   a. primary sex organs   **d.** external genitalia

   b. accessory glands   **e.** the perineum

   c. secondary sex organs

3. The male gonads are the

    a. scrotum

    b. penis

    c. prostate

    d. ductus deferens

    e. testes

4. The medical term that refers to the area between the thighs is the

    a. perineum

    b. raphae

    c. spermatic cord

    d. genitalia

    e. varicocele

5. The distinct ridge in the scrotum is called the

    a. dartos

    b. raphe

    c. hydrocele

    d. epididymis

    e. cavernosa

C. Explain spermatogenesis. Demonstrate your knowledge of spermatogenesis by selecting the correct answer to the following questions. **LO 7.1**

1. The major androgen of the male reproductive system:

    a. estrogen

    b. testosterone

    c. semen

    d. cortisone

    e. spermatid

2. That which suspends each testis in the scrotum is the

    a. spermatic cord

    b. ductus deferens

    c. dartos muscle

    d. interstitial cells

    e. tunica

3. After meiosis, the four daughter cells eventually differentiate in:

    a. spermatids

    b. spermatozoa

    c. germ cells

    d. flagella

    e. oocytes

4. How many chromosomes are found in a sperm cell?

    a. 15

    b. 20

    c. 23

    d. 35

    e. 43

5. The term that is the plural form of sperm:

    a. spermatic

    b. spermatozoon

    c. spermatid

    d. spermatogenesis

    e. spermatozoa

D. Roots. The following medical terms all share the same root/combining form. Employ your knowledge of the other elements to determine the correct term for the sentence. Use the provided terms to fill in the blanks. **LO 7.5, 7.6, 7.7**

cryptorchism	orchitis	epididymoorchitis	orchiopexy	orchiectomy	anorchism

1. Patient has inflammation of the epididymis and testicle on the right side. Diagnosis: _____

2. Patient was born without testes. Diagnosis: _____

3. Patient had one diseased testicle removed. Procedure: _____

4. Patient had testicular torsion repaired. Procedure: _____

5. Patient has inflammation of both testicles. Diagnosis: _____

6. Patient was born with an undescended right testicle. Diagnosis: _____

E. Proper documentation. Patients will explain procedures and conditions in common language. Can you interpret what they communicate into proper medical terminology? **LO 7.6, 7.7, 7.8**

1. "I had a surgery so that I can't get a woman pregnant." His procedure was a _____.

2. "I have to get up a lot in the night to urinate." He is complaining of _____.

3. "I was unable to retract my foreskin." He had the condition _____.

4. "My husband had his entire prostate removed." His surgical procedure was a _____.

5. "My son was born with an undescended testicle." The child has _____.

F. Abbreviations are another form of precise communication. Demonstrate that you know the meanings of the abbreviations in this exercise. Select the best answer. **LO 7.5, 7.6, 7.9**

1. Which of the following is a diagnosis for a type of prostate disease?

   a. BPH   c. PSA

   b. TURP   d. LCC-ST

2. Which of the following can produce *condylomata acuminata*?

   a. STD   c. ED

   b. UTI   d. TUIP

3. The abbreviation *DRE* relates to a:

   a. disorder of the penis

   b. structure of the male reproductive system

   c. diagnostic procedure

   d. medication to treat prostate cancer

2014 Nucleus Medical Media

G. Deconstruction. Deconstruction of medical terms is a tool for analyzing the meaning. In the following chart, you are given a medical term. Deconstruct the term into its prefix, root (or combining form) and suffix. Write the element and its meaning in the appropriate column and the meaning of the term in the last column. If the term does not have a word element, write n/a. The first one is done for you. **LO 7.2, 7.6**

Term	Prefix	Meaning of Prefix	Root/ Combining Form	Meaning of Root/Combing Form	Suffix	Meaning of Suffix	Meaning of Term
phimosis	1. n/a	2. n/a	3. phim	4. muzzle	5. -osis	6. condition	7. Condition in which the prepuce cannot be retracted
hyperplasia	8.	9.	10.	11.	12.	13.	14.
epididymis	15.	16.	17.	18.	19.	20.	21.
teratoma	22.	23.	24.	25.	26.	27.	28.
cavernosa	29.	30.	31.	32.	33.	34.	35.

H. Disorder or disease. Complete the diagnosis documentation for the following patients. Fill in the blanks with the correct medical term for the disorder or disease mentioned in each statement. **LO 7.6**

1. Excess fluid has collected in the space between the visceral and parietal layers of the tunica vaginalis of the patient's right testis:

   hydro _____.

2. Noncancerous enlargement compressing the prostatic urethra is: benign _____ plasia.

3. Marked curvature of the erect penis caused by fibrous tissue is _____ disease.

4. Opening of the urethra is on the dorsum of the penis: _____ spadias.

5. Veins in the spermatic cord become tortuous and dilated: varico _____.

6. Opening of the urethra is on the undersurface of the penis instead of at the head of the glans: hypo _____.

7. Yeast infection of the glans and foreskin is _____ itis.

8. Foreskin is tight and cannot be retracted over the glans for cleaning: _____ sis.

9. Inflammation of the epididymis is _____ itis.

I. **Trace the pathway taken by a sperm cell from the testes to its ejaculation.** Number the following terms in the correct order. Fill in the blanks. **LO 7.1**

_____ **a.** epididymis

_____ **b.** urethra

_____ **c.** testis

_____ **d.** seminiferous tubules

_____ **e.** ejaculatory duct

_____ **f.** ductus deferens

_____ **g.** penis

J. **Pronunciation is important whether you are saying the word or listening to a word from a coworker.** Identify the proper pronunciation of the following medical terms. **LO 7.3, 7.4, 7.6**

1. The correct pronunciation for the process of maturing from child to young adult

    a. li-**BEE**-doh   **b.** lye-bee-**DOO**   **c.** **PYU**-ber-tee   **d.** poo-**BURR**-tee

    Correctly spell the term: _____

2. The correct pronunciation for varicose veins of the spermatic cord

    a. **AN**-ork-ism   **b.** an-**OR**-kizm   **c.** **VAIR**-oh-koh-**SEE**-al   **d.** **VAIR**-ih-koh-seal

    Correctly spell the term: _____

3. The correct pronunciation for inflammation of the prostate

    a. pross-tah-**TIE**-tis   **b.** pross-**TAY**-tis   **c.** **PRAY**-stay-ties   **d.** **PRO**-stay-tis

    Correctly spell the term: _____

4. The correct pronunciation for the hormone present in many tissues, but first isolated from the prostate gland

    a. **AN**-droh-jen   **b.** **AND**-rah-jen   **c.** **PROS**-tah-**GLAN**-din   **d.** **PROS**-tay-gleh-**DAN**

    Correctly spell the term: _____

5. The correct pronunciation for the area between thighs, extending from the coccyx to the pubis

    a. **PER**-ih-**NEE**-um   **b.** **JEN**-ih-tal   **c.** **GOHN**-ads   **d.** **SKROHT**-um

    Correctly spell the term: _____

2014 Nucleus Medical Media

Case Reports

A. **After reading the following Case Report, correctly answer the following questions.** The answers to the questions may not be in the Case Report itself but can be found in the chapter content.

Dr. Helinski, the emergency physician on duty, has referred Joseph Davis to a surgeon for repair of his condition, and it is your duty to obtain from the patient's insurance company preapproval for the surgery. You must be prepared to furnish answers to the following questions the insurance company will ask. Fill in the blanks. **LO 7.6, 7.7, 7.8**

 ## Case Report (CR) 7.1

You are

. . . an EMT-P working in the Emergency Department at Fulwood Medical Center.

Your patient is

. . . Joseph Davis, a 17-year-old high school senior.

He is brought in by his mother at 0400 hrs. He complains of sudden onset of pain in his left **testicle** 3 hours earlier that woke him up. The pain is intense and has made him vomit. VS: T 99.2°F, P 88, R 15, BP 130/70. Examination reveals his left testicle to be enlarged, warm, and tender. His abdomen is normal to palpation.

At your request, Dr. Helinski, the emergency physician on duty, examines him immediately. He diagnoses a **torsion** of the patient's left testicle.

Joseph Davis presented with typical symptoms and signs of testicular torsion. The affected testis rapidly became painful, tender, swollen, and inflamed. Emergency surgery was performed, and the testis and cord were manually untwisted through an incision in the scrotum. The testis was stitched to surrounding tissues to prevent a recurrence.

---

1. What is the patient's diagnosis? _____

2. Is this condition the result of an accident? _____

3. What procedure is the surgeon going to perform? _____

B. **After reading the following Case Report, correctly answer the following questions.** The answers to the questions may not be in the Case Report itself but can be found in the chapter content. **LO 7.3, 7.5, 7.6, 7.8, 7.9, 7.10**

 ## Case Report (CR) 7.2

You are

. . . a surgical technologist (LCC-ST) working with **urologist** Phillip Johnson, MD, in the **Urology** Clinic at Fulwood Medical Center.

Your patient is

. . . Mr. Ronald Detrick, a 60-year-old man who has been referred to the Urology Clinic c/o having to get out of bed to urinate four or five times at night.

Mr. Detrick has difficulty starting urination, has a weak stream, and feels he is not emptying his bladder completely. His symptoms have been gradually worsening over the past year. He has lost interest in sex. His physical examination is unremarkable except that **DRE reveals a** diffusely enlarged prostate with no nodules.

---

1. Based on your occupation, which of the following tasks would you likely assist Dr. Johnson with?

   a. Performing transillumination to assess a hydrocele.

   b. Swabbing urethral opening to send to lab for assessment.

   c. Gathering the necessary equipment for a vasectomy.

   d. Retracting the foreskin of a patient with phimosis.

2. What does the abbreviation *c/o* stand for?

   a. complains on

   b. complains of

   c. chronic opinion

   d. claims opinion

3. Provide the words that DRE stands for.

   D= _____ R= _____ E= _____

4. Based on Mr. Detrick's symptoms and the results of the DRE, correctly predict the diagnosis Dr. Johnson will make.

   a. Fungal infection phimosis

   b. Epididymitis with orchitis

   c. Benign prostatic hyperplasia

   d. Type I prostatitis

   e. Cancer of the prostate

5. Provide the medical term that correctly documents Mr. Detrick's statement that he has *". . . to get out of bed to urinate four or five times at night."* _____

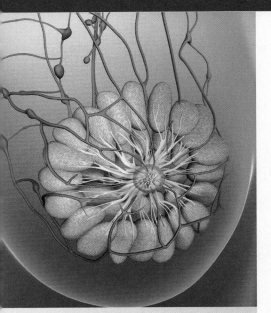

2014 Nucleus Medical Media

Female Reproductive System

The Languages of Gynecology and Obstetrics

Chapter Learning Outcomes

Upon completion of this chapter, you will be able to:

LO 8.1 Identify and describe the anatomy and physiology of the female reproductive system.

LO 8.2 Use roots, combining forms, suffixes, and prefixes to construct and analyze medical terms related to the female reproductive system.

LO 8.3 Spell medical terms related to the female reproductive system.

LO 8.4 Pronounce medical terms related to the female reproductive system.

LO 8.5 Describe diagnostic procedures utilized in gynecology and obstetrics.

LO 8.6 Identify and describe disorders and pathological conditions in gynecology and obstetrics.

LO 8.8 Describe the therapeutic procedures and pharmacologic agents used in gynecology and obstetrics.

LO 8.8 Apply knowledge of medical terms relating to obstetrics and gynecology accurately in documentation, medical records, and communication.

LO 8.9 Identify and correctly use abbreviations of terms used in gynecology and obstetrics.

LO 8.10 Identify health professionals involved in obstetrics and gynecology accurately.

The health professionals you will find involved in the care of women at different times in their lives include the following:

- **Gynecologists** are physicians who are specialists in diseases of the female reproductive tract.
- **Obstetricians** are physicians who are specialists in the care of women during pregnancy and childbirth.
- **Neonatologists** are physicians who are pediatric subspecialists in disorders of the newborn, particularly ill or premature infants.
- **Perinatologists** are physicians who are obstetric subspecialists in the care of mothers with high-risk pregnancies and fetuses at higher-than-normal risk for complications.
- **Certified midwives/nurse-midwives** are independent practitioners who provide care to mothers during pregnancy, delivery, and birth, and to mothers and newborn infants for 6 weeks after birth.
- **Obstetrical-gynecological nurse practitioners** are registered nurses who have acquired skills in the management of health and illness for women throughout their life cycle.

Section 8.1 External Genitalia and Vagina

External Genitalia

Both the female and male reproductive systems are dormant until **puberty,** when the gonads (ovaries in the female and testes in the male) begin to secrete significant quantities of sex hormones (estrogen and progesterone in the female, androgens in the male). In the female, the external genitalia become more prominent, pubic hair develops, the vagina becomes lubricated, and breast enlargement occurs. Understanding the anatomy and physiology of the mature external genitalia and vagina is an important introduction to the female reproductive system. The area between the thighs extending from the coccyx to the **pubis** is called the **perineum.** The female external genitalia occupy most of the perineum and are collectively called the **vulva** *(Figure 8.1a).* The structures of the vulva include the:

- **Mons pubis**—a mound of skin and adipose tissue overlying the symphysis pubis. In **postpubescent** females, it is covered with **pubic** hair.

- **Labia majora**—a pair of thick folds of skin, connective tissue, and adipose tissue. In postpubescent females, their outer surface is covered with coarse hair, and the inner surface has numerous sweat and sebaceous glands.

- **Labia minora**—a pair of thin folds of hairless skin immediately internal to the labia majora. Sebaceous glands are present on these folds, together with melanocytes *(see Chapter 4)* that give the folds a dark melanin pigmentation. Anteriorly, the labia minora join together to form the prepuce (hood) of the clitoris. Posteriorly they merge with the labia majora.

- **Clitoris**—a small erectile body capped with a glans. It has two corpora cavernosa surrounded by connective tissue. The clitoris contains many sensory nerve receptors.

Deep to the labia majora on either side of the vaginal orifice is an erectile body called the **vestibular bulb** *(Figure 8.1b).* The two bulbs become congested with blood and more sensitive during sexual arousal. Posterior to the vestibular bulbs on each side of the **vaginal** orifice is a pea-sized **greater vestibular gland (Bartholin gland).** These glands secrete mucin, which lubricates the vagina. Secretion is increased during sexual arousal and intercourse.

> **Did you know...**
>
> - **Obstetrics (OB)** is the medical specialty for the care of women during pregnancy and the **postpartum** period.
> - **Gynecology (GYN)** is the medical specialty for the care of the female reproductive system.

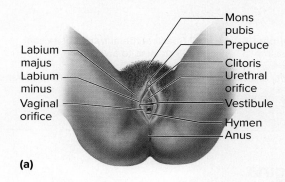

Labium majus
Labium minus
Vaginal orifice
Mons pubis
Prepuce
Clitoris
Urethral orifice
Vestibule
Hymen
Anus

(a)

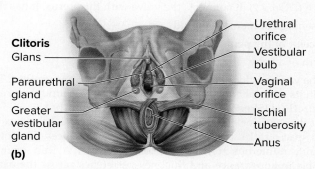

Clitoris
Glans
Paraurethral gland
Greater vestibular gland
Urethral orifice
Vestibular bulb
Vaginal orifice
Ischial tuberosity
Anus

(b)

▲ **Figure 8.1 Female perineum and vulva.** [a] Surface anatomy. [b] Subcutaneous structures.

WORD	PRONUNCIATION	ELEMENTS		DEFINITION
clitoris	**KLIT**-oh-ris		Greek *clitoris*	Erectile organ of the vulva
greater vestibular gland (also known as Bartholin gland)	**GRATE**-ur ves-**TIB**-you-lar GLAND		Casper Bartholin the Younger, 1655–1738, Danish anatomist	Pea-sized glands on the posterolateral walls of the vagina that secrete mucus
gynecology	guy-nih-**KOL**-oh-jee	S/ R/CF	-logy *study of* gynec/o- *female*	Medical specialty for the care of the female reproductive system
gynecologist	guy-nih-**KOL**-oh-jist	S/	-logist *specialist*	Specialist in gynecology
labium labia (pl)	**LAY**-bee-um **LAY**-bee-ah		Greek *lip*	Fold of the vulva
majus majora (pl)	**MAY**-jus **MAY**-jor-ah		Latin *greater*	Bigger or greater; for example, labia majora
minus minora (pl)	**MY**-nus **MY**-nor-ah		Latin *smaller*	Smaller or lesser; for example, labia minora
mons pubis	MONZ **PYU**-bis		**mons** Latin *mountain* **pubis** Latin *pubic bone*	Fleshy pad with pubic hair, overlying the pubic bone
obstetrics (OB)	ob-**STET**-riks		Latin *a midwife*	Medical specialty for the care of women during pregnancy and the postpartum period
obstetrician	ob-steh-**TRISH**-un	S/ R/	-ician *expert, specialist* obstetr- *midwifery*	Medical specialist in obstetrics
perineum	**PER**-ih-**NEE**-um		Latin *perineum*	Area between the thighs, extending from the coccyx to the pubis
perineal (adj)	**PER**-ih-**NEE**-al	S/ R/CF	-al *pertaining to* perin/e- *perineum*	Pertaining to the perineum
postpubescent	post-pyu-**BESS**-ent	S/ P/ R/	-ent *pertaining to, end result* post- *after* -pubesc- *to reach puberty*	After the period of puberty
puberty	**PYU**-ber-tee	S/ R/	-ty *quality, state* puber- *growing up*	Process of maturing from child to young adult capable of reproducing
pubis pubic (adj)	**PYU**-bis **PYU**-bik	S/ R/	Latin *pubic bone* -ic *pertaining to* pub- *pubis*	Bony front arch of the pelvis of the hip; also called pubic bone Pertaining to the pubis
vestibule vestibular (adj)	**VES**-tih-byul ves-**TIB**-you-lar	S/ R/	Latin *entrance* -ar *pertaining to* vestibul- *vestibule*	Space at the entrance of a canal Pertaining to a vestibule
vestibular bulb	ves-**TIB**-you-lar BULB		Latin *bulb, onion*	Structure on each side of the entrance to the vagina
vulva	**VUL**-vah		Latin *a wrapper or covering*	Female external genitalia
vulvar (adj)		S/	-ar *pertaining to*	Pertaining to the vulva

The Vagina

The **vagina,** or birth canal, is a fibromuscular tube, 4 to 5 inches (10 to 13 cm) in length (*Figure 8.2*). It connects the vulva with the uterus. It has three main functions:

- Discharge of menstrual fluid
- Receipt of the penis and semen
- Birth of a baby

The vagina is located between the rectum and the urethra. The urethra is embedded in its anterior wall. In the wall of the vagina around the urethra are several small **paraurethral (Skene) glands** that open into the urethra.

At its posterior end, the vagina extends beyond the cervix of the uterus to form blind spaces called the anterior and posterior **fornices.** The lower end of the vagina contains numerous transverse folds, or **rugae.** A thin membranous fold, highly variable in appearance and thickness, stretches across the external opening of the vagina to form the **hymen.** The intact hymen contains one or two openings to allow the escape of menstrual fluid.

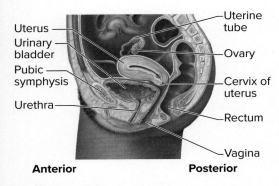

Uterus
Urinary bladder
Pubic symphysis
Urethra

Uterine tube
Ovary
Cervix of uterus
Rectum
Vagina

Anterior   **Posterior**

▲ **Figure 8.2** Female reproductive organs.

WORD	PRONUNCIATION	ELEMENTS		DEFINITION
fornix **fornices (pl)**	**FOR**-niks **FOR**-nih-seez		Latin *arch, vault*	Arch-shaped, blind-ended part of the vagina behind and around the cervix
hymen	**HIGH**-men		Greek *membrane*	Thin membrane partly occluding the vaginal orifice
paraurethral glands **(also known as Skene glands)**	**PAR**-ah-you-**REE**-thral GLANDZ SKEEN GLANDZ	S/ P/ R/	**-al** *pertaining to* **para-** *alongside* **-urethr-** *urethra* Alexander Skene, 1838–1900, New York gynecologist	Glands in the anterior wall of the vagina that secrete mucin to lubricate the vagina
ruga **rugae (pl)**	**ROO**-gah **ROO**-jee		Latin *a wrinkle*	A fold, ridge, or crease
vagina **vaginal (adj)**	vah-**JIE**-nah **VAJ**-in-al	S/ R/	Latin *a sheath* **-al** *pertaining to* **vagin-** *vagina*	Female genital canal extending from the uterus to the vulva Pertaining to the vagina
vulvovaginal (adj)	**VUL**-voh-**VAJ**-ih-nal	S/ R/CF R/	**-al** *pertaining to* **vulv/o-** *vulva* **-vagin-** *vagina*	Pertaining to the vulva and vagina

Check Point Section 8.1

A. Latin and Greek terms cannot be further deconstructed into prefix, root, or suffix. *You must know them for what they are. Match the meaning in the left column with the correct medical term in the right column.* **LO 8.1**

_____ **1.** A covering or wrapper

_____ **2.** Mountain

_____ **3.** Lesser

_____ **4.** Lip

a. labia

b. vulva

c. minora

d. mons

Section 8.2 Ovaries, Uterine Tubes, and Uterus

Anatomy of the Female Reproductive Tract

Ovaries

The female gonads, the primary sex organs, are the ovaries. The female internal accessory organs include a pair of uterine (fallopian) tubes, a uterus, and a vagina. Women are born with all the eggs (ova) that they will release, but it is not until puberty that the eggs mature and start to leave the ovary. The ovarian hormones, estrogen and progesterone, are involved in menstruation and pregnancy (PGY). The pituitary gland at the base of the brain produces other hormones that control the functions of the ovaries, uterus, and breast *(see Chapter 17)*. These complex interactions are the core of the human reproductive system and an essential part of understanding the human body. Each **ovary** is an almond-shaped organ located in a shallow depression (ovarian fossa) in the lateral wall of the pelvic cavity *(Figure 8.3)*. The ovary is about 1 inch (2.5 cm) long and ½ inch (1.3 cm) in diameter. It is enclosed in a capsule called the *tunica albuginea*. Each ovary is held in place by ligaments that attach it to the pelvic wall and uterus.

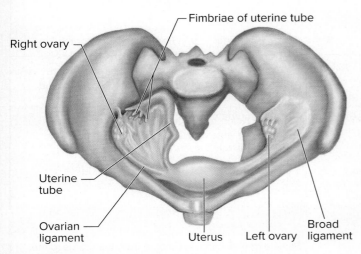

Figure 8.3 **Ovaries.** The ovaries are located on each side against the lateral walls of the pelvic cavity. The right uterine tube is retracted to reveal the ovarian ligament.

Uterine (Fallopian) Tubes

Each uterine tube is a canal about 4 inches (10 cm) long, extending from the uterus and opening to the abdominal cavity near the ovary. The tubes are supported by the broad ligaments. Each tube has four areas:

- **infundibulum**—ovarian end, the outer one-third flares out into a funnel-shaped, with fingerlike folds called **fimbriae** (*see Figure 8.3*). At ovulation, the fimbriae enclose the ovary
- **ampulla**—widened area, typically the site of fertilization
- **isthmus**—the inner one-third of each tube approaching the uterus
- **uterine**—extends from isthmus into the uterus

The wall of the tube has an inner layer of mucosal cells that secrete mucus, some of which are ciliated. The cilia beat toward the uterus and transport the egg down the uterine tube with peristaltic contractions, a journey that takes 3 or 4 days.

The **adnexa** of the uterus are the uterine tubes, the broad ligaments, and the ovaries.

Uterus

The uterus is a thick-walled, muscular organ in the pelvic cavity. It normally tilts forward **(anteverted)** over the urinary bladder. Anatomically, it is divided into three regions:

- **Fundus**—the broad, curved upper region between the lateral attachments of the uterine tubes.
- **Body**—the midportion.
- **Cervix**—the cylindrical inferior portion that projects into the vagina.

The cavity of the uterus is triangular, with its upper two corners receiving the openings of the uterine tubes. Its lower end communicates with the vagina through the cervical canal, which has an **internal os** from the lumen and an **internal os** into the vagina (*see Figure 8.4*).

The cervical canal contains mucous glands; secretions of mucus help prevent the spread of infection from the vagina. The uterus is supported by the muscular floor of the pelvic outlet and by ligaments that extend to the pelvic wall from the uterus and cervix.

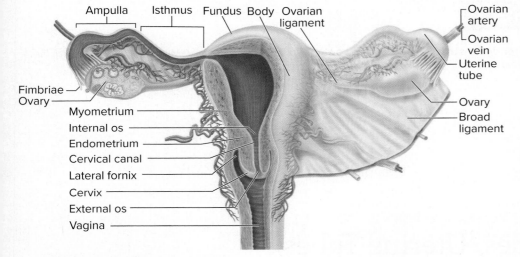

Figure 8.4 **Female reproductive tract.**

The wall of the uterus has three layers. From the outside, these are the:

- **Perimetrium**—a continuation of the broad ligament.
- **Myometrium**—a thick layer of smooth muscle.
- **Endometrium**—the lining that sheds in menstruation.

WORD	PRONUNCIATION		ELEMENTS	DEFINITION
adnexa (pl) adnexum (sing)	ad-**NEK**-sa ad-**NEK**-sum	S/ R/	-um *structure* adnex- *connected parts*	Parts accessory to an organ or structure
			Latin *connected parts*	
adnexal (adj)	ad-**NEK**-sal	S/	-al *pertaining to*	Pertaining to accessory structures; for example, structures alongside the uterus, uterine tubes, and ovaries
anteverted	an-teh-**VERT**-ed	S/ P/ R/	-ed *pertaining to* ante- *before, forward* -vert- *to turn*	Tilted forward
anteversion	an-teh-**VER**-shun	S/	-ion *condition, process*	Forward tilting of the uterus
endometrium	**EN**-doh-**MEE**-tree-um	S/ P/ R/CF	-um *structure* endo- *within, inside* -metr/i- *uterus*	Inner lining of the uterus
endometrial (adj)	**EN**-doh-**MEE**-tree-al	S/	-ial *pertaining to*	Pertaining to the inner lining of the uterus
fimbria fimbriae (pl)	**FIM**-bree-ah **FIM**-bree-ee		Latin *fringe*	A fringe-like structure on the surface of a cell or a microorganism
fundus	**FUN**-dus		Latin *bottom*	Part farthest from the opening of a hollow organ
infundibulum infundibula (pl)	**IN**-fun-**DIB**-you-lum **IN**-fun-**DIB**-you-lah		Latin *funnel*	Funnel-shaped structure
isthmus	**IS**-mus		Greek *isthmus*	Part connecting two larger parts; in this case, the uterus to the uterine tube
myometrium	my-oh-**MEE**-tree-um	S/ R/CF R/CF	-um *tissue* my/o- *muscle* -metr/i- *uterus*	Muscle wall of the uterus
os	OS		Latin *mouth*	Opening into a canal; for example, the cervix
ovary ovaries (pl)	**OH**-va-ree **OH**-vah-rees		Latin *egg*	One of the paired female egg-producing glands
ovarian (adj)	oh-**VAIR**-ee-an	S/ R/	-an *pertaining to* ovari- *ovary*	Pertaining to the ovary
perimetrium	per-ih-**MEE**-tree-um	S/ P/ R/CF	-um *structure* peri- *around* -metr/i- *uterus*	The covering of the uterus; part of the peritoneum
uterus uterine (adj)	**YOU**-ter-us **YOU**-ter-ine	S/ R/	Latin *womb* -ine *pertaining to, substance* uter- *uterus*	Organ in which an egg develops into a fetus Pertaining to the uterus
uterine tubes (also called **fallopian tubes**)	**YOU**-ter-ine TUBES fah-**LOH**-pee-an TUBES			Tubes connected from the uterus to the abdominal cavity. Carry the ovum from the ovary to the uterus.

Oogenesis and Ovulation

During prenatal development, small groups of cells within the female fetus's ovarian cortex form around 2 million **follicles.** In each group of cells, there is a single large cell, the primary **oocyte,** surrounded by a layer of **follicular cells.** Many of these follicular cells degenerate. Under normal circumstances, there are no further changes within ovarian follicles until puberty.

At puberty, some 400,000 primary oocytes remain, each containing 23 pairs of chromosomes. They undergo meiosis to produce secondary oocytes, each containing 23 single chromosomes. As they mature, the follicular cells form a fluid-filled **primary follicle,** in which the oocyte is located *(Figure 8.5).* **Oogenesis** begins in the fetal period and ends at menopause *(see Figure 8.6).* Surrounding the oocyte (egg) and lining the fluid-filled **antrum** of the follicle are **granulosa cells** that secrete estrogen.

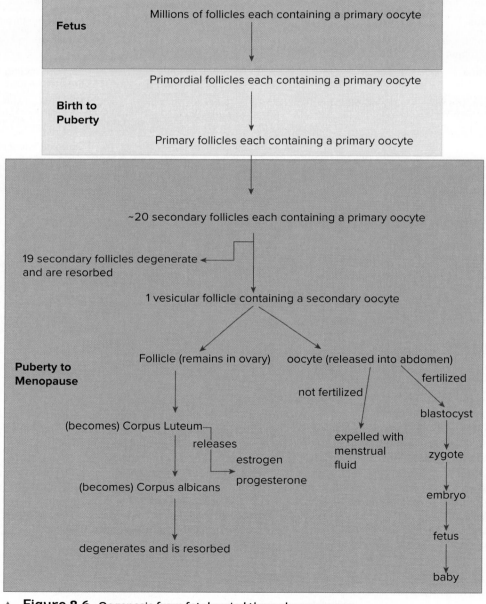

Developmental Sequence

Primordial follicles
Primary follicles
Secondary follicle
Oocyte
Mature follicle
Oocyte
Suspensory ligament and blood vessels
Ovarian ligament

Corpus albicans
Corpus luteum
Ovulated oocyte

▲ **Figure 8.5** Oogenesis.
The development of the oocyte begins with the primordial follicles.

Ovulation

At the beginning of the menstrual cycle, as many as 20 primary follicles can start the maturing process, but only one develops fully. The remainder degenerate. By the midpoint of the menstrual cycle, the mature follicle bulges out on the surface of the ovary and ruptures **(ovulation).** The oocyte and lining cells from the follicle can either be taken into the uterine tube or fall into the pelvic cavity and degenerate.

During the time that the follicles are developing and maturing, the endometrium is undergoing cyclical changes that are under the influence of hormones. The first phase occurs for 5 days and is the shedding of the endometrial lining. After this phase, the endometrial lining begins to rebuild in preparation to protect and nourish the fertilized egg. In the final phase, the endometrium becomes rich in blood supply and in the development of glands. If the ovum is unfertilized, then the uterine cycle starts over again, beginning with the shedding of the endometrium.

Fetus
Millions of follicles each containing a primary oocyte

Birth to Puberty
Primordial follicles each containing a primary oocyte
Primary follicles each containing a primary oocyte

Puberty to Menopause
~20 secondary follicles each containing a primary oocyte

19 secondary follicles degenerate and are resorbed

1 vesicular follicle containing a secondary oocyte

Follicle (remains in ovary)
oocyte (released into abdomen)

not fertilized
fertilized

(becomes) Corpus Luteum
releases
estrogen
progesterone

expelled with menstrual fluid

blastocyst

(becomes) Corpus albicans

zygote

embryo

degenerates and is resorbed

fetus

baby

▲ **Figure 8.6** Oogenesis from fetal period through menopause.

Ovarian Hormones

The ovaries of the sexually mature female secrete **estrogens** and **progesterone.**

Estrogens are produced in the ovarian follicles. Their sexual functions are to:

1. Convert girls into sexually mature women through the onset of breast development, the growth of pubic hair, and the establishment of menstruation.

2. Participate in the menstrual cycle *(see Figure 8.7).*

3. Participate in pregnancy when that occurs.

Progesterone is produced by the corpus luteum of the ovary and by the adrenal glands *(see Chapter 17).* Its sexual functions are to:

1. Prepare the lining of the uterus for implantation of the egg *(see Figure 8.7).*

2. Inhibit lactation during pregnancy.

3. Produce menstrual bleeding if pregnancy does not occur.

The synthesis and secretion of estrogen is stimulated by **follicle-stimulating hormone (FSH)** from the pituitary gland. FSH is controlled by the hypothalamic **gonadotropin-releasing hormone (GnRH).** Progesterone production is stimulated by **luteinizing hormone (LH)** from the pituitary gland, which is also stimulated by GnRH.

The ovaries also secrete small amounts of androgens, male hormones.

The Uterine (Menstrual) Cycle

The menstrual cycle averages 28 days in length. It begins with a 2-week follicular phase. The beginning of the cycle is recognized by physiologists as menstruation, which occurs during the first 3 to 5 days.

After menstruation ends, the uterus starts to replace the endometrial tissue lost during menstruation. The developing ovarian follicles mature, and one of them ovulates around day 14. Around this time, the fimbriae of the uterine tube envelope the ovaries and, in time with the mother's heartbeat, caress the released ovum to guide it into the uterine tube.

After ovulation, in the postovulatory phase, the endometrial lining continues to grow. The residual ovarian follicle becomes a **corpus luteum** containing **lutein** cells that are involved in progesterone production. Around day 24, the corpus luteum **involutes.** By day 26, it is an inactive scar called a **corpus albicans.** At this time, the arteries supplying the endometrium of the uterus contract. This leads to ischemia, tissue necrosis, and the start of menstruation.

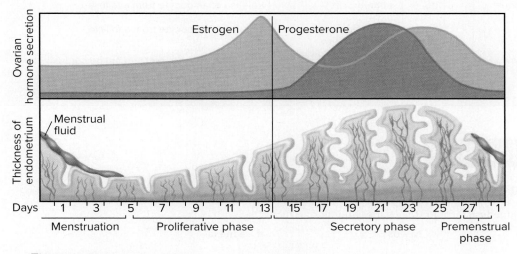

▲ **Figure 8.7** Menstrual cycle.

WORD	PRONUNCIATION	ELEMENTS		DEFINITION
antrum	**AN**-trum		Greek *cave*	A nearly closed cavity or chamber
corpus albicans corpus luteum	**KOR**-pus **AL**-bih-kanz **KOR**-pus **LOO**-tee-um		**albicans** Latin *white* **corpus** Latin *body* **luteum** Latin *yellow*	An atrophied corpus luteum Yellow structure formed at the site of a ruptured ovarian follicle
estrogen	**ESS**-troh-gen	S/ R/CF	**-gen** *create, produce* **estr/o** *woman*	Generic term for hormones that stimulate female secondary sex characteristics
follicle	**FOLL**-ih-kull		Latin *small sac*	Spherical mass of cells containing a cavity, such as a hair follicle
follicular (adj)	fo-**LIK**-you-lar	S/ R/	**-ar** *pertaining to* **follicul-** *follicle*	Pertaining to a follicle
gonadotropin	**GO**-nad-oh-**TROH**-pin	S/ R/CF	**-tropin** *nourishing* **gonad/o-** *gonad*	Hormone capable of promoting gonad function
granulosa cell	gran-you-**LOH**-sah SELL	S/ R/	**-osa** *like* **granul-** *small grain*	Cell lining the ovarian follicle
involution involute (verb)	in-voh-**LOO**-shun in-vol-**LUTE**	S/ P/ R/	**-ion** *process* **in-** *in* **-volut-** *shrink*	A decrease in size or vigor
menopause	**MEN**-oh-paws	R/CF R/	**men/o** *menses* **pause** *cessation*	Permanent ending of menstrual periods.
menses menstruation menstruate (verb) menstrual (adj)	**MEN**-seez men-stru-**A**-shun **MEN**-stru-ate **MEN**-stru-al	 S/ R/ S/ S/	Latin *month* **-ation** *action* **menstru-** *menses* **-ate** *pertaining to* **-al** *pertaining to*	Monthly uterine bleeding Monthly uterine bleeding The act of menstruation Pertaining to menstruation
oocyte oogenesis (**Note:** The *genesis* R/CF is used most often in a suffix position.)	**OH**-oh-site oh-oh-**JEN**-eh-sis	S/ R/CF R/CF	**-cyte** *cell* **o/o-** *egg* **-genesis** *form, create*	Female egg cell Development of female egg cell
ovulation ovulate (verb)	**OV**-you-**LAY**-shun **OV**-you-late	S/ R/ S/	**-ation** *process* **ovul-** *egg* **-ate** *composed of, pertaining to*	Release of an oocyte from a follicle To release an oocyte from a follicle
progesterone (**Note:** two suffixes)	pro-**JESS**-ter-own	S/ S/ P/ R/	**-one** *hormone* **-er-** *agent* **pro-** *before* **-gest-** *pregnancy*	A steroid hormone released by the corpus luteum and involved in the menstrual cycle, pregnancy, and the development of an embryo

Check Point Section 8.2

A. Demonstrate your understanding of the language of *gynecology*. *Select the correct answer that completes each statement.* **LO 8.1**

1. What is the "collective" (as a group) medical term for the ovaries and uterine tubes?
   a. infundibulum   b. fossa   c. os   d. adnexa

2. Another name for the uterine tube is the _____ tube.
   a. cervical   b. os   c. fallopian   d. ovarian

3. The fingerlike folds that envelope the ovary are the:
   a. os   b. adnexa   c. fimbriae   d. ampulla

4. The opening of a canal is the:
   a. os   b. cervix   c. infundibulum   d. fundus

5. In the term *anteversion,* the prefix means:

   a. to turn   **b.** before, forward   **c.** within   **d.** pertaining to

6. In the term *endometrium,* the prefix means:

   a. outer   **b.** inner   **c.** surrounding   **d.** structure   **e.** around

B. Apply your knowledge *of the female reproductive system by choosing the correct answer:* **LO 8.1**

1. The permanent ending of menstrual periods is:

   a. menopause   **b.** amenorrhea   **c.** involution

2. The release of a female egg is called:

   a. oogenesis   **b.** ovulation   **c.** involution

3. Which is the correct spelling for the term?

   a. ooginesis   **b.** oogenisis   **c.** oogenesis

C. Describe the events and structures of oogenesis and ovulation. *Select the answer that correctly completes each statement.* **LO 8.1**

1. At which stage of human growth are follicles developed?

   a. puberty   **b.** menopause   **c.** fetal   **d.** childhood

2. Oocytes are contained in a:

   a. follicle   **b.** corpus albicans   **c.** corpus luteum   **d.** zygote

3. The fluid-filled area of the follicle is the:

   a. corpus luteum   **b.** antrum   **c.** oocyte   **d.** granulosum

D. Construct these medical terms. *Given the definition, fill in the blank with the missing word element.* **LO 8.1, 8.2**

1. A decrease in size or vigor   in/ _____ /ion

2. Hormone that prepares the uterus for pregnancy   _____ /gest/er/one

3. The act of menstruation   menstru/ _____

4. Hormone that promotes female secondary sex characteristics   _____ / _____ /gen

5. Development of female egg cell   _____ /genesis

6. Pertaining to a follicle   follicul/ _____

Section 8.3   Disorders of the Female Reproductive Tract

Disorders of External Genitalia and Vagina

Bacterial vaginosis is the most common cause of **vaginitis** in women of childbearing age. In bacterial vaginosis, the different types of invading bacteria outnumber the normal bacteria of the vagina. The main symptom is an abnormal vaginal discharge with a fishlike odor. Diagnosis is made by laboratory examination of a specimen taken by vaginal swab.

Toxic shock syndrome is a life-threatening illness caused by toxins circulating in the bloodstream. Certain rare strains of bacteria produce these toxins. In the most common form of toxic shock syndrome, the bacteria are in the vagina of women, and their growth is encouraged by the presence of a superabsorbent **tampon** that is not changed frequently.

Vulvovaginal candidiasis is a common cause of genital itching or burning, with a "cottage-cheese" **vaginal** discharge. It is caused by an overgrowth of the yeast fungus called *Candida* and can occur after taking antibiotics. Recent research has found that it is associated with vitamin D deficiency. Diagnosis is made by microscopic examination of a specimen taken by a vaginal swab.

Allergic and irritative causes of **vulvovaginitis** can be caused by vaginal hygiene products, spermicides, detergents, and synthetic underwear.

Vulvodynia is a chronic, lasting, severe pain around the vaginal orifice, which feels raw. Painful intercourse (**dyspareunia**) is common. The vulva may look normal or be slightly swollen. The etiology is unknown.

Word Analysis and Definition: Disorders of External Genitalia and Vagina

S = Suffix   P = Prefix   R = Root   R/CF = Combining Form

WORD	PRONUNCIATION		ELEMENTS	DEFINITION
Candida candidiasis (also called **thrush**)	**KAN**-did-ah kan-dih-**DIE**-ah-sis	S/ R/	Latin *dazzling white* -iasis *state of, condition* candid- *Candida, a yeast*	A yeastlike fungus Infection with the yeastlike fungus *Candida*
dyspareunia	dis-pah-**RUE**-nee-ah	S/ P/ R/	-ia *condition* dys- *painful* -pareun- *lying beside, sexual intercourse*	Pain during sexual intercourse
vulvodynia	vul-voh-**DIN**-ee-uh	S/ R/CF	-dynia *pain* vulv/o- *vulva*	Chronic vulvar pain
vulvovaginitis	**VUL**-voh-vaj-ih-**NIE**-tis	S/ R/CF R/	-itis *inflammation* vulv/o- *vulva* -vagin- *vagina*	Inflammation of the vagina and vulva

Sexually Transmitted Diseases

According to the **Centers for Disease Control and Prevention (CDC)**, 15 million cases of sexually transmitted diseases **(STDs)** are reported annually in the United States, with adolescents and young adults being at the greatest risk. Some of the common STDs are described as follows:

Chlamydia infection is known as the "silent" disease because infected women and men have no symptoms. When there are signs, a vaginal or penile discharge and irritation with dysuria are common. It can be passed on to a newborn during childbirth, causing eye infections or pneumonia. It is a reason why antibiotic eyedrops are given to newborns.

Gonorrhea is spread by unprotected sex and can be passed on to a baby in childbirth, causing a serious eye infection. This is another reason why newborns are given eyedrops. Symptoms in both male and female adults may not be present. In the female, they can include a vaginal discharge, bleeding, and dysuria. Gonorrhea is also a cause of PID.

Chancre

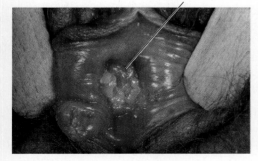

Syphilis, caused by a **spirochete,** is transmitted sexually and can then spread through the bloodstream to every organ in the body. It is also transmitted among intravenous drug users who share needles. **Primary syphilis** begins 10 to 90 days after infection as an ulcer, a **chancre,** at the place of infection *(Figure 8.8)*. Four to 10 weeks later, if the primary syphilis is not treated, **secondary syphilis** appears as a rash on the hands and soles of the feet, with swollen glands and muscle and joint pain. **Tertiary syphilis** can occur years after the primary infection and can cause permanent damage to the brain with dementia. Because primary syphilis is curable with penicillin or other antibiotics, tertiary syphilis is rarely seen today. A pregnant woman with untreated syphilis can transmit the infection to her fetus before birth.

Chancroid is an ulcerative disease (not caused by a spirochete) and is without systemwide effects, unlike syphilis. It develops as a chancre with swollen, tender lymph nodes in the groin.

Trichomoniasis ("trich") is caused by the parasite *Trichomonas vaginalis.* Men can carry the infection in their urethra and almost never have symptoms. The vagina is the common site of infection in women. It can produce a frothy yellow-green discharge with irritation

▲ **Figure 8.8** Chancre of primary syphilis in female. CNRI/Science Source

and itching of the vulva. It is called a "ping-pong" infection because if both partners are not treated, the infection will be given back and forth to the partners.

Molluscum contagiosum is caused by a virus that can be sexually transmitted; the resulting tumors are small, shiny bumps that have a milky-white fluid inside *(Figure 8.9)*. They can disappear and reappear anywhere on the body. Molluscum contagiosum is often seen in children and is not sexually transmitted in such cases.

Pelvic inflammatory disease (PID) is caused by the upward movement of microorganisms from the cervix and vagina into the uterus, uterine tubes, and ovaries. It is often caused by chlamydia and gonorrhea; however recent studies suggest that it may be associated with other bacteria.

Genital herpes simplex is a disease caused by the virus **herpes simplex type 2 (HSV-2)** *(Figure 8.10)*. The sores are painful, and the disease can present with fever; joint pains; and enlarged, tender lymph nodes. The genital sores can recur throughout life. After the initial infection, the virus remains dormant in the dorsal root ganglia of nerves. Blisters around the mouth ("cold sores") are caused by a related virus, **herpes simplex type 1 (HSV-1)**.

Herpes of the newborn occurs when a pregnant woman with genital herpes sores delivers her baby vaginally and transmits the virus to the baby *(Figure 8.11)*. Because the baby's immune system is not well developed, the infection is destructive and can be fatal. If there is evidence of genital herpes lesions in the mother, the fetus should be delivered by cesarean section (C-section).

Human papilloma virus (HPV) causes genital warts in both men and women *(Figure 8.12)* and can also cause changes to the cells in the cervix. Some strains of the virus can increase a woman's risk for **cervical** cancer.

Medications such as podophyllin, trichloracetic acid, and *Aldara* cream can be applied to the warts, and cryotherapy or laser therapy also can be used. Because of the sites of the warts around the genitalia, condoms cannot provide complete protection.

Human immunodeficiency virus (HIV) is a virus that attacks the immune system and can lead to **acquired immunodeficiency syndrome (AIDS)**. Because HIV is carried in body fluids, it is transmitted during unprotected sex. Sharing needles can spread the virus. The virus also can pass from an infected pregnant woman to her unborn child, and she must take medications to protect the baby.

Symptoms often do not appear until years after the initial infection. The initial symptoms of HIV are similar to the flu. A person is diagnosed HIV-positive using a blood test that identifies antibodies to the virus **(ELISA)**, with a confirmatory western blot that identifies the specific antibody proteins. The CDC considers an HIV-infected person with a CD4 count below 200 to have AIDS, whether the person is sick or well; CD4 cells, also known as helper T cells, play key roles in the body's defense mechanisms.

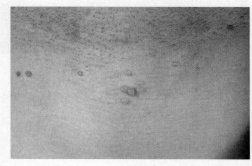

▲ **Figure 8.9** Molluscum contagiosum.
Biophoto Associates/ScienceSource

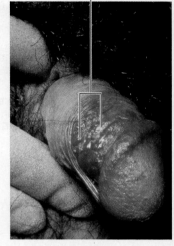

Vesicles

▲ **Figure 8.10** Genital herpes simplex in male.
Biophoto Associates/ScienceSource

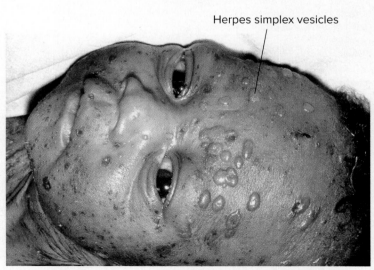

Herpes simplex vesicles

▲ **Figure 8.11** Premature baby born with herpes simplex infection.
Dr. M.A. Ansary/Science Source

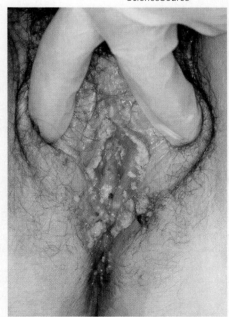

▲ **Figure 8.12** HPV in the female vulva.
Joe Miller/Centers for DiseaseControl and Prevention

Word Analysis and Definition: Sexually Transmitted Diseases

S = Suffix   P = Prefix   R = Root   R/CF = Combining Form

WORD	PRONUNCIATION		ELEMENTS	DEFINITION
acquired immunodeficiency syndrome (AIDS)	ah-**KWIRED** **IM**-you-noh-de-**FISH**-en-see **SIN**-drome	S/ R/CF R/ P/ R/	**acquired** Latin *obtain* **-ency** *condition* **immun/o-** *immune response* **-defici-** *lacking, inadequate* **syn-** *together* **-drome** *running*	Infection with the HIV virus
chancre	**SHAN**-ker		Latin *cancer*	Primary lesion of syphilis
chancroid	**SHAN**-kroyd	S/ R	**-oid** *resembling* **chancr-** *chancre*	Infectious, painful, ulcerative STD not related to syphilis
chlamydia	klah-**MID**-ee-ah		Latin *cloak*	A species of bacteria causing an STD
gonorrhea	gon-oh-**REE**-ah	S/ R/CF	**-rrhea** *flow or discharge* **gon/o-** *seed*	Specific contagious sexually transmitted infection
herpes simplex virus (HSV)	**HER**-peez **SIM**-pleks **VIE**-rus	R/	**herpes** Greek *spreading skin eruption* **virus** *poison*	An infection that manifests with painful, watery blisters on the skin and mucous membranes
human immunodeficiency virus (HIV)	**HYU**-man **IM**-you-noh-dee-**FISH**-en-see **VIE**-rus	S/ R/CF R/ R/	**human** Latin *human being* **-ency** *condition* **immun/o-** *immune response* **-defici-** *lacking, inadequate* **virus** *poison*	Etiologic agent of AIDS
human papilloma virus (HPV)	**HYU**-man pap-ih-**LOH**-mah **VIE**-rus	S/ R/ R/	**human** Latin *human being* **-oma** *tumor* **papill-** *pimple* **virus** *poison*	An infection that causes warts on the skin and genitalia and can increase the risk for cervical cancer
molluscum contagiosum (**Note:** The "s" in contagiosum is added to make the word flow.)	moh-**LUS**-kum kon-**TAY**-jee-oh-sum	S/ R/	**-um** *structure* **mollusc-** *soft* Latin *to touch closely*	STD caused by a virus
opportunistic infection (**Note:** This term contains two suffixes.)	**OP**-or-tyu-**NIS**-tik in-**FEK**-shun	S/ S/ R/ S/ R/	**-ic** *pertaining to* **-ist-** *specialist in* **opportun-** *take advantage of* **-ion** *action, condition, process* **infect-** *corrupt, internal invasion, infection*	An infection that causes disease when the immune system is compromised for other reasons
spirochete	**SPY**-roh-keet	S/ R/CF	**-chete** *hair* **spir/o-** *spiral*	Spiral-shaped bacterium causing an STD (syphilis)
syphilis	**SIF**-ih-lis		Possibly from Latin poem "Syphilis Sive Morbus Gallicus," by Fracastorius Alteration	Sexually transmitted disease caused by a spirochete
Trichomonas trichomoniasis	trik-oh-**MOH**-nas **TRIK**-oh-moh-**NIE**-ah-sis	S/ R/CF R/	**-iasis** *condition* **trich/o-** *hair, flagellum* **-mon-** *single*	A parasite causing an STD Infection with *Trichomonas vaginalis*

HIV damages the immune system, so infections will develop that the body would normally cope with easily. These are **opportunistic infections** and include herpes simplex, candidiasis, syphilis, and tuberculosis.

Disorders of the Ovaries

Ovarian Cysts and Cancer

An ovarian cyst is a fluid-filled sac in the ovary. Most cysts are normal and are called *functional cysts.* They follow ovulation and disappear within 3 months.

Polycystic ovarian syndrome (PCOS), in which multiple follicular cysts form in both ovaries *(Figure 8.13).* Because of the repeated cyst formation, no egg matures and is released, ovulation does not occur, and progesterone is not produced. Without progesterone, the menstrual cycle is irregular or absent.

The cysts produce androgens, which prevent ovulation and produce acne, the male-pattern hair loss from the front of the scalp, and weight gain. In addition, women with PCOS make too much insulin, which interferes with normal fat metabolism and prevents it being used for energy. This leads to difficulty in losing weight and causes patches of dark skin. Women with PCOS are also at increased risk for endometrial cancer, type 2 diabetes, high blood cholesterol, hypertension, and heart disease.

Ovarian cancer is the second most common gynecologic cancer after endometrial cancer, but it accounts for more deaths than any other gynecologic malignancy. Symptoms develop late and are usually vague, making early diagnosis difficult. A mass in the abdomen may be detected during routine pelvic examination.

Disorders of the Uterus and Uterine Tubes

Primary amenorrhea occurs when a girl has not menstruated by age 16. This can occur with or without other signs of puberty. There are numerous possible causes: drastic weight loss from malnutrition; dieting; bulimia or anorexia nervosa *(see Chapter 18);* extreme exercise, as in some young gymnasts; extreme obesity; chronic illness; congenital abnormalities of the uterus or vagina; and congenital hormonal disorders.

Secondary amenorrhea occurs when a woman who has menstruated normally then misses three or more periods in a row and is not in her **menopause.** The causes include pregnancy (by far the most common cause); ovarian disorders such as PCOS; excessive weight loss; low body fat percentage; excessive exercise (e.g., in marathon runners); certain drugs, including antidepressants; and stress.

Primary dysmenorrhea, or **premenstrual syndrome (PMS),** refers to pain or discomfort associated with menstruation. The pain can begin 1 or 2 days before menses, peak on the first day of flow, and then slowly subside. The pain can be cramping or aching and be associated with headache, diarrhea or constipation, and urinary frequency.

Secondary dysmenorrhea is pain associated with disorders such as infection in the genital tract or endometriosis.

Endometriosis is said to affect 1 in 10 American women of childbearing age. The endometrium becomes implanted outside the uterus on the uterine (fallopian) tubes, the ovaries, and the pelvic peritoneum. The displaced endometrium continues to go through its monthly cycle. It thickens and bleeds, but because there is nowhere for the blood to go, it leads to cysts and scar tissue and produces pain. The etiology of **endometriosis** is unknown.

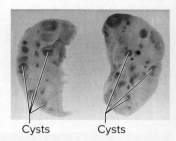

Cysts   Cysts

▲ **Figure 8.13**
Polycystic ovary. Biophoto Associates/ScienceSource

WORD	PRONUNCIATION	ELEMENTS		DEFINITION
amenorrhea	a-men-oh-**REE**-ah	S/ P/ R/CF	-rrhea *flow or discharge* a- *without* -men/o- *month, menses*	Absence or abnormal cessation of menstrual flow
dysmenorrhea	dis-men-oh-**REE**-ah	S/ P/ R/CF	-rrhea *flow or discharge* dys- *painful or difficult* -men/o- *month, menses*	Painful and difficult menstruation
endometriosis	EN-doh-mee-tree-OH-sis	S/ P/ R/CF	-osis *condition* endo- *within, inside* -metr/i- *uterus*	Endometrial tissue in the abdomen outside the uterus
polycystic	pol-ee-**SIS**-tik	S/ P/ R/	-ic *pertaining to* poly- *many* -cyst- *cyst*	Composed of many cysts
premenstrual	pre-**MEN**-stru-al	P/ S/ R/	pre- *before* -al *pertaining to* -menstru- *menses*	Occurring before menstruation

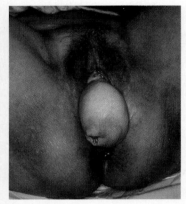

▲ **Figure 8.14 Complete prolapse of the uterus, which protrudes outside the vaginal canal.** Scott Camazine/SueTrainor/Science Source

Leiomyoma

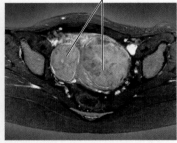

▲ **Figure 8.15** Leiomyomas (fibroids). In this sectioned uterus, a smaller rounded leiomyoma is present, causing a small, rounded bulge in the uterine wall. The larger mass at the top is another leiomyoma projecting from the surface into the uterine cavity. Zephyr/Science Source

Uterine Prolapse

The uterus is normally supported by the muscles, ligaments, and connective tissue of the pelvic floor. Difficult childbirth can weaken these tissues, so the uterus can descend into the vaginal canal. Aging, obesity, lack of exercise, chronic coughing, and chronic constipation also are thought to play a role in the development of the **prolapse** (*Figure 8.14*).

If the uterus is tilted backward toward the rectum, its position would be **retroverted,** a condition found in 20% of women.

Uterine prolapse can be accompanied by prolapse of the bladder and anterior vaginal wall, called a **cystocele,** or of the rectum and posterior wall of the vagina, called a **rectocele.** Signs and symptoms of prolapse include incontinence, pelvic pressure, difficulty with inserting tampons, and seeing or feeling a bulge coming out of the vagina.

Uterine Fibroids

Fibroids are noncancerous growths of the uterus that appear during childbearing years. Three out of four women have them, but only one out of four women has symptoms from them.

The symptoms they can produce include:

- **Menorrhagia**—abnormally long, heavy menstrual bleeding.
- **Metrorrhagia**—irregular bleeding between menstrual periods.
- **Polymenorrhea**—too frequent periods (occur more often than every 21 days) and no ovulation in the cycle.
- **Pelvic pressure**—low-back pain, urinary incontinence, and frequency.

Uterine fibroids are also called **fibromyomas, leiomyomas,** or **myomas** (*Figure 8.15*). They arise in the myometrium, producing a pale, firm, rubbery mass separate from the surrounding tissue. They vary in size from seedlings to large masses that distort the uterus. They can protrude into the uterine cavity, causing menorrhagia, or project outside the uterus and press on the bladder or rectum to produce symptoms.

Other Causes of Uterine Bleeding

Dysfunctional uterine bleeding (DUB) is a term applied when no cause can be found for a patient's menorrhagia.

Endometrial polyps are benign extensions of the endometrium that can cause irregular and heavy bleeding. They can be removed by hysteroscopy or D&C.

Menopause

Menopause is diagnosed when a woman has not menstruated for a year and is not pregnant; she is in the "change of life." In this normal, natural, biological process of reproductive aging, levels of estrogen and progesterone start to decline around the age of 40. For most women, menstruation ceases between the ages of 45 and 55. Significant quantities of estrogen and progesterone are no longer secreted, so the endometrial lining of the uterus cannot grow and be shed as in a normal menstrual period.

Without estrogen and progesterone, the uterus, vagina, and breasts atrophy, and more bone is lost than is replaced. Blood vessels constrict and dilate in response to changing hormone levels and can cause hot flashes.

WORD	PRONUNCIATION		ELEMENTS	DEFINITION
cystocele	SIS-toh-seal	S/ R/CF	-cele *swelling, hernia* cyst/o- *bladder*	Hernia of the bladder into the vagina
dysfunctional	dis-FUNK-shun-al	S/ P/ R/	-al *pertaining to* dys- *painful, difficult* -function- *perform*	Having difficulty in performing
fibroid	FIE-broyd	S/ R/	-oid *resembling* fibr- *fiber*	Uterine tumor resembling fibrous tissue
fibromyoma (also called fibroid)	FIE-broh-my-OH-mah	S/ R/CF R/	-oma *tumor, mass* fibr/o- *fiber* -my- *muscle*	Benign neoplasm derived from smooth muscle containing fibrous tissue
leiomyoma (also called fibroid)	LIE-oh-my-OH-mah	S/ R/CF R/	-oma *tumor, mass* lei/o- *smooth* -my- *muscle*	Benign neoplasm derived from smooth muscle
menopause (Note: This term has no suffix, only a combining form and a root.)	MEN-oh-paws	R/CF R/	men/o- *month, menses* -pause *cessation*	Permanent ending of menstrual periods
menopausal (adj)	men-oh-PAWS-al	S/	-al *pertaining to*	Pertaining to menopause
menorrhagia	men-oh-RAY-jee-ah	S/ R/CF	-rrhagia *excessive flow, discharge* men/o- *menses*	Excessive menstrual bleeding
metrorrhagia	MEH-troh-RAY-jee-ah	S/ R/CF	-rrhagia *excessive flow, discharge* metr/o- *uterus*	Irregular uterine bleeding between menses
myoma	my-OH-mah	S/ R/	-oma *tumor, mass* my- *muscle*	Benign tumor of muscle
polymenorrhea	POL-ee-men-oh-REE-ah	S/ P/ R/CF	-rrhea *flow* poly- *many* men/o- *menses*	More than normal frequency of menses
prolapse	proh-LAPS		Latin *a falling*	The falling or slipping of a body part from its normal position
rectocele	REK-toh-seal	S/ R/CF	-cele *swelling, hernia* rect/o- *rectum*	Hernia of the rectum into the vagina
retroversion	reh-troh-VER-shun	S/ P/ R/	-ion *process, condition* retro- *backward* -vers- *turned*	The tipping backward of the uterus
retroverted	reh-troh-VERT-ed	S/	-ed *pertaining to*	Tilted backward

Endometrial Cancer

Endometrial cancer is the fourth most common cancer in women (after lung, breast, and colon cancer). Forty thousand new cases are diagnosed each year, mostly in women between the ages of 60 and 70. The most common symptom is vaginal bleeding after menopause. It also can cause a vaginal discharge, pelvic pain, and dyspareunia. Higher levels than normal of estrogen are thought to be a risk factor for endometrial cancer.

Cervical Cancer

Cervical cancer is less common than endometrial cancer, but 50% of cases occur between ages 35 and 55. In 2020 it is estimated that 13,800 cases of invasive cervical cancer will be diagnosed in the United States.

Early cervical cancer produces no symptoms or signs and may be found on a routine Pap test (see below). In the precancerous stage, abnormal cells **(dysplasia)** are found only in the outer layer of the cervix.

Thirteen types of human papilloma virus can convert these **dysplastic** cells to cancer cells. A vaccine has been developed that makes people immune to two of the most common types of HPV.

Uterine (Fallopian) Tubes

Salpingitis is an inflammation of the uterine (fallopian) tubes and is part of pelvic inflammatory disease. A bacterial infection, often from an STD, spreads from the vagina through the cervix and uterus. Symptoms are lower abdominal pain, fever, and a vaginal discharge.

Female Infertility

Infertility is the inability to become pregnant after 1 year of unprotected intercourse. It affects 10% to 15% of all couples. The causes of infertility are due to:

- The female factor alone in 35%
- The male factor alone in 30%
- Male and female factors in 20%
- Unknown factors in 15%

In women, fertility begins to decrease as early as age 30, and pregnancy rates are very low after age 44.

Causes of Infertility in the Female

- **Infrequent ovulation** is responsible in 20% of female infertility problems when both ovulation and menses occur at intervals of longer than 1 month. Bulimia, anorexia nervosa, rapid weight loss, excessive exercise training, low body weight, obesity, and polycystic ovarian syndrome are among the causes.
- **Scarring of the uterine tubes** is responsible for 30% of female infertility problems. Scarring can result from previous surgery, previous tubal pregnancy, pelvic inflammatory disease, or endometriosis. The scarring blocks the sperm from reaching the egg.
- **Structural abnormalities** of the uterus are responsible for 20% of female infertility problems. Fibroid tumors; uterine polyps; and scarring from infections, abortions, and miscarriages can all produce abnormalities of the uterus. These abnormalities also block the sperm from reaching the egg.

Word Analysis and Definition: Female Infertility

S = Suffix   P = Prefix   R = Root   R/CF = Combining Form

WORD	PRONUNCIATION	ELEMENTS		DEFINITION
dysplasia	dis-**PLAY**-zee-ah	S/ P/ R/	-ia *condition* dys- *painful, difficult* -plas- *molding*	Abnormal tissue formation
dysplastic (adj)	dis-**PLAS**-tic	S/	-tic *pertaining to*	Pertaining to abnormal tissue function
infertility infertile (adj)	in-fer-**TIL**-ih-tee in-**FER**-tile	S/ P/ R/	-ity *condition* in- *not* -fertil- *able to conceive*	Inability to conceive over a long period of time
salpingitis	sal-pin-**JIE**-tis	S/ R/	-itis *inflammation* salping- *tube*	Inflammation of the uterine tube

Check Point Section 8.3

 Case Report (CR) 8.1

You are

. . . a **registered nurse (RN)** working in the Emergency Department at Fulwood Medical Center.

Your patient is

. . . Ms. Lara Baker, a 32-year-old single mother who works in the billing department of the medical center. You have been asked to take her VS. For the past couple of days, she has had muscle aches and a feeling of general uneasiness that she had thought were due to her heavy menstrual period. In the past 3 hours, she has developed a severe headache with nausea and vomiting. A diffuse rash over her trunk that looks like sunburn is now spreading to her upper arms and thighs.

VS: T 104.2°F, P 120 and irregular, R 20, BP 86/50. As you took her VS, you noted that she did not seem to understand where she was. She was unable to pass urine for a urine specimen.

For this patient, the treatment she receives in the next few minutes is vital for her survival. You have your supervising nurse and the emergency physician come to see her immediately. As you participate in this patient's care, clear communication among the team members is essential.

During the nursing assessment, the receiving ICU nurse found a tampon. She was admitted to intensive care. The **tampon** was removed and cultured, IV fluids and antibiotics were administered, and her kidney and liver functions were monitored. The causative organism was *Staphylococcus aureus.* She recovered well but had a second episode 6 months later.

A. After reading Case Report (CR) 8.1, answer the following questions. *For multiple choice questions, select the correct answer. For multiple choice questions, select the correct answer. For the fill-in-the-blank questions, enter the correct term.* **LO 8.6, 8.8**

1. From Case Report 8.1, what was the diagnosis?

   a. vulvodynia

   b. toxic shock syndrome

   c. dyspareunia

2. Is the causative agent for the patient's condition bacterial or viral? _____

3. How would you classify her body temperature?

   a. high

   b. low

   c. normal

B. Disease. *Test your knowledge of diseases. Anyone working in a gynecology clinic or internal medicine practice will have patients diagnosed with sexually transmitted diseases. Make the correct association between the name of the STD and its description by matching the statement in the left column with the medical term in the right column.* **LO 8.6**

_____	**1.** "Silent disease"	**a.** secondary syphilis
_____	**2.** Chancre appears at the place of infection	**b.** trichomoniasis
_____	**3.** Female symptoms include dysuria and vaginal discharge	**c.** chlamydia
_____	**4.** Chlamydia or gonorrhea can cause this	**d.** primary syphilis
_____	**5.** Can cause dementia if untreated	**e.** pelvic inflammatory disease
_____	**6.** Appears as a rash with joint pain	**f.** tertiary syphilis
_____	**7.** "Ping-pong" infection	**g.** chancroid
_____	**8.** Ulcerative disease not caused by a spirochete	**h.** gonorrhea

C. Sexually transmitted diseases have different causative agents. *Use the provided word bank to fill in the blanks.* **LO 8.6**

trichomoniasis	molluscum contagiosum	syphilis	gonorrhea

1. This disease is caused by a spirochete. _____

2. A virus is responsible for causing this disease. _____

3. This disease is caused by a parasite. _____

4. This disease is caused by bacteria. _____

D. Disease. *Continue working with the medical terminology for sexually transmitted diseases. Make the correct association between the description of the disease in the left column and its medical term listed in the right column.* **LO 8.6**

_____ 1. Causes cold sores around the mouth   **a.** herpes simplex type 2

_____ 2. Infection with this virus can lead to AIDS   **b.** AIDS

_____ 3. Causes painful genital sores   **c.** herpes of the newborn

_____ 4. Increases risk for cervical cancer   **d.** HPV

_____ 5. Infections that would not normally develop in healthy persons   **e.** herpes simplex type 1

_____ 6. Diagnosed when CD4 count is less than 200   **f.** opportunistic

_____ 7. Transmitted during vaginal delivery   **g.** HIV

E. Apply your knowledge of the *language of gynecology* by choosing the correct answer to the following questions. *Choose the best answer.* **LO 8.8**

1. The *gynecologic malignancy* that accounts for the most deaths is

    a. cervical cancer   **b.** breast cancer   **c.** ovarian cancer

2. Secondary amenorrhea is a disorder in which

    a. a woman experiences painful menstruation

    b. a female has not had her first period by age 16

    c. the endometrium is implanted outside of the uterus

    d. a woman who has normally menstruated misses three periods in a row and is not in menopause

    e. the uterine tubes become infected and inflamed due to an infection that started in the vagina

F. Critical thinking. *Use Case Report (CR) 8.2 along with the reading to answer the following questions.* **LO 8.6, 8.8, 8.9**

Case Report (CR) 8.2

You are

. . . a certified health education specialist **(CHES)** employed by Fulwood Medical Center.

Your patient is

. . . Ms. Claire Marcos, a 21-year-old student referred to you by Anna Rusack, MD, a gynecologist.

Ms. Marcos has been diagnosed with **polycystic ovarian syndrome (PCOS),** and your task is to develop a program of self-care as part of her overall plan of therapy.

From her medical record, you see that she has presented with irregular, often missed menstrual periods since the beginning of puberty; persistent acne; patches of dark skin on the back of her neck and under her arms; loss of hair from the front of her scalp; and inability to control her weight. She is 5 feet 4 inches and weighs 150 pounds.

Her self-care program is to include exercise, diet, and regular use of birth control medication and metformin to lower insulin levels and help reduce her weight.

---

1. Ms. Marcos's ovaries were enlarged due to:

   a. cancer   **b.** endometriosis   **c.** cysts   **d.** testosterone

2. The abbreviation for her condition is:

   a. PMS   **b.** FSH   **c.** GnRH   **d.** PCOS

3. A consequence of her condition is that she does not:

   a. create oocytes   **b.** release oocytes   **c.** produce testosterone   **d.** have an appetite

4. Her condition is associated with what other condition?

   a. heart disease   **b.** peptic ulcer   **c.** decreased fat storage   **d.** hematuria

G. Build the *language of gynecology* by completing the medical term with the correct element. *Fill in the blanks.* **LO 8.2, 8.6**

1. benign neoplasm derived from smooth muscle   leio/ _____ /oma

2. irregular bleeding between menses   metro/ _____

3. permanent ending of menstrual periods   _____ /pause

4. uterine tumor resembling fibrous tissue   _____ /oid

*Note: Although the suffix **-oma** means tumor (or mass), it is not necessarily a malignancy. Fibromyomas, leiomyomas, and myomas are all benign neoplasms or tumors. This is an important distinction for coders especially to note.*

H. Proofread the following sentences for errors in documentation. *It may be an error of fact and/or spelling. Rewrite the correct form of the misspelled word. Fill in the blank.* **LO 8.1, 8.6**

1. Cervixal cancer is more common than endometrial cancer.

   _____

2. The most common symptom of endometrial cancer is vaginal bleeding after menopause.

   _____

3. Displasia is abnormal tissue formation.

   _____

4. A routine Pap test can detect the precancerus stage of cervical cancer.

   _____

I. Discuss female infertility. *Select the best answer that completes each statement.* **LO 8.6**

1. Statistically speaking, the most common cause of infertility in the female is:

   a. scarring of the uterine tubes   **c.** uterine polyps

   b. infrequent ovulation   **d.** fibroid tumors

2. In order to be diagnosed with infertility, a female must be unable to conceive for a minimum of:

   a. 3 months   **c.** 1 year

   b. 6 months   **d.** 2 years

3. Infertility due to sperm being blocked from reaching the egg can result from:

   a. anorexia   **c.** excessive exercising

   b. endometriosis   **d.** bulimia

Section 8.4 Procedures and Pharmacology-Gynecology

Gynecologic Diagnostic Procedures

Palpation is routinely used to feel the structures of the reproductive system.

Laparoscopy directly examines the uterus, fallopian tubes, and ovaries through a **laparoscope** inserted into the abdominal cavity through a small incision in the abdominal wall. Carbon dioxide can be pumped through the laparoscope to inflate the abdominal cavity so that the pelvic organs can be seen more clearly.

Cervical biopsy is a procedure to remove tissue from the cervix for pathological testing for precancerous lesions or cervical cancer.

Colposcopy uses an instrument with a magnifying lens and a light called a **colposcope** to examine the lining of the vagina and cervical canal. Both colposcopy and cervical biopsy are often performed because a Pap test result was abnormal.

Hysteroscopy is the examination of the inside of the uterus using a thin, flexible, lighted tube called a **hysteroscope** to look for abnormalities of the cervical canal and endometrium.

Hysterosalpingography is a procedure in which x-rays (**hysterosalpingograms**) are taken after a radiopaque dye is injected through the cervix into the uterus through a slender catheter to outline the interior of the uterus and fallopian tubes (*see Figure 8.16*). It can be used to help define the cause of female infertility or to confirm that a sterilization procedure to block the uterine tubes is successful.

Endometrial biopsy—biopsy of the lining of the uterus—is performed to determine the cause of abnormal uterine bleeding and to check the effects of hormones on the endometrium.

Dilation and curettage (D and C) is a surgical procedure in which the cervix is dilated so that the cervical canal and uterine endometrium can be scraped to remove abnormal tissues for pathological examination.

Loop electrosurgical excision procedure (LEEP) uses a wire loop heated by electricity to remove tissue from the vagina and cervix for pathological examination.

After a complete history and physical examination, including vagina and pelvic organs, other diagnostic tools to determine the cause(s) for infertility include:

- **Hormone blood levels** of progesterone, estrogens, and FSH.
- **Hysterosalpingogram,** in which x-rays of the uterus and uterine tubes are taken after dye is injected into the uterus through a slender catheter (*Figure 8.16*).
- **Ultrasound** of the abdomen, which can show the shape and size of the uterus, and vaginal ultrasound, which can show the shape and size of the ovaries.

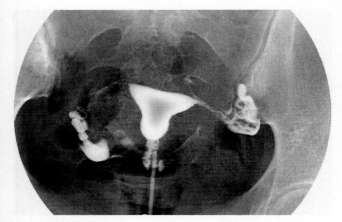

▲ **Figure 8.16** Hysterosalpingogram of a normal uterus, uterine tubes, and ovaries.
Du Cane Medical ImagingLtd/Science Source

- **Hysteroscopy,** which can visualize the inside of the uterus and be used to take an endometrial biopsy and remove polyps or fibroids.
- **Laparoscopy,** which allows inspection of the outside of the uterus and ovaries and removal of any scar tissue blocking tubes.
- **Postcoital testing,** in which the cervix is examined soon after unprotected intercourse to see if sperm can travel through into the uterus.

Ultrasound exams are performed as transabdominal or transvaginal depending on what is being evaluated. These exams are used to look for possible causes of pelvic pain, locate an intrauterine device (IUD), or look for possible reasons for infertility.

A **swab** from the vagina, mouth, throat, rectum, or area around cervix is used to determine the presence of a STI. The swab is sent to a laboratory for testing.

Hysteroscopy has multiple purposes such as visualizing an IUD or removing scar tissue.

Pap Test

Pap test screens for cervical cancer. In a Pap test, the doctor brushes cells from the cervix (*Figure 8.17*). The cells are smeared onto a slide or rinsed into a special liquid and sent to the laboratory for examination. This test enables abnormal cells (see *Figure 8.18*), precancerous or cancerous, to be detected. It is the most successful and accurate test for early detection of abnormalities. Current screening guidelines were last updated in March 2012 by the National Cancer Institute, the American Cancer Society, and other national organizations. According to the guidelines, a Pap test should be scheduled as follows:

- **Initial Pap test**—at age 21.
- **Age 21 to 29**—every 3 years.
- **Age 30 to 65**—Pap and HPV cotesting every 5 years or Pap alone every 3 years.
- **Age 65 onward**—continue screening if risk factors are present including HIV infection, **immunosuppression,** previous treatment for precancerous cervical lesion or cervical cancer. Schedule individually with your doctor.
- **Any abnormal result** at any age mandates working out the best schedule for follow-up testing with your doctor.
- A Pap test is best performed 10 to 20 days after the first day of the **last menstrual period (LMP).**

More than 90% of abnormal Papanicolaou **(Pap)** smears are caused by HPV infections. A vaccine is now available that can prevent lasting infections from the two HPV strains that cause 70% of cervical cancers and another two strains that cause 90% of genital warts.

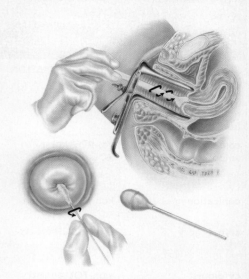

▲ **Figure 8.17** Pap smear being performed.

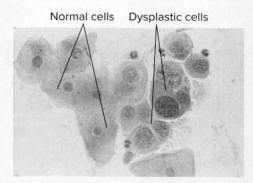

Normal cells   Dysplastic cells

▲ **Figure 8.18** Abnormal pap smear with dysplastic cells. Parviz M. Pour/Science Source

Word Analysis and Definition: Gynecologic Diagnostic Procedures

S = Suffix   P = Prefix   R = Root   R/CF = Combining Form

WORD	PRONUNCIATION		ELEMENTS	DEFINITION
biopsy (Note: The "o" in the root bio is dropped from the spelling.)	BIE-op-see	S/ R/CF	-opsy to view bi/o- life	Removal of living tissue for laboratory examination
colposcopy colposcope	kol-POS-koh-pee KOL-poh-scope	S/ R/CF S/	-scopy to view colp/o- vagina -scope instrument for viewing	Examination of vagina and cervix with an endoscope Endoscope to view the vagina and cervix
conization	koh-nih-ZAY-shun	S/ R/	-ation process coniz- cone	Surgical excision of a cone-shaped piece of tissue
cryosurgery	cry-oh-SUR-jer-ee	S/ P/ R/	-ery process of cryo- icy, cold -surg- operate	Use of liquid nitrogen or argon gas to freeze and kill tissue
cytologist	sigh-TOL-oh-jist	S/ R/CF	-logist specialist cyt/o- cell	Specialist in the study of cells
curette curettage	kyu-RET kyu-reh-TAHZH	S/ R/	French cleanse -age related to curett- to cleanse	Instrument with sharpened edges for scraping Scraping of the interior of a cavity
dilation	die-LAY-shun		Latin to spread out	Artificial enlargement of an opening or hollow structure
excision	eck-SIZH-un	S/ R/	-ion action excis- cut out	Surgical removal of part or all of a structure
hysterosalpingogram hysteroscope hysteroscopy	HIS-ter-oh-sal-PING-oh-gram HIS-ter-oh-skope his-ter-OS-koh-pee	S/ R/CF R/CF S/ S/	-gram a record hyster/o- uterus -salping/o- uterine tube -scope instrument for viewing -scopy to view	Radiograph of uterus and uterine tubes after injection of contrast material Endoscope to visually examine the uterine cavity Visual examination of the uterine cavity
immunosuppression	IM-you-noh-suh-PRESH-un	S/ R/CF R/	-ion process immun/o- immune response -suppress- press under	Suppression of the immune system
laparoscope laparoscopy	LAP-ah-roh-skope lap-ah-ROS-koh-pee	S/ R/CF S/	-scope instrument for viewing lapar/o- abdomen -scopy to view	Endoscope to view the contents of the abdomen Endoscopic examination of the contents of the abdomen
palpate (verb) palpation (noun)	PAL-pate pal-PAY-shun	S/ R/	Latin to touch -ion process, action palpat- touch, stroke	To examine with the fingers and hands Examination using the fingers and hands
Pap test	PAP TEST		George Papanicolaou 1883–1962, Greek-US physician and cytologist	Examination of cells taken from the cervix
postcoital	post-KOH-ih-tal	S/ P/ R/	-al pertaining to post- after -coit- sexual intercourse	After sexual intercourse
screen screening	SKREEN SKREEN-ing	S/ R/	Middle English screne -ing process screen- a system for separating	A test to determine the presence or absence of a disease A testing process that determines the presence or absence of a disease
swab	SWOB		Old English to sweep	Wad of cotton
ultrasound	ULL-trah-sound	P/ R/	ultra- higher -sound noise	Very high frequency sound waves

Gynecologic Therapeutic Procedures

Gynecologic surgical procedures can take place in the office or an operating room.

In office procedures include those for cervical cancer. Treatment for cervical cancer depends on the stage of the cancer. In preinvasive cancer, when it is only in the outer layer of the lining of the cervix, treatment can include:

- **Conization.** A cone-shaped piece of tissue from around the abnormality is removed with a scalpel.
- **Loop electrosurgical excision procedure (LEEP).** A wire loop carries an electrical current to slice off cells from the mouth of the cervix.
- **Laser surgery.** A laser beam is used to kill precancerous and cancerous cells.
- **Cryosurgery.** Freezing is used to kill the precancerous and cancerous cells.

Dilation and curettage (D&C) involves dilating the entrance to the uterus through the cervix so that a thin instrument can be inserted to scrape or suction away the lining of the uterus and take tissue samples.

Endometrial ablation is a heat-generating tool or a laser removes or destroys the lining of the uterus and prevents or reduces menstruation. Endometrial ablation is used only in women who do not plan to have future children.

Surgery can be performed via **laparotomy, laparoscopy. Robot-assisted laparoscopic** surgery uses using sophisticated robotic surgical tools through a laparoscope.

Gynecologic surgeries performed in an operating room can be approached via the abdomen, vagina, or laparoscopically.

Hysterectomy—removal of the uterus—is performed because of uterine fibroids, uterine cancer, and endometriosis.

- **Radical hysterectomy** removes the whole uterus, the cervix, and the top of the vagina; ovaries also may be removed.
- **Total hysterectomy** is removal of the whole uterus and cervix.
- **Subtotal hysterectomy** is removal of the upper uterus, leaving the cervix in place.

Oophorectomy is surgical removal of one or both ovaries.

Treatment of rectocele, cystocele and prolapse of other pelvic organs depends on the severity of symptoms. Physical therapy is a nonsurgical option directed at strengthening pelvic floor muscles. Another nonsurgical option is an individually fitted vaginal **pessary** inserted into the vagina which supports pelvic organs. **Sacral colpopexy** surgery treats pelvic organ prolapse by suspending the vaginal vault to the sacral promontory using a graft or surgical mesh.

Colporrhaphy is surgical repair of a vaginal wall because of a **cystocele** (protrusion of the urinary bladder into the vagina) or a **rectocele** (protrusion of the rectum into the vagina).

A **salpingectomy** may be necessary in a woman who has salpingitis that has developed into a pelvic abscess.

Tubal ligation prevents future pregnancies.

Treatment options for fibroids are numerous and include:

- **Expectant management,** or watchful waiting.
- **Myomectomy,** removal of the fibroids surgically, leaving the uterus in place.
- **Hormone therapy,** which uses **GnRH agonists** to cause estrogen and progesterone levels to fall so that menstruation stops and fibroids shrink.
- **Hysterectomy,** major surgery that is performed by many gynecologists as a last resort.

Endometrial cancer is staged at the time of any surgical procedure into four groups, depending on its localization to the uterus or its spread outside. Surgery is the most common treatment. If the cancer has spread to other parts of the body, progesterone therapy, radiation therapy, and chemotherapy are used.

Infertility treatment is directed at the underlying cause. If the cause of infertility is infrequent ovulation, the patient can be treated with hormones to stimulate release of the egg. These hormones include clomiphene citrate and injectable forms of FSH, LH, and GnRH.

Surgical procedures to initiate pregnancy include:

- **Intrauterine insemination.** Sperm are inserted directly into the uterus via a special catheter.
- **In vitro fertilization (IVF).** Eggs and sperm are combined in a laboratory dish, and two resulting embryos are placed inside the uterus. This can result in twins.

WORD	PRONUNCIATION		ELEMENTS	DEFINITION
ablation	ab-**LAY**-shun	S/ P/ R/	**-ion** *action* **ab-** *away from* **-lat-** *to take*	Removal of tissue to destroy its function
colpopexy	**KOL**-poh-pek-see	S/ R/CF	**-pexy** *surgical fixation* **colp/o-** *vagina*	Surgical fixation of the vagina
colporrhaphy	col-**POR**-ah-fee	R/CF R/	**colp/o-** *vagina* **-rrhaphy** *suture*	Suture of a rupture of the vagina
conization	koh-nih-**ZAY**-shun	S/ R/	**-ation** *process* **coniz-** *cone*	Surgical excision of a cone-shaped piece of tissue
cryosurgery	cry-oh-**SUR**-jer-ee	S/ R/CF R/	**-ery** *process of* **cry/o-** *icy, cold* **-surg-** *operate*	Use of liquid nitrogen or argon gas in a probe to freeze and kill abnormal tissue
curette curettage	kyu-**RET** kyu-reh-**TAHZH**	S/ R/	French *cleanse* **-age** *related to* **curett-** *to cleanse*	Scoop-shaped instrument for scraping the interior of a cavity or removing new growths Scraping of the interior of a cavity
electrosurgical	ee-**LEK**-troh-SUR-ji-kal	S/ R/CF R	**-ical** *pertaining to* **electr/o-** *electric, electricity* **-surg-** *operate*	Use of electrical current to remove tissue
hysterectomy	his-ter-**EK**-toh-mee	S/ R/	**-ectomy** *surgical excision* **hyster-** *uterus*	Surgical removal of the uterus
in vitro fertilization (IVF)	IN **VEE**-troh **FER**-til-eye-**ZAY**-shun	S/ R/	**in vitro** Latin *in glass* **-ization** *process of creating* **fertil-** *able to conceive*	Process of combining sperm and egg in a laboratory dish and placing the resulting embryos inside the uterus
insemination inseminate (verb)	in-sem-ih-**NAY**-shun in-**SEM**-ih-nate	S/ P/ R/ S/	**-ation** *process* **in-** *in* **-semin-** *scatter seed* **-ate** *process*	Introduction of semen into the vagina semen into the vagina
ligature ligate (verb) ligation (noun)	**LIG**-ah-chur **LIE**-gate lie-**GAY**-shun	S/ S/ R/	Latin *band, tie* **-ate** *process* **-tion** *process* **ligat-** *tie up*	Thread or wire tied around a tubal structure to close it Use of a tie to close a tube Tie off a structure, such as a bleeding blood vessel
myomectomy	my-oh-**MEK**-toh-mee	S/ R/ R/	**-ectomy** *surgical excision* **my-** *muscle* **-om-** *tumor*	Surgical removal of a fibroid
oophorectomy	**OH**-oh-for-**EK**-toh-mee	S/ R/	**-ectomy** *surgical excision* **oophor-** *ovary*	Surgical removal of the ovary(ies)
pessary	**PESS**-ah-ree		Greek *an oval stone*	Appliance inserted into the vagina to support the uterus
salpingectomy	sal-pin-**JEK**-toh-mee	S/ R/	**-ectomy** *surgical excision* **salping-** *fallopian tube*	Surgical removal of uterine tube(s)
vestibulectomy	vess-tib-you-**LEK**-toe-me	S/ R/	**-ectomy** *surgical excision* **vestibul-** *entrance*	Surgical excision of the vulva

Gynecologic Pharmacology

Hormone replacement therapy (HRT)—medications to relieve menopausal symptoms by replacement of diminished circulating estrogen and progesterone hormones—have to be given in effective forms. Estrogen when taken orally is converted by the liver to estrone, a weaker estrogen. When estrogen, as **synthetic estradiol,** is used **transdermally** as a patch, gel, or vaginal pessary, it enters the bloodstream as a more effective **bioidentical** estrogen with fewer side effects. Similarly, **micronized** bioidentical progesterone is more effective and has fewer side effects than synthetic **progestin.** However, long-term hormone therapy, as it is now called, is no longer routinely recommended. When taken for more than a few years, it increases the risk of breast cancer.

Hormone therapy can be used the treatment of fibroids. **GnRH agonists** to cause estrogen and progesterone levels to fall so that menstruation stops, and fibroids shrink.

If the cause of infertility is infrequent ovulation, the patient can be treated with hormones to stimulate release of the egg. These hormones include clomiphene citrate and injectable forms of FSH, LH, and GnRH.

Bacterial vaginosis is treated with antibiotics such as clindamycin. Vulvovaginal candidiasis can be treated by applying miconazole (*Monistat*) or clotrimazole (*Desenex*) vaginally, and, if necessary, taking fluconazole (*Diflucan*) orally.

Treatment for STDs

- Trichomoniasis infection of the vagina can be treated with a single oral dose of metronidazole (*Flagyl*) or tinidazole (*Tindamax*). Because it is a "ping-pong" infection between partners, both individuals should be treated.

- Treatment for chlamydia is with oral antibiotics such as doxycycline, erythromycin, or azithromycin.

- Gonorrhea can be treated with a single dose of the antibiotic ceftriaxone. Its causative agent, *Neisseria gonorrhoeae,* is developing resistance to antibiotics.

- Antibiotics such as azithromycin and ceftriaxone are effective in the treatment of **chancroid.**

- The lesions of molluscum contagiosum are treated with podophyllin ointment, or liquid nitrogen and laser surgery can be used.

There is no cure for genital herpes. Three antiviral medications can provide clinical benefit by limiting the replication of the virus. These are acyclovir (*Zovirax*), valacyclovir (*Valtrex*), and famcyclovir (*Famvir*). In people who have recurrent outbreaks, medication taken every day can reduce the recurrences by 70% to 80%.

The HPV vaccine (*Gardasil*) is offered to girls and women aged 9 to 26 and to boys and men of the same age group.

There is no cure for HIV or AIDS, but combinations of anti-HIV medications are taken to stop the replication of the virus in the cells of the body and stop the progression of the disease. Development of resistance to the drugs is a problem.

Word Analysis and Definition: Gynecologic Pharmacology

S = Suffix   P = Prefix   R = Root   R/CF = Combining Form

WORD	PRONUNCIATION	ELEMENTS		DEFINITION
estradiol	ess-trah-**DIE**-ol	S/ R/	-diol *chemical name* estra- *woman*	The most potent natural estrogen
synthetic	sin-**THET**-ik	S/ P/ R/	-ic *pertaining to* syn- *together* -thet- *arrange*	Built up or put together from simpler compounds
transdermal	trans-**DER**-mal	S/ P/ R/	-al *pertaining to* trans- *across* -derm- *skin*	Going across or through the skin
bioidentical	**BIE**-oh-igh-**DEN**-ti-kul	R/CF	identical Latin *the same* bio- *life*	The same as to what is produced in the body
micronized	**MY**-krohn-ized	S/	micron one-millionth of a meter -ize *affected in a certain way*	To reduce into a powder in which the particles are a few microns in length

Check Point Section 8.4

A. Define gynecologic diagnostic procedures. *It is important to correctly use diagnostic terms when communicating verbally with health care professionals and documenting care of your patients. Choose the correct answer to complete each statement.* **LO 8.5**

1. The term **palpate** means to:

   a. smell   **b.** touch   **c.** excise   **d.** incise

2. A diagnostic test for infertility in which the cervix is viewed after unprotected sexual intercourse:

   a. hysteroscopy   **b.** biopsy   **c.** postcoital testing   **d.** ultrasound

3. The injection of dye followed by an x-ray of the uterus and uterine tubes is termed:

   a. hysterosalpingography   **b.** postcoital testing   **c.** mammography   **d.** endometrial biopsy

4. A **colposcope** is used to:

   a. view the vagina and cervical canal   **b.** x-ray the uterus   **c.** view the internal os of the cervix   **d.** remove cells from the uterus

B. The Pap test is an important diagnostic test for women. *Test your understanding of this diagnostic test by answering these questions. Select the correct answer for each question.* **LO 8.5**

1. How often should a 30–40-year-old woman have a Pap test on its own?

   a. annually   **b.** biannually   **c.** every three years   **d.** every five years

2. What causes the majority of abnormal Pap smears?

   a. improper specimen collection

   b. poor hygiene

   c. infection by the human papilloma virus

   d. overgrowth of yeast in vagina

3. The optimal time to perform a Pap smear is _____ days after the last menstrual period.

   a. 2–3   **b.** 4–6   **c.** 8–12   **d.** 10–20

C. Construct medical terms. *Complete medical terms related to gynecologic diagnostic procedures. Be precise! Fill in the blanks.* **LO 8.8**

1. Use of very high frequency sound waves   _____ /sound

2. Specialist in the study of the anatomy, physiology and pathology of the cell   cyt/o/ _____

3. Visual inspection of the uterine cavity using an endoscope   hyster/o/ _____

D. Apply your knowledge of the language of gynecology. *Match the word element in the first column with its correct meaning in the second column.* **LO 8.1, 8.2, 8.8**

	Term		Meaning
_____	1. *oophor-*		**a.** to cleanse
_____	2. *-ectomy*		**b.** uterine tube
_____	3. *hyster/o*		**c.** vagina
_____	4. *-pexy*		**d.** uterus
_____	5. *salping/o*		**e.** surgical removal
_____	6. *semin-*		**f.** surgical fixation
_____	7. *curette-*		**g.** scatter seed
_____	8. *colp/o*		**h.** ovary

E. Demonstrate your knowledge of gynecologic pharmacology. *Select the correct answer that completes the sentence or answers the question.* **LO 8.8**

1. A pharmacologic method to treat vulvodynia is:

   a. transdermal estradiol   **b.** micronized bioidentical progesterone   **c.** topical anesthetic cream   **d.** *Gardasil injection*

2. A medication used to promote ovulation:

   a. clomiphene   **b.** podophyllin ointment   **c.** Minipill   **d.** acyclovir

3. Miconazole and clotrimazole are used to treat:

   a. chlamydia   **b.** vulvodynia   **c.** infertility   **d.** fungal infections

4. An increased risk of breast cancer is seen with which type of long-term pharmacologic therapy?

   a. pessary   **b.** antibiotic   **c.** hormone   **d.** antiviral

5. Which type of medication is used to reduce, not cure, herpes outbreaks?

   a. metronidazole   **b.** liquid nitrogen   **c.** valacyclovir   **d.** Gardasil

Section 8.5 Obstetrics: Pregnancy and Childbirth

Conception

When released from the ovary, an egg takes 72 hours to reach the uterus, but it must be **fertilized** *(Figure 8.19)* within 12 to 24 hours to survive. Therefore, **fertilization** must normally take place in the distal third of the uterine tube.

Between 200 million and 600 million sperm are deposited in the vagina near the cervix. Many are destroyed by the acidity in the vagina or just drain out. Others fail to get through the cervical mucus. Approximately half the survivors will go up the wrong uterine tube. The journey through the uterus into the uterine tube takes about an hour. Some 2,000 to 3,000 sperm reach the egg. Several of these penetrate the outer layers of the egg and clear the path for the one sperm that will penetrate all the way into the egg cytoplasm to fertilize it *(see Figure 8.19)* and produce a **zygote**.

Implantation

While still in the uterine tube, the **zygote** divides, producing a ball of cells called a **morula**. Within the morula, a fluid-filled cavity develops, and the morula becomes a **blastocyst**. A week after fertilization, the blastocyst enters the uterine cavity and burrows into the endometrium **(implantation)**. A group of cells in the blastocyst, the inner cell mass, differentiate into the germ layers and form the embryo. Other cells from the blastocyst, together with endometrial cells, form the **placenta.**

   Twins (and other multiple births) can be produced in two ways:

- **Dizygotic** twins are produced when two eggs are released by the ovary and fertilized by two separate sperm. They can be of different sexes and are only as genetically similar as other siblings would be.

- **Monozygotic** twins are produced when a single egg is fertilized and later two inner cell masses form within a single blastocyst, each producing an embryo. These twins share a single placenta, are genetically identical, are the same sex, and look alike.

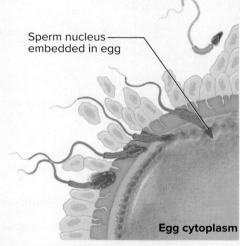

Sperm nucleus embedded in egg

Egg cytoplasm

▲ **Figure 8.19** Fertilization.
Kibble, Medical Physiology: TheBig Picture

WORD	PRONUNCIATION	ELEMENTS		DEFINITION
blastocyst	**BLAS**-toh-sist	S/ R/CF	-cyst *bladder* blast/o- *germ cell*	The developing embryo during the first 2 weeks
conception	kon-**SEP**-shun		Latin *something received*	Fertilization of the egg by sperm to form a zygote
dizygotic	die-zie-**GOT**-ik	S/ P/ R/	-ic *pertaining to* di- *two* -zygot- *yoked together*	Twins from two separate zygotes
fertilize fertilization	**FER**-til-ize **FER**-til-eye-**ZAY**-shun	S/ R/	Latin *make fruitful* -ation *process* fertiliz- *make fruitful*	To penetrate an oocyte with a sperm so as to impregnate Union of a male sperm and a female egg
implantation	im-plan-**TAY**-shun	S/ P/ R/	-ation *process* im- *in* -plant- *to plant*	Attachment of a fertilized egg to the endometrium
monozygotic	**MON**-oh-zie-**GOT**-ik	S/ P/ R/	-ic *pertaining to* mono- *one* -zygot- *yoked together*	Twins from a single zygote
morula	**MOR**-you-lah		Latin *mulberry*	Ball of cells formed from divisions of a zygote
placenta	plah-**SEN**-tah		Latin *a cake*	Organ that allows metabolic interchange between the mother and fetus
placental (adj)	plah-**SEN**-tal	S/ R/	-al *pertaining to* placent- *placenta*	Pertaining to the placenta
zygote	**ZIE**-goht		Greek *joined together*	Cell resulting from the union of the sperm and egg

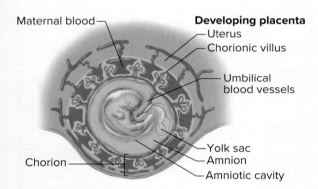

Maternal blood
Developing placenta
Uterus
Chorionic villus
Umbilical blood vessels
Chorion
Yolk sac
Amnion
Amniotic cavity

▲ **Figure 8.20** Embryo at 4.5 weeks.

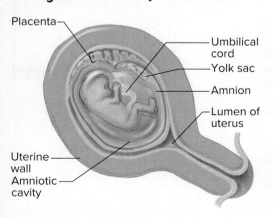

Placenta
Umbilical cord
Yolk sac
Amnion
Lumen of uterus
Uterine wall
Amniotic cavity

▲ **Figure 8.21** Embryo and placenta at 13.5 weeks.

Development of Embryo, Fetus, and Placenta

Embryo

From week 2 until week 8 is the **embryonic period,** in which most of the external structures and internal organs of the **embryo** are formed, together with the placenta, umbilical cord, **amnion, yolk sac,** and **chorion** *(Figure 8.20).* The amnion is a fluid-filled sac that protects the embryo. The yolk sac is a small sac arising from the ventral surface of the embryo. It contributes to the formation of the digestive tract and produces blood cells and future sex germ cells. The chorion forms the placenta by penetrating deeply into the endometrium. At the eighth week, all the organ systems are present; the embryo is just over 1 inch long and is now called a **fetus.**

The Placenta

The **placenta** is a disc of tissue that increases in size as pregnancy proceeds *(Figure 8.21).* The surface facing the fetus is smooth and gives rise to the **umbilical cord,** which contains two arteries and one vein. The surface attached to the uterine wall consists of treelike structures called **chorionic villi.** The cells of the **villi** keep the maternal and fetal circulations largely separate, but they are very thin and allow an exchange of gases, nutrients, and waste products to occur.

The functions of the placenta are to:

- **Transport nutrients** (such as glucose, amino acids, fatty acids, minerals) from mother to fetus.
- **Transport nitrogenous wastes** (such as ammonia, urea, creatinine) from fetus to mother, who can excrete them.
- **Transport oxygen** from mother to fetus and carbon dioxide from fetus to mother, who can excrete it.
- **Transport maternal antibodies** to the fetus.
- **Secrete hormones** (such as estrogen and progesterone) and allow maternal hormones to pass to the fetus.

Unfortunately, some undesirable items and many medications also can cross the placenta. These include the HIV and rubella viruses and the bacteria that cause syphilis. Alcohol, nicotine, carbon monoxide from smoking, and drugs (e.g., heroin and cocaine) all have bad effects on the fetus.

Fetus

The **fetal period** lasts from the eighth week until birth. At the eighth week, the heart is beating. By the twelfth week, the bones have begun to calcify, and the external genitalia can be differentiated as male or female. In the fourth month, downy hair called **lanugo** appears over the body. In the fifth month, skeletal muscles become active, and the baby's movements are felt between 16 and 22 weeks of gestation (*Figure 8.22*). A protective substance called **vernix caseosa** covers the skin. In the sixth and seventh months, weight gain is increased, and body fat is deposited.

At 38 weeks, the baby is at full term and ready for birth.

The length of **pregnancy,** the gestation, is often considered to be 40 weeks, which is the time from a woman's last menstrual period to birth. However, the woman does not become pregnant until she ovulates 2 weeks after her last period, so gestation is really 38 weeks. Gestation is also divided into **trimesters**. The first trimester is up to week 12, the second from week 13 to 24, and the third from week 25 to birth.

A pregnant woman is described as a **gravida**. A woman in her first pregnancy is a **primigravida**. A woman in her second pregnancy is a gravida 2. **Parity** relates to outcome of the pregnancy: Deliveries after the 20th week are numbered successively as **para** 1, 2, 3, and so on. **Abortus** refers to losses of pregnancy before the 20th week. The total of abortus and paras equals a woman's gravidity.

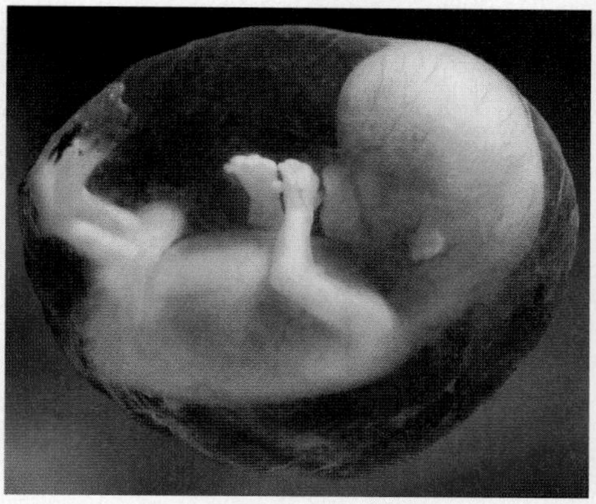

▲ **Figure 8.22** Developing fetus at **20 weeks.** Steve Allen/Brand XPictures/Getty Images

Word Analysis and Definition: Development of Embryo, Fetus, and Placenta

S = Suffix   P = Prefix   R = Root   R/CF = Combining Form

WORD	PRONUNCIATION		ELEMENTS	DEFINITION
abortion	ah-**BOR**-shun	S/ R/	**-ion** *action, process* **abort-** *fail at onset*	Spontaneous or induced expulsion of an embryo or fetus from the uterus
abortus	ah-**BOR**-tus	S/	**-us** *pertaining to*	Product of abortion
amnion	**AM**-nee-on		Greek *membrane around fetus*	Membrane around the fetus that contains amniotic fluid
amniotic (adj)	am-nee-**OT**-ik	S/ R/CF	**-tic** *pertaining to* **amni/o-** *amnion*	Pertaining to the amnion
chorion	**KOH**-ree-on		Greek *membrane*	The fetal membrane that forms the placenta
chorionic (adj)	koh-ree-**ON**-ik	S/ R/	**-ic** *pertaining to* **chorion-** *chorion*	Pertaining to the chorion
chorionic villus	koh-ree-**ON**-ik **VILL**-us		**villus** Latin *shaggy hair*	Vascular process of the embryonic chorion to form the placenta
embryo	**EM**-bree-oh		Greek *a young one*	Developing organism from conception until the end of the second month
embryonic (adj)	em-bree-**ON**-ic	S/ R/CF	**-nic** *pertaining to* **embry/o-** *embryo*	Pertaining to the embryo
fetus	**FEE**-tus		Latin *offspring*	Human organism from the end of the eighth week after conception to birth
fetal (adj)	**FEE**-tal	S/ R/	**-al** *pertaining to* **fet-** *fetus*	Pertaining to the fetus
gravid (adj) gravida primigravida	**GRAV**-id **GRAV**-ih-dah pree-mih-**GRAV**-ih-dah	P/ R/	Latin *pregnant* Latin *pregnant woman* **primi-** *first* **-gravida** *pregnant woman*	Pregnant A pregnant woman First pregnancy
lanugo	la-**NYU**-go		Latin *wool*	Fine, soft hair on the fetal body
parity para	**PAIR**-ih-tee **PAH**-rah		Latin *to bear* Latin *bring forth*	Number of deliveries Abbreviation for number of deliveries
pregnancy pregnant (adj)	**PREG**-nan-see **PREG**-nant		Latin *with child*	State of being pregnant Female containing an embryo or fetus
trimester	**TRY**-mes-ter		Latin *of 3 months' duration*	One-third of the length of a full-term pregnancy
umbilicus umbilical (adj)	um-**BIL**-ih-kus um-**BIL**-ih-kal	S/ R/	Latin *navel* **-al** *pertaining to* **umbilic-** *umbilicus*	Pit in the abdomen where the umbilical cord entered the fetus Pertaining to the umbilicus or the center of the abdomen
vernix caseosa	**VER**-niks kay-see-**OH**-sah		**vernix** Latin *varnish* **caseosa** Latin *cheese*	Cheesy substance covering skin of the fetus
villus villi (pl)	**VILL**-us **VILL**-eye		Latin *shaggy hair*	Thin, hairlike projection of a mucous membrane lining a cavity
yolk sac	YOKE SACK		**yolk** Latin *yellow* **sac** Latin *pouch or bag*	Source of blood cells and future sex cells for the fetus

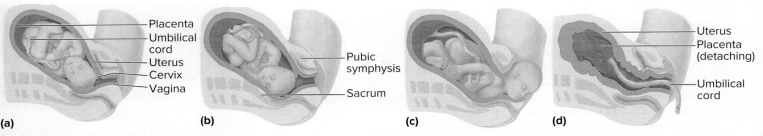

(a)   (b)   (c)   (d)

▲ **Figure 8.23** The stages of childbirth. (a) First stage: early dilation of cervix. (b) First stage: late dilation of cervix. (c) Second stage: expulsion of the fetus. (d) Third stage: expulsion of the placenta.

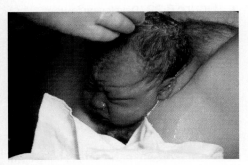

▲ **Figure 8.24** Delivery of head.
Petit Format/Science Source

Pregnancy and Childbirth

Hormones of Pregnancy

Human chorionic gonadotropin (hCG) is secreted by the blastocyst and the placenta. Its presence in the mother's blood and urine is the basis for laboratory and home pregnancy tests. It can be detected as early as 9 or 10 days after conception. hCG stimulates the growth of the corpus luteum and its production of estrogen and progesterone.

Estrogen stimulates the mother's uterus to enlarge and her breasts to increase to twice their normal size. It makes the pelvic joints and ligaments more flexible so that the pelvic outlet widens for childbirth.

Progesterone is secreted by the corpus luteum and the placenta. It suppresses further ovulation, prevents menstruation, stimulates the proliferation of the endometrium to support the implantation, and inhibits contractions of the uterine muscle.

Follicle-stimulating hormone (FSH) and **luteinizing hormone (LH)** from the pituitary gland stimulate the maintenance of the corpus luteum and its estrogen and progesterone production.

Labor and Childbirth

Labor contractions begin about 30 minutes apart. They have to be intermittent because each contraction shuts down the maternal blood supply to the placenta and therefore shuts down the blood supply to the fetus. Labor pains are due to ischemia of the **myometrium.**

Labor is divided into three stages, each of which is usually longer in a **primipara** (first-time birth) than in a **multipara** (two or more births).

First Stage of Labor—Dilation of the Cervix

This is the longest stage. It can be a few hours in a multipara to more than 1 day in a primipara. **Dilation** is widening of the cervical canal to the same diameter as the baby's head *(Figure 8.23a and b)*. At the same time, the wall of the cervix becomes thinner, a process called **effacement.** During dilation, the fetal membranes rupture, and the "waters break" as amniotic fluid is released.

Second Stage of Labor—Expulsion of the Fetus

As the uterus continues to contract, additional pain is generated by the stretching of the cervix and vagina by the baby's head. When the head reaches the vaginal opening and stretches the vulva, the head is said to be **crowning** *(Figure 8.24)*. This process is sometimes helped by performing an **episiotomy,** an incision in the perineum to prevent tearing.

After the baby is delivered, the umbilical cord is clamped in two places and cut between the two clamps.

Third Stage of Labor—Expulsion of the Placenta

After the baby is delivered, the uterus continues to contract. It pushes the placenta off the uterine wall and expels it out of the vagina. This usually takes 5 to 15 minutes; after 30 minutes the placenta is said to be **retained** and may have to be removed manually by the obstetrician.

Postpartum

The 6 weeks **postpartum** (after the birth) are called the **puerperium.** The uterus shrinks (involution) through self-digestion **(autolysis)** of uterine cells by their own lysosomal enzymes. This generates a vaginal discharge called **lochia** that lasts about 10 days.

Word Analysis and Definition: Pregnancy and Childbirth

WORD	PRONUNCIATION	ELEMENTS		DEFINITION
autolysis	awe-**TOL**-ih-sis	P/ R/	auto- *self* -lysis *destruction*	Self-destruction of cells by enzymes within the cells
crowning	**KROWN**-ing	S/ R/	-ing *doing, quality of* crown- *crown*	During childbirth, when the maximum diameter of the baby's head comes through the vulvar ring
dilation	die-**LAY**-shun	S/ R/	-ion *process* dilat- *open out*	Stretching or enlarging of an opening
effacement	ee-**FACE**-ment	S/ R/	-ment *resulting state* efface- *wipe out*	Thinning of the cervix during labor
episiotomy	eh-peez-ee-**OT**-oh-mee	S/ R/CF	-tomy *surgical incision* episi/o- *vulva*	Surgical incision of the vulva
human chorionic gonadotropin	**HYU**-man koh-ree-**ON**-ik **GOH**-nad-oh-**TROH**-pin	S/ R/ S/ R/CF	human Latin *human being* -ic *pertaining to* chorion- *chorion* -tropin *nourishing* gonad/o- *gonad*	Hormone secreted by the blastocyst and the placenta to maintain pregnancy
labor	**LAY**-bore		Latin *toil, suffering*	Process of expulsion of the fetus
lochia	**LOW**-kee-uh		Greek *relating to childbirth*	Vaginal discharge following childbirth
multipara	mul-**TIP**-ah-ruh	P/ R/	multi- *many* -para *to bring forth*	Woman who has given birth to two or more children
postpartum	post-**PAR**-tum	P/ R/	post- *after* -partum *childbirth*	After childbirth
primipara	pree-**MIP**-ah-ruh	P/ R/	primi- *first* -para *to bring forth*	Woman who has given birth for the first time
puerperium (**Note:** This term is composed only of roots.)	pyu-er-**PEE**-ree-um	R/ R/	puer- *child* -perium *bringing forth*	Six-week period after birth in which the uterus involutes

Check Point Section 8.5

A. Tracing the pathway of embryo implantation. *You are given the terminology—put it in the correct order of the implantation process.* **LO 8.1**

morula	embryo
blastocyst	zygote
fertilization	egg

1. _____   4. _____

2. _____   5. _____

3. _____   6. _____

B. Terminology challenge. *Fill in the blanks with the correct term being described.* **LO 8.1**

1. Cell resulting from the union of a sperm and an egg: _____.

2. Twins that originated from one fertilized egg: _____.

3. Twins that originated from two fertilized eggs: _____.

C. Precision in documentation includes using the correct form (noun, verb, adjective) of the medical term. *Practice precision in this written **language of obstetrics**. Fill in the blanks.* **LO 8.1, 8.3**

amnion   amniotic

1. The _____ will be punctured in order to withdraw the _____ fluid.

embryo   embryonic

2. The _____ stage of gestation means the _____ has formed all major organ systems in the first 8 weeks of human development.

umbilical   umbilicus

3. The medical term for the navel is the _____. The _____ cord enters the fetus in the abdomen.

D. Several of these elements you have seen before, and you will certainly see them again in other terms. *Learn each once, and recognize it all the time. Choose the best answer to the questions.* **LO 8.1, 8.2**

1. The term that contains the prefix meaning *many* is
   a. primipara
   b. lochia
   c. multipara
   d. biopsy

2. The term that contains the suffix meaning *incision* is
   a. episiotomy
   b. curette
   c. dilation
   d. palpation

3. The term that contains the suffix meaning *to bring forth* is
   a. primipara
   b. involution
   c. effacement
   d. follicular

4. The term that contains the root meaning *child* is
   a. lochia
   b. multipara
   c. puerperium
   d. crowning

5. The term that contains the suffix meaning *process* is
   a. effacement
   b. episiotomy
   c. dilation
   d. coital

6. The term that contains the prefix meaning *first* is
   a. multipara
   b. puerperium
   c. primipara
   d. zygote

7. The term that contains the prefix meaning *self* is
   a. multipara
   b. autolysis
   c. lochia
   d. postpartum

8. The term that contains the prefix meaning *after* is
   a. primipara
   b. postpartum
   c. multipara
   d. lochia

E. Review the text regarding pregnancy and childbirth. *Select all answers that correctly complete each statement.* **LO 8.1, 8.9**

1. The hormones involved in pregnancy and childbirth are:
   a. FSH   b. LH   c. progesterone   d. BMT   e. MRI   f. HCG   g. estrogen   h. insulin

2. The first stage of labor:
   a. is dilation of the cervix.
   b. is the shortest stage of labor.
   c. includes the process of effacement.
   d. includes the rupture of the fetal membranes.
   e. can be shorter in multipara and longer in primipara.

Section 8.6 Disorders of Pregnancy and Childbirth

Ectopic Pregnancy

If the uterine tube is obstructed, the fertilized egg will be prevented from moving into the uterus and will continue its development in the uterine tube. This is called an **ectopic pregnancy.** Tubal disorders that cause ectopic pregnancy include previous salpingitis, pelvic inflammatory disease (PID), and endometriosis.

High Risk Pregnancy

A **perinatologist** is an obstetrician specializing in caring for mothers with a high-risk pregnancy and for fetuses at higher-than-normal risk. A high-risk pregnancy can occur in mothers with pre-existing conditions such as diabetes or high blood pressure. It can also develop during the pregnancy, for example, preeclampsia or placental disorders.

Preeclampsia and Eclampsia

Preeclampsia is a sudden, abnormal increase in blood pressure after the 20th week of pregnancy, with proteinuria and edema.

    Eclampsia is a life-threatening condition, characterized by the signs and symptoms of preeclampsia and with the addition of convulsions. Management involves immediate admission to the hospital with control of the mother's blood pressure. The baby is delivered as soon as the mother is stabilized, regardless of maturity.

Amniotic Fluid Abnormalities

Amniotic fluid abnormalities occur in the second trimester. Normally, the fetus breathes in and swallows amniotic fluid to promote development of the gastrointestinal tract and lungs.

- **Oligohydramnios** is too little amniotic fluid. It is associated with an increase in the risk of birth defects and poor fetal growth. Its etiology is unknown.

- **Polyhydramnios** is too much amniotic fluid. It causes abdominal discomfort and breathing difficulties for the mother. It also is associated with **preterm delivery,** placental problems, and fetal growth problems.

Gestational Diabetes Mellitus

In some pregnant women, the amount of insulin they can produce decreases. This leads to **gestational diabetes mellitus (GDM)** and increased risk of preeclampsia. For the neonate, it increases the risk of **perinatal mortality.** Later in life, both mother and child are at increased risk for developing type 2 diabetes and obesity.

Hyperemesis Gravidarum

Eighty percent of pregnant women experience some degree of "morning sickness." It is at its worst between 2 and 12 weeks and resolves in the second trimester. For a few women, nausea and vomiting persist. This is **hyperemesis gravidarum.** Severe cases may have to be admitted to the hospital for intravenous (IV) fluids.

Did you know...

- Preeclampsia threatens the life of both mother and fetus.

- For the neonate, preeclampsia increases the risk of **perinatal mortality.**

- **Teratogenesis** is the production of fetal abnormalities—**congenital malformations**—caused by a chemical agent taken by the mother early in pregnancy, including alcohol.

WORD	PRONUNCIATION	ELEMENTS		DEFINITION
congenital	kon-**JEN**-ih-tal	S/ P/ R/	-al *pertaining to* con- *together, with* -genit- *bring forth*	Present at birth, either inherited or due to an event during gestation up to the moment of birth
eclampsia	eh-**KLAMP**-see-uh		Greek *a shining forth*	Convulsions in a patient with preeclampsia
ectopic	ek-**TOP**-ik	S/ R/	-ic *pertaining to* ectop- *on the outside, displaced*	Out of place, not in a normal position
hyperemesis gravidarum	high-per-**EM**-eh-sis gra-vih-**DAR**-um	P/ R/	hyper- *excessive* -emesis *vomiting* gravidarum Latin *pregnant woman*	Excessive vomiting due to pregnancy
malformation	mal-for-**MAY**-shun	S/ P/ R/	-ion *process* mal- *bad* -format- *to form*	Failure of proper development
mortality	mor-**TAL**-ih-tee	S/ S/ R/	-al- *pertaining to* -ity *condition, state* mort- *death*	Fatal outcome or death rate
oligohydramnios	**OL**-ih-goh-high-**DRAM**-nee-os	P/ R/ R/	oligo- *too little, scanty* -hydr- *water* -amnios *amnion*	Too little amniotic fluid
polyhydramnios	**POL**-ee-high-**DRAM**-nee-os	P/	poly- *many*	Too much amniotic fluid
perinatal	per-ih-**NAY**-tal	S/ P/ R/	-al *pertaining to* peri- *around* -nat- *birth*	Around the time of birth
perinatologist	**PER**-ih-nay-**TOL**-o-jist	R/CF S/	-nat/o- *birth* -logist *one who studies, specialist*	Obstetrician who specializes
preeclampsia	pree-eh-**KLAMP**-see-uh	S/ P/ R/	-ia *condition* pre- *before* -eclamps- *shining forth*	Hypertension, edema, and proteinuria during pregnancy
preterm	**PREE**-term	P/ R/	pre- *before* -term *normal gestation*	Baby delivered before 37 weeks of gestation
premature (syn)	pree-mah-**TYUR**	R/	-mature *ripe, ready*	Occurring before the expected time; for example, an infant born before 37 weeks of gestation
teratogen	**TER**-ah-toh-jen	S/ R/CF	-gen *produce, create* terat/o- *monster, malformed fetus*	Agent that produces fetal deformities
teratogenesis	**TER**-ah-toh-**JEN**-eh-sis	S/	-genesis *form, create*	Process involved in producing fetal deformities
teratogenic (adj)	**TER**-ah-toh-**JEN**-ik	S/	-ic *pertaining to*	Capable of producing fetal deformities

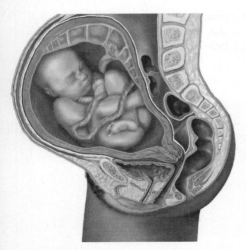

▲ **Figure 8.25** Breech presentation.

Disorders of Childbirth

Fetal distress due to lack of oxygen is an uncommon complication of labor but is detrimental if not recognized.

Abnormal position of fetus occurs when the baby at the beginning of labor is not in a head-first **(vertex)** presentation facing rearward. Abnormal positions include:

- **Breech.** The buttocks present *(Figure 8.25)*.
- **Face.** The face instead of the top of the head presents.
- **Shoulder.** The shoulder and upper back are trying to exit the uterus first.

Nuchal cord is the condition of having the cord wrapped around the baby's neck during delivery. This occurs in 20% of deliveries.

Prolapsed umbilical cord occurs when the cord precedes the baby down the birth canal. Pressure on the cord can cut off the baby's blood supply, which is still being provided through the umbilical arteries.

Premature rupture of the membranes (PROM) occurs in 10% of normal pregnancies and increases the risk of infection of the uterus and fetus.

Gestational Classification

Every **neonate** (newborn) is one of the following:

- **Premature**—less than 37 weeks gestation.
- **Full-term**—between 37 and 42 weeks gestation.
- **Postmature**—longer than 42 weeks gestation *(Figure 8.26)*.

Neonatologists are **pediatricians** that care for premature neonates or have other illnesses occurring at birth. **Prematurity** occurs in about 8% of newborns. The earlier the baby is born, the more life-threatening problems occur.

Because their lungs are underdeveloped, premature babies can develop **respiratory distress syndrome (RDS),** also called **hyaline membrane disease.** The premature baby's lungs are not mature enough to produce **surfactant,** a mixture of lipids and proteins that keeps the alveoli from collapsing.

If their brains are underdeveloped, premature newborns can have inconsistent breathing with **apnea.** They are susceptible to bleeding into the brain. Their immune systems have low levels of antibodies to provide protection from infection.

An immature liver can impair the excretion of bilirubin *(see Chapter 5)*, and premature babies become jaundiced. High levels of bilirubin can produce **kernicterus,** in which deposits of bilirubin in the brain cause brain damage.

Postmaturity is much less common than prematurity. Its etiology is unknown, but the placenta begins to shrink and is less able to supply sufficient nutrients to the baby. This leads to hypoglycemia; loss of subcutaneous fat; dry, peeling skin; and, if oxygen is lacking, fetal distress. The baby can pass stools **(meconium)** into the amniotic fluid. In its distress, the baby can take deep gasping breaths and inhale the meconium fluid. This leads to **meconium aspiration syndrome (MAS)** and respiratory difficulty at birth.

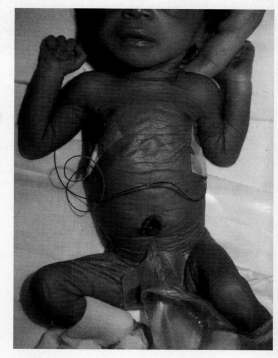

▲ **Figure 8.26** **Postmature infant.**
Image appears with permission from VisualDx

Placental Disorders

Placenta abruptio is separation of the placenta from the uterine wall before delivery of the baby. The baby's oxygen supply is cut off, and fetal distress appears quickly. It is an obstetric (OB) emergency, and usually a C-section is indicated.

Placenta previa occurs when the placenta is positioned over the internal os of the cervix. The placenta may separate from the uterine wall during stage one of labor and the cervix starts to dilate.

Retained placenta is a low-lying placenta between the baby's head and the internal os of the cervix. It can cause severe bleeding during labor. The expulsion of the placenta *(Figure 8.27)* can happen naturally. The result of retained placenta is heavy uterine bleeding called **postpartum hemorrhage (PPH).** Manual removal of the retained product may be necessary under spinal, epidural, or general anesthesia.

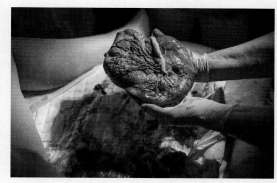

▲ **Figure 8.27** **Placenta (afterbirth).** AzmanL/ Getty Images

WORD	PRONUNCIATION		ELEMENTS	DEFINITION
abruptio	ab-**RUP**-shee-oh		Latin *to break off*	Placenta abruptio is the premature detachment of the placenta
apnea	**AP**-nee-ah		Greek *lack of breath*	Absence of spontaneous respiration
breech	BREECH		Old English *trousers*	Buttocks-first presentation of fetus at delivery
distress	dis-**TRESS**		Latin *circumstance causing anxiety or hardship*	State that is causing pain or suffering
hyaline membrane disease	**HIGH**-ah-line **MEM**-brain diz-**EEZ**	P/ R/	**hyaline** Greek *glassy* **membrane** Latin *a skin* **dis-** *without* **-ease** *comfort*	Respiratory distress syndrome of the newborn
kernicterus	ker-**NIK**-ter-us	R/ R/	**kern-** *nucleus* **-icterus** *jaundice*	Bilirubin staining of the basal nuclei of the brain
meconium meconium aspiration syndrome	meh-**KOH**-nee-um meh-**KOH**-nee-um AS-pih-**RAY**-shun **SIN**-drome	S/ R/ P/ R/	Greek *a little poppy* **-ion** *process* **aspirat-** *to breathe* **syn-** *together* **-drome** *running*	The first bowel movement of the newborn Condition that occurs when the fetus passes the first bowel movement in the amniotic fluid and then inhales it into its lungs
neonate neonatal (adj) (*Note: The "e" is dropped as it is followed by another vowel, "a."*) neonatologist	**NEE**-oh-nate **NEE**-oh-**NAY**-tal **NEE**-oh-nay-**TOL**-oh-jist	R/CF R/CF S/ R/ R/CF S/	**neo-** *new* **-nat/e** *born* **-al** *pertaining to* **-nat-** *born* **-nat/o-** *birth* **-logist** *one who studies, specialist*	A newborn infant Pertaining to the newborn infant or the newborn period Medical specialist in disorders of the newborn
nuchal cord	**NYU**-kul KORD		French *the back (nape) of the neck*	Loop of umbilical cord around the fetal neck
pediatrics pediatrician	pee-dee-**AT**-riks **PEE**-dee-ah-**TRISH**-an	S/ R/ R/ S/	**-ics** *knowledge* **-iatr-** *medical treatment* **ped-** *child* **-ician** *expert*	Medical specialty of treating children during development from birth through adolescence Medical specialist in disorders of childhood and adolescence
postmature (adj) postmaturity (noun)	post-mah-**TYUR** post-mah-**TYUR**-ih-tee	P/ R/CF S/	**post-** *after* **matur/e** *ripe, ready* **-ity** *condition*	Pertaining to an infant born after 42 weeks of gestation Condition of being postmature
premature (adj) prematurity (noun) preemie (informal)	pree-mah-**TYUR** pree-mah-**TYUR**-ih-tee **PREE**-mee	P/ R/CF S/	**pre-** *before, in front of* **-mature** *ripe, ready* **-ity** *condition*	Occurring before the expected time; for example, when an infant is born before 37 weeks of gestation Condition of being premature Premature baby
previa	**PREE**-vee-ah	P/ R/	**pre-** *before, in front of* **-via** *the way*	Anything that blocks the fetus during its birth; for example, an abnormally situated placenta, placenta previa
surfactant	sir-**FAK**-tant		surface active agent	A protein and fat compound that creates surface tension to hold the lung alveolar walls apart
vertex	**VER**-teks		Latin *whorl*	Topmost point of the vault of the skull

A. After reading Case Report (CR) 8.3, answer the following questions. *Choose the best answer.* **LO 8.6, 8.8**

Case Report (CR) 8.3

You are

. . . an obstetric assistant working with Garry Joiner, MD, an obstetrician at Fulwood Medical Center.

Your patient is

. . . Mrs. Gloria Maggay, a 29-year-old housekeeper.

Mrs. Maggay's last menstrual period (**LMP**) was 8 weeks ago, and she has a positive home pregnancy test. This is her first pregnancy. She has breast tenderness and mild nausea. For the past 2 days, she has had some cramping and right-sided, lower abdominal pain, and this morning she had vaginal spotting. Her VS are T 99°F, P 80, R 14, BP 130/70.

While you are waiting for Dr. Joiner to come and examine Mrs. Maggay, she complains of feeling faint and has a sharp, severe pain in her lower abdomen on the right side. Her pulse rate has increased to 92. You need to recognize what is happening. Mrs. Maggay's symptoms are those of an ectopic pregnancy. The sudden increase in the pain and the rise in pulse rate can indicate that the tube has ruptured and is hemorrhaging into the abdominal cavity. The gynecologist should see her immediately and, if necessary, take her to the **operating room (OR)** for laparoscopic surgery to stop the bleeding and evacuate the products of conception.

1. Which of the following symptoms did Mrs. Maggay develop while she was in the office?

    a. decreased pulse rate   **b.** vaginal spotting   **c.** severe right-sided abdominal pain   **d.** mild nausea

2. Mrs. Maggay is most liking suffering from:

    a. fertilized egg implanted in a uterine tube   **b.** endometrial tissue occurring outside of the uterus

    c. prolapsed uterus   **d.** rupture of the appendix

B. Define the meaning of the word elements. *Select the correct answer that completes each statement.* **LO 8.3, 8.6**

1. The word element that means **scanty:**
    a. *poly-*   **b.** *hyper-*   **c.** *oligo-*   **d.** *ectop-*   **e.** *-amnios*

2. The word element *terat-* means:
    a. four   **b.** condition of   **c.** death   **d.** monster   **e.** shining forth

3. The word element *-emesis* means:
    a. excessive   **b.** tension   **c.** vomiting   **d.** bleeding   **e.** nausea

C. Elements. *Real familiarity with obstetrical and reproductive terms means you can look at an element and identify it as either a prefix (P), root (R), or suffix (S). Identify each element by writing its type and meaning in the appropriate columns. The first one is done for you. Fill in the blanks.* **LO 8.2, 8.6**

Element	Type	Meaning	Element	Type	Meaning
1. *post*	P	after	5. *mature*		
2. *ity*			6. *pre*		
3. *kern*			7. *dis*		
4. *syn*					

D. Describe the disorders of childbirth. *Match the disorder in the first column with its correct description in the second column.* **LO 8.6**

	Term		Meaning
_____	1. prolapsed umbilical cord	a.	cord is wrapped around the baby's neck during delivery
_____	2. placenta previa	b.	cord comes before the baby during delivery
_____	3. kernicterus	c.	brain damage due to bilirubin deposits
_____	4. nuchal cord	d.	separation of the placenta from the uterine wall before delivery
_____	5. placenta abruptio	e.	placenta is positioned over the internal os of the cervix

Section 8.7 Procedures and Pharmacology-Obstetrics

Contraception

Contraception is the prevention of pregnancy. Common methods of contraception include the following.

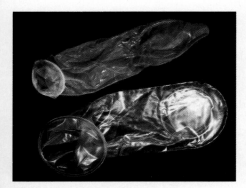

▲ **Figure 8.28** **Male and female condoms.** Scott Camazine/Science Source

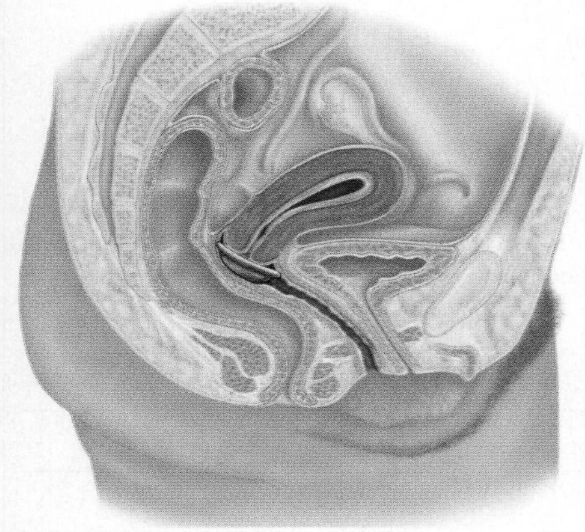

▲ **Figure 8.29** Diaphragm.

Behavioral Methods

- **Abstinence** is reliable if followed consistently.
- **Rhythm method** avoids intercourse near the time of expected ovulation, which is difficult to determine. It has a 25% failure rate.
- **Coitus interruptus** involves the male withdrawing his penis before ejaculation. There is a 20% failure rate.

Barrier Methods

- **Male condom**—a sheath of latex or rubber rolled on over the erect penis. There is a 14% to 15% failure rate for pregnancy.
- **Female condom**—a polyurethane sheath that fits into the vagina with a ring at one end to go over the cervix and a larger diameter at the other end to go over the vulva *(Figure 8.28)*. There is a 2% failure rate for pregnancy. Both male and female condoms help protect against STDs.
- **Diaphragm** *(Figure 8.29)* **and cervical cap**—a latex or rubber dome inserted into the vagina and placed over the cervix. When used with a **spermicide,** they have a 5% to 10% failure rate for pregnancy.
- **Spermicidal foam and gel**—inserted into the vagina. Used on their own, they have a 25% failure rate.
- **Sponge**—a spermicidal-coated polyurethane barrier placed in the vagina to inhibit sperm. It has a 10% failure rate.

Intrauterine Devices

Intrauterine devices (IUDs) are small plastic devices that are flexible and T-shaped that are placed high in the uterus. There are two types of IUDs: copper and hormonal.

It is the copper that is wrapped around the IUD *(ParaGard)* that impairs the ability of sperm to move, making it difficult for it to reach the egg. It can be left in place for 5–10 years.

Hormonal IUDs *(Kileena, Liletta, Mirena,* and *Skyla)* release progestin which thickens cervical mucus making it difficult for sperm to enter the uterus and fertilize an egg. It can be left in place for 3–5 years.

Hormonal Methods

- **Oral contraceptives** (birth control pills) utilize a mixture of estrogen and progesterone to prevent follicular development and ovulation *(Figure 8.30)*. They are taken orally and have a 5% failure rate, usually due to inconsistent pill taking.
- **Estrogen/progestin patches** deliver the hormones transdermally. Some are applied monthly, some weekly. Their failure rate is approximately 9% when reapplied at the correct time.
- **Injected progestins,** such as *Depo-Provera,* are given by injection every 3 months. Their failure rate is less than 1%.
- **Implanted progestins,** such as *Nexplanon,* are contained in porous silicone tubes that are inserted under the skin and slowly release the progestin for up to 5 years. Their failure rate is less than 1%.
- **Morning-after pills,** such as Plan B, contain large doses of progestins to inhibit or delay ovulation. They are a backup when taken within 72 hours of unprotected intercourse.
- **Mifepristone,** when taken with a prostaglandin, induces a miscarriage.

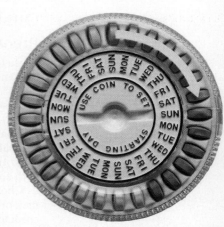

▲ **Figure 8.30** Oral contraceptives.
Don Farrall/Photodisc/GettyImages

Surgical Methods

- **Tubal ligation** ("getting your tubes tied") is performed with laparoscopy. Both uterine tubes are cut, a segment is removed, and the ends are tied off and cauterized shut. Failure rate is less than 1%. A **tubal anastomosis** is the procedure of rejoining the tubes if there is a subsequent change of mind.
- **Vasectomy** in the male is discussed in *Chapter 7.*

Word Analysis and Definition: Contraception

S = Suffix   P = Prefix   R = Root   R/CF = Combining Form

WORD	PRONUNCIATION		ELEMENTS	DEFINITION
abstinence	**AB**-stih-nens	S/	**-ence** *forming, quality of, state of*	Choosing to not participate in a behavior, in this case, sexual intercourse
		P/	**ab-** *away from*	
		R/	**-stin-** *partition*	
anastomosis	ah-**NAS**-to-**MOH**-sis	S/	**-osis** *condition*	A surgically made union between two tubular structures
anastomoses (pl)		R/	**anastom-** *join together*	
coitus	**KOH**-it-us		Latin *come together*	Sexual intercourse
condom	**KON**-dom		Old English *sheath or cover*	A sheath or cover for the penis or vagina to prevent conception and infection
contraception	kon-trah-**SEP**-shun	S/	**-ion** *process*	Prevention of pregnancy
		P/	**contra-** *against*	
		R/	**-cept-** *receive*	
contraceptive	kon-trah-**SEP**-tiv	S/	**-ive** *quality of*	An agent that prevents conception
diaphragm (*Note:* **Diaphragm** also is the term for the muscle that separates the thoracic and abdominal cavities.)	**DIE**-ah-fram		Greek *partition or wall*	A ring and dome-shaped material inserted in the vagina to prevent pregnancy
intrauterine	**IN**-trah-**YOU**-ter-ine	S/	**-ine** *pertaining to*	Pertaining to the inside of the uterus
		P/	**intra-** *inside, within*	
		R/	**-uter-** *uterus*	
ligature	**LIG**-ah-chur		Latin *band, tie*	Thread or wire tied around a tubal structure to close it
ligation	lie-**GAY**-shun	S/	**-ion** *process*	Use of a tie to close a tube
		R/	**ligat-** *tie up*	
progestin	pro-**JESS**-tin	S/	**-in** *chemical compound*	A synthetic form of progesterone
		P/	**pro-** *before*	
		R/	**-gest-** *produce, pregnancy*	
spermicide	**SPER**-mih-side	S/	**-cide** *to kill*	Agent that destroys sperm
		R/CF	**sperm/i-** *sperm*	
spermicidal (adj)	**SPER**-mih-**SIDE**-al	S/	**-cidal** *pertaining to killing*	Pertaining to the destruction of sperm

Obstetric Diagnostic Procedures

Prenatal Screening Tests

These tests can help determine if the pregnancy is at a higher risk for the baby to have a specific problem; the test does not diagnose a problem, only whether it is more or less likely. There is no risk of miscarriage from these tests.

First trimester screening is done between the 11th and 13th weeks of pregnancy. It combines maternal blood testing for human chorionic gonadotropin (hCG) (the pregnancy hormone) and **pregnancy-associated plasma protein A (PAPP-A)** with an ultrasound measurement of the back of the baby's neck **(nuchal translucency—NT).** Women with higher than average NT measurements and/or higher or lower than average hCG or PAPP-A values *might* be at risk for having a baby with Down Syndrome or with another rare chromosomal problem, Trisomy 18.

Chorionic villus sampling (CVS) also uses ultrasound guidance to insert a needle through the abdomen or a catheter through the cervix to obtain a sample of placental tissue that can be tested for fetal chromosomal abnormalities. The main advantage of CVS is that it can be performed between 9 and 13 weeks of pregnancy, earlier than amniocentesis (*see below*).

Second trimester screening is done between the 15th and 18th weeks of gestation. Called the **quad screen,** it measures the levels of four substances in a pregnant woman's blood: alpha-fetoprotein (AFP), hCG, unconjugated estriol, and dimeric inhibin. These chemicals are made by the placenta and fetus. Women with high or low levels of these substances *may* be at risk for having a baby with Down Syndrome, Trisomy 18, a neural tube defect (*see Chapter 9*) such as spina bifida, or an abdominal wall defect in which abdominal contents protrude through the abdominal wall.

Cystic fibrosis screening is a blood test to determine the presence of the gene that causes CF. Both parents have to be carriers of the gene for the baby to be at risk for CF.

2-D ultrasound can be used to show most of the organs and bones of the baby in utero. In addition to the screenings described above, ultrasound can be used between 18 and 20 weeks of pregnancy to provide a detailed picture of the baby's anatomy, its size, and growth. A 3-D ultrasound creates a 3-D image of the fetus using specialized probes and computer software. A 4-D ultrasound provides 3-D imaging in real time. Ultrasound carries no known risks and is the most frequently used method of prenatal screening.

Diagnostic Tests

Diagnostic tests, as distinct from screening tests, can confirm the presence of the congenital anomaly suggested by the screening test.

Amniocentesis uses ultrasound guidance to insert a thin needle through the abdominal wall into the amniotic sac around the baby to remove a small amount of amniotic fluid. This fluid contains fetal skin fibroblasts that can be tested for abnormalities. Amniocentesis is performed between 15 and 20 weeks to diagnose chromosome abnormalities and neural tube defects.

Therapeutic Procedures

During labor, there is electronic fetal heart monitoring to determine whether the baby is in distress. Treatment is to give the mother oxygen or increase IV fluids. If distress persists, the baby is delivered as quickly as possible by **forceps extraction,** vacuum extractor, or **cesarean section (C-section).**

WORD	PRONUNCIATION	ELEMENTS		DEFINITION
amniocentesis	**AM**-nee-oh-sen**TEE**-sis	S/ R/CF	-centesis *puncture* amni/o- *amnion*	Removal of amniotic fluid for diagnostic purposes
cesarean section (C-section) (syn)	seh-**ZAH**-ree-an **SEK**-shun		Roman law under the Caesars required that pregnant women who died be cut open and the fetus extracted	Extraction of the fetus through an incision in the abdomen and uterine wall
diagnostic	die-ag-**NOS**-tik	S/ P/ R/	-tic *pertaining to* dia- *complete* -gnos- *recognize an abnormal condition*	Pertaining to establishing the cause of a disease
estrogen estriol	**ES**-troh-jen **ESS**-tree-ol	S/ R/CF R/CF S/	-gen *create* estr/o- *woman* estr/i- *woman* -ol *chemical name*	Generic term for hormones that stimulate secondary sex characteristics One of the three main estrogens
forceps extraction	**FOR**-seps ek-**STRAK**-shun		**forceps** Latin *a pair of tongs* **extraction** Latin *to draw out*	Assisted delivery of the baby by an instrument that grasps the head of the baby
gonadotropin	**GO**-nad-oh-**TROH**-pin	S/ R/CF	-tropin *nourishing* gonad/o *gonad*	Hormone capable of promoting gonad function
maternal	mah-**TER**-nal	S/ R/	-al *pertaining to* matern- *mother*	Pertaining to, or derived from, the mother
neural neural tube	**NYU**-ral **NYU**-ral TYUB	S/ R/	-al *pertaining to* neur- *nerve*	Pertaining to any structure composed of nerve cells Embryologic tubelike structure that forms the brain and spinal cord
nuchal	**NYU**-kul		French *the back (nape) of the neck*	The back (nape) of the neck
prenatal	pree-**NAY**-tal	S/ P/ R/	-al *pertaining to* pre- *before* -nat- *born*	Before birth
quad screen	**KWAD SKREEN**		**quad** *four* **screen** *test*	Measurement of the levels of four substances in mother's blood that *may* indicate a fetal birth defect
translucent	tranz-**LOO**-sent	S/ P/ R/	-ent *pertaining to* trans- *across, through* -luc- *light*	Allowing light to pass through

Check Point Section 8.7

A. Review the medical terms relating to methods of contraception. *With critical thinking, you will be able to answer the following questions using these terms. Select the correct answer that completes each statement or answers each question.* **LO 8.8**

1. The prefix in the medical term **contraception** means:

   a. receive   b. process   c. against   d. before

2. The medical term that has a word element that means *chemical compound* is:

   a. spermicidal   b. coitus   c. progestin   d. diaphragm

3. Which of the following is considered to be a barrier method of contraception?

   a. intrauterine device   b. diaphragm   c. implanted progestins   d. birth control pill

4. A pill that induces miscarriage is:

   a. IUD   b. MRI   c. RU-486   d. PCOS

5. An agent that destroys sperm is a:

   a. progestin   b. spermicidal   c. spermicide   d. condom

B. Describe the meaning of abbreviations related to obstetrical screening tests. *Given the abbreviation, choose its correct description.* **LO 8.5, 8.9**

1. PAPP-A is used to screen for:

   a. spina bifida   **b.** fetal alcohol syndrome   **c.** Down syndrome   **d.** cystic fibrosis

2. An abnormally high or low hCG level may indicate which disorder?

   a. nuchal translucency   **b.** spina bifida   **c.** fetal alcohol syndrome   **d.** cystic fibrosis

3. How is NT measured?

   a. maternal blood testing   **b.** fetal blood testing   **c.** amniocentesis   **d.** ultrasound

C. Construct medical terms related to obstetrics. *Given the definition, complete the described medical terms by inputting the correct word element.* **LO 8.2, 8.8**

1. Hormone capable of promoting gonad function: gonad/o/_____

2. To puncture the amniotic sac: amni/o/ _____

3. Pertaining to the mother: _____ /al

4. Allowing light to pass through: _____ /luc/ent

5. Pertaining to a nerve: _____ /al

Section 8.8   The Breast Anatomy and Disorders

The Breast

Until the relatively recent introduction of bottles filled with liquid supplied by cows or soybeans, the milk produced by the female breast was essential for the survival of the human species. Nourishment of the infant remains the breast's major function.

Anatomy of the Breast

The breasts of males and females are identical until puberty, when ovarian hormones stimulate the development of the breast in females. Adult males still have main milk ducts in their breasts.

Each adult female breast has a **body** located over the pectoralis major muscle and an **axillary tail** extending toward the armpit. The **nipple** projects from the breast and contains multiple openings of the main milk ducts. The reddish-brown **areola** surrounds the nipple. The small bumps on its surface are **areolar glands.** These are sebaceous glands, the secretions of which prevent chapping and cracking during breastfeeding.

Internally, the breasts are supported by **suspensory ligaments** that extend from the skin to the fascia overlying the pectoralis major muscle *(Figure 8.31)*.

The **nonlactating breast** consists mostly of adipose and connective tissues. It has a system of ducts that branch through the connective tissue and converge on the nipple.

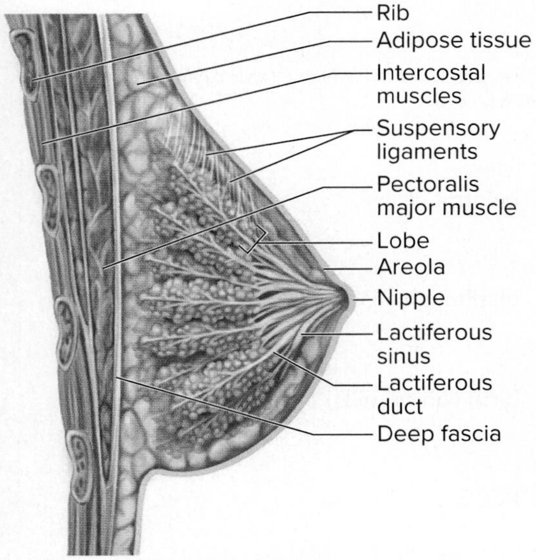

Mammary Gland

When the **mammary gland** develops during pregnancy, it is divided into 15 to 20 lobes that contain the secretory **alveoli** that produce milk. Each lobe is drained by the main milk ducts, called **lactiferous ducts** *(see Figure 8.31)*. Immediately before opening onto the nipple, each lactiferous duct dilates to form a **lactiferous sinus** in which milk is stored before being released from the nipple.

Labels: Rib, Adipose tissue, Intercostal muscles, Suspensory ligaments, Pectoralis major muscle, Lobe, Areola, Nipple, Lactiferous sinus, Lactiferous duct, Deep fascia

▲ **Figure 8.31** Anatomy of lactating breast.

Lactation

When the mammary gland develops during pregnancy, high estrogen levels cause the lactiferous ducts to grow and branch, and progesterone stimulates the budding of alveoli at the ends of the ducts. The alveoli are formed in grapelike clusters. The percentage of adipose and connective tissue diminishes.

In late pregnancy, the alveoli and ducts contain **colostrum.** This secretion contains more protein but less fat than human milk, but it also contains high levels of **immunoglobulins** *(see Chapter 12)* to give the newborn infant protection from infections. Colostrum is replaced by milk 2 or 3 days after the baby's birth, and this replacement is complete by day 5.

Milk production is mainly controlled by **prolactin,** a hormone from the pituitary gland. The other essential stimulus to milk production is the baby's sucking *(Figure 8.32),* which stimulates prolactin production. In addition, the **sucking reflex** stimulates the pituitary gland to produce **oxytocin** *(see Chapter 17),* which causes milk to be ejected from the alveoli into the duct system, and helps to form a bond between mother and child.

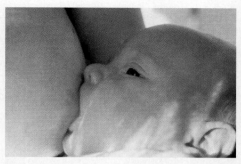

▲ **Figure 8.32** **Breastfeeding.** Ascent/PKSMedia/EyeWire/Getty Images

Word Analysis and Definition: Breast Anatomy

S = Suffix   P = Prefix   R = Root   R/CF = Combining Form

WORD	PRONUNCIATION		ELEMENTS	DEFINITION
alveolus alveoli (pl)	al-**VEE**-oh-lus al-**VEE**-oh-lie		Latin *small hollow or cavity*	Small empty sac or space
areola areolar (adj)	ah-**REE**-oh-luh ah-**REE**-oh-lar	S/ R/	Latin *small area* -ar *pertaining to* **areol-** *area around the nipple*	Circular reddish area surrounding the nipple Pertaining to the areola
colostrum	koh-**LOSS**-trum		Latin *foremilk*	The first breast secretion at the end of pregnancy
duct	DUKT		Latin *to lead*	A tube to carry fluid or gas
lactation	lak-**TAY**-shun	S/ R/CF	-ation *process* **lact/i-** *milk*	Production of milk
lactiferous (adj) lactate (verb)	lak-**TIF**-er-us	S/ R/	-ous *pertaining to* **-fer-** *to bear, carry*	Pertaining to or yielding milk
mammary	**MAM**-ah-ree	S/ R/	-ary *pertaining to* **mamm-** *breast*	Relating to the lactating breast
nipple	**NIP**-el		Old English *small nose*	Projection from the breast into which the lactiferous ducts open
oxytocin	**OK**-see-**TOH**-sin	S/ R/CF R/	-in *chemical compound* **ox/y-** *oxygen* **-toc-** *labor, birth*	Pituitary hormone that stimulates the uterus to contract and causes breast milk to be ejected from the alveoli into the duct system
prolactin	pro-**LAK**-tin	S/ P/ R/	-in *chemical compound* **pro-** *before* **-lact-** *milk*	Pituitary hormone that stimulates production of milk

Disorders of the Breast

Mastitis, inflammation of the breast, can occur in association with breastfeeding if the nipple or areola is cracked or traumatized. It is usually segmental in one of the lobes of the breast and responds well to antibiotics. It is not an indication for stopping breastfeeding.

Mastalgia (breast pain) is the most common benign breast disorder. The pain can be associated with breast tenderness and be part of PMS (premenstrual syndrome).

Nipple discharge, particularly if it is from one breast and bloody, is an indication of an underlying disorder such as breast cancer and warrants investigation.

Fibroadenomas are circumscribed, small, benign tumors that can be either cystic or solid and can be multiple.

Fibrocystic disease of the breast presents as a dense, irregular cobblestone consistency of the breast, often with intermittent breast discomfort *(Figure 8.33).* It occurs in over 60% of all women and is considered by many doctors as a normal variant.

Galactorrhea is the production of milk when a woman is not breastfeeding. Sometimes the cause cannot be found, but it can occur in association with hormone therapy, antidepressants, tumor of the

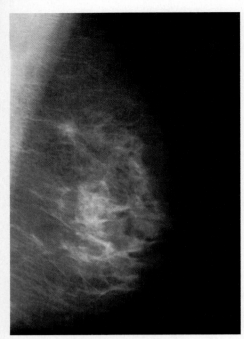

▲ **Figure 8.33** Mammogram showing fibrocystic disease of the breast.
ALIX/Phanie/Science Source

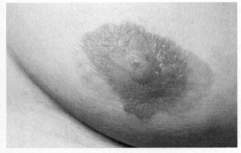

▲ **Figure 8.34** Paget disease of the nipple is associated with breast cancer.
Wellcome Photo Library

Did you know...

- Sixteen percent of female cancers are breast cancer.
- Risk factors for developing breast cancer include stress, being sedentary, and night shift work.

pituitary gland *(see Chapter 17),* and use of street drugs such as opiates and marijuana. In most cases, the milk production ceases with time.

Gynecomastia, enlargement of the breast, can be unilateral or bilateral and occur in both sexes. It is usually associated with either liver disease, marijuana, or drug therapy such as estrogens, calcium channel blockers, and antineoplastic drugs. It remits or disappears after the drug is withdrawn.

Breast cancer affects one in eight women in their lifetime. Risk factors include a family history, particularly if a woman carries either of the breast cancer **genes,** *BRCA1* or *BRCA2;* the use of postmenopausal estrogen therapy; and an early menarche and late menopause. Breast cancer does not have a singular cause. It is thought to be caused by the interaction of genes and exposure to environmental risk factors.

Jobs associated with the occurrence of breast cancer include flight attendants, health care providers, and sales and retail work. Women with a breast implant are at risk for developing Breast Implant Associated Lymphoma (BIA-LCL), a type of non-Hodgkin's lymphoma *(see Chapter 20).* Breast cancer occurs rarely in men.

Most breast cancers occur in the upper and outer quadrant of the breast, and symptoms include:

- A lump or thickening in the breast.
- Change in size, shape, or appearance of the breast.
- Dimpling of the skin of the breast.
- Pitting of the skin of the breast.
- Bloody discharge from the nipple.
- Peeling, flaking, redness, or scaling of the nipple and areola (**Paget's disease of the breast**).

Paget's disease of the breast *(see Figure 8.34)* occurs in 5% of breast cancers. The nipple and areola become scaly, red, flaky, and itchy due to cancer cells collecting there. The underlying cancer is usually found in the ducts of the nipple. The 19th-century British surgeon Sir James Paget first reported the relationship between the changes in the nipple and breast cancer.

Breast cancer can **metastasize** to lymph nodes, lungs, liver, bone, brain, and skin.

Word Analysis and Definition: Disorders of the Breast

S = Suffix   P = Prefix   R = Root   R/CF = Combining Form

WORD	PRONUNCIATION	ELEMENTS		DEFINITION
fibroadenoma	FIE-broh-ad-en-OH-mah	S/ R/CF R/	-oma *tumor* fibr/o- *fiber* -aden- *gland*	Benign tumor containing much fibrous tissue
fibrocystic disease	fie-broh-SIS-tik diz-EEZ	S/ R/CF R/	-ic *pertaining to* fibr/o- *fiber* -cyst- *cyst*	Benign breast disease with multiple tiny lumps and cysts
galactorrhea	gah-LAK-toh-REE-ah	S/ R/CF	-rrhea *flow* galact/o- *milk*	Abnormal flow of milk from the breasts
gynecomastia	GUY-nih-koh-MAS-tee-ah	S/ R/CF R/	-ia *condition* gynec/o- *female* -mast- *breast*	Enlargement of the breast
mastalgia	mass-TAL-jee-uh	S/ R/	-algia *pain* mast- *breast*	Pain in the breast
mastitis	mass-TIE-tis	S/ R/	-itis *inflammation* mast- *breast*	Inflammation of the breast
Paget's disease of the breast	PA-jet		Sir James Paget, 1814–1899, English surgeon	Changes in the nipple when associated with breast cancer

Check Point Section 8.8

A. Spelling your documentation correctly is a mark of an educated professional. *Read the following statements and insert the correctly spelled term in the blanks.* **LO 8.1, 8.3**

1. (Prolectin/Prolactin) _____ is the pituitary hormone that stimulates production of milk.

2. The circular, reddish area surrounding the nipple is the (aireola/areola) _____.

3. (Oxitocin/Oxytocin) _____ is the pituitary hormone that stimulates the uterus to contract.

4. The first breast secretion at the end of pregnancy is known as (colestrium/colostrum) _____.

5. The projection from the breast into which the milk ducts open is the (nippel/nipple) _____.

6. (Laktiferous/Lactiferous) _____ means *pertaining to or yielding milk.*

7. The areolar glands are (cebaceous/sebaceous) _____ glands.

B. Find the one false statement in the following choices. *Choose T if the statement is True. Choose F if the statement is False.* **LO 8.1**

1. The lactiferous ducts produce milk.   T   F

2. In late pregnancy, the alveoli and ducts contain colostrum.   T   F

3. High levels of immunoglobulins are in breast milk.   T   F

4. Milk production is mainly controlled by prolactin.   T   F

5. The sucking reflex produces estrogen.   T   F

6. Milk flows from the lactiferous duct to the lactiferous sinus to the nipple.   T   F

C. Build your knowledge of suffixes, which always provide a big clue to the meaning of a medical term. *Review all the terms in the section; then answer the following questions. All of these questions can be answered by analyzing the elements in each term. Fill in the blank.* **LO 8.6**

1. Pain in the breast: _____

2. Inflammation of the breast: _____

3. A small, benign tumor of the breast: _____

4. Enlargement of the breast: _____

5. Benign breast disease with multiple tiny bumps and cysts: _____

D. Deconstruct medical terms to understand their meanings. *Fill in the blank.* **LO 8.2, 8.6**

1. The suffix in the term **galactorrhea** means: _____

2. The root in the term **mastalgia** means: _____

3. The combining form in the term **galactorrhea** means: _____

4. The suffix in the term **mastitis** means: _____

5. The suffix in the term **gynecomastia** means: _____

Section 8.9 Procedures and Pharmacology of the Breast

Diagnostic Procedures

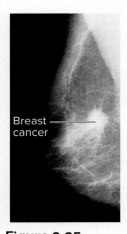

▲ **Figure 8.35**
Mammogram showing breast cancer. UHB Trust/The ImageBank/Getty Images

Breast self-examination (BSE) on a monthly basis has been shown to be of questionable value. It is recommended by the American College of Obstetricians and Gynecologists (**ACOG**) and the American Medical Association (**AMA**) but neither recommended nor discouraged by the American Cancer Society (**ACS**), the National Cancer Institute (**NCI**), and other organizations.

However, many breast cancers are discovered as a lump by the patient during a self-examination. Another 40% are discovered on routine **mammogram** *(Figure 8.33)*. Routine **mammography** reduces breast cancer mortality by 25% to 30% *(Figure 8.35)*. However, it has a false positive rate of 7% and a false negative rate of 10%.

- **2-D mammography** takes two images of the breast, one from the side and one from the top.

- **3-D mammography** takes multiple x-ray images that are taken when camera moves in an arc over the breast. A computer combines the images to recreate a 3-D image of the breast. As of 2020, the ACS does not recommend a 3-D mammogram over a 2-D mammogram.

- Ultrasound, magnetic resonance imaging (MRI), and positron emission mammography (PEM) *(see Chapter 21)* are adjuncts to routine 2-D or 3-D mammography for further evaluation of suspicious lesions.

The pathology report on breast cancer cells will include results of a hormone receptor **assay.** A breast cancer is called **estrogen-receptor-positive (ER-positive)** if its cells have receptors for estrogen that promote their growth. A breast cancer is called **progesterone-receptor-positive** if its cells have receptors for progesterone that can promote their growth. Approximately two-thirds of breast cancers test positive for hormone receptors. The pathology report also will tell if the breast cancer cells have too many copies of the **gene HER2**. If the breast cancer cells are negative for both hormone receptors and HER2, it is called a **triple negative** breast cancer.

Stereotactic biopsy, a needle biopsy performed during mammography, and **excisional biopsy,** surgical removal of a tumor with a surrounding margin of normal breast tissue, provide material for a pathological diagnosis.

Staging of breast cancer (**TNM**) is based on the size of the tumor in the breast (T), the status of the lymph nodes in the axilla (N), and the metastatic spread to distant sites (M) *(see Chapter 20)*.

Therapeutic Procedures

Surgical treatments for breast cancer include the following:

- **Lumpectomy** and **quadrantectomy** are breast-conserving surgical procedures.
- **Simple mastectomy** removes the whole breast.
- **Modified radical mastectomy** removes the whole breast and the axillary lymph nodes, but the muscle is left intact.
- **Radical mastectomy** is complete removal of all breast tissue, the underlying pectoralis major muscle, and all associated lymph nodes.

    Radiation therapy uses high energy rays or particles to destroy cancer cells. **External beam radiation** is delivered from a machine outside the body. **Internal radiation (brachytherapy)** uses **radioactive** seeds or pellets placed inside the body for a short time at the site of the lesion.

    Suction **lipectomy (liposuction)** is the insertion of a metal tube into an incision of the skin, and then suction is applied and fat tissue is aspirated and removed. This technique is used to treat excess breast tissue in gynecomastia. It also is used for other areas of the body not related to disorders of the breast.

Pharmacology

Chemotherapy is a systemic therapy affecting the whole body by going through the bloodstream to destroy any cancer cells; unfortunately it also affects other body cells, producing side effects (*see Chapter 20*). There are numerous chemotherapy drugs that are used to treat breast cancer which are often used in combination. Examples of these medications include but are not limited to 5-fluoro-uracil (*5-FU*), capecitabine, carboplatin (*Paraplatin*), cyclophosphamide (*Cytoxan*), docetaxel (*Taxotere*), doxorubicin (*Adriamycin*), methotrexate sodium, paclitaxel (*Taxol*), and pertuzmab.

    In 2019 the US FDA approved the first immunotherapy treatment. It is a combination of atezolizumab (*Tecentriq*) and nab-paclitaxel (*Abraxane*) for people with advanced triple negative breast cancer.

    Women with stage IV cancers are treated with chemotherapy and other types of medications including hormone therapy (tamoxifen) and target therapy such as ribociclib (*Kisquali*). Numerous standard chemotherapy regimens use combinations of the drugs.

    Selective estrogen receptor modulator (SERM) medications include tamoxifen (*Soltamox* or *Novadex*), raloxifene (*Evista*), and toremifene (*Fareston*). These medications block estrogen from attaching to the estrogen receptors of ER-positive breast cancer cells, either slowing the growth of or killing the cancer cells.

    For breast cancer cells that produce excessive amounts of HER2, *Herceptin* blocks this production, causing the cancer cells to die.

Word Analysis and Definition: Diagnostic and Therapeutic Procedures and Pharmacology of the Breast

S = Suffix   P = Prefix   R = Root   R/CF = Combining Form

WORD	PRONUNCIATION		ELEMENTS	DEFINITION
assay	**ASS**-ay		French *to try*	Analysis of concentration of drugs or other biological markers
brachytherapy	brak-kee-**THAIR**-ah-pee	P/ R/	brachy- *short* -therapy *treatment*	Radiation therapy in which the source of irradiation is implanted in the tissue to be treated
chemotherapy	**KEE**-moh-**THAIR**-ah-pee	R/CF R/	chem/o- *chemical* -therapy *treatment*	Treatment using chemical agents
lipectomy	lip-**EK**-toh-mee	S/ R/	-ectomy *surgical excision* lip- *fatty tissue*	Surgical removal of adipose tissue
lumpectomy	lump-**EK**-toh-mee	S/ R/	-ectomy *surgical excision* lump- *piece*	Removal of a lesion with preservation of surrounding tissue
mammogram	**MAM**-oh-gram	S/ R/CF	-gram *a record* mamm/o- *breast*	The record produced by x-ray imaging of the breast
mammography	mah-**MOG**-rah-fee	S/	-graphy *process of recording*	Process of x-ray imaging of the breast
mastectomy	mass-**TEK**-toh-mee	S/ R/	-ectomy *surgical excision* mast- *breast*	Surgical excision of the breast
quadrantectomy	kwad-ran-**TEK**-toh-mee	S/ R/	-ectomy *surgical excision* quadrant- *quarter*	Surgical excision of a quadrant of the breast
radiation	ray-dee-**AY**-shun	S/ R/	-ation *process* radi- *radiation*	The sending forth of x-rays or other rays for treatment or diagnosis
radical	**RAD**-ih-kal		Latin *root*	Extensive or thorough
stereotactic	**STER**-ee-oh-**TAK**-tik	S/ R/CF R/	-ic *pertaining to* stere/o- *three-dimensional* -tact- *orderly arrangement*	Pertaining to a precise three-dimensional method to locate a lesion

Check Point Section 8.9

A. As a health care professional, you must know the proper use of each medical term. *Use the words provided below to correctly complete each sentence. Fill in the blanks.* **LO 8.5, 8.8**

mammography   mammogram   quadrantectomy   mastectomy

1. Mrs. Rivera makes a yearly checkup with her gynecologist to include a _____.

2. This year, the radiologist responsible for evaluating Mrs. Rivera's _____ tests noted an abnormal area in her right breast.

3. After several diagnostic tests, it was determined that Mrs. Rivera should have one-fourth of her breast removed, medically termed as a _____.

4. The pathologist reported her findings and the surgeon deemed it necessary to remove Mrs. Rivera's entire right breast along with the pectoralis major muscle and associated lymph nodes. Mrs. Rivera was advised to have a radical _____.

Table 8.1 Abbreviations

Abbreviation	Meaning	Abbreviation	Meaning
ACOG	American College of Obstetricians and Gynecologists	HPV	human papilloma virus
ACS	American College of Surgeons	HRT	hormone replacement therapy
AIDS	acquired immunodeficiency syndrome	HSV	herpes simplex virus
AMA	American Medical Association	IUD	intrauterine device
BIA-		IVF	in vitro fertilization
ALCL	Breast Implant-Associated Anaplastic Large Cell Lymphoma	LEEP	loop electrosurgical excision procedure
BRCA1		LH	luteinizing hormone
BRCA2	breast cancer genes	LMP	last menstrual period
BSE	breast-self examination	MAS	meconium aspiration syndrome
CDC	Centers for Disease Control and Prevention	NCI	National Cancer Institute
C-section	cesarean section	NT	nuchal translucency
CVS	chorionic villus sampling	OB	obstetrics
D and C	dilation and curettage	Pap	Papanicolaou—a Greek gynecologist
DNA	deoxyribonucleic acid	PAPP-A	pregnancy-associatedplasma protein A
DUB	dysfunctional uterine bleeding	PCOS	polycystic ovarian syndrome
ELISA	enzyme-linked immunosorbent assay	PEM	Positron emission mammography
ER-		PGY	pregnancy
positive	Estrogen-receptor-positive	PID	pelvic inflammatory disease
FP	alpha-fetoprotein	PMS	premenstrual syndrome
FSH	follicle-stimulating hormone	PPH	postpartum hemorrhage
GDM	gestational diabetes mellitus	PROM	premature rupture of the membranes
GnRH	gonadotropin-releasing hormone	RDS	respiratory distress syndrome
GYN	gynecology	RU-486	mifepristone
hCG	human chorionic gonadotropin	SERM	selective estrogen receptor modulator
HER2	Human Growth Factor Receptor 2	STD	sexually transmitted disease
HIV	human immunodeficiency virus	TNM	tumor, nodes, metastasis

Table 8.2 Comparison of common female reproductive system disorders

Disorder or Disease	Signs and Symptoms	Diagnostic Tests	Treatment
Bacterial vaginosis	Fishy odor, pelvic discomfort. No inflammation	Observe discharge, measure pH of discharge, and office-based microscopy	Metronidazole (*Flagyl*) or Tinidazole (*Tindamax*)
Cystocele	Sense that something is bulging through the vaginal opening, difficulty emptying the bladder, feeling of heaviness in the pelvic area	Pelvic exam	Watchful waiting, Kegel exercises, vaginal pessary, surgery
Dysmenorrhea	Pelvic pain, cramping during menstruation	Pelvic exam, transvaginal ultrasound	NSAIDs, hormonal contraceptives
Trichomoniasis	Green or yellow, frothy discharge; foul odor; vaginal pain or soreness	Observe discharge, measure pH of discharge, and office-based microscopy	Metronidazole (*Flagyl*) or Tinidazole (*Tindamax*)
Vulvodynia	Discomfort with sexual intercourse	Rule out other causes of pain (bacterial or fungal infection)	Avoid irritants (soaps, perfumes), biofeedback *(see Chapter 18)*, topical creams, medications to decrease nerve sensitivity. Vulvectomy as a last resort
Vulvovaginal candidiasis	White, thick, cheesy, or curdy discharge; vulvar itching or burning; no odor. Red, swollen vulva	Observe discharge, measure pH of discharge, and office-based microscopy	Topical clotrimazole or miconazole

Female Reproductive System

Challenge Your Knowledge

A. Language of gynecology. Demonstrate your knowledge of gynecologic terminology by answering the following multiple-choice questions. Choose the correct answer. **LO 8.1, 8.5, 8.6**

1. The mons pubis, labia majora and minora, and clitoris are collectively called the
   - a. prepuce
   - b. hymen
   - c. vulva
   - d. vaginosis
   - e. antrum

2. This procedure can be used to visualize the inside of the uterus, take a biopsy, and/or remove polyps or fibroids:
   - a. cytoscopy
   - b. hysteroscopy
   - c. ureteroscopy
   - d. bronchoscopy
   - e. thoracoscopy

3. Painful intercourse is called
   - a. salpingitis
   - b. dyspnea
   - c. hyperemesis
   - d. dyspareunia
   - e. candidiasis

4. The thin membrane that partially occludes the vagina is called the
   - a. fornix
   - b. mons
   - c. vestibule
   - d. hymen
   - e. clitoris

5. Irregular bleeding between menstrual periods is called
   - a. amenorrhea
   - b. metrorrhagia
   - c. polymenorrhea
   - d. dysmenorrhea
   - e. menorrhagia

6. The ovaries in the female and testes in the male can both be called
   - a. adnexa
   - b. ova
   - c. fornices
   - d. rugae
   - e. gonads

7. Which of the following is an STD?
   - a. toxic shock syndrome
   - b. vulvovaginal candidiasis
   - c. dyspareunia
   - d. all of these
   - e. none of these

8. Human immunodeficiency virus (HIV) damages the immune system, so infections will develop that the body would otherwise cope with easily. These infections are called
   - a. bacterial
   - b. staph
   - c. opportunistic
   - d. strep
   - e. viral

9. Chronic, lasting, severe pain around the vaginal orifice is a condition called
   - a. vulvitis
   - b. vaginitis
   - c. vulvodynia
   - d. candidiasis
   - e. endometriosis

10. Inflammation of the uterine tubes is called
    - a. ureteritis
    - b. uveitis
    - c. hyperemesis
    - d. endometriosis
    - e. salpingitis

11. The process of egg formation is called
    - a. oophorectomy
    - b. ova
    - c. oogenesis
    - d. oophocentesis
    - e. ovulation

12. Estrogen, progesterone, and androgen are all
    - a. antigens
    - b. enzymes
    - c. hormones
    - d. antibiotics
    - e. vitamins

B. **Latin and Greek terms cannot be further deconstructed into prefix, root, combining form, or suffix.** You must know them for what they are. Test your knowledge of these terms with this exercise. Match the medical term in the first column with the correct meaning in the second column. **LO 8.1, 8.2**

_____ 1. fornix   a. fringe

_____ 2. menses   b. membrane

_____ 3. ruga   c. egg

_____ 4. chancre   d. month

_____ 5. os   e. sheath

_____ 6. hymen   f. wrapper or covering

_____ 7. ovary   g. arch, vault

_____ 8. vagina   h. mouth

_____ 9. vulva   i. ridge or crease

_____ 10. fimbria   j. cancer

C. **Deconstruction.** Deconstruction of medical terms is a tool for analyzing the meaning. In the following chart, you are given a medical term. Deconstruct the term into its prefix, root (or combining form), and suffix. Write the element and its meaning in the appropriate column and the meaning of the term in the last column. If the term does not have a word element, write n/a. *The first one is done for you.* **LO 8.1, 8.2**

Medical Term	Prefix	Meaning of Prefix	Root/ Combining Form	Meaning of Root/ Combining Form	Suffix	Meaning of Suffix	Meaning of Term
mammary	1. n/a	2. n/a	3. mamm	4. breast	5. ary	6. pertaining to	7. Pertaining to the breast
neonatal	8.	9.	10.	11.	12.	13.	14.
primigravada	15.	16.	17.	18.	19.	20.	21.
postpartum	22.	23.	24.	25.	26.	27.	28.
endometrium	29.	30.	31.	32.	33.	34.	35.

D. **Plurals of some medical terms can be difficult to convert from the singular because there are so many different rules for plurals.** Practice makes perfect in your ability to form the correct plural of the term. Fill in the plural column. **LO 8.3**

Singular Term	Plural Term
cilium	1.
fimbria	2.
fornix	3.
infundibulum	4.
labium	5.
majus	6.
minus	7.
ovary	8.
ovum	9.
ruga	10.

E. **Trace the pathway of conception.** The following phrases describe the process of fertilization. Order the items A to H to indicate the correct order of their occurrence. **LO 8.1**

_____ **1.** Nuclei of male and female cells unite.

_____ **2.** Morula becomes a blastocyst.

_____ **3.** Inner cell mass differentiates and forms embryo.

_____ **4.** Zygote produces morula.

_____ **5.** Ovary releases egg.

_____ **6.** All organ systems are present; embryo becomes fetus.

_____ **7.** Blastocyst implants in the endometrium.

_____ **8.** Zygote is formed.

F. **Language of obstetrics.** Pregnancy has its own associated set of obstetric terms. Apply your knowledge of obstetric terms to answering the following questions. Circle the correct answer. **LO 8.1, 8.5, 8.6**

1. The *nuchal cord* is

   a. only present in ectopic pregnancy

   b. wrapped around the baby's neck during delivery

   c. a congenital malformation

   d. only present in breech births

   e. present in 50% of births

2. What keeps the maternal and fetal blood circulations separated?

   a. umbilical cord

   b. amnion

   c. yolk sac

   d. cells of the villi

   e. placenta

3. A test for chromosomal abnormalities and genetic birth defects is

    a. teratogenesis   **d.** labor

    b. hyperemesis   **e.** amniocentesis

    c. dilation

4. When the head is just starting to push out of the vaginal opening, it is said to be

    a. effacing   **d.** ovulating

    b. crowning   **e.** none of these

    c. dilating

5. Which undesirable item can cross the placenta into the fetus?

    a. rubella virus   **d.** glucose

    b. oxygen   **e.** hormones

    c. maternal antibodies

6. The pit in the abdomen where the umbilical cord enters the fetus is the

    a. meatus   **d.** a and b

    b. navel   **e.** none of these

    c. yolk sac

7. Postpartum vaginal discharge is called

    a. puerperium   **d.** amniocentesis

    b. lochia   **e.** oligohydramnios

    c. polyhydramnios

G. **Language of obstetrics.** Pregnancy has its own associated set of obstetric terms. Apply your knowledge of obstetric terms to answering the following questions. Circle the correct answer. **LO 8.1**

1. Where does fertilization actually take place?

    a. left ovary   **d.** proximal third of the uterine tube

    b. distal third of the uterine tube   **e.** uterus

    c. right ovary

2. During the first stage of labor, what is the process in which the wall of the cervix becomes thinner?

    a. crowning   **d.** autolysis

    b. effacement   **e.** involution

    c. delivery

3. What is the term for a fertilized egg's development in the uterine tube instead of the uterus?

    a. preeclampsia   **d.** ectopic

    b. postpartum   **e.** endometriosis

    c. eclampsia

4. The protective layer covering the skin of the fetus in utero is the

   a. estrogen   d. chorion

   b. lanugo   e. morula

   c. vernix caseosa

5. A woman who has given birth for the first time is

   a. multipara   d. postpartum

   b. gravidarum   e. puerperium

   c. primipara

H. Describe the events and structures of ovulation. Match the medical term in the first column with the correct meaning in the second column. **LO 8.1**

_____ 1. After menses ends, uterus replaces this   a. uterine cycle

_____ 2. Formed where ovarian follicle ruptures   b. fimbriae

_____ 3. Envelope the ovary   c. lutein

_____ 4. The first 14 days of menses   d. corpus albicans

_____ 5. Averages 28 days in length   e. follicular phase

_____ 6. Inactive scar   f. postovulatory phase

_____ 7. Mature ovarian follicle does this   g. corpus luteum

_____ 8. Cells involved in progesterone production   h. endometrial tissue

_____ 9. Period of time after ovulation   i. ruptures

I. Patient documentation. The following mammogram report for a patient contains terminology you should understand after reading this chapter. Answer the questions about the report by filling in the blanks. **LO 8.5, 8.6, 8.7, 8.8**

Exam: Diagnostic bilateral mammogram

Reason for exam: Discomfort in both breasts

The glandular tissue is heterogeneously dense. There are scattered fibroglandular densities bilaterally. There is a benign-appearing curvilinear area of glandular tissue in the right lower inner breast. There are a few faint calcifications in the lower inner left breast and in the central left breast. Magnification views were performed of the left breast calcifications in two positions, and they have an appearance most consistent with benign process. There is no associated mass or distortion.

Impression: Heterogeneously dense glandular tissue with focal glandular density in the medial aspect of the right breast and faint calcifications in the left breast. Probably benign.

Recommendation: Comparison with prior films. If prior films are not available, recommend follow-up mammogram in 6 months. Findings were submitted to the patient in writing.

1. The term that means *pertaining to two sides:* _____

2. A density is found in the middle of the (right/left) breast: _____

3. Calcifications are found in the (right/left) breast: _____

4. Does this patient have signs of malignancies? _____

5. The medical term for discomfort in the breast: _____

J. **Pronunciation is important whether you are saying the word or listening to a word from a coworker.** Identify the proper pronunciation of the following medical terms. **LO 8.4, 8.5, 8.6, 8.7, 8.10**

1. The correct pronunciation for a condition of pain during sexual intercourse

   a. **DIS**-pair-you-nee-ah

   b. dis-pah-**RUE**-nee-ah

   c. dis-**YOU**-ree-ah

   d. **DIS**-your-**EE**-ah

   Correctly spell the term: _____

2. The correct pronunciation for the human organism from the end of the eighth week after conception to birth

   a. nee-oh-**NATE**

   b. **EM**-bree-oh

   c. **ZIE**-goht

   d. **FEE**-tus

   Correctly spell the term: _____

3. The correct pronunciation for an endoscope to view the vagina and cervix

   a. **KOL**-poh-scope

   b. col-**POR**-ah-fee

   c. kyu-**REH**-rahzh

   d. **KOH**-nih-**ZAY**-shun

   Correctly spell the term: _____

4. The correct pronunciation for the specialist that cares for a mother with a high-risk pregnancy

    a. PER-ee-**NAY**-tol-oh-guest

    b. PER-ih-nay-**TOL**-oh-jist

    c. PEE-dee-ah-**TRISH**-an

    d. pee-**DEE**-ah-tis-**EE**-an

Correctly spell the term: _____

5. The correct pronunciation for the first bowel movement of the newborn

    a. KERN-ict-er-us

    b. ker-**NIK**-ter-us

    c. meh-**KOH**-nee-um

    d. meek-**OH**-nee-yum

Correctly spell the term: _____

Case Reports

A. After reading the following Case Report, correctly answer the following questions. The answers to the questions may not be in the Case Report itself but can be found in the chapter content. **LO 8.3, 8.5, 8.6, 8.8, 8.9**

 ## Case Report (CR) 8.4

You are...

a registered nurse (RN) working in the labor and delivery unit at Fulwood Medical Center.

Your patient is

. . . Ms. Mukta Pathak, a 28-year-old a **gravid 2, para1** mother who is 38 weeks along in her pregnancy. You are assisting Dorothy Brown, CNM, in the delivery of a baby. Ms. Brown palpated the abdomen and notes that the baby is in breech position to. She asks you to assist in pressing on the abdomen to turn the baby into proper position. Ms. Brown also calls the radiology department for sonographers to assist in determining the position of the baby.

Pressing on the abdomen is successful, and the **ultrasound** confirms that the baby is in proper position. A few hours later, Ms. Pathak is fully effaced, and it is time to deliver the baby. The neonate is born with a loosely-wrapped **nuchal cord**, to which Ms. Brown corrects. Upon delivery, Mr. Pathak assists with the cutting of the umbilical cord, and a crying neonate is passed to you. You remove the **vernix caseosa** and begin the assessment of the neonate.

---

1. By date of the pregnancy the neonate will:

    a. lack surfactant   **c.** have subcutaneous fat deposits

    b. will have dry, leathery skin   **d.** passed meconium into amnion

2. Ms. Pathak has been pregnant _____ time(s) and has _____ child(ren).

3. What is Ms. Brown's occupation? (provide one term in each blank) _____

_____

_____

4. It is safe for ultrasound to be used as a diagnostic tool because it:

    a. lacks radiation to view tissues and structures

    b. provides a very small amount of radiation

    c. the dose of radiation is given for a small amount of time

5. A nuchal cord means that the _____ cord was wrapped around the neonate's _____.

6. The vernix caseosa is a normal substance to remove.   True   False

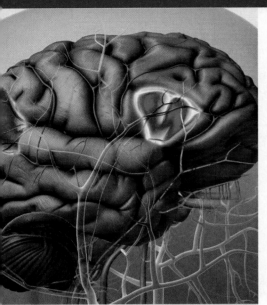

2014 Nucleus Medical Media

CHAPTER

9

Nervous System
The Language of Neurology

Chapter Sections

9.1 Functions and Structure of the Nervous System

9.2 The Brain and Cranial Nerves

9.3 Disorders of the Brain and Cranial Nerves

9.4 Disorders of the Spinal Cord and Peripheral Nerves

9.5 Procedures and Pharmacology

Chapter Learning Outcomes

Upon completion of this chapter, you will be able to:

LO 9.1 Identify and describe the anatomy and physiology of the nervous system.

LO 9.2 Use roots, combining forms, suffixes, and prefixes to construct and analyze medical terms related to the nervous system.

LO 9.3 Spell medical terms related to the nervous system.

LO 9.4 Pronounce medical terms related to the nervous system.

LO 9.5 Describe diagnostic procedures utilized in neurology.

LO 9.6 Identify and describe disorders and pathological conditions related to the nervous system.

LO 9.7 Describe the therapeutic procedures and pharmacologic agents used in neurology.

LO 9.8 Apply knowledge of medical terms relating to neurology to documentation, medical records, and communication.

LO 9.9 Identify and correctly use abbreviations of terms used in neurology.

LO 9.10 Identify health professionals involved in the care of neurological patients.

The health professionals involved in the diagnosis and treatment of patients with problems in the nervous system include:

- **Neurologists,** who are medical doctors who specialize in disorders of the nervous system.
- **Neurosurgeons,** who are medical doctors who perform surgical procedures on the nervous system.
- **Electroneurodiagnostic technicians** (also called EEG technicians), who are professionals who operate specialized equipment that measures the electrical activity of the brain, spinal cord, and peripheral nervous system.

Section 9.1 Functions and Structure of the Nervous System

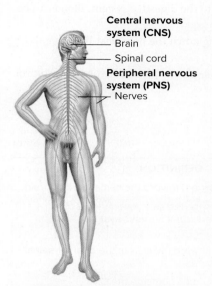

▲ Figure 9.1 The nervous system.

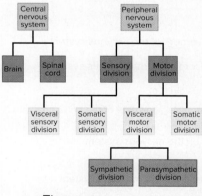

▲ Figure 9.2 Components of the nervous system.

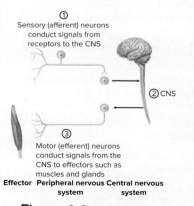

▲ Figure 9.3 Afferent and efferent neurons.

Functions of the Nervous System

Every time you stop to smell the roses, touch a petal, bend down, cut a stem, carry it indoors, place it in a vase, and admire its color, a wide range of sensations and actions are interpreted and controlled by your nervous system. The trillions of cells in your body must communicate and work together for you to function effectively. All this is done through your nervous system, and it is essential that you understand how this system operates. You can then understand how your body functions and maintains its homeostasis to respond to changes in your internal and external environments.

1. **Sensory input** to the brain comes from receptors all over the body at both the conscious and subconscious levels. Seeing the rose, touching it, smelling it, and noting your body position as you bend are external stimuli of which you are aware. Inside your body, internal stimuli about the amount of oxygen and carbon dioxide in your blood and other homeostatic variables are being continually processed at the subconscious level.

2. **Motor input** from the brain stimulates the skeletal muscles to contract and enables you to bend down, cut a stem, or move in any way. Smooth muscle in the walls of blood vessels contracts when stimulated by the nervous system. The production of sweat, saliva, and digestive enzymes is controlled by the nervous system.

3. **Evaluation and integration** occur in the brain to process the sensory input, initiate a motor response, and store the event in memory.

4. **Homeostasis** is maintained by the nervous system taking in internal sensory input and, for example, responding by stimulating the heart to deliver the correct volume of blood for oxygenation and removal of waste products.

5. **Mental activity** occurs in the brain so that you can think, feel, understand, respond, and remember.

Divisions (Components) of the Nervous System

The nervous system has two major anatomical subdivisions *(Figure 9.2):*

1. The **central nervous system** (CNS), consisting of the brain and spinal cord.

2. The **peripheral nervous system** (PNS) consisting of all the **neurons, nerves, ganglia,** and **plexuses** outside the central nervous system. It includes 12 pairs of cranial nerves originating from the brain and 31 pairs of spinal nerves originating from the spinal cord.

The PNS, in turn, is further subdivided into

a. **Sensory division,** in which sensory nerves (**afferent nerves**) carry messages toward the spinal cord and brain from sense organs *(Figure 9.3).* **Visceral nerves** carry signals from the viscera in the thoracic and abdominal cavities; for example, the heart and lungs and the stomach and intestines. **Somatic nerves** carry signals from the skin, muscles, bones, and joints.

b. Motor division, in which motor nerves (**efferent nerves**) carry messages away from the brain and spinal cord to muscles and organs.

    i. The visceral motor division is called the **autonomic nervous system (ANS).** It carries signals to glands and to cardiac and smooth muscle. It operates at a subconscious level outside voluntary control. It has two subdivisions:

        (1) The **sympathetic division** arouses the body for action; for example, by increasing the heart and respiratory rates to increase oxygen supply to brain and muscles. At the same time, it slows digestion, so less blood flow is needed to the digestive system. Blood can be directed where it is needed more.

        (2) The **parasympathetic division** calms the body, slowing down the heartbeat but stimulating digestion.

    ii. The **somatic motor division** carries signals to the skeletal muscles and is under voluntary control.

Word Analysis and Definition: Components of the Nervous System

S = Suffix   P = Prefix   R = Root   R/CF = Combining Form

WORD	PRONUNCIATION	ELEMENTS		DEFINITION
afferent	**AF**-eh-rent		Latin *to bring to*	Conducting impulses inward *toward* the spinal cord or brain
autonomic	awe-toh-**NOM**-ik	S/ P/ R/	**-ic** *pertaining to* **auto-** *self* **-nom-** *law*	Not voluntary; pertaining to the self-governing visceral motor division of the peripheral nervous system
efferent	**EF**-eh-rent		Latin *to bring away from*	Conducting impulses outward *away from* the brain or spinal cord
ganglion ganglia (pl)	**GANG**-lee-on **GANG**-lee-ah		Greek *swelling*	Collection of nerve cell bodies outside the CNS
motor	**MOH**-tor		Latin *to move*	Pertaining to nerves that send impulses out to cause muscles to contract or glands to secrete
nerve nervous (adj)	NERV **NER**-vus	S/ R/	Latin *nerve* **-ous** *pertaining to* **nerv-** *nerve*	A cord of fibers in connective tissue that conduct impulses Pertaining to nerves
neurology	nyu-**ROL**-oh-jee	S/ R/CF	**-logy** *study of* **neur/o-** *nerve*	Medical specialty of disorders of the nervous system
neurologist	nyu-**ROL**-oh-jist	S/	**-logist** *one who studies, specialist*	Medical specialist in disorders of the nervous system
neurologic (adj)	**NYUR**-oh-**LOJ**-ik	S/	**-ic** *pertaining to*	Pertaining to the nervous system
neuron	**NYUR**-on		Greek *nerve*	Technical term for a nerve cell; consists of the cell body with its dendrites and axons
neurosurgeon	**NYU**-roh-**SUR**-jun	S/ R/CF R/	**-eon** *one who does* **neur/o-** *nerve* **-surg-** *operate*	Specialist in operating on the nervous system
neurosurgery	**NYU**-roh-**SUR**-jer-ee	S/	**-ery** *process of*	Medical specialty in surgery of the nervous system
parasympathetic (**Note:** This term has two prefixes.)	par-ah-sim-pah-**THET**-ik	S/ P/ P/ R/	**-ic** *pertaining to* **para-** *beside* **-sym-** *together* **-pathet-** *suffering*	Pertaining to division of autonomic nervous system; has opposite effects of the sympathetic division
peripheral	peh-**RIF**-er-al	S/ R/	**-al** *pertaining to* **peripher-** *outer part*	Pertaining to the periphery or external boundary
plexus plexuses (pl)	**PLEK**-sus **PLEK**-sus-ez		Latin *braid*	A weblike network of joined nerves
sensory	**SEN**-soh-ree	S/ R/	**-ory** *having the function of* **sens-** *feel*	Having the function of sensation; relate *to structures of the nervous system that carry impulses to the brain*
somatic	soh-**MAT**-ik	S/ R/	**-ic** *pertaining to* **somat-** *body*	Pertaining to a division of the peripheral nervous system serving the skeletal muscles
sympathetic	sim-pah-**THET**-ik	S/ P/ R/	**-ic** *pertaining to* **sym-** *together* **-pathet-** *suffering*	Pertaining to the part of the autonomic nervous system operating at the unconscious level
visceral	**VISS**-er-al	S/ R/	**-al** *pertaining to* **viscer-** *internal organs*	Pertaining to the internal organs

Cells of the Nervous System

Neurons (nerve cells) receive stimuli and transmit impulses to other neurons or to receptors in other organs. Each neuron consists of a **cell body** and two types of processes or extensions, called **axons** and **dendrites** *(Figure 9.4)*.

Dendrites are short, highly branched extensions of the neuron's cell body. They conduct impulses toward the cell body. The more dendrites a neuron has, the more impulses it can receive from other neurons.

A single axon, or nerve fiber, arises from the cell body and carries impulses away from the cell body. Each axon has a constant diameter but can range in length from a few millimeters to a meter. The axon is covered in a fatty **myelin** sheath that is covered by a membrane called the **neurilemma.** The myelin sheath, like the plastic covering of electrical wire, enables the nerve impulse to travel faster.

The axon terminates in a network of small branches. Each branch ends in a **synaptic terminal** that forms a **synapse** (junction) with a dendrite from another neuron or with a receptor on a muscle cell or gland cell *(Figure 9.5)*. The synaptic terminals contain vesicles full of **neurotransmitters** that cross the synapse to stimulate or inhibit the receptor on a dendrite of another neuron or the cell of a muscle or gland. Examples of neurotransmitters are:

- **Acetylcholine**—stimulates muscle cells to contract.

- **Norepinephrine**—found in many areas of the brain and spinal cord; has a stimulatory effect that is increased by cocaine and amphetamines.

- **Serotonin**—found in many areas of the brain and spinal cord; is involved with mood, anxiety, and sleep.

- **Dopamine**—confined to small areas of the brain; plays a role in movement, memory, pleasurable reward, behavior and cognition, mood, and learning.

- **Endorphins**—found in areas around the brainstem; are the body's natural pain relievers.

Groups of cell bodies outside the CNS cluster together to form ganglia, and axons collect together to form nerves. Groups of nerves collect together to form a **plexus,** in which nerve fibers from different spinal nerves are sorted and recombined so that all the fibers (motor and sensory) going to a specific body part are located in a single nerve. The three plexuses are the **cervical plexus** to the neck, the **brachial plexus** to the arm, and the **lumbosacral plexus** to the pelvis and legs. *Figure 9.6* shows an example of a plexus, the brachial plexus, in which spinal nerves **C5** to **T1** unite to form three **trunks** that go on to supply the motor and sensory functions of the arm.

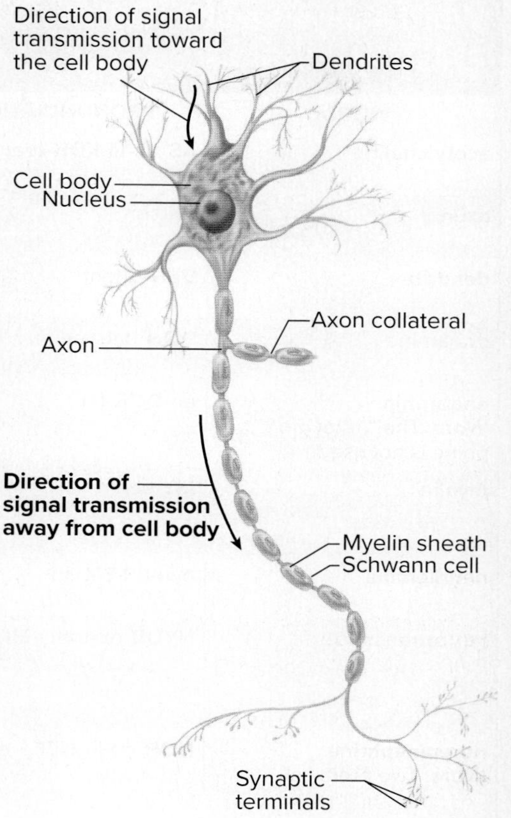

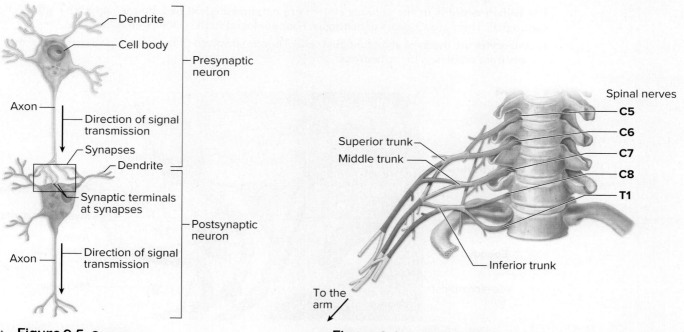

▲ **Figure 9.4** Neuron.

▲ **Figure 9.5** Synapse.

▲ **Figure 9.6** Brachial plexus.

WORD	PRONUNCIATION	ELEMENTS		DEFINITION
acetylcholine	**AS**-eh-til-**KOH**-leen	R/ R/	**acetyl-** *acetyl* **-choline** *choline*	Parasympathetic neurotransmitter
axon	**AK**-son		Greek *axis*	Single process of a nerve cell carrying nervous impulses away from the cell body
dendrite	**DEN**-dright		Greek *looking like a tree*	Branched extension of the nerve cell body that receives nervous stimuli
dopamine	**DOH**-pah-meen		Precursor of norepinephrine	Neurotransmitter in some specific small areas of the brain
endorphin (**Note:** The "m" of morphine is not used.)	en-**DOR**-fin	P/ R/	**end-** *within* **-morphin** *morphine*	Natural substance in the brain for pain relief
myelin	**MY**-eh-lin	S/ R/	**-in** *substance, chemical compound* **myel-** *spinal cord*	Material of the sheath around the axon of a nerve
neurilemma	nyu-ri-**LEM**-ah	S/ R/CF	**-lemma** *covering* **neur/i-** *nerve*	Covering of a nerve around the myelin sheath
neurotransmitter	**NYUR**-oh-trans-**MIT**-er	S/ P/ R/CF R/	**-er** *agent* **-trans-** *across* **neur/o-** *nerve* **-mitt-** *to send*	Chemical agent that relays messages from one nerve cell to the next
norepinephrine (**Note:** Two prefixes)	**NOR**-ep-ih-**NEF**-rin	S/ P/ P/ R/	**-ine** *pertaining to* **nor-** *normal* **-epi-** *upon, above* **-nephr-** *kidney*	Parasympathetic neurotransmitter
serotonin	ser-oh-**TOH**-nin	S/ R/CF R/	**-in** *chemical compound* **ser/o-** *serum, serous* **-ton-** *tension*	Neurotransmitter in the central and peripheral nervous systems
synapse synaptic (adj)	**SIN**-aps sih-**NAP**-tik	P/ R/	**syn-** *together* **-apse** *clasp*	Junction between two nerve cells, or a nerve fiber and its target cell; where electrical impulses are transmitted between the cells

Neuroglia

The trillion neurons in the nervous system are outnumbered 50 to 1 by the supportive **glial** cells (**neuroglia**). There are six types of neuroglia. Four are found in the CNS *(Figure 9.7)*:

1. **Astrocytes** are the most abundant glial cells. They are involved in the transportation of water and salts from capillaries to the neurons.

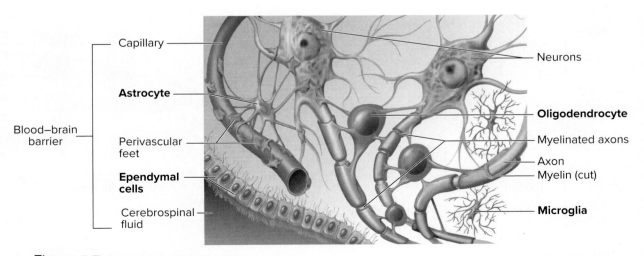

▲ **Figure 9.7** Neuroglial cells in the CNS.

2. **Oligodendrocytes** form the myelin sheaths around axons in the brain and spinal cord. Axons that have myelin sheaths are called *myelinated axons*. Bundles of these axons appear white and create the **white matter** of the brain and spinal cord. Neuron cell bodies, dendrites, and synapses appear gray and create the **gray matter.**

3. **Microglia** phagocytose bacteria and cell debris.

4. **Ependymal cells** line the central canal of the spinal cord and the ventricles of the brain. They help regulate the composition of the **cerebrospinal fluid (CSF).**

Two types of neuroglial cells are found in the PNS:

1. **Neurolemmocytes (Schwann cells)** form the myelin sheaths of the peripheral nerves that speed up signal conduction in the nerve fiber.

2. **Satellite cells** are found around the neuron cell bodies. Their function is unknown.

The **blood–brain barrier (BBB)** is a physical barrier between the capillaries that supply the CNS and most parts of the CNS. Astrocytes and the tight junctions between endothelial cells of the capillaries work together to prevent foreign substances, toxins, and infection from reaching the brain. Many medications are unable to pass this barrier, but alcohol gets through, producing its buzz and problems with coordination and cognition.

Word Analysis and Definition: Neuroglia

S = Suffix   P = Prefix   R = Root   R/CF = Combining Form

WORD	PRONUNCIATION		ELEMENTS	DEFINITION
astrocyte	**ASS**-troh-site	S/ R/CF	**-cyte** *cell* **astr/o-** *star*	Star-shaped connective tissue cell in the nervous system
blood–brain barrier (BBB)	BLUD BRAYN **BAIR**-ee-er		**blood** Old English *fluid connective tissue* **brain** Old English *organ that controls the functions of the body* **barrier** Old French *obstacle, gatekeeper*	A selective mechanism that protects the brain from toxins and infections
cerebrospinal	**SER**-eh-broh-**SPY**-nal	S/ R/CF R/	**-al** *pertaining to* **cerebr/o-** *brain* **-spin-** *spinal cord*	Pertaining to the brain and spinal cord
cerebrospinal fluid (CSF)	**SER**-eh-broh-**SPY**-nal **FLU**-id	R/	**fluid** *flowing*	Fluid formed in the ventricles of the brain; surrounds the brain and spinal cord
ependyma ependymal (adj)	ep-**EN**-dih-mah ep-**EN**-dih-mal		Greek *garment*	Membrane lining the central canal of the spinal cord and the ventricles of the brain
glia glial (adj) microglia	**GLEE**-ah **GLEE**-al my-**KROH**-glee-ah	 P/ R/	Greek *glue* **micro-** *small* **-glia** *glue, supportive tissue of the nervous system*	Connective tissue that holds a structure together Small nervous tissue cells that are phagocytes
neuroglia	nyur-**OH**-glee-ah	R/CF	**neur/o-** *nerve*	Connective tissue holding nervous tissue together
gray matter	GRAY **MATT**-er		**gray** Old English *color between white and black* **matter** Latin *a physical substance*	Regions of the brain and spinal cord occupied by cell bodies and dendrites
neurolemmocyte (same as Schwann cell)	**NYUR**-oh-**LEM**-oh-site SHWANN SELL	S/ R/CF R/CF	**-cyte** *cell* **neur/o-** *nerve* **-lemm/o** *rind, husk* Theodor Schwann, German anatomist, 1810–1882	Connective tissue cell of the peripheral nervous system that forms a myelin sheath
oligodendrocyte	**OL**-ih-goh-**DEN**- droh-site	S/ P/ R/CF	**-cyte** *cell* **oligo-** *scanty* **-dendr/o-** *treelike*	Connective tissue cell of the central nervous system that forms a myelin sheath
white matter	WITE **MATT**-er		**white** Old English *color opposite of black* **matter** Latin *a physical substance*	Regions of the brain and spinal cord occupied by bundles of axons

A. The nervous system has two major anatomical subdivisions, each with specialized functions. *Keep in mind that there are systems and divisions of systems. Use the precise* **language of neurology** *to answer the following questions.* **LO 9.1**

1. This division carries signals to the skeletal muscles and is under voluntary control:

    a. somatic motor division   **b.** somatic sensory division   **c.** autonomic motor division   **d.** autonomic sensory division

2. This system consists of the brain and spinal cord:

    a. central nervous system   **b.** peripheral nervous system

3. This division carries messages to the brain from the sensory organs:

    a. somatic motor division   **b.** somatic sensory division   **c.** autonomic motor division   **d.** autonomic sensory division

4. The visceral motor division is also called the

    a. peripheral   **b.** somatic   **c.** autonomic   **d.** ganglionic

5. This division arouses the body for action:

    a. parasympathic   **b.** sympathetic   **c.** somatic

6. This system consists of neurons, nerves, ganglia, and plexuses:

    a. central nervous system   **b.** peripheral nervous system

7. This division calms the body and slows the heartbeat:

    a. parasympathic   **b.** sympathetic   **c.** somatic

8. This division has efferent nerves to carry messages from the brain to muscles and organs:

    a. motor   **b.** sensory

B. Spelling is very important for every medical term. *Choose the correct spelling in the* **language of neurology.** **LO 9.1, 9.3**

1. Junction between two nerve cells:

    a. synapses   **b.** sinapse   **c.** synapse

2. The material of the sheath around a nerve axon:

    a. myelin   **b.** myalin   **c.** myeline

3. Branched extension of the nerve cell body that receives an impulse:

    a. denderite   **b.** dendrite   **c.** dendryte

4. Chemical agent that relays messages:

    a. neutrontransmitter   **b.** neurontransmiter   **c.** neurotransmitter

5. Covering of a nerve around the sheath:

    a. neurelemma   **b.** neurilemmia   **c.** neurilemma

C. Using the terms relating to the cells of the nervous system, fill in the blanks in the following questions and statements. **LO 9.1, 9.3**

1. The neurotransmitter that is a natural pain reliever. _____

2. Which part of the neuron carries impulses away from the cell body? _____

3. Which term comes from the Greek language meaning *looking like a tree*? _____

D. Identify the correct meaning for each element. *Knowing the definitions of elements is your key to unlocking the meaning of medical terms. Match the element in the left column with its correct meaning in the right column.* **LO 9.2**

_____ 1. *oligo-*

_____ 2. *glia*

_____ 3. *cerebr/o*

_____ 4. *astr/o*

_____ 5. *spin*

_____ 6. *-cyte*

_____ 7. *dendr/o*

a. cell

b. spinal cord

c. treelike

d. scanty

e. brain

f. glue

g. star

Section 9.2 The Brain and Cranial Nerves

Brain

Smelling the roses, seeing them, and touching them are recognized and interpreted in the brain, as are all sensations. The actions of bending down, cutting the rose stem, walking into the house, and placing it in a vase originate in the brain, as do all our voluntary actions. The integration of a sensory stimulus with a motor response occurs in the brain. The brain is the control center for many of the body's functions. The brain carries out the higher mental functions, such as reasoning, planning, forming ideas, and all aspects of memory. The adult brain weighs about 3 pounds. Its size and weight are proportional to body size, not intelligence.

The brain is divided into three major regions: the **cerebrum,** the **brainstem,** and the **cerebellum.**

The cerebrum is about 80% of the brain and consists of two **cerebral hemispheres** that are anatomically mirror images of each other *(Figure 9.8).* They are separated by a deep longitudinal fissure, at the bottom of which they are connected by a bridge of nerve fibers called the **corpus callosum.**

On the surface of the cerebrum, numerous ridges **(gyri)** are separated by grooves called **sulci.**

Each cerebral hemisphere is divided into four **lobes** *(see Figure 9.8a):*

1. The **frontal lobe** is located behind the forehead. It forms the anterior part of the hemisphere. It is responsible for memory, intellect, concentration, problem solving, emotion, and the planning and execution of behavior, including voluntary motor control of muscles.

2. The **parietal lobe,** located above the ear, is posterior to the frontal lobe. The parietal lobe receives and interprets sensations of pain, pressure, touch, temperature, and body part awareness.

3. The **temporal lobe,** located behind the ear, is below the frontal and parietal lobes. The temporal lobe is involved in interpreting sensory experiences, sounds, and spoken words.

4. The **occipital lobe,** located at the back of the head, forms the posterior part of the hemisphere. The occipital lobe interprets visual images and the written word.

The cerebral hemispheres are covered by a thin layer of gray matter (unmyelinated nerve fibers) called the **cerebral cortex.** It is folded into the gyri, sulci, and fissures and contains 70% of all the neurons in the nervous system. Below the cerebral cortex is a mass of white matter, in which bundles of myelinated nerve fibers connect the neurons of the cortex to the rest of the nervous system.

The **brain stem** relays sensory impulses from peripheral nerves to higher brain centers. It also controls vital cardiovascular and respiratory functions.

The **cerebellum,** the most posterior area of the brain, coordinates skeletal muscle activity to maintain the body's posture and balance.

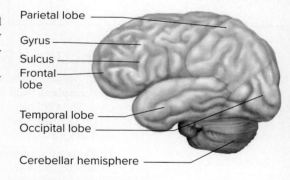

Parietal lobe

Gyrus

Sulcus

Frontal lobe

Temporal lobe

Occipital lobe

Cerebellar hemisphere

(a) View from left side

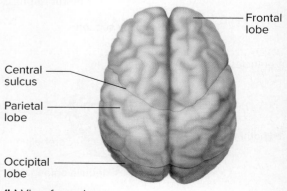

Frontal lobe

Central sulcus

Parietal lobe

Occipital lobe

(b) View from above

▲ **Figure 9.8** Brain.

Word Analysis and Definition: The Brain

S = Suffix   P = Prefix   R = Root   R/CF = Combining Form

WORD	PRONUNCIATION		ELEMENTS	DEFINITION
brainstem	**BRAYN**-stem		brain Old English *brain* stem Old English *support*	Region of the brain that includes the thalamus, pineal gland, pons, fourth ventricle, and medulla oblongata
cerebellum	ser-eh-**BELL**-um	S/ R/	**-um** *structure* **cerebell-** *little brain*	The most posterior area of the brain
cerebrum cerebral (adj)	**SER**-eh-brum **SER**-eh-bral *or* ser-**EE**-bral	S/ R/	Latin *brain* **-al** *pertaining to* **cerebr-** *brain*	The major portion of the brain divided into two hemi-spheres (cerebral hemispheres) separated by a fissure Pertaining to the brain
corpus callosum	**KOR**-pus kah-**LOH**-sum	S/ R/	corpus Latin *body* **-um** *structure* **callos-** *thickening*	Bridge of nerve fibers connecting the two cerebral hemispheres
cortex cortical (adj)	**KOR**-teks **KOR**-tih-kal		Latin *shell*	Gray covering of cerebral hemispheres
frontal lobe	**FRON**-tal LOBE	S/ R/	**-al** *pertaining to* **front-** *forehead* lobe Greek *lobe*	Area of brain behind the forehead
gyrus gyri (pl)	**JIE**-rus **JIE**-ree		Greek *circle*	Rounded elevation on the surface of the cerebral hemispheres
occipital lobe	ok-**SIP**-it-al LOBE	S/ R/	**-al** *pertaining to* **occipit-** *back of head* lobe Greek *lobe*	Posterior area of cerebral hemispheres
parietal lobe	pah-**RYE**-eh-tal LOBE	S/ R/	**-al** *pertaining to* **pariet-** *wall* lobe Greek *lobe*	Area of brain above the ear
sulcus sulci (pl)	**SUL**-cuss **SUL**-sigh		Latin *furrow, ditch*	Groove on the surface of the cerebral hemispheres that separates gyri
temporal lobe	**TEM**-por-al LOBE	S/ R/	**-al** *pertaining to* **tempor-** *temple, side of head* lobe Greek *lobe*	Posterior two-thirds of cerebral hemispheres

Functional Brain Regions

Deep inside each cerebral hemisphere are spaces called **ventricles.** They contain the watery **cerebrospinal fluid (CSF),** which circulates through the ventricles and around the brain and spinal cord. The CSF helps protect, cushion, and provide nutrition for the brain and spinal cord.

Underneath the cerebral hemispheres and the ventricles are important regions of the brain *(Figures 9.9 and 9.10):*

1. **Thalamus**—receives all sensory impulses and channels them to the appropriate region of the cortex for interpretation. As the sensory fibers carrying impulses pass through the thalamus, they **decussate** (cross over) so that the impulses from the left side of the body go to the right brain, and impulses coming from the right side of the body go to the left brain. Similarly, motor impulses coming from the right brain decussate and supply the left side of the body, and motor impulses coming from the left brain decussate and supply the right side of the body. If a lesion caused by a stroke is in the right brain, the left side of the body will be affected, and vice versa.

2. The **hypothalamus** regulates
   a. Blood pressure
   b. Body temperature
   c. Water and electrolyte balance
   d. Hunger and body weight
   e. Sleep and wakefulness
   f. Movements and secretions of the digestive tract

3. The **basal nuclei** are collections of gray matter lateral to the thalamus that aid in controlling the amplitude of our voluntary muscular movements and posture, as well as playing a part in emotion and cognition.

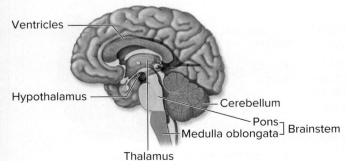

Midsagittal section

Ventricles — Hypothalamus — Cerebellum — Pons — Medulla oblongata — Brainstem — Thalamus

▲ **Figure 9.9** Lateral view of functional regions of brain.

4. The **limbic system** controls emotional experience, fear, anger, pleasure, and sadness.
5. The **brainstem** *(Figure 9.9)* contains two major areas:
   a. The **pons** *(Figure 9.9)*, which relays sensory impulses from peripheral nerves to higher brain centers.
   b. The **medulla oblongata** *(Figure 9.9)*, within which nuclei of gray matter form centers to control vital visceral activities, such as:
      i. **Cardiac center**—regulates heart rate.
      ii. **Respiratory center**—regulates breathing.
      iii. **Vasomotor center**—regulates vasoconstriction and vasodilation of blood vessels.
      iv. **Reticular formation**—responds to sensory impulses by arousing the cerebral cortex into wakefulness.

The most posterior area of the brain, the cerebellum *(Figures 9.9 and 9.10)*, coordinates skeletal muscle activity to maintain posture and balance.

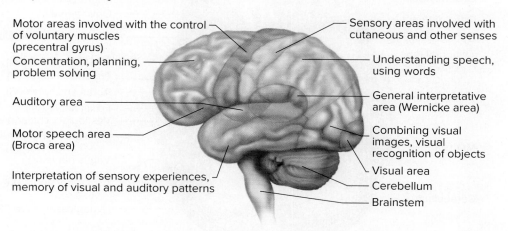

Motor areas involved with the control of voluntary muscles (precentral gyrus)
Concentration, planning, problem solving
Auditory area
Motor speech area (Broca area)
Interpretation of sensory experiences, memory of visual and auditory patterns
Sensory areas involved with cutaneous and other senses
Understanding speech, using words
General interpretative area (Wernicke area)
Combining visual images, visual recognition of objects
Visual area
Cerebellum
Brainstem

▲ **Figure 9.10** Cerebral cortex, functional regions.

Word Analysis and Definition: Brain Regions

S = Suffix   P = Prefix   R = Root   R/CF = Combining Form

WORD	PRONUNCIATION		ELEMENTS	DEFINITION
brainstem	**BRAYN**-stem		**brain** Old English *brain* **stem** Old English *support*	Region of the brain that includes the thalamus, pineal gland, pons, fourth ventricle, and medulla oblongata
decussate	**DEH**-keh-sayt		Latin *to make in the form of a cross*	Cross over like the arms of an "X"
hypothalamus	high-poh-**THAL**-ah-muss	S/ P/ R/	-us *pertaining to* hypo- *below* -thalam- *thalamus*	Area of gray matter forming part of the walls and floor of the third ventricle
hypothalamic (adj)	high-poh-tha-**LAM**-ik	S/	-ic *pertaining to*	Pertaining to the hypothalamus
limbic	**LIM**-bic		Latin *border*	Pertaining to the limbic system, which controls vital functions of breathing, heartbeat, and blood pressure
medulla oblongata	meh-**DULL**-ah ob-lon-**GAH**-tah	R/ S/ R/	**medulla** *middle* -ata *place* **oblong-** *elongated*	Most posterior subdivision of the brainstem, continuation of the spinal cord
pons	PONZ		Latin *bridge*	Relays sensory information from the peripheral nerves to different areas of the brain
reticulum	reh-**TIK**-you-lum	S/ R/	-um *structure* **reticul-** *fine net*	Fine network of cells in the medulla oblongata
reticular (adj)	reh-**TIK**-you-lar	S/	-ar *pertaining to*	Pertaining to the reticulum
thalamus	**THAL**-ah-mus		Greek *inner room*	Relays sensory information to the cerebral cortex
ventricle ventricular (adj)	**VEN**-trih-kel ven-**TRIK**-you-lar	S/ R/	Latin *belly* -ar *pertaining to* **ventricul-** *ventricle*	A cavity of the heart or brain Pertaining to a ventricle

Table 9.1 Mnemonic for the Cranial Nerves

Oh	(olfactory–I)
once	(optic–II)
one	(oculomotor–III)
takes	(trochlear–IV)
the	(trigeminal–V)
anatomy	(abducens–VI)
final	(facial–VII)
very	(vestibulocochlear–VIII)
good	(glossopharyngeal–IX)
vacations	(vagus–X)
are	(accessory–XI)
heavenly!	(hypoglossal–XII)

Cranial Nerves

To function, the brain must communicate with the rest of the body, and it does this through the spinal cord and the **cranial nerves.** Twelve pairs of cranial nerves arise from the base of the brain (*Figure 9.11*). A mnemonic to help you remember their names is in *Table 9.1*.

The two pairs of nerves for smell and vision contain only sensory fibers. The other 10 pairs are mixed nerves containing sensory, motor, and parasympathetic fibers. The cranial nerves have, from front to back, both names and numbers. The latter are always written in Roman numerals (*Table 9.2*).

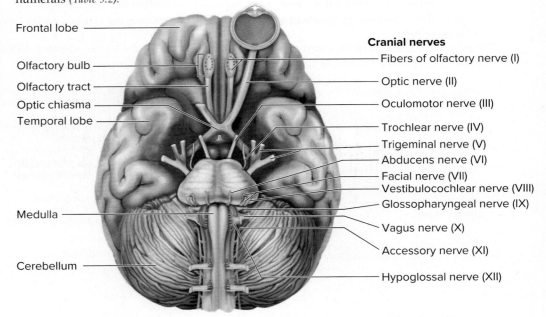

▶ **Figure 9.11 Cranial nerves.** Base of brain showing origins of the 12 cranial nerves.

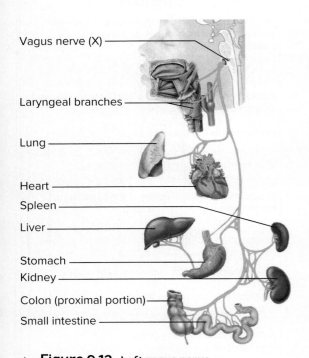

▲ **Figure 9.12 Left vagus nerve.**

Table 9.2 Cranial Nerves

Roman Numeral	Name	Description
I	**Olfactory** nerves	Sensory nerves for smell
II	**Optic** nerves	Sensory nerves for vision
III	**Oculomotor** nerves	Predominantly motor nerves for eye movement and pupil size
IV	**Trochlear** nerves	Predominantly motor nerves for eye movement
V	**Trigeminal** nerves	Sensory and motor nerves responsible for face, nose, and mouth sensations and for chewing
VI	**Abducens** nerves	Predominantly motor nerves responsible for eye movement
VII	**Facial** nerves	Mixed nerves associated with taste (sensory), facial expression (motor), and production of tears and saliva (parasympathetic fibers of motor nerves)
VIII	**Vestibulocochlear (auditory)** nerves	Predominantly sensory nerves associated with hearing and balance
IX	**Glossopharyngeal** nerves	Mixed nerves for sensation and swallowing in the pharynx
X	**Vagus** nerves	Mixed sensory and parasympathetic nerves supplying the pharynx, larynx (speech), and the viscera of the thorax and abdomen (*Figure 9.12*)
XI	**Accessory** nerves	Predominantly motor nerves supplying neck muscles, pharynx, and larynx
XII	**Hypoglossal** nerves	Predominantly motor nerves that move the tongue in speaking, chewing, and swallowing

WORD	PRONUNCIATION	ELEMENTS		DEFINITION
abducens	ab-**DYU**-senz		Latin *abduct, draw away from*	Sixth (VI) cranial nerve; responsible for eye movement
accessory	ak-**SESS**-oh-ree		Latin *move toward*	Eleventh (XI) cranial nerve; supplying neck muscles, pharynx, and larynx
auditory	**AW**-dih-tor-ee	S/ R/	**-ory** *having the function of* **audit-** *hearing*	Pertaining to the sense of or the organs of hearing
cranial	**KRAY**-nee-al	S/ R/	**-al** *pertaining to* **crani-** *skull, cranium*	Pertaining to the skull
facial	**FAY**-shal		Latin *face*	Seventh (VII) cranial nerve; supplying the forehead, nose, eyes, mouth, and jaws
glossopharyngeal	**GLOSS**-oh-fah-**RIN**-jee-al	S/ R/CF R/	**-eal** *pertaining to* **gloss/o-** *tongue* **-pharyng-** *pharynx*	Ninth (IX) cranial nerve; supplying the tongue and pharynx
hypoglossal	high-poh-**GLOSS**-al	S/ P/ R/	**-al** *pertaining to* **hypo-** *below, under* **-gloss** *tongue*	Twelfth (XII) cranial nerve; supplying muscles of the tongue
oculomotor	**OK**-you-loh-**MOH**-tor	S/ R/CF R/	**-or** *doer* **ocul/o-** *eye* **-mot-** *move*	Third (III) cranial nerve; moves the eye
olfactory	ol-**FAK**-toh-ree	S/ R/	**-ory** *having the function of* **olfact-** *smell*	First (I) cranial nerve; carries information related to the sense of smell
optic	**OP**-tik	S/ R/	**-ic** *pertaining to* **opt-** *eye*	Second (II) cranial nerve; carries visual information
trigeminal	try-**GEM**-in-al	S/ P/ R/	**-al** *pertaining to* **tri-** *three* **-gemin-** *double, twin*	Fifth (V) cranial nerve, with its three different branches supplying the face
trochlear	**TROHK**-lee-ar	S/ R/	**-ar** *pertaining to* **trochle-** *pulley*	Fourth (IV) cranial nerve; supplies one muscle of the eye
vagus	**VAY**-gus		Latin *to wander*	Tenth (X) cranial nerve; supplies many different organs throughout the body
vestibulocochlear (**Note:** This term starts with a combining form, not a prefix.)	ves-**TIB**-you-loh-**KOK**-lee-ar	S/ R/CF R/	**-ar** *pertaining to* **vestibul/o-** *vestibule of inner ear* **-cochle-** *cochlea*	Eighth (VIII) cranial nerve; carrying information for the senses of hearing and balance

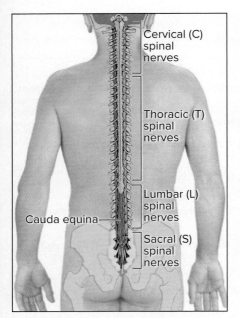

▲ **Figure 9.13** Spinal cord regions.

Cervical (C) spinal nerves

Thoracic (T) spinal nerves

Lumbar (L) spinal nerves

Cauda equina

Sacral (S) spinal nerves

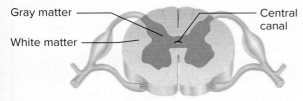

Gray matter

White matter

Central canal

▲ **Figure 9.14** Cross-section of spinal cord.

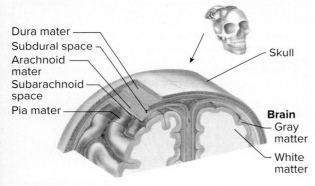

Dura mater
Subdural space
Arachnoid mater
Subarachnoid space
Pia mater

Skull

Brain
Gray matter
White matter

▲ **Figure 9.15** Meninges of the brain.

Spinal Cord and Meninges

Spinal Cord

This part of the central nervous system consists of 31 segments, each of which gives rise to a pair of spinal nerves. These are the major link between the brain and the peripheral nervous system and are a pathway for sensory and motor impulses. The spinal cord occupies the upper two-thirds of the vertebral canal, extending from the base of the skull to the first lumbar vertebra. From here, a group of nerve fibers continues down the vertebral canal and is called the **cauda equina.** The spinal cord is divided into four regions *(Figure 9.13)*:

1. The **cervical region** is continuous with the medulla oblongata. It contains the motor neurons that supply the neck, shoulders, and upper limbs through eight pairs of cervical spinal nerves (**C1–C8**).

2. The **thoracic region** contains the motor neurons that supply the thoracic cage, rib movement, vertebral column movement, and postural back muscles through 12 pairs of thoracic spinal nerves (**T1–T12**).

3. The **lumbar region** supplies the hips and front of the lower limbs through five pairs of lumbar nerves (**L1–L5**).

4. The **sacral region** supplies the buttocks, genitalia, and backs of the legs through five sacral nerves (**S1–S5**) and one coccygeal nerve.

A cross-section of the spinal cord *(Figure 9.14)* reveals that it has a core of gray matter shaped like a butterfly surrounded by white matter. In the center of the gray matter is the central canal that contains CSF. The gray matter contains the axons of sensory neurons bringing impulses into the cord and the neurons of motor nerves that send impulses out to skeletal muscles.

The white matter contains myelinated nerve fibers organized into **tracts** that conduct either sensory impulses up the cord to the brain or motor impulses down the cord from the brain.

All individual spinal nerves except C1 supply a specific segment of skin called a **dermatome.** Each spinal nerve, except for C1, exits and enters the spinal cord through an **intervertebral** space. Cervical nerve one passes between a space between the skull and the first vertebra.

Meninges

The brain and spinal cord are protected by the cranium and the vertebrae, cushioned by the CSF, and covered by the **meninges** *(Figure 9.15)*. The meninges have three layers:

1. **Dura mater**—the outermost layer, composed of tough connective tissue attached to the inner surface of the cranium but separated from the vertebral canal by the **epidural space,** into which **epidural** injections are introduced.

2. **Arachnoid mater**—a thin web over the brain and spinal cord. The CSF is contained in the **subarachnoid space** between the arachnoid and pia mater.

3. **Pia mater**—the innermost layer of the meninges, attached to the surface of the brain and spinal cord. It supplies nerves and blood vessels that nourish the outer cells of the brain and spinal cord.

Word Analysis and Definition: Spinal Cord and Meninges

S = Suffix   P = Prefix   R = Root   R/CF = Combining Form

WORD	PRONUNCIATION	ELEMENTS		DEFINITION
arachnoid mater	ah-**RAK**-noyd **MAY**-ter	S/ R/ R/	**-oid** *resembling* **arachn-** *cobweb, spider* **mater** *mother*	Weblike middle layer of the three meninges
cauda equina (***Note:*** Both these terms are stand-alone combining forms.)	**KAW**-dah eh-**KWIE**-nah	R/CF R/CF	**caud/a** *tail* **equin/a** *horse*	Bundle of spinal nerves in the vertebral canal below the ending of the spinal cord
cervical (***Note:*** Cervical also is used to refer to a region of the uterus.)	**SER**-vih-kal	S/ R/	**-al** *pertaining to* **cervic-** *neck*	Pertaining to the neck region
dermatome	**DER**-mah-tome	S/ R/CF	**-tome** *instrument to cut* **derm/a-** *skin*	The area of skin supplied by a single spinal nerve; alternatively, an instrument used for cutting thin slices
dura mater (***Note:*** Both terms are stand-alone roots.)	**DYU**-rah **MAY**-ter	R/CF R/	**dur/a** *hard* **mater** *mother*	Hard, fibrous outer layer of the meninges
epidural epidural space	ep-ih-**DYU**-ral ep-ih-**DYU**-ral SPASE	S/ P/ R/	**-al** *pertaining to* **epi-** *above* **-dur-** *dura mater*	Above the dura Space between the dura mater and the wall of the vertebral canal or skull
intervertebral	**IN**-ter-**VER**-teh-bral	S/ P/ R/	**-al** *pertaining to* **inter-** *between* **-vertebr-** *vertebra*	The space between two vertebrae
lumbar	**LUM**-bar		Latin *loins*	Pertaining to the region in the back and sides between the ribs and pelvis
meninges	meh-**NIN**-jeez		Greek *membrane*	Three-layered covering of the brain and spinal cord
pia mater (***Note:*** Both these terms are stand-alone roots.)	**PEE**-ah **MAY**-ter	R/ R/	**pia** *delicate* **mater** *mother*	Delicate inner layer of the meninges
sacral	**SAY**-kral	S/ R/	**-al** *pertaining to* **sacr-** *sacrum*	In the neighborhood of the sacrum
subarachnoid space	sub-ah-**RAK**-noyd SPASE	S/ P/ R/	**-oid** *resembling* **sub-** *under* **-arachn-** *cobweb, spider*	Space between the pia mater and the arachnoid mater
thoracic	thor-**ASS**-ik	S/ R/	**-ic** *pertaining to* **thorac-** *chest*	Pertaining to the chest (thorax)
tract	TRAKT		Latin *draw out*	Bundle of nerve fibers with common origin and destination

Check Point Section 9.2

A. Roots. *The lobes of the cerebral hemispheres share a common suffix -al, meaning pertaining to. It is the root that describes the exact location of the lobe in the cerebral hemispheres. Use your knowledge of roots to understand the anatomical location of the lobes. Fill in the blanks.* **LO 9.1**

1. The cerebral lobe located above the ear: _____ /al.   The root means _____ .

2. The cerebral lobe located behind the forehead: _____ /al. The root means _____ .

3. The most posterior cerebral lobe: _____ /al. The root means: _____ .

B. Describe the structure of the cerebrum. *Identify the cerebral structures being described. Fill in the blanks.* **LO 9.1, 9.3**

1. Elevation or "wrinkle" of the cerebrum:

   singular form _____

   plural form _____ .

2. Gray covering of the cerebrum: _____ .

3. Shallow indention of the cerebrum:

   singular form _____

   plural form _____ .

C. Latin and Greek terms cannot be deconstructed into prefix, root, and suffix. *You must know them for what they are. Test your knowledge of these terms with the following exercise. Match the terms in the left column to their correct meaning in the right column.* **LO 9.1**

_____ 1. thalamus   **a.** bridge

_____ 2. decussate   **b.** inner room

_____ 3. limbic   **c.** border

_____ 4. pons   **d.** cross over

D. Identify the areas of the brain that control the body's involuntary actions. *Fill in the blanks.* **LO 9.1**

cardiac   **respiratory**   **vasomotor**   **reticular formation**   **medulla oblongata**

1. What is the center of the brain that controls vital and visceral activity?

   _____

2. What part of the brain regulates heartbeat?

   _____

3. What responds to sensory impulses by arousing the cerebral cortex into wakefulness?

   _____

4. Where in the brain is breathing regulated?

   _____

5. What regulates vasoconstriction and vasodilation of blood vessels?

   _____

E. Elements. *Continue your work with elements to help build your knowledge of the language of neurology. One element in each of the following medical terms is set in bold. Identify the type of element (prefix, root, root/combining form, suffix) in the first column; then write the meaning of the element in the second column, and the function of the nerve: sensory, motor, or mixed (meaning both sensory and motor functions) in the right column. Fill in the chart.* **LO 9.1, 9.2**

Medical Term	Type of Element	Meaning of Element	Function
*glosso***pharynge***al*	1.	2.	3.
tri*geminal*	4.	5.	6.
audit*ory*	7.	8.	9.
olfact*ory*	10.	11.	12.

F. Place the meninges in order from superficial to deep. *Place a "1" in the blank for the most superficial layer and "3" for the deepest layer.* **LO 9.1**

_____ arachnoid mater

_____ pia mater

_____ dura mater

Section 9.3 Disorders of the Brain and Cranial Nerves

Disorders of the Brain

Dementia

Dementia is *not* a normal part of aging and is *not* a specific disease. It is a term used for a collection of symptoms that can be caused by a number of disorders affecting the brain.

Alzheimer disease is the most common form of dementia. It affects 10% of the population over 65% and 50% of the population over 85. Neurons in the areas of the brain associated with memory and **cognition** are replaced by abnormal clumps and tangles of a protein *(Figure 9.16)*.

Vascular dementia is the second most common form of dementia. It can come on gradually when arteries supplying the brain become arteriosclerotic (narrowed or blocked), depriving the brain of oxygen, or can occur suddenly after a **stroke** *(see Chapter 7)*.

Confusion is used to describe people who cannot process information normally. For example, they cannot answer questions appropriately, understand where they are, or remember important facts. Confusion is often part of dementia or delirium.

Delirium is the sudden onset of disorientation, an inability to think clearly or pay attention. There is a change in the level of **consciousness,** varying from increased wakefulness to drowsiness. It is a mental state, not a disease. It can be part of dementia or a stroke.

Other conditions causing dementia are often treatable. They include:

- **Reactions to medications** (e.g., sedatives, antiarthritics). Remove or lower the dose of the medication.
- **Metabolic abnormalities** (e.g., hypoglycemia). Correct the metabolic abnormality.
- **Nutritional deficiencies** (e.g., vitamins B_1 and B_6). Remedy the nutritional deficiency.
- **Emotional problems** (e.g., depression in the elderly). Use behavioral therapy or antidepressives.
- **Infections** (e.g., AIDS, encephalitis). Treat the underlying infection.

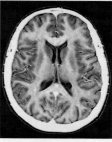

(a)

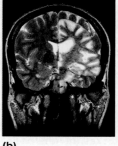

(b)

▲ **Figure 9.16** **Brain sections.** (*a*) MRI scan of normal brain. (*b*) MRI scan of Alzheimer disease showing cerebral atrophy (yellow). Medical Body Scans/Science Source; Jessica Wilson/Medical Body Scans/Science Source

Word Analysis and Definition: Disorders of the Brain

S = Suffix   P = Prefix   R = Root   R/CF = Combining Form

WORD	PRONUNCIATION		ELEMENTS	DEFINITION
Alzheimer disease	**OLTS**-high-mer diz-**EEZ**		Alois Alzheimer, German neurologist, 1864–1915	Common form of dementia; brain tissue has protein clumps and tangles
cognition	kog-**NIH**-shun		Latin *knowledge*	Process of acquiring knowledge through thinking, learning, and memory
cognitive (adj)	**KOG**-nih-tiv	S/	-ive *nature of, quality of pertaining to*	Pertaining to the mental activities of thinking and learning
		R/	cognit- *thinking*	
confusion	kon-**FEW**-zhun	S/	-ion *action, condition*	Mental state in which environmental stimuli are not processed appropriately
		R/	confus- *bewildered*	
conscious consciousness	**KON**-shus **KON**-shus-ness	S/	Latin *to be aware* -ness *quality, state*	Having present knowledge of oneself and one's surroundings The state of being aware of and responsive to the environment
		R/	conscious- *aware*	
unconscious	un-**KON**-shus	P/	un- *not*	Not conscious, lacking awareness
delirium	deh-**LIR**-ee-um	S/	-um *structure*	Acute altered state of consciousness with agitation and disorientation; condition is reversible
		R/	deliri- *confusion, disorientation*	
dementia	dee-**MEN**-shee-ah	S/	-ia *condition*	Chronic, progressive, irreversible loss of the mind's cognitive and intellectual functions
		P/	de- *without*	
		R/	-ment- *mind*	

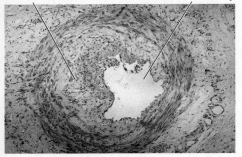

Atherosclerosis   Residual lumen of artery

(a)

Cerebrovascular Accidents (CVAs) or Strokes

A **stroke** (also known as a **cerebrovascular accident,** or **CVA**) occurs when the blood supply to a part of the brain is suddenly interrupted and thus brain cells are deprived of oxygen *(see Chapter 10).* Some cells die; others are left badly damaged. With timely treatment, the damaged cells can be saved. There are two types of stroke:

1. **Ischemic strokes** account for 90% of all strokes and are caused by:

   a. **Atherosclerosis**—plaque in the wall of a cerebral artery *(Figure 9.17a).*

   b. **Embolism**—blood clot in a cerebral artery originating from elsewhere in the body *(Figure 9.17b).*

   c. **Microangiopathy**—occlusion of small cerebral arteries.

2. **Hemorrhagic strokes (intracerebral hemorrhage)** occur when a blood vessel in the brain bursts or when a cerebral **aneurysm** or **arteriovenous malformation** (**AVM**) ruptures.

Symptoms of Strokes

The symptoms of a stroke can include the sudden onset of numbness or weakness, especially on one side of the body; difficulty in walking, balance, or coordination; trouble speaking or understanding speech; trouble seeing in one or both eyes; dizziness; confusion; and severe headache. A method to remember common warning signs of stroke is to use the acronym FAST:

Face—Ask the person to smile. Does one side of the Face droop?

Arms—Ask the person to raise both arms. Does one Arm drift downward?

Speech—Ask the person to repeat a simple phrase. Is his or her Speech slurred or strange?

Time—If any of the previous signs is present, Time to call 911 immediately.

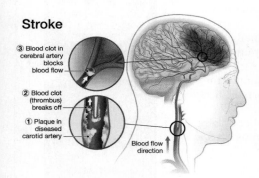

Stroke

③ Blood clot in cerebral artery blocks blood flow

② Blood clot (thrombus) breaks off

① Plaque in diseased carotid artery

Blood flow direction

(b)

▲ **Figure 9.17** **Causes of ischemic strokes.** (*a*) Atherosclerosis in a cerebral artery leaving a small, residual lumen. (*b*) Embolus blocking an artery. Healthy tissue is on the left (tan); blood-starved tissue is on the right (gray). Wellcome Photo Library; Axel_Kock/Shutterstock

Disability after Strokes

Although stroke is a disease of the brain, it can affect the whole body. A common residual disability is complete paralysis of one side of the body, called **hemiplegia.** If one side of the body is weak rather than paralyzed, the disability is called **hemiparesis.** Problems with forming and understanding speech and problems with awareness, attention, learning, judgment, and memory can remain after a stroke. Stroke patients may have difficulty controlling their emotions and may experience depression. All of these disabilities require well-planned rehabilitation.

Transient Ischemic Attack

Transient ischemic attacks (TIAs) are short-term, small strokes with symptoms lasting for less than 24 hours. If neurologic symptoms persist for more than 24 hours, then it is a full-blown stroke with brain cell damage and death.

The most frequent cause is a small **embolus** that occludes a small artery in the brain. Often, the embolus arises from a clot in the atrium in atrial fibrillation or from an atherosclerotic plaque in a carotid artery. If the impairment of blood supply lasts more than a few minutes, the affected nerve cells can die and cause permanent neurologic deficit.

Did you know...

- Risk factors for **ischemic strokes** are hypertension, diabetes mellitus, high cholesterol levels, cigarettes, and obesity.

- Risk factors for **hemorrhagic strokes** are hypertension, cerebral arteriovenous malformations, and cerebral aneurysms.

- More than 10% of people who have a TIA will have a stroke within 3 months.

WORD	PRONUNCIATION	ELEMENTS		DEFINITION
aneurysm aneurysmal (adj)	**AN**-yur-izm		Greek *dilation*	Circumscribed dilation of an artery or cardiac chamber
arteriovenous malformation	ar-**TEER**-ee-oh-**VEE**-nus mal-for-**MAY**-shun	S/ R/CF R/ S/ P/ R/	-ous *pertaining to* arteri/o- *artery* -ven- *vein* -ion *process* mal- *bad* -format- *to form*	An abnormal communication between an artery and a vein
cerebrovascular accident (*Note:* also known as a stroke)	**SER**-eh-broh-**VAS**-cyoo-lar **AK**-si-dent STROHK	S/ R/CF R/	-ar *pertaining to* cerebr/o- *brain* -vascul- *blood vessel* French *accident, what comes by chance*	Acute clinical event caused by an impaired cerebral circulation
embolus emboli (pl)	**EM**-boh-lus		Greek *plug, stopped*	Detached piece of thrombus, a mass of bacteria, quantity of air, or foreign body that blocks a blood vessel
hemiparesis	**HEM**-ee-pah-**REE**-sis	P/ R/	hemi- *half* -paresis *weakness*	Weakness of one side of the body
hemiplegia hemiplegic (adj)	hem-ee-**PLEE**-jee-ah hem-ee-**PLEE**-jik	S/ P/ R/ S/	-ia *condition* hemi- *half* -pleg- *paralysis* -ic *pertaining to*	Paralysis of one side of the body Pertaining to or suffering from hemiplegia
ischemia ischemic (adj)	is-**KEE**-mee-ah is-**KEE**-mik	S/ R/ S/	-emia *blood condition* isch- *to keep back* -emic *in the blood*	Lack of blood supply to a tissue Pertaining to or affected by ischemia
microangiopathy	**MY**-kroh-an-jee-**OP**-ah-thee	S/ P/ R/CF	-pathy *disease* micro- *small* -angi/o- *blood vessel*	Disease of the very small blood vessels (capillaries)

Cerebral Palsy

Definition

Cerebral palsy (CP) is the term used to describe the motor **impairment** resulting from brain damage in an infant or young child, regardless of the cause or the effect on the child. It is not hereditary. In congenital CP, the cause is often unknown but can be brain malformations or maternal use of cocaine; CP developed at birth or in the neonatal period is usually related to an incident causing hypoxia of the brain. Cerebral palsy causes delay in the development of normal milestones in infancy and childhood.

The medical terminology of the classification and effects of CP is important, and it is used in many other conditions, including the after effects of strokes. The technical terms that follow are labels used to describe the type and extent of a problem. They do not describe the individual.

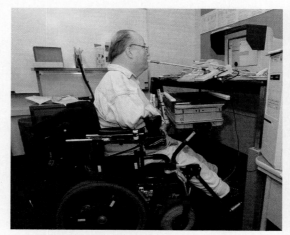

▲ **Figure 9.18** Quadriplegia.
Scott J. Ferrell/Getty Images

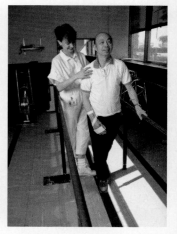

▲ **Figure 9.19** Hemiplegia.
James Prince/Science Source

Classification by Number of Limbs Impaired

- **Quadriplegia (tetraplegia).** All four limbs are involved *(Figure 9.18)*.
- **Diplegia.** Paralysis of corresponding parts (e.g., both arms) on both sides of the body.
- **Hemiplegia.** The arm and leg of one side of the body are affected *(Figure 9.19)*.
- **Monoplegia.** Only one limb is affected, usually an arm *(Figure 9.20)*.
- **Paraplegia.** Both lower extremities are involved *(Figure 9.21)*.
- **Triplegia.** Three limbs are involved.

Classification by Movement Disorder

- **Spastic**—pertaining to tight muscles that are resistant to being stretched. They can become overactive when used and produce **clonic** movements.
- **Athetoid**—pertaining to difficulty in controlling and coordinating movements, leading to involuntary writhing movements in constant motion.
- **Ataxic**—pertaining to a poor sense of balance and depth perception, leading to a staggering walk and unsteady hands.

Combined Classifications

- The classifications of movement disorder and number of limbs involved are combined, for example, **spastic diplegia.**

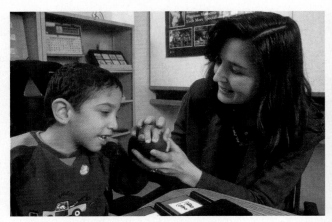

▲ **Figure 9.20** **Monoplegia.** David Grossman/Science Source

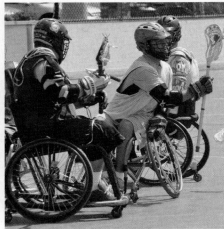

▲ **Figure 9.21** Paraplegia.
The Washington Post/Getty Images

Word Analysis and Definition: Cerebral Palsy

S = Suffix   P = Prefix   R = Root   R/CF = Combining Form

WORD	PRONUNCIATION	ELEMENTS		DEFINITION
ataxia	a-**TAK**-see-ah	S/ P/ R/	-ia *condition* a- *without* -tax- *coordination*	Inability to coordinate muscle activity, leading to jerky movements
ataxic (adj)	a-**TAK**-sik	S/	-ic *pertaining to*	Pertaining to or suffering from ataxia
athetosis	ath-eh-**TOH**-sis **ATH**-eh-toyd	S/ R/ S/	-osis *condition* athet- *uncontrolled,* *without position*	Slow, writhing involuntary movements
athetoid (adj)			-oid *resembling*	Resembling athetosis
clonic	**KLON**-ik		Greek *turmoil*	Alternating muscular contraction and relaxation
diplegia	die-**PLEE**-jee-ah	S/ P/ R/	-ia *condition* di- *two* -pleg- *paralysis*	Paralysis of corresponding parts on both sides of the body (e.g., both arms)
diplegic (adj)	die-**PLEE**-jik	S/	-ic *pertaining to*	Pertaining to or suffering from diplegia
impairment	im-**PAIR**-ment	S/ R/	-ment *action, state* impair- *worsen*	Diminishing of normal function
monoplegia	**MON**-oh-**PLEE**-jee-ah	S/ P/ R/	-ia *condition* mono- *one* -pleg- *paralysis*	Paralysis of one limb
monoplegic (adj)	**MON**-oh-**PLEE**-jik	S/	-ic *pertaining to*	Pertaining to or suffering from monoplegia
palsy	**PAWL**-zee		Latin *paralysis*	Paralysis or paresis from brain damage
paraplegia	**PAIR**-ah-**PLEE**-jee-ah	S/ P/ R/	-ia *condition* para- *abnormal, beside* -pleg- *paralysis*	Paralysis of both lower extremities
paraplegic (adj)	**PAIR**-ah-**PLEE**-jik	S/	-ic *pertaining to*	Pertaining to or suffering from paraplegia
quadriplegia	kwad-rih-**PLEE**-jee-ah kwad-rih-**PLEE**-jik	S/ P/ R/	-ia *condition* quadri- *four* -pleg- *paralysis*	Paralysis of all four limbs
quadriplegic (adj)		S/	-ic *pertaining to*	Pertaining to or suffering from quadriplegia
spasm	SPAZM		Greek *spasm*	Sudden involuntary contraction of a muscle group
spastic (adj)	**SPAS**-tik	S/ R/	-ic *pertaining to* spast- *tight*	Increased muscle tone on movement Pertaining to or suffering from increased muscle tone on movement
tetraplegia	teh-trah-**PLEE**-jee-ah	S/ P/ R/	-ia *condition* tetra- *four* -pleg- *paralysis*	Paralysis of four limbs
tetraplegic (adj)	teh-trah-**PLEE**-jik	S/	-ic *pertaining to*	Pertaining to or suffering from tetraplegia
triplegia	trie-**PLEE**-jee-ah	S/ P/ R/	-ia *condition* tri- *three* -pleg- *paralysis*	Paralysis of three limbs
triplegic (adj)	trie-**PLEE**-jik	S/	-ic *pertaining to*	Pertaining to or suffering from triplegia

Epilepsy

Epilepsy is a chronic disorder in which clusters of neurons in the brain discharge their electrical signals in an abnormal rhythm. This disturbed electrical activity (a **seizure**) can cause strange sensations and behavior, convulsions, and loss of consciousness.

The causes of epilepsy are numerous, from abnormal brain development to brain damage.

In 2017, the **International League Against Epilepsy** revised its classifications based on the onset of the seizure.

1. **Focal seizures,** previously termed partial seizures, occur when the epileptic activity is in one area of the brain only. For example, in a partial seizure the only symptom of an epileptic attack could be a series of involuntary jerking movements of a single limb.

Did you know...

- Between 1% and 3% of the population will develop some form of epilepsy.
- Two-thirds of epileptic patients are manageable with medication.
- Status epilepticus is a medical emergency.
- First-aid treatment of a seizure is to ease the person to the floor and turn them onto their side. Do not try to keep the limbs from moving.

2. **Generalized onset seizures** occur in both hemispheres of the brain. Examples include:

    a. **Absence seizures,** previously known as **"petit mal,"** are most common in children ages 4 to 14 but may continue through adult life. The child stares vacantly for less than 10 seconds, apparently out of contact with surroundings. The child may be accused of daydreaming. Recovery is quick.

    b. **Tonic-clonic seizures,** previously called **"grand mal,"** are dramatic. The person experiences a **loss of consciousness (LOC),** breathing stops, the muscles stiffen, and the jaw clenches. This "tonic" phase lasts for 30 to 60 seconds. It is followed by the "clonic" phase, in which the whole body shakes with a series of violent, rhythmic jerkings of the limbs. The seizures last for about one to three minutes, and consciousness returns.

    c. **Febrile seizures** are triggered by a high fever in infants age 6 months to 5 years. Very few of these infants go on to develop epilepsy.

3. **Unknown onset seizures** are those that the practitioner is unsure of its onset. It serves as a temporary classification until the practitioner is able to determine its onset type.

    Status epilepticus occurs when the brain is in a state of persistent seizure. It is defined as one continuous seizure lasting more than 10 minutes or three recurrent seizures without the person regaining consciousness between them. Many physicians believe that 5 minutes in this state is sufficient to damage neurons. Status epilepticus is a medical emergency and requires maintenance of the airway, breathing, and circulation and the **intravenous (IV)** administration of diazepam and anticonvulsant drugs.

    Seizures may be followed by a **postictal state** period of diminished function in the area of the brain surrounding the seizure focus. Symptoms include confusion, muscle soreness, and headache.

    Syncope and cataplexy are symptoms of other conditions that resemble symptoms of epilepsy.

- **Syncope** (fainting or passing out) is a temporary loss of consciousness and posture. It is usually due to hypotension and the associated deficient oxygen supply (hypoxia) to the brain. This disorder is called **neurally mediated syncope (NMS).** In adults, it may be associated with cardiac arrhythmias and other diseases.

- **Cataplexy,** the sudden loss of voluntary muscle tone with brief episodes of total paralysis associated **narcolepsy.** Sleep-paralysis, excessive daytime sleepiness, and hallucinations are also symptoms of narcolepsy.

Word Analysis and Definition: Epilepsy

S = Suffix   P = Prefix   R = Root   R/CF = Combining Form

WORD	PRONUNCIATION		ELEMENTS	DEFINITION
absence seizure (**Note:** Formerly referred to as "petit mal")	**AB**-sens **SEE**-zhur	P/ R/ S/ R/	**ab-** *away from* **-sence** *to feel* **-ure** *process* **seiz-** *to convulse*	A brief seizure characterized by absence of activity and occasionally clonic movements
epilepsy	**EP**-ih-**LEP**-see		Greek *seizure*	Chronic brain disorder due to paroxysmal excessive neuronal discharges
febrile	**FEB**-ril or **FEB**-rile or **FEE**-bril		Latin *febris*	Pertaining to or having a fever
postictal	post-**IK**-tal	S/ P/ R/	**-al** *pertaining to* **post-** *after* **-ict-** *seizure*	Occurring after a seizure
status epilepticus	**STAT**-us ep-ih-**LEP**-tik-us	S/ R/ S/ R/	**-us** *pertaining to* **stat-** *standing still* **-ic-** *pertaining to* **epilept-** *seizure*	A recurrent state of seizure activity lasting longer than a specific time frame (usually 30 minutes)
tic	TIK		French *tic*	Sudden, involuntary, repeated contraction of muscles
tonic-clonic seizure (**Note:** Formerly referred to as "grand mal")	**TON**-ik-**KLON**-ik **SEE**-zhur	S/	**-ic** *pertaining to*	Generalized seizure due to epileptic activity in all or most of the brain
tonic **clonic** **seizure**	**TON**-ik **KLON**-ik **SEE**-zhur	R/ R/ S/ R/	**ton-** *pressure, tension* **clon-** *violent action* **-ure** *process* **seiz-** *to grab, convulse*	Muscular contraction in a continuous state Relating to muscle movements showing contraction and relaxation in rapid succession An epileptic attack

Other Brain Disorders

Movement Disorder

Parkinson disease is caused by the degeneration of neurons in the basic ganglia that produce a neurotransmitter called **dopamine.** Motor symptoms of abnormal movements, **tremor** of the hands, rigidity, a shuffling or **festinant** (hastening, falling-forward) gait, and weak voice appear. The symptoms gradually increase in severity. The cause is unknown, and there is no cure.

Huntington disease (also known as **Huntington chorea**) is a hereditary disorder starting with mild personality changes between the ages of 30 and 50. Involuntary, irregular, jerky (**choreic**) movements and muscle weakness follow, and dementia occurs in the later stages. A gene defect is on chromosome 4, but there is no known cure.

Tourette syndrome (TS) and other **tic disorders** are characterized by episodes of involuntary, rapid, repetitive, fixed movements of individual muscle groups. They occur with varying frequency and are associated with meaningless vocal sounds or meaningful words and phrases.

Neoplasm

Brain tumors are most often secondary tumors that have metastasized from cancers in the lung, breast, skin, or kidney. **Primary brain tumors** arise from any of the glial cells and are called **gliomas** (*Figure 9.22*). The most malignant form of glioma is called **glioblastoma multiforme.**

Headaches

A headache (**cephalalgia**) is classified into either being primary or secondary. Secondary headaches occur for the first time in relation to another disorder.

Primary headaches include:

- **Migraine** produces an intense throbbing, pulsating pain usually in one area of the head, often with nausea and vomiting. It can be preceded by an **aura,** visual disturbances such as flashing lights, or temporary loss of vision. It occurs three times as often in women as men.

- **Tension-type** was previously known as a tension headache, ordinary headache, and muscle contraction headache. The exact cause of this type of headache is unknown. Patient will report increased tenderness with palpation of head and neck muscles.

- **Trigeminal autonomic cephalalgias** consist of **cluster headaches,** among other headache types, with intense unilateral pain in the supraorbital, orbital, and/or temporal regions. Attacks occur in series that may last for weeks or months (cluster periods).

- **Other primary headache disorders** are those that do not fit the previous categories and occur without a secondary cause. Examples of this category of headaches include headaches due to cough, exercise, or cold-stimulus.

Infections of the Brain

Brain abscess is most often a direct spread of infection from sinusitis, otitis media, or mastoiditis (*see Chapter 16*). It also can be a result of bloodborne pathogens from lung or dental infections.

Creutzfeldt-Jakob disease (CJD) produces a rapid deterioration of mental function with difficulty in coordination of muscle movement. Some cases are linked to the consumption of beef from cattle with **mad cow disease (bovine spongiform encephalopathy, or BSE).** Damage to the brain is thought to be caused by an abnormal infectious protein called a **prion.**

Encephalitis is inflammation of the **parenchyma** of the brain. It is usually caused by a virus such as human immunodeficiency virus (HIV), West Nile virus, herpes simplex, or the childhood diseases of measles, mumps, chickenpox, and rubella. It occurs most often in the elderly, those with compromised immune systems (*see Chapter 15*), and children.

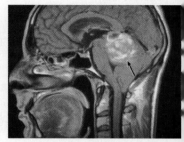

▲ **Figure 9.22** MRI shows a glioma (arrow). Simon Fraser/ Science Source

Word Analysis and Definition: Brain Disorders

S = Suffix   P = Prefix   R = Root   R/CF = Combining Form

WORD	PRONUNCIATION		ELEMENTS	DEFINITION
aura	AWE-rah		Greek *breath of air*	Sensory experience preceding an epileptic seizure or a migraine headache
bovine spongiform encephalopathy (also called *mad cow disease*)	BOH-vine SPON-jee-form en-sef-ah-LOP-ah-thee	S/ R/ S/ R/CF S/ P/ R/CF	-ine *pertaining to* bov- *cattle* -form *appearance of* spong/i- *sponge* -pathy *disease* en- *in* -cephal/o- *head*	Disease of cattle (mad cow disease) that can be transmitted to humans, causing Creutzfeldt-Jakob disease
cataplexy	KAT-ah-plek-see	P/ R/	cata- *down* -plexy *stroke*	*Sudden loss of muscle tone with brief paralysis*
cephalalgia	sef-uh-LAL-jee-uh	S/ R/	-algia *pain* cephal- *head*	Pertaining to pain in the head
chorea choreic (adj)	kor-EE-ah kor-EE-ik	S/ R/	Greek *dance* -ic *pertaining to* chore- *dance*	Involuntary, irregular spasms of limb and facial muscles
Creutzfeldt-Jakob disease	KROITS-felt-YAK-op diz-EEZ		Hans Creutzfeldt, 1885–1964, and Alfons Jakob, 1884–1931, German neuropsychiatrists	Progressive incurable neurologic disease caused by infectious prions
festinant	FES-tih-nant		Latin *to hasten*	Shuffling, falling-forward gait
glioblastoma multiforme	GLIE-oh-blas-TOH-mah MULL-tih-FOR-mee	S/ R/CF R/ P/ S/	-oma *tumor* gli/o- *glue* -blast- *germ cell* multi- *many* -forme *appearance of*	A malignant form of brain cancer
glioma	glie-OH-mah	S/ R/	-oma *tumor, mass* gli- *glue*	Tumor arising in a glial cell
Huntington disease Huntington chorea (syn)	HUN-ting-ton diz-EEZ kor-EE-ah		George Huntington, U.S. physician, 1851–1916 chorea Greek *dance*	Progressive inherited, degenerative, incurable neurologic disease
migraine	MY-grain	P/ R/	mi- *derived from hemi; half* -graine *head pain*	Paroxysmal severe headache confined to one side of the head
narcolepsy	NAR-coh-lep-see	S/ R/CF	-lepsy *seizure* narc/o- *stupor*	Condition with frequent incidents of sudden, involuntary deep sleep
parenchyma	pah-RENG-kih-mah		Greek *to pour in beside*	Characteristic functional cells of a gland or organ that are supported by the connective tissue framework
Parkinson disease	PAR-kin-son diz-EEZ		James Parkinson, British physician, 1755–1824	Disease of muscular rigidity, tremors, and a masklike facial expression
prion	PREE-on		derived from *protein-infectious particle*	Small infectious protein particle
Reye syndrome	RAY SIN-drome		R. Douglas Reye, 1912–1977, Australian pathologist	Encephalopathy and liver damage in children following an acute viral illness; linked to aspirin use
syncope	SIN-koh-peh		Greek *cutting short*	Temporary loss of consciousness and postural tone due to diminished cerebral blood flow
Tourette syndrome	tur-ET SIN-drome		Georges Gilles de la Tourette, French neurologist, 1857–1904	Disorder of multiple motor and vocal tics
tremor	TREM-or		Latin *to shake*	Small, shaking, involuntary, repetitive movements of hands, extremities, neck, or jaw

Traumatic Brain Injury

Traumatic brain injury (TBI) are events that cause damage to the brain. A bump, blow, or jolt to the head, and penetrating head injury can cause a TBI. Over 1 million people are seen by medical doctors each year following a blow to the head. Of these, 50,000 to 100,000 will have prolonged problems affecting their work and their **activities of daily living (ADLs).** These injuries can occur during combat situations, but they also occur in sports, such as boxing, ice hockey, and American football, which are all sports that often involve severe contact injuries to the head.

If you are driving your car at 50 miles per hour and are hit head-on, your brain goes from 50 miles per hour to zero instantly. Your soft brain tissue is propelled forward and squished against the front of your hard skull **(coup).** Then the brain and the rest of your body rebound backward. The soft brain is then squished against the back of your rigid skull **(contrecoup).** The squished front and back areas are at least bruised. This bruise is called a **contusion** *(Figure 9.23).*

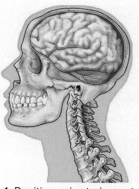
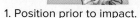
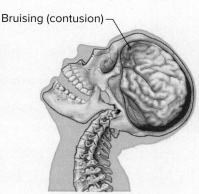
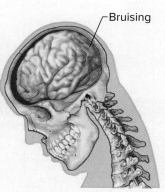
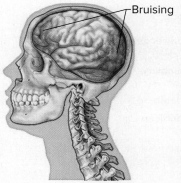

Bruising (contusion)

Bruising

Bruising

1. Position prior to impact.

2. Impact from the front.

3. Contrecoup action.

4. Subsequent coup-contrecoup injury.

▲ **Figure 9.23** Contusions caused by back-and-forth movement of brain in skull.

If the process is more severe, blood vessels tear and blood flows into the brain. In addition, the brain itself can tear and cut brain connections and signals. In any injury, brain swelling can occur. Because the skull is hard and rigid, it cannot expand to cope with this extra volume. So the soft brain tissue is compressed, and some areas can stop working.

A mild head injury is called a **concussion.** You may feel dazed or have a period of confusion during which you do not recall the event that caused the concussion. In more severe cases, you may lose consciousness for a brief period of time and have no memory of the event. Repeated concussions have a cumulative effect, with loss of mental ability (as in many American football players) and/or traumatically induced Parkinson disease (as happened with professional boxer Muhammad Ali).

In more severe TBIs, the symptoms will depend on the area of the brain damaged. Some symptoms, such as difficulty with memory or concentration, irritability, aggression, **insomnia,** posttraumatic stress disorder (PTSD), or depression, can be long-term. Traumatic brain injury has become a signature wound of the wars in Iraq and Afghanistan.

Shaken baby syndrome (SBS), also referred to as **abusive head trauma (AHT),** is a type of TBI produced when a baby is violently shaken. The baby has weak neck muscles and a heavy head. Shaking makes the brain bounce back and forth in the skull, leading to severe brain damage. Other injuries include retinal hemorrhages, subdural hematoma, damage to the spinal cord, and fractures of the ribs and limb bones. This syndrome usually occurs in children younger than 2 years.

Commonalities of Brain Injury

Cerebral edema is excess accumulation of water in the intra- or extracellular spaces of the brain. It is associated with trauma, tumors, inflammation, toxins (such as aspirin in **Reye syndrome**), ischemia, and malignant hypertension.

The residual effects of brain damage, whether due to trauma or stroke, have terminology:

- **Impairment** is a deviation from normal function; for example, not being able to control an unwanted muscle movement.
- **Disability** is a restriction in the ability to perform a normal activity of daily living (ADL), for example, a 3-year-old who cannot walk independently.
- **Handicap** is defined as having a disadvantage that prevents a child or adult from achieving a normal role in society commensurate with age and sociocultural setting; for example, a 16-year-old who cannot take care of personal toiletry and hygienic needs.

WORD	PRONUNCIATION	ELEMENTS		DEFINITION
activities of daily living	ak-**TIV**-ih-teez of **DAY**-lee **LIV**-ing	S/ R/ S/ R/ S/ R/	-ity *condition, state* activ- *movement* -ly *every* dai- *day* -ing *quality of* liv- *life*	Daily routines for mobility and personal care: bathing, dressing, eating, and moving
concussion	kon-**KUSH**-un	S/ R/	-ion *action, condition* concuss- *shake violently*	Mild head injury
contusion	kon-**TOO**-zhun	S/ R/	-ion *action, condition* contus- *bruise*	Bruising of a tissue, including the brain
coup	KOO		French *a blow*	Injury to the brain occurring directly under the skull at the point of impact
contrecoup	**KON**-treh-koo		French *counterblow*	Injury to the brain at a point directly opposite the point of original contact
disability	dis-ah-**BILL**-ih-tee	P/ R/	dis- *away from* -ability *competence*	Diminished capacity to perform certain activities or functions
edema	ee-**DEE**-mah		Greek *swelling*	Excessive collection of fluid in cells and tissues
handicap	**HAND**-ee-cap		French *assess before a race*	Condition that interferes with a person's ability to function normally
insomnia	in-**SOM**-nee-ah	S/ P/ R/	-ia *condition* in- *not* -somn- *sleep*	Inability to sleep
Reye syndrome	RYE **SIN**-drome		R. Douglas Reye, 1912–1977, Australian pathologist	Encephalopathy and liver damage in children following an acute viral illness; linked to aspirin use

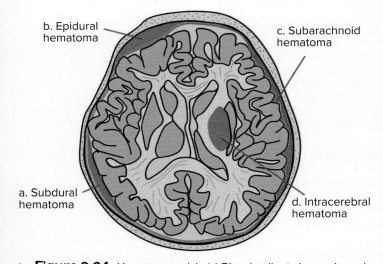

Intracranial hemorrhage

b. Epidural hematoma

c. Subarachnoid hematoma

a. Subdural hematoma

d. Intracerebral hematoma

▲ **Figure 9.24** Hematomas. (*a*)–(*c*) Blood collects in meningeal spaces, putting pressure on brain tissue.
(*d*) Hemorrhagic stroke. Blood collects within brain tissue and compresses ventricle. Songkram Chotik-anuchit/Shutterstock

Disorders of the Meninges

Intracranial hemorrhages are often the result of head trauma. Hematomas form as blood fills the space.

Subdural hematoma is bleeding into the subdural space outside the brain (*Figure 9.24a*). Most subdural hematomas are associated with closed head injuries and bleeding from broken veins caused by violent rotational movement of the head. They have been seen following roller-coaster rides with high-speed turns that jerk and whip the head. Although the blood accumulation is slow, the bleeding must be stopped surgically.

Epidural hematoma is a pooling of blood in the epidural space outside the brain (*Figure 9.24b*). Most are associated with a fractured skull and bleeding from an artery that lies in the meninges. If the bleeding is not stopped surgically by **ligating** (tying off) the blood vessel, brain compression with severe neurologic injury or death can occur.

Spontaneous **subarachnoid hemorrhage** (*Figure 9.24c*) can be preceded by a sudden "thunderclap" severe headache, followed by nausea and vomiting. The blood collects between the pia mater and the arachnoid mater. It is commonly caused by the bursting of a blood vessel at the surface of the brain.

Meningitis is inflammation of the meninges covering the brain and spinal cord. Viral meningitis is the most common form and occurs at all ages. Bacterial meningitis is more common in the very young or very old. **Meningococcal meningitis** is contagious, spread through droplet infection by coughing and sneezing and through close living conditions, as in college dormitories. Vaccines are available to prevent most causes of meningitis (*see Chapter 12*).

Meningioma is a tumor originating in the arachnoid cells of the meninges, most commonly overlying the cerebral hemispheres. It is usually benign and produces a slow-growing, focal, spherical tumor. Symptoms can take years to develop. Surgical resection is usually curative.

Disorders of the Cranial Nerves

Bell palsy is a disorder of the seventh cranial nerve (facial nerve), causing a sudden onset of weakness or paralysis of facial muscles on one side of the face *(Figure 9.25)*. Common symptoms are a **hemifacial** inability to smile, whistle, or grimace; drooping of the mouth with drooling of saliva; and inability to close the eye on the affected side. Early treatment with steroids and supportive measures is essential. The facial nerve also can be affected by trauma or tumors.

Trigeminal neuralgia (tic douloureux) is intermittent, shooting pain in the area of the face and head innervated by the fifth cranial nerve. The pain is abrupt (sudden), unilateral, and often severe, and can affect any area of the face from the crown of the head to the jaw. Chewing or touching the affected area causes pain.

Horner syndrome presents with a unilateral droopy eyelid (ptosis), small pupil, and decrease in perspiration on the face. It can occur in lung cancer and injuries to the head, neck, and cervical spinal cord *(Figure 9.26)*. The signs of Horner syndrome are due to the blocking of the sympathetic pathway to the eye.

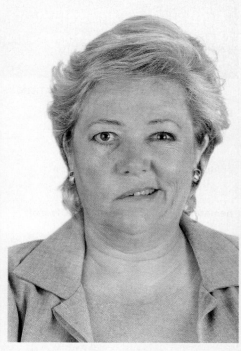

▲ **Figure 9.25** Bell palsy of right side of face. Jo Ann Snover/Shutterstock

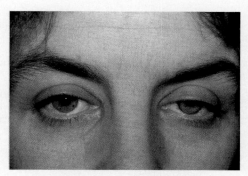

▲ **Figure 9.26** Horner syndrome showing ptosis and small pupil of left eye. Science Photo Library/Science Source

Word Analysis and Definition: Disorders of the Meninges and Cranial Nerves

S = Suffix   P = Prefix   R = Root   R/CF = Combining Form

WORD	PRONUNCIATION		ELEMENTS	DEFINITION
Bell palsy	BELL **PAWL**-zee		Charles Bell, 1774–1842, Scottish surgeon, anatomist, and physiologist **palsy** Latin *paralysis*	Paresis or paralysis of one side of face
epidural	ep-ih-**DYU**-ral	S/ P/ R/	-al *pertaining to* epi- *above* -dur- *dura mater*	Above the dura
hematoma	hee-mah-**TOH**-mah	S/ R/	-oma *tumor, mass* hemat- *blood*	Collection of blood that has escaped from the blood vessels into tissue
hemifacial	hem-ee-**FAY**-shal	S/ P/ R/	-al *pertaining to* hemi- *half* -faci- *face*	Pertaining to one side of the face
Horner syndrome	**HOR**-ner **SIN**-drome	P/ R/	Johann Friedrich Horner, 1831–1886, Swiss ophthalmologist syn- *together* -drome *running*	Disorder of the sympathetic nerves to the face and eye Combination of symptoms and signs associated with a particular disease process
meningioma	meh-**NIN**-jee-**OH**-mah	S/ R/CF	-oma *tumor, mass* mening/i- *meninges*	Tumor arising from the arachnoid layer of the meninges
meningococcal	meh-nin-goh-**KOK**-al	S/ R/CF R/	-al *pertaining to* mening/i- *meninges* -cocc- *spherical bacterium*	Pertaining to the *meningococcus* bacterium
meningitis	men-in-**JIE**-tis	S/	-itis *infection*	Inflammation of the membranes surrounding the brain or spinal cord
neuralgia	nyur-**AL**-jee-ah	S/ R/	-algia *pain* neur- *nerve*	Pain in the distribution of a nerve
subdural	sub-**DUR**-al	S/ P/ R/	-al *pertaining to* sub- *under* -dur- *dura mater*	Located in the space between the dura mater and arachnoid membrane
tic douloureux trigeminal neuralgia (syn)	TIK duh-luh-**RUE**		douloureux French *painful tic*	Painful, sudden, spasmodic, involuntary contractions of the facial muscles supplied by the trigeminal nerve

Check Point Section 9.3

A. Deconstruct medical terms and define their meanings. *Multiple choice. Choose the letter that best completes each sentence.* **LO 9.2, 9.6**

1. The prefix in the term **dementia** means:

   a. only   **b.** without   **c.** together   **d.** into

2. The suffix in the term **delirium** means:

   a. condition   **b.** structure   **c.** disease   **d.** aware

B. Explain disorders of the brain. *Match each disorder with its correct description.* **LO 9.6**

_____ **1.** delirium

_____ **2.** Alzheimer disease

_____ **3.** confusion

_____ **4.** vascular dementia

a. common form of dementia due to protein clumps and tangles

b. dementia due to decreased blood flow to the brain

c. altered state of consciousness with agitation and disorientation

d. condition in which a person cannot properly process information

C. Use the terms related to cerebrovascular accidents to complete the clinic note presented below. *Replace the words in italics with the correct medical terms related to cerebrovascular accidents.* **LO 9.6, 9.8**

Mrs. Jacobson presents to the ED with her son. Her son was visiting when she began to slur her speech and the right side of her face appeared droopy. The physician suspects that Mrs. Jacobson has had a **(1)** *stroke*. Upon examination, the patient exhibits **(2)** *weakness* in her left hand grip as well as her left leg. A **(3)** *surgeon that specialized in treatment of disorders of the nervous system* is consulted. An MRI is performed and it is determined that the patient has an **(4)** *abnormal connection between a cerebral artery and vein* that has ruptured. She is immediately sent to surgery to place a clip on the ruptured vessel.

1. _____ .

2. Left-sided _____ .

3. _____ .

4. _____   _____ .

D. Deconstruct medical terms to decipher their meaning. *Being able to pick out the word elements and define them will help you determine the meaning of the entire medical term. Select the correct answer for each question.* **LO 9.2, 9.6**

1. The prefix in the term **hemiparesis** means:

   a. blood vessel   **b.** paralysis   **c.** weakness   **d.** half

2. The suffix in the term **malformation** means:

   a. process   **b.** structure   **c.** pertaining to   **d.** bad

3. The root in the term **arteriovenous** that means *vein* is:

   a. *arteri/o*   **b.** *ven/o*   **c.** *ven*   **d.** *ous*

4. The root/combining form in the term **cerebrovascular** that means *brain* is:

   a. *cerebr/o*   **b.** *vascul*   **c.** *vascul/a*   **d.** *ar*

E. Deconstruct medical terms to determine their meaning. *Multiple choice. Choose the correct answer.* **LO 9.2, 9.6**

1. The prefix in the term **monoplegia** means:

   a. one   **b.** two   **c.** three   **d.** four   **e.** five

2. The root in the term **quadriplegia** means:

   a. two   **b.** four   **c.** paralysis   **d.** weakness

3. The suffix in the term **triplegia** means:

   a. one   **b.** three   **c.** pertaining to   **d.** condition of

F. In practice, you will find that some people will use the new terms for seizures, and some will use the older traditional terms. It is important that you know both. *Fill in the blank with the correct term.* **LO 9.6**

1. A tonic-clonic seizure is traditionally known as a _____ mal seizure.

2. An absence seizure is traditionally known as a _____ mal seizure.

G. Match the signs of a brain disorder with their corresponding condition. **LO 9.6**

_____ **1.** infant with high fever   **a.** absence seizure

_____ **2.** child appears to be daydreaming   **b.** postictal state

_____ **3.** transient neurologic deficit after a seizure   **c.** febrile seizure

H. Based on the given scenario, determine the specific type of primary headache with which the patient is likely suffering. *Fill in the blanks.* **LO 9.6**

1. Patient complains of intense pain on only one side of the head. The patient states that the pain is mainly around and above her eye. She states that the headache occurs in a pattern in which it occurs for 2 weeks, stops for 1 week, and then repeats. This is a _____ headache.

2. Patient complains of a headache that occurs 5 minutes after he begins to run. Headache due to _____.

3. Patient states she has been experiencing intense headaches that cause her nausea and vomiting. Just prior to the headache, she sees bright flashing lights. She has had three of these type headaches in the last two months. This is a _____ headache.

I. Write the abbreviation that is described in the following sentences. *Fill in the blanks.* **LO 9.9**

1. An infant is brought to the emergency department after being shaken by the parent. The infant is very sleepy and does not respond to painful stimuli. The infant may be suffering from _____.

2. After suffering a stroke, the patient is no longer able to brush her hair or teeth. She has an injury that is affecting her _____.

3. The goal keeper for the high school soccer team slid into the goal post head first and lost consciousness. She will be sent to the emergency department to be evaluated for the presence of a _____.

J. Identify the correct definitions of common medical terms. *From the given definition, choose the correct term.* **LO 9.6**

1. A restriction in the ability to perform activities of daily living:
   a. disability   **b.** impairment   **c.** handicap   **d.** contusion

2. A deviation from normal function:
   a. disability   **b.** impairment   **c.** handicap   **d.** contusion

K. Deconstruct the terms into their basic elements. **LO 9.2**

1. In the term **hematoma,** the meaning of the suffix is:
   a. meninges   **b.** spherical   **c.** mass   **d.** blood   **e.** bruise

2. In the term **hemifacial,** the prefix means:
   a. half   **b.** pertaining to   **c.** face   **d.** blood   **e.** nerve

3. In the term **meningitis,** the word part that means inflammation is the:
   a. prefix   **b.** root   **c.** suffix

L. Based on the given scenario, determine what disorder the person is likely to have. **LO 9.6, 9.8**

1. Mr. Turner brings his 3-year-old son to the pediatrician. The father has noticed that his son's right eyelid is drooping and the pupil of the right eye remains small, even when the pupil of the left is large. The pediatrician may suspect that the child is suffering from:
   a. Huntington disease   **b.** Parkinson disease   **c.** Horner syndrome   **d.** Bell palsy

Section 9.4 Disorders of the Spinal Cord and Peripheral Nerves

Disorders of the Myelin Sheath of Nerve Fibers

There are many disorders of the nervous system that affect the spinal cord and the peripheral nerves without affecting the brain. When the myelin sheath surrounding nerve fibers is damaged, nerves do not conduct impulses normally. **Demyelination,** the destruction of an area of the myelin sheath, can occur in the PNS caused by inflammation, vitamin B_{12} deficiency, poisons, and some medications.

Guillain-Barré syndrome is a disorder of the peripheral nerves in which the body makes antibodies against myelin, leading to loss of nerve conduction, muscle weakness, and **paresthesias** (changes in sensation). Treatment is with corticosteroids, and recovery of neurologic function is slow.

Demyelination of nerve fibers in the brain, spinal cord, and optic nerves also can occur. **Multiple sclerosis (MS)** is a chronic, progressive disorder and the most common of the demyelination disorders. MS is a chronic, progressive disorder. **Intermittent** myelin damage and scarring slow nerve impulses *(Figure 9.27)*. This leads to muscle weakness, pain, numbness, and vision loss. Because different nerve fibers are affected at different times, MS symptoms often worsen (**exacerbations**) or show partial or complete reduction (**remissions**). MS has an average age of onset between 18 and 35 years and is more common in women. Its cause is unknown, but it is thought to be an autoimmune disease.

Other causes of demyelination in the CNS are injury, ischemia, toxic agents such as chemotherapy or radiotherapy, and congenital disorders such as **Tay-Sachs disease. Tay-Sachs disease** is a rare genetic condition caused by the absence of an enzyme that breaks down fatty substances, causing a buildup of fats in neurons in the brain, resulting in damage in the brain tissue. The most common form has onset in infancy but can appear in children and adults. Infantile signs include blindness, sensitivity to sound, hypotonia, and seizures. After viral infections or vaccinations, **postinfectious encephalomyelitis** is a demyelination process, as is **HIV encephalitis,** which is seen in up to 30% of patients with AIDS.

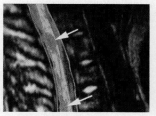

▲ **Figure 9.27 Multiple sclerosis.** Note areas of the spinal cord where myelin sheath has been destroyed (arrows). Normal spinal cord is yellow. James Cavallini/Science Source

Word Analysis and Definition: Disorders of the Myelin Sheath

S = Suffix   P = Prefix   R = Root   R/CF = Combining Form

WORD	PRONUNCIATION	ELEMENTS		DEFINITION
demyelination	dee-**MY**-eh-lin-**A**-shun	S/ P/ R/	-ation *process* de- *away from, without* -myelin- *myelin*	Process of losing the myelin sheath of a nerve fiber
encephalitis encephalomyelitis	en-**SEF**-ah-**LIE**-tis en-**SEF**-ah-loh-**MY**-eh-**LIE**-tis	S/ R/ R/CF R/	-itis *inflammation* encephal- *brain* encephal/o- *brain* -myel- *spinal cord*	Inflammation of brain cells and tissues Inflammation of the brain and spinal cord
exacerbation (contrast remission)	ek-zas-er-**BAY**-shun	S/ R/	-ation *process* exacerb- *increase, aggravate*	Period when there is an increase in the severity of a disease
Guillain-Barré syndrome	**GEE**-yan-bah-**RAY** **SIN**-drome		Georges Guillain, 1876–1961, and Jean-Alexandre Barré, 1880–1967, French neurologists	Disorder in which the body makes antibodies against myelin, disrupting nerve conduction
intermittent	**IN**-ter-**MIT**-ent	S/ P/ R/	-ent *end result* inter- *between* -mitt- *send*	Alternately ceasing and beginning again
paresthesia paresthesias (pl)	par-es-**THEE**-ze-ah	S/ P/ R/	-ia *condition* par(a)- *abnormal* -esthes- *sensation, feeling*	Abnormal sensation; for example, tingling, burning, prickling
remission (contrast exacerbation)	ree-**MISH**-un	S/ P/ R/	-ion *action, condition* re- *back* -miss- *send*	Period when there is a lessening or absence of the symptoms of a disease
Tay-Sachs disease	TAY SACKS diz-**EEZ**		Waren Tay, 1843–1927, English ophthalmologist and Bernard Sachs, 1858–1944, American neurologist	Disease in which fat buildup in neurons of the brain and spinal cord causing their destruction

Disorders of the Spinal Cord

Trauma

Approximately, half a million people in the United States have **spinal cord injuries (SCIs).** About 17,000 new injuries occur each year; 80% involve males. Quadriplegia is slightly more common than paraplegia (see definitions on page 289).

Because of its anatomy with nerve fibers and tracts going up and down, to and from the brain, injury to the spinal cord results in loss of function below the injury. For example, if the cord is injured in the thoracic region, the arms function normally, but the legs can be **paralyzed.** Both muscle control and sensation are lost.

The spinal cord is injured in three ways (*Figure 9.28*):

1. **Severed** if the spinal cord is severed, the loss is permanent.

2. **Contused** contusions can cause temporary loss lasting days, weeks, or months.

3. The spinal cord can acutely become compressed by a broken or dislocated vertebra, bleeding, or swelling.

In an acute injury, the first goal of treatment is to prevent further damage, which is why you see football players being carried off the field strapped to a board and carefully padded to prevent even slight shifting of the spine.

Compression of the cord also can occur slowly from a tumor in the cord or spine and can also be due to a **herniated** disc. Cancer or osteoporosis can cause a vertebra to collapse and compress the cord.

- **Cervical spondylosis** is a disorder in which the discs and vertebrae in the neck degenerate, narrow the spinal canal, and compress the spinal cord and/or the spinal nerve roots.

- In **syringomyelia,** fluid-filled cavities grow in the spinal cord and compress nerves that detect pain and temperature. There is no specific cure.

Other Disorders

Acute transverse myelitis is a localized disorder of the spinal cord that blocks transmission of impulses up and down the spinal cord. People who have **Lyme disease,** syphilis, or tuberculosis or those who inject heroin or amphetamines intravenously are at risk of developing this disorder. The disorder causes loss of sensation, muscle **paralysis,** and loss of bladder and bowel control. There is no specific treatment. Most people recover completely.

Subacute combined degeneration of the spinal cord is due to a deficiency of vitamin B_{12}. The sensory nerve fibers in the spinal cord degenerate, producing weakness, clumsiness, tingling, and loss of the position sense as to where limbs are. Treatment is injections of vitamin B_{12}.

Poliomyelitis (polio) is an acute infectious disease, occurring mostly in children, that is caused by the poliovirus. The virus can be asymptomatic in the nasopharynx and gastrointestinal (GI) tract. When it spreads to the nervous system, it replicates in the spinal cord and destroys motor neurons. Symptoms are progressive muscle **paralysis.** Poliomyelitis is preventable by vaccination and has almost been eradicated in the world.

Postpolio syndrome (PPS), in which people develop tired, painful, and weak muscles many years after recovery from polio, is classified as a motor neuron disorder.

Motor neuron disorders occur when motor nerves in the spinal cord and brain progressively deteriorate. This leads to muscle weakness that can progress to paralysis. **Amyotrophic lateral sclerosis (ALS,** or Lou Gehrig disease) and its variants, **progressive muscular atrophy** and **primary lateral sclerosis,** are examples. There is no cure.

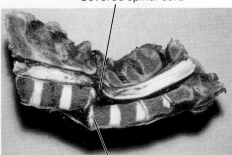

Severed spinal cord

(a) Fracture-dislocation of vertebra

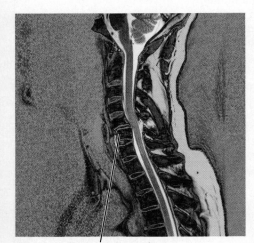

(b) Fractured vertebra

▲ **Figure 9.28** Spinal cord injuries. (*a*) Severed spinal cord from fracture-dislocation of vertebra. (*b*) Compressed spinal cord with vertebral fracture.
Wellcome Photo Library; Simon Fraser/Newcastle Hospitals NHS/Science Photo Library/Science Source

WORD	PRONUNCIATION	ELEMENTS		DEFINITION
acute	ah-**KYOOT**		Latin *sharp*	Having a rapid onset and duration
amyotrophic	a-my-oh-**TROH**-fik	S/ P/ R/CF R/	**-ic** *pertaining to* **a-** *without* **-my/o-** *muscle* **-troph-** *nourishment, development*	Pertaining to muscular atrophy
atrophy	**AT**-roh-fee	P/ R/	**a-** *without* **-trophy** *nourishment, development*	Wasting or diminished volume of a tissue or organ
compression	kom-**PRESH**-un	S/ P/ R/	**-ion** *action* **com-** *together* **-press-** *squeeze*	A squeezing together so as to increase density and/or decrease a dimension of a structure
hernia (noun)	**HER**-nee-ah		Latin *rupture*	Protrusion of a structure through the tissue that normally contains it
herniation	**HER**-nee-**AY**-shun	S/ R/	**-ation** *process* **herni-** *rupture*	Protrusion of an anatomical structure from its normal location
herniate (verb)	**HER**-nee-ate	S/	**-ate** *composed of*	To protrude
Lyme disease	LIME diz-**EEZ**		Named in 1977 after a group of children in Lyme, Connecticut who acquired the disease.	Disease transmitted by the bite of an infected deer tick
myelitis	**MY**-eh-**LIE**-tis	S/ R/	**-itis** *inflammation* **myel-** *spinal cord*	Inflammation of the spinal cord
paralyze (verb)	**PAIR**-ah-lize	P/ R/	**para-** *abnormal* **-lyze** *destroy*	To make incapable of movement
paralysis	pah-**RAL**-ih-sis	S/	**-lysis** *destruction*	Loss of voluntary movement
paralytic (adj)	pair-ah-**LYT**-ic	S/	**-lytic** *loosen*	Pertaining to or suffering from paralysis
poliomyelitis	**POH**-lee-oh-**MY**-eh-**LIE**-tis	S/ P/ R/	**-itis** *inflammation* **polio-** *gray matter* **-myel-** *spinal cord*	Inflammation of the gray matter of the spinal cord, leading to paralysis of the limbs and muscles of respiration
polio (abbrev)				
postpolio syndrome	post-**POH**-lee-oh **SIN**-drome	P/ P/ R/	**post-** *after* **syn-** *together* **-drome** *running*	Progressive muscle weakness in a person previously affected by polio
spondylosis	spon-dih-**LOH**-sis	S/ R/	**-osis** *condition* **spondyl-** *vertebra*	Degenerative osteoarthritis of the spine
subacute	sub-ah-**KYOOT**	S/	Latin *sharp* **sub-** *below, under, slightly, underneath*	Less than rapid onset and duration of a condition, but not a long term disease
syringomyelia	sih-**RING**-oh-my-**EE**-lee-ah	S/ R/CF R/	**-ia** *condition* **syring/o-** *tube, pipe* **-myel-** *spinal cord*	Abnormal longitudinal cavities in the spinal cord that cause paresthesias and muscle weakness

Disorders of the Peripheral Nerves

The term **neuropathy** is used here as any disorder affecting one or more peripheral nerves.

Mononeuropathy is damage to a single peripheral nerve. Prolonged pressure on a nerve that runs close to the surface over a bony prominence is a common cause. Examples are:

- **Carpal tunnel syndrome.** The median nerve at the wrist is compressed between the wrist bones and a strong overlying ligament. Numbness, pain, and tingling of the thumb side of the hand are the symptoms. Incision of the ligament relieves the pressure.

- **Ulnar nerve palsy.** Nerve damage occurs as the ulnar nerve crosses too close to the surface over the humerus at the back of the elbow. Pins-and-needles sensation and weakness in the hand result. Hitting the ulnar nerve is the cause of pain when you hit your "funny bone."

- **Peroneal nerve palsy.** Nerve damage occurs as the peroneal nerve passes too close to the surface near the back of the knee. Compression of the nerve occurs in people who are bedridden or strapped in a wheelchair.

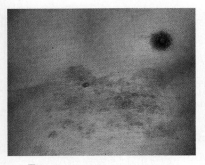

▲ **Figure 9.29** **Herpes zoster (shingles).** Martin Dr Baumgartner/ imageBROKER/Shutterstock

Polyneuropathy is damage to, and the simultaneous malfunction of, many peripheral nerves throughout the body.

Symptoms of acute polyneuropathy include muscle weakness and a pins-and-needles sensation or loss of sensation. The symptoms begin suddenly in the legs and work upward to the arms.

In **diabetic chronic polyneuropathy,** only sensation is affected, most commonly in the feet. Pins and needles, numbness, and a burning sensation are prominent.

When people with a neuropathy are unable to sense pain, they can injure a joint many times without feeling it. The joint malfunctions and can progress to being permanently destroyed. Joints involved in this **neuropathic joint disease** are called **Charcot joints.**

Herpes zoster (shingles) is an infection of peripheral nerves arising from a reactivation of the primary virus infection in childhood with **chickenpox (varicella).** During the primary infection of chickenpox, the virus gains entry into sensory dorsal root ganglia. Later in life, for unknown reasons, the virus can produce the painful, unilateral **dermatome** rash of shingles *(Figure 9.29).*

Postherpetic neuralgia is acute dermatome pain persisting after the acute rash of shingles has subsided. It is debilitating and very difficult to treat.

Neuromuscular junction disorders occur where nerves connect with muscle fibers and interfere with the **neurotransmitter acetylcholine.** Examples are:

- **Myasthenia gravis,** in which the immune system produces antibodies that attack the acetylcholine receptors on the muscle cells. The common symptoms are drooping eyelids; weak eye muscles, causing double vision; difficulty talking and swallowing; and muscle weakness in the limbs.

- **Botulism,** a rare, life-threatening food poisoning caused by toxins from the bacterium **Clostridium botulinum.** These **neurotoxins** paralyze the muscles. Botulism can develop from ingesting food containing the toxin or from a wound infected with *Clostridium botulinum.*

- Certain **insecticides (organophosphates)** and nerve gases used in chemical warfare that act on neuromuscular junctions.

- Nerve **compression** occurring when the space around a nerve is constricted. The pinched nerve becomes **edematous** and later fibrotic and produces pain and **paresthesias.** Examples are **sciatica,** when the **sciatic** nerve is compressed in the lower spine, and **carpal tunnel syndrome,** when the median nerve is compressed at the wrist.

Congenital Anomalies of the Nervous System

Some of the most devastating **congenital neurologic anomalies** develop in the first 8 to 10 weeks of gestation, when the nervous system is in its early stages of formation. These malformations can be detected by using ultrasonography and amniocentesis *(see Chapter 8).* Many can be prevented by the mother taking 4 mg/day of folic acid before conception and during early pregnancy.

A **teratogen** is an agent that can cause malformations of an embryo or fetus *(see Chapter 8).* It can be a chemical, virus, or radiation. Some teratogens are encountered in the workplace and include textile dyes, photographic chemicals, semiconductor materials, lead, mercury, and cadmium. One of the early uses of the drug thalidomide was to control morning sickness in pregnancy, but it caused severe limb and other deformities in the baby.

Anencephaly is absence of the cerebral hemispheres and is always fatal *(Figure 9.30).*

Microcephaly, decreased head size, is associated with small cerebral hemispheres and with moderate to severe motor and intellectual disability. One cause of microcephaly is an infection during pregnancy with the Zika virus. This virus is carried by an aggressive mosquito that can bite in the daytime or at night, and also can be passed from an infected person to another person during sex.

Hydrocephalus, ventricular enlargement in the cerebral hemispheres with excessive CSF, is usually due to an obstruction that prevents the CSF from exiting the ventricles to circulate around the spinal cord *(Figure 9.31).*

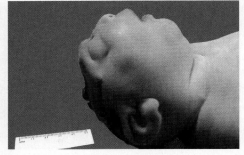

▲ **Figure 9.30** **Newborn with anencephaly.** McGraw Hill

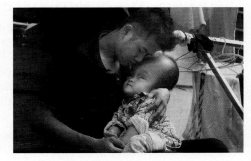

▲ **Figure 9.31** **Infant with hydrocephalus.** Imaginechina Limited/ AlamyStock Photo

WORD	PRONUNCIATION		ELEMENTS	DEFINITION
botulism	**BOT**-you-lizm		Latin *sausage*	Caused by the neurotoxin produced by *Clostridium botulinum*
carpal	**KAR**-pal	S/ R/	-al *pertaining to* **carp-** *wrist*	Pertaining to the wrist
carpal tunnel syndrome	**KAR**-pal **TON**-nell **SIN**-drome	 P/ R/	**tunnel** English *tube, pipe* **syn-** *together* -**drome** *running*	Compression of the median nerve in the wrist causing numbness, pain and tingling in the fingers and thumb
Charcot joint	**SHAR**-koh JOYNT		Jean-Martin Charcot, 1825–1893, French neurologist	Bone and joint destruction secondary to a neuropathy and loss of sensation
chickenpox varicella (syn)	**CHICK**-en-pocks **VAIR**-uh-**SELL**-uh		Disease originally considered a "chicken" (not dangerous) version of smallpox	Acute, contagious viral disease
Clostridium botulinum	klos-**TRID**-ee-um bot-you-**LIE**-num			Bacterium that causes botulism
herpes zoster shingles (syn)	**HER**-pees **ZOS**-ter **SHING**-guls		**herpes** Greek *spreading skin eruption* **zoster** Greek *girdle*	Painful eruption of vesicles that follows a dermatome or nerve root on one side of the body
myasthenia gravis	my-as-**THEE**-nee-ah **GRA**-vis	S/ R/ P/ R/ R/	-ia *condition* **my-** *muscle* -a- *without* -sthen- *strength* **gravis** *serious*	Disorder of fluctuating muscle weakness
neuralgia	nyu-**RAL**-jee-ah	S/ R/	-algia *pain* **neur-** *nerve*	Pain in the distribution of a nerve
neuromuscular	**NYUR**-oh-**MUSS**-kyu-lar	S/ R/CF R/	-ar *pertaining to* **neur/o-** *nerve* -muscul- *muscle*	Pertaining to both nerves and muscles
neuropathy	nyu-**ROP**-ah-thee	S/ R/CF	-pathy *disease* **neur/o-** *nerve*	Any disease of the nervous system
neuropathic (adj) mononeuropathy polyneuropathy	nyur-oh-**PATH**-ik **MON**-oh-nyu-**ROP**-ah-thee **POL**-ee-nyu-**ROP**-ah-thee	S/ P/ P/	-ic *pertaining to* **mono-** *one* **poly-** *many*	Pertaining to a disease of the nervous system Disorder affecting a single nerve Disorder affecting many nerves
neurotoxin	**NYUR**-oh-tock-sin	R/CF R/	**neur/o-** *nerve* -toxin *poison*	Agent that poisons the nervous system
peroneal	pair-uh-**NEE**-al	S/ R/	-eal *pertaining to* **peron-** *fibula*	Pertaining to the lateral part (fibula) of the lower leg, or the nerve named after it
postherpetic	**POST**-her-**PET**-ik	S/ P/ R/	-ic *pertaining to* **post-** *after* -herpet- *herpes*	Pertaining to after herpes infection
sciatica sciatic (adj)	sigh-**AT**-ih-kah sigh-**AT**-ik		Greek *related to the hip joint*	Pain from compression of L5 or S1 nerve roots Pertaining to the sciatic nerve or sciatica
ulnar	**UL**-nar	S/ R/	-ar *pertaining to* **uln-** *ulna*	Pertaining to the ulna (medial forearm bone) or any of the structures (artery, vein, nerve) named after it
varicella	**VAIR**-uh-**SELL**-uh		Latin *a tiny spot*	An acute infectious disease caused by the varicella-zoster virus

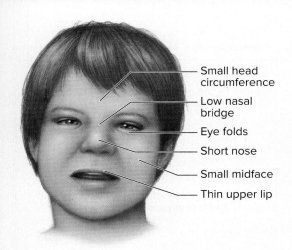

- Small head circumference
- Low nasal bridge
- Eye folds
- Short nose
- Small midface
- Thin upper lip

▲ **Figure 9.32** Fetal alcohol syndrome.

Fetal alcohol syndrome (FAS) can occur when a pregnant woman drinks alcohol. The child born with FAS has a small head, narrow eyes, and a flat face and nose (*Figure 9.32*). Intellect and growth are impaired. Fetal alcohol syndrome is a cause of intellectual disability.

Spina bifida occulta—small partial defect in the vertebral arch. The spinal cord or meninges do not protrude. Often the only sign is a tuft of hair on the skin overlying the defect.

Spina bifida cystica—no vertebral arch is formed. The spinal cord and meninges protrude through the opening and may or may not be covered with a thin layer of skin (*see Figure 9.33a and b*).

Meningocele—protrusion of the meninges only.

Meningomyelocele—protrusion of the meninges and spinal cord; paralysis of the lower limbs may be present.

The defect must be closed promptly to preserve spinal cord function and prevent infection. The cause of spina bifida is not known.

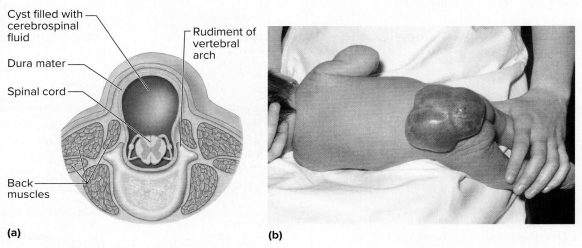

Cyst filled with cerebrospinal fluid

Dura mater

Spinal cord

Back muscles

Rudiment of vertebral arch

(a)

(b)

▲ **Figure 9.33** **Spina bifida cystica.** (*a*) cross section of spinal cord in spina bifida cystica. (*b*) Child with spina bifida cystica. (b) Biophoto Associates/Science Source

Word Analysis and Definition: Congenital Anomalies

S = Suffix   P = Prefix   R = Root   R/CF = Combining Form

WORD	PRONUNCIATION	ELEMENTS		DEFINITION
anencephaly	**AN**-en-**SEF**-ah-lee	S/ P/ R/	**-y** *condition* **an-** *without* **-encephal-** *brain*	Born without cerebral hemispheres
anomaly	ah-**NOM**-ah-lee		Greek *abnormality*	A structural abnormality
hydrocephalus	**HIGH**-droh-**SEF**-ah-lus	S/ R/CF R/	**-us** *pertaining to* **hydr/o-** *water* **-cephal-** *head*	Enlarged head due to excess CSF in the cerebral ventricles
meningocele	meh-**NING**-oh-seal	S/ R/CF	**-cele** *hernia* **mening/o-** *meninges*	Protrusion of the meninges from the spinal cord or brain through a defect in the vertebral column or cranium
meningomyelocele (**Note:** also referred to as *myelomeningocele*)	meh-**NING**-oh-**MY**-el-oh-seal	R/CF	**-myel/o-** *spinal cord*	Protrusion of the spinal cord and meninges through a defect in the vertebral arch of one or more vertebrae
microcephaly	**MY**-kroh-**SEF**-ah-lee	S/ P/ R/	**-y** *condition* **micro-** *small* **-cephal-** *head*	An abnormally small head
spina bifida	**SPY**-nah **BIH**-fih-dah	R/CF P/ R/	**spin/a** *spine* **bi-** *two* **-fida** *split*	Failure of one or more vertebral arches to close during fetal development
spina bifida cystica	**SPY**-nah **BIH**-fih-dah **SIS**-tik-ah	S/ R/	**-ica** *pertaining to* **cyst-** *cyst*	Meninges and spinal cord protrude through the absent vertebral arch and have the appearance of a cyst
spina bifida occulta	**SPY**-nah **BIH**-fih-dah oh-**KUL**-tah	R/	**occulta** *hidden*	The deformity of the vertebral arch is not apparent from the skin surface
teratogen	teh-**RAT**-eh-jen	S/ R/CF	**-gen** *produce, create* **terat/o-** *monster, malformed fetus*	Agent that produces fetal deformities
teratogenic (adj) (**Note:** Has two suffixes.)	teh-**RAT**-eh-**JEN**-ik	S/	**-ic** *pertaining to*	Capable of producing fetal deformities

Check Point Section 9.4

A. Test yourself on the elements and terms related to disorders of the myelin sheath of nerve fibers. *Choose the best answer.* **LO 9.2, 9.6**

1. **Guillain-Barré syndrome** disrupts
   - **a.** nerve conduction
   - **b.** blood flow
   - **c.** metabolism

2. In the term **paresthesia,** the prefix means
   - **a.** between
   - **b.** abnormal
   - **c.** many

3. **Remission** is the opposite of
   - **a.** intermittence
   - **b.** exacerbation
   - **c.** demyelination

4. The element gravis suggests
   - **a.** deep
   - **b.** serious
   - **c.** minor

5. In the term **demyelination,** the prefix means
   - **a.** away from
   - **b.** in front of
   - **c.** in between

6. **Encephalomyelitis** is inflammation of the
   - **a.** brain
   - **b.** spinal cord
   - **c.** brain and spinal cord

B. Identify the meaning of the basic word elements. *Match the word element in the first column to its correct meaning in the second column.* **LO 9.2**

_____	**1.** *a-*	**a.** abnormal
_____	**2.** *-ic*	**b.** destruction
_____	**3.** *my/o*	**c.** pertaining to
_____	**4.** *spondyl-*	**d.** without
_____	**5.** *-ia*	**e.** vertebra
_____	**6.** *-lysis*	**f.** condition of
_____	**7.** *para-*	**g.** muscle

C. Complete the definition with the correct medical language. *Fill in the blanks.* **LO 9.2**

1. Disorder affecting the nervous system   neuro/ _____

2. Agent that poisons the nervous system   neuro/ _____

3. Disorder affecting a single nerve   _____ /neuro/pathy

4. Pertaining to the lateral side of the lower leg   _____ /eal

D. Search and find the correct term for the element you are given. *Choose the best answer.* **LO 9.2, 9.6**

1. Find the term with the prefix meaning *without:*

 a. hydrocephalus   **b.** anencephaly   **c.** impairment

2. Find the term with the root meaning *cyst:*

 a. meningocele   **b.** cystica   **c.** teratogen

3. Find the term with the root meaning *monster:*

 a. teratogen   **b.** spina   **c.** myelomeningocele

4. Find the term with the root meaning *split:*

 a. bifida   **b.** occulta   **c.** cystica

5. Find the term with the root meaning *head:*

 a. anomaly   **b.** hydrocephalus   **c.** meningocele

6. Find the term with the root meaning *hidden:*

 a. spina bifida   **b.** spina bifida cystica   **c.** spina bifida occulta

7. Find the term with the combining form meaning *water:*

 a. teratogenic   **b.** hydrocephalus   **c.** myelomeningocele

8. Find the term with the suffix meaning *hernia:*

 a. meningocele   **b.** hydrocephalus   **c.** anomaly

9. Find the term with the combining form meaning *spinal cord:*

 a. meningomyelocele   **b.** cystocele   **c.** meningocele

10. Find the term with the prefix meaning *small:*

 a. anencephaly   **b.** teratogenic   **c.** microcephaly

Section 9.5 Procedures and Pharmacology

Diagnostic Procedures in Neurology

To obtain a specimen of CSF, a **lumbar puncture (LP)** or **spinal tap** is performed *(Figure 9.34)*. A needle is inserted through the skin, back muscles, spinal ligaments of an intervertebral space, epidural space, dura mater, and arachnoid mater into the subarachnoid space. The CSF is then aspirated. Laboratory examination of the CSF that shows white blood cells suggests meningitis. High protein levels indicate meningitis or damage to the brain or spinal cord. Blood suggests a brain hemorrhage or a traumatic tap.

Electroencephalography records the brain's electrical activity and helps identify seizure disorders, sleep disturbances, degenerative brain disorders, and brain damage.

Computed tomography (CT), a computer-enhanced x-ray technique, generates images of slices of the brain and can detect a wide range of brain and spinal cord disorders, including tumors, areas of dead brain tissue due to stroke, and birth defects.

Magnetic resonance imaging (MRI) produces highly detailed anatomical images of most neurologic disorders, including strokes, brain tumors, and myelin sheath damage.

Magnetic resonance angiography uses an injection of a radiopaque dye to produce images of blood vessels of the head and neck during MRI.

Cerebral angiography is an invasive procedure in which a radiopaque dye is injected into the blood vessels of the neck and brain. It can detect blood vessels that are partially or completely blocked, aneurysms, or arteriovenous malformations.

Cerebral arteriography can determine the site of bleeding in hemorrhagic strokes.

Color Doppler ultrasonography uses high-frequency sound (ultrasound) waves to show different rates of blood flow through the arteries of the neck or the base of the brain. This evaluates TIAs and the risk of a full-blown stroke.

Echoencephalography uses ultrasound waves to produce an image of the brain in children under the age of 2 because their skulls are thin enough for the waves to pass through them.

Positron emission tomography (PET) involves attaching radioactive molecules onto a substance necessary for brain function (for example, the sugar glucose). As the molecules circulate in the brain, the radioactive labels give off positively charged signals that can be recorded *(Figure 9.35)*.

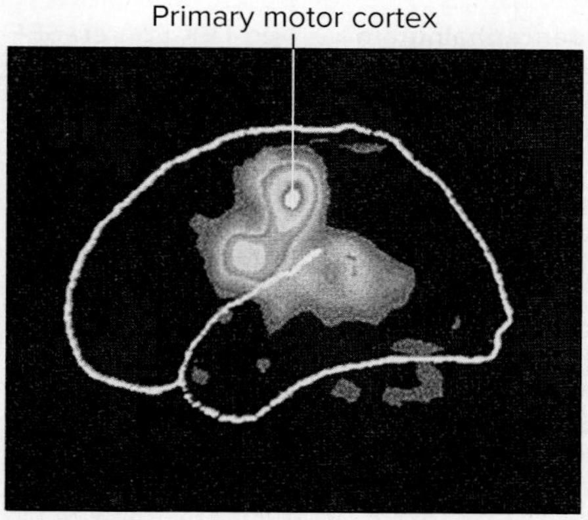

Myelography is the use of x-rays of the spinal cord that are taken after a radiopaque dye has been injected into the CSF by spinal tap. It has been replaced by MRI when that is available.

Evoked responses are a procedure in which stimuli for vision, sound, and touch are used to activate specific areas of the brain and their responses are measured with EEG or PET scans. This provides information about how that specific area of the brain is functioning in disorders such as MS.

Electromyography (EMG) involves placing small needles into a muscle to record its electrical activity at rest and during contraction. It is used to provide information in disorders of muscles, peripheral nerves, and the **neuromuscular** junction.

Nerve conduction studies measure the speed at which motor or sensory nerves conduct impulses. The studies exclude disorders of the brain, spinal cord, and muscles and focus on the peripheral nerves.

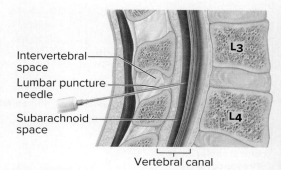

Intervertebral space

Lumbar puncture needle

Subarachnoid space

L3

L4

Vertebral canal

▲ **Figure 9.34** Lumbar puncture (spinal tap).

Primary motor cortex

▲ **Figure 9.35** PET scan of the brain showing the motor cortex. Marcus E. Raichle

WORD	PRONUNCIATION	ELEMENTS		DEFINITION
angiography	an-jee-**OG**-rah-fee	S/	-graphy *process of recording*	Process of recording the image of blood vessels after injection of contrast material
		R/CF	angi/o- *blood vessel*	
arteriography	ar-teer-ee-**OG**-rah-fee	S/	-graphy *process of recording*	X-ray visualization of an artery after injection of contrast material
		R/CF	arteri/o- *artery*	
Doppler	**DOP**-ler		Johann Christian Doppler, 1803–1853, Austrian mathematician and physicist	Diagnostic instrument that sends an ultrasonic beam into the body
Doppler ultrasonography	**DOP**-ler **UL**-trah-soh-**NOG**-rah-fee	S/	-graphy *process of recording*	Imaging that detects direction, velocity, and turbulence of blood flow; used in workup of stroke patients
		P/	ultra- *beyond*	
		R/CF	-son/o- *sound*	
color Doppler ultrasonography				Computer-generated color image to show directions of blood flow
echoencephalography	**EK**-oh-en-sef-ah-**LOG**-rah-fee	S/	-graphy *process of recording*	Use of ultrasound in the diagnosis of intracranial lesions
		R/CF	ech/o- *sound wave*	
		R/CF	-encephal/o- *brain*	
electroencephalogram (EEG)	ee-**LEK**-troh-en-**SEF**-ah-loh-gram	S/	-gram *recording*	Record of the electrical activity of the brain
		R/CF	electr/o- *electricity*	
		R/CF	-encephal/o- *brain*	
electroencephalograph	ee-**LEK**-troh-en-**SEF**-ah-loh-graf	S/	-graph *to write, record*	Device used to record the electrical activity of the brain
electroencephalography	ee-**LEK**-troh-en-**SEF**-ah-**LOG**-rah-fee	S/	-graphy *process of recording*	The process of recording the electrical activity of the brain
electromyography	ee-**LEK**-troh-my-**OG**-rah-fee	S/	-graphy *process of recording*	Recording of electrical activity in muscle
		R/CF	electr/o- *electricity*	
		R/CF	-my/o- *muscle*	
myelography	my-eh-**LOG**-rah-fee	S/	-graphy *process of recording*	Radiography of the spinal cord and nerve roots after injection of contrast medium into the subarachnoid space
		R/CF	myel/o- *spinal cord*	
nerve conduction study	NERV kon-**DUK**-shun **STUD**-ee	R/	nerve *nerve*	Procedure to measure the speed at which an electrical impulse travels along a nerve
		S/	-ion *action*	
		P/	con- *with, together*	
		R/	-duct- *lead*	
		R/	study *inquiry*	

Therapeutic Procedures

Craniotomy is the surgical removal of part of a skull bone (the bone flap) to expose the brain for surgery.

Cranioplasty is the repair of a bone defect in the skull, often the result of craniotomy. Cranioplasty uses titanium mesh, plates, and perhaps bone cement.

Microvascular decompression (MVD) is a surgery to treat an artery or vein that is pressing a cranial nerve, for example, the trigeminal nerve. After the craniotomy, the blood vessel is moved off the cranial nerve, followed by a sponge wrapped around the nerve.

Deep brain stimulation is the surgical placement of electrodes deep into specific areas of the brain to deliver electrical stimulations to treat the tremors of Parkinson disease, essential tremor, or multiple sclerosis.

Endoscopic pituitary surgery utilizes an approach through the inside of the nose to remove pituitary tumors.

Endovascular coiling blocks the blood flow to an aneurysm.

Flow diversion uses **stents** placed via a catheter to maintain blood flow through a blood vessel where blockage or an aneurysm has occurred.

Treatment of many acute ischemic strokes is by **thrombolysis** using clot busters such as **tissue plasminogen activator (tPA)** within 4½ hours of the stroke, with supportive measures followed by rehabilitation.

Treatment for TIA is directed at the underlying cause. **Carotid endarterectomy** may be necessary if a carotid artery is significantly occluded with plaque.

A **shunt** is used in hydrocephalus to drain the excess CSF from the ventricles to either the peritoneal cavity or an atrium of the heart.

Botulinum toxin (BoTox) injections are used in the treatment of migraines, spasticity, and neuralgias.

Treatment of Cerebral Palsy

A multidisciplinary team of health professionals is required to develop an individualized treatment plan and to involve the patients, families, teachers, and caregivers in decision making and planning.

Physical therapy is designed to prevent muscles from becoming weak or rigidly fixed with **contractures,** to improve motor development, and to facilitate independence. Speech therapy and psychotherapy complement physical therapy.

A variety of devices and mechanical aids ranging from muscle braces to motorized wheelchairs help overcome physical limitations.

Treatment of Gliomas

Treatment is a combination of surgery, radiotherapy, and chemotherapy. The combination is necessary because even if you remove 99% of a tumor, there will be up to 1 billion cells remaining. A more recent therapy, **brachytherapy,** implants small radioactive pellets directly into the tumor. The radiation is released over time.

Word Analysis and Definition: Therapeutic Procedures

S = Suffix   P = Prefix   R = Root   R/CF = Combining Form

WORD	PRONUNCIATION	ELEMENTS		DEFINITION
Botox	**BOH**-tox		Botulinum toxin	Neurotoxin injected into muscles to prevent the muscles from contracting
brachytherapy	brah-kee-**THAIR**-ah-pee	P/ R/CF	**brachy-** *short* **-therapy** *medical treatment*	Radiation therapy in which the source of irradiation is implanted in the tissue to be treated
cranium	**KRAY**-nee-um		Greek *skull*	The bony container of the brain, excluding the face
cranioplasty	**KRAY**-nee-oh-**PLAS**-tee	S/ R/CF	**-plasty** *surgical repair* **crani/o-** *skull*	Repair of a bone defect in the skull
craniotomy	**KRAY**-nee-**OT**-oh-mee	S/	**-tomy** *surgical incision*	Surgical removal of part of a skull bone to expose the brain for surgery
endovascular	**EN**-doh-**VAS**-kyu-lar	S/ P/ R/	**-ar** *pertaining to* **endo-** *inside* **-vascul-** *blood vessel*	Relating to the inside of a blood vessel
shunt	SHUNT		**Middle English** *divert*	A bypass or diversion of fluid

Pharmacology of the Nervous System

The transmission of impulses from one neuron to another and from a neuron to a cell is achieved by neurotransmitters at synaptic connections. Drugs that affect the nervous system, called *psychoactive drugs,* target this synaptic mechanism.

Psychoactive drugs are able to change mood, behavior, cognition, and anxiety. They can be classified into several families:

1. **Stimulants**—caffeine, nicotine, amphetamines, and cocaine—enhance the **stimulation** provided by the sympathetic nervous system. They cause the level of dopamine to rise in the synapses, leading to the pleasurable effects associated with these drugs.

2. **Sedatives**—ethanol (beverage alcohol), barbiturates, and meprobamate—decrease the sensitivity of the postsynaptic neurons to quiet the nervous excitement. They also act on the sleep centers to induce sleep.

3. Inhaled anesthetics such as isoflurane act similarly to, but are more powerful than, sedatives.

4. Opiates—morphine, codeine, heroin, methadone, and oxycodone—depress nerve transmission in the synapses of sensory pathways of the brain and spinal cord. They also inhibit centers in the brain controlling coughing, breathing, and intestinal motility. Codeine is used in cough medicines. Constipation is a side effect of all these drugs. Opiates are **addictive** because they produce tolerance and physical dependence.

5. Opiate **antagonists,** such as naloxone and naltrexone, prevent opiates from acting in the synapses. They can be used in drug overdoses and to help a person recovering from heroin addiction stay drug-free.

6. **Tranquilizers,** such as chlorpromazine, haloperidol, and the benzodiazepines (*Librium, Valium, Xanax*), act like sedatives but without their sleep-inducing effect.

7. Antidepressants all increase the amount of serotonin at the synapses, where it is a neurotransmitter. Antidepressants are used to treat neuropathic pain migraines. Amitriptyline, sertraline (*Zoloft*) and fluoxetine (*Prozac*) are examples.

8. **Psychedelics** distort sensory perceptions, particularly sight and sound. They can be natural plant products, such as mescaline, psilocybin, and dimethyltryptamine. They also can be synthetic, such as **lysergic acid diethylamide (LSD), methylenedioxymethamphetamine (MDMA** or "ecstasy"), and **phencyclidine (PCP** or "angel dust"). They increase the amount of serotonin in the synaptic junctions, and some have an additional amphetamine stimulation.

9. **Marijuana** has the active ingredient **tetrahydrocannabinol (THC).** It produces the drowsiness of sedatives like alcohol, the dulling of pain like opiates, and, in high doses, the perception distortions of the psychedelics. Unlike the case with opiates or sedatives, **tolerance** does not occur.

Medications have crossover to other conditions. Anticonvulsants used to treat epilepsy may be used to treat neuropathic pain. Beta blockers used to treat high blood pressure (hypertension) also treat migraines.

Medications to treat epilepsy are based on the type of seizure. If one medication is ineffective, then another medication can be added. Carbamazepine (*Tegretol*) is often a first choice. Other medications include pregabalin (*Lyrica*), valproic acid (*Depakote*), brivaracetam (*Briviact*), and lacosamide (*Vimpat*).

Spasticity is treated with skeletal muscle relaxants baclofen, benzodiazepines such as diazepam, and botulinum toxins.

Migraines can be treated for acute episodes or preventively. Acute episode medications range from NSAIDs, caffeine, beta blockers, antidepressants, and triptans such as frovatriptan (*Frova*), rizatriptan (*Maxalt*), and sumatriptan (*Imitrex*). Preventative medications such as botulinum toxins, erenumab-aooe (*Aimovig),* galcanezumab-gnlm (*Emgality*), and ubrogepant (*Ubrelvy*) have proven effective.

Antibiotics are used to treat acute bacterial infections that cause encephalitis and meningitis. A culture of the CSF obtained via lumbar puncture determines the choice of antibiotic by identifying the type of bacteria present. There is no treatment for viral meningitis; viral meningitis is typically mild and the duration of illness is short.

Medications to treat multiple sclerosis are categorized as those that slow the progression of the disease, symptoms such as bladder problems, fatigue, depression, and pain. Medical marijuana may help with spasticity and bladder problems.

WORD	PRONUNCIATION	ELEMENTS		DEFINITION
addiction	ah-**DIK**-shun	P/ R/ S/	ad- *to* -dict- *consent, surrender* -ion *condition, action*	Habitual psychologic and physiologic dependence on a substance or practice
addictive	ah-**DIK**-tiv	S/	-ive *quality of, pertaining to*	Pertaining to or causing addiction
antagonism	an-**TAG**-oh-nizm	S/ P/ R/	-ism *process, action* ant- *against* -agon- *contest against*	Situation of opposing
antagonist	an-**TAG**-oh-nist	S/	-ist *agent*	An opposing structure, agent, disease, or process
antiepileptic	**AN**-tee-eh-pih-**LEP**-tik	S/ P/ R/	-tic *pertaining to* anti- *against* -epilep- *seizure*	A pharmacologic agent capable of preventing or arresting epilepsy
psychedelic	sigh-keh-**DEL**-ik	S/ R/CF R/	-ic *pertaining to* psych/e- *mind, soul* -del- *visible*	Agent that intensifies sensory perception
psychoactive	sigh-koh-**AK**-tiv	S/ R/CF R/	-ive *quality of, pertaining to* psych/o- *mind, soul* -act- *to do*	Able to alter mood, behavior, and/or cognition
sedative	**SED**-ah-tiv	S/ R/	-ive *quality of, pertaining to* sedat- *to calm*	Agent that calms nervous excitement
sedation	seh-**DAY**-shun	S/	-ion *condition, action*	State of being calmed
stimulant stimulate (verb) stimulation	**STIM**-you-lant **STIM**-you-late stim-you-**LAY**-shun	S/ R/ S/	-ant *forming* stimul- *excite, strengthen* -ation *process*	Agent that excites or strengthens functional activity Arousal to increased functional activity
tolerance	**TOL**-er-ants	S/ R/	-ance *state of, condition* toler- *endure*	The capacity to become accustomed to a stimulus or drug
tranquilizer	**TRANG**-kwih-lie-zer	S/ R/	-izer *affects in a particular way* tranquil- *calm*	Agent that calms without sedating or depressing

Pain Management

Pain persisting longer than 3 months is said to be **chronic.** It can be caused by cancer, arthritis, fibromyalgia, low-back or neck problems, headache, or injuries that have not healed. Normal activities can be restricted or be impossible.

In 2016, the cost of chronic pain was estimated to be $560 billion due to medical costs, lost work productivity, and disability programs. In modern health care, chronic pain management has become essential and often uses a multidisciplinary approach. Pain management is now a board-certified subspecialty for **anesthesiologists.**

Medications are the cornerstone of pain management, and the following can be used depending on the severity of the pain:

- Mild pain. **Analgesics,** such as acetaminophen, and **nonsteroidal anti-inflammatory drugs (NSAIDs),** such as ibuprofen, are used. A study published in 2017 of 28,947 Danish patients showed that patients taking NSAIDs had a 31% increased risk of having cardiac arrest.

- Moderate pain. **Opiate** medications in combination with acetaminophen or NSAIDs are used. Some opiates used in combination medications are codeine, hydrocodone, and oxycodone. Examples are hydrocodone/acetaminophen (*Vicodin*), oxycodone/acetaminophen (*Percocet*), and oxycodone/aspirin (*Percodan*). These opiate medications are addictive, and are frequently abused and sold on the street.

- Severe pain. Higher doses of opiates are used, often not as combination products. These include **morphine,** fentanyl, and oxy- and hydromorphone. The opiates can be taken orally, by patch, sublingually, by intravenous (IV) infusion, or by continuous delivery systems. These oral opiates are also addictive and are sold on the street.

- **Buprenorphine** is an opioid that has recently been recommended for treatment in chronic pain. It provides analgesia with less risk for abuse and addiction. It is a controlled substance (*see Chapter 22*) and there are strict federal regulations on the qualifications of physicians allowed to prescribe it.

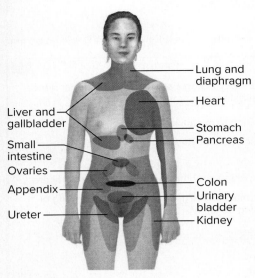

Liver and gallbladder — Lung and diaphragm — Heart — Stomach — Pancreas — Small intestine — Ovaries — Appendix — Colon — Urinary bladder — Ureter — Kidney

▲ **Figure 9.36** Referred pain.

Central sensitization pain is a new concept describing how neurons in the spinal cord sending messages to the brain become excitable. They exaggerate the pain response in tissues they supply. The input can be somatic from skeletal muscles (as in fibromyalgia) or visceral (as in irritable bowel syndrome).

Interventional pain management, particularly for pain originating in the spine and spinal nerves, is being increasingly used. Examples are:

- **Epidural or facet nerve blocks.** Anesthetic or anti-inflammatory agents are injected into an area surrounding the pain-generating nerve.
- **Radiofrequency (RF) nerve ablation.** A probe heats the area around a pain-generating spinal nerve and temporarily deactivates it.
- **Spinal infusion pump.** Pain medications such as morphine are delivered through an indwelling catheter into the **intrathecal** CSF surrounding the spinal cord. A pump delivery device is inserted under the skin of the abdomen.

Phantom limb pain occurs following the amputation of a limb or part of a limb. Any stimulation of the remaining intact portion of the sensory pathway coming originally from the limb is interpreted by the brain as coming from the original limb. The pain can be severe and debilitating or just an insatiable urge to scratch an itch.

Referred pain occurs when pain in the viscera is felt in the skin or other superficial sites *(Figure 9.36)*. An example is the pain of a heart attack felt along the front of the left shoulder and down the underside of the left arm. This is because spinal cord segments T1 to T5 receive sensory input from the heart, as well as from the skin of the shoulder and arm. This input is transmitted to the brain. The brain cannot distinguish the true source of the pain. It assumes it is coming from the skin, which has more pain receptors than the heart and is injured more often.

Word Analysis and Definition: Pain Management

S = Suffix   P = Prefix   R = Root   R/CF = Combining Form

WORD	PRONUNCIATION	ELEMENTS		DEFINITION
ablation	ab-**LAY**-shun	S/ P/ R/	-ion *action, condition* ab- *away from* -lat- *to take*	Removal of tissue to destroy its function
analgesia	an-al-**JEE**-zee-ah	S/ P/ R/	-ia *condition* an- *without* -alges- *sensation of pain*	State in which pain is reduced
analgesic	an-al-**JEE**-zik	S/	-ic *pertaining to*	Substance that produces analgesia
anesthesia	an-es-**THEE**-zee-ah	P/ R/CF	an- *without* -esthesi/a *sensation, feeling*	Complete loss of sensation
anesthesiologist	**AN**-es-thee-zee-**OL**-oh-jist	S/ P/ R/CF	-logist *one who studies, specialist* an- *without* -esthesi/o- *feeling, sensation*	Medical specialist in anesthesia
anesthesiology	**AN**-es-thee-zee-**OL**-oh-jee	S/	-logy *study of*	Medical specialty of anesthesia
anesthetic	an-es-**THET**-ik	S/ P/ R/	-ic *pertaining to* an- *without* -esthet- *sensation, perception*	An agent that causes absence of feeling or sensation
facet	**FAS**-et		French *little face*	Small area, in this case around a pain-generating nerve
intrathecal	**IN**-trah-**THEE**-kal	S/ P/ R/	-al *pertaining to* intra- *within* -thec- *sheath*	Within the subarachnoid or subdural space
morphine	**MOR**-feen		Latin *god dreams*	Derivative of opium used as an analgesic or sedative
opiate	**OH**-pee-ate		Latin *bringing sleep*	A drug derived from opium

Check Point Section 9.5

A. Create medical terms common to diagnostic procedures in neurology. *Given the definition, complete the medical term it is defining using word elements related to diagnostic terms in neurology. Fill in the blanks.* **LO 9.2, 9.5**

1. The machine that creates the record of the electrical activity of the brain. electro/encephalo/_____

2. The process of recording arteries. arterio/_____

3. The use of high-frequency sound waves to view blood flow. Doppler ultra/_____ /graphy

4. Process of recording the spinal cord. _____ /graphy

5. Process of recording the electrical activity of the muscle. electro/_____ /graphy

B. Demonstrate understanding of word elements in medical terms. *This exercise uses layman's terms and asks you to replace those words the medical term they are describing. Fill in the blanks.* **LO 9.7, 9.8**

A 27 year old male is brought to the emergency department by paramedics. The male is unconscious. The paramedics report that he was involved in an altercation at a bar when he was struck in the head with a barstool. He was immediately brought to the operating room where the (1) *surgical expert in the treatment of neurological conditions* performed a (2) *procedure in which part of the skull was removed.* A large clot was removed from the subdural space. The wound was closed and the patient was admitted to the surgical ICU. The injury to skull shattered several areas of the (3) *bones that cover the brain*, and therefore the patient will require a (4) *repair of defect of the skull* at a later date when he becomes medically stable

1. The medical term that replaces the italicized words: _____

2. The medical term that replaces the italicized words: _____

3. The medical term that replaces the italicized words: _____

4. The medical term that replaces the italicized words: _____

C. Deconstruct this *language of neurology* into its basic elements to help understand the meaning of the term. *Write the elements between the slashes. A combining vowel will have a space to enter it in. The first one is done for you. Every term does not need every element, so you will have some blanks.* **LO 9.2, 9.7**

1. antagonist   _____ant_____/_____agon_____/_____ist_____

2. addiction   _____/_____/_____

3. tranquilizer   _____/_____/_____

4. stimulant   _____/_____/_____

5. psychedelic   _____/_____/_____

6. tolerance   _____/_____/_____

7. psychoactive   _____/_____/_____

D. Define the element. *Write the meaning of each element to see how it will aid you in understanding the meaning of the complete term. Fill in the blank.* **LO 9.2**

1. *an-* _____.

2. *intra-* _____.

3. *thec-* _____.

4. *-ia* _____.

5. *ab-* _____.

E. The language of pain management is specific. *It is important to use medical terms related to pain management correctly. Choose the correct answer for each question.* **LO 9.7, 9.10**

1. A medical specialist in area of pain management is a(n):

   a. neurologist   **b.** anesthesiologist   **c.** analgesic   **d.** urologist

2. A medication indicated for *moderate* pain is:

   a. codeine   **b.** ibuprofen   **c.** morphine   **d.** fentanyl

3. A medication that blocks all sensation, including pain:

   a. analgesic   **b.** anesthetic

4. A medication that blocks pain but allows other sensations to be felt:

   a. analgesic   **b.** anesthetic

Table 9.1 Chapter 9 Abbreviations

Abbreviation	Meaning	Abbreviation	Meaning
ADLs	activities of daily living	MDMA	methylenedioxymethamphetamine (ecstasy)
AHT	abusive head trauma	MRI	magnetic resonance imaging
ALS	amyotrophic lateral sclerosis	MS	multiple sclerosis
ANS	autonomic nervous system	NMS	neurally mediated syncope
AVM	arteriovenous malformation	NSAIDs	nonsteroidal anti-inflammatory drugs
BBB	blood–brain barrier	PCP	phencyclidine (angel dust)
BSE	bovine spongiform encephalopathy	PET	positron emission tomography
C1–C8	cervical spinal nerves	PNS	peripheral nervous system
C5	fifth cervical vertebra or nerve	polio	poliomyelitis
CJD	Creutzfeldt Jakob disease	PPS	postpoliomyelitis syndrome
CNS	central nervous system	PTSD	posttraumatic stress disorder
CP	cerebral palsy	RF	radiofrequency
CSF	cerebrospinal fluid	S1–S5	sacral nerves
CT	computed tomography	SBS	shaken baby syndrome
CVA	cerebrovascular accident	SCI	spinal cord injury
EEG	electroencephalogram	T1	first thoracic vertebra or nerve
EMG	electromyography	T1–T12	thoracic spinal nerves
FAS	fetal alcohol syndrome	TB	tuberculosis
GI	gastrointestinal	TBI	traumatic brain injury
IV	intravenous	THC	tetrahydrocannabinol (marijuana)
L1–L5	lumbar nerves	TIA	transient ischemic attack
LOC	loss of consciousness	TS	Tourette syndrome
LP	lumbar puncture	VEP	visual evoked potential
LSD	lysergic acid diethylamide		

Table 9.2 Comparison of Common Neurologic Disorders

Disorder	Signs and Symptoms	Diagnostic Tests	Treatment
Bacterial meningitis	Headache, neck stiffness, fever, altered mental status, rash	Lumbar puncture to obtain CSF—increased neutrophil count	Antibiotics, corticosteroids
Concussion	Headaches, dizziness, confusion, may have loss of consciousness	Immediate concussion evaluation; repeat in 24–48 hours. Consider CT or MRI of head if there is a loss of consciousness	Physical rest and avoid digital screens for 24–48 hours
Subarachnoid hemorrhage	Sudden, severe headache. May have nausea and vomiting, or loss of consciousness	Lumbar puncture—presence of blood can indicate subarachnoid hemorrhage CT scan, MRI	Craniotomy for access to site of bleeding. Bleeding is stopped by placing a metal clip near the aneurysm.

Nervous System

Challenge Your Knowledge

A. **Construct the proper medical terms for the statements.** You have an assortment of prefixes, roots, combining forms, and suffixes with which to construct your terms. Fill in the blanks. **LO 9.2, 9.6**

hydro	lepsy	esthesia
narco	lysis	a
algia	occulta	para
neur	itis	post
an	trophy	

1. Recurring episodes of falling asleep during the day: _____

2. Complete loss of sensation: _____

3. Pain in the distribution of a nerve: _____

4. Wasting away of tissue: _____

5. Derived from a word meaning *hidden:* _____

B. **Similar but different.** The following medical terms contain a similar root, but the suffixes change the meaning of the terms. Use the correct form of these terms in the following sentences. Fill in the blanks. **LO 91, 9.10**

neurosurgery	neurologic	neurologist	neurosurgeon	neurology

The _____ from the Fulwood _____ Department referred the patient to

a _____ for surgical consultation. The patient's _____ condition was deteriorating

rapidly, and she would probably need _____.

C. **Identify the elements in each medical term and unlock the meaning of the word.** Fill in the chart. If the word does not have a particular word element, write n/a. **LO 9.2, 9.6**

Medical Term	Meaning of Prefix	Meaning of Root/Combining Form	Meaning of Suffix	Meaning of the Term
dementia	1.	2.	3.	4.
sympathy	5.	6.	7.	8.
confusion	9.	10.	11.	12.
hemiparesis	13.	14.	15.	16.
hypothalamic	17.	18.	19.	20.
anesthetic	21.	22.	23.	24.
cataplexy	25.	26.	27.	28.

D. Diseases and disorders. The Fulwood Neurology Clinic treats patients with varied diseases and disorders of the nervous system. Are you familiar enough with their terminology and symptoms to match the correct disease or disorder with the appropriate statement for each patient? Select the correct choice. **LO 9.6**

1. Patient has had a hemorrhagic stroke. Another name for this is:

    a. intercranial hemorrhage   **b.** intercerebral hemorrhage   **c.** intracerebral hemorrhage

2. Patient bumped head on low doorway:

    a. concussion   **b.** seizure   **c.** convulsion

3. Patient has inflammation of the parenchyma of the brain:

    a. meningitis   **b.** encephalitis   **c.** vasculitis

4. Infection of the peripheral nerves arising from a reactivation of the chickenpox (varicella) virus is:

    a. herpes simplex   **b.** shingles   **c.** post herpetic neuralgia

5. Infant has motor impairment resulting from brain damage at birth:

    a. Bell palsy   **b.** cerebral palsy   **c.** palsy

6. Patient had very bad dental infection that resulted in bloodborne pathogens lodging in her brain:

    a. brain tumor   **b.** brain abscess   **c.** brain hematoma

7. Patient complains of intermittent, shooting pain in the area of the face and head:

    a. trigeminal neuralgia   **b.** peripheral neuropathy   **c.** neuritis

E. Abbreviations are helpful only if you know what they are meant to communicate. Write the correct abbreviation for each described condition, structure, or procedure. **LO 9.9**

1. This system is composed of the brain and the spinal cord.

_____

2. The neurologist ordered a test to evaluate the electrical activity of the brain.

_____

3. The infant's condition of monoplegia was due to a reduction of oxygen delivered to her brain during her birth.

_____

F. Plurals. Refresh your memory on the rules for plurals. Precision in communication depends on this. The singular form is given; circle the best answer for the plural form. **LO 9.1, 9.3**

1. ganglion: **a.** ganglius   **b.** ganglia   **c.** gangli

2. plexus: **a.** plexuses   **b.** plexuia   **c.** plexui

3. sulcus: **a.** sulces   **b.** sulci   **c.** sulcia

4. gyrus: **a.** gyri   **b.** gryia   **c.** gryuses

G. **Word Elements remain the core of a medical term.** Reinforce your knowledge of these elements with this exercise. Match the correct word element in the left column to its meaning in the right column. **LO 9.2**

_____ **1.** *-pathy*   **a.** hearing

_____ **2.** *cephal/o*   **b.** muscle

_____ **3.** *alges*   **c.** sleep

_____ **4.** *syring/o*   **d.** blood vessel

_____ **5.** *audit*   **e.** tube, pipe

_____ **6.** *-trophy*   **f.** disease

_____ **7.** *my/o*   **g.** development

_____ **8.** *pleg*   **h.** head

_____ **9.** *somn*   **i.** sensation of pain

_____ **10.** *angi/o*   **j.** paralysis

H. **Medical language.** The nervous system is a complicated one and has a large range of vocabulary. Assess your knowledge of the nervous system by selecting the correct answer in the following questions. **LO 9.2**

1. The area of the brain that controls emotional experience, fear, anger, pleasure, and sadness:

a. cerebral cortex   **b.** corpus callosum   **c.** central sulcus   **d.** limbic system

2. Astrocytes, oligodendrocytes, microglia, ependymal, Schwann, and satellite are all terms relating to:

a. capillaries   **b.** tumors   **c.** hematomas   **d.** neuroglia   **e.** ganglia

3. Body temperature is regulated by the:

a. thalamus   **b.** hypothalamus   **c.** limbic system   **d.** pons   **e.** cerebellum

4. Centers that control vital visceral activities are located in the:

a. pons   **b.** corpus   **c.** medulla oblongata   **d.** hypothalamus   **e.** CSF

I. **Latin and Greek terms do not deconstruct like some medical terms.** Test your knowledge of these terms with this exercise. Match the terms in the left column to their correct meaning in the right column. **LO 9.1**

_____ **1.** gyrus   **a.** bridge

_____ **2.** sulcus   **b.** circle

_____ **3.** efferent   **c.** brain

_____ **4.** cerebrum   **d.** ditch, furrow

_____ **5.** pons   **e.** away from

J. Medical language. The nervous system is a complicated one and has a large range of vocabulary. Assess your knowledge of the nervous system by selecting the correct answer to the following questions. **LO 9.1, 9.6, 9.7, 9.9**

1. An agent capable of preventing or arresting epilepsy is called an:

   a. antidiuretic   **b.** antibiotic   **c.** antiepileptic   **d.** antidepressant   **e.** antibody

2. Administration of tPA is for:

   a. ALS   **b.** thrombolysis   **c.** seizures   **d.** dementia   **e.** meningitis

3. **Hypoglossal** refers to structures that can be found under the:

   a. diaphragm   **b.** tongue   **c.** jawbone   **d.** bronchus   **e.** alveoli

4. In simple terms, a **synapse** is a:

   a. malformation   **b.** birth defect   **c.** junction   **d.** seizure   **e.** vesicle

5. Implantation of radioactive pellets directly into a tumor is called:

   a. bradytherapy   **b.** bradycardia   **c.** brachytherapy   **d.** brachial plexus   **e.** none of the above

6. A condition a child is born with that was caused by his/her mother's consumption of alcohol. The child has a small head, narrow eyes, and a flat face and nose.

   a. MDMA   **b.** LOC   **c.** NMS   **d.** VEP   **e.** FAS

7. The groove that separates gyri is called:

   a. gyrus   **b.** cortex   **c.** fissure   **d.** sulcus   **e.** dermatome

8. The cerebral hemispheres are covered by a thin layer of gray matter called the:

   a. basal ganglia   **b.** corpus callosum   **c.** frontal lobe   **d.** cerebral cortex   **e.** cerebellum

9. The abbreviation for a short-term, small stroke is:

   a. EEG   **b.** HACE   **c.** TIA   **d.** PET   **e.** SBS

10. The medical term that means *pertaining to or caused by a seizure* is:

    a. clonic   **b.** ictal   **c.** tonic   **d.** visceral   **e.** synaptic

K. **Test-taking strategy practice.** Use your knowledge of medical terminology to insert the correct term in the appropriate statement. Not all answers will be used, and no answer will be used more than once. **LO 9.1, 9.6**

hemiplegia	somatic	afferent
meningitis	meningioma	quadriplegia
festinant	microcephaly	visceral
neurotransmitters	dendrite	dementia

1. _____ nerves carry signals from major organs such as the heart, lungs, stomach, and intestines.

2. An abnormally small head: _____

3. A process or extension of a neuron: _____

4. Shuffling gait: _____

5. Loss of the mind's cognitive functions: _____

6. Paralysis of all four limbs: _____

7. Chemicals that cross the synapse to another neuron: _____

8. _____ nerves carry signals from the skin, muscles, bones, and joints.

L. **Analyze the following diagnostic procedures on the basis of their elements alone; then answer the questions.** Fill in the blanks. **LO 9.5**

1. **echoencephalography**

   The combining form _____ tells me this is a diagnostic procedure on the _____.

2. **electromyography**

   The combining form _____ tells me this is a diagnostic procedure on the _____.

3. **myelography**

   The combining form _____ tells me this is a diagnostic procedure on the _____.

4. **electroencephalography**

   The combining form _____ tells me this is a diagnostic procedure on the _____.

5. Each of the four procedures listed previously ends with the suffix _____, which means

   _____.

Use the terms in questions 1 to 5 to identify (define) the statements in questions 6 through 8. (Hint: In some cases you are asked for the *record*, and in some cases you are asked for the *recording*.) Be precise! Fill in the blanks.

6. Recording of electrical activity in muscle: _____

7. Radiography of the spinal cord and nerve roots after injection of contrast medium into the subarachnoid space:

   _____

8. Record of the electrical activity of the brain: _____

M. **Diagnostic testing.** You are responsible for scheduling diagnostic procedures for patients in the Neurology Clinic at Fulwood Medical Center. Practice your *language of neurology* by scheduling these patients appropriately, using the following procedures. **LO 9.7**

CT scan	angiography
myelography	magnetic resonance imaging
evoked responses	nerve conduction studies
electromyography	electroencephalogram
lumbar puncture or spinal tap	magnetic resonance angiography

Patient Needs/Symptoms:	Schedule Patient for:
1. Dr. Solis would like to measure the speed at which a patient's motor nerves conduct impulses.	
2. Doctor has ordered a recording of the electrical activity of the patient's brain.	
3. Dr. Solis suspects a tumor and needs to see a highly detailed anatomical image of the brain.	
4. Patient needs x-rays of the spinal cord taken after dye has been injected into it.	
5. Dr. Solis wants a sample of the patient's CSF.	
6. Patient has to schedule a study with contrast to image the cerebral blood vessels.	
7. Patient has a blocked carotid artery.	
8. Patient has possibly had a stroke; study will be looking for areas of dead brain tissue.	
9. Sensory stimuli will be used to activate specific areas of the brain and measure responses with EEG.	
10. Doctor wants to test and record the electrical activity of a patient's muscle at rest and during contractions.	

N. **Pronunciation is important whether you are saying the word or listening to a word from a coworker.** Identify the proper pronunciation of the following medical terms. **LO 9.3, 9.4, 9.6, 9.7**

1. The correct pronunciation for an agent that causes an absence of feeling:

    a. ANAL-jeh-zik   b. an-al-**JEE**-zik   c. **AN**-eh-thet-ik   d. an-es-**THET**-ik

    Correctly spell the term: _____

2. The correct pronunciation for the failure of one or more vertebral arches to close during fetal development:

    a. SPY-na **BYE**-fih-day b. **SPY**-nah **BIH**-fih-dah c. **MAY**-nin-go-sell   d. meh-**NING**-oh-seal

    Correctly spell the term: _____

3. The correct pronunciation for a pharmacologic agent capable of preventing or arresting epilepsy:

    a. sed-**AY**-tiv   b. **SED**-ah-tiv   c. **AN**-tee-eh-pih-**LEP**-tik d. **AN**-tee-**PIE**-lep-**TIK**

    Correctly spell the term: _____

4. The correct pronunciation for the disorder described as a degenerative osteoarthritis of the spine:

    e. spon-dih-**LOH**-sis   f. spond-**ILL**-oh-**SIS**   g. **NEE**-ralj-**EE**-ah   h. nyu-**RAL**-jee-ah

    Correctly spell the term: _____

5. The correct pronunciation for the time occurring after a seizure:

    a. post-**IK**-tal   b. pah-**STICK**-tal   c. **TON**-ik   d. tone-**IK**

    Correctly spell the term: _____

Case Report

A. **Review this chapter's Case Report 9.1.** *Utilize the language of neurology and previous chapters to correctly answer each question. Fill in the blanks.* **LO 9.5, 9.6, 9.8, 9.9, 9.10**

Case Report (CR) 9.1

You are

. . . an **electroneurodiagnostic technician** working with Gregory Solis, MD, a **neurosurgeon** at Fulwood Medical Center.

Your patient is

. . . Ms. Roberta Gaston, a 39-year-old woman, who has been referred by Raul Cardenas, MD, a **neurologist,** for evaluation for possible **neurosurgery.**

Ms. Gaston has had **epileptic seizures** since the age of 16. She has **generalized tonic-clonic seizures** occurring once a week. She also has daily minor spells when she stops interacting with her surroundings and blinks rhythmically for about 20 seconds, after which she returns to normal. Numerous **antiepileptic** drugs, including phenobarbital, valproic acid, and phenytoin, have been tried with no relief. She is not able to work and is cared for by her parents.

Her neurologic examination is normal. Her **EEG** shows diffuse spike-and-wave discharges with a left-sided frontal predominance. Her **CT** is normal. An **MRI** shows a 20-mm diameter mass adjacent to the anterior horn of her left **ventricle.** Continuous EEG/video monitoring shows **ictal** activity in the left frontal lobe. Dr. Solis performed a surgical resection of the mass, which was a **glioma.** Ms. Gaston has been seizure-free since the surgery a year ago.

---

1. Which diagnostic test revealed the cause of Ms. Gaston's seizures? (provide the term, not the abbreviation)

   _____

2. Which specialist will treat the cause of the seizures? _____

3. What is the current name for her "minor spells?" (two words, provide plural form) seizures? _____

4. Which diagnostic test came back as normal? (provide the abbreviation) _____

5. Were the medications effective in controlling the seizures? _____

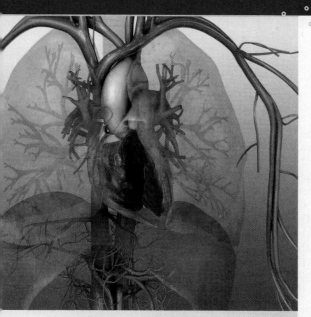

2014 Nucleus Medical Media

Cardiovascular System
The Language of Cardiology

Chapter Sections

Chapter Learning Outcomes

Upon completion of this chapter, you will be able to:

LO 10.1   Identify and describe the anatomy and physiology of the cardiovascular system.

LO 10.2   Use roots, combining forms, suffixes, and prefixes to construct and analyze medical terms related to the cardiovascular system.

LO 10.3   Spell medical terms related to the cardiovascular system.

LO 10.4   Pronounce medical terms related to the cardiovascular system.

LO 10.5   Describe diagnostic procedures utilized in cardiology.

LO 10.6   Identify and describe disorders and pathological conditions related to the cardiovascular system.

LO 10.7   Describe the therapeutic procedures and pharmacologic agents used in cardiology.

LO 10.8   Apply knowledge of medical terms relating to cardiology to documentation, medical records, and communication.

LO 10.9   Identify and correctly use abbreviations of terms used in cardiology.

LO 10.10 Identify health professionals involved in the care of cardiology patients.

The health professionals involved in the diagnosis and treatment of cardiovascular problems include:

- **Cardiologists,** medical doctors who specialize in disorders of the cardiovascular system.
- **Cardiovascular surgeons,** medical doctors who specialize in surgery of the heart and peripheral blood vessels.
- **Cardiovascular nurses,** who have extensive additional training and experience in treating patients with heart disease and often work in intensive care units, cardiovascular surgery, and cardiac clinics.
- **Cardiovascular technologists** and **technicians,** who assist physicians in the diagnosis and treatment of cardiovascular disorders.
- **Cardiac sonographers** or **echocardiographers,** who are technologists who use **ultrasound** to observe the heart chambers, valves, and blood vessels.
- **Perfusionists,** manage the heart-lung bypass machine during cardiac surgeries.
- **Phlebotomists,** who assist physicians by drawing patient blood samples for laboratory testing.

Section 10.1 The Heart

Position of the Heart
Location of the Heart

If you have a healthy heart rate of 60 beats per minute and you live to be 80 years old, your heart will beat (contract and relax) at least 2,522,880,000 times. Your heart pumps approximately 2,000 gallons of blood each day. In 80 years of life, it will have pumped a total of 58,400,000 gallons of blood. If your heart is unable to maintain this ability to pump blood for just a few minutes, your life is in danger. The heart is roughly the size of a fist and weighs around 10 ounces. It is a blunt cone that points down and to the left. The heart lies obliquely between the lungs, with one-third of its mass behind the **sternum** and two-thirds to the left of the sternum (*Figure 10.1a*). The **apex** can normally be palpated in the fifth **intercostal** space, between the fifth and sixth ribs. The base of the heart lies behind the sternum and the second intercostal space, between the second and third ribs. The region of the thoracic cavity in which the heart lies is called the **mediastinum** (*Figure 10.1b*).

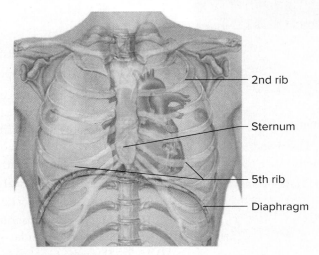

(a) Relationship of heart to sternum

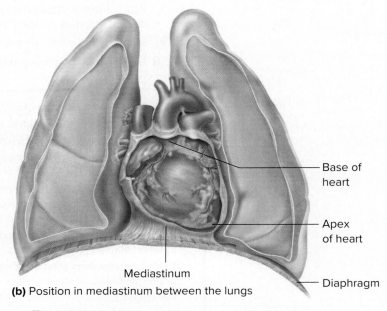

(b) Position in mediastinum between the lungs

▲ **Figure 10.1** **Position of heart in thoracic cavity.**

Functions and Structure of the Heart

Functions of the Heart

1. **Pumping blood.** Contractions of the heart generate the pressure to produce movement of blood through the blood vessels.

2. **Routing blood.** The heart can be described as two pumps. A pump on the right side of the heart sends blood through the **pulmonary** circulation of the lungs and back to the pump on the left side, which sends blood through the **systemic** circulation of the body. The valves of the heart ensure this one-way flow of blood.

3. **Regulating blood supply.** The changing metabolic needs of tissues and organs (for example, when you exercise) are met by changes in the rate and force of the heart's contraction.

Structure of the Heart

The heart wall consists of three layers *(Figure 10.2)*:

1. **Endocardium**—a single layer of cells over a thin layer of connective tissue lining the heart.

2. **Myocardium**—**cardiac** muscle cells that enable the heart to contract.

3. **Epicardium**—a thin serous membrane that is the inner layer of the pericardium.

   The **pericardium** is a connective tissue sac that surrounds and protects the heart. It consists of an inner **visceral** layer **(epicardium)** and outer **parietal** layer, between which is the **pericardial** cavity. This cavity contains a lubricant fluid that allows the heart to beat with very little friction around it.

Blood Supply to Heart Muscle

Because the heart beats continually and strongly, it requires an abundant supply of oxygen and nutrients. To meet this need, the cardiac muscle has its own blood circulation, the **coronary circulation** *(Figure 10.3)*.

Immediately above the aortic valve in the root of the aorta, the right and left **coronary arteries** exit from the aorta and divide into branches to begin the coronary circulation.

After the blood has flowed through the arteries into the capillaries of the myocardium, 80% drains into veins that flow into the right atrium and 20% flows into the right ventricle. There, the deoxygenated blood mixes with the deoxygenated blood from the rest of the body.

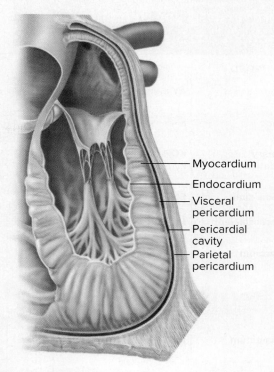

▲ **Figure 10.2** Heart wall.

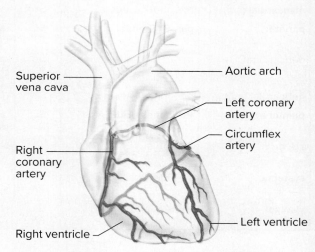

▲ **Figure 10.3** Coronary arterial circulation.

WORD	PRONUNCIATION	ELEMENTS		DEFINITION
apex	**AY**-peks		Latin *summit or tip*	Tip or end of cone-shaped structure, such as the heart
cardiac	**KAR**-dee-ak	S/ R/	-ac *pertaining to* cardi- *heart*	Pertaining to the heart
coronary circulation	**KOR**-oh-nair-ee **SER**-kyu-**LAY**-shun	S/ R/	-ary *pertaining to* coron- *crown* Latin *to encircle*	Blood flow through the vessels supplying the heart
endocardium	**EN**-doh-**KAR**-dee-um	S/ P/	-um *structure* endo- *inside*	The inside lining of the heart Pertaining to the endocardium
endocardial (adj)	**EN**-doh-**KAR**-dee-al	R/ S/	-cardi- *heart* -al *pertaining to*	
epicardium	**EP**-ih-**KAR**-dee-um	S/ P/ R/	-um *structure* epi- *upon, above* -cardi- *heart*	The outer layer of the heart wall
intercostal	**IN**-ter-**KOS**-tal	S/ P/ R/	-al *pertaining to* inter- *between* -cost- *rib*	The space between two ribs
mediastinum	**MEE**-dee-ass-**TIE**-num	S/ P/ R/	-um *structure* media- *middle* -stin- *partition*	Area between the lungs containing the heart, aorta, venae cavae, esophagus, and trachea
myocardium	**MY**-oh-**KAR**-dee-um	S/ R/CF R/	-um *structure* my/o- *muscle* -cardi- *heart*	All the heart muscle
myocardial (adj)	**MY**-oh-**KAR**-dee-al	S/	-al *pertaining to*	Pertaining to the myocardium
parietal	pah-**RYE**-eh-tal	S/ R/	-al *pertaining to* pariet- *wall*	Pertaining to the outer layer of the pericardium and other body cavities
pericardium	per-ih-**KAR**-dee-um	S/ P/ R/	-um *structure* peri- *around* -cardi- *heart*	Structure around the heart Pertaining to the pericardium
pericardial (adj)	per-ih-**KAR**-dee-al	S/	-al *pertaining to*	
pulmonary	**PULL**-moh-**NAIR**-ee	S/ R/	-ary *pertaining to* pulmon- *lung*	Pertaining to the lungs and their blood supply
sternum	**STIR**-num		Latin *chest*	Long, flat bone forming the center of the anterior wall of the chest
systemic	sis-**TEM**-ik	S/ R/	-ic *pertaining to* system- *body as a whole*	Relating to the entire organism
visceral	**VISS**-er-al	S/ R/	-al *pertaining to* viscer- *an organ*	Pertaining to the internal organs

Blood Flow through the Heart

The heart has four chambers (*Figure 10.4b*):

1. Right **atrium**
2. Right **ventricle**
3. Left atrium
4. Left ventricle

   The right and left sides of the heart are separated by the cardiac **septum,** which can be described in two sections:

- The right and left atria are separated by a thin muscle wall called the **interatrial** septum.
- The right and left ventricles are separated by a thicker muscle wall called the **interventricular** septum.

   In addition, the **atrioventricular (AV)** septum is located between and behind the right atrium and left ventricle.

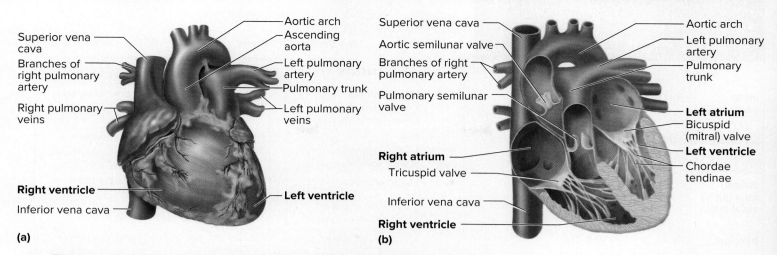

(a)
Superior vena cava
Branches of right pulmonary artery
Right pulmonary veins
Right ventricle
Inferior vena cava
Aortic arch
Ascending aorta
Left pulmonary artery
Pulmonary trunk
Left pulmonary veins
Left ventricle

(b)
Superior vena cava
Aortic semilunar valve
Branches of right pulmonary artery
Pulmonary semilunar valve
Right atrium
Tricuspid valve
Inferior vena cava
Right ventricle
Aortic arch
Left pulmonary artery
Pulmonary trunk
Left atrium
Bicuspid (mitral) valve
Left ventricle
Chordae tendinae

▲ **Figure 10.4** External (*a*) and internal (*b*) anatomy of the heart: frontal view.

Blood circulates around the body (through the systemic circulation) to unload oxygen and nutrients and pick up carbon dioxide and metabolic waste products. This deoxygenated blood returns to the heart via the **superior and inferior venae cavae.** These large veins open into the right atrium. When the right atrium contracts, the blood flows through the **tricuspid valve** into the right ventricle. The tricuspid valve then shuts so when the right ventricle contracts, blood cannot flow back into the atrium.

When the right ventricle contracts, the blood is pushed out through the **semilunar pulmonary valve** into the **pulmonary trunk** (*Figure 10.4a and b*) to begin the pulmonary circulation. The pulmonary valve then shuts to prevent blood flowing back into the ventricle. The pulmonary trunk divides into two arteries; the right pulmonary artery goes to the right lung and the left pulmonary artery goes to the left lung. In the lungs, carbon dioxide is unloaded, and oxygen is picked up from the air by the blood. The oxygen-rich blood is returned to the heart by the pulmonary veins (*Figure 10.4a and b*).

The blood from the pulmonary veins flows into the left atrium. When the atrium contracts, the blood flows through the **mitral** (or **bicuspid**) valve into the left ventricle. The bicuspid valve then shuts so that blood cannot flow back into the left atrium when the ventricle contracts. The bicuspid and tricuspid valves are anchored to the floor of the ventricles by stringlike **chordae tendineae** (*see Figure 10.4b*).

When the left ventricle contracts, the oxygenated blood is forced out under pressure through the **aortic** semilunar valve into the **aorta,** to return to circulating round the body in the systemic circulation (*Figure 10.5*). The aortic valve then shuts so blood cannot flow back into the left ventricle. The four valves all allow the blood to flow only in one direction.

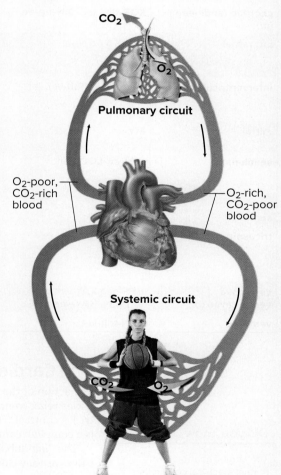

CO_2
O_2
Pulmonary circuit
O_2-poor, CO_2-rich blood
O_2-rich, CO_2-poor blood
Systemic circuit
CO_2
O_2

▲ **Figure 10.5** General schematic of the cardiovascular circulation. Sergey Ryzhov/ Shutterstock

Did you know...

The pulmonary circulation is the only place in the body where deoxygenated blood is carried in arteries and oxygenated blood is carried in veins.

WORD	PRONUNCIATION	ELEMENTS		DEFINITION
aorta aortic (adj)	ay-**OR**-tuh ay-**OR**-tic	 S/ R/	Greek *lift up* -ic *pertaining to* aort- *aorta*	Main trunk of the systemic arterial system Pertaining to the aorta
atrioventricular (AV)	**AY**-tree-oh-ven-**TRIK**-you-lar	S/ R/CF R/	-ar *pertaining to* atri/o- *entrance, atrium* -ventricul- *ventricle*	Pertaining to both the atrium and the ventricle
atrium atria (pl) atrial (adj)	**AY**-tree-um **AY**-tree-ah **AY**-tree-al	 S/ R/	Latin *entrance* -al *pertaining to* atri- *entrance, atrium*	Chamber where blood enters the heart on both right and left sides Pertaining to the atrium
bicuspid	by-**KUSS**-pid	S/ P/ R/	-id *having a particular quality* bi- *two* -cusp- *point*	Having two points; a bicuspid heart valve has two flaps
chordae tendineae (pl)	**KOR**-dee ten-**DIN**-ee-ee		chorda Latin *cord* tendinea Latin *tendons*	Tendinous cords attaching the bicuspid and tricuspid valves to the heart wall
interatrial	**IN**-ter-**AY**-tree-al	S/ P/ R/	-al *pertaining to* inter- *between* -atri- *atrium, entrance*	Between the atria of the heart
interventricular	**IN**-ter-ven-**TRIK**-you-lar	S/ P/ R/	-ar *pertaining to* inter- *between* -ventricul- *ventricle*	Between the ventricles of the heart
mitral	**MY**-tral		Latin *turban*	Shaped like the headdress of a Catholic bishop
semilunar	sem-ee-**LOO**-nar	S/ P/ R/	-ar *pertaining to* semi- *half* -lun- *moon*	Appears like a half moon
septum septa (pl)	**SEP**-tum **SEP**-tah		Latin *partition*	A wall dividing two cavities
tricuspid	try-**KUSS**-pid	S/ P/ R/	-id *having a particular quality* tri- *three* -cusp- *point*	Having three points; a tricuspid heart valve has three flaps
vena cava venae cavae (pl)	**VEE**-nah **KAY**-vah **VEE**-nee **KAY**-vee	R/CF R/	ven/a *vein* cava *cave*	One of the two largest veins in the body
ventricle	**VEN**-trih-kel		Latin *small belly*	Chamber of the heart or brain

The Cardiac Cycle

The action of the four heart chambers is coordinated. When the atria contract (atrial **systole**), the ventricles relax (ventricular **diastole,** or ventricular filling). When the atria relax (atrial diastole), the ventricles contract (ventricular systole). Then the atria and ventricles all relax briefly. This series of events is a complete cardiac cycle, or heartbeat.

The "*lub*-dub, *lub*-dub" sounds heard through the stethoscope are made by the snap of the heart valves as they close.

Electrical Properties of the Heart

As the cardiac muscles contract, they generate a small electrical current. Because the muscle cells are coupled together electrically, they stimulate their neighbor cells so that the myocardium of the atria, and that of the ventricles, each acts as a *single* unit.

Did you know...

The normal heartbeat with normal electrical conduction through the heart leading to a ventricular rate of around 60 to 90 beats per minute is called **sinus rhythm.**

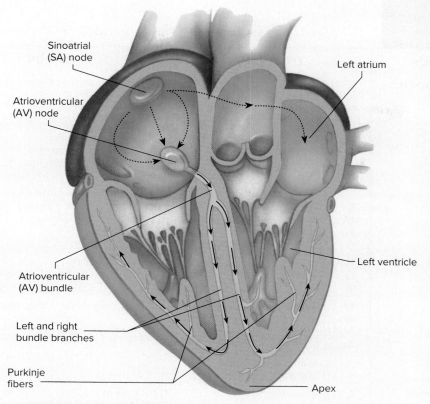

Sinoatrial
(SA) node

Atrioventricular
(AV) node

Atrioventricular
(AV) bundle

Left and right
bundle branches

Purkinje
fibers

Left atrium

Left ventricle

Apex

▲ **Figure 10.6** Cardiac conduction system.

To keep the heart beating in a rhythm, a **conduction system** is in place. It consists of five components *(Figure 10.6)*:

1. A small region of specialized muscle cells in the right atrium initiates the electrical current and, therefore, the heartbeat. This area is called the **sinoatrial (SA) node.** It is the **pacemaker** of heart rhythm.

2. Electrical signals from the SA node spread out through the atria and then come back together at the **atrioventricular (AV) node.** This is the electrical gateway to the ventricles, and normally electrical currents cannot get to the ventricles by any other route. The AV node delays impulses to ensure that the atria have ejected their blood into the ventricles before the ventricles contract.

3. Electrical signals leave the AV node to reach the ventricles through the **AV bundle** (**bundle of His**).

4. This *AV* bundle divides into the right and left **bundle branches,** which supply the two ventricles.

5. From the two bundle branches, **Purkinje fibers** spread through the ventricular myocardium and distribute the electrical stimuli to cause contraction of the ventricular myocardium.

Word Analysis and Definition: Cardiac Cycle

S = Suffix   P = Prefix   R = Root   R/CF = Combining Form

WORD	PRONUNCIATION	ELEMENTS		DEFINITION
atrioventricular	AY-tree-oh-ven-TRIK-you-lar	S/ R/CF R/	-ar *pertaining to* atri/o- *entrance, atrium* -ventricul- *ventricle*	Pertaining to both the atrium and ventricle
AV bundle bundle of His (syn) AV node	AY-VEE BUN-del BUN-del OV HISS AY-VEE NODE		(bundle) Old English *to bind* (His) Wilhelm His Jr., 1863–1934, Swiss cardiologist and anatomist	Pathway for electrical signals to be transmitted to the ventricles Part of the heart's conduction system that receives the electrical impulse that traveled from the atria, delays it, and then sends it to AV bundle
conduction	kon-DUCK-shun	S/ P/ R/	-ion *process* con- *together, with* -duct- *lead*	Process of transmitting energy
diastole diastolic (adj)	die-AS-toh-lee die-as-TOL-ik	S/ R/	Greek *dilation* -ic *pertaining to* diastol- *dilate*	Relaxation of heart cavities, during which they fill with blood Pertaining to relaxation of the heart cavities
pacemaker	PACE-may-ker	S/ R/	-maker *one who makes* pace- *step, pace*	Device that regulates cardiac electrical activity
Purkinje fibers	per-KIN-jee FIE-bers		Johannes von Purkinje, 1787–1869, Bohemian anatomist and physiologist	Network of nerve fibers in the myocardium
sinoatrial node	sigh-noh-AY-tree-al NODE	S/ R/CF R/	-al *pertaining to* sin/o- *sinus* -atri- *entrance, atrium*	The center of modified cardiac muscle fibers in the wall of the right atrium that acts as the pacemaker for the heart rhythm
sinus rhythm	SIGH-nus RITH-um		sinus Latin *channel, cavity* rhythm Greek *to flow*	The normal (optimal) heart rhythm arising from the sinoatrial node
systole systolic (adj)	SIS-toh-lee sis-TOL-ik	S/ R/	Greek *contraction* -ic *pertaining to* systol- *contract*	Contraction of the heart muscle Pertaining to contraction of the heart muscle

Check Point Section 10.1

A. Define the words in bold using the correct medical term. *Use the terms related to the function and structure of the heart to correctly answer the questions. Fill in the blanks.* **LO 10.1**

1. With the exception of the cranial and spinal cavities, all other cavities are lined with a double-walled serous membrane. The inner layer touches the **organ,** the outer layer forms the **wall** of the cavity.

    Which medical term means pertaining to an *organ?* _____.

    Which medical term means pertaining to a *wall?* _____.

2. The right side of the heart pumps blood through arteries to the **lungs** to pick up oxygen. The left side of the heart pumps blood through arteries to deliver oxygenated blood to the organs of each body **system.**

    The right side of the heart pumps blood to the _____ circulation.

    The left side of the heart pumps blood to the _____ circulation.

B. Construct medical terms. *Provide the correct prefix to the term to correctly complete each sentence.* **LO 10.1**

1. The **inside** of the heart is termed the _____ /cardium.

2. The **muscular** part of the heart is termed the _____ /cardium.

3. The **outer** layer of the heart is termed the _____ /cardium.

C. Plurals of medical terms follow certain established rules. *Apply these rules and change the singular forms into plurals.* **LO 10.1, 10.3**

1. Singular: **atrium** Plural: _____

2. Singular: **septum** Plural: _____

3. Singular: **vena cava** Plural: _____

4. Singular: **ventricle** Plural: _____

D. Describe the blood flow through the heart. *Given the name of the blood vessel, describe how it interacts with the heart chambers. Match the term in the first column with its proper description in the second column.* **LO 10.1**

Blood Vessel	Interaction with the Heart
_____ 1. aorta	**a.** receives blood from the right ventricle
_____ 2. venae cavae	**b.** receives blood from the left ventricle
_____ 3. pulmonary arteries	**c.** empties blood into the left atrium
_____ 4. pulmonary veins	**d.** empties blood into the right atrium

E. Place in order the electrical events of the heart. *In the list below, number the events as they normally occur in the heart. Start with 1 for the first event, through 5 for the last event.* **LO 10.1**

_____ AV bundle

_____ SA node

_____ Purkinje fibers

_____ AV node

_____ bundle branches

F. Define the events of the cardiac cycle. *From the provided definition, give the correct term it is describing. Fill in the blanks.* **LO 10.1**

1. Period of time when the heart chamber is contracting. _____

2. Period of time when the heart chamber is filling with blood. _____

Section 10.2 Circulatory Systems

Blood Circulation Systems

There are two major **circulations:** the **pulmonary** and the **systemic.**

Pulmonary Circulation

Deoxygenated blood from the body flows into the right atrium of the heart and then into the right ventricle, which pumps it out into the pulmonary trunk *(Figure 10.7)*. This trunk branches into the right pulmonary **artery** to the right lung and the left pulmonary artery to the left lung. Gas exchange occurs between the air in the lungs and blood *(see Chapter 13)*. Carbon dioxide is removed from the blood and excreted into the air. Oxygen is taken into the blood from the air in the lungs.

The blood exits each lung through two pulmonary veins. All four pulmonary veins take blood into the left atrium of the heart.

Did you know...

The peripheral circulation
- Transports oxygen, nutrients, hormones, and enzymes to the cells and carries carbon dioxide and waste products to the lungs, liver, and kidney for excretion.
- Maintains homeostasis by enabling cells to meet their metabolic needs and maintains a steady flow of blood and blood pressure in the tissues.

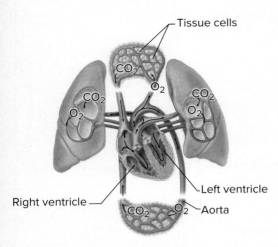

▲ **Figure 10.7** Systemic and pulmonary circulations.

Systemic Arterial Circulation

The systemic circulation (*Figures 10.7 and 10.8*) refers to the process wherein oxygenated blood enters the left side of the heart from the pulmonary veins. The blood passes through the left atrium into the left ventricle. The ventricle pumps it out into the **aorta,** which takes the blood to all areas of the body. The **coronary circulation** takes blood to and away from the myocardium. The **peripheral** vessels are those that carry blood to and from the other body tissues.

The aorta is described in four parts:

1. **Ascending aorta,** which gives rise to the coronary circulation. Right and left coronary arteries branch from it to supply the myocardium.

2. **Aortic arch** *(Figure 10.8),* which has three main branches:
   a. **Brachiocephalic artery,** a short artery that divides into two arteries:
      i. **Right common carotid artery,** which supplies the right side of the head, brain, and neck.
      ii. **Right subclavian artery,** which supplies the right upper limb.
   b. **Left common carotid artery,** which supplies the left side of the head, brain, and neck. The right and left common carotid arteries divide into two branches:
      i. The **internal carotid** artery, which enters the cranial cavity through a foramen in the base of the skull and supplies the brain.
      ii. The **external carotid** artery, which supplies the neck and face.
   c. **Left subclavian artery,** which supplies the left upper limb.

3. **Thoracic aorta,** which has two major groups of branches:
   a. **Visceral** branches—small **bronchial arteries** that supply the bronchi and bronchioles *(see Chapter 13),* the esophagus, and the pericardium.
   b. **Parietal** branches—**intercostal arteries** that supply the chest wall and a **phrenic artery** that supplies the diaphragm.

4. **Abdominal aorta,** which has two major groups of branches:
   a. **Visceral branches** that supply the abdominal organs:
      i **Celiac trunk,** which supplies the stomach, liver, gallbladder, pancreas, and spleen.
      ii. **Superior mesenteric artery,** which supplies the small intestine and part of the large intestine.
      iii. **Inferior mesenteric artery,** which supplies the remainder of the large intestine.
      iv. Paired **renal arteries,** which supply the kidneys and adrenal glands.
      v. Paired **gonadal arteries,** which supply the testes or ovaries.
   b. Four pairs of **lumbar** arteries that supply the abdominal wall.
   At the level of the fifth lumbar vertebra (at the top of the pelvis), the aorta divides into the right and left **common iliac arteries.** Visceral branches from these arteries supply the urinary bladder, uterus, and vagina. The common iliac arteries give off an internal iliac artery to supply the pelvis. The common iliac artery becomes the external iliac artery and then the femoral artery as it goes down the thigh and supplies the lower limb. The pulse that can be felt in the back of the knee is from the **popliteal artery.**

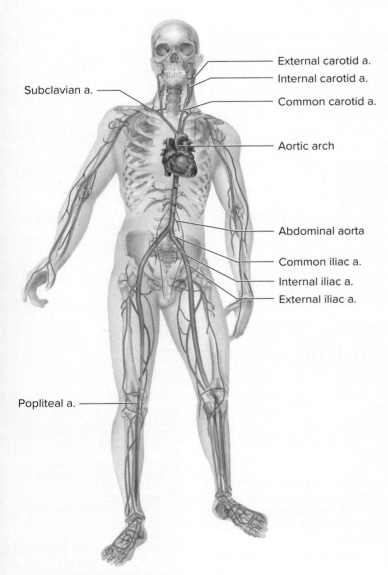

▲ **Figure 10.8** The major systemic arteries.
(*a.* = artery)

WORD	PRONUNCIATION		ELEMENTS	DEFINITION
artery	**AR**-ter-ee		Greek *artery*	Thick-walled blood vessel carrying blood away from the heart
bronchus bronchi (pl) bronchial	**BRONG**-kus **BRONG**-key-al	S/ R/CF	Latin *windpipe* al *pertaining to* **bronch/i** *bronchus*	One of the two subdivisions of the trachea Pertaining to the bronchi
brachiocephalic	**BRAY**-kee-oh-seh-**FAL**-ik	S/ R/CF R/	-ic *pertaining to* **brachi/o**- *arm* **-cephal**- *head*	Pertaining to the head and arm, as an artery supplying blood to both
carotid	kah-**ROT**-id		Greek *carotid artery*	Main artery of the neck
circulation	**SER**-kyu-**LAY**-shun		Latin *to encircle*	Continuous movement of blood through the heart and blood vessels
gonad gonadal (adj)	**GO**-nad go-**NAD**-al		Greek *seed*	Testis or ovary Pertaining to a testis or ovary
iliac	**ILL**-ee-ak		Latin *groin, flank*	Pertaining to, or near, the ilium (pelvic bone)
lumbar	**LUM**-bar		Latin *loin*	Relating to the region in the back and sides between the ribs and pelvis
mesentery mesenteric (adj)	**MESS**-en-ter-ee **MESS**-enter-ree	P/ R/CF S/	mes- *middle* **-enter/o** *intestine* -ic *pertaining to*	A double layer peritoneum enclosing the abdominal viscera Pertaining to the mesentery
peripheral	peh-**RIF**-er-al	S/ R/	-al *pertaining to* **peripher**- *outer part*	Pertaining to a part of the body away from a central point. For example, the peripheral circulation is away from the heart
popliteal	pop-**LIT**-ee-al	S/ R/CF	-al *pertaining to* **poplit/e**- *back of knee*	Pertaining to the back of the knee
pulmonary	**PULL**-moh-**NAIR**-ee	S/ R/	-ary *pertaining to* **pulmon**- *lung*	Pertaining to the lungs and their blood supply
renal	**REE**-nal	S/ R/	-al *pertaining to* **ren**- *kidney*	Pertaining to the kidney
subclavian	sub-**CLAY**-vee-an	S/ P/ R/	-ian *one who does* sub- *under* **-clav**- *clavicle*	Underneath and behind the clavicle
visceral	**VISS**-er-al	S/ R/	-al *pertaining to* **viscer**- *an organ*	Pertaining to the internal organs

Blood Vessels in the Circulations

Arterioles, Capillaries, and Venules

As the arteries branch farther away from the heart and distribute blood to specific organs, they become smaller, muscular vessels called **arterioles.** By contracting and relaxing, these arterioles are the primary controllers by which the body directs the relative amounts of blood that organs and structures receive.

From there, the blood flows into **capillaries** and **capillary beds** *(Figure 10.9)*. There are approximately 10 billion capillaries in the body. Each capillary consists of only a single layer of **endothelium** supported by a thin connective tissue basement membrane. Between the overlapping **endothelial** cells are thin slits through which larger water-soluble substances can pass. Red blood cells flow through the small capillaries in single file.

From the capillaries, tiny **venules** accept the blood and merge to form **veins.** The veins form reservoirs for blood; at any moment 60% to 70% of the total blood volume is contained in the venules and veins.

The circulatory system exists to serve the capillaries because capillaries are the only place where water and materials are exchanged between the blood and tissue fluids.

Diffusion is the means by which this capillary exchange occurs. Nutrients and oxygen diffuse from a higher concentration in the capillaries to a lower concentration in the **interstitial** fluid around the cells. Waste products diffuse from a higher concentration in the interstitial fluid to a lower concentration in the capillaries.

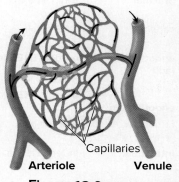

Capillaries

Arteriole   Venule

▲ **Figure 10.9** Capillary bed.

Systemic Venous Circulation

There are three major types of veins (*Figure 10.10*):

1. **Superficial**—such as those you can see under the skin of your arms and hands.

2. **Deep**—running parallel to arteries and draining the same tissues that the arteries supply.

3. **Venous sinuses**—in the head and heart and having specific functions.

In the lower limb, the superficial veins merge to form the **saphenous vein.** The deep veins form the **femoral vein.** They join together with veins from the pelvis to form the **common iliac vein.** The right and left common iliac veins form the **inferior vena cava (IVC).**

Veins draining the abdominal organs merge into the **hepatic portal vein,** which delivers nutrients from the stomach and intestines to the liver. Within the liver, the nutrients are either stored or converted into chemicals that can be used by other cells in the body. The blood leaves the liver in **hepatic veins** that drain into the IVC.

In the upper limb, the superficial veins merge to form the **axillary vein.** The deep veins alongside the limb arteries empty into the **brachial veins.** These also flow into the axillary vein.

As the axillary vein passes behind the clavicle, its name changes to the **subclavian vein.**

In the head and neck, the superficial veins outside the skull drain into the right and left **external jugular veins.** Inside the cranial cavity, **venous sinuses** around the brain drain into the right and left **internal jugular veins.**

The external jugular veins empty into the subclavian veins. The internal jugular veins join with the subclavian veins on each side to form the **brachiocephalic veins.** The right and left brachiocephalic veins join together to form the superior vena cava (SVC). The SVC empties into the right atrium.

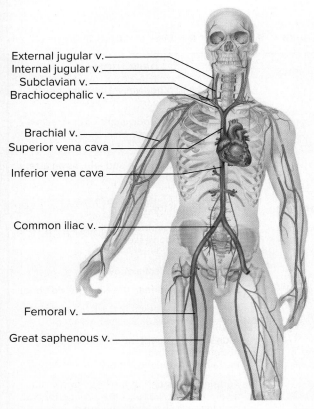

External jugular v.
Internal jugular v.
Subclavian v.
Brachiocephalic v.

Brachial v.
Superior vena cava

Inferior vena cava

Common iliac v.

Femoral v.

Great saphenous v.

▲ **Figure 10.10** **The major systemic veins.** (*v.* = vein)

Word Analysis and Definition: Blood Vessels in the Circulations

S = Suffix   P = Prefix   R = Root   R/CF = Combining Form

WORD	PRONUNCIATION		ELEMENTS	DEFINITION
arteriole	ar-**TEER**-ee-ole	S/ R/	-ole *small* arteri- *artery*	Small terminal artery leading into the capillary network
axilla axillary (adj)	**AK**-sill-ah **AK**-sil-air-ee	 S/ R/	Latin *armpit* -ary *pertaining to* axill- *armpit*	Medical name for the armpit Pertaining to the axilla
brachial	**BRAY**-kee-al	S/ R/	-al *pertaining to* brachi- *arm*	Pertaining to the arm
capillary	**KAP**-ih-lair-ee	S/ R/	-ary *pertaining to* capill- *hairlike structure*	Minute blood vessel between the arterial and venous systems
endothelial (adj) endothelium	en-doh-**THEE**-lee-al en-doh-**THEE**-lee-um	S/ P/ R/ S/	-al *pertaining to* endo- *inside, within* -theli- *lining* -um *structure*	A type of epithelial cell that lines the inside of blood vessels, lymphatic vessels, and the heart Tissue found lining the inside of blood vessels and lymphatic vessels
femoral	**FEM**-oh-ral	S/ R/	-al *pertaining to* femor- *femur*	Pertaining to the femur
interstitial	in-ter-**STISH**-al	S/ R/	-ial *pertaining to* interstit- *spaces within tissues*	Pertaining to spaces between cells in a tissue or organ
jugular	**JUG**-you-lar	S/ R/	-ar *pertaining to* jugul- *throat*	Pertaining to the throat
saphenous	**SAF**-ih-nus		Arabic *hidden, concealed*	Relating to the saphenous vein in the thigh
vein venous (adj) venule	VANE **VEE**-nuss **VEN**-yule	 S/ R/ S/	Latin *vein* -ous *pertaining to* ven- *vein* -ule *small*	Blood vessel carrying blood toward the heart Pertaining to venous blood or the venous circulation Small vein leading from the capillary network

Blood Vessel Function Related to Structure

Except for the capillaries and venules, all the blood vessel walls show a basic structure of three layers *(Figure 10.11)*:

1. **Tunica intima** (interna)—the innermost layer of endothelial cells, with thin layers of fibrous and elastic connective tissue supporting them.

2. Tunica **media**—a middle layer of smooth muscle cells arranged circularly around the blood vessel. A membrane of elastic tissue separates the tunica media from the outer layer of the wall.

3. Tunica **adventitia** (externa)—an outer connective tissue layer of varying density and thickness.

The larger arteries near the heart, the aorta and its major branches, have to cope with large quantities of blood and fluctuating pressures between systole and diastole. Therefore, these arteries have a large number of elastic fibers and a relatively small number of muscle fibers.

The functions of the medium-sized and smaller arteries are to regulate the blood supply to the different regions of the body and to ensure that the blood pressure in the arteries is at an appropriate level. The tunica media of these arteries contains 25 to 40 layers of smooth muscle to enable the muscles to contract (**vasoconstriction**) and to relax (**vasodilation**) to increase flow.

The function of the veins is to return the blood from the periphery to the heart in a low-pressure system. For example, by the time blood reaches the venules, its pressure has dropped from the 120 mm Hg of systole to around 15 mm Hg. By the time the blood is in the venae cavae, the **central venous pressure (CVP)** is down to around 4 to 5 mm Hg.

Veins have a much thinner tunica media than arteries, with few muscle cells and elastic fibers *(Figure 10.11)*. They have a larger lumen and a thick tunica adventitia that merges with the connective tissue of surrounding structures. In the limbs, the veins are surrounded and massaged by muscles to squeeze the blood along the veins. One-way valves in the veins allow the blood to flow toward the heart but not away from the heart. They are shaped like and function like the semilunar valves of the heart.

Space Medicine

Normally, gravity helps the blood circulate in the lower limbs. When astronauts are weightless for long periods of time, blood pools in the central and upper areas of the body, and there appears to be an excess blood volume. The kidney compensates by excreting more fluid, leading to a 10% to 20% decrease in blood volume and a low blood pressure. Astronauts compensate for this by wearing lower-body suction suits, which apply a vacuum force to draw blood into the lower limbs.

Arterial Pulses

The pulse is always part of a clinical examination because it can show heart rate, rhythm, and the state of the arterial wall by **palpation**. There are nine locations on each side of the body where large arteries are close to the surface and can be palpated *(Figure 10.12)*.

The most easily accessible is the **radial artery** at the wrist, where the pulse is usually taken. The **brachial artery** at the elbow is also used for taking blood pressure readings. All the pulse sites can be used as **pressure points** to temporarily reduce arterial bleeding in an emergency.

The two pulses that can be palpated in the feet are the **pedal** pulses, one in each foot.

Blood Pressure

Blood pressure (BP) is the force the blood exerts on arterial walls as it is pumped around the circulatory system by the left ventricle.

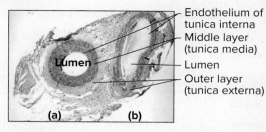

▲ **Figure 10.11** Anatomy of an artery and vein. (a) Artery. (b) Vein. CNRI/Science Source

Labels:
- Endothelium of tunica interna
- Middle layer (tunica media)
- Lumen
- Outer layer (tunica externa)
- Lumen
- (a)
- (b)

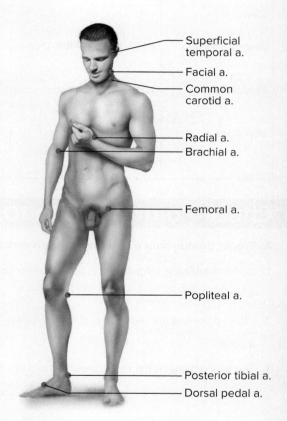

▲ **Figure 10.12** Arterial pulses. (*a.* = artery)

Labels:
- Superficial temporal a.
- Facial a.
- Common carotid a.
- Radial a.
- Brachial a.
- Femoral a.
- Popliteal a.
- Posterior tibial a.
- Dorsal pedal a.

> **Did you know...**
>
> - All blood vessel walls have three layers.
> - **Vital signs (VS)** measure temperature (T), pulse rate (P), respiration rate (R), and blood pressure (BP) to assess cardiorespiratory function.

Word Analysis and Definition: Blood Vessel Function Related to Structure

S = Suffix   P = Prefix   R = Root   R/CF = Combining Form

WORD	PRONUNCIATION		ELEMENTS	DEFINITION
adventitia	ad-ven-**TISH**-ah		Latin *from outside*	Outer layer of connective tissue covering blood vessels or organs
intima	**IN**-tih-ma		Latin *inmost*	Inner layer of a structure, particularly a blood vessel
media	**MEE**-dee-ah		Latin *middle*	Middle layer of a structure, particularly a blood vessel
pedal	**PEED**-al	S/ R/	-al *pertaining to* ped- *foot*	Pertaining to the foot
radial	**RAY**-dee-al	S/ R/	-al *pertaining to* radi- *radius (forearm bone)*	Pertaining to the forearm
tunica	**TYU**-nih-kah		Latin *coat*	A layer in the wall of a blood vessel or other tubular structure
vasoconstriction	**VAY**-soh-con-**STRIK**-shun	S/ R/CF R/	-ion *process* vas/o- *blood vessel* -constrict- *narrow*	Reduction in diameter of a blood vessel
vasodilation	**VAY**-soh-die-**LAY**-shun	S/ R/CF R/	-ion *process* vas/o- *blood vessel* -dilat- *open up*	Increase in diameter of a blood vessel
vital signs	**VIE**-tal SIGNS		**vital** Latin *life* **signs** Latin *mark*	A procedure during a physical examination in which temperature, pulse rate, respiration rate, and blood pressure are measured to assess general health and cardiorespiratory function

Check Point Section 10.2

A. Proper pronunciation of terms is key to verbal communication. *Choose the answer that correctly completes each statement.* **LO 10.4**

1. In the combining form *brachi/o,* the vowel *i* is pronounced like the vowel in:

   a. key   **b.** eye   **c.** sick   **d.** rate

2. When pronouncing the term *popliteal,* emphasis is put on the syllable:

   a. pop   **b.** lit   **c.** ee   **d.** al

3. The first syllable in the term *carotid* sounds like the first syllable in the term:

   a. cat   **b.** carrot   **c.** cousin   **d.** cake

B. Blood travels through the body in a system of connected tubes called blood vessels. *Below are sentences that describe this system. Use the words provided to correctly fill in the blanks.* **LO 10.2**

   circulation   peripheral   artery   pulmonary

The body has a system that moves blood to all of the organs. This system that delivers blood to the body's organs is called the systemic (1) _____. This circulation delivers oxygen-rich blood to the (2) _____ organs which include the arms and legs. The (3) _____ system delivers blood to the lungs to pick up oxygen and get rid of carbon dioxide. Any vessel that carries blood away from the heart is called an (4) _____.

C. Use the medical terminology of the circulatory system. *Select the correct answer to complete each statement.* **LO 10.1**

1. The blood exits each lung through the

   a. vena cava   **b.** pulmonary veins   **c.** aorta   **d.** pulmonary arteries

2. The *coronary circulation* arises in the

   a. thoracic aorta   **b.** carotid arteries   **c.** ascending aorta   **d.** subclavian arteries

3. *Carbon dioxide* is removed from the blood and excreted through

    a. sweat   **b.** lymph   **c.** urine   **d.** air

4. *Deoxygenated blood* from the body flows into the

    a. right atrium   **b.** right ventricle   **c.** left atrium   **d.** left ventricle

5. *Gas exchange* occurs between the air in the lungs and the

    a. heart   **b.** blood   **c.** ventricles   **d.** windpipe

6. The pulse that can be felt at the back of the knee is from the

    a. aorta   **b.** popliteal vein   **c.** carotid artery   **d.** popliteal artery

7. The _____ arteries supply the chest wall.

    a. phrenic   **b.** visceral   **c.** intercostal   **d.** mesenteric

8. This circulation takes blood to all areas of the body

    a. coronary   **b.** pulmonary   **c.** cardiovascular   **d.** systemic

9. The *subclavian* artery is located

    a. above the heart   **b.** below the stomach   **c.** above the neck   **d.** below the collarbone

10. The _____ circulation takes blood to the lungs to become oxygenated.

    a. systemic   **b.** pulmonary   **c.** coronary   **d.** carotid

D. Identify the meanings of the word elements. *Choose the correct answer that relates to the definitions of word elements.* **LO 10.1, 10.2**

1. Identify a suffix listed below that means *small:*

    a. *-ary*   **b.** *-ial*   **c.** *-ery*   **d.** *-ule*

2. In the term **femoral,** the root is

    a. *-al*   **b.** *fem-*   **c.** *fem/o*   **d.** *femor-*   **e.** *-oral*

3. The root *jugul-* means

    a. neck   **b.** head   **c.** throat   **d.** large

E. Identify the medical term for each of the following descriptions. *Fill in the blanks.* **LO 10.1**

1. Write the term that means *small vein:* _____.

2. Write the term that means *small artery:* _____.

3. The only type of vessel where diffusion of gases between tissues and blood takes place (singular): _____.

4. The two large veins in the neck are the _____ veins.

F. Match the definition in the left column with the correct medical term in the right column. LO 10.1

_____	1. Pertaining to the forearm	**a.** radial
_____	2. Reduction in diameter of a blood vessel	**b.** vasodilation
_____	3. Inner layer of a structure	**c.** adventitia
_____	4. Latin for *coat*	**d.** pedal
_____	5. Outer tissue covering of an organ	**e.** vasoconstriction
_____	6. Middle layer of a structure	**f.** media
_____	7. Pertaining to the foot	**g.** intima
_____	8. Increase in diameter of a blood vessel	**h.** tunica

Section 10.3 Disorders of the Heart and Circulatory System

Disorders of the Heart

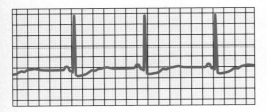

▲ **Figure 10.13** Bradycardia.

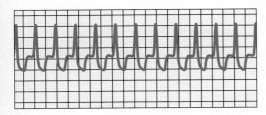

▲ **Figure 10.14** Tachycardia.

Abnormal Heart Rhythms

Every different structure within the heart may not function properly. When the heart is beating outside of normal sinus rhythm, the condition is termed **arrhythmia** or **dysrhythmia** (these two terms are synonyms). The normal rate of heartbeat is 60 to 100 beats per minute. A heart rate slower than 60 is called **bradycardia** *(Figure 10.13)*. A heart rate faster than 100 is called **tachycardia** *(Figure 10.14)*.

There are four common types of **arrhythmias (dysrhythmias),** abnormal or irregular heartbeats:

1. **Premature beats** may originate in either the atrium or the ventricle, or both. They may occur in individuals of all ages and could be associated with caffeine and stress.

2. **Atrial fibrillation** (**A-fib**) occurs when the two atria quiver rather than contract in an organized fashion to pump blood into the ventricle. This causes blood to pool in the atria and sometimes clot. **Paroxysmal atrial tachycardia (PAT)** presents with periods of rapid, regular heartbeats that originate in the atrium. The episodes begin and end abruptly. The heart rate speeds up to 160 to 200 beats per minute.

3. **Ventricular arrhythmias** consist of several types. **Ventricular tachycardia** is a rapid heartbeat arising in the ventricles. **Premature ventricular contractions (PVCs)** occur when extra impulses arise from a ventricle. **Ventricular fibrillation (V-fib)** is characterized by erratic ventricular contractions. The ventricles quiver and beat ineffectively instead of pumping.

4. **Heart block** occurs when interference in cardiac electrical conduction causes the contractions of the atria to fail to coordinate with the contractions of the ventricles.

Palpitations are unpleasant sensations of a rapid or irregular heartbeat that last a few seconds or minutes. They can be brought on by exercise, anxiety, and stimulants like caffeine. Occasionally, they can be caused by an arrhythmia.

Word Analysis and Definition: Abnormal Heart Rhythms

S = Suffix   P = Prefix   R = Root   R/CF = Combining Form

WORD	PRONUNCIATION	ELEMENTS		DEFINITION
arrhythmia (note the double "rr")	ah-**RITH**-mee-ah	S/ P/ R/	**-ia** *condition* **a-** *without* **-rrhythm-** *rhythm*	An abnormal heart rhythm
bradycardia	brad-ee-**KAR**-dee-ah	S/ P/ R/	**-ia** *condition* **brady-** *slow* **-card-** *heart*	Slow heart rate (below 60 beats per minute)
dysrhythmia	dis-**RITH**-mee-ah	S/ P/ R/	**-ia** *condition* **dys-** *bad* **-rhythm-** *rhythm*	An abnormal heart rhythm
fibrillation	fih-brih-**LAY**-shun	S/ R/	**-ation** *process* **fibrill-** *small fiber*	Uncontrolled quivering or twitching of the heart muscle
palpitation	pal-pih-**TAY**-shun	S/ R/	**-ation** *process* **palpit-** *throb*	Forcible, rapid beat of the heart felt by the patient
paroxysmal	par-ok-**SIZ**-mal	S/ R/	**-al** *pertaining to* **paroxysm-** *irritation*	Occurring in sharp, spasmodic episodes
tachycardia	tak-ih-**KAR**-dee-ah	S/ P/ R/	**-ia** *condition* **tachy-** *rapid* **-card-** *heart*	Rapid heart rate (above 100 beats per minute)

Disorders of the Heart Valves

Heart valves can **malfunction** in two basic ways:

1. **Stenosis** occurs when the valve does not open fully, and its opening is narrowed (constricted). Blood cannot flow freely through the valve and accumulates behind the valve.

2. **Incompetence** or **insufficiency** occurs when the valve cannot close fully, and blood can **regurgitate** (flow back) through the valve to the chamber from which it started.

Mitral valve stenosis can occur following rheumatic fever. Because the blood cannot flow freely through the valve, the left atrium becomes dilated. Eventually, **chronic heart failure** results.

Mitral valve incompetence occurs when there is leakage back through the valve as the left ventricle contracts. The left atrium becomes dilated. Again, chronic heart failure results.

Mitral valve prolapse (**MVP**) occurs when the cusps of the valve bulge back into the left atrium when the left ventricle contracts, thus allowing blood to flow back into the atrium (*Figure 10.15*).

Aortic valve stenosis is common in the elderly when the valves become calcified due to **atherosclerosis.** Blood flow into the systemic circuit is diminished, leading to dizziness and fainting. The left ventricle dilates, hypertrophies, and ultimately fails.

Aortic valve incompetence initially produces few symptoms other than a murmur, but eventually the left ventricle fails.

Rheumatic fever is an inflammatory disease. If a sore throat caused by group A beta-hemolytic *streptococcus* (*see Chapter 13*) is not treated with a complete course of antibiotics, antibodies to the bacteria can develop and attack normal tissue. Multiple joints are inflamed, and endocarditis can affect the function of the heart valves—particularly the mitral and aortic valves.

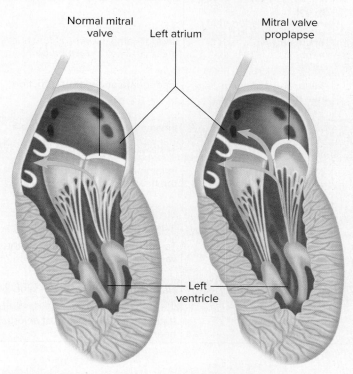

Normal mitral valve — Left atrium — Mitral valve proplapse — Left ventricle

▲ **Figure 10.15** Mitral valve. (a) Normal. (b) Mitral valve prolapse.

Disorders of the Heart Wall

Endocarditis is inflammation of the lining of the heart. It is usually secondary to an infection elsewhere. Intravenous drug users and people with damaged heart valves are at high risk for endocarditis.

Myocarditis is inflammation of the heart muscle. It can be bacterial, viral, or fungal in origin or a complication of other diseases, such as influenza.

Pericarditis is inflammation of the covering of the heart. The inflammation causes an **exudate** (pericardial **effusion**) to be released into the pericardial space. This interferes with the heart's ability to contract and expand normally, and cardiac output falls—a condition called **cardiac tamponade.**

Cardiomyopathy is a weakening of the heart muscle that causes it to pump inadequately. The etiology can be viral, idiopathic (when the cause is unknown), or alcoholic. It causes **cardiomegaly** and heart failure.

WORD	PRONUNCIATION	ELEMENTS		DEFINITION
cardiomegaly	KAR-dee-oh-MEG-ah-lee	S/ R/CF	-megaly *enlargement* cardi/o- *heart*	Enlargement of the heart
cardiomyopathy	KAR-dee-oh-my-OP-ah-thee	S/ R/CF R/CF	-pathy *disease* cardi/o- *heart* -my/o- *muscle*	Disease of heart muscle, the myocardium
cor pulmonale	KOR pul-moh-NAH-lee	R/ S/ R/	cor *heart* -ale *pertaining to* pulmon- *lung*	Right-sided heart failure arising from chronic lung disease
effusion	eh-FYU-shun		Latin *pouring out*	Collection of fluid that has escaped from blood vessels into a cavity or tissues
endocarditis	EN-doh-kar-DIE-tis	S/ P/ R/	-itis *inflammation* endo- *within* -card- *heart*	Inflammation of the lining of the heart
exudate	EKS-you-date	S/ P/ R/	-ate *process, composed of* ex- *out of* -ud- *sweat*	Fluid that has come out of a tissue or its capillaries because of inflammation or injury
incompetence	in-KOM-peh-tense	S/ P/ R/	-ence *quality of* in- *not* -compet- *strive together*	Failure of valves to close completely
insufficiency	in-suh-FISH-en-see	S/ P/ R/CF	-ency *quality of* in- *not* -suffic/i- *enough*	Lack of completeness of function; in the heart, failure of a valve to close properly
malfunction	mal-FUNK-shun	S/ P/ R/	-ion *action, condition* mal- *bad, inadequate* -funct- *perform*	Inadequate or abnormal function
myocarditis	MY-oh-kar-DIE-tis	S/ R/CF R/	-itis *inflammation* my/o- *muscle* -card- *heart*	Inflammation of the heart muscle
pericarditis	PER-ih-kar-DIE-tis	S/ P/ R/	-itis *inflammation* peri- *around* -card- *heart*	Inflammation of the pericardium, the covering of the heart
prolapse	proh-LAPS		Latin *a falling*	The falling or slipping of a body part from its normal position
regurgitate	ree-GUR-jih-tate	S/ P/ R/	-ate *pertaining to* re- *back* -gurgit- *flood*	To flow backward; in this case, through a heart valve
stenosis	steh-NOH-sis	S/ R/CF	-sis *abnormal condition* sten/o- *narrow*	Narrowing of a canal or passage, as in the narrowing of a heart valve
tamponade	tam-poh-NAID	S/ R/	-ade *process* tampon- *plug*	Pathologic compression of an organ such as the heart

Coronary Artery Disease (CAD)

The arteries supplying the myocardium become narrowed by atherosclerotic **plaques,** called **atheroma.** As the atheroma increases, the lumen of the artery becomes increasingly narrow *(compare Figure 10.16a and b).* The blood supplied to the cardiac muscle by the artery is reduced. Platelet aggregation can occur on the plaque to form a blood clot (**coronary thrombosis**). **Atherosclerosis** is the most common form of **arteriosclerosis** (hardening of the arteries) and can lead to **arteriosclerotic heart disease (ASHD).**

Angina pectoris, pain in the chest on exertion, is often the first symptom of reduced oxygen supply to the myocardium.

When blood flow in any of the coronary arteries is blocked (**occluded**), **myocardial ischemia** occurs. If ischemia is not reversed within 4 to 6 hours, the myocardial cells die, resulting in a condition called **myocardial infarction.** The area of **necrosis** becomes **fibrotic** (stiff), which decreases the ability of the heart to pump blood.

Cardiogenic shock occurs when the heart fails to pump effectively and organs and tissues are **perfused** inadequately. The pulse is weak and rapid, and **blood pressure** (**BP**) drops. The patient becomes pale, cold, sweaty, and anxious.

The other form of circulatory shock is **hypovolemic shock,** in which there is a loss of blood volume, often from hemorrhage or dehydration.

Cardiac arrest is the sudden cessation of cardiac activity resulting from **anoxia.**

Death is recorded by a flat ECG line as in **asystole.**

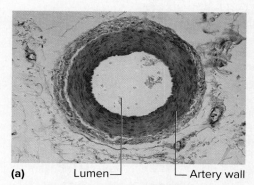

(a) Lumen — Artery wall

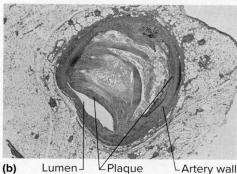

(b) Lumen — Plaque — Artery wall

▲ **Figure 10.16** Arterial structure.
(a) Normal coronary artery. (b) Advanced atherosclerosis with narrowed lumen.
Ed Reschke/Stone/Getty Images

WORD	PRONUNCIATION		ELEMENTS	DEFINITION
angina pectoris	an-**JUH**-nuh **PEK**-tor-iss		**angina** Greek *strangling* **pectoris** Latin *chest*	Condition of severe pain in the chest due to coronary heart disease
anoxia	an-**OK**-see-ah	S/ P/ R/	**-ia** *condition* **an-** *without* **-ox-** *oxygen*	Without oxygen
anoxic (adj)	an-**OK**-sik	S/	**-ic** *pertaining to*	Pertaining to or suffering from a lack of oxygen
arteriosclerosis	ar-**TEER**-ee-oh-skler-**OH**-sis	S/ R/CF R/CF	**-sis** *abnormal condition* **arteri/o-** *artery* **-scler/o-** *hardness*	Hardening of the arteries
arteriosclerotic (adj)	ar-**TEER**-ee-oh-skler-**OT**-ik	S/	**-tic** *pertaining to*	Pertaining to or suffering from arteriosclerosis
asystole	ay-**SIS**-toh-lee	P/ R/	**a-** *without* **-systole** *contraction*	Absence of contractions of the heart
atheroma	ath-er-**ROH**-mah	S/ R/	**-oma** *tumor* **ather-** *porridge, gruel*	Lipid deposit in the lining of an artery
atherosclerosis	**ATH**-er-oh-skler-**OH**-sis	S/ R/CF R/CF	**-sis** *abnormal condition* **ather/o-** *porridge, gruel* **-scler/o-** *hardness*	Atheroma in arteries
cardiogenic	**KAR**-dee-oh-**JEN**-ik	S/ R/CF	**-genic** *creation, producing* **cardi/o-** *heart*	Of cardiac origin
fibrosis	fie-**BROH**-sis	S/ R/CF	**-sis** *condition* **fibr/o-** *fiber*	Repair of dead tissue cells by formation of fibrous tissue
fibrotic (adj)	fie-**BROT**-ik	S/	**-tic** *pertaining to*	Pertaining to fibrosis
hypovolemic	**HIGH**-poh-voh-**LEE**-mik	S/ P/ R/	**-emic** *in the blood* **hypo-** *below* **-vol-** *volume*	Having decreased blood volume in the body
infarct	in-**FARKT**	P/ R/	**in-** *in* **-farct** *stuff*	Area of cell death resulting from an infarction
infarction	in-**FARK**-shun	S/	**-ion** *process*	Sudden blockage of an artery
ischemia	is-**KEE**-mee-ah	S/ R/	**-emia** *blood condition* **isch-** *to keep back*	Lack of blood supply to a tissue
ischemic (adj)	is-**KEE**-mik	S/	**-emic** *in the blood*	Pertaining to or affected by ischemia
necrosis	neh-**KROH**-sis	S/ R/	**-osis** *condition* **necr-** *death*	Pathologic death of tissue or cells
necrotic (adj)	neh-**KROT**-ik	S/ R/CF	**-tic** *pertaining to* **necr/o-** *death*	Affected by necrosis
occlude (verb) occlusion (noun)	ok-**KLUDE** ok-**KLU**-zhun	 S/ R/	Latin *to close* **-ion** *process* **occlus-** *to close*	To close, plug, or completely obstruct A complete obstruction
perfuse (verb)	per-**FYUSE**		Latin *to pour*	To force blood to flow through a lumen or a vascular bed
perfusion (noun)	per-**FYU**-shun	S/ R/	**-ion** *action, condition* **perfus-** *to pour*	The act of perfusing
plaque	PLAK		French *a plate*	Patch of abnormal tissue
sedentary	sed-en-**TAIR**-ee	S/ R/	**-ary** *pertaining to* **sedent-** *sitting*	Accustomed to little exercise or movement
thrombosis	throm-**BOH**-sis	S/ R/	**-osis** *abnormal condition* **thromb-** *clot*	Formation of a clot (thrombus)

Hypertensive Heart Disease

Hypertension (HTN) is the most common cardiovascular disorder in this country, affecting more than 20% of the adult population. It results from a prolonged elevated blood pressure (BP) throughout the vascular system. The high pressure forces the ventricles to work harder to pump blood. Eventually, the myocardium becomes strained and less efficient. It is the major cause of heart failure, stroke, and kidney failure.

High BP is currently defined as a BP reading at or above 120/80 mm **Hg** (mercury). A normal BP is below 120/80 mm Hg. The first number, or **systolic** reading, reflects the BP when the heart is contracting. The second number, or **diastolic** reading, reflects BP when the heart is relaxed between contractions.

Primary (essential) hypertension is the most common type of hypertension. Its etiology is unknown. Its risk factors are:

- Being overweight
- Stress
- Lack of exercise
- Using tobacco
- Using alcohol

Secondary hypertension results from other diseases, such as kidney disease, atherosclerosis, and hyperthyroidism.

Malignant hypertension is a rare, severe, life-threatening form of hypertension in which the BP reading can be greater than 200/120 mm Hg. Aggressive intervention is indicated to reduce the blood pressure.

Prehypertension, with a systolic pressure between 120 and 139 mm Hg and a diastolic pressure between 80 and 90 mm Hg, may indicate an increased risk for cardiovascular disease.

Congestive Heart Failure (CHF)

Congestive heart failure occurs with the inability of the heart to supply enough cardiac output to meet the body's metabolic needs. The patient shows **shortness of breath** (**SOB**) and **orthopnea.**

The most common conditions leading to CHF are:

- Cardiac ischemia
- Cardiomyopathy
- Chronic lung disease
- Valvular regurgitation
- Severe hypertension
- Aortic stenosis

Congenital Heart Disease (CHD)

Congenital heart disease is the result of abnormal development of the heart in the fetus.
Common congenital defects include:

- **Atrial septal defect (ASD).** A hole in the interatrial septum allows blood to **shunt** from the higher-pressure left atrium to the lower-pressure right atrium.
- **Ventricular septal defect (VSD).** A hole in the interventricular septum allows blood to shunt from the higher-pressure left ventricle to the lower-pressure right ventricle *(see Figure 10.17a)*.
- **Patent ductus arteriosus (PDA).** The ductus arteriosus is a normal blood vessel in the fetus that usually closes within 24 hours of birth. When the artery remains open (patent), blood can shunt from the aorta to the pulmonary artery, and the higher pressure causes damage to the lungs *(Figure 10.17b)*.
- **Coarctation of the aorta.** This is a narrowing of the aorta shortly after the artery to the left arm branches from the aorta. It causes **hypertension** in the arms behind the narrowing and **hypotension** in the lower limbs and organs like the kidney below the narrowing.
- **Tetralogy of Fallot (TOF).** This is a **syndrome** with four congenital heart defects. All these congenital abnormalities can be surgically repaired.

Normal heart

Ventricular septal defect

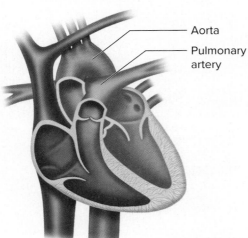

Normal heart

Patent ductus arteriosus

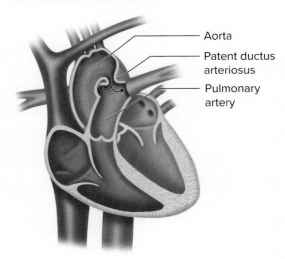

▲ **Figure 10.17** Congenital heart defects.

WORD	PRONUNCIATION	ELEMENTS		DEFINITION
coarctation	koh-ark-**TAY**-shun	S/ R/	**-ation** *process* **coarct-** *press together*	Constriction stenosis, particularly of the aorta
congenital	kon-**JEN**-ih-tal	S/ P/ R/	**-al** *pertaining to* **con-** *together, with* **-genit-** *bring forth*	Present at birth, either inherited or due to an event during gestation up to the moment of birth
defect	**DEE**-fect		Latin *to lack*	An absence, malformation, or imperfection
hypertension	**HIGH**-per-**TEN**-shun	S/ P/ R/	**-ion** *action, condition* **hyper-** *excessive* **-tens-** *pressure*	Persistent high arterial blood pressure
hypertensive (adj) hypotension prehypertension	**HIGH**-per-**TEN**-siv **HIGH**-poh-**TEN**-shun pree-**HIGH**-per-**TEN**-shun	S/ P/ P/	**-ive** *quality of* **hypo-** *low, below* **pre-** *before*	Suffering from hypertension Persistent low arterial blood pressure Precursor to hypertension
orthopnea	or-**THOP**-nee-ah	S/ R/CF	**-pnea** *breathe* **orth/o-** *straight*	Difficulty in breathing when lying flat
orthopneic (adj)	or-**THOP**-nee-ik	S/	**-ic** *pertaining to*	Pertaining to or affected by orthopnea
patent ductus arteriosus	**PAY**-tent **DUK**-tus ar-**TEER**-ee-oh-sus		**patent** Latin *lie open* **ductus** Latin *leading* **arteriosus** Latin *like an artery*	An open, direct channel between the aorta and the pulmonary artery
shunt	SHUNT		Middle English *divert*	A bypass or diversion of fluid; in this case, blood
syndrome	**SIN**-drohm	P/ R/	**syn-** *together* **-drome** *running*	Combination of signs and symptoms associated with a particular disease process
tetralogy of Fallot (TOF)	teh-**TRAL**-oh-jee OV fah-**LOH**	S/ P/	**-logy** *study of* **tetra-** *four* Etienne-Louis Fallot, 1850–1911, French physician	Set of four congenital heart defects occurring together

Circulatory Disorders

Disorders of Veins

Phlebitis is an inflammation of a vein. There are many causes for phlebitis, including venous infections and the presence of an intravenous (IV) catheter.

Thrombophlebitis is an inflammation of the lining of a vein (tunica intima), allowing clots (thrombi) to form.

Deep vein thrombosis (DVT) is thrombus formation in a deep vein, often due to reduced blood flow. Risk factors include immobility, surgery, prolonged travel, and contraception (estrogen). The increased pressure in the capillaries due to back pressure from the blocked blood flow in the veins causes an increase in the flow of fluid from the capillaries to the interstitial spaces. The collection of fluid is called **edema.**

A major complication of thrombus formation is that a piece of the clot can break off and be carried in the bloodstream to lodge in a blood vessel in another organ and block blood flow. The piece that breaks off is called an **embolus** or **thromboembolism.** It often lodges in the lungs, producing pulmonary embolus *(see Chapter 13).*

Varicose veins are superficial veins that have lost their elasticity and appear swollen and tortuous *(Figure 10.18).* Their valves become incompetent, and blood flows backward and pools. Smaller, more superficial varicose veins are called **spider veins.** Varicose veins are associated with a family history, obesity, and prolonged standing. **Collateral** circulations develop to take the blood through alternative routes.

Disorders of Arteries

Peripheral vascular disease (PVD) is a general term describing all the disorders of the systemic arterial and venous systems.

An **aneurysm** is a localized dilation of an artery as a result of a localized weakness of the vessel wall. Common sites occur along the aorta, mostly the abdominal aorta. They can rupture, leading to severe bleeding and hypovolemic shock.

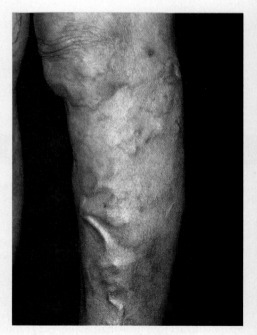

▲ **Figure 10.18** Varicose veins of leg.
Dr. P. Marazzi/Science Source

Intracranial aneurysms, particularly at the base of the brain, are an important cause of bleeds into the cranial cavity *(see Chapter 9).*

Thromboangiitis obliterans (Buerger disease) is an inflammatory disease of the arteries with clot formation, usually in the legs. The occlusion of arteries and impaired circulation leads to intermittent claudication.

Carotid artery disease affects the two major arteries supplying the brain. They can be involved in **arteriosclerosis** and the deposition of plaque, which puts the patient at risk for a stroke.

Word Analysis and Definition: Circulatory Disorders

S = Suffix   P = Prefix   R = Root   R/CF = Combining Form

WORD	PRONUNCIATION	ELEMENTS		DEFINITION
aneurysm	**AN**-yur-izm		Greek *dilation*	Circumscribed dilation of an artery or cardiac chamber
claudication	klaw-dih-**KAY**-shun	S/ R/	-ation *process* claudic- *limping*	Intermittent leg pain and limping
collateral	koh-**LAT**-er-al	S/ P/ R/	-al *pertaining to* col- *before* -later- *at the side*	Situated at the side, often to bypass an obstruction
edema edematous (adj) pitting edema	ee-**DEE**-mah ee-**DEM**-ah-tus **PIT**-ing ee-**DEE**-mah	 S/ R/	Greek *swelling* -tous *pertaining to* edema- *swelling,* *edema*	Excessive accumulation of fluid in cells and tissues Pertaining to or marked by edema Edema that maintains indentations made by applying pressure to the area for a time
embolus emboli (pl)	**EM**-boh-lus		Greek *plug, stopped*	Detached piece of thrombus, a mass of bacteria, quantity of air, or foreign body that blocks a blood vessel
peripheral	peh-**RIF**-er-al	S/ R/	-al *pertaining to* peripher- *outer part*	Pertaining to the periphery or an external boundary
phlebitis	fleh-**BIE**-tis	S/ R/	-itis *inflammation* phleb- *vein*	Inflammation of a vein
thromboembolism	**THROM**-boh-**EM**-boh-lizm	S/ R/CF R/	-ism *condition* thromb/o- *clot* -embol- *plug*	A piece of detached blood clot (embolus) blocking a distant blood vessel
thrombophlebitis	**THROM**-boh-fleh-**BIE**-tis	S/ R/CF R/	-itis *inflammation* thromb/o- *clot* -phleb- *vein*	Inflammation of a vein with clot formation
thrombus thrombosis	**THROM**-bus throm-**BOH**-sis	S/ R/ S/	-us *pertaining to* thromb- *clot* -osis *condition*	A clot attached to a diseased blood vessel or heart lining Formation of a thrombus

Check Point Section 10.3

A. The definitions for the medical terms relating to abnormal heart rhythms are given to you—construct each term by providing the missing word element. *Fill in the blanks with the missing prefix or root.* **LO 10.2, 10.6**

1. Forcible, rapid beat of the heart: _____ /ation

2. Uncontrolled heart muscle twitching: _____ /ation

3. Sharp, spasmodic episode: _____ /al

4. Rapid heart rate (greater than 100 beats per minute): _____ /card/ia

5. Slow heart rate (less than 60 beats per minute): _____ /card/ia

6. Abnormal heart rhythm: _____ /rrhythm/ia

B. Use your knowledge of the *language of cardiology* to match the description in the left column with the correct medical term in the right column. *Match the term to its correct meaning.* **LO 10.6**

_____ 1. Weakening of heart muscle

_____ 2. Inflammation that causes exudates

_____ 3. Cusps of valve bulge back into atrium

_____ 4. Constricted valve opening

_____ 5. Failure of right ventricle to pump properly

_____ 6. Cardiomyopathy can be the cause

_____ 7. Causes valve regurgitation

_____ 8. Inflammatory disease that affects the heart

a. incompetence

b. cardiomegaly

c. cor pulmonale

d. pericarditis

e. rheumatic fever

f. cardiomyopathy

g. prolapse

h. stenosis

C. Consult the text content related to coronary artery disease for the best medical terms to complete the following sentences in patient documentation. *Fill in the blank with the correct term. Use the words in parentheses as a hint to the correct medical term to use.* **LO 10.6, 10.8**

1. His _____ (little exercise or movement) lifestyle, coupled with obesity, increases his risk factors for a heart attack.

2. After the myocardial infarction, the area of the myocardium became _____ (stiff).

3. _____ (absence of heart contractions) occurred at 2251 hrs, and the patient was pronounced dead.

4. Angioplasty showed a large clot _____ (complete obstruction) her left coronary artery.

5. The prolonged period of ischemia led to tissue _____ (death).

6. Cardiogenic shock occurred, and the patient's tissues were not _____ (forcing blood through a vascular bed or lumen) adequately.

D. Abbreviations need to be used carefully so that you communicate exactly what is necessary. *Match the abbreviation to the correct condition described.* **LO 10.1, 10.6, 10.9**

_____ 1. ASD

_____ 2. TOF

_____ 3. VSD

_____ 4. PDA

_____ 5. CHF

_____ 6. BP

_____ 7. HTN

a. force of blood pushing on the vessel walls

b. artery remains open instead of normally closing after birth

c. chronic elevated blood pressure

d. congenital heart defect that is made up of four congenital abnormalities

e. abnormal opening between the atria

f. abnormal opening between the ventricles

g. heart is unable to pump enough blood to meet the body's needs

E. Apply the language of the cardiovascular system. *Select the best answer to complete each statement.* **LO 10.2, 10.6**

1. The suffix tells you that **thrombophlebitis** is a(n)

    a. puncture   b. inflammation   c. excision   d. vein

2. **Collateral** means

    a. at the front   b. in the middle   c. at the side

3. The combining form *phleb/o-* means

    a. artery   b. vein   c. capillary

4. The combining form *scler/o-* describes a

    a. softening   b. clotting   c. hardening   d. constriction

5. The symptom of **edema** is a

    a. rash   **b.** swelling   **c.** lesion

6. Aneurysm describes a blood vessel that is

    a. dilated   **b.** constricted   **c.** collapsed   **d.** obstructed

7. The roots tell you that **thromboembolism** is a(n)

    a. clot or plug   **b.** tear or rupture   **c.** swelling or lesion   **d.** vein or artery

8. The combining form *thromb/o-* means

    a. clot   **b.** lump   **c.** plug   **d.** vein

Section 10.4 Procedures and Pharmacology

Cardiovascular Diagnostic Tests

Blood Tests

Lipid profile helps determine the risk of CAD and comprises:

- **Total cholesterol**
- **High-density lipoprotein (HDL)** ("good cholesterol")
- **Low-density lipoprotein (LDL)** ("bad cholesterol")
- **Triglycerides**

The following are chemical indicators used as risk factors in the diagnosis and monitoring of cardiovascular diseases:

- **B-type natriuretic peptide (BNP),** a brain hormone, is used to diagnose and monitor congestive heart failure and to predict the course of end-stage heart failure.
- **C-reactive protein (CRP),** produced by the endothelial cells of arteries, when elevated, has been identified as a risk factor for atherosclerosis and CAD.
- **Homocysteine** is an amino acid in the blood. Elevated levels are related to a higher risk of CAD, stroke, and peripheral vascular disease.
- **Creatine kinase (CK)** is an enzyme released into the blood by dead myocardial cells in MI.
- **Troponin I and T** are part of a protein complex in muscle that is released into the blood during myocardial injury. Troponin I is found in heart muscle but not in skeletal muscle. Its presence in blood is therefore a highly sensitive indicator of a recent MI. Both CK and Troponin I and T are used to confirm a suspected MI.

Word Analysis and Definition: Cardiovascular Diagnostic Tests

S = Suffix   P = Prefix   R = Root   R/CF = Combining Form

WORD	PRONUNCIATION		ELEMENTS	DEFINITION
cholesterol	koh-**LESS**-ter-ol	S/ R/CF	-sterol *steroid* chol/e- *bile*	Steroid formed in liver cells which circulates in the plasma
creatine kinase	**KREE**-ah-teen **KI**-nase	S/ R/ S/ R/	-ine *pertaining to* creat- *flesh* -ase *enzyme* kin- *motion*	Enzyme elevated in the plasma following heart muscle damage
homocysteine	ho-moh-**SIS**-teen	P/ R/	homo- *same* cysteine *an amino acid*	An amino acid similar to cysteine
lipid	**LIP**-id		**Greek** *fat*	General term for all types of fatty compounds
lipoprotein	**LIE**-poh-pro-teen	R/CF R/	lip/o- *fat* -protein *protein*	Molecules made of combinations of fat and protein
natriuretic peptide	**NAH**-tree-you-**RET**-ik **PEP**-tide	S/ R/CF R/ S/ R/	-ic *pertaining to* natr/i *sodium* -uret- *ureter* -ide *particular quality* pept- *amino acid*	Protein that increases the excretion of sodium by the kidney
profile	**PRO**-file	S/ R/	pro- *forward* -file *contour, line*	A set of characteristics which determine the structure of a group
triglyceride	try-**GLISS**-eh-ride	S/ P/ R/	-ide *having a particular quality* tri- *three* -glycer- *glycerol*	Any of a group of fats containing three fatty acids
troponin	**TROH**-po-nin	S/ R/	-onin *chemical substance* trop(h)- *nourishment*	A protein complex found in myocardial muscle fibers and released into the blood within 4 hours of myocardial damage

Cardiovascular Diagnostic Procedures

Auscultation via a **stethoscope** is used to listen to the sounds of the heart during the cardiac cycle. A **murmur** can be heard when blood flows against a restriction, such as a stenosed or incompetent valve.

- A **bruit** can be auscultated over an area of restricted blood flow, such as a plaque in an artery.

Arterial blood pressure is measured with a **sphygmomanometer** and a stethoscope.

Electrocardiography is the process of recording the electricity passing through the heart muscle by using electrodes placed on the skin. The electrodes are connected to an electrocardiograph, which then amplifies the electrical changes to record an **electrocardiogram (ECG or EKG)** in the form of five waves *(Figure 10.19)*. The waves are labeled P, Q, R, S, and T.

Smaller single-lead electrograph devices are used like the Holter monitor. The data from the electrograph is sent electronically to the company. Patients use an app to record their symptoms and activity. Certified Cardiographic Technicians (CCT) create a report for the cardiologist based on the data from the electrograph and patient's diary.

Smartphone apps providing at home ECGs are being evaluated for their effectiveness compared to a standard 12-lead ECG.

Implantable loop recorders are inserted into the skin above the heart. They record the ECG for up to 3 years. They are indicated for infrequent arrhythmias.

Cardiac stress testing is an exercise tolerance test to raise your heart rate and monitor the effect on cardiac function. **Nuclear imaging** of the heart, using an injection of a radioactive substance, can be used with the stress test.

A **Holter monitor** is a continuous ECG recorded on a digital recording device as you work, play, and rest for 24 to 48 hours. The patient keeps a diary of all symptoms and activities so that the data on the monitor can be correlated with symptoms and activities.

Persantine/thallium exercise testing is used for people unable to engage in physical exercise. It combines nuclear imaging with a drug that increases the demand on the heart.

Echocardiography uses ultrasound waves to study cardiac function at rest. The test is performed by a cardiac **sonographer,** who places a **transducer** on the patient's chest. A stress echocardiogram is performed after the patient has exercised on a treadmill.

Transesophageal echocardiography (TEE) involves insertion of a small probe into the esophagus to record the anatomy and function of heart valves.

Did you know...

Noninvasive monitoring of the electrical activity of the heart is performed by using **electrodes.**

Did you know...

- Devices like an **ECG** or **Holter** can provide an automated interpretation of heart rhythms.
- However, it is necessary that cardiologists or other health care providers provide the final interpretation of the test.

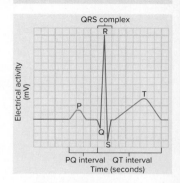

▲ **Figure 10.19** Normal electrocardiogram.

An **event monitor** is used for patients whose symptoms occur sporadically. A monitor is held over the chest when an event occurs. The data are stored and transmitted by telephone to a monitoring station.

An **ambulatory blood pressure monitor** provides a record of your BP over a 24-hour period as you go about your daily activities.

Electron beam tomography (EBT) is a scan that identifies calcium deposits in arteries.

Cardiac catheterization detects patterns of pressures and blood flows in the heart. A thin tube is guided into the heart under x-ray guidance after being inserted into a vein or artery.

Coronary angiogram *(Figure 10.20)* uses a contrast dye injected during cardiac catheterization to identify coronary artery blockages.

Homan's sign is a quick evaluation for the presence of a DVT in the presence of other clinical signs.

A **venogram** is a radiograph (x-ray record) of a vein. It is used to view the blood flow through the veins.

Color Doppler ultrasonography uses high-frequency sound (ultrasound) waves to evaluate cardiac valve function and to show different rates of blood flow through the heart and blood vessels.

CT scans and **MRIs** provide images of the heart anatomy including heart valves and coronary arteries.

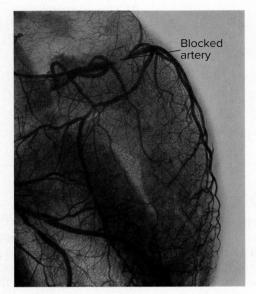

Blocked artery

▲ **Figure 10.20** Coronary angiogram showing blocked artery. SPL/Science Source

WORD	PRONUNCIATION	ELEMENTS		DEFINITION
angiogram	**AN**-jee-oh-gram	S/ R/CF	-gram *a record* angio- *blood vessel*	Radiograph obtained after injection of radiopaque contrast material into blood vessels
auscultation	aws-kul-**TAY**-shun	S/ R/	-ation *process* auscult- *listen to*	Diagnostic method of listening to body sounds with a stethoscope
catheter	**KATH**-eh-ter		**Greek** *to send down*	Hollow tube that allows passage of fluid into or out of a body cavity, organ, or blood vessel
catheterize (verb) catheterization (*Note:* 3 suffixes)	**KATH**-eh-ter-**RIZE**	S/ S/ R/ S/	-ize *action* -er- *agent* cathet- *catheter* -ation *process*	To introduce a catheter Introduction of a catheter
Doppler	**DOP**-ler		Johann Christian Doppler, 1803–1853 Austrian physicist	Diagnostic instrument that sends an ultrasonic beam into the body
ultrasonography	**ULL**-trah-soh-**NOG**-rah-fee	S/ P/ R/CF	-graphy *process of recording* ultra- *beyond* -son/o *sound*	Imaging that detects direction, velocity and turbulence of blood flow
electrocardiogram	ee-**LEK**-troh-**KAR**-dee-oh-gram	S/ R/CF R/CF	-gram *record* electro- *electricity* -cardi/o- *heart*	Record of the electrical signals of the heart
electrocardiograph	ee-**LEK**-troh-**KAR**-dee-oh-graph	S/	-graph- *to record*	Machine that makes the electrocardiogram
electrocardiography	ee-**LEK**-troh-**KAR**-dee-**OG**-rah-fee	S/	-graphy *process of recording*	The process of making an electrocardiogram
echocardiogram	**ECK**-oh-**KAR**-dee-oh-gram	S/ R/CF R/CF	-gram *record* ech/o- *sound wave* -cardi/o *heart*	Ultrasound recording of heart function
murmur	**MUR**-mur		**Latin** *low voice*	Abnormal sound heard on auscultation of the heart or blood vessels
sphygmomanometer	**SFIG**-moh-mah-**NOM**-ih-ter	S/ R/CF R/CF	-meter *instrument to measure* sphygmo- *pulse* -man/o- *pressure*	Instrument to measure arterial blood pressure
tomography	toe-**MOG**-rah-fee	S/ R/CF	-graphy *process of recording* tom/o *section, slice*	Radiographic image of a selected slice of tissue
venogram	**VEE**-no-gram	S/ R/CF	-gram *a record* ven/o- *vein*	Radiograph of vein after injection of radiopaque image

Cardiovascular Treatment Procedures

Cardiologists treat heart problems that do not require surgery: catheterization, stent placement, and angioplasty.

Cardiovascular surgeons perform surgeries on the heart: coronary artery bypass grafting (CABG), heart valve dysfunction, correction of congenital heart defects.

The most immediate need in the treatment of MI is to provide perfusion to get blood and oxygen to the affected myocardium. This can be attempted in several ways:

1. **Clot-busting drugs (thrombolysis)**. Streptokinase or tissue plasminogen activator (**tPA**) are injected within a few hours of the MI to dissolve the thrombus.

2. **Angioplasty** also called **percutaneous transluminal coronary angioplasty (PTCA)**. A balloon-tipped catheter is guided to the site of the blockage and inflated to expand the artery from the inside by compressing the plaque against the walls of the artery.

3. **Stent placement.** To reduce the likelihood that the artery will close up again (occlude), a wire mesh tube, or stent (*Figure 10.21*), is placed inside the vessel. Some stents (**drug-eluting** stents) are covered with a special medication to help keep the artery open.

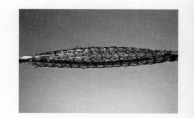

▲ **Figure 10.21** Stent.
Clouds Hill Imaging Ltd./Science Source

4. **Angioplasty, Laser** has a catheter with a laser tip. Instead of compressing the artery, the laser opens the blocked artery.

5. **Rotational atherectomy.** A high-speed rotational device is used to "sand" away calcified plaque.

6. **Coronary artery bypass graft (CABG).** Cardiovascular surgeons perform this procedure, mostly used for people with extensive disease in several arteries: healthy blood vessels harvested from the leg, chest, or arm detour blood around blocked coronary arteries. The procedure is performed by a perfusionist using a heart-lung machine that pumps the recipient's blood through the machine to oxygenate it while surgery is performed. More recently, the procedure is being performed "off-pump" with the heart still beating.

7. **Heart transplant,** in which the heart of a recently deceased person (donor) is transplanted to the recipient after the recipient's diseased heart has been removed. The immune characteristics of the donor and recipient have to be a close match.

Procedures used in cardiology to treat arrhythmias:

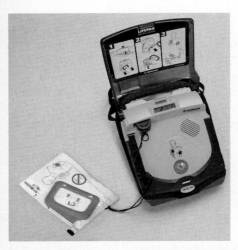

▲ **Figure 10.22** **Automated external defibrillator (AED).**

Rick Brady/McGraw-Hill Education

- **Cardioversion,** which uses a therapeutic dose of electrical current to the heart synchronized to a specific moment in the electrical cycle (at the QRS complex) to convert an abnormally fast heart rate or cardiac arrhythmia to a normal rhythm.

- **Defibrillation,** which uses a nonsynchronized electrical shock to terminate ventricular fibrillation or pulseless ventricular tachycardia and revert to a normal rhythm. It is not effective for asystole.

- **Radiofrequency ablation,** which uses a catheter with an electrode in its tip guided into the heart to destroy the cells from which abnormal cardiac rhythms are originating.

- **Artificial pacemakers,** which consist of a battery, electronic circuits, and computer memory to generate electronic signals. The signals are carried along thin, insulated wires to the heart muscle. The most common need for a pacemaker is a very slow heart rate (bradycardia).

- **Implantable cardioverter/defibrillator (ICD),** which senses abnormal rhythms and gives the heart a small electrical shock to return the rhythm to normal.

- **Automated external defibrillators (AEDs)** *(Figure 10.22),* which send an electrical shock to the heart to restore a normal contraction rhythm.

A prolapsed or incompetent heart valve can often be repaired. There are two valve replacement options:

1. **A mechanical (prosthetic) valve.** Various models and designs are made from different metal alloys and plastics.

2. **Tissue valves.** This can come from a pig (porcine) or cow (bovine). Occasionally, a tissue valve can come from a human donor, or a valve can be constructed of tissue from the patient's own pericardium.

Treatments for Stroke

Ischemic strokes (caused by clots) tPa treatment remains the gold standard. Mechanical thrombectomy is an option to remove large vessel occlusion. A catheter is inserted in the artery of the groin to the area of the clot. The device grabs the clot; suction may also be used.

Hemorrhagic (ruptured blood vessel) catheter inserted into artery is threaded to ruptured blood vessel; a coil is inserted stopping the bleeding. Surgery may be required.

Treatments for Peripheral Vascular Disorders

1. **Varicose veins** can be treated with laser technology and **sclerotherapy,** where solutions that scar (**sclerose**) the veins are injected into them.

2. **Peripheral angioplasty** is the use of a balloon to open a peripheral artery in the leg or abdomen and is often used with stenting. It is occasionally used to treat venous stenosis.

3. **Lifestyle changes** to treat or prevent peripheral vascular disease include stopping smoking, regular exercise, healthy diet, and maintaining a healthy weight.

WORD	PRONUNCIATION	ELEMENTS		DEFINITION
ablation	ab-**LAY**-shun	S/ R/	-ion *process* ablat- *take away*	Removal of a tissue to destroy its function
angioplasty	**AN**-jee-oh-**PLAS**-tee	S/ R/CF	-plasty *surgical repair* angi/o- *blood vessel*	Recanalization of a blood vessel by surgery
atherectomy	ath-er-**EK**-toh-mee	S/ R/	-ectomy *excision* ather- *porridge, gruel*	Surgical removal of the atheroma
cardiologist cardiology	kar-dee-**OL**-oh-jist kar-dee-**OL**-oh-jee	S/ R/CF S/	-logist *specialist* cardi/o- *heart* -logy *study of*	A medical specialist in diagnosis and treatment of the heart (cardiology) Medical specialty of diseases of the heart
cardiopulmonary resuscitation	**KAR**-dee-oh-**PUL**-moh-nair-ee ree-sus-ih-**TAY**-shun	S/ R/CF R/ S/ R/	-ary *pertaining to* cardi/o- *heart* -pulmon- *lung* -ation *process* resuscit- *revival from apparent death*	The attempt to restore cardiac and pulmonary function
cardioversion cardioverter	**KAR**-dee-oh-**VER**-shun **KAR**-dee-oh-**VER**-ter	S/ R/CF R/ R/	-ion *action, process* cardi/o- *heart* -vers- *turn* -verter *that which turns*	Restoration of a normal heart rhythm by electrical shock Device used to generate the electrical shock to the heart
defibrillation defibrillator	dee-fib-rih-**LAY**-shun dee-**FIB**-rih-lay-tor	S/ P/ R/ S/	-ation *process* de- *without, away from* -fibrill- *small fiber* -ator *instrument*	Restoration of uncontrolled twitching of cardiac muscle fibers to normal rhythm Instrument for defibrillation
implantable	im-**PLAN**-tah-bul	S/ P/ R/	-able *capable of* im- *in* -plant- *insert*	Able to be inserted into tissues
laser	**LAY**-zer		acronym for **L**ight **A**mplification by **S**timulated **E**mission of **R**adiation	Intense, narrow beam of monochromatic light
prosthesis prosthetic (adj)	**PROS**-thee-sis pros-**THET**-ik	 S/ R/	Greek *an addition* -ic *pertaining to* prosthet- *addition*	A manufactured substitute for a missing or diseased part of the body Pertaining to a prosthesis
sclerotherapy sclerose (verb) sclerosis (noun)	**SKLAIR**-oh-**THAIR**-ah-pee skleh-**ROZE** skleh-**ROH**-sis	R/CF R/ S/ S/	scler/o- *hardness* -therapy *treatment* -ose *full of* -osis *condition*	To collapse a vein by injecting a solution into it to harden it To harden or thicken Thickening or hardening of a tissue
stent	STENT		Charles Stent, 1807–1885, English dentist	Wire mesh tube used to keep arteries open
thrombolysis	throm-**BOL**-eye-sis	S/ R/CF	- lysis *dissolve* thromb/o- *clot*	Dissolving a thrombus (clot)

Cardiovascular Drugs

Beta Blockers

Beta blockers diminish the effects of **epinephrine** and other stress hormones *(see Chapter 17)*. All beta blockers are approved for the treatment of hypertension. Specific beta blockers are approved for treatment of:

- angina
- atrial arrhythmias
- coronary artery disease
- heart failure
- hypertension
- early posttraumatic stress disorder *(see Chapter 9)*

Beta blockers are also sometimes used in the prevention of migraines. There are some 20 different beta-blocking agents altogether.

The **renin-angiotensin** system is a complex biological system between the heart, brain, blood vessels, and kidneys. It plays an important role in the pathology of hypertension, cardiovascular disease, chronic kidney disease, and diabetic nephropathy *(see Chapter 17)*. The potent chemical angiotensin II is formed in the blood from angiotensin I by the angiotensin converting enzyme (**ACE**). Angiotensin II causes blood vessels to contract and narrow, leading to hypertension.

ACE inhibitors inhibit, or slow, the activity of the angiotensin converting enzyme (ACE). This action decreases the formation of angiotensin II, so blood vessels dilate more and blood pressure falls. Some 10 different ACE inhibitors have been approved to control hypertension, treat heart failure, prevent strokes, and improve survival rates after heart attacks.

Angiotensin receptor blockers (**ARBs**) block the interaction between angiotensin and the angiotensin receptors on the muscles in the wall of blood vessels, allowing blood vessels to dilate. They are used when patients are unable to tolerate ACE inhibitors because of persistent cough or, more rarely, angioedema.

Calcium channel blockers (**CCBs**) inhibit the flow of calcium through channels in cardiac muscles and in the muscles in the walls of blood vessels. This leads to a decrease in muscle contraction and dilation of the blood vessels. More than 20 CCBs have been approved to treat hypertension (particularly in elderly patients), angina, arrhythmias, and Raynaud disease. Diltiazem (*Cardizem, Tiazac,* others) verapamil (*Calan, Verelan*) are antihypertensives that work differently than those ending in -dipine. A high mortality rate has been reported among people who take the drugs over an extended dosage period.

Cholesterol Lowering Drugs

Cholesterol Lowering Drugs are a class of drugs that block the enzyme in the liver that is responsible for making **cholesterol,** an essential component in all cell membranes that is necessary for the production of bile acids, steroid hormones, and Vitamin D. However, the body's production of cholesterol also contributes to the development of atherosclerosis. Seven statins are approved by the **FDA** for use; they vary in their potency to decrease cholesterol levels. Examples include atorvastatin (*Lipitor*), lovastatin (*Mevacor*), rosuvastatin (*Crestor*), simvastatin (*Zocor*), and pravastatin (*Pravachol*).

One new drug, Omega-3-acid esters (*Lovaza*), lowers very high triglyceride levels. Another new drug, Evolocumab (*Repatha, Praluent*) decreases LDL levels in the blood. A study published in 2020 suggests that evolocumab may reduce the risk of a myocardial infarction.

Other Cardiovascular Drugs

Chronotropic drugs alter the heart rate. Epinephrine (adrenaline), norepinephrine (noradrenaline), and atropine increase the heart rate. Quinidine (*Quinidex*), procainamide (*Pronestyl*), lidocaine (*Xylocaine*), and propranolol (*Inderal*) slow the heart.

Inotropic drugs alter the contractions of the myocardium. Digitalis and its derivatives, digoxin and digitoxin, increase the strength of contractions of the myocardium, thus leading to increased cardiac output.

Dromotropic drugs affect the conduction speed in the atrioventricular (**AV**) node and subsequently the rate of conduction of electrical impulses in the heart. A calcium channel blocker, such as verapamil, slows the speed of conduction through the cardiac neural system and has a negative dromotropic effect.

Anticoagulants reduce susceptibility to thrombus formation. These include aspirin, warfarin (*Coumadin*), heparin and a low molecular weight heparin named dalteparin (*Fragmin*), and new thrombin inhibitors *(see Chapter 11)* such as dabigatran etexilate (*Pradaxa*) and rivaroxaban (*Xarelto*).

- **Streptokinase,** which is derived from hemolytic streptococci, dissolves the fibrin in blood clots. If administered intravenously within 3 to 4 hours of a heart attack caused by a clot, it can be effective in dissolving the clot.

- **Tissue plasminogen activator (tPA)** binds strongly to fibrin and dissolves clots that have caused heart attacks. It is similar in effect and use to streptokinase. Reteplase (*Retavase*) and urokinase (*Abbokinase*) are forms of tPA.

Table 10.1 Anti-hypertensive Medications

Medication	Suffix	Examples
Beta-blockers	-olol	atenolol (*Tenormin*)
		carvedilol (*Coreg*)
		labetalol (*Normodyne*)
		metoprolol (*Lopressor*)
		pinidolol (*Visken*)
		propanolol (*Inderal*)
Calcium channel blocker	-dipine (several)	amlodipine (*Norvasc*)
		nicardipine
		nifedipine (*Adalat CC, Procardia*)
ACE—inhibitors	-pril	captopril
		enalapril (*Vasotec*)
		ramipril (*Altace*)
Angiotensin receptor blockers	-sartan	azilsartan (*Edarbi*)
		eprosartan
		olmesartan (*Benicar*)

Word Analysis and Definition: Cardiovascular Drugs

S = Suffix   P = Prefix   R = Root   R/CF = Combining Form

WORD	PRONUNCIATION		ELEMENTS	DEFINITION
beta blocker	**BAY**-tah **BLOK**-er	S/ R/	**beta** Greek *second letter in Greek alphabet* **-er** *agent* **block-** *to obstruct*	A beta-adrenergic blocking agent used in the treatment of cardiac arrhythmias, hypertension, and other diseases
chronotropic	**KRONE**-oh-**TROH**-pik	S/ R/CF	**-tropic** *change* **chron/o-** *time*	Affecting the heart rate
diuretic	die-you-**RET**-ik	S/ P/ R/	**-ic** *pertaining to* **di-** *from* **dia-** *throughout* **-uret-** *urine, urination*	Agent that acts on the kidney to increase urine output
dromotropic	**DROH**-moh-**TROH**-pik	S/ R/CF	**-tropic** *change* **drom/o-** *race, a running*	Affecting the rate of conduction in the AV node, and subsequently the heart rate
inhibit	in-**HIB**-it		Latin *to keep back*	To curb or restrain
inotropic	**IN**-oh-**TROH**-pik	S/ R/CF	**-tropic** *change* **in/o-** *sinew*	Affecting the contractility of cardiac muscle
statin	**STAT**-in		Latin *condition, state*	A drug used to lower cholesterol in the bloodstream

Check Point Section 10.4

A. Describe blood tests that aid in the diagnosis of heart disease. *Match the term in the first column with its correct description in the second column.* **LO 10.5, 10.9**

Term	Meaning
_____ 1. CK	**a.** "good" cholesterol
_____ 2. HDL	**b.** "bad" cholesterol
_____ 3. LDL	**c.** used to diagnose and monitor congestive heart failure
_____ 4. BNP	**d.** produced by the endothelial cells of the arteries
_____ 5. CRP	**e.** enzyme released by dead myocardial cells

B. Build your language of cardiology by completing the following documentation. *There is only one best answer for each blank. Fill in the blanks.* **LO 10.5**

electrode   electrocardiogram   electrocardiograph   electrocardiography

The patient was scheduled for (1) _____ today. The CVT attached the (2) _____ to the patient's chest and proceeded to turn on the (3) _____. Unfortunately, a malfunction of the machine prevented him from obtaining the (4) _____. This study will have to be rescheduled for the patient.

C. Build your language of cardiology by completing the following documentation. *There is only one best answer for each blank. Fill in the blanks.* **LO 10.5, 10.7**

catheter   catheterization   catheterize

The cardiologist performed coronary artery (1) _____ to determine if the patient had any coronary artery blockage. A cardiac (2) _____ was inserted into the patient's left coronary artery. The cardiologist will also (3) _____ right coronary artery to determine if a blockage exists there.

D. Determine the treatment for the condition. *From the given information, determine the treatment that would be appropriate to treat the cardiovascular disease.* **LO 10.7**

1. A person suffers a cardiac arrest at a college. The students use a device that shocks the heart. What is the device they will use?

   a. Automated external defibrillator   **b.** Stent placement   **c.** Radiofrequency ablation   **d.** Pacemaker

2. Mr. Rosares arrives at the emergency department with chest pain. When asked, he states that the chest pain started one hour ago. The cardiologist determines that he has a clot occluding one of his coronary arteries. Which procedure will the cardiologist likely choose?

   a. Defibrillation   **b.** Heart transplant   **c.** Thrombolysis   **d.** Cardioversion

E. Determine the type of condition that is treated with a particular procedure. *Choose the primary condition that the procedure would be used to treat.* **LO 10.7**

1. Coronary artery bypass grafting

   a. Arrhythmia   **b.** Occluded coronary artery

2. Radiofrequency ablation

   a. Arrhythmia   **b.** Occluded coronary artery

3. Cardioversion

   a. Arrhythmia   **b.** Occluded coronary artery

F. Abbreviations are commonly used in verbal communication and written documentation. *From the definition, identify the correct abbreviation. Use the provided abbreviations below. Fill in the blanks.* **LO 10.7, 10.9**

ACE   ARB   AV   CCB   FDA   tPA

1. The organization responsible for approving drugs for use in the United States: _____

2. The medication that dissolves clots: _____

3. Dromotropic medications work by affecting the _____ node.

4. This medication reduces blood pressure by blocking an enzyme from functioning: _____

5. The medication _____ blocks angiotensin receptors on muscles, thus reducing blood pressure.

6. A reduction in heart muscle contractility can be achieved through the use of _____.

G. Construct terms using word elements. *The roots/combining forms are important when describing the effects of cardiac medications. Given the definition, provide the missing combining form element. Enter it as one term, for example: sclero* (**LO 10.2, 10.7**)

1. A medication that slows down the rate of conduction through the heart: _____ /tropic

2. A medication that affects the heart rate: _____ /tropic

3. A medication that affects the contractility of the heart: _____ /tropic

Table 10.2 Chapter 10 Abbreviations

Abbreviation	Meaning
ABI	ankle/brachial index
ACE	angiotensin converting enzyme
AED	automated external defibrillator
A-fib	atrial fibrillation
ARB	angiotensin receptor blocker
ASD	atrial septal defect
ASHD	arteriosclerotic heart disease
AV	atrioventricular
BNP	B-type natriuretic peptide
BP	blood pressure
CABG	coronary artery bypass graft
CAD	coronary artery disease
CCB	calcium channel blocker
CHD	congenital heart disease
CHF	congestive heart failure
CK	creatine kinase
CPR	cardiopulmonary resuscitation
CRP	C-reactive protein
CVT	cardiovascular technician
DVT	deep vein thrombosis
ECG/EKG	electrocardiogram

Abbreviation	Meaning
FDA	Food and Drug Administration
HDL	high-density lipoprotein
HTN	hypertension
ICD	implantable cardioverter/defibrillator
IVC	inferior vena cava
LDL	low-density lipoprotein
MI	myocardial infarction
PAT	paroxysmal atrial tachycardia
PDA	patent ductus arteriosus
PTCA	percutaneous transluminal coronary angioplasty
PVC	premature ventricular contraction
PVD	peripheral vascular disease
SA	sinoatrial
SOB	shortness of breath
STAT	immediately
SVC	superior vena cava
TOF	tetralogy of Fallot
tPA	tissue plasminogen activator
V-fib	ventricular fibrillation
VSD	ventricular septal defect

Table 10.3 Comparison of common cardiovascular disorders

Disorder or Disease	Signs and Symptoms	Diagnostic Tests	Treatment
Stroke— The symptoms for both types of strokes are the same	**F**ace drooping **A**rm weakness **S**peech slurred Time to call 911	Physical exam Neurologic exam CT scan or MRI, which may include an angiogram, ECG Blood tests	
Hemorrhagic Stroke			Insert catheter with coil. The coil is inserted at the site of vessel rupture Surgery may be required for complicated ruptures
Ischemic Stroke			tPA if patient arrives to hospital within 3 hours of onset of symptoms Blood clot removal
Thrombophlebitis		Ultrasound Blood test	NSAIDs, heat compression Blood thinning medications Clot-dissolving medications, Compression stockings
Mitral valve regurgitation	Fatigue, palpitations, shortness of breath	Auscultation—murmur, echocardiography, ECG, exercise or stress test, MRI	Depends on severity—watchful waiting, medications to treat symptoms, valve replacement
Ventricular septal defect	Increased respiratory rate, baby has trouble eating	Auscultation—murmur, echocardiography	Surgery—place patch over defect or a piece of the pericardium

2014 Nucleus Medical Media

Cardiovascular System

Challenge Your Knowledge

A. **Diagnostic tests may yield results that indicate a procedure should be performed.** Match up the following cardiac procedures.
LO 10.7, 10.8, 10.9

1. to reduce occlusion of an artery, this may be inserted

2. donor to recipient

3. arrhythmia is converted back to normal rhythm

4. clot-busting drug therapy

5. surgical removal of the lipid deposit in an artery

6. catheter with electrode destroys abnormal cells

7. healthy blood vessels are harvested to detour blood around blocked vessels

8. high-speed rotational device "sands away" plaque

9. artery-cleaning angioplasty

a. radiofrequency ablation

b. rotational atherectomy

c. atherectomy

d. stent

e. transplant

f. CABG

g. defibrillation

h. PTCA

i. thrombolysis

B. **Choose the professional whose primary job is described.** Write the term described. **LO 10.10**

cardiologist   cardiovascular technician   phlebotomist   sonographer

1. obtain venous blood used for diagnostic testing: _____

2. diagnose and treat heart conditions: _____

3. perform cardiac tests ordered by physicians: _____

4. person who specializes in obtaining ultrasounds of body structures: _____

C. **Abbreviations are present throughout medical documentation, and you must be absolutely certain you are interpreting them correctly.** Fill in the correct abbreviation in the following patient documentation. All of the abbreviations contain some combination of the following letters. You will have to use some letters more than once. **LO 10.9**

A   C   D   F   H   I   M   P   S   V   O

1. Studies show that the patient has a hole in the interventricular septum, allowing blood to shunt from the higher-pressure left ventricle to the lower-pressure right ventricle. The abbreviation for the diagnosis is _____.

2. The pediatric cardiologist was called to the Neonatal Unit because the baby's fetal blood vessel had not closed normally. The baby was diagnosed with _____.

3. The patient's arterial vessels have become dangerously narrowed due to his _____, and an angioplasty will be scheduled.

4. Due to her sedentary lifestyle, obesity, hypertension, and smoking history, the patient is at great risk for _____.

5. This patient's left ventricle is failing because it cannot pump out the blood it receives. He is going into _____.

6. An infant male was born with tetralogy of Fallot (_____). This is a form of _____.

7. This patient's ischemic attack resulted in occlusion of her coronary artery, and a (surgical procedure) _____ followed.

D. Translate from layman's language to medical terminology. Provide a medical term for every underlined word or phrase. Fill in the blanks. **LO 10.6**

1. If any of the <u>heart</u> (_____) arteries become <u>blocked</u> (_____), the blood supply to a part of the <u>heart muscle</u> (_____) is cut off and the cells supplied by that artery are <u>dead</u> (_____) within minutes.

2. Aortic valve <u>narrowing</u> (_____) is common in the elderly and may need to be replaced with a <u>mechanical</u> (_____) valve. This often occurs as a consequence of <u>lipid deposits in the lining of an artery</u> (_____).

3. The <u>cause</u> (_____) of weakening of the <u>heart muscle</u> (_____) can be viral, <u>unknown</u> (_____), or alcoholic.

4. <u>Inflammation of the lining of a vein</u> (_____) allows <u>clots</u> (_____) to form.

E. The cardiac cycle can be heard through the stethoscope. Apply the correct terms in the appropriate place to describe what happens in the chambers of the heart during the cardiac cycle. One term you will use twice. Three terms you will not use at all. **LO 10.1**

atrial diastole	relax	heartbeat	atrial systole	ventricular systole
atria	ventricular diastole	contraction	contract	murmur

1. When the atria _____, called _____ (atrial emptying), the ventricles _____, called _____ (or ventricular filling).

2. When the atria relax, called _____, the ventricles _____, called _____.

3. Then the atria and ventricles all relax briefly. This series of events is the complete cardiac cycle or _____.

F. Build your knowledge of the heart's location and function by selecting the correct answers to the following questions: **LO 10.1**

1. Which of the following is *NOT* a function of the heart?

   a. pulmonary circulation

   b. maintaining respiration

   c. systemic circulation

   d. regulating blood supply

   e. pumping blood

2. The heart lies in the thoracic cavity between the lungs in an area called the

   a. sternum

   b. mediastinum

   c. ventricle

   d. atrium

   e. vena cava

3. If the *base* of the heart is the upper end of the heart, what is the tip (or other end) of the heart called?

   a. tricuspid

   b. atrium

   c. aorta

   d. semilunar

   e. apex

4. What is responsible for ensuring the one-way flow of blood in the heart?

   a. blood vessels

   b. pulmonary circulation

   c. coronary circulation

   d. valves

   e. blood pressure

G.   Test your knowledge of the cardiovascular system by selecting the correct answer. LO 10.1, 10.6, 10.9

1. The long, flat bone forming the center of the anterior wall of the chest is the

   a. mediastinum

   b. sternum

   c. myocardium

   d. apex

   e. pericardium

2. The area of cell death caused by the sudden blockage of a blood vessel is termed

   a. fibrosis

   b. infarct

   c. coronary

   d. sinus

   e. visceral

3. The term **sinus rhythm** refers to

   a. the AV node

   b. normal heartbeat

   c. dysrhythmias

   d. arrhythmias

   e. a pacemaker

4. Pathologic compression of the heart is known as

   a. endocarditis

   b. prolapse

   c. tamponade

   d. regurgitation

   e. effusion

5. The abbreviations that represent cardiac diagnoses are

   a. SOB and EKG

   b. MI and PAT

   c. CPR and CVT

   d. STAT and SA

   e. AED and ID

6. What is the purpose of the four valves in the heart?

   a. Blood flows in only one direction.

   b. Blood gets oxygenated.

   c. The heart muscle can rest between beats.

   d. They prevent infection.

   e. They are the gateway to the heart.

7. In the term **cardioversion,** the suffix -ion means

   a. a structure

   b. a process

   c. to pour

   d. pertaining to

   e. small

H. Test your knowledge of the cardiovascular system with the following questions. LO 10.1, 10.6

1. Tissue for heart valves can come from
   a. rabbits
   b. monkeys
   c. occasionally humans
   d. dogs
   e. horses

2. Abnormality in valve closure produces
   a. exudate
   b. infarct
   c. murmur
   d. necrosis
   e. fibrillation

3. The cordlike tendons that anchor the mitral and tricuspid heart valves to the floor of the ventricles are
   a. semilunar
   b. intraventricular
   c. mesenteric
   d. chordae tendineae
   e. fibrotic

4. The pacemaker of heart rhythm is the
   a. AV node
   b. bundle branch
   c. SA node
   d. coronary sinus
   e. PVC

5. Vessels that take blood away from the heart are termed
   a. veins
   b. capillaries
   c. arteries
   d. tendons
   e. muscles

6. Which of the following terms does NOT apply to blood vessels?
   a. arterioles
   b. venules
   c. hilum
   d. veins
   e. arteries

7. The term **visceral** pertains to
   a. an artery
   b. a vein
   c. a capillary
   d. the aorta
   e. an internal organ

8. Capillary exchange occurs by
   a. infusion
   b. transfusion
   c. perfusion
   d. diffusion
   e. effusion

9. The circulatory system that takes blood to the lungs to pick up oxygen and get rid of carbon dioxide is the
   a. coronary
   b. pulmonary
   c. systemic

I. Challenge your knowledge of medical terminology and provide the correct answers to the following questions. **LO 10.1, 10.3, 10.6, 10.7**

1. A *flat line* on an ECG is called _____.

2. *Death of tissue* is _____.

3. *Arrhythmia* is another term for _____.

4. An *abnormal sound* in the closure of a heart valve is a _____.

5. A medication that *affects the heart rate* is called a _____.

6. *Medications that lower cholesterol* are also called _____.

7. A *bypass* or diversion of fluid is _____.

8. A *hollow tube* that allows passage of fluid into or out of a body cavity is _____.

9. An agent that *increases* urine output is a _____.

10. *The main artery* in the neck is the _____.

J. Form medical terms to fill in the blanks. **LO 10.1, 10.5, 10.6, 10.7, 10.9**

1. A _____ is a specialist in the study of the heart.

2. In the abbreviation CPR, the "C" stands for _____.

3. The abbreviation ECG stands for _____.

4. The study of the heart is the specialty called _____.

5. The term that means *pertaining to the heart and blood vessels* is _____.

6. The instrument used for taking an ECG is _____.

7. The device that measures blood pressure is _____.

K. The following procedures could all be performed by a cardiovascular surgeon. Deconstruct each medical term into its elements. Fill in the blanks. **LO 10.2, 10.7**

1. ablation: _____/_____/_____

P   R/CF   S

2. angioplasty: _____/_____/_____

P   R/CF   S

3. defibrillation: _____/_____/_____

P   R/CF   S

4. sclerotherapy: _____/_____/_____

P   R/CF   S

5. atherectomy: _____/_____/_____

P   R/CF   S

L. Use your knowledge of cardiac pharmacology and insert the correct medical term for the drugs defined. Fill in the blanks with the class of drugs being described. **LO 10.7**

1. class of drugs that block the enzyme in the liver responsible for making cholesterol: _____

2. alter the contractions of the myocardium: _____

3. reduce susceptibility to clot formation: _____

4. stimulate urinary fluid loss to lessen fluid volume the heart has to cope with: _____

5. alter the heart rate: _____

M. Using your knowledge of the terminology in the following report, choose the correct answer for the following questions. LO 10.1, 10.6

CHEST X-RAY REPORT

The left ventricle is slightly enlarged. Right atrium and right ventricle appear to be dilated. There is tortuosity of the thoracic aorta, with arteriosclerosis. The hilar and interstitial structures are somewhat accentuated. There are large pericardial fat pads. Tricuspid and pulmonic valves appear normal but are not well seen. Mitral valve appears grossly normal for age. Aortic valve appears grossly normal for age.

1. Where are the pericardial fat pads?

   a. in the heart   **d.** beside the heart

   b. around the heart   **e.** above the heart

   c. below the heart

2. Which two heart chambers have a somewhat similar appearance?

   a. right and left ventricle   **d.** right atrium and left ventricle

   b. right and left atrium   **e.** right atrium and right ventricle

   c. left atrium and right ventricle

3. What is another spelling and pronunciation for *dilation?*

   a. dillation   **d.** diletation

   b. dilatation   **e.** dilletation

   c. dillatation

4. **Interstitial** means

   a. space between the cells of a structure or organ   **d.** membrane between the cells of a structure or organ

   b. cavity between the cells of a structure or organ   **e.** wall between the cells of a structure or organ

   c. fluid between the cells of a structure or organ

N. Procedures. You have passed your certification examination and have been hired as the coder for the Cardiology Department at Fulwood Medical Center. You are coding the claims for the following tests performed in the department. How much do you know about cardiology testing? Match the letter to the numbered blank. **LO 10.5, 10.7, 10.9**

_____ 1. Thallium testing

_____ 2. EKG, also known as

_____ 3. Continuous ECG recorded digitally

_____ 4. Cardiac stress testing

_____ 5. TEE

_____ 6. Helps determine risk of CAD

_____ 7. Event tracker

_____ 8. Sound waves study heart function

_____ 9. Electron beam CT

_____ 10. Cardiac catheterization

_____ 11. Radioactive substance injected

_____ 12. X-ray record of a vein

_____ 13. Dye injected to find heart blockage

a. venogram

b. through esophagus to record heart valves

c. echocardiography

d. detects patterns of pressure in the heart

e. used when people are unable to do physical exercise

f. coronary angiogram

g. exercise tolerance test

h. sporadic symptoms

i. lipid profile

j. ECG

k. Holter monitor

l. identifies calcium in arteries

m. nuclear imaging

O. Identify the elements in each medical term and unlock the meaning of the word. Fill in the chart. If the word does not have a particular word element, write n/a. **LO 10.2**

Medical Term	Meaning of Prefix	Meaning of Root/ Combining Form	Meaning of Suffix	Meaning of the Term
incompetence	1.	2.	3.	4.
dysrhythmia	5.	6.	7.	8.
arteriole	9.	10.	11.	12.
mediastinum	13.	14.	15.	16.
venogram	17.	18.	19.	20.
inotropic	21.	22.	23.	24.
chronotropic	25.	26.	27.	28.

P. Pronunciation is important whether you are saying the word or listening to a word from a coworker. Identify the proper pronunciation of the following medical terms. Then correctly spell the term. **LO 10.1, 10.3, 10.4, 10.5, 10.6, 10.7**

1. The correct pronunciation for a small vein leading away from a capillary network

    a. vay-**NYOU**-el

    b. veen-**UHL**

    c. **VEN**-yule

    d. **VANE**-yule-ah

    Correctly spell the term: _____

2. The correct pronunciation for an agent that affects the heart rate

    a. **IN**-oh-**TROH**-pik

    b. **IN**-oh-troop-**IK**

    c. **DROH**-moh-**TROH**-pik

    d. **DRUM**-oh-troop-**IK**

    Correctly spell the term: _____

3. The correct pronunciation for anenzyme elevated in the plasma following heart muscle damage

   a. **KREE**-ah-teen **KI**-nase

   b. creat-in-**KI**-nase

   c. try-**GLISS**-eh-ride

   d. try-**GLICE**-er-ide

   Correctly spell the term: _____

4. The correct pronunciation for the surgical removal of the atheroma

   a. an-**JEEO**-plast-er-**EE**

   b. **AN**-jee-oh-**PLAS**-tee

   c. ath-er-**EK**-toh-mee

   d. **ATHREK**-to-mee

   Correctly spell the term: _____

5. The correct pronunciation for referring to the repair of dead tissue cells by formation of fibrous tissue

   a. is-**KEE**-mik

   b. **ICE**-keh-mik

   c. fie-**BROT**-ik

   d. fib-**ROW**-tick

   Correctly spell the term: _____

Q. **Build your *language of cardiology* by completing the following documentation.** *There is only one best answer for each blank.* **LO 10.10**

cardiology   cardiovascular   cardiologist   cardiac

The **(1)** _____ Department sent a specialist to examine the patient in the Emergency Room. The **(2)** _____ ordered a cardiac catheterization, which showed three obstructed arteries in the patient's heart, so the **(3)** _____ surgeon was notified immediately to perform **(4)** _____ surgery.

R. **Describe the health care professionals specific to the care of the heart.** *Match the health care professional in the first column with its correct description in the second column.* **LO 10.10**

Term	Meaning
_____ 1. echocardiographer	a. medical doctor specializing in surgery of the heart and peripheral blood vessels
_____ 2. phlebotomist	b. technician who uses ultrasound to observe the structures of the heart
_____ 3. cardiologist	c. assists physicians in the diagnosis and treatment of cardiovascular disorders
_____ 4. cardiovascular surgeon	d. draws patient blood samples for laboratory testing
_____ 5. cardiovascular technician	e. medical doctor specializing in disorders of the cardiovascular system

Case Reports

A. **After reading the following Case Report, correctly answer the following questions.** The answers to the questions may not be in the Case Report itself but can be found in the chapter content. **LO 10.3, 10.5, 10.6, 10.8, 10.9, 10.10**

Case Report (CR) 10.1

You are

. . . a **cardiovascular technologist (CVT)** employed by the **Cardiology** Department at Fulwood Medical Center. Dr. Wang, MD has called you to the Emergency Department **STAT** to take an **ECG.**

Your patient is

. . . Mr. Flank Johnson. From his medical records, you see that he is the 64-year-old owner of a printing company.

Eight months ago, Mr. Johnson had a left total hip replacement. In the past 3 months, he has returned to his daily workouts. This morning, while riding his exercise bike, he felt tightness in his chest. He kept on cycling and developed pain in the center of his chest radiating down his left arm and up into his jaw. He became **diaphoretic.** His personal trainer called 911.

You perform the ECG, and the automatic report indicated that Mr. Johnson was having a **MI** affecting the anterior wall of his left ventricle. You immediately use the call system to summon help.

As you are removing the electrodes, Mr. Johnson complains that he is feeling faint and has shortness of breath.

---

1. Mr. Johnson's first symptom was:

    a. diaphoresis

    b. angina

    c. claudication

    d. palpitations

2. Which of Mr. John's symptoms is a classic symptom of an MI?

    a. feeling short of breath

    b. feeling faint

    c. diaphoresis

    d. pain in left arm and jaw

3. When it comes to the ECG report, Dr. Wang will:

    a. evaluate it and interpret it.

    b. rely on the automated report.

    c. ask you to interpret it for him.

    d. hold treatment until cardiologist interprets it.

4. The cause of the MI is likely due to:

    a. increased physical activity.

    b. an atrial arrhythmia.

    c. an occluded coronary artery.

    d. uncontrolled hypertension.

5. As Dr. Wang is treating the MI, he will call for which type of specialist?

    a. neurologist

    b. pulmonologist

    c. cardiologist

    d. cardiovascular surgeon

    e. perfusionist

6. Provide the meaning of each abbreviation found in Case Report 10.1: (provide one word for each blank)

    a. ECG: _____ _____ _____

    b. MI: _____ _____

    c. STAT: _____

    d. CVT: _____ _____ _____

B. **After reading the following Case Report, correctly answer the following questions.** The answers to the questions may not be in the Case Report itself but can be found in the chapter content. **LO 10.1, 10.3, 10.5, 10.6, 10.8, 10.9, 10.10**

📁 Case Report (CR) 10.2

Mrs. Martha Jones, who had been referred to Dr. Bannerjee's cardiovascular clinic, has several circulatory problems related to her diabetes and obesity. She was diagnosed previously with hypertension, CAD, and diabetic retinopathy. She now has severe pain in her legs when walking.

Her ankle/brachial index (ABI), which measures the ratio of the blood pressure in her ankle to that in her arm, showed significant blockage of blood flow. Doppler studies confirmed this. This blockage produces the pain when walking (intermittent claudication). It is due to arteriosclerosis of the large arteries in her legs. Angiograms showed several atherosclerotic areas in her popliteal artery.

The ulcers on the edges of her big toes result from thickening of the walls of her capillaries and arterioles and the resulting poor circulation to her feet. Again, this is due to her diabetes.

In the venous system of her legs, the tender cordlike lesion is due to thrombophlebitis of a superficial vein in her left leg.

Pain in the calf on flexion of the ankle (Homans sign) indicates that she may have deep vein thrombosis **DVT**. A venogram confirmed this diagnosis.

---

1. Provide the medical terms that describe: (provide one word for each blank)

    a. DVT: _____ _____ _____

    b. CAD: _____ _____ _____

2. Provide the medical term that describes the words "pain while walking." _____

3. Which of the following statements are true regarding Doppler studies?

    a. It shows blood flow through vessel.

    b. It uses radiation to provide the image.

    c. The study is completed by a phlebotomist.

    d. The results are part of an evaluation for pericarditis.

4. Which of the following would confirm the diagnosis of a DVT?

    a. venogram

    b. auscultation

    c. catheterization

    d. exercise test

5. Mrs. Jones's vessel that has atherosclerosis is found on the posterior side of her:

    a. arm

    b. thigh

    c. knee

    d. groin

6. Dr. Bannergee is which type of specialist?

    a. internist

    b. cardiologist

    c. cardiovascular surgeon

    d. family practice physician

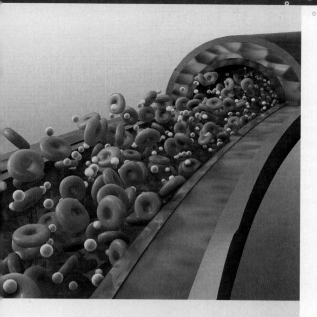

Chapter Learning Outcomes

Upon completion of this chapter, you will be able to:

LO 11.1 Identify and describe the anatomy and physiology of the blood and its related components.

LO 11.2 Use roots, combining forms, suffixes, and prefixes to construct and analyze medical terms related to hematology.

LO 11.3 Spell medical terms related to hematology.

LO 11.4 Pronounce medical terms related to the hematology.

LO 11.5 Describe diagnostic procedures utilized in hematology.

LO 11.6 Identify and describe disorders and pathological conditions related to blood.

LO 11.7 Describe the therapeutic procedures and pharmacologic agents used in hematology.

LO 11.8 Apply knowledge of medical terms relating to hematology to documentation, medical records, and communication.

LO 11.9 Identify and correctly use abbreviations of terms used in hematology.

LO 11.10 Identify health professionals involved in the care of hematology patients.

Health professionals involved in the diagnosis and treatment of patients with problems with the blood system including

- **Hematologist**—a medical specialist in the field of hematology. They treat blood disorders including anemia, hemophilia, and other clotting disorders. They perform blood marrow aspirations to diagnose blood disorders.
- **Infusion therapy nurse**—administers iron transfusions to patients with severe anemia.

Section 11.1 Components of Blood

Components of Blood

The study of the blood and its disorders—the red and white blood cells within the blood, their proportions, and overall cell health—is called **hematology.** A **hematologist** is a medical specialist trained in this area. Blood is a type of connective tissue and consists of cells contained in a liquid matrix.

Blood volume varies with body size and the amount of adipose tissue. An average-size adult has about 5 L (liters) (10 pints) of blood, which represents some 8% of body weight.

If a specimen of blood is collected in a tube and centrifuged, the cells of the blood are packed into the bottom of the tube *(Figure 11.1).* These cells are called the formed elements of blood and consist of 99% red blood cells (**RBCs**), together with white blood cells (**WBCs**) and platelets. The blood sample is normally about 45% formed elements.

The **hematocrit (Hct)** is the percentage of total blood volume composed of red blood cells. The red blood cells can account for 40% to 54% of the total blood volume in normal males and 38% to 47% in females.

Plasma is the remaining 55% of the blood sample. It is a clear, yellowish liquid that is 91% water. Plasma is the fluid noncellular part of blood. Plasma is a **colloid,** a liquid that contains suspended particles, most of which are the plasma proteins named:

- **Albumin**—makes up 58% of the proteins.

- **Globulin**—makes up 38% of the plasma proteins. Antibodies are globulins *(see Chapter 12).*

- **Fibrinogen**—makes up 4% of the plasma proteins and is part of the mechanism for blood clotting *(see Lesson 11.4).*

    Nutrients, waste products, hormones, and **enzymes** are dissolved in plasma for transportation.

When blood is allowed to clot and the solid clot is removed, **serum** is left. Serum is identical to plasma except for the absence of clotting proteins.

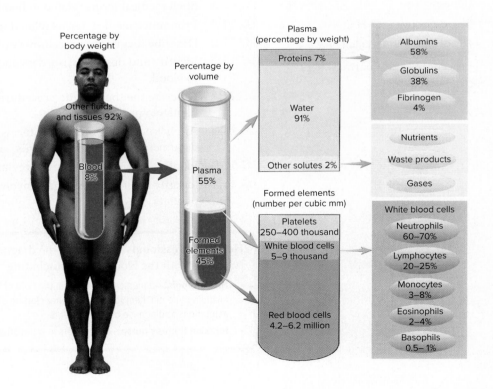

▲ **Figure 11.1** **Components of blood.** Hattie Young/Science Source

WORD	PRONUNCIATION		ELEMENTS	DEFINITION
albumin	al-**BYU**-min		Latin *white of an egg*	Simple, soluble protein
colloid	**COLL**-oyd	S/ R/	-oid *appearance of* coll- *glue*	Liquid containing suspended particles
fibrin fibrinogen	**FIE**-brin fie-**BRIN**-oh-jen	S/ R/CF	Latin *fiber* -gen *create, produce* fibrin/o- *fibrin*	Stringy protein fiber that is a component of a blood clot Precursor of fibrin in blood-clotting process
globulin	**GLOB**-you-lin		Latin *globule*	Family of blood proteins
hematocrit hematology hematologist	hee-**MAT**-oh-krit he-mah-**TOL**-oh-jee he-mah-**TOL**-oh-jist	S/ R/CF S/ S/	-crit *to separate* hemat/o- *blood* -logy *study of* -logist *specialist*	Percentage of red blood cells in the blood Medical specialty in the disorders of blood Specialist in hematology
hemoglobin	**HEE**-moh-**GLOH**-bin	R/CF R/	hem/o- *blood* -globin *protein*	Red-pigmented protein that is the main component of red blood cells
index indices (pl)	**IN**-deks **IN**-dih-seez		Latin *one that points out*	A standard indicator of measurement relating one component to another
microcytic	my-kroh-**SIT**-ik	S/ P/ R/	-ic *pertaining to* micro- *small* -cyt- *cell*	Pertaining to a small cell
plasma	**PLAZ**-mah		Greek *something formed*	Fluid, noncellular component of blood
serum	**SEER**-um		Latin *whey*	Fluid remaining after removal of cells and fibrin clot

Functions of Blood

The functions of blood are to:

1. **Maintain the body's homeostasis** *(see Chapter 4).*
2. **Maintain body temperature.** Warm blood is transported from the interior of the body to its surface, where heat is released from the blood.
3. **Transport nutrients, vitamins, and minerals** from the digestive system and storage areas to organs and cells where they are needed. Examples of nutrients are glucose and amino acids *(see Chapter 5).*
4. **Transport waste products** from cells and organs to the liver and kidneys for detoxification and excretion. Examples are **creatinine, urea,** bilirubin, and lactic acid *(see Chapter 5).*
5. **Transport hormones** from endocrine glands to the target cells. Examples are insulin and thyroxin *(see Chapter 17).*
6. **Transport gases** to and from the lungs and cells. Examples are oxygen and carbon dioxide *(see Chapter 13).*
7. **Protect against foreign substances.** Cells and chemicals in the blood are an important part of the immune system for dealing with microorganisms and toxins *(see Chapter 12).*
8. **Form clots.** Clots provide protection against blood loss and are the first step in tissue repair and restoration of normal function.
9. **Regulate pH and osmosis.**

Hydrogen ion concentration is measured by using a **pH** scale to show the balance between **acid** and **alkaline** in any solution. Pure water is the neutral solution and has a pH of 7.0. Solutions with a pH less than 7.0 are acidic. Solutions with a pH greater than 7.0 are alkaline (or basic). Blood has a pH between 7.35 and 7.45 and must be maintained within that range for life to continue. **Buffer** systems in the blood are used to maintain the correct pH range. Examples of buffer systems are bicarbonate and phosphate.

Osmosis is the passage of water through a selectively permeable membrane, such as a cell membrane, from the "more watery" side to the "less watery" side. All cells exchange water by osmosis, and red blood cells exchange 100 times their own volume across the cell membrane every second.

Viscosity, the resistance of a fluid to flow, is an important element that affects the blood's ability to flow through blood vessels. Whole blood is five times as **viscous** as water. If the viscosity decreases because red blood cells are deficient (as in **anemia**), blood flows more easily and puts a strain on the heart because of the increased amount of blood being returned to it in a unit of time.

> **Did you know...**
>
> Failure to maintain the normal pH range of the blood between 7.35 and 7.45 can cause paralysis and death.

WORD	PRONUNCIATION		ELEMENTS	DEFINITION
acid	**ASS**-id		Latin *sour*	Substance with a pH below 7.0
alkaline (basic (syn))	**AL**-kah-line	S/ R/	**-ine** *pertaining to, substance* **alkal-** *base*	Substance with a pH above 7.0
buffer	**BUFF**-er		Latin *cushion*	Substance that resists a change in pH
creatinine	kree-**AT**-ih-neen	S/ R/	**-ine** *pertaining to, substance* **creatin-** *creatine*	Breakdown product of the skeletal muscle protein creatine
homeostasis	hoh-mee-oh-**STAY**-sis	S/ R/CF	**-stasis** *control* **home/o-** *the same*	Stability or equilibrium of a system or the body's internal environment
osmosis	oz-**MOH**-sis	S/ R/	**-sis** *process* **osmo-** *push*	The passage of water across a cell membrane
urea	you-**REE**-ah		Greek *urine*	End product of nitrogen metabolism
viscous viscosity	**VISS**-kus vis-**KOS**-ih-tee	S/ R/CF	Latin *sticky* **-sity** *condition, state* **visc/o-** *resistance to flow*	Sticky; resistant to flowing The resistance of a fluid to flow

Check Point Section 11.1

A. Know your elements—they will increase your medical vocabulary! *Match the element to its correct meaning.* **LO 11.1, 11.2**

_____ **1.** *-oid*

_____ **2.** *-gen*

_____ **3.** *hem/o*

_____ **4.** *-crit*

_____ **5.** *coll*

_____ **6.** *globin*

a. protein

b. blood

c. glue

d. create, produce

e. appearance of

f. to separate

B. Identify the medical term being described below. *Fill in the blanks.* **LO 11.1**

1. A substance that resists a change in pH _____.

2. A substance with a pH greater than 7.0 _____.

3. A substance with a pH less than 7.0 _____.

4. Movement of water across a cell membrane _____.

5. Resistance of a fluid to flow _____.

C. Deconstruct medical terms to decipher their meaning. *Identify where the slash would occur to deconstruct terms into their word elements. Choose the correct answer for each term.* **LO 11.1, 11.2**

1. viscosity

    a. vis/co/sity   **b.** visc/osity   **c.** visc/o/sity   **d.** viscos/ity

2. alkaline

    a. alkal/ine   **b.** al/ka/line   **c.** alkl/aline   **d.** al/kal/ine

3. osmosis

    a. o/sm/o/sis   **b.** os/mo/sis   **c.** osm/o/sis   **d.** osmo/sis

4. homeostasis

    a. homeo/stas/is   **b.** home/o/stasis   **c.** homeo/sta/sis   **d.** ho/meo/stas/is

Section 11.2 Red Blood Cells (Erythrocytes)

Structure and Function of Red Blood Cells

Structure of Red Blood Cells

In your bloodstream at this moment are approximately 25 trillion RBCs. Approximately, 2.5 million of them are being destroyed every second. This means that 1% of your RBCs are destroyed and replaced every day of your life. Each RBC is a **biconcave** disc with edges that are thicker than the center *(Figure 11.2)*. This biconcave shape gives the disc a larger surface area than if it were a sphere. The biconcave surface area enables a more rapid flow of gases into and out of the RBC.

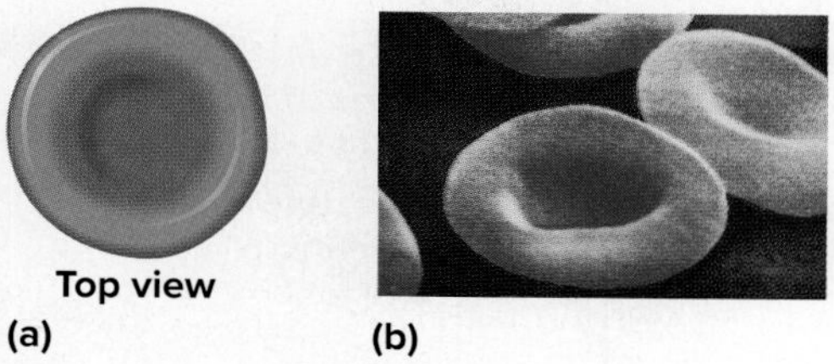

The main component of RBCs is **hemoglobin (Hb)**, which gives the cell its red color. Hemoglobin occupies about one-third of the total cell volume and is composed of the iron-containing pigment **heme** bound to a protein called globin. The rest of the red blood cell consists of the cell membrane, water, electrolytes, and enzymes. Mature RBCs do not have a nucleus.

RBCs are unable to move themselves and are dependent on the heart and blood to move them around the body.

Top view
(a)   **(b)**

▲ **Figure 11.2** **RBCs.** Bill Longcore/Science Source

Function of Red Blood Cells

The functions of the RBCs are to

1. **Transport oxygen (O$_2$)** from the lungs to cells all over the body. Oxygen is transported in combination with hemoglobin (**oxyhemoglobin**).

2. **Transport carbon dioxide (CO$_2$)** from the tissue cells to the lungs for excretion.

3. **Transport nitric oxide (NO),** a gas produced by cells lining the blood vessels that signals smooth muscle to relax and is also a transmitter of signals between nerve cells.

Life History of Red Blood Cells

Red blood cell formation (**erythropoiesis**) occurs in the spaces in bones filled with red bone marrow. **Hematopoietic stem cells** become nucleated **erythroblasts** and then nonnucleated **reticulocytes,** which are released into the bloodstream. In approximately 5 days, the reticulocytes mature into **erythrocytes.**

A hormone, **erythropoietin,** produced by the kidneys and liver, controls the rate of RBC production. A lack of oxygen in the blood triggers the release of erythropoietin, which travels in the blood to the red bone marrow to stimulate RBC production.

RBC production is also influenced by the availability of iron, the B vitamins B$_{12}$ and folic acid, and amino acids through absorption from the digestive tract *(Figure 11.3)*.

The average life span of an RBC is 120 days, during which time the cell has circulated through the body about 75,000 times. With age, the cells become more fragile, and squeezing through tiny capillaries ruptures them. **Macrophages** in the liver and spleen take up the hemoglobin that is released and break it down into its components heme and globin. The heme is broken down into iron and into a rust-colored pigment called bilirubin.

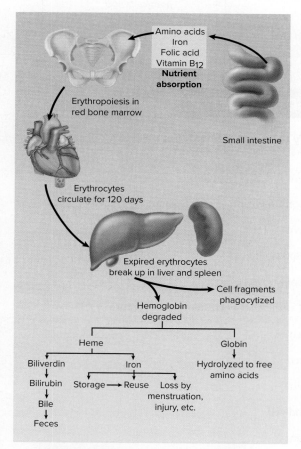

Amino acids
Iron
Folic acid
Vitamin B$_{12}$
Nutrient absorption

Erythropoiesis in red bone marrow

Small intestine

Erythrocytes circulate for 120 days

Expired erythrocytes break up in liver and spleen

Cell fragments phagocytized

Hemoglobin degraded

Heme   Globin

Biliverdin   Iron   Hydrolyzed to free amino acids

Bilirubin   Storage → Reuse   Loss by menstruation, injury, etc.

Bile

Feces

▲ **Figure 11.3** **Life and death of RBCs.**

S = Suffix   P = Prefix   R = Root   R/CF = Combining Form

WORD	PRONUNCIATION	ELEMENTS		DEFINITION
biconcave	**BIE**-kon-**KAVE**	P/ R/	**bi-** two, double **-concave** arched, hollow	Having a hollowed surface on both sides of a structure
erythroblast	eh-**RITH**-roh-blast	S/ R/CF	**-blast** germ cell **erythr/o-** red	Precursor to a red blood cell
erythrocyte	eh-**RITH**-roh-site	S/ R/CF	**-cyte** cell **erythr/o-** red	Another name for a red blood cell
erythropoiesis	eh-**RITH**-roh-poy-**EE**-sis	S/ R/CF	**-poiesis** to make **erythr/o-** red	The formation of red blood cells
erythropoietin	eh-**RITH**-roh-**POY**-ee-tin	S/	**-poietin** the maker	Protein secreted by the kidney that stimulates red blood cell production
hematopoietic	**HEE**-mah-toh-poy-**ET**-ik	S/ S/ R/CF	**-ic** pertaining to **-poiet-** the making **hemat/o-** blood	Pertaining to the making of red blood cells
heme	HEEM		Greek blood	The iron-based component of hemoglobin that carries oxygen
hemoglobin	**HEE**-moh-**GLOH**-bin	R/CF R/	**hem/o-** blood **-globin** protein	Red-pigmented protein that is the main component of red blood cells
macrophage	**MAK**-roh-fayj	P/ R/CF	**macro-** large **-phag/e** to eat	Large white blood cell that removes bacteria, foreign particles, and dead cells
oxyhemoglobin	**OK**-see-**HEE**-moh-**GLOH**-bin	R/CF R/CF R/	**ox/y-** oxygen **-hem/o-** blood **-globin** protein	Hemoglobin in combination with oxygen
reticulocyte	ri-**TIK**-you-loh-site	S/ R/CF	**-cyte** cell **reticul/o-** netlike	Immature red blood cell

Check Point Section 11.2

A. Given the definition, identify the word element. *One word in the definition is in bold; find the element in the term that has the same meaning. The first one is done for you. Fill in the blanks.* **LO 11.1, 11.2**

1. **macrophage:**   Element ____*macro*____ = ____*large*____

   Definition: **large** white blood cell that removes bacteria and dead cells

2. **erythroblast:**   Element _____ = _____

   Definition: **precursor** to red blood cell

3. **biconcave:**   Element _____ = _____

   Definition: having a hollowed surface on **both** sides of a structure

4. **erythropoiesis:**   Element _____ = _____

   Definition: the **formation** of red blood cells

5. **reticulocyte:**   Element _____ = _____

   Definition: immature red blood **cell**

6. **erythropoietin:**   Element _____ = _____

   Definition: protein that is secreted by kidney and stimulates **red blood cell** production

7. **hematopoietic:**   Element _____ = _____

   Definition: **pertaining to** the making of red blood cells

Section 11.3 White Blood Cells (Leukocytes)

Types of White Blood Cells

Granulocytes

1. **Neutrophils** *(Figure 11.4)* are normally 50% to 70% of the total WBC count. They are also called **polymorphonuclear leukocytes (PMNLs).** These cells phagocytize bacteria, fungi, and some viruses and secrete a group of enzymes called lysozymes, which destroy some bacteria.

2. **Eosinophils** *(Figure 11.5)* are normally 2% to 4% of the total WBC count. They are mobile cells that leave the bloodstream to enter tissue undergoing an allergic response.

3. **Basophils** *(Figure 11.6)* are normally less than 1% of the total WBC count. Basophils migrate to damaged tissues, where they release histamine (which increases blood flow) and **heparin** (which prevents blood clotting).

Because of their granular cytoplasm surrounding a nucleus, the above three types of WBCs are called **granulocytes.** Their granules are the sites for production of enzymes and chemicals.

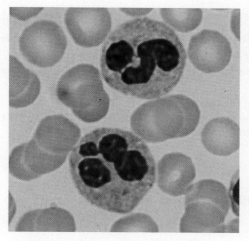

▲ **Figure 11.4** **Neutrophils are granulocytes.** Ed Reschke/Stone/Getty Images

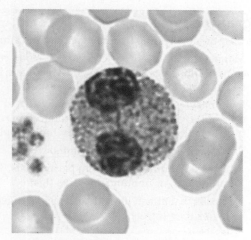

▲ **Figure 11.5** **Eosinophils are granulocytes.** Ed Reschke

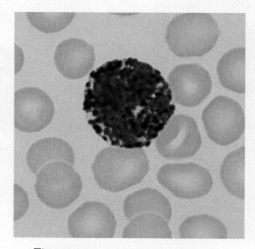

▲ **Figure 11.6** **Basophils are granulocytes.** Ed Reschke/Stone/Getty Images

WORD	PRONUNCIATION	ELEMENTS		DEFINITION
basophil	**BAY**-so-fill	S/ R/CF	**-phil** *attraction* **bas/o-** *base*	A basophil's granules attract a basic blue stain in the laboratory
eosinophil	ee-oh-**SIN**-oh-fill	S/ R/CF	**-phil** *attraction* **eosin/o-** *dawn*	An eosinophil's granules attract a rosy-red color on staining
granulocyte	**GRAN**-you-loh-site	S/ R/CF	**-cyte** *cell* **granul/o-** *small grain*	A white blood cell that contains multiple small granules in its cytoplasm
heparin	**HEP**-ah-rin	S/ R/	**-in** *chemical* **hepar-** *liver*	An anticoagulant secreted particularly by liver cells
leukocyte (**Note:** alternative spelling **leucocyte**)	**LOO**-koh-site	S/ R/CF	**-cyte** *cell* **leuk/o-** *white*	Another term for a white blood cell
neutrophil	**NEW**-troh-fill	S/ R/CF	**-phil** *attraction* **neutr/o-** *neutral*	A neutrophil's granules take up purple stain equally whether the stain is acid or alkaline
polymorphonuclear	**POL**-ee-more-foh-**NEW**-klee-ar	S/ P/ R/CF R/	**-ar** *pertaining to* **poly-** *many* **-morph/o-** *shape* **-nucle-** *nucleus*	White blood cell with a multilobed nucleus

Agranulocytes

Because monocytes and lymphocytes have no granules in their cytoplasm, they are called **agranulocytes.**

1. **Monocytes** *(Figure 11.7)* are the largest blood cell and are normally 3% to 8% of the total WBC count. Monocytes leave the bloodstream and become macrophages that phagocytize bacteria, dead neutrophils, and dead cells in the tissues.

2. **Lymphocytes** *(Figure 11.8)* are normally 25% to 35% of the total WBC count. They are the smallest type of WBC. Lymphocytes are produced in red bone marrow and migrate through the bloodstream to lymphatic tissues—lymph nodes, tonsils, spleen, and thymus—where they proliferate.

There are two main types of lymphocyte:

a. **B cells** that differentiate into plasma cells. These are stimulated by bacteria or toxins to produce **antibodies,** or **immunoglobulins (Igs).**

b. **T cells** that attach directly to foreign antigen-bearing cells such as bacteria, which they kill with toxins they secrete.

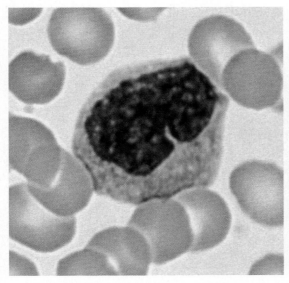

▲ **Figure 11.7** Monocytes are agranulocytes.
Ed Reschke/Stone/Getty Images

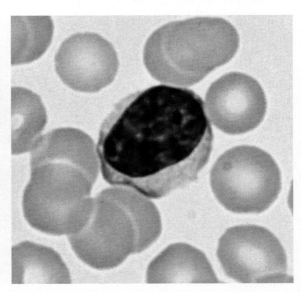

▲ **Figure 11.8** Lymphocytes are agranulocytes.
Ed Reschke/Stone/Getty Images

Word Analysis and Definition: Agranulocytes

S = Suffix   P = Prefix   R = Root   R/CF = Combining Form

WORD	PRONUNCIATION	ELEMENTS		DEFINITION
agranulocyte	ay-**GRAN**-you-loh-site	S/ P/ R/CF	**-cyte** *cell* **a-** *without, not* **-granul/o-** *granule*	A white blood cell without any granules in its cytoplasm
antibody antibodies (pl)	**AN**-tih-body **AN**-tih-bod-ee	P/ R/	**anti-** *against* **-body** *substance*	Protein produced in response to an antigen
immunoglobulin	**IM**-you-noh-**GLOB**-you-lin	S/ R/CF R/	**-in** *chemical* **immun/o-** *immune response* **-globul-** *protein*	Specific protein evoked by an antigen; all antibodies are immunoglobulins
lymphocyte	**LIM**-foh-site	S/ R/CF	**-cyte** *cell* **lymph/o** *lymph*	Small white blood cell with a large nucleus

Check Point Section 11.3

A. Define the meaning of word elements related to the functions of white blood cells. *Fill in the blanks with the correct definition.* **LO 11.1, 11.2**

1. The root in the medical term **heparin** means _____.

2. The suffix that means *attraction* is _____.

3. The prefix that means *many* is _____.

B. Using the medical terms related to the functions of white blood cells, match the correct term in column one to its meaning in column two. LO 11.1

_____ **1.** eosinophil

_____ **2.** leucocyte

_____ **3.** basophil

_____ **4.** heparin

_____ **5.** polymorphonuclear

a. anticoagulant secreted by liver cells

b. white blood cell with a multilobed nucleus

c. white blood cell

d. releases histamine in damaged tissues

e. involved in an allergic response

C. Use the medical terminology learned in this lesson to answer the questions. *Select the correct answer to correctly complete each statement.* **LO 11.1**

1. In the term **agranulocyte,** there is an element meaning
   a. within
   b. alongside
   c. under
   d. without, not
   e. beside

2. In the term **agranulocyte,** there is a term meaning
   a. blue
   b. behind
   c. cell
   d. against
   e. deficient

3. In the term **immunoglobulin,** there is an element meaning
   a. protein
   b. many
   c. against
   d. liquid
   e. black

4. The correct plural of **antibody** is
   a. antibodys
   b. antibodies
   c. antibodyies
   d. antebodyies
   e. antybodies

1. Because monocytes and lymphocytes have no granules in their cytoplasm, they are called *agranulocytes*.   T   F
2. Monocytes are the largest blood cell.   T   F
3. A lymphocyte is a white blood cell.   T   F
4. B cells and T cells are types of monocytes.   T   F
5. Lymphocytes are the smallest type of white blood cell.   T   F

Section 11.4 Blood Groups and Hemostasis

Red Cell Antigens

On the surfaces of red blood cells are molecules called **antigens.** In the plasma, antibodies are present. Each antibody can combine with only a specific antigen. If the plasma antibodies combine with a red cell antigen, bridges are formed that connect the red cells together. This is called **agglutination,** or clumping, of the cells. Hemolysis (rupture) of the cells also occurs.

The antigens on the surfaces of the cells have been categorized into groups, of which two are the most important. These are the ABO and Rhesus (Rh) blood groups.

ABO Blood Group

Figure 11.9 shows the different combinations of antigens and antibodies in the different blood types. The two major antigens on the cell surface are antigen A and antigen B.

A person with only antigen A has *type A* blood.

A person with only antigen B has *type B* blood.

A person with both antigen A and antigen B has *type AB* blood and is a universal recipient who can receive blood from any other type in the ABO system.

A person with neither antigen has *type O* blood and is a universal donor, able to give blood to any other person no matter what that person's blood type is.

Rhesus (Rh) Blood Group

If an **Rh** antigen is present on an RBC surface, the blood is said to be Rh-positive (Rh$^+$). If there is no Rh antigen on the surface, the blood is Rh-negative (Rh$^-$). The presence or absence of Rh antigen is inherited. The antigen is named the **Rhesus factor** because it was first found on the red blood cell of a rhesus monkey.

If an Rh-negative person receives a transfusion of Rh-positive blood, anti-Rh antibodies will be produced. This can cause RBC agglutination and hemolysis.

If an Rh-negative woman and an Rh-positive man conceive an Rh-positive child *(Figure 11.10a)*, the placenta normally prevents maternal and fetal blood from mixing. However, at birth or during a miscarriage, fetal cells can enter the mother's bloodstream. These Rh-positive cells stimulate the mother's tissues to produce Rh-antibodies *(Figure 11.10b)*.

If the mother becomes pregnant with a second Rh-positive fetus, her Rh-antibodies can cross the placenta and agglutinate and hemolyze the fetal RBCs *(Figure 11.10c)*. This causes hemolytic disease of the newborn (**HDN,** or **erythroblastosis fetalis**).

Hemolytic disease of the newborn due to Rh-incompatibility can be prevented. The Rh-negative mother should be given Rh immune globulin (RhoGAM) during pregnancy, or soon after giving birth to an Rh-positive child.

Other causes of hemolytic disease of the newborn include ABO incompatibility, incompatibility in other blood group systems, hereditary **spherocytosis,** and some infections acquired before birth.

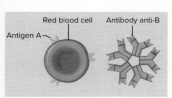

(a) Type A blood

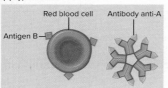

(b) Type B blood

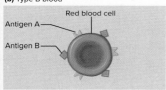

(c) Type AB blood

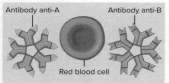

(d) Type O blood

▲ **Figure 11.9** ABO blood types.

Did you know...

- All blood groups are inherited.
- Rh factor is an antigen on the surface of a red blood cell.

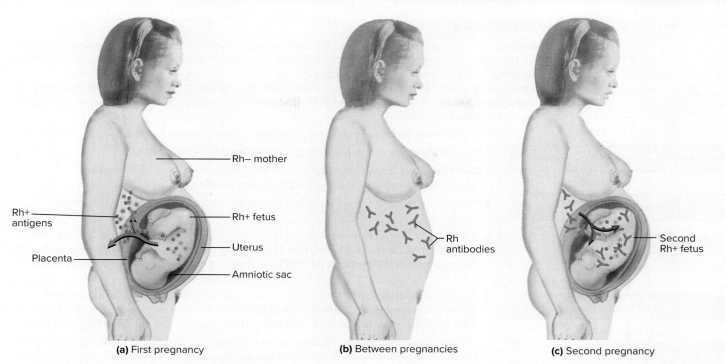

- Rh– mother
- Rh+ antigens
- Rh+ fetus
- Uterus
- Placenta
- Amniotic sac

(a) First pregnancy

- Rh antibodies

(b) Between pregnancies

- Second Rh+ fetus

(c) Second pregnancy

▲ **Figure 11.10** Hemolytic disease of the newborn.

Word Analysis and Definition: Rhesus Blood Group

S = Suffix   P = Prefix   R = Root   R/CF = Combining Form

WORD	PRONUNCIATION	ELEMENTS		DEFINITION
agglutination	ah-glue-tih-**NAY**-shun	S/ P/ R/	-ation *process* ag- *to* -glutin- *glue*	Process by which cells or other particles adhere to each other to form clumps
antibody	**AN**-tih-bod-ee	P/ R/	anti- *against* -body *substance*	Protein produced in response to an antigen
antigen	**AN**-tih-jen	P/ S/	anti- *against* -gen *to produce*	Any substance that can trigger an immune response
erythroblastosis fetalis	eh-**RITH**-ro-blas-**TOH**-sis fee-**TAH**-lis	S/ R/CF S/ S/ S/ R/	-osis *condition* erythr/o- *red* -blast- *germ cell, immature cell* -is *belonging to* -al- *pertaining to* fet- *fetus*	Hemolytic disease of the newborn due to Rh incompatibility
Rhesus factor	**REE**-sus **FAK**-tor	 R/	**Rhesus** Greek *mythical king of Thrace* factor *maker*	Antigen on red blood cells of Rh-positive (Rh⁺) individuals. It was first identified in the blood of a rhesus monkey
spherocytosis	**SFEER**-oh-sigh-**TOH**-sis	S/ R/CF R/	-osis *condition* spher/o- *sphere* -cyt- *cell*	Presence of spherocytes in blood

Hemostasis

Hemostasis, the control of bleeding, is a vital issue in maintaining homeostasis, the state of equilibrium of the body. Uncontrolled bleeding can take the body out of balance by decreasing blood volume and lowering blood pressure, leading to death.

Platelets (also called **thrombocytes**) play a key role in hemostasis. They are minute fragments of large bone marrow cells called **megakaryocytes.** They have no nucleus. Platelet granules secrete chemicals that are critical to hemostasis:

- **Coagulation factors**—proteins and enzymes—that initiate the process.
- **Vasoconstrictors** that cause constriction in injured blood vessels.
- **Chemicals** that attract neutrophils and monocytes to sites of inflammation.
  Hemostasis is achieved through a three-step mechanism:

1. **Vascular spasm**—an immediate but temporary constriction of the injured blood vessel.
2. **Platelet plug formation**—an accumulation of platelets that bind themselves together and adhere to surrounding tissues. The binding and adhesion of platelets is mediated through **von Willebrand factor (vWF),** a protein produced by the cells lining blood vessels.
3. **Blood coagulation**—the process beginning with the production of molecules that make **prothrombin** and **thrombin** and finishing with the formation of a blood clot that traps blood cells, platelets, and tissue fluid in a network of fibrin *(Figures 11.11).*

After a blood clot forms, platelets adhere to strands of fibrin and contract to pull the fibers closer together. As the blood clot shrinks, it pulls the edges of the broken blood vessel together. **Fibroblasts** invade the clot to produce a fibrous connective tissue that seals the blood vessel.

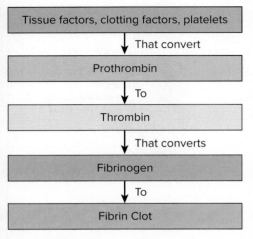

▲ **Figure 11.11** Blood coagulation.

Word Analysis and Definition: Hemostasis

S = Suffix   P = Prefix   R = Root   R/CF = Combining Form

WORD	PRONUNCIATION	ELEMENTS		DEFINITION
anticoagulant	**AN**-tee-koh-**AG**-you-lant	S/ P/	-ant *forming* anti- *against*	Substance that prevents clotting
coagulant coagulation	koh-**AG**-you-lant koh-ag-you-**LAY**-shun	R/ S/	-coagul- *clump* -ation *process*	Substance that induces clotting The process of blood clotting
fibroblast	**FIE**-broh-blast	S/ R/CF	-blast *immature cell* fibr/o- *fiber*	Cell that forms collagen fibers
hemostasis (**Note:** Homeostasis has a very different meaning.)	hee-moh-**STAY**-sis	S/ R/CF	-stasis *control, stop* hem/o- *blood*	Controlling or stopping bleeding
megakaryocyte	**MEG**-ah-**KAIR**-ee-oh-site	S/ P/ R/CF	-cyte *cell* mega- *enormous* -kary/o- *nucleus*	Large cell with large nucleus. Parts of the cytoplasm break off to form platelets
platelet thrombocyte (syn)	**PLAYT**-let	S/ R/	-let *small* plate- *flat*	Cell fragment involved in the clotting process
prothrombin	proh-**THROM**-bin	S/ P/ R/	-in *substance* pro- *before* -thromb- *clot*	Protein formed by the liver and converted to thrombin in the blood-clotting mechanism
thrombin thrombocyte (also called **platelet**) thrombus thrombosis	**THROM**-bin **THROM**-boh-site **THROM**-bus throm-**BOH**-sis	 S/ R/CF S/ S/ R/	Greek *clot* -cyte *cell* thromb/o- *clot* -us *pertaining to* -osis *condition* thromb- *clot*	Enzyme that forms fibrin Another name for a platelet A clot attached to a blood vessel or heart lining Formation of a thrombus

The flowchart in the figure reads:

Tissue factors, clotting factors, platelets
↓ That convert
Prothrombin
↓ To
Thrombin
↓ That converts
Fibrinogen
↓ To
Fibrin Clot

A. Place the steps of hemostasis in the correct order. *There are three steps to hemostasis. Place them in order, with the first step being "1" and the last step being "3."* **LO 11.1**

_____ platelet plug

_____ vascular spasm

_____ blood coagulation

B. Use the language of hematology to answer the following questions. *Fill in each blank with the correct medical term relating to hemostasis.* **LO 11.1, 11.3**

1. A cell that forms collagen fibers: _____.

2. A platelet is a fragment of a: _____.

3. The process of forming a clot: _____

C. Match the elements in the first column with the correct meanings in the second column. **LO 11.9**

_____ **1.** *anti-*   **a.** condition

_____ **2.** *-stasis*   **b.** substance

_____ **3.** *glutin*   **c.** control

_____ **4.** *-ation*   **d.** glue

_____ **5.** *-osis*   **e.** against

_____ **6.** *-in*   **f.** process

D. Identify the components of blood typing. *Choose the correct term in the parentheses that completes each statement.* **LO 11.1**

1. It is the (antigen/antibody) on the erythrocyte that determines a person's blood type.

2. It is the (red blood cells/plasma) that contains antibodies that seek out antigens.

3. A person with type B blood has B (antigens/antibodies).

4. A person with type A blood has anti-B (antigens/antibodies).

5. A person with type O blood has no (anti-A antibodies/antigens).

E. Deconstruct medical terms to determine their meanings. *Using the terms relating to rhesus factor, identify the meanings of the word elements.* **LO 11.6**

1. In the medical term **erythroblastosis fetalis,** the condition affects which component of the blood?

   a. white blood cells   **b.** plasma   **c.** coagulation   **d.** red blood cells

2. In the medical condition **erythroblastosis fetalis,** who is harmed: the mother or the baby?

   a. mother   **b.** baby

F. Explain the disorder erythroblastosis fetalis. *Choose the correct answer for each question regarding this condition.* **LO 11.6**

1. In order for this disorder to occur, the mother must have blood that is:

   a. type A   **b.** type B   **c.** type O   **d.** Rh−   **e.** Rh+

2. The trigger for this condition to occur is a baby with blood that is:

   a. type A   **b.** type B   **c.** type O   **d.** Rh−   **e.** Rh+

3. It is impossible for the first child to have this condition.

   a. True   **b.** False

Section 11.5 Disorders of Blood Cells

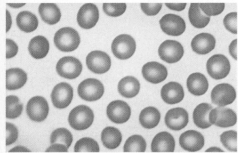

(a)   1200×

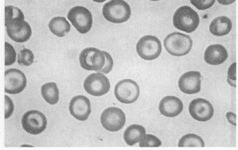

(b)   1000×

▲ **Figure 11.12** **Red blood cells.**
(a) Normal RBCs. (b) Hypochromic
RBCs. Ed Reschke

Did you know...

- Anemia reduces the oxygen-
  carrying capacity of blood.
- Hemolysis liberates
  hemoglobin from red blood
  cells.

Disorders of Red Blood Cells

Anemia is a reduction in the number of RBCs or in the amount of hemoglobin each RBC contains *(Figure 11.12)*. Both of these conditions reduce the oxygen-carrying capacity of the blood and produce the symptoms of shortness of breath (**SOB**) and fatigue. They also produce **pallor** (paleness of the skin) because of the deficiency of the red-colored oxyhemoglobin, the combination of oxygen and hemoglobin, and the red blood cells are **hypochromic** *(Figure 11.12b)*

There are several types of anemia:

- **Iron-deficiency anemia** can be caused by blood loss, such as gastrointestinal bleeding or heavy menstruation; lack of iron in the diet; inability to absorb iron from the small intestine; and pregnancy.
- **Pernicious anemia (PA)** is due to vitamin B_{12} deficiency. This is caused by a shortage of *intrinsic factor (see Chapter 5)*, which is normally secreted by cells in the lining of the stomach and binds with vitamin B_{12}; this complex is absorbed into the bloodstream. Without vitamin B_{12}, hemoglobin cannot be formed. The RBCs decrease in number and in hemoglobin concentration and increase in size (**macrocytic**).
- **Sickle cell anemia** (also called *sickle cell disease*) is a genetic disorder found most commonly in African Americans, Africans, and some Mediterranean populations. It results from the production of an abnormal hemoglobin that causes the RBCs to form a rigid sickle cell shape *(Figure 11.13)*. The abnormal cells are sticky, clump together (**agglutinate**), and block small capillaries. This causes intense pain in the **hypoxic** tissues (a sickle cell crisis) and can cause stroke and kidney and heart failure.

  There is a minor form of the disease, sickle cell trait, in which symptoms rarely occur and do not progress to the full-blown disease.
- **Hemolytic anemia** is due to excessive destruction of normal and abnormal RBCs. **Hemolysis** can be caused by such toxic substances as snake and spider venoms, mushroom toxins, and drug reactions. Trauma to RBCs by hemodialysis or heart-lung machines can produce a hemolytic anemia.
- **Aplastic anemia** is a condition in which the bone marrow is unable to produce sufficient new cells of all types—red cells, white cells, and platelets. It can be associated with exposure to radiation, benzene, and certain drugs.
- **Hemoglobinopathies,** such as sickle cell disease and **thalassemia,** with their inherited abnormal hemoglobins, also cause hemolysis of RBCs. Hemolysis also can occur through incompatible blood transfusions or maternal-fetal incompatibilities *(see Lesson 11.5)*. Jaundice is a complication.
- **Polycythemia vera** is an overproduction of RBCs and WBCs due to an unknown cause.
- **Poikilocytosis** is a categorical term referring to the presence of irregular-shaped red blood cells. Examples include **spherocytes** and sickle cells.

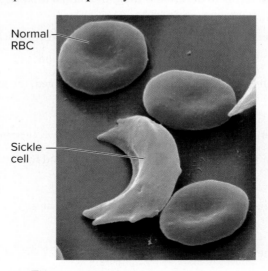

Normal RBC

Sickle cell

▲ **Figure 11.13** **Sickle cell anemia.** Eye of
Science/Science Source

WORD	PRONUNCIATION		ELEMENTS	DEFINITION
agglutinate	ah-**GLUE**-tin-ate	S/ P/ R/	-ate *composed of, pertaining to* ag- *to* -glutin- *stick together, glue*	Stick together to form clumps
anemia anemic (adj)	ah-**NEE**-me-ah ah-**NEE**-mik	P/ S/ S/	an- *without* -emia *blood* -emic *pertaining to a* *condition of the blood*	Decreased number of red blood cells Pertaining to or suffering from anemia
aplastic anemia	ay-**PLAS**-tik ah-**NEE**-mee-ah	S/ P/ R/ S/ P/	-tic *pertaining to* a- *without* -plas- *formation* -emia *blood* an- *without, lack of*	Condition in which the bone marrow is unable to produce sufficient red cells, white cells, and platelets
hemoglobinopathy	**HEE**-moh-**GLOH**-bih-**NOP**-ah-thee	S/ R/CF R/CF	-pathy *disease* hem/o- *blood* -globin/o- *protein*	Disease caused by the presence of an abnormal hemoglobin in the red blood cells
hemolysis hemolytic (adj)	hee-**MOL**-ih-sis hee-moh-**LIT**-ik	S/ R/CF S/ R/	-lysis *destruction* hem/o- *blood* -ic *pertaining to* -lyt- *destroy*	Destruction of red blood cells so that hemoglobin is liberated Pertaining to the process of destruction of red blood cells
hypochromic	high-poh-**CROH**-mik	S/ P/ R/	-ic *pertaining to* hypo- *deficient, below* -chrom- *color*	Pale in color, as in RBCs when hemoglobin is deficient
hypoxia (**Note:** The surplus "o" is not used.) hypoxic (adj)	high-**POK**-see-ah high-**POK**-sik	S/ P/ R/ S/	-ia *condition* hypo- *deficient* -ox- *oxygen* -ic *pertaining to*	Below normal levels of oxygen in tissues, gases, or blood Deficient in oxygen
incompatible	in-kom-**PAT**-ih-bul	S/ P/ R/	-ible *can do* in- *not* -compat- *blood tolerate*	Substances that interfere with each other physiologically
macrocyte macrocytic (adj) microcytic	**MAK**-roh-site mak-roh-**SIT**-ik my-kroh-**SIT**-ik	R/CF P/ S/ R/ P/	cyt/e *cell* macro- *large* -ic *pertaining to* -cyt- *cell* micro- *small*	Large red blood cell Pertaining to macrocytes Pertaining to a small cell
pallor	**PAL**-or		Latin *paleness*	Paleness of the skin or a red blood cell
pernicious anemia (PA)	per-**NISH**-us ah-**NEE**-mee-ah	 S/ P/	**pernicious** Latin *destructive* -emia *blood* an- *without, lack of*	Chronic anemia due to lack of vitamin B$_{12}$
poikilocytic (adj) poikilocytosis	**POY**-kee-loh-**SIT**-ik **POY**-kee-loh-sigh-**TOH**-sis	S/ P/ R/ S/	-ic *pertaining to* poikilo- *irregular* -cyt- *cell* -osis *condition*	Pertaining to an irregular-shaped red blood cell A condition of irregular-shaped red blood cells
polycythemia vera	**POL**-ee-sigh-**THEE**-mee-ah **VEH**-rah	S/ P/ R/	-hemia *blood condition* poly- *many, much* -cyt- *cell* **vera** Latin *truth*	Chronic disease with bone marrow hyperplasia and increase in number of red blood cells and in blood volume
spherocyte spherocytosis	**SFEER**-oh-site **SFEER**-oh-sigh-**TOH**-sis	S/ R/CF S/ R/	-cyte *cell* spher/o- *sphere* -osis *condition* -cyt- *cell*	A spherical cell Presence of spherocytes in blood
thalassemia	thal-ah-**SEE**-mee-ah	S/ R/	-emia *blood condition* thalass- *sea*	Group of inherited blood disorders that produce a hemolytic anemia and occur in people living around the Mediterranean Sea

Disorders of White Blood Cells

Normally a cubic millimeter (**mm³**) of blood contains 5,000 to 10,000 white blood cells. **Leukocytosis** is defined as a total WBC count of normal cells exceeding 10,000/mm³ due to any cause.

Causes of leukocytosis are:

- **Neutrophilia,** an increase in the number and percentage of neutrophils. This can be due to bacterial infections, for example, appendicitis or bacterial pneumonia.

- **Eosinophilia,** an increase in the number of eosinophils. This occurs with allergic reactions or parasitic infection.

- **Basophilia,** which occurs when there is an increase in basophils. Basophilia can be caused by allergic reactions or infection due to tuberculosis, chicken pox, and influenza.

Leukocytosis is the presence of too many white blood cells. **Leukopenia** results when the WBC count drops below 5,000 cells/mm³ of blood. Leukopenia is most often associated with **neutropenia,** but it also can be associated with decreases in the other white blood cells. This condition reduces the body's ability to fight infection.

Monocytosis is a condition in which there is an increase in monocytes. This condition occurs in cases of chronic infection and autoimmune diseases. **Monocytopenia** is a decrease in monocytes, which can arise from chemotherapy.

Lymphocytosis is an increase in the number of lymphocytes. This condition can be caused by infection, HIV/AIDs, and **mononucleosis.** AIDS also can lead to **lymphocytopenia,** as can hepatitis, influenza, and tuberculosis.

Leukemia is cancer of the hematopoietic tissues and produces a high number of leukocytes and their **precursors** in the WBC count. As the **leukemic** cells proliferate, they take over the bone marrow and cause a deficiency of normal RBCs, WBCs, and **platelets.** This makes the patient anemic and vulnerable to infection and bleeding.

Myeloid leukemia is characterized by uncontrolled production of granulocytes and their precursors *(Figure 11.14)* and starts in the bone marrow. It can be in an acute or chronic form.

Lymphoid leukemia is characterized by uncontrolled production of lymphocytes. It can be in an acute or chronic form. **Acute lymphoblastic leukemia (ALL)** is the most common form of childhood cancer and is curable with modern treatments, such as chemotherapy and bone marrow and umbilical cord **stem cell** transplants.

Pancytopenia occurs when the erythrocytes (RBCs), leukocytes (WBCs), and thrombocytes (**platelets**) in the circulating blood are all markedly reduced. This can occur with cancer chemotherapy.

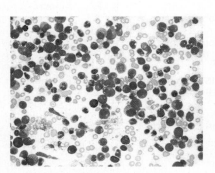

▲ **Figure 11.14** Myeloid leukemia.
Jose Luis Calvo/Shutterstock

WORD	PRONUNCIATION	ELEMENTS		DEFINITION
basophilia	**BAY**-so-**FILL**-ee-ah	S/ R/CF	**-philia** *attraction* **bas/o-** *base*	Condition of increased basophil cells
eosinophilia	ee-oh-**SIN**-o-**FILL**-ee-ah	S/ R/CF	**-philia** *attraction* **eosin/o-** *dawn*	Condition of increased eosinophil cells
leukemia leukemic (adj) leukopenia	loo-**KEE**-mee-ah loo-**KEE**-mik loo-koh-**PEE**-nee-ah	S/ R/ S/ S/	**-emia** *a blood condition* **leuk-** *white* **-emic** *pertaining to a blood condition* **-penia** *deficiency*	Disease when the blood is taken over by white blood cells and their precursors Pertaining to or affected by leukemia A deficient number of white blood cells
leukocytosis	**LOO**-koh-sigh-**TOH**-sis	S/ R/CF R/	**-osis** *condition* **leuk/o-** *white* **-cyt-** *cell*	An excessive number of white blood cells
lymphocytopenia	**LIM**-foh-sigh-toh-**PEE**-nee-ah	S/ R/CF R/CF	**-penia** *deficiency* **lymph/o-** *lymph* **-cyt/o-** *cell*	Condition of decreased lymphocytes in the blood
lymphocytosis	**LIM**-foh-sigh-**TOH**-sis	S/ R/CF R/	**-osis** *condition* **lymph/o-** *lymph* **-cyt-** *cell*	Condition of increased lymphocytes in the blood
lymphoid lymphoid leukemia	**LIM**-foyd **LIM**-foyd loo-**KEE**-mee-ah	S/ R/ S/ R/	**-oid** *resembling* **lymph-** *lymph* **-emia** *blood condition* **leuk-** *white*	Resembling lymphatic tissue Malignant disease marked by an uncontrolled production of lymphocytes
monocytosis monocytopenia	**MON**-oh-sigh-**TOH**-sis **MON**-oh-sigh-toh-**PEE**-nee-ah	S/ P/ R/CF S/	**-osis** *condition* **mono-** *single* **-cyt/o-** *cell* **-penia** *deficiency*	Increased number of monocytes in the blood Decreased number of monocytes in the blood
mononucleosis	**MON**-oh-nyu-klee-**OH**-sis	S/ P/ R/	**-osis** *condition* **mono-** *single* **-nucle-** *nucleus*	Presence of large numbers of mononuclear leukocytes
myeloid myeloid leukemia	**MY**-eh-loyd **MY**-eh-loyd loo-**KEE**-mee-ah	S/ R/ S/ R/	**-oid** *resembling* **myel-** *bone marrow* **-emia** *blood condition* **leuk-** *white*	Resembling cells derived from bone marrow Leukemia that begins with cells in the bone marrow and moves into the blood
neutrophilia neutropenia	**NEW**-troh-**FILL**-ee-ah **NEW**-troh-**PEE**-nee-ah	S/ R/CF S/	**-philia** *attraction* **neutr/o-** *neutral* **-penia** *deficiency*	An excess number of neutrophils A deficiency of neutrophils
pancytopenia	**PAN**-sigh-toh-**PEE**-nee-ah	S/ P/ R/CF	**-penia** *deficiency* **pan-** *all* **-cyt/o-** *cell*	Deficiency of all types of blood cells
precursor	pree-**KUR**-sir	P/ R/	**pre-** *before, in front of* **-cursor** *run*	Cell or substance formed earlier in the development of the cell or substance
stem cell	STEM SELL		**stem** Old English *stalk of a plant*	Undifferentiated cell found in a differentiated tissue that can divide to yield the specialized cells in that tissue

Disorders of Coagulation (Coagulopathies)

Hemophilia in its classical form (hemophilia A) is a disease that males inherit from their mothers and is due to a deficiency of a coagulation factor, called factor VIII. The disorder causes painful bleeding into skin, joints, and muscles. Concentrated factor VIII is given intravenously to reduce the symptoms.

Von Willebrand disease (vWD) is a deficiency of vonWillebrand factor, causing increased amount of time needed to form a clot.

Disseminated intravascular coagulation (DIC) occurs when the clotting mechanism is activated simultaneously throughout the cardiovascular system. The trigger is usually a severe bacterial infection. Small clots form and obstruct blood flow into tissues and organs, particularly the kidney, leading to renal failure. As the clotting mechanisms are overwhelmed, severe bleeding occurs.

Thrombus formation (**thrombosis**) is a clot that attaches to diseased or damaged areas on the walls of blood vessels or the heart. If part of the thrombus breaks loose and moves through the circulation, it is called an **embolus.**

Purpura is bleeding into the skin from small arterioles that produces a larger individual lesion than petechiae from capillary bleeding *(Figure 11.15)*. **Bruises** (or **hematomas**) are **extravasations** of blood from all types of blood vessels.

Thrombocytopenia is a low platelet count (below $100,000/mm^3$ of blood). It occurs when bone marrow is destroyed by radiation, chemotherapy, or leukemia. Small capillary hemorrhages called **petechiae** and bruises can be seen in the skin. **Idiopathic (immunologic) thrombocytopenic purpura (ITP)** is an acute self-limiting form of the disease usually seen in children.

Thrombotic thrombocytopenic purpura (TTP) and **hemolytic-uremic syndrome (HUS)** are acute, potentially fatal disorders in which loose strands of fibrin are deposited in numerous small blood vessels. This causes damage to platelets and RBCs, causing thrombocytopenia and hemolytic anemia.

Henoch-Schönlein purpura (anaphylactoid purpura) is a disorder involving purpura, joint pain, and **glomerulonephritis** *(see Chapter 6)*. The etiology is unknown. Most cases resolve spontaneously.

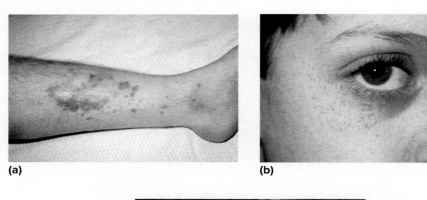

(a) (b)

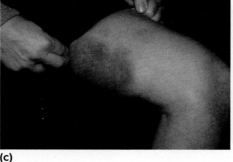

(c)

▲ **Figure 11.15** **Subsurface bleeding.** (a) Purpura. (b) Pinpoint petechiae. (c) Bruises.
Mediscan/Alamy Stock Photo Dr. P. Marazzi/Science Source Paul Cox/Alamy Stock Photo

Word Analysis and Definition: Disorders of Coagulation

S = Suffix   P = Prefix   R = Root   R/CF = Combining Form

WORD	PRONUNCIATION	ELEMENTS		DEFINITION
coagulopathy coagulopathies (pl)	koh-ag-you-**LOP**-ah-thee	S/ R/CF	**-pathy** *disease* **coagul/o-** *clotting*	Disorder of blood clotting
disseminate	dih-**SEM**-in-ate	S/ P/ R/	**-ate** *composed of, pertaining to* **dis-** *apart* **-semin-** *scatter seed*	Widely scatter throughout the body or an organ
embolus	**EM**-boh-lus		Greek *plug, stopper*	Detached piece of thrombus, a mass of bacteria, quantity of air, or foreign body that blocks a blood vessel
extravasate	eks-**TRAV**-ah-sate	S/ P/ R/	**-ate** *composed of, pertaining to* **extra-** *out of, outside* **-vas-** *blood vessel*	To ooze out from a vessel into the tissues
hematoma bruise (syn)	hee-mah-**TOH**-mah BROOZ	S/ R/	**-oma** *mass, tumor* **hemat-** *blood* Old English *to bruise*	Collection of blood that has escaped from the blood vessels into tissue
hemophilia	hee-moh-**FILL**-ee-ah	S/ R/CF	**-philia** *attraction* **hem/o-** *blood*	An inherited disease from a deficiency of clotting factor VIII
petechia petechiae (pl)	peh-**TEE**-kee-ah peh-**TEE**-kee-ee		Latin *spot on the skin*	Pinpoint capillary hemorrhagic spot in the skin
purpura	**PUR**-pyu-rah		Greek *purple*	Skin hemorrhages that are red initially and then turn purple
thrombocytopenia	**THROM**-boh-sigh-toh-**PEE**-nee-ah	S/ R/CF R/CF	**-penia** *deficiency* **thromb/o-** *clot* **-cyt/o-** *cell*	Deficiency of platelets in circulating blood

Check Point Section 11.5

A. Define word elements pertaining to hematology. *If you can remember the meaning of word elements, you can define the medical term.*
LO 11.2

1. The suffix that means *attraction* is:

    a. *-osis*   **b.** *-penia*   **c.** *-ic*   **d.** *-philia*

2. The combining form that means *white* is:

    a. *neutr/o*   **b.** *leuk/o*   **c.** *cyt/o*   **d.** *bas/o*

3. The suffix *–penia* means:

    a. deficiency   **b.** excessive   **c.** one   **d.** white

B. Fill in the blank with the correct medical term related to disorders of coagulation. LO 11.6

1. A decrease in the number of thrombocytes in the circulating blood: _____.

2. A thrombus that has detached and lodged in another blood vessel: _____.

3. A pinpoint hemorrhage: _____.

C. Match the term in the first column to its correct definition in the second column. LO 11.5

_____ **1.** hematoma

_____ **2.** extravasate

_____ **3.** petechia

_____ **4.** purpura

_____ **5.** disseminate

a. widely scatter throughout the body

b. bleeding into the skin from arterioles

c. escape from a blood vessel

d. collection of blood that has escaped from a blood vessel

e. small capillary hemorrhage

D. Choose the correct abbreviation. _From the given description, choose the correct abbreviation of the described conditions._ **LO 11.5**

1. Loose strands of fibrin are deposited in numerous small blood vessels:

  a. DIC   **b.** ITP   **c.** TTP   **d.** vWD

2. Deficiency of factor vWF:

  a. DIC   **b.** ITP   **c.** TTP   **d.** vWD

Section 11.6 Procedures and Pharmacology

Diagnostic Procedures

A **complete blood count (CBC)** measures the following:

- The number of red blood cells (RBC count)
- The amount of hemoglobin in the blood
- The percentage of the blood composed of red blood cells (hematocrit)
- Average red blood cell size **(MCV)**
- Hemoglobin amount per red blood cell **(MCH)**
- Amount of hemoglobin relative to the size of the red blood cell **(MCHC)**
- The number of white blood cells (WBC count)
- The types of white blood cells (WBC differential)
- Platelet count

    Serum iron is the amount of iron in the blood.

    Serum ferritin is the amount in the blood of the iron–protein complex that regulates iron storage and transport.

    Erythrocyte sedimentation rate (ESR) is a nonspecific measure of inflammation.

    Bone marrow is found inside the larger bones and contains cells that produce RBCs, WBCs, and platelets. **Bone marrow biopsy** and **aspiration** are performed in the investigation of anemias, polycythemia, cancers (to determine if the cancer has spread to the bones), and bone marrow diseases.

    Prothrombin time (PT), partial thromboplastin time (PTT), and **International Normalized Ratio (INR)** are used to evaluate bleeding and clotting disorders and to monitor anticoagulation therapies _(see Lesson 11.4)._

    A **Monospot test** is used to diagnose infectious mononucleosis caused by the Epstein-Barr virus. It detects the presence of antibodies that the body developed in response to external antigens.

Therapeutic Procedures

A **transfusion** of blood or packed red blood cells *(Figure 11.16)* replaces lost red blood cells to restore the blood's oxygen-carrying capacity. During **autologous** donation and transfusion, people donate their own blood ahead of time to be given to them if necessary during a surgical procedure.

Bone marrow transplant is the transfer of bone marrow from a healthy, compatible bone marrow donor to a patient with aplastic anemia, leukemia, lymphoma, multiple myeloma, or other disease.

Hematopoietic stem cells are found in the bone marrow and are capable of generating all our blood cells such as red cells, white cells, and platelets. In hematology, clinical trials to treat hemophilia and thalassemia with **gene therapy** are underway using **allogenic** cells from a **compatible** donor.

Gene therapy is an experimental technique to treat or prevent disease by replacing a **mutated** gene with a healthy copy, by inactivating a mutated gene that is functioning improperly, or by introducing a new gene into the body.

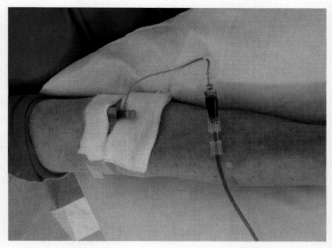

▲ **Figure 11.16** Patient receiving blood transfusion.
Dave Moyer

Word Analysis and Definition: Diagnostic and Therapeutic Procedures

S = Suffix   P = Prefix   R = Root   R/CF = Combining Form

WORD	PRONUNCIATION		ELEMENTS	DEFINITION
allogen	**AL**-oh-jen	P/ S/	**allo-** *different* **-gen** *to produce*	Antigen from someone else in the same species
allogenic (adj)	al-oh-**JEN**-ik	S/	**-ic** *pertaining to*	Pertaining to an allogen
aspiration	**AS**-pih-**RAY**-shun	S/ R/	**-ion** *process* **aspirat-** *to breathe*	Removal by suction of fluid or gas from a body cavity
autologous	awe-**TOL**-oh-gus	P/ R/	**auto-** *self, same* **-logous** *relation*	Blood transfusion with the same person as donor and recipient
compatible	kom-**PAT**-ih-bul	S/ P/ R/	**-ible** *able to* **com-** *with* **-pat-** *lie together*	Able to exist together with something else
corpuscle	**KOR**-pus-ul	S/ R/	**-cle** *small (can also be cule)* **corpus-** *body*	A blood cell
corpuscular (adj)	kor-**PUS**-kyu-lar	S/ S/	**-ar** *pertaining to* **-cul-** *small*	Pertaining to corpuscle
ferritin	**FER**-ih-tin	S/ R/	**-in** *chemical* **ferrit-** *iron*	Iron—protein complex that regulates iron storage and transport
gene	JEEN		Greek *birth*	Functional unit of heredity
Monospot test (Trade name)	**MON**-oh-spot TEST			Detects heterophile antibodies in infectious mononucleosis
mutate (verb) mutation	**MYU**-tayt myu-**TAY**-shun	S/ R/	Latin *to change* **-ion** *action, condition, process* **mutat-** *change*	Change the chemistry of a gene Change in the chemistry of a gene
transfusion	trans-**FYU**-zhun	P/ R/	**trans-** *across* **-fusion** *to pour*	Transfer of blood or a blood component from donor to recipient
transplant	**TRANZ**-plant	P/ R/	**trans-** *across* **-plant** *plant*	The tissue or organ used or the act of transferring tissue from one person to another

Pharmacology

Anticoagulants used to reduce or prevent blood clotting include:

- **Aspirin,** which reduces platelet **adherence** and is used in small 81 mg doses to reduce the incidence of heart attack.
- **Heparin,** which prevents prothrombin and fibrin formation and is given **parenterally;** its dose is monitored by **activated partial thromboplastin time** (aPTT).
- **Warfarin** *(Coumadin),* which inhibits the synthesis of prothrombin and others to act as an anticoagulant. It is given by mouth and its dose is monitored by **prothrombin times** (PTs), which are reported as an **International Normalized Ratio** (INR).
- **Dabigatran etexilate** *(Pradaxa),* inhibits the activation of prothrombin, and **rivaroxaban** *(Xarelto),* which inhibits the direct **synthesis** of thrombin, are given by mouth to reduce the risk of **embolism** and stroke in patients with nonvalvular atrial fibrillation *(see Chapter 10).* **Idarucizumab** *(Praxbind injection)* is available for patients using *Pradaxa* when reversal of its anticoagulant effects is needed for emergency surgery, for urgent procedures, or in life-threatening or uncontrolled bleeding.
- **Streptokinase,** derived from hemolytic streptococci, which dissolves the fibrin in blood clots. Given intravenously within 3 to 4 hours of a heart attack, it is often effective in dissolving a clot that has caused the heart attack.

Recombinant Factor VIII, developed through **recombinant DNA** technology, is the main medication used to treat hemophilia A. It is given intravenously through a vein in the arm or a port in the chest. **Desmopressin acetate** *(DDAVP)* is a synthetic version of **vasopressin** that helps stop bleeding in patients with mild hemophilia.

Pernicious anemia is treated initially with injections of vitamin B_{12}, and then the vitamin B_{12} can be given through a nasal gel.

Eltrombopag *(Promacta)* is available for pediatric patients with idiopathic thrombocytopenic purpura (ITP) who have not responded to corticosteroids, immunoglobulins, or splenectomy.

Most **leukemias** in both adults and children are treated with **chemotherapy,** often with added radiation therapy and a stem cell transplant.

Word Analysis and Definition: Pharmacology

S = Suffix   P = Prefix   R = Root   R/CF = Combining Form

WORD	PRONUNCIATION		ELEMENTS	DEFINITION
adhere adherence	add-**HEER** add-**HEER**-ents	S/ R/	Latin *to stick to* -ence *forming, quality of* adher- *stick to*	To stick to something The act of sticking to something
chemotherapy	**KEE**-moh-**THAIR**-ah-pee	R/CF R/	chem/o- *chemical* therapy *treatment*	Treatment using chemical agents
embolism	**EM**-boh-lizm		Greek *a plug or patch*	A plug of tissue or air from afar that obstructs a blood vessel
parenteral	pah-**REN**-ter-al	S/ P/ R/	-al *pertaining to* par- *abnormal* -enter- *intestine*	Administering medication by any means other than the GI tract
recombinant DNA	ree-**KOM**-bin-ant **DEE**-en-a	S/ P/ R/	-ant *forming* re- *again* -combin- *combine*	Deoxyribonucleic acid (DNA) altered by inserting a new sequence of DNA into the chain
streptokinase	strep-toh-**KIE**-nase	P/ R/	strepto- *curved* -kinase *enzyme*	An enzyme that dissolves clots
vasopressin (also called antidiuretic hormone)	vay-soh-**PRESS**-in	S/ R/CF R/	-in *chemical compound* vas/o- *blood vessel* -press- *close, press*	Pituitary hormone that constricts blood vessels and decreases urinary output

Check Point Section 11.6

 Case Report (CR) 11.1

You are

. . . an **emergency medical technician (EMT)** employed in the Fulwood Medical Center Emergency Department.

Your patient is

. . . Janis Tierney, a 17-year-old high school student.

Ms. Tierney presents with fainting at school. She is pale. Her pulse is 90. Blood pressure (BP) is 100/60.

She tells you that she is having a menstrual period with excessive bleeding. Her physical examination is otherwise unremarkable. She has a history of easy bruising and recurrent nosebleeds and an episode of severe bleeding after a tooth extraction. Laboratory tests reveal that she has a deficiency of **von Willebrand factor (vWF).** Her platelets are unable to stick together or adhere to the wall of an injured blood vessel, and a platelet plug cannot form in the lining of her uterus to help end her menstrual flow.

Von Willebrand disease (vWD) is the most common hereditary bleeding disorder. It affects at least 1% of the population and both sexes equally.

A. Refer to the above Case Report along with the other text material to answer the following questions. *Select the answer that correctly completes each statement.* **LO 11.6, 11.8**

1. Because Ms. Tierney has a deficiency in vWF, she is unable to:

   a. produce fibrinogen

   b. coagulate her blood

   c. form a platelet plug

   d. create a vascular spasm

2. Her excessive loss of blood is causing her heart rate to:

   a. stay within normal limits

   b. increase

   c. decrease

3. Her abnormal blood pressure is related to:

   a. stress

   b. recurrent nose bleeds

   c. loss of blood

   d. her tooth extraction

Case Report (CR) 11.2

You are

. . . a medical assistant working with Susan Lee, MD, a primary care physician at Fulwood Medical Center.

Your patient is

. . . Mrs. Luisa Sosin, a 47-year-old woman who presented a week ago with fatigue, lethargy, and muscle weakness. Physical examination revealed **pallor** of her skin, a pulse rate of 100, and a respiratory rate of 20. Dr. Lee referred her for extensive blood work. Dr. Lee also determined that the patient had been taking aspirin and other **nonsteroidal anti-inflammatory drugs (NSAIDs)** for the past 6 months for low-back pain.

You are responsible for documenting her investigation and care. She is your next patient, and you are reviewing the laboratory report above.

Because Mrs. Luisa Sosin was deficient in iron and hemoglobin, her RBCs were small (microcytic) and lacked the red color of oxyhemoglobin, and some were irregular-shaped (poikilocytic) rather than the normal, round shape. The volume of each cell, mean corpuscular volume (MCV), and the amount of hemoglobin in each cell, mean corpuscular hemoglobin (MCH), were decreased. The amount of iron in her blood (serum iron) and the amount of ferritin in her serum were decreased. Her total iron-binding capacity was raised because the shortage of iron resulted in an increased availability of the protein to which iron is bound in the bloodstream.

B. Use the above Case Report to answer the following questions. LO 11.6, 11.8

1. If a term means deficient in, what element would it start with? _____

2. What is the opposite of microcytic? _____

3. The condition in which the bone marrow is unable to produce sufficient red cells, white cells, and platelets is _____.

4. Mrs. Sosin's pallor is due to an abnormality in which type of blood cell? (use the 3-letter abbreviation) _____

C. Match each pathology with the definition. LO 11.6

_____	1. Neutrophilia	**a.** Decreased number of monocytes in the blood
_____	2. Eosinophilia	**b.** an increase in the number of eosinophils. This occurs with allergic reactions or parasitic infection
_____	3. Basophilia	**c.** increase in the number of lymphocytes. This condition can be caused by infection, HIV/AIDs, and mononucleosis
_____	4. Leukopenia	**d.** an increase in basophils. Basophilia can be caused by allergic reactions or infection due to tuberculosis, chicken pox, and influenza
_____	5. Monocytosis	**e.** an increase in the number and percentage of neutrophils caused by bacterial infections
_____	6. Lymphocytosis	**f.** WBC count drops below 5,000 cells/mm3 of blood
_____	7. Leukemia	**g.** erythrocytes (RBCs), leukocytes (WBCs), and thrombocytes (platelets) in the circulating blood are all markedly reduced
_____	8. Monocytopenia	**h.** cancer of the hematopoietic tissues decrease in monocytes, which can arise from hemotherapy
_____	9. Pancytopenia	**i.** an increase in monocytes. This condition occurs in cases of chronic infection and autoimmune diseases

D. Identify the action of medications as they relate to hematology. *Select the correct answer to correctly complete each statement.* **LO 11.7**

1. Dissolves fibrin in clots:

   a. *Coumadin*

   b. *Pradaxa*

   c. Streptokinase

   d. *Xarelto*

2. Decreases platelet adherence:

   a. *Coumadin*

   b. Aspirin

   c. Streptokinase

   d. *Promacta*

3. Prevents the activation of prothrombin: (choose all that apply)

   a. Vasopressin

   b. *Pradaxa*

   c. Heparin

   d. *Xarelto*

4. **Inhibits the direct synthesis of thrombin: (choose all that apply)**

   a. *Pradaxa*

   b. Streptokinase

   c. *Xarelto*

   d. Heparin

5. Reverses the effects of *Pradaxa:*

   a. *Promacta*

   b. *Praxbind*

   c. *Coumadin*

   d. *Desmopressin*

E. Identify the meaning of the word parts as they relate to hematology. *Select the answer that correctly completes each statement.* **LO 11.1**

1. The word element that means **different:**

   a. *allo-*   b. *trans-*   c. *corpus-*   d. *-gen*

2. The word part *ferrit-* means:

   a. blood   b. cell   c. iron   d. protein

F. Interpret abbreviations. *Given the abbreviation, choose what the diagnostic test is measuring.* **LO 11.5**

1. WBC differential

   a. number of leukocytes

   b. measure of inflammation

   c. types of leukocytes

   d. average red blood cell size

2. PT

   a. evaluates bleeding and clotting disorders

   b. hemoglobin amount per erythrocyte

   c. counts the number of platelets

   d. determines presence of bone cancer

3. MCH

   a. measures amount of iron in the blood

   b. determines amount of hemoglobin per erythrocyte

   c. measures the various blood cell components

   d. used to monitor anticoagulation therapies

G. Match the therapy In the first column to the disorder it treats in the second column. LO 11.7

_____ 1. Vitamin B_{12}

_____ 2. *Promacta* (eltrombopag)

_____ 3. desmopressin acetate

_____ 4. Recombinant Factor VIII

a. idiopathic thrombocytopenic purpura

b. mild hemophilia

c. pernicious anemia

d. hemophilia A

Table 11.1 Chapter 11 Abbreviations

Abbreviation	Meaning	Abbreviation	Meaning
ALL	acute lymphoblastic leukemia	MCHC	mean corpuscular hemoglobin concentration; the average concentration of hemoglobin in a given volume of red blood cells
CBC	complete blood count		
CO_2	carbon dioxide	MCV	mean corpuscular volume; the average volume of a red blood cell
DIC	disseminated intravascular coagulation		
dL	deciliter; one tenth of a liter	mm^3	cubic millimeter
EBV	Epstein–Barr virus	NO	nitric oxide
ESR	erythrocyte sedimentation rate	NSAID	nonsteroidal anti-inflammatory drug
fL	femtoliter; one quadrillionth of a liter	O2	oxygen
		PA	pernicious anemia
Hb	hemoglobin; also may be written as Hgb	pg	picogram; one-trillionth of a gram
Hct	hematocrit	PT	prothrombin time
HDN	hemolytic disease of the newborn (erythroblastosis fetalis)	PTT	partial thromboplastin time
		RBC	red blood cell
HUS	hemolytic uremic syndrome	Rh	rhesus
INR	International Normalized Ratio	RhoGAM	rhesus immune globulin
		SOB	shortness of breath
ITP	idiopathic (or immunologic) thrombocytopenic purpura	TIBC	total iron binding capacity; the amount of iron needed to saturate transferrin, the protein that transports iron in the blood
L	liter		
mcg	microgram; one-millionth of a gram; sometimes written as mg		
		TTP	thrombotic thrombocytopenic purpura
MCH	mean corpuscular hemoglobin; the average amount of hemoglobin in the average red blood cell	vWD	von Willebrand disease
		vWF	von Willebrand factor
MCH	mean corpuscular hemoglobin	WBC	white blood cell

Table 11.2 Common disorders of the blood system

Disorder or Disease	Signs and Symptoms	Diagnostic Tests	Treatment
Thalassemia	Usually diagnosed at birth Fatigue, weakness, pallor	Prenatal—amniocentesis CBC, hemoglobin tests	Moderate to severe—blood transfusions. Medications: deferasirox (*Exjade, Jadenu*) or deferiprone (*Ferriprox*)
Sickle cell anemia	Yellowing of skin and eyes, fatigue, painful swelling of hands and feet	Blood test at birth	*Voxelotor, Crizanlizumab-tmca*, blood transfusion
Erythroblastosis fetalis	Baby has yellowing of umbilical cord, skin and eyes. May have enlarged liver or spleen	Ultrasound of fetus, evaluating size of liver and spleen; amniocentesis. At birth, umbilical cord blood to determine blood type, RBC count	Prevented by mother receiving Rho(D) immune globulin at 28 weeks of pregnancy Treatment for baby: phototherapy, blood transfusion
Acute myeloid leukemia	Fatigue, weight loss, fever, night sweats, bruising	CBC, bone marrow biopsy	Chemotherapy, radiation, stem cell transplant

Blood

Challenge Your Knowledge

A. **True or false.** The following statements about blood are either true or false. *Choose T if the statement is true. Choose F if the statement is false.* **LO 11.1**

1. The formed elements of blood are RBCs, WBCs, platelets, and serum.   T   F
2. Buffer systems in the blood maintain the correct pH range.   T   F
3. Serum is identical to plasma except for the absence of clotting proteins.   T   F
4. Sickle cell anemia is a genetic disorder.   T   F
5. All cells exchange water by thrombosis.   T   F
6. Plasma is the fluid, noncellular part of blood.   T   F
7. The bloodstream is a liquid transport system.   T   F
8. Whole blood is less viscous than water.   T   F
9. Monocytes are the largest blood cells.   T   F
10. Erythropoiesis occurs in bone spaces filled with red bone marrow.   T   F

B. **Medical terms may be similar in appearance.** You need to use your knowledge of prefixes, roots, and suffixes to help determine the difference between similar terms. Using the following terms, correctly insert them into the following paragraph. Use the italicized words as a hint as to which term goes into the blank. **LO 11.1, 11.6**

erythrocyte   erythroblast   erythroblastosis   erythropoiesis   erythropoietin

The *immature RBC* (1) (_____) undergoes *the process of formation* (2) (_____) in the red bone marrow.

Too many immature cells result in a condition known as (3) _____. A mature RBC is called an (4) _____.

The hormone (5) _____ controls the rate of RBC production.

C. **Pharmacology of blood clotting.** Anyone working with patients must know about prescribed drugs and their function. Match the drug action in the first column with the correct drug in the second column. **LO 11.7**

_____ 1. Dissolves fibrin in blood clots   a. heparin

_____ 2. Reduces platelet adherence   b. Xarelto

_____ 3. Prevents prothrombin and fibrin formation   c. Coumadin

_____ 4. Inhibits formation of prothrombin   d. streptokinase

_____ 5. Inhibits synthesis of thrombin   e. aspirin

D. How well do you understand what you read? First, read the paragraph aloud to check your pronunciation. Enter the term found in the paragraph in the left column of the chart next to its correct meaning. **LO 11.3**

When a lab tech takes a blood sample, he spins it in a centrifuge. Formed elements are separated from the colloidal suspension and are packed into the bottom of the tube. The patient's hematocrit can be determined from this test. Whole blood contains all the formed elements. Transfusions can be done with either whole blood or only certain portions of the formed elements—only transfusing RBCs or platelets, for instance. The remaining part (55%) of a blood sample is the plasma, which is mostly water. Plasma provides the fluid transport for the formed elements as well as nutrients, hormones, and enzymes for body cells. Waste cell products dissolve in plasma and are excreted through the kidneys and liver.

Term	Meaning
1.	percentage of RBCs in the blood
2.	liquid containing particles that do not settle
3.	introduction of blood or a blood component into a vein
4.	something life sustaining
5.	blood clotting cell
6.	instrument for separating a blood sample
7.	liquid transport system
8.	erythrocyte

E. List the different blood types in the ABO blood group. Be sure to note which type is the "universal donor" and which type is the "universal recipient." Fill in the blanks. **LO 11.1**

The two major antigens on the cell surface are antigen A and antigen B.

1. A person with only antigen A has type _____ blood.

2. A person with only antigen B has type _____ blood.

3. A person with *both* antigen A and antigen B has type _____ blood.

4. A person with *neither* antigen A nor antigen B has type _____ blood.

5. Because the blood type in question 4 has *neither* antigen, it is compatible with any blood type; therefore, it is the universal (donor/recipient) _____.

6. Because the blood type in question 3 has *both* antigens, it is the universal (donor/recipient) _____.

F.   Build medical terms from the following group of elements. The definition is given to you; fill in the medical term. You will not use every element, and some you may use twice. Fill in the blanks. **LO 11.2**

Use a combination of these elements to complete the terms:

ic	micro	auto	osis	hypo	crit	ox
ary	cyte	thrombo	macro	ar	erythro	cyt

1. Another name for an RBC   erythro/ _____
2. Pertaining to a small cell   _____ /cyt/ _____
3. Blood transfusion with the same person as both donor and recipient   _____ /logous
4. Large RBC   _____ /cyte
5. Percentage of RBCs in blood   hemato/ _____
6. Same as a platelet   _____ /cyte
7. Formation of a clot   thromb/ _____

G.   Test your knowledge of blood, blood groups, and Rh factor by choosing the correct answer to the following questions. Select the answer that correctly completes each sentence. **LO 11.1**

1. A person with both antigen A and antigen B will have

   a. blood type O

   b. blood type A

   c. blood type B

   d. blood type AB

   e. blood type B–

2. Where are antibodies synthesized after birth?

   a. in the heart

   b. in the blood

   c. in the arteries

   d. in the plasma

   e. in the veins

3. What normally prevents maternal and fetal blood from mixing during pregnancy?

   a. cell membranes

   b. the peritoneum

   c. the placenta

   d. the amniotic sac

   e. the matrix

4. Blood is said to be Rh-positive if

   a. the Rh antigen is present on the RBC surface

   b. the Rh antibody is present in the blood type

   c. the Rh antibody is present in the plasma

   d. the Rh antigen is present on the WBCs

   e. the blood type is AB

5. **Agglutination** occurs when

   a. you have not been vaccinated

   b. you are given the wrong blood type

   c. your antibodies are low

   d. your hematocrit is high

   e. you are Rh-positive

6. The term **transfusion** is used only for

   a. plasma

   b. whole blood

   c. blood or a blood component

   d. saline solution

   e. intravenous (IV) antibiotics

H. **Multiple choice.** Use the *language of hematology* to answer the following questions. Remember that in the case of multiple choice, there is only one best answer. **LO 11.1, 11.5, 11.6, 11.7**

1. Blood volume varies with

   a. your body size

   b. your weight

   c. the amount of your connective tissue

   d. the amount of your erythrocytes

   e. your height

2. The percentage of erythrocytes in a blood sample is called the

   a. hemoglobin

   b. hematocrit

   c. hematemesis

   d. hemolysis

   e. hemostasis

3. In the term **hypochromic,** the root means

   a. blood

   b. center

   c. color

   d. glue

   e. air

4. How many types of leukocytes also qualify as granulocytes?

   a. one

   b. two

   c. three

   d. four

   e. five

5. **Myeloid leukemia** is a disorder of

   a. erythrocytes

   b. leukocytes

   c. platelets

   d. plasma

   e. hemoglobin

6. In the term **erythrocyte,** the combining form means

   a. yellow

   b. red

   c. white

   d. black

   e. blue

7. **Heparin** is an

   a. antidepressant

   b. antihistamine

   c. antibody

   d. anticoagulant

   e. antibiotic

8. Which of these terms cannot be connected with blood?

   a. liquid matrix

   b. complete blood count

   c. formed elements

   d. infusion

   e. transfusion

9. The largest leukocyte is

   a. monocyte

   b. macrophage

   c. eosinophil

   d. basophil

   e. neutrophil

10. What is plasma minus its protein fibrinogen?

   a. hemoglobin

   b. antithrombin

   c. plasmin

   d. serum

   e. a formed element

I. **There are many diseases associated with the various components of blood.** Select the correct answer in the following descriptions; then, on the blanks, write in which blood component is associated with the disease you circled. Use RBC, WBC, and P (for platelet) for blood component notations. **LO 11.1, 11.6, 11.9**

Blood Component

1. Chronic bleeding from the gastrointestinal tract can cause

   a. iron-deficiency anemia   **b.** pernicious anemia   **c.** sickle cell anemia   _____

2. A deficiency of a specific protein of the factor VIII complex is

   a. thrombus   **b.** von Willebrand disease   **c.** iron-deficiency anemia   _____

3. Cancer of the hematopoietic tissues is called

   a. leukemia   **b.** lukemia   **c.** lukemmia   _____

4. A disease resulting from vitamin B_{12} deficiency is

   a. pernicious anemia   **b.** hemolytic anemia   **c.** polycythemia vera   _____

5. A disease males inherit from their mothers is

   a. hemmaphilia   **b.** hemophilia   **c.** hemmophilia   _____

6. A hereditary disease found mostly in people of African descent is

   a. sickle cell anemia   **b.** iron-deficiency anemia   **c.** polycythemia vera   _____

7. In this disease, numerous small clots form and obstruct blood flow into organs:

   a. DIC   **b.** vWD   **c.** EBV   _____

8. This is seen in viral infections such as influenza:

   a. leukopenia   **b.** leukocytosis   **c.** leukemia   _____

9. Low blood cell count that produces a tendency to bleed is

   a. thrombocitopenia   **b.** thrombocytopenia   **c.** thrombocytopennia   _____

10. Destruction of blood cells by toxic substances is

   a. polycythemia vera   **b.** hemolytic anemia   **c.** pernicious anemia   _____

J. **Demonstrate your knowledge of word elements by deconstructing the following medical terms.** Place each word element from the medical term to its correct type. If the term does not have a particular element, write n/a. **LO 11.2**

Term	Prefix	Root/Combining Form	Suffix
agranulocyte	1.	2.	3.
hypochromic	4.	5.	6.
monocytosis	7.	8.	9.
poikilocytic	10.	11.	12.
precursor	13.	14.	15.
microcytic	16.	17.	18.
pancytopenia	19.	20.	21.

K. **Write the terms next to the appropriate statement that follows.** Fill in the blanks. **LO 11.3**

1. That which comes before something _____

2. Pertaining to a small cell _____

3. Decreased number of erythrocytes _____

4. Pigmented protein in erythrocytes _____

5. Excessively high leukocyte count _____

6. Deficiency of all formed elements in the blood _____

7. Increase in the number of monocytes in the blood _____

8. Pertaining to an erythrocyte of irregular shape _____

L. **With the possible exception of the appendix, everything in the body has a function.** The functions are listed as follows. Assign each a letter for the blood component that performs the function. **LO 11.1**

Functions

a. A function of an erythrocyte

b. A function of a leukocyte

c. A function of a platelet

d. A function of plasma

Assign one of the previous functions to each of the following statements. Fill in the blank with the correct letter that corresponds to each function.

1. Transport oxygen _____
2. Help maintain hemostasis _____
3. Migrate to damaged tissues and release histamine _____
4. Carry nutrients, hormones, and enzymes to cells _____
5. Dissolve cellular waste products _____
6. Secrete lysozymes _____
7. Transport carbon dioxide _____
8. Seal off injury and hemorrhage _____
9. Provide fluid environment to formed elements _____
10. Transport nitric oxide _____

M. **Pronunciation is important whether you are saying the word or listening to a word from a coworker.** Identify the proper pronunciation of the following medical terms. Correctly spell the term. **LO 11.2, 11.3, 11.4, 11.6, 11.7**

1. The correct pronunciation for a specific white blood cell's granules attracting rosy-red dye

a. ee-oh-**SIN**-oh-fill

b. ees-**SIN**-oh-fill

c. **GRAN**-you-loh-site

d. **GRAIN**-yule-oh-site

Correctly spell the term: _____

2. The correct pronunciation for a white blood cell without any granules in its cytoplasm

    a. IN-oh-**TROH**-pik

    b. IN-oh-troop-**IK**

    c. ay-**GRAIN**-yule-oh-site

    d. ay-**GRAN**-you-loh-site

    Correctly spell the term: _____

3. The correct pronunciation for the transfer of blood or a blood component from donor to recipient

    a. TRANZ-plant

    b. TRAINZ-plant

    c. trans-**FYU**-zhun

    d. tray-nuhs-**FYU**-zhun

    Correctly spell the term: _____

4. The correct pronunciation for sticking together to form clumps

    a. threw-mob-**OH**-sis

    b. throm-**BOH**-sis

    c. ah-**GLUE**-tin-ate

    d. ah-**GLUE**-tine-eate

    Correctly spell the term: _____

5. The correct pronunciation for referring to the repair of dead tissue cells by formation of fibrous tissue

    a. hoh-mee-oh-**STAY**-sis

    b. home-oh-**STAU**-sis

    c. hee-moh-**STAY**-sis

    d. heh-moh-**STAY**-sees

    Correctly spell the term: _____

Case Report

A. **After reading the following Case Report, correctly answer the following questions.** The answers to the questions may not be in the Case Report itself but can be found in the chapter content. **LO 11.5, 11.6, 11.8, 11.9**

Case Report (CR) 11.3

You are

. . . a laboratory technician reviewing a peripheral blood smear.

Your patient is

. . . Mrs. Latisha Masters, a 27-year-old student.

Mrs. Masters presented with a 5-day history of fatigue, low-grade fever, and sore throat. Physical examination showed tonsillitis with bilateral, enlarged, tender cervical lymph nodes and an enlarged spleen.

The WBC count you performed showed 9,200 cells per cubic millimeter. The peripheral smear you are looking at is reported as showing the presence of atypical mononuclear cells with abundant cytoplasm.

Latisha Masters' blood smear indicated a diagnosis of **infectious mononucleosis.** caused by the **Epstein-Barr virus (EBV).** This virus infects white blood cells. A positive **heterophile reaction (Monospot test)** was present. Infectious mononucleosis This condition occurs in the 15- to 25-year-old population. Its cause, the EBV, is a very common virus, a member of the herpes virus family. The EBV and is transmitted by exchange of saliva, as in kissing. In patients with symptoms compatible with infectious mononucleosis., a positive Monospot test is diagnostic.

---

1. What is the name of the cell you counted?

   a. erythrocyte

   b. leukocyte

   c. thrombocyte

2. What caused Mrs. Masters' condition?

   a. Bacterium

   b. Virus

   c. Fungus

3. Which diagnostic test would confirm the diagnosis?

   a. Monospot test

   b. Peripheral smear

   c. Complete blood count

   d. Prothrombin time

4. Provide the abbreviation for the specific cause of her condition: _____

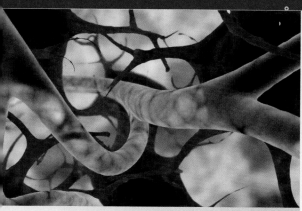

2014 Nucleus Medical Media

Chapter Sections

Lymphatic and Immune Systems

The Language of Immunology

Chapter Learning Outcomes

Upon completion of this chapter, you will be able to:

LO 12.1 Identify and describe the anatomy and physiology of the lymphatic and immune system.

LO 12.2 Use roots, combining forms, suffixes, and prefixes to construct and analyze medical terms related to lymphatic and immune system.

LO 12.3 Spell medical terms related to the lymphatic and immune system.

LO 12.4 Pronounce medical terms related to the lymphatic and immune system.

LO 12.5 Describe diagnostic procedures utilized in immunology.

LO 12.6 Identify and describe disorders and pathological conditions related to the lymphatic and immune system.

LO 12.7 Describe the therapeutic procedures and pharmacologic agents used in the lymphatic and immune system.

LO 12.8 Apply knowledge of medical terms relating to lymphatic and immune system to documentation, medical records, and communication.

LO 12.9 Identify and correctly use abbreviations of terms used in lymphatic and immune system.

LO 12.10 Identify health professionals involved in the care of patients with immune disorders.

The health professionals involved in the diagnosis and treatment of problems with the lymphatic and immune systems include:

- **Immunologists** and **allergists,** who are physicians who specialize in immune system disorders, such as allergies, asthma, and immunodeficiency and autoimmune diseases.
- **Epidemiologists,** who are medical scientists involved in the study of epidemic diseases and how they are transmitted and controlled.
- **Medical** or **laboratory technicians,** who perform testing procedures on blood, body fluids, and other tissues using microscopes, computers, and other equipment.

Section 12.1 Lymphatic System

Lymphatic System

As part of your defense mechanisms, the lymphatic system and its fluid provide surveillance and protection against foreign materials. The body has three lines of defense mechanisms against foreign organisms **(pathogens)**, cells **(cancer)**, and molecules **(pollutants** and **allergens):**

1. **Physical mechanisms**—the skin and mucous membranes, chemicals in perspiration, saliva and tears, hairs in the nostrils, cilia and mucus to protect the lungs. These are described in the individual body system chapters.

2. **Cellular mechanisms**—based on defensive cells **(lymphocytes)** that directly attack suspicious cells such as cancer cells, transplanted tissue cells, or cells infected with viruses or **parasites.** This is the basis for the lymphatic system.

3. **Humoral defense mechanisms**—based on **antibodies** that are found in body fluids and bind to bacteria, **toxins,** and extracellular viruses, tagging them for destruction. This is the basis for the **immune** system.

The lymphatic system *(Figure 12.1)* **has three components:**

1. A network of thin **lymphatic capillaries and vessels,** similar to blood vessels, that penetrates into the interstitial spaces of nearly every tissue in the body except cartilage, bone, red bone marrow, and the central nervous system (CNS).

2. A group of tissues and organs that produce **immune cells.**

3. **Lymph,** a clear colorless fluid similar to blood plasma but whose composition varies from place to place in the body. It flows through the network of lymphatic capillaries and vessels.

The lymphatic system has three functions:

1. To **absorb** excess interstitial fluid and return it to the bloodstream.

2. To **remove** foreign chemicals, cells, and debris from the tissues.

3. To **absorb** dietary lipids from the small intestine *(see Chapter 5).*

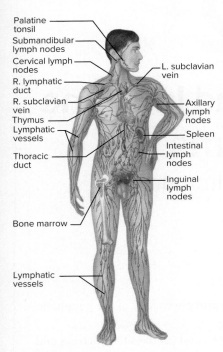

▲ **Figure 12.1** **The lymphatic system.**
(R. = right; L. = left)

The lymphatic network begins with **lymphatic capillaries,** which are closed-ended tubes nestled among blood capillary networks *(Figure 12.2).* The lymphatic capillaries are designed to let interstitial fluid enter, and the interstitial fluid becomes lymph. In addition, bacteria, viruses, cellular debris, and traveling cancer cells can enter the lymphatic capillaries with the interstitial fluid. The lymphatic capillaries converge to form the larger lymphatic collecting vessels. These resemble small veins and have one-way valves in their lumen. They travel alongside veins and arteries.

The larger lymphatic collecting vessels merge into **lymphatic trunks** that drain lymph from a major body region. In turn, these lymphatic trunks merge into two large **lymphatic ducts:**

1. The **right lymphatic duct** receives lymph from the right arm, right side of the thorax, and right side of the head and drains into the **right subclavian vein** *(Figure 12.1).*

2. The **thoracic duct** on the left, the largest lymphatic vessel, receives lymph from both sides of the body below the diaphragm and from the left arm, left side of the head, and left thorax. It begins in the abdomen at the level of the second lumbar vertebra (L2) and passes up through the diaphragm and mediastinum to empty into the **left subclavian vein** *(Figure 12.1).*

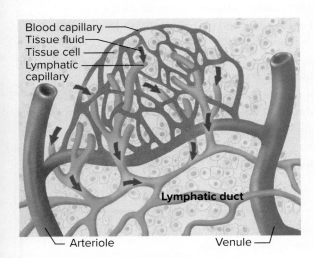

▲ **Figure 12.2** **Lymphatic flow.**

WORD	PRONUNCIATION		ELEMENTS	DEFINITION
allergen (**Note:** The duplicate letter "g" is deleted to better form the word.)	**AL**-er-jen	S/ R/ R/	-gen *to produce* all- *different, strange* -erg- *work*	Substance producing a hypersensitivity (allergic) reaction
allergic (adj) allergy	ah-**LER**-jic **AL**-er-jee	S/ S/	-ic *pertaining to* -ergy *process of working*	Pertaining to or suffering from an allergy Hypersensitivity to a particular allergen
antibody antibodies (pl)	**AN**-tih-bod-ee **AN**-tih-bod-ees	P/ R/	anti- *against* -body *substance, body*	Protein produced in response to an antigen
humoral	**HYU**-mor-al	S/ R/	-al *pertaining to* humor- *fluid*	Defense mechanism arising from antibodies in the blood
immune (adj) immunity	im-**YUNE** im-**YOU**-nih-tee	S/ R/	Latin *protected from* -ity *condition* immun- *immune response*	Protected from an infectious disease State of being protected
immunology immunologist	im-you-**NOL**-oh-jee im-you-**NOL**-oh-jist	S/ R/CF S/	-logy *study of* immun/o- *immune response* -logist *one who studies, specialist*	The science and practice of immunity and allergy Medical specialist in immunology
immunize (verb) immunization immunoglobulin	**IM**-you-nize im-you-nih-**ZAY**-shun **IM**-you-noh-**GLOB**-you-lin	S/ R/ S/ S/ R/CF R/	-ize *affect in a specific way* immun- *immune response* -ization *process of affecting in a specific way* -in *chemical compound* immun/o- *immune response* -globul- *protein*	Make resistant to an infectious disease Administration of an agent to provide immunity Specific protein evoked by an antigen; all antibodies are immunoglobulins
lymph lymphatic (adj) lymphocyte	LIMF lim-**FAT**-ik **LIM**-foh-site	S/ R/ S/ R/CF	Latin *clear spring water* -atic *pertaining to* lymph- *lymph* -cyte *cell* lymph/o- *lymph*	A clear fluid collected from tissues and transported by lymph vessels to the venous circulation Pertaining to lymph or the lymphatic system Small white blood cell with a nucleus
node	NOHD		Latin *a knot*	A circumscribed mass of tissue
parasite	**PAR**-ah-site		Greek *a guest*	An organism that attaches itself to, lives on or in, and derives its nutrition from another species
pathogen	**PATH**-oh-jen	S/ R/CF	-gen *to produce* path/o- *disease*	A disease-causing microorganism
pollutant	poh-**LOO**-tant	S/ R/	-ant *pertaining to* pollut- *unclean*	Substance that makes an environment unclean or impure
toxin toxic (adj) toxicity (contains two suffixes)	**TOK**-sin **TOK**-sick toks-**ISS**-ih-tee	S/ R/ S/	Greek *poison* -ic *pertaining to* tox- *poison* -ity *state, condition*	Poisonous substance formed by a cell or organism Pertaining to a toxin, poisonous The state of being poisonous

Lymphatic Nodes, Tissues, and Cells

Lymph Nodes

At irregular intervals, the lymphatic collecting vessels enter into the part of the lymphatic network called **lymph nodes** (*Figure 12.3*). There are hundreds of lymph nodes stationed all over the body. They are especially concentrated in the neck, axilla, and groin. Their functions are to filter impurities from the lymph and alert the immune system to the presence of pathogens.

The lymph moves slowly through the node (*Figure 12.3*), which filters the lymph and removes any foreign matter. On its journey back to the bloodstream, lymph passes through several nodes and becomes cleansed of most foreign matter. **Macrophages** in the lymph nodes ingest and break down the foreign matter and display fragments of it to **T cells** (*see the following section*). This alerts the immune system to the

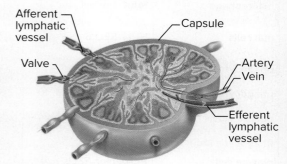

▲ **Figure 12.3** Lymph node.

presence of an invader. Lymph leaves the nodes again when it enters into the efferent collecting vessels. All these lymph vessels move lymph toward the thoracic cavity.

Lymphatic Tissues and Cells

Many organs have a sprinkling of lymphocytes in their connective tissues and mucous membranes, particularly in passages that open to the exterior—the respiratory, digestive, urinary, and reproductive tracts—where invaders have access to the body.

In some organs, lymphocytes and other cells form dense clusters called **lymphatic follicles.** These are constant features in the tonsils, the adenoids, and the ileum.

Lymphatic tissues are composed of a variety of cells that include:

1. **T lymphocytes (T cells).** The "T" stands for *thymus,* where they mature.

   T lymphocytes make up 75% to 85% of body lymphocytes. There are several types of T cells:

   a. **Cytotoxic or "killer" T cells** destroy target cells. Their cell membrane holds a **coreceptor** that can recognize a specific antigen. Coreceptors are named with the letters **"CD" (cluster of differentiation)** followed by a number, for these cells, CD8.

   b. **Helper T cells** contain the CD4 coreceptor and are called CD4 cells. They begin the defensive response against a specific antigen.

   c. **Memory T cells** arise from cytotoxic T lymphocytes that have previously destroyed a foreign cell. If they encounter the same antigen, they can now quickly kill it without initiation by a helper T cell.

   d. **Suppressor T cells** suppress activation of the immune system. Failure of these cells to function properly may result in autoimmune diseases.

2. **B lymphocytes (B cells).** These cells mature in the bone marrow. B lymphocytes make up 15% to 25% of lymphocytes. They are activated by helper T cells, respond to a specific antigen, and cause the production of antibodies called **immunoglobulins (Ig).** The mature B cells are called **plasma cells** and secrete large quantities of antibodies that immobilize, neutralize, and prepare the specific antigen for destruction.

3. **Null cells.** These are large granular lymphocytes that are natural killer cells but lack the specific surface markers of the T and B lymphocytes.

4. **Macrophages.** These cells develop from monocytes *(see Chapter 11)* that have migrated from blood. They ingest and destroy tissue debris, bacteria, and other foreign matter **(phagocytosis).**

Word Analysis and Definition: Lymphatic Nodes, Tissues, and Cells

S = Suffix   P = Prefix   R = Root   R/CF = Combining Form

WORD	PRONUNCIATION		ELEMENTS	DEFINITION
coreceptor	koh-ree-**SEP**-tor	S/ P/ R/	-or *a doer* co- *with, together* -recept- *receive*	Cell surface protein to enhance the sensitivity of an antigen receptor
cytotoxic (adj)	sigh-toh-**TOK**-sik	S/ R/CF	-toxic *able to kill* cyt/o- *cell*	Agent able to destroy cells
follicle	**FOLL**-ih-kull		Latin *a small sac*	Spherical mass of cells containing a cavity, or a small cul-de-sac such as a hair follicle
macrophage	**MAK**-roh-fayj	S/ P/	-phage *to eat* macro- *large*	Large white blood cell (WBC) that removes bacteria, foreign particles, and dead cells
null cells	NULL SELLS		**null** Latin *none*	Lymphocytes with no surface markers, unlike T cells or B cells
phagocyte	**FAG**-oh-site	S/ R/CF	-cyte *cell* phag/o- *to eat*	Blood cell that ingests and destroys foreign particles and cells
phagocytize (verb)	**FAG**-oh-site-ize	S/ R/	-ize *action* -cyt- *cell*	Ingest foreign particles and cells
phagocytosis	**FAG**-oh-sigh-**TOH**-sis	S/	-osis *condition*	Process of ingestion and destruction of foreign particles and cells
phagocytic (adj)	fag-oh-**SIT**-ik	S/	-ic *pertaining to*	Pertaining to phagocytes or phagocytosis
plasma cell	**PLAZ**-mah SELL		**plasma** Greek *something formed*	Cell derived from B lymphocytes and active in formation of antibodies

Lymphatic Organs

Spleen

The **spleen,** a highly vascular and spongy organ, is the largest lymphatic organ. It is located in the left upper quadrant of the abdomen below the diaphragm and lateral to the kidney *(Figure 12.4)*. It is the only organ the body can live without.

The spleen contains two basic types of tissue:

1. **White pulp**—which is a part of the immune system that produces T cells, B cells, and macrophages. The blood passing through the spleen is monitored for antigens. Antibodies are produced, and the foreign matter is removed.

2. **Red pulp**—which acts as a **reservoir** for erythrocytes, platelets, and macrophages that remove old and defective erythrocytes.

Thus, the functions of the spleen are to:

- **Produce** T cells, B cells, and macrophages.
- **Phagocytize** bacteria and other foreign materials.
- **Initiate an immune response** to produce antibodies when antigens are found in the blood.
- **Phagocytize** old, defective erythrocytes and platelets (hemolysis).
- **Serve as a reservoir** for erythrocytes and platelets.

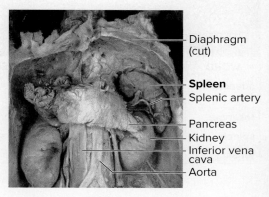

▲ **Figure 12.4** **Position of spleen.**
Dennis Strete/McGraw Hill

Tonsils

The **tonsils** *(see Chapter 13)* are two masses of lymphatic tissue located at the entrance to the oropharynx, where they entrap inhaled and ingested pathogens. **Adenoids** are similar tissue on the posterior wall of the nasopharynx *(see Chapter 13)*. The tonsils and adenoids form lymphocytes and antibodies, trap bacteria and viruses, and drain them into the tonsillar lymph nodes for elimination. They can become infected themselves.

Thymus Gland

The thymus gland has both endocrine *(see Chapter 17)* and lymphatic functions. T cells develop and mature in it and are released into the bloodstream. The thymus is largest in infancy and childhood *(Figure 12.5a and b)* and reaches its maximum size at puberty. It then regresses into a small structure in the adult *(Figure 12.5b)* and is eventually replaced by fibrous and adipose tissue.

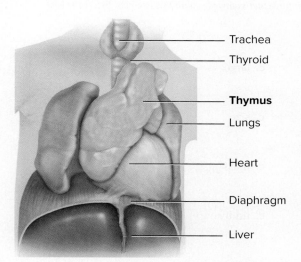

▲ **Figure 12.5(a)** **Large thymus in an infant.**

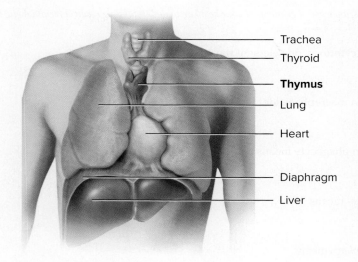

▲ **Figure 12.5(b)** **Adult thymus.**

WORD	PRONUNCIATION	ELEMENTS		DEFINITION
adenoid	**ADD**-eh-noyd	S/ R/	**-oid** *resemble* **aden-** *gland*	Single mass of lymphoid tissue in the midline at the back of the throat
reservoir	**REZER** -vwhar		**French** *collection place*	A cavity that stores fluids
spleen	SPLEEN		Greek *spleen*	Vascular, lymphatic organ in the left upper quadrant of the abdomen
tonsil	**TON**-sill		Latin *tonsil*	Mass of lymphoid tissue on either side of the throat at the back of the tongue

Check Point Section 12.1

A. Build the correct medical terms that match the definitions given. *If the term does not have a particular word element, leave it empty. Fill in the blanks.* **LO 12.1, 12.2**

1. substance that makes the environment unclean or impure:

_____ / _____ / _____
P   R/CF   S

2. make resistant to infectious disease:

_____ / _____ / _____
P   R/CF   S

3. the basis of humoral defense mechanisms:

_____ / _____ / _____
P   R/CF   S

B. Elements. *Knowledge of elements is your best key to understanding medical terminology. Reinforce that knowledge with this exercise. Select the best choice.* **LO 12.1, 12.2**

1. In the term **cytotoxic,** one element means

   a. to eat   **b.** able to kill   **c.** large

2. The prefix in **macrophage** identifies

   a. color   **b.** location   **c.** size

3. The suffix in **phagocyte** means

   a. cyst   **b.** cell   **c.** mass

4. The prefix *co-* means

   a. next to   **b.** with   **c.** under

5. The suffix *-phage* means

   a. flow   **b.** eat   **c.** produce

6. This suffix means condition:

   a. *-osis*   **b.** *-ize*   **c.** *-ic*

C. Identify the correct answer that contains all the lymphatic organs. *Select the best choice.* **LO 12.1**

1. Which of the following is a list of only lymphatic organs?

    a. liver, spleen, thyroid gland

    b. spleen, lungs, kidney

    c. tonsils, spleen, parathyroid gland

    d. thymus gland, spleen, lymph vessels and nodes

    e. gallbladder, spleen, thyroid gland

D. The spleen is a very important organ in the body. *Select T if the statement is True. Select F if the statement is False.* **LO 12.1**

	T	F
1. The spleen is a highly vascular and spongy organ.	T	F
2. The spleen is the largest of the lymphatic organs.	T	F
3. The spleen is located in the right upper quadrant of the body.	T	F
4. The spleen contains white pulp and red pulp.	T	F
5. The spleen serves as a reservoir for RBCs and platelets.	T	F

E. This exercise describes the "where" of lymphatic tissue—you need to supply the term that is the "what." "*What am I?*" *Identify the correct medical term for each of the following questions.* **(LO 12.1, 12.3)**

1. I am located below the diaphragm and lateral to the kidney. _____

2. I am located at the entrance to the oropharynx, where I trap pathogens. _____

3. I am located on the posterior wall of the nasopharynx. _____

4. I am located in the chest cavity. _____

Section 12.2 Immune System

The Immune System

The study of the immune system is called immunology. The medical specialist involved in the study and research of the immune system and in treating disorders of the immune system is called an immunologist. The immune system is not an organ system but a group of specialized cells in different parts of the body that recognize foreign substances and neutralize them. It is the third line of defense listed at the beginning of this chapter. When the immune system is functioning correctly, it protects the body against bacteria, viruses, cancer cells, and foreign substances. When the immune system is weak, it allows pathogens (including the viruses that cause common colds and "flu") and cancer cells to successfully invade the body.

   T lymphocytes and B lymphocytes protect the body through adaptive immunity.

- Receptors on the surface of T cells and B cells recognize specific nonself (foreign) antigens.

- Antigens are molecules that trigger an immune response. Each antigen has a unique structure that is recognized by the immune system.

- **Haptens** are small, foreign molecules that attach themselves to host molecules to form large, unique complexes that the immune system can recognize as foreign. Haptens are found in cosmetics, detergents, industrial chemicals, poison ivy, and animal dander.

Three characteristics distinguish immunity from the first two lines of defense:

1. **Specificity.** The immune response is directed against a particular pathogen. Immunity to one pathogen does not confer immunity to others. Specificity has one disadvantage. If a virus or a bacterium changes a component of its genetic code, it will lead to a change in the structure and/or physiology of the microorganism, which then is no longer recognized by the immune system. This **mutation** occurs, for example, in bacteria in response to antibiotics and in HIV's response to anti-HIV drugs (development of **resistance**).

2. **Memory.** When exposure to the same identical pathogen occurs again, the immune system recognizes the pathogen and has its responses ready to act quickly.

3. **Discrimination.** The immune system learns to recognize agents **(antigens)** that represent **"self"** and agents that are **"nonself"** (foreign). Most of this recognition is developed prior to birth. A variety of disorders occur when this discrimination breaks down. They are known as **autoimmune** disorders.

Word Analysis and Definition: Immune System

S = Suffix   P = Prefix   R = Root   R/CF = Combining Form

WORD	PRONUNCIATION		ELEMENTS	DEFINITION
antigen	**AN**-tih-jen	P/ S/	anti- *against* -gen *produce, create*	Substance capable of triggering an immune response
autoimmune	aw-toh-im-**YUNE**	P/ R/	auto- *self, same* -immune *immune response*	Immune reaction directed against a person's own tissue
discrimination	**DIS**-krim-ih-**NAY**-shun	S/ P/ R/	-ation *process* dis- *away from, apart* -crimin- *distinguish*	Ability to distinguish between different things
hapten	**HAP**-ten		Greek *to fasten or bind*	Small molecule that has to bind to a larger molecule to form an antigen
mutate (verb) mutation	**MYU**-tayt myu-**TAY**-shun	 S/ R/	Latin *to change* -ion *action, condition, process* mutat- *change*	To make a change in the chemistry of a gene Change in the chemistry of a gene
resistance resistant (adj)	ree-**ZIS**-tants ree-**ZIS**-tant	S/ R/ S/	-ance *state of, condition* resist- *to withstand* -ant *pertaining to*	Ability of an organism to withstand the effects of an antagonistic agent Able to resist
specific (adj) specificity (*Note:* two suffixes)	speh-**SIF**-ik spes-ih-**FIS**-ih-tee	S/ R/ S/	-ic *pertaining to* specif- *species* -ity *condition, state*	Relating to a particular entity State of having a fixed relation to a particular entity

Immunity

Immunity is classified biologically into two types, though both mechanisms often respond to the same antigen:

1. **Cellular (cell-mediated) immunity** is a direct form of defense based on the actions of lymphocytes to attack foreign and diseased cells and destroy them.

   The many different types of T cells, B cells, and macrophages described in the previous lesson of this chapter are involved in this style of attack.

2. **Humoral (antibody-mediated) immunity** is an indirect form of attack that employs antibodies produced by plasma cells, which have been developed from B cells. The antibodies bind to an antigen and thus tag them for destruction.

   These antibodies are called **immunoglobulins (Igs),** defensive gamma globulins in the blood plasma and body secretions. There are five classes of antibodies (immunoglobulins):

   • **IgG** makes up about 80% of the antibodies. It is found in plasma and tissue fluids. It crosses the placenta to give the fetus some immunity.

   • **IgA** makes up about 13% of the antibodies. It is found in exocrine secretions such as breast milk, tears, saliva, nasal secretions, intestinal juices, bile, and urine.

Did you know...

• The immune system is thought to be able to produce some 2 million different antibodies.

• Antibodies do not actively destroy an antigen. They render it harmless and mark it for destruction by phagocytes.

- **IgM** makes up about 6% of antibodies. It develops in response to antigens in food or bacteria.
- **IgD** is found on the surface of B cells and acts as a receptor for antigens.
- **IgE** is found in exocrine secretions along with IgA and also in the serum.

Once released by plasma cells, the antibodies function in several ways to make antigens harmless, including:

- **Neutralization.** An antibody binds to the antigen and masks it.
- **Agglutination.** An antibody binds to two or more bacteria to prevent them from spreading through the tissues.
- **Precipitation.** Antibodies create an antigen–antibody complex that is too heavy to stay in solution. The complex precipitates (drops out of solution) and can be ingested and destroyed by phagocytes.
- **Complement fixation.** The complement system is a group of 20 or more proteins continually present in blood plasma; IgG and IgM bind to foreign cells, initiating the **binding of complement** to the cell and leading to its destruction. Complement fixation is the major defense mechanism against bacteria and mismatched blood cells.

Based on the production or acquisition of antibodies, four classes of immunity can be described:

1. **Natural active immunity**—the production of your own antibodies as a result of normal maturation, pregnancy, or an infection.
2. **Artificial active immunity**—the production of your own antibodies as a result of **vaccination** or **immunization.** A **vaccine** consists of either killed or **attenuated** (weakened) pathogens (antigens).
3. **Natural passive immunity**—a temporary immunity that results from acquiring antibodies from another individual. This occurs for the fetus through the placenta (IgG) or for the infant through breast milk (IgA).
4. **Artificial passive immunity**—a temporary immunity that results from the injection of an **immune serum** from another individual or an animal. Immune serum is used to treat snakebite, tetanus, and rabies.

Definition of Terms

- **Immunity** is protection from an infectious disease. If you are immune to a disease, you can be exposed to it without becoming infected.
- A **vaccine** is a product that stimulates a person's immune system to produce immunity to a specific disease, protecting that person from that disease. Vaccines are administered through needle injections, by mouth, or by nasal spray.
- **Vaccination** is the act of introducing a vaccine into the body to produce immunity to a specific disease.
- **Immunization** is the process by which a person becomes protected against a disease through vaccination. This term is often used interchangeably with vaccination or **inoculation.**

These definitions are provided by the U.S. Centers for Disease Control and Protection.

S = Suffix   P = Prefix   R = Root   R/CF = Combining Form

WORD	PRONUNCIATION	ELEMENTS		DEFINITION
agglutination	ah-glue-tih-**NAY**-shun	S/	-ation *process*	Process by which cells or other particles adhere to each other to form clumps
		R/	**glutin-** *sticking together, clumping*	
		P/	**ag-**	Stick together to form clumps
agglutinate (verb)	ah-**GLUE**-tin-ate	S/	-ate *composed of, pertaining to*	
attenuate	ah-**TEN**-you-ate	S/	-ate *composed of, pertaining to*	Weaken the ability of an organism to produce disease
		R/	**attenu-** *to weaken*	
attenuated (adj)	ah-**TEN**-you-ay-ted	S/	-ated *process*	Weakened
complement	**KOM**-pleh-ment		Latin *that which completes*	Group of proteins in serum that finish off the work of antibodies to destroy bacteria and other cells
humoral immunity	**HYU**-mor-al	S/	-al *pertaining to*	Defense mechanism arising from antibodies in the blood
	im-**YOU**-nih-tee	R/	**humor-** *fluid*	
		S/	-ity *condition*	
		R/	**immun-** *immune response*	
immune serum (also called **antiserum**)	im-**YUNE SEER**-um		**immune** Latin *protected from*	Serum taken from another human or animal that has antibodies to a disease
			serum Latin *whey*	
vaccine	vak-**SEEN**		Latin *relating to a cow*	Preparation to generate active immunity
vaccinate (verb)	**VAK**-sin-ate	S/	-ate *composed of, pertaining to*	To administer a vaccine
		R/	**vaccin-** *giving a vaccine*	
vaccination	vak-sih-**NAY**-shun	S/	-ation *process*	Administration of a vaccine

Check Point Section 12.2

A. Build your knowledge of elements and their meaning by matching the element in the left column with the definition in the right column. LO 12.2

_____ 1. *crimin*   a. species

_____ 2. *-ity*   b. away from

_____ 3. *specif*   c. distinguish

_____ 4. *anti-*   d. process

_____ 5. *dis-*   e. pertaining to

_____ 6. *-ation*   f. condition, state

_____ 7. *-ic*   g. produce, create

_____ 8. *-gen*   h. against

B. Identify the meanings of the word elements. *Knowing the meanings of the word elements will help you to define medical terms. Select the answer that correctly completes each statement.* **LO 12.2**

1. The root *attenu-* means:

   a. clumping   **b.** inject   **c.** fluid   **d.** weaken

2. The suffix *-ity* means:

   a. source   **b.** process   **c.** condition   **d.** pertaining to

C. Relate the name of the four classes of immunity to how it creates an immunity. *Select the answer that correctly completes each statement.* **LO 12.1**

1. If the source of the immunity originates with an injection or a fluid that is inhaled or swallowed, then it is termed to be:

   a. natural   **b.** artificial

2. If the person creates his or her antibodies after exposure, then the immunity is termed:

   a. active   **b.** passive

3. If the source of the immunity originates within a person's own body or from a mother to her baby, then the immunity is termed:

   a. natural   **b.** artificial

4. If a person is given antibodies, then the immunity is termed:

   a. active   **b.** passive

Section 12.3   Disorders of the Lymphatic and Immune System

Disorders of the Lymphatic System

Physicians routinely palpate accessible lymph nodes in the neck **(cervical nodes)**, axillae **(axillary nodes)**, and groin **(inguinal nodes)** for enlargement and tenderness. Their presence indicates disease in the tissues drained by the lymph nodes. Cancerous lymph nodes are enlarged, firm, and usually painless.

Infections in the lymph nodes cause them to be swollen and tender to the touch, a condition called **lymphadenitis.** All lymph node enlargements are collectively called **lymphadenopathy.**

Lymphoma is a malignant neoplasm of the lymphatic organs, usually the lymph nodes. The disorder usually presents as an enlarged, nontender lymph node, often in the neck or axilla.

Lymphomas are grouped into two categories:

1. **Hodgkin lymphoma**—characterized by the presence of abnormal, cancerous B cells called **Reed-Sternberg cells.** These are large cells with two nuclei resembling the eyes of an owl. The cancer spreads in an orderly manner to adjoining lymph nodes. This enables the disease to be staged, depending on how far it has spread.

2. **Non-Hodgkin lymphomas**—occur much more frequently than Hodgkin lymphoma. They include some 30 different disease entities in 10 different subtypes.

Tonsillitis, inflammation of the tonsils and adenoids, occurs mostly in the first years of life. The infection can be viral or bacterial (usually streptococcal). It produces enlarged, tender lymph nodes under the jaw *(Figure 12.6)*.

Splenomegaly, an enlarged spleen, is not a disease in itself but the result of an underlying disorder. However, when the spleen enlarges, it traps and removes an excessive number of blood cells and platelets **(hypersplenism)** and reduces the number of blood cells and platelets in the bloodstream.

The potential causes of splenomegaly are numerous and include infections such as infectious mononucleosis, lymphomas, anemias such as sickle cell anemia, and storage diseases such as Gaucher disease.

Ruptured spleen is a common complication from car accidents or other trauma when the abdomen and rib cage are damaged. Intra-abdominal bleeding from the ruptured spleen can be extensive, with a dramatic fall in blood pressure (BP).

Lymphedema is localized, nonpitting fluid retention caused by a compromised lymphatic system, often after surgery, radiation therapy, or removal of lymph nodes to determine the presence of cancer cells. It also can be primary, where the cause is unknown.

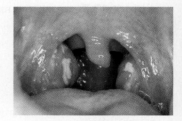

▲ **Figure 12.6** **Tonsillitis.** Open mouth and throat of a 15-year-old girl with inflamed tonsils. They are flecked with infected white patches due to tonsillitis, an infection usually caused by streptococci bacteria.
Dr. P. Marazzi/Science Source

WORD	PRONUNCIATION%	ELEMENTS		DEFINITION
Hodgkin lymphoma	HOJ-kin lim-FOH-muh	S/ R/	Thomas Hodgkin, 1798–1866, British physician -oma *tumor, mass* lymph- *lymph*	Disease marked by chronic enlargement of lymph nodes spreading to other nodes in an orderly way
hypersplenism (*Note:* the one "e.")	high-per-SPLEN-izm	S/ P/ R/	-ism *condition, process* hyper- *excessive* -splen- *spleen*	Condition in which the spleen removes blood components at an excessive rate
lymphadenitis lymphadenopathy	lim-FAD-eh-NIE-tis lim-FAD-eh-NOP-ah-thee	S/ S/ R/CF	-itis *inflammation* -pathy *disease* lymphaden/o- *lymph node*	Inflammation of a lymph node Any disease process affecting a lymph node
lymphedema	LIMF-eh-DEE-mah	R/ S/	lymph- *lymph* -edema *edema*	Tissue swelling due to lymphatic obstruction
lymphoma	lim-FOH-mah	S/ R/	-oma *tumor* lymph- *lymph*	Any neoplasm of lymphatic tissue
splenectomy (*Note:* The "ee" in spleen becomes "e" for easier pronunciation.)	sple-NEK-toh-mee	S/ R/	-ectomy *surgical excision* splen- *spleen*	Surgical removal of the spleen
splenomegaly	sple-noh-MEG-ah-lee	S/ R/CF	-megaly *enlargement* splen/o- *spleen*	Enlarged spleen
tonsillectomy	ton-sih-LEK-toh-mee	S/ R/	-ectomy *surgical excision* tonsill- *tonsil*	Surgical removal of the tonsils
tonsillitis	ton-sih-LIE-tis	S/	-itis *inflammation*	Inflammation of the tonsils

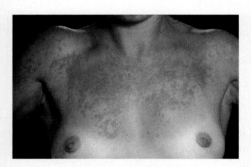

▲ **Figure 12.7** **Sun allergy.** BSIP/Science Source

Disorders of the Immune System

Hypersensitivity is an excessive immune response to an antigen that would normally be tolerated. Hypersensitivity includes:

- **Allergies,** which are reactions to environmental antigens such as pollens, molds, and dusts; to foods such as peanuts, shellfish, and eggs; to plants such as poison ivy; to sunlight (*Figure 12.7*); and to drugs such as penicillin, as well as asthmatic reactions to inhaled antigens (see following text).
- Abnormal reactions to your *own* tissues (**autoimmune disorders**).
- Reactions to tissues **transplanted** from *another* person (**alloimmune disorders**).

In most allergic (hypersensitivity) reactions, **allergens** (antigens) bind to IgE on the membranes of basophils and mast cells (*see Chapter 11*) and, within seconds of exposure, stimulate the cells to produce **histamine.** This triggers vasodilation, increased capillary permeability, and smooth muscle spasms. The symptoms produced by these changes include edema; mucus hypersecretion and congestion; watery eyes; hives (**urticaria**); and sometimes cramps, diarrhea, and vomiting.

Anaphylaxis is an acute, immediate, and severe allergic reaction. It can be relieved by antihistamines.

Anaphylactic shock is more severe and is characterized by dyspnea due to bronchiole constriction, circulatory shock, and sometimes death. It is a life-threatening medical emergency and requires immediate epinephrine and circulatory support.

Asthma is triggered by allergens (as listed earlier) and by air pollutants, drugs, and emotions. These all stimulate plasma cells to secrete IgE, which binds to cells in the respiratory mucosa and releases a mixture of histamine and interleukins. Within minutes, the bronchioles constrict spasmodically (bronchospasm), leading to the wheezing and coughing of asthma.

Autoimmune disorders are an overvigorous response of the immune system in which the immune system fails to distinguish self-antigens from foreign antigens. These self-antigens produce **autoantibodies** that attack the body's own tissues. This type of response occurs, for example, in lupus erythematosus, type 1 diabetes, multiple sclerosis, rheumatoid arthritis, and psoriasis.

Immunodeficiency disorders are a deficient response of the immune system in which it fails to respond vigorously enough. They are in three categories:

1. **Congenital** (inborn)—caused by a genetic abnormality that is often sex-linked, with boys affected more often than girls. An example from among the 20 or more congenital immunodeficiency diseases is **inherited combined immunodeficiency disease,** in which there is an absence of both T cells and B cells. Affected children are very susceptible to opportunistic infections and must live in protective sterile enclosures.

2. **Immunosuppression**—a common side effect of corticosteroids in treatment to prevent transplant rejection and in chemotherapy treatment for cancer. These drugs reduce the numbers of all lymphocytes, making it possible for opportunistic infections to invade the body.

3. **Acquired immunodeficiency**—a result of diseases such as acquired immunodeficiency syndrome (AIDS) that involve a severely depressed immune system from infection with the human immunodeficiency virus (HIV).

Immunology of Transplantation

The success of any organ **transplantation** is based on control of the recipient's immune system to prevent rejection of the **allograft,** tissue from another individual of the same species.

Transplant immunity is designed to cause rejection, and both cellular and humoral defense mechanisms are involved. To try to prevent this, the recipient and donor must match at both the human lymphocyte antigen (HLA) and blood group system (ABO) *(see Chapter 11)* types. A combination of immunosuppressive drugs is used to control graft rejection, but the drugs have adverse side effects on the recipient. One combination is corticosteroids with cyclosporine or FK506. Other drugs are in clinical trials.

Word Analysis and Definition: Disorders of the Immune System

S = Suffix   P = Prefix   R = Root   R/CF = Combining Form

WORD	PRONUNCIATION		ELEMENTS	DEFINITION
allogen	**AL**-oh-jen	P/ R/	**allo-** *strange, different* **-gen** *producing*	Antigen from someone else in the same species
allogenic (adj)	al-oh-**JEN**-ik	S/	**-ic** *pertaining to*	Pertaining to allogen
allograft	**AL**-oh-graft	R/	**-graft** *tissue for transplant*	Tissue graft from another person or cadaver
alloimmune	**AL**-oh-im-**YUNE**	P/ R/	**allo-** *strange, different* **-immune** *immune response*	Reaction directed against foreign tissue
anaphylaxis	**AN**-ah-fih-**LAK**-sis	P/ R/	**ana-** *away from* **-phylaxis** *protection*	Immediate severe allergic response
anaphylactic (adj)	**AN**-ah-fih-**LAK**-tik	S/ R/	**-tic** *pertaining to* **-phylac-** *protect*	Pertaining to anaphylaxis
autoantibody autoantibodies (pl)	**AW**-toh-**AN**-tih-bod-ee **AW**-toh-**AN**-tih-bod-ees	P/ P/ R/	**auto-** *self, same* **-anti-** *against* **-body** *substance, body*	An antibody that reacts with a person's own cells and tissues
histamine antihistamine	**HISS**-tah-meen an-tee-**HISS**-tah-meen	S/ R/ P/	**-amine** *nitrogen containing* **hist-** *derived from histidine* **anti-** *against*	Compound liberated in tissues as a result of injury or an allergic response Drug used to treat allergic symptoms because of its action antagonistic to histamine
hypersensitivity	**HIGH**-per-sen-sih-**TIV**-ih-tee	S/ P/ R/	**-ity** *condition* **hyper-** *excessive* **-sensitiv-** *feeling*	Exaggerated abnormal reaction to an allergen
immunodeficiency	**IM**-you-noh-dee-**FISH**-en-see	S/ R/CF R/	**-ency** *quality* **immun/o-** *immune response* **-defici-** *failure*	Failure of the immune system
immunosuppression	**IM**-you-noh-suh-**PRESH**-un	S/ R/CF R/	**-ion** *process* **immun/o-** *immune response* **-suppress-** *pressed under*	Suppression of the immune response by an outside agent, such as a drug
transplant	**TRANZ**-plant	P/ R/	**trans-** *across* **-plant** *plant*	The tissue or organ used, or the act of transferring tissue from one person to another
transplantation	**TRANZ**-plan-**TAY**-shun	S/	**-ation** *process, action*	The moving of tissue or an organ from one person or place to another
urticaria	ur-tih-**KARE**-ee-ah		Latin *nettle*	Rash of itchy wheals (hives)

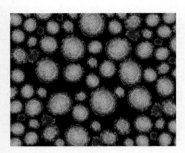

Viral Infections

Viruses are the smallest of the microorganisms. Viruses spread from person to person through coughs, sneezes, and unwashed hands.

Viruses cause specific childhood diseases like measles (rubeola), German measles (rubella), chickenpox (varicella), and mumps. They cause upper respiratory infections (see *Chapter 13*), including modern respiratory infections like **severe acute respiratory syndrome (SARS), avian influenza** (bird flu), and **West Nile virus (WNV).** WNV is a seasonal **epidemic** in North America that flares up in the summer and fall.

Influenza (Flu)

There are three types of **influenza** viruses that infect humans. Types A and B cause seasonal **epidemics** and spread through respiratory droplets. Symptoms include fever, malaise, cough, headaches, and sore throat.

Coronavirus

A coronavirus (**CoV**) (*Figure 12.8*) is a type of virus. A new type of coronavirus emerged in 2002 that was associated with a severe acute respiratory syndrome (**SARS**); SARS-associated coronavirus (**SARS-CoV**).

Coronavirus 2019 (**COVID 19**) is a previously unrecorded (**novel**) CoV associated with severe respiratory illness (**SARS-CoV-2**) classified as a pneumonia.

As of 2020, research reports that COVID-19 infected people with no symptoms have low levels of IgM; severe, symptomatic people have high levels of IgA, which is found in mucous membranes. Severity of illness may be due to cytokine storm syndrome causing a **hyperimmune** response. SARS-CoV-2 is actively being researched for its effects on the human body.

HIV and AIDS

Human immunodeficiency virus (HIV) is one of a group of **viruses** known as **retroviruses.** Like other viruses, it can replicate only inside a living host cell; HIV invades helper T (CD4) cells and cells in the upper respiratory tract and CNS. Inside the cell, the virus generates new deoxyribonucleic acid (DNA) and can stay **dormant** in the cell for months or years. When it is activated, the new viruses emerge from the dying host cell and attack more CD4 cells. This dormant phase **(incubation)** can range from a few months to 12 years.

The CD4 cells are the central coordinators for the immune response. As the virus destroys more and more cells, the CD4 count falls, and antibodies cannot be produced. Symptoms appear, including chills, fever, night sweats, fatigue, weight loss, and lymphadenitis.

When CD4 cells are very low, **opportunistic infections** by bacteria, viruses, and fungi can occur. These infections include toxoplasmosis, pneumocystis, tuberculosis, herpes simplex, cytomegalovirus, and candidiasis. If human immunodeficiency virus (HIV) invades the brain, it causes dementia. Cancers also can invade, and a form of malignancy called **Kaposi sarcoma** (*Figure 12.9*) is often seen in association with acquired immunodeficiency syndrome (AIDS).

HIV is found in blood, semen, vaginal secretions, saliva, tears, and the breast milk of infected mothers.

The most common means of transmission of HIV are:

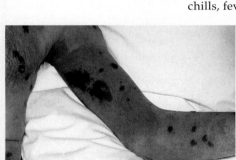

▲ **Figure 12.9** Lesions of Kaposi **sarcoma.** SPL/Science Source

- **Sexual intercourse** (vaginal, oral, anal).
- **Sharing of needles** for drug use.
- **Contaminated blood products.** (All donated blood is now tested for HIV.)
- **Transplacental** (from an infected mother to her fetus).

The virus survives poorly outside the human body. It is destroyed by laundering, dishwashing, chlorination, disinfectants, alcohol, and germicidal skin cleansers.

In the United States, the number of new HIV diagnoses declined about 19% from 2005 to 2014, but diagnoses have increased among certain groups and in certain geographical regions so new infections continue to occur (*Figure 12.10*).

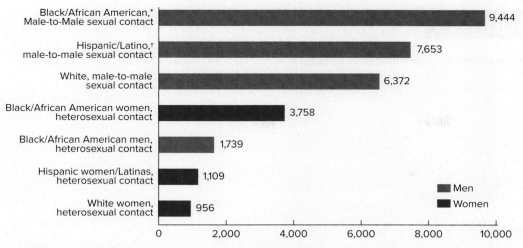

▲ **Figure 12.10** **HIV diagnoses.** New HIV diagnoses in the United States for the most-affected subpopulations 2018.

Word Analysis and Definition: Viral Infections				
		S = Suffix P = Prefix R = Root R/CF = Combining Form		
WORD	**PRONUNCIATION**	**ELEMENTS**		**DEFINITION**
dormant	**DOR**-mant	S/	**-ant** *forming*	Inactive
		R/	**dorm-** *sleep*	
endemic	en-**DEM**-ik	S/	**-ic** *pertaining to*	Pertaining to a disease always present in a community
		P/	**en-** *in*	
		R/	**-dem-** *the people*	
epidemic	ep-ih-**DEM**-ik	P/	**epi-** *above, upon*	Pertaining to an outbreak in a community of a disease or a health-related behavior
pandemic	pan-**DEM**-ik	P/	**pan-** *all*	Pertaining to a disease attacking the population of a very large area
hyperimmune	**HIGH**-per-im-**YUNE**	P/	**hyper-** *excessive*	An increased titer of antibodies in response to an antigen
		R/	**immun-** *immune response*	
incubation	in-kyu-**BAY**-shun	S/	**-ation** *process*	Process to develop an infection
		R/	**incub-** *sit on, hatch*	
influenza	in-flew-**EN**-zah		Latin *caused by the influence of the heavenly bodies*	Acute viral infection of upper and lower respiratory tracts
novel	**NOV**-el		Old French *new, fresh*	Not previously identified
opportunistic	**OP**-or-tyu-**NIS**-tik	S/	**-ic** *pertaining to*	An organism or a disease in a host with lowered resistance
		S/	**-ist-** *agent*	
		R/	**opportun-** *take advantage of*	
retrovirus	**REH**-troh-**VIE**-rus	P/	**retro-** *backward*	Virus that replicates in a host cell by converting its ribonucleic acid (RNA) core into deoxyribonucleic acid (DNA)
		R/	**-virus** *poison*	
sarcoma	sar-**KOH**-mah	S/	**-oma** *tumor, mass*	A malignant tumor originating in connective tissue
		R/	**sarc-** *flesh*	
Kaposi sarcoma	ka-**POH**-see sar-**KOH**-mah		Moritz Kaposi, 1837–1902, Hungarian dermatologist	A malignancy often seen in AIDS patients
virus	**VIE**-rus		**Latin** *poison*	Group of infectious agents that require living cells for growth and reproduction
viral (adj)	**VIE**-ral	S/	**-al** *pertaining to*	Pertaining to or caused by a virus
		R/	**vir-** *virus*	

Check Point Section 12.3

A. Deconstruct medical terms into their elements. *Deconstruct each term using the slashed lines.* **LO 12.2, 12.6**

1. lymphedema: _____ / _____
            R   S

2. tonsillitis: _____ / _____
            R   S

3. lymphadenitis: _____ / _____
            R   S

4. hypersplenism: _____ / _____ / _____
            P   R   S

B. Use the terms related to disorders of the lymphatic system above that is described by each statement. **LO 12.6**

1. Write the term that means *tumor of lymphatic tissue:* _____

2. Write the term that means *any neoplasm of lymph tissue:* _____

3. The term that means *tissue swelling that occurs as a result of obstructed lymphatics:* _____

4. The term that means *inflammation of a lymph node:* _____

Case Report (CR) 12.1

You are

. . . a laboratory technician working the night shift at Fulwood Medical Center.

Your patient is

. . . Mr. Michael Cowan, a 40-year-old homeless man and drug addict, who has presented to the Emergency Department with a high fever for which no cause is obvious on clinical examination.

You are called to the Emergency Room to take blood from Mr. Cowan. You have inserted the needle into an antecubital vein, and he starts jerking his arm around and trying to get off the gurney. In the struggle, the needle comes out of the vein and pricks your hand through your glove.

As you immediately *flush* and *clean* the wound, *report* the incident, seek *immediate medical attention,* and go through your *initial medical evaluation,* it is essential that you have knowledge about your immune system and its response to the potential infection. Then you can make *informed decisions* about your treatment and future employment.

C. Analyze Case Report 12.1, then answer the following questions. **LO 12.6, 12.7, 12.8**

1. What is the purpose of flushing the wound?

  a. Hydrate the skin   **c.** Remove pathogens from the wound

  b. Replace any lost blood   **d.** Water is a natural antibiotic

2. Mr. Cowan's high fever is most likely due to:

  a. an infection   **b.** heatstroke   **c.** an allergic reaction   **d.** cardiac arrest

3. If you have been exposed to a pathogen, your body will react to it by creating:

  a. haptens   **b.** erythrocytes   **c.** mutations   **d.** antibodies

D. Build more medical vocabulary for immunology. *Complete the construction of the medical term by using the following elements to fill in the blanks.* **LO 12.2, 12.6**

| hyper | defici | phylaxis | auto | suppress | graft |
| ion | anti | sensitiv | trans | allo | gen |

1. Exaggerated, abnormal reaction to an antigen _____ / _____/ity

2. Suppression of the immune response caused by an outside agent immuno/ _____ / _____

3. Immediate, severe, allergic response ana/_____

4. Skin from another person or cadaver allo/_____

5. Failure of the immune system immuno/_____/ency

6. Transferring tissue or an organ from one person to another _____/plant

7. Antigen from someone else in the same species allo/_____

8. Reaction against foreign tissue _____/immune

9. Drug used to treat allergic symptoms _____/histamine

 ## Case Report (CR) 12.2

You are

. . . a medical assistant working with Henry Vandenberg, MD, in the AIDS Clinic at Fulwood Medical Center.

Your patient is

. . . Mr. Eugene Holman, a 40-year-old male who is known to be **HIV-positive (HIV+)** and has been receiving treatment with efavirenz, zidovudine, and lamivudine.

In the past couple of months, Mr. Holman has not been taking his medication regularly. In the previous week, he has noticed a progressive shortness of breath and a nonproductive cough. Vital signs are T 102°, P 120, R 32, BP 110/60. He is anxious and dyspneic but not cyanotic. His breath sounds are clear, with no rales or rhonchi heard. You have called Dr. Vandenberg to see him.

Mr. Holman's chest x-ray shows bilateral, diffuse, fluffy infiltrates spreading out from the hila. Bronchial **lavage** with laboratory examination shows *Pneumocystis jiroveci.* His CD4 count is 140. Mr. Holman has developed an **opportunistic** infection, which is probably due to *Pneumocystis jiroveci.*

E. Analyze Case Report 12.2 and then answer the following questions. *Select the answer that correctly completes each statement.* **LO 12.6**

1. Mr. Holman developed an opportunistic infection because:

   a. the pathogen is potent
   c. he forgets to take his medication

   b. he is homeless
   d. his immune system is compromised

2. The diagnostic test that determined the reason for the infection was:

   a. breath sounds b. bronchial lavage c. CD4 count d. chest x-ray

1. In the term **viral,** the root means:

   a. pertaining to   **b.** cancer   **c.** process   **d.** virus

2. In the term **sarcoma,** the root means:

   a. cancer   **b.** flesh   **c.** tumor   **d.** inflammation

3. In the term **dormant,** the suffix means:

   a. forming   **b.** take advantage   **c.** pertaining to   **d.** sleep

Section 12.4 Procedures and Pharmacology

Diagnostic Procedures

Immunoassays use the antibody–antigen reaction to produce a measurable response.

Immunodiagnostics uses an antigen–antibody reaction as a diagnostic tool. A tool can contain either an antigen or the antibody. A test is positive based on the presence or quantity of the antibody–antigen reaction. The antigen or antibody used in the test can be **conjugated** with a radiolabel, **fluorescent** label, or a color-forming enzyme.

Enzyme-linked immunosorbent assay (ELISA). ELISA uses antibodies conjugated to enzymes linked to color-changing dyes to detect specific antibody and chemicals. ELISA is used to diagnose HIV, West Nile virus, malaria, tuberculosis, and rotavirus in feces, as well as in drug screening.

Fluorescent immunoassay tests use a fluorescent labeled antibody to attach to antigen. When exposed to a specific light, the antibody–antigen reaction fluoresces; can diagnose Lyme disease, Strep A, and several autoimmune diseases.

Lateral—flow immunoassay—an antibody is placed on a membrane, the specimen (e.g., urine, serum) flows across the membrane, antigens react with antibodies. An area of the strip contains chemical that changes color when the antibody–antigen reaction flows through it. Used to diagnose Strep A and pregnancy.

In **agglutination tests,** a particle such as a latex bead or a **bacterium** is coupled to the pathogen specific antigen or antibody creating a particle complex. If the target antibody or antigen is present in the specimen (e.g., serum, urine, CSF), it attaches to the particle complex and produces agglutination.

High blood levels of IgA are found in multiple myeloma, autoimmune diseases such as rheumatoid arthritis and systemic lupus erythematosus *(see Chapter 15),* and cirrhosis of the liver *(see Chapter 5).* Low levels of IgA occur in some types of leukemia *(see Chapter 11)* and in nephrotic syndrome *(see Chapter 6).*

Diagnostic tests for allergies include:

- **nasal smears** to check the amount of eosinophils in the nose.

- **skin tests** to measure the level of IgE antibodies in response to allergens that are injected under the skin or applied with a small scratch. A reaction appears as a small red area.

- **blood tests** measure IgE antibodies to specific allergens in the blood. A **radioallergosorbent test (RAST)** uses a **radioimmunoassay** to detect the specific IgE antibodies, but is now little used.

- **Challenge testing** is performed by an allergist, who administers a very small amount of an allergen orally or by inhalation and monitors its effect.

Diagnostic procedures to evaluate enlarged lymph nodes for Reed-Sternberg cells to look for cells, x-rays, computed tomography (CT) and magnetic resonance imaging (MRI) scans, **lymphangiogram,** and bone marrow biopsy.

Viral Testing

Nucleic acid amplification tests (NAATs) detect a virus's genetic material; can be part of diagnosis for hepatitis, upper respiratory tract infection, COVID-19.

Antigen tests detect viral proteins; part of diagnosis for hepatitis, COVID-19 *(Figure 12.11).*

Antibody or serology tests look for antibodies in your blood to determine indicating a viral past infection; used as part of diagnosis of hepatitis, HIV, and COVID-19.

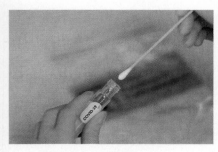

▲ **Figure 12.11 Swab sample.** Sample is sent for COVID testing. Horth Rasur/ Shutterstock

WORD	PRONUNCIATION	ELEMENTS		DEFINITION
bacterium bacteria (pl)	bak-**TEER**-ee-um bak-**TEER**-ee-ah		Greek *a staff*	A unicellular microorganism that multiplies by cell division
complex	**KOM**-pleks		Latin *woven together*	A stable combination of two or more compounds in the body
conjugate	**KON**-joo-gate	S/ P/ R/	-ate *composed of, pertaining to* con- *together* -jug- *yoke*	To join together, usually in pairs
fluoresce	flor-**ESS**		Greek *bright color*	Emit a bright-colored light when irradiated with ultraviolet or violet-blue rays
fluorescence fluorescent (adj)	flor-**ESS**-ens flor-**ESS**-ent	S/ S/	-ence *quality of* -ent *forming*	Property of glowing in ultraviolet light Produced by fluorescence
immunoassay	**IM**-you-no-**ASS**-ay	R/CF R/	immun/o- *immune* -assay *evaluate*	Biochemical test that uses the reaction of an antibody to its antigen to measure the amount of a substance in a liquid
immunodiagnostics	**IM**-you-no-die-ag-**NOSS**-tiks	S/ R/CF R/	-ics *pertaining to* immun/o- *immune* -diagnost- *decision*	A diagnostic process using antigen–antibody reactions
lymphangiogram	lim-**FAN**-jee-oh-gram	S/ R/CF	-gram *recording* lymphangi/o- *lymphatic vessels*	Radiographic images of lymph vessels and nodes following injection of contrast material
radioallergosorbent	**RAY**-dee-oh-ah-**LUR**-go-**SOAR**-bent	S/ R/CF R/CF R/	-ent *end result* radi/o- *radiation* -allerg/o- *allergy* -sorb- *suck in*	A radioimmunoassay to detect IgE-bound allergens responsible for tissue hypersensitivity
radioimmunoassay	**RAY**-dee-oh-im-you-no-**ASS**-ay	R/CF R/	-immun/o- *immune* -assay *evaluate*	Immunoassay of a substance that has been radioactively labeled
serum	**SEER**-um		Latin *whey*	Fluid remaining after removal of cells and fibrin clot
serology	seer-**OL**-oh-jee	S/	-logy *study of*	Study of the reaction between antigens and antibodies in serum

Therapeutic Procedures and Drugs for the Lymphatic and Immune Systems

Lymphatic Therapy

Careful observation to **chemotherapy, radiation,** and **bone marrow transplantation** are considered based on the rate of growth of cancer cells of Hodgkin and Non-Hodgkin's lymphoma.

Regional lymphadenectomy removes a several lymph nodes from an area.

Radical lymphadenectomy removes all the lymph nodes from an area to detect presence of cancer cells.

Compression garments and treatments, and massage are used for lymphedema. There is no cure.

Antibiotics treat strep throat and tonsillitis. Recurrent tonsillitis may be treated with a **tonsillectomy.**

Splenectomy is most performed for a ruptured spleen and painful splenomegaly.

Immunotherapy

Immunotherapy, also called **biologic therapy,** is designed to boost the body's natural defenses against cancer by using substances either made in the laboratory or made by the body to enhance or restore immune system function. This form of therapy can stop or slow the growth of cancer cells, and stop cancer from metastasizing.

The types of immunotherapy include:

- **Monoclonal antibodies,** made in the laboratory, can attach to cancer cells to flag them so that macrophages in the body's immune system can recognize and destroy them. Two pathways inside cells that cancers use to evade the immune system have been identified and named PD-1/PD-L1 and CTLA-4. These pathways can be blocked with antibodies called **immune checkpoint inhibitors** to allow the body's immune system to respond to the cancer. Immune checkpoint inhibitors ipilimumab *(Yervoy)*, nivolumab *(Opdivo)*, and pembrolizumab *(Keytruda)* have been shown to improve overall patient survival in advanced melanoma.

- **Interferons** are a nonspecific immunotherapy mostly given at the same time as other cancer treatments such as chemotherapy or radiation therapy. An interferon called **interferon alpha** made in a laboratory is the most common type of interferon used in cancer treatment.
- **Interleukins** are also a nonspecific immunotherapy used to treat kidney and skin cancers, including melanoma.

Human immunoglobulins are given by injection to confer passive (temporary) immunity that provides immediate protection lasting several weeks. There are two types:

- **Human normal immunoglobulin (HNIG)** made from the plasma of about 1,000 unselected donors to provide antibodies against hepatitis A, rubella, measles, and other viruses found in the general population.
- **Hyperimmune specific immunoglobulins** are made from selected donors and provide antibodies individually against hepatitis B, varicella zoster, rabies, tetanus, and cytomegalovirus.

Immunosuppressant Drugs

Immunosuppressant drugs inhibit or prevent activity of the immune system and are used to prevent the rejection of transplanted organs and tissues, treat autoimmune diseases, and help control long-term allergic asthma. There are four main types of immunosuppressant drugs:

- **Glucocorticoids,** which suppress cell-mediated immunity and protect through T-cells and macrophages, and by stimulating cells to secrete **cytokines.**
- **Cytostatics,** which inhibit cell division. Cyclophosphamide *(Cytoxan)*, a nitrogen mustard **alkylating** agent, is probably the most potent immunosuppressant. Methotrexate, an **antimetabolite,** interferes with the **synthesis** of nucleic acids and is used in the treatment of autoimmune diseases. Azathioprine **(***Imuran***)** is the main immunosuppressive **cytotoxic** substance and is used to control transplant rejection reactions.
- **Antibodies** can be used as quick immunosuppressive therapy and are described above in sections on monoclonal antibodies and immunoglobulins.
- **Calcineurin** is a phosphatase that stimulates the growth and differentiation of T cells. **Calcineurin inhibitors** such as cyclosporin *(Sandimmune)*, tacrolimus *(Prograf)*, and sirolimus *(Rapamune)* are used in the prevention and treatment of transplant rejection reactions.

HIV Drugs

Antiretroviral treatment (ART) medications do not cure HIV, instead decreases the amount of HIV in the blood, letting infected people live a longer healthier life and decrease risk of passing HIV to another person. Medication must be taken daily else the amount of HIV in the blood will increase.

Initial regimens of three or more classes of antiretroviral drugs. Combination medications deliver this combination in one tablet: bictegravir/tenofovir alafenamide/emtricitabine *(Biktarvy)*, and dolutegravir/abacavir/lamivudine *(Triumeq)*.

Influenza Drugs

Oseltamivir phosphate *(Tamiflu)* can be used to prevent the flu or to treat the flu within 48 hours of the onset of symptoms.

Zanamivir (*Relenza***)** is orally inhaled white powder that can be taken to prevent influenza infection during a flu outbreak.

Word Analysis and Definition: Therapeutic Procedures and Drugs

S = Suffix   P = Prefix   R = Root   R/CF = Combining Form

WORD	PRONUNCIATION	ELEMENTS		DEFINITION
alkylation	al-kih-**LAY**-shun	S/ R/	-ation *process* alkyl- *alkali*	Introduction of a side chain into a compound
antimetabolite	**AN**-tih-meh-**TAB**- oh-lite	S/ P/ R/	-ite *resembling* anti- *against* -metabol- *change*	A substance that antagonizes another substance
antiretroviral	**AN**-tee-**RET**-roh-**VIE**-ral	P/ P/ R/ S/	anti- *against* -retro- *backward* -vir- *virus* -al *pertaining to*	Drug that fights infection by a virus
biologic	**BI**-oh-**LOJ**-ik	S/ R/CF R/	-ic *pertaining to* bio- *life* -log- *study of*	Pertaining to the study of life and living organisms
calcineurin	kal-see-**NYUR**-in	S/ R/CF R/	-in *chemical* calc/i *calcium* -neur- *nerve*	A chemical that stimulates the growth and differentiation of T-cells
compression	kom-**PRESH**-un	S/ P/ R/	-ion *action* com- *together* -press- *squeeze*	A squeezing together to increase density and/or decrease a dimension of a structure
cytokine	**SIGH**-toh-kine	S/ R/CF	-kine *movement* cyt/o- *cell*	A hormone-like protein that regulates the intensity of an immune response
cytostatic	**SIGH**-toh-**STAT**-ik	S/ R/CF R/	-ic *pertaining to* cyt/o- *cell* -stat- *stop*	Inhibiting cell division
cytotoxic	**SIGH**-toh-**TOK**-sik	S/	-toxic *able to kill*	Destructive to cells
immunoglobulin	**IM**-you-noh-**GLOB**-you-lin	S/ R/CF R/	-in *chemical* immun/o- *immune response* -globul- *protein*	Specific protein (antibody) generated by an antigen
immunotherapy	**IM**-you-noh-**THAIR**-ah-pee	R/CF R/	immun/o- *immune response* -therapy *treatment*	Treatment to boost immune system function
inhibitor	in-**HIB**-ih-tor	S/ R/	-or *that which does* inhibit- *restrain*	An agent that restrains a chemical action
interferon	in-ter-**FEER**-on	S/ P/ R/	-on *term* inter- *between* -fer- *to strike*	A small protein produced by T-cells in response to infection
interleukin	**IN**-ter-**LOO**-kin	S/ P/ R/	-in *chemical* inter- *between* -leuk- *white*	A group of cytokines synthesized by white blood cells
monoclonal	**MON**-oh-**KLOH**-nal	S/ P/ R/	-al *pertaining to* mono- *one* -clon- *cutting used for propagation*	Derived in the laboratory from a protein from a single colony of cells
splenectomy (*Note:* The "ee" in spleen becomes "e" for easier pronunciation.)	sple-**NEK**-toh-mee	S/ R/	-ectomy *surgical excision* splen- *spleen*	Surgical removal of the spleen
tonsillectomy	ton-sih-**LEK**-toh-mee	S/ R/	-ectomy *surgical excision* tonsill- *tonsil*	Surgical removal of the tonsils

A. Immunoglobulin (Ig) levels are used to support the diagnosis of lymphatic system disorders. *Match the Ig levels in the first column with the condition it is associated with in the second column.* **LO 12.5**

_____ 1. increased IgE antibodies   a. HIV infection

_____ 2. increased IgG antibodies   b. leukemia

_____ 3. decreased IgG antibodies   c. parasitic infections

B. Choose the correct test used in the diagnosis of conditions caused by immune system disorders. **LO 12.5**

1. The test used to detect the presence of HIV infection:

     a. ELISA   b. RAST   c. challenge testing   d. Ig levels

2. Patient inhales allergens to see if they cause an allergic reaction:

     a. skin test   b. blood test   c. challenge testing   d. agglutination testing

3. Measures the amount of antibody present in cerebrospinal fluid or serum:

     a. RAST   b. complement fixation test   c. ELISA   d. challenge testing

C. Identify the action of the drug based on a word element that it contains. *Being able to pick out and define word elements can help you determine the meaning of the word. Select the answer that correctly completes each statement.* **LO 12.7**

1. A medication that would provide antibodies to persons to prevent viral infections:

     a. cytostatic   b. glucocorticoid   c. human normal immunoglobulin   d. monoclonal antibodies

2. A medication that would inhibit cell division:

     a. cytostatic   b. calcineurin   c. interleukin   d. interferon

D. Categorize medications of immunotherapy. *Match the medication in the first column with the disorder it is used to treat in the second column.* **LO 12.7**

_____ 1. interleukin   a. treat kidney and skin cancers

_____ 2. interferons   b. flag cancer cells for macrophages

_____ 3. monoclonal antibodies   c. given alongside chemotherapy and radiation therapy

E. Categorize immunosuppressant drugs. *Match the medication in the first column with the disorder it is used to treat in the second column.* **LO 12.7**

_____ 1. methotrexate   a. interferes with nucleic acids as a means to treat autoimmune diseases

_____ 2. tacrolimus (*Prograf*)   b. inhibits cell division

_____ 3. glucocorticoid   c. suppresses cell-mediated immunity

_____ 4. cyclophosphamide (*Cytoxan*)   d. prevents and treats transplant rejection reactions

Table 12.1 Chapter 12 Abbreviations

Abbreviation	Meaning
AIDS	acquired immunodeficiency syndrome
B cells	B lymphocytes
CD	cluster of differentiation
CMV	cytomegalovirus
CoV	coronavirus
COVID 19	coronavirus 2019
HIV	human immunodeficiency virus
Ig	immunoglobulin
IgA	immunoglobulin A

Abbreviation	Meaning
IgD	immunoglobulin D
IgE	immunoglobulin E
IgG	immunoglobulin G
IgM	immunoglobulin M
SARS	severe acute respiratory syndrome
SARS-CoV	coronavirus associated with severe acute respiratory syndrome
SARS-CoV-2	(the second) coronavirus associated with severe acute respiratory syndrome
T cells	T lymphocytes

Table 12.2 Common disorders and diseases of the lymphatic and immune systems

Disorder or Disease	Signs and Symptoms	Diagnostic Tests	Treatment
Asthma	Shortness of breath, wheezing, cyanosis	Arterial blood gas, measure eosinophil level. Pulmonary function test when not in asthma attack	Bronchodilators, steroids. Oxygen when needed
HIV	Low CD4 count, may have Kaposi sarcoma lesions	HIV-1/2 antigen/antibody immunoassay; CD4 lymphocyte count	Antiretroviral medications
Influenza	Fever, cough, chills, fatigue	Rapid influenza antigen test or rapid influenza diagnostic test	Rest, fluids, oseltamivir phosphate (*Tamiflu*)

Lymphatic and Immune Systems

Challenge Your Knowledge

A. **Latin and Greek elements cannot be deconstructed into prefix, root, or suffix.** You must know them for what they are. Test your knowledge of these elements with this exercise. Match the meaning in the left column with the correct medical term in the right column. **LO 12.1**

_____ 1. protected from	**a.** conjugate
_____ 2. that which completes	**b.** hapten
_____ 3. none	**c.** lymph
_____ 4. to fasten or bind	**d.** assay
_____ 5. to join	**e.** mutate
_____ 6. a knot	**f.** complement
_____ 7. to change	**g.** edema
_____ 8. to evaluate	**h.** immune
_____ 9. swelling	**i.** null
_____ 10. clear fluid	**j.** node

B. **Language of immunology.** Challenge your knowledge of the immune system and employ the *language of immunology* to answer the following questions. Choose the correct answer. **LO 12.1, 12.3, 12.6, 12.7**

1. Choose the correct pair of spellings:

   a. tonsel   tonselectomy

   b. tonsil   tonsillectomy

   c. tonssil   tonsilectomy

   d. tonsill   tonsilectomy

   e. tonnsil   tonsillectomy

2. This triggers vasodilation in an allergic response:

   a. interferon

   b. complement fixation

   c. histamine

   d. hormones

   e. antihistamine

3. The largest lymphatic vessel is the

   a. thoracic duct

   b. lymph node

   c. spleen

   d. lymphatic duct

   e. aorta

4. Kaposi sarcoma is a form of

   a. lymphadenitis

   b. malignancy

   c. lymphadenopathy

   d. lung cancer

   e. lymphoma

5. Ingestion and destruction of tissue debris and bacteria is called

    a. lymphadenitis

    b. phagocytosis

    c. lymphadenopathy

    d. agglutination

    e. osmosis

6. A life-threatening medical emergency that cannot be relieved by antihistamines is

    a. asthma

    b. Kaposi sarcoma

    c. anaphylactic shock

    d. urticaria

    e. lymphadenitis

7. An allergic reaction is one of

    a. hypoglycemia

    b. hypersensitivity

    c. hypotension

    d. hyperglycemia

    e. hypertension

8. White pulp and red pulp can be found in the

    a. lymph nodes

    b. spleen

    c. lymph vessels

    d. kidney

    e. thymus

C. **Language of immunology.** Challenge your knowledge of the immune system and employ the *language of immunology* to answer the following questions. Circle the correct choice. **LO 12.1, 12.6, 12.7**

1. Which disease is likely to cause enlarged lymph nodes under the jaw?

    a. tonsillitis

    b. lymphoma

    c. hypersplenism

    d. asthma

    e. urticaria

2. Abnormal, cancerous B cells are known as

    a. macrophages   **d.** killer cells

    b. osteoblasts   **e.** phagocytes

    c. Reed-Sternberg cells

3. Lymph nodes accessible for palpation are in the

    a. neck   **d.** all of these

    b. axilla   **e.** only A and C

    c. groin

4. Immunosuppressive drugs are given after

    a. organ transplant

    b. anaphylactic shock

    c. retrovirus

    d. opportunistic infection

    e. viral load count

5. Serum used to treat a snake bite is an example of

    a. natural active immunity

    b. artificial active immunity

    c. natural passive immunity

    d. artificial passive immunity

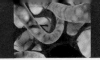

D. Correct spelling of medical terms is *always important*. Listed below are two examples of medical terms for which a variation of the term is not always spelled the same as the original term. Fill in the blanks with the correctly spelled medical terms. **LO 12.1, 12.6, 12.7**

Example 1:

Lymphatic organ in LUQ of abdomen   1. _____

Excision/removal of this organ   2. _____

Enlargement of this organ due to an underlying disorder   3. _____

Example 2:

Lymphoid tissue on either side of the throat   4. _____

Inflammation of this tissue   5. _____

Removal of this tissue   6. _____

E. Construct the entire term by entering the prefix *on* the line. Fill in the blanks. **LO 12.2**

1. Reaction directed against foreign tissue   _____/immune

2. Substance produced in response to an antigen   _____/body

3. Surface protein that enhances sensitivity of antigen receptor   _____/recept/or

4. Spleen removes blood components at an excessive rate   _____splen/ism

5. Virus that converts its RNA core to DNA in a host cell   _____/virus

F. Suffixes. Construct new terms using your knowledge of word elements from this and previous chapters. Take a basic root/combining form, add a variety of suffixes, and change the meaning different ways to form six new terms. Fill in the chart, then fill in the blanks. **LO 12.2, 12.8, 12.10**

Root/Combining Form	Suffix	Meaning of Term
lymph	1.	Neoplasm of lymphatic tissue
lymphaden	2.	Inflammation of a lymph node
lympho	3.	Small white blood cell with large nucleus
lymphaden	4.	Removal of a lymph node
lymph	5.	Pertaining to lymph
lymphadeno	6.	Any disease process affecting a lymph node

7. Which of the previous terms would be found in a surgeon's dictation? _____

8. Which of the previous terms would a pathologist use? _____

9. Which of the previous terms would an oncologist use in dictation? _____

G. Immune system. Build your knowledge of the immune system and its components by correctly matching the definition in the left column with the medical term in the right column. Fill in the blanks. **LO 12.1, 12.5, 12.6, 12.7**

_____ 1. Molecule that triggers an immune response   a. mutation

_____ 2. Major defense mechanism against bacteria   b. agglutination

_____ 3. Preparation for active development of antibodies   c. hapten

_____ 4. Weakened ability to produce disease   d. hypersensitivity

_____ 5. Change in the chemistry of a gene   e. immunoglobulins

_____ 6. Often appears after surgery or radiation therapy   f. antigen

_____ 7. Excessive immune response to an antigen   g. lymphedema

_____ 8. Small molecule has to bind to a larger molecule   h. attenuate

_____ 9. Cells clumping together   i. vaccine

_____ 10. Antibodies produced by humoral immunity   j. complement fixation

H. Elements. With the exception of Greek and Latin terms that do not deconstruct, most medical terms from any body system can typically be reduced into their basic elements for analysis. Deconstruct the following medical terms into their basic elements to analyze the meanings for the _language of immunology_. The first one is done for you. Fill in the table. **LO 12.2**

Medical Term	Prefix	Root/ Combining Form	Suffix
coreceptor	_co_	_recept_	_or_
interleukin	1.	2.	3.
dormant		4.	5.
hypersplenism	6.	7.	8.
tonsillitis		9.	10.
anaphylaxis	11.	12.	13.
retrovirus		14.	15.

I. Pronunciation is important whether you are saying the word or listening to a word from a coworker. Identify the proper pronunciation of the following medical terms. Correctly spell the term. **LO 12.3, 12.4, 12.5, 12.6, 12.7**

1. The correct pronunciation for having a property of glowing in ultraviolet light

     a. **RAY**-dee-oh- im-**YUNE**-ass-ay

     b. **RAY**-dee-oh-im-you-no-**ASS**-ay

     c. **FLOR**-ess-ent

     d. flor-**ESS**-ens

     Correctly spell the term: _____

2014 Nucleus Medical Media

2. The correct pronunciation for the surgical removal of the spleen

    a. ton-sigh-**LEK**-tuh-mee

    b. ton-sih-**LEK**-toh-mee

    c. sple-**NEK**-toh-mee

    d. splee-**NEK**-toh-mee

    Correctly spell the term: _____

3. The correct pronunciation for a malignant tumor originating in connective tissue

    a. **SAR**-koh-mah

    b. sark-oh-**MOH**

    c. try-**GLISS**-eh-ride

    d. try-**GLICE**-er-ide

    Correctly spell the term: _____

4. The correct pronunciation for a disease-causing organism

    a. tok-**SIK**

    b. **TOK**-sik

    c. **PATH**-oh-jen

    d. path-**OH**-jen

    Correctly spell the term: _____

5. The correct pronunciation for the term that means to ingest foreign particles and cells

    a. **SIGH**-tuh-tok-sik

    b. sigh-toh-**TOK**-sik

    c. **FAYG**-oh-site-ize

    d. **FAG**-oh-site-ize

    Correctly spell the term: _____

Case Reports

A. Read Case Report 12.3 and answer the following questions. LO 12.8

 Case Report (CR) 12.3

You are

. . . a medical assistant working with Susan Lee, MD, in her primary care clinic at Fulwood Medical Center.

Your patient is

. . . Ms. Anna Clemons, a 20-year-old waitress, who is a new patient. She has noticed a lump in her right neck. On questioning, you find that she has lost about 8 pounds in weight in the past couple of months, has felt tired, and has had some night sweats.

Her vital signs (VS) are normal. There are two firm, enlarged lymph nodes in her right neck. Physical examination is otherwise unremarkable, and there is no evidence of infection in her head, throat, or upper respiratory tract.

Ms. Clemons has cancerous nodes in her neck. They were not caused by metastatic cancer but by a cancer of the lymph nodes called Hodgkin lymphoma.

1. What outward sign does the patient have?

   a. infection

   b. cancerous nodes

   c. weight loss

   d. tachycardia

2. What is the patient's chief complaint?

   a. feeling tired

   b. shortness of breath

   c. fever

   d. headache

3. Did the patient present with an increased body temperature?

   a. yes

   b. no

4. What is the medical term for enlarged lymph nodes?

   a. immunosuppression

   b. lymphadenopathy

   c. lymphedema

   d. cytokine

5. What findings were present on physical examination?

   a. hypertension

   b. pain

   c. swelling

   d. enlarged cervical lymph nodes

   e. edema

6. The cancerous nodes were not caused by *metastatic cancer*. What does this mean?

   a. it started at the nodes

   b. the cancer is congenital

   c. the cancer spread from another location

   d. it is incurable

7. What are some of the diagnostic tests used to confirm this disease? (Choose all correct answers)

   a. lymph node biopsy

   b. lymphangiogram

   c. chemotherapy

   d. radiation

8. What is the surgical procedure to remove malignant lymph nodes? _____

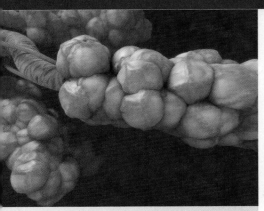

2014 Nucleus Medical Media

CHAPTER
13

Respiratory System
The Language of Pulmonology

Chapter Sections

Chapter Learning Outcomes

Upon completion of this chapter, you will be able to:

LO 13.1 Identify and describe the anatomy and physiology of the respiratory system.

LO 13.2 Use roots, combining forms, suffixes, and prefixes to construct and analyze medical terms related to the respiratory system.

LO 13.3 Spell medical terms related to the respiratory system.

LO 13.4 Pronounce medical terms related to the respiratory system.

LO 13.5 Describe diagnostic procedures utilized in pulmonology.

LO 13.6 Identify and describe disorders and pathological conditions related to the respiratory system.

LO 13.7 Describe the therapeutic procedures and pharmacologic agents used in the respiratory system.

LO 13.8 Apply knowledge of medical terms relating to pulmonology to documentation, medical records, and communication.

LO 13.9 Identify and correctly use abbreviations of terms used in pulmonology.

LO 13.10 Identify health professionals involved in the care of respiratory patients.

Health professionals involved in the diagnosis and treatment of respiratory problems include:

- **Pulmonologists,** physicians who specialize in the diagnosis and treatment of respiratory disorders.

- **Thoracic surgeons,** physicians who specialize in the surgical treatment of lung/pulmonary problems.

- **Registered respiratory therapists (RRTs)** or **respiratory care practitioners,** who exercise independent clinical judgment in evaluating, treating, and caring for patients who have respiratory disorders. They also supervise RTs.

- **Respiratory therapy technicians (RTs),** who assist physicians and RRTs in evaluating, monitoring, and treating patients with respiratory disorders.

Section 13.1 Respiratory System

Structure and Functions of the Respiratory System

It sounds like a good scheme. Humans and animals can breathe in oxygen (O_2) and breathe out carbon dioxide (CO_2); plants and trees can breathe in CO_2 and breathe out O_2 and nature stays in balance. Unfortunately, we humans have generated increasing amounts of CO_2 in the air by burning coal, oil, and natural gas and cutting down forests to disturb the balance. In addition, we have created organic and inorganic chemicals and small particles of solid matter in the air that can damage our respiratory tract and be taken into our bodies to cause cancer, brain damage, and birth defects. These materials are called pollutants. This section will start the process of understanding how we breathe and lead to how the above mentioned, leads to pathology. The **respiratory tract** *(Figure 13.1)* has six connected elements:

1. **Nose**
2. **Pharynx**
3. **Larynx**
4. **Trachea**
5. **Bronchi** and **bronchioles**
6. **Alveoli**

Respiration is the exchange of gases. Respiration is the transport of **O_2** from the outside air to tissue cells and the transport of **CO_2** in the opposite direction.
Respiration has four components:

1. **Ventilation,** which is the movement of air and its gases into and out of the lungs (inspiration and expiration).
2. **Pulmonary exchange of gases** between air in the alveoli and pulmonary capillaries (external respiration).
3. **Gas transport** from the pulmonary capillaries through the arterial system to the peripheral capillaries in tissues and the transport of gases back to the lung capillaries through the venous system.
4. **Peripheral gas exchange** between tissue capillaries and tissue cells for use in cellular metabolism (internal respiration) *(see Chapter 3).*

The five **functions** of the respiratory system are:

1. **Exchange of gases.** All the body cells need O_2 and produce CO_2. The respiratory system allows O_2 from the air to enter the blood and CO_2 to leave the blood and enter the air.
2. **Regulation of blood pH.** This is accomplished by changing blood CO_2 levels *(see Chapter 3).*
3. **Protection.** The respiratory system uses nasal hair, cilia lining the airways, and mucus formed throughout the system to protect against foreign bodies and against some microorganisms.
4. **Voice production.** Movement of air across the vocal cords makes speech and other sounds possible.
5. **Olfaction.** The 12 million receptor cells for smell are in a patch of epithelium the size of a quarter that is in the extreme superior region of the nasal cavity, the **olfactory region** *(Figure 13.2).* Each cell has 10 to 20 hairlike structures called **cilia** that project into the nasal cavity covered in a thin mucous film. Because the olfactory region is right at the top of the nose, you often have to sniff the air right up there to stimulate the sense of smell. A dog has 4 billion receptor cells, which is why dogs can be trained to sniff for drugs, explosives, and dead bodies.

Many of your sensations of taste are influenced by your sense of smell. For example, without its aroma, coffee tastes only bitter. The same is true for peppermint. This is why, when you have a cold, much of your sense of taste is lost.

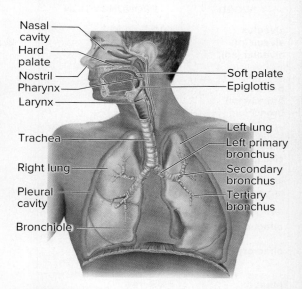

▲ **Figure 13.1 The respiratory system.** Lankford, T. Randall. Integrated science for health students. Virginia: Reston, 1979.

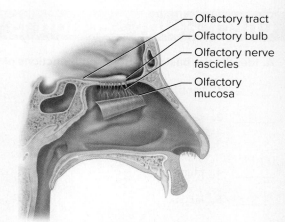

▲ **Figure 13.2 Olfactory region of nose.**

S = Suffix   P = Prefix   R = Root   R/CF = Combining Form

WORD	PRONUNCIATION		ELEMENTS	DEFINITION
alveolus alveoli (pl) alveolar (adj)	al-**VEE**-oh-lus al-**VEE**-oh-lee al-**VEE**-oh-lar	S/ R/	Latin *hollow sac* -ar *pertaining to* alveol- *alveolus*	Tiny air sac terminal element of the respiratory tract Pertaining to the alveoli
bronchus bronchi (pl) bronchiole	**BRONG**-kuss **BRONG**-key **BRONG**-key-ole	S/ R/	Greek *windpipe* -ole *small* bronchi- *bronchus*	One of two subdivisions of the trachea Increasingly smaller subdivisions of bronchi
cilium cilia (pl)	**SILL**-ee-um **SILL**-ee-ah		Latin *eyelash*	Hairlike motile projection from the surface of a cell
larynx laryngeal (adj)	**LAIR**-inks lah-**RIN**-jee-al	S/ R/	Greek *larynx* -eal *pertaining to* laryng- *larynx*	Organ of voice production Pertaining to the larynx
olfaction olfactory (adj)	ol-**FAK**-shun ol-**FAK**-toh-ree	S/ R/ S/	-ion *action, process* olfact- *smell* -ory *having the function of*	Sense of smell Carries information related to the sense of smell
pharynx pharyngeal (adj)	**FAIR**-inks fah-**RIN**-jee-al	S/ R/	Greek *throat* -eal *pertaining to* pharyng- *pharynx*	Air tube from the back of the nose to the larynx Pertaining to the pharynx
respiration respiratory (adj)	**RES**-pih-**RAY**-shun **RES**-pir-ah-**TOR** -ee		Latin *breathing*	Fundamental process of life used to exchange oxygen and carbon dioxide Pertaining to respiration
thorax thoracic (adj)	**THOR**-acks thor-**ASS**-ik	S/ R/	Greek *breastplate* -ic *pertaining to* thorac- *chest*	The trunk between the abdomen and neck Pertaining to the thorax
trachea	**TRAY**-kee-ah		Greek *windpipe*	Air tube from the larynx to the bronchi
ventilation	ven-tih-**LAY**-shun	S/ R/	-ation *process* ventil- *wind*	Movement of gases into and out of the lungs

Check Point Section 13.1

A. Identify the basic structures and functions of the respiratory system. *Match each term on the left with its definition on the right.* **LO 13.1**

_____ **1.** ventilation

_____ **2.** respiration

_____ **3.** olfaction

_____ **4.** pharynx

_____ **5.** larynx

_____ **6.** trachea

a. organ that produces the voice

b. organ that connects the mouth with the larynx

c. sense of smell

d. movement of gases in and out of the lungs

e. organ that connects the larynx to the bronchi

f. exchange of gases

Section 13.2 Upper Respiratory Tract

Structure and Functions of the Nose

The upper respiratory tract consists of the nose, pharynx, and larynx. It is the first site that brings air and its pollutants inside your body. As a health professional, you must understand the roles of the upper respiratory tract in trying to protect you, as well as enabling you to live by transporting O_2 into and CO_2 out of your body. When you breathe in air through your nose, the air goes through the nostrils (**nares**) into the **vestibule** of the **nasal cavity.** The nares are guarded by internal (guard) hairs to prevent the entry of large particles.

The nasal cavity is divided by the nasal **septum** into right and left compartments. On the medial wall of each nasal cavity, three bony ridges called **conchae (turbinate bones)** stick out into each cavity. Beneath each concha is a passageway called a **meatus** *(Figure 13.3).* The palate *(see Chapter 14)* forms the floor of the nose.

The nasal cavity is lined with a mucous membrane (mucosa) containing goblet cells that secrete mucus. Mucus forms a protective layer that can trap particles of dust and solid pollutants.

The **paranasal,** frontal, and maxillary **sinuses** open into the nose. Because they are hollow, the functions of these sinuses are to reduce the weight of the skull and to act as resonating chambers for the sounds of the voice. If your sinuses are congested, your voice loses its normal quality.

The following are functions of the nose:

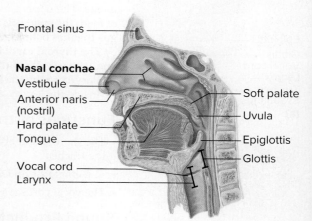

▲ **Figure 13.3** **Upper respiratory tract.**

- **Passageway for air.** The palate is the floor of the nasal cavity that separates it from the mouth and enables you to breathe even with food in your mouth.
- **Air cleanser.** The hairs in the vestibule trap some of the large particles in the air.
- **Air moisturizer.** Moisture from nasal mucus and from tears that drain into the cavity through the nasolacrimal duct *(see Chapter 16)* is added to the air.
- **Air warmer.** The blood flowing through the nasal cavity beneath the mucous membrane also warms the air. This prevents damage from the cold to the more fragile lower respiratory passages.
- **Sense of smell (olfaction).** The olfactory region recognizes some 4,000 separate smells.

Structure and Functions of the Pharynx

The **pharynx** is a muscular funnel that receives air from the nasal cavity and food and drink from the oral cavity. It is divided into three regions *(Figure 13.4):*

1. **Nasopharynx**—located at the back of the nose, above the soft palate and uvula. It is lined with a mucous membrane that includes goblet cells, which produce mucus. Mucus, including any trapped debris, is moved from the nasal cavity through the nasopharynx and swallowed. The posterior surface contains the **pharyngeal tonsil (adenoid).** Only air moves through this region.

2. **Oropharynx**—located below the soft palate and above the epiglottis. It contains two sets of tonsils called the *palatine* and *lingual* tonsils. Air, food, and drink all pass through this region.

3. **Laryngopharynx**—located below the tip of the epiglottis. This is the pathway to the esophagus. During swallowing, the epiglottis shuts off the trachea so that food cannot enter it. Only food and drink pass through the laryngopharynx.

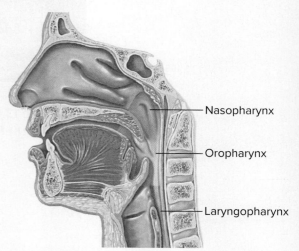

▲ **Figure 13.4** **Regions of pharynx.**

Structure and Functions of the Larynx

The flow of inhaled air moves on from the pharynx to the **larynx** *(Figure 13.5a)*, an enlargement of the airway located between the oropharynx and the trachea. The upper opening into it from the oropharynx is called the **glottis.**

The larynx has an outer casing of nine **cartilages** connected to one another by muscles and ligaments. The uppermost cartilage, the leaf-shaped **epiglottis,** guards the glottis. During the swallowing of food, the epiglottis is pushed down by the tongue to close the glottis and direct food into the esophagus that lies behind it.

The **thyroid cartilage,** or "Adam's apple," is the largest cartilage in the body and forms the anterior and lateral walls of the larynx. Below the thyroid cartilage the ring-shaped **cricoid** cartilage connects the larynx to the trachea *(Figure 13.5b)*.

Inside the larynx are the **true vocal cords** *(Figure 13.5b)*. **Intrinsic** muscles control the cords.

Functions of the Larynx

- The thyroid and cricoid cartilages maintain an open passage for the movement of air to and from the trachea.
- The epiglottis and vestibular folds prevent food and drink from entering the larynx *(Figure 13.5b)*.
- The vocal cords *(Figure 13.5a)* are the source of sound production.

Sound Production

Air moving past the vocal cords makes them vibrate to produce sound. The force of the air moving past the vocal cords determines the loudness of the sound. The intrinsic muscles of the cords pull them closer together with varying degrees of tautness. A high-pitched sound is produced by taut cords *(Figure 13.6b)* and a lower pitch by more relaxed cords *(Figure 13.6a)*.

The male vocal cords are longer and thicker than the female, vibrate more slowly, and produce lower-pitched sounds.

The crude sounds produced by the larynx are transformed into words by the actions of the pharynx, tongue, teeth, and lips.

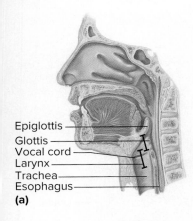

Epiglottis
Glottis
Vocal cord
Larynx
Trachea
Esophagus

(a)

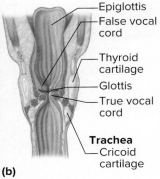

Epiglottis
False vocal cord
Thyroid cartilage
Glottis
True vocal cord
Trachea
Cricoid cartilage

(b)

▲ **Figure 13.5** **Larynx.**
(*a*) Location. (*b*) Structure.

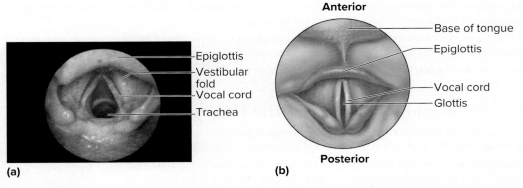

Epiglottis
Vestibular fold
Vocal cord
Trachea

(a)

Anterior

Base of tongue
Epiglottis
Vocal cord
Glottis

Posterior

(b)

▲ **Figure 13.6** **View of larynx.** (*a*) Using laryngoscope. (*b*) Vocal cords pulled close and taut.
CNRI/Science Source

Word Analysis and Definition: Structure and Function of the Nose, Pharynx, and Larynx

S = Suffix   P = Prefix   R = Root   R/CF = Combining Form

WORD	PRONUNCIATION		ELEMENTS	DEFINITION
adenoid	ADD-eh-noyd	S/ R/	-oid *resembling* aden- *gland*	Single mass of lymphoid tissue in midline at the back of the throat
concha conchae (pl)	KON-kah KON-kee		Latin *shell*	Shell-shaped bone on the lateral wall of the nasal cavity
cricoid	CRY-koyd		Latin *a ring*	Ring-shaped cartilage in the larynx
glottis epiglottis	GLOT-is ep-ih-GLOT-is	S/ P/ R/	Greek *opening of larynx* -is *pertaining to* epi- *above* -glott- *opening of larynx*	The opening from the oropharynx into the larynx Leaf-shaped plate of cartilage that shuts off the larynx during swallowing
intrinsic	in-TRIN-sik		Latin *on the inside*	Any muscle whose origin and insertion are entirely within the structure under consideration; for example, inside the vocal cords or the eye
laryngopharynx	lah-RING-oh-FAIR-inks	R/CF R/	laryng/o- *larynx* -pharynx *pharynx*	Region of the pharynx below the epiglottis that includes the larynx
larynx	LAIR-inks		Greek *larynx*	Organ of voice production
meatus	mee-AY-tus		Latin *a passage*	Passage or channel; also used to denote the external opening of a passage
naris nares (pl) nasal paranasal	NAH-ris NAH-reez NAY-zal PAIR-ah-NAY-zal	S/ R/ P/	-al *pertaining to* nas- *nose* para- *adjacent to*	Nostril Pertaining to the nose Adjacent to the nose
nasopharynx nasopharyngeal (adj)	NAY-zoh-FAIR-inks NAY-zoh-fair-IN-jee-al	R/CF R/ S/ R/	nas/o- *nose* -pharynx *pharynx* -eal *pertaining to* -pharyng- *pharynx*	Region of the pharynx at the back of the nose above the soft palate Pertaining to the nasopharynx
oropharynx oropharyngeal (adj)	OR-oh-FAIR-inks OR-oh-fair-IN-jee-al	R/CF R/ S/ R/	or/o- *mouth* -pharynx *pharynx* -eal *pertaining to* -pharyng- *pharynx*	Region at the back of the mouth between the soft palate and the tip of the epiglottis Pertaining to the oropharynx
pharynx pharyngeal (adj)	FAIR-inks fair-IN-jee-al	S/ R/ S/	Greek *throat* pharyng- *pharynx* -eal *pertaining to*	Air tube from the back of the nose to the larynx Pertaining to the pharynx
sinus	SIGH-nus		Latin *cavity*	Cavity or hollow space in a bone or other tissue
thyroid	THIGH-royd		Greek *an oblong shield*	Gland in the neck, or a cartilage of the larynx
tonsil	TON-sill		Latin *tonsil*	Inflammation of the tonsils
turbinate	TUR-bin-ate		Latin *shaped like a top*	Another name for the nasal conchae on the medial walls of the nasal cavity
vocal	VOH-kal	S/ R/	-al *pertaining to* voc- *voice*	Pertaining to the voice

Check Point Section 13.2

A. Greek and Latin terms. *Not all terms can be deconstructed into word parts. Identify the definitions of the following terms related to the language of pulmonology.* **LO 13.1**

_____ 1. concha   **a.** a passage

_____ 2. sinus   **b.** shell

_____ 3. pharynx   **c.** nostril

_____ 4. meatus   **d.** throat

_____ 5. naris   **e.** cavity

B. The pharynx is divided into three regions. *List the three regions in descending order from the back of the nose down.* **LO 13.1**

1. _____

2. _____

3. _____

Deconstruct. *For long or short medical terms, deconstruction into word elements is your key to solving the meaning of the term. If there is no particular element, leave the space blank.* **LO 13.1, 13.2**

1. adenoid

Rewrite this term, and slash all its elements:

_____ / _____ / _____
        P   R/CF   S

2. nasopharyngeal

Rewrite this term, and slash all its elements:

_____ / _____ / _____
        P   R/CF   S

3. pharyngeal

Rewrite this term, and slash all its elements:

_____ / _____ / _____
        P   R/CF   S

4. laryngopharynx

Rewrite this term, and slash all its elements:

_____ / _____ / _____
        P   R/CF   S

Trachea

Once the air you inhale has passed through the upper airway and many of the pollutants and impurities have been filtered out and swallowed into the digestive system, there remains the major need of getting O_2 into the blood and removing CO_2 from the blood. To do these, the inhaled air passes down the trachea, through the bronchi and bronchioles, and into the alveoli of the lungs, where these exchanges can occur. These structures form the lower respiratory tract. The flow of inhaled air now moves into the **trachea** (wind-pipe). This is a rigid tube that descends from the larynx to divide into the two main bronchi *(Figure 13.7a)*. The rigidity of the trachea is produced by 16 to 20 C-shaped rings of cartilage that form its anterior and lateral walls *(Figure 13.7b)*. The open part of the "C" faces posteriorly and is closed by the **trachealis** muscle. The trachea divides into the two primary (main) bronchi for the right and left lungs *(Figure 13.7a)*.

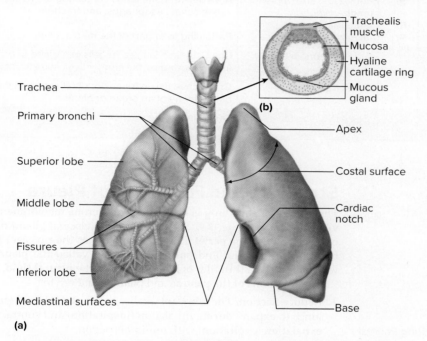

Trachealis muscle
Mucosa
Hyaline cartilage ring
Mucous gland
(b)

Trachea
Primary bronchi
Superior lobe
Middle lobe
Fissures
Inferior lobe
Mediastinal surfaces

Apex
Costal surface
Cardiac notch
Base

(a)

▲ **Figure 13.7** **Lower respiratory tract.** (*a*) Gross anatomy. (*b*) Cross-section of the trachea to show the C-shaped tracheal cartilage.

Structure of the Lungs

The two lungs are the main organs of respiration and are located in the thoracic cavity. Each lung is a soft, spongy, conical organ with its base resting on the **diaphragm.** Its apex lies above and behind the clavicle. Its outer, convex costal surface presses against the rib cage. Its inner, concave surface lies alongside the **mediastinum.**

The right lung has three **lobes:** superior, middle, and inferior. The left lung has two lobes: superior and inferior *(see Figure 13.7a)*. The lobes are separated from each other by **fissures.** The heart makes a concave impression in the left lung, known as the *cardiac notch.*

Each lung receives its bronchus, blood vessels, lymphatic vessels, and nerves through its **hilum** *(Figure 13.8)*. The lung's specific functional cells are called the lung **parenchyma** and are

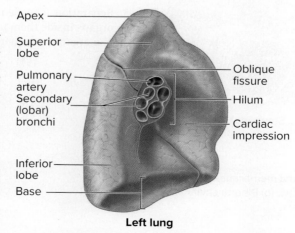

Apex
Superior lobe
Pulmonary artery
Secondary (lobar) bronchi
Inferior lobe
Base

Oblique fissure
Hilum
Cardiac impression

Left lung

▲ **Figure 13.8** Left lung hilum: medial surface.

supported by a thin connective tissue framework called the **stroma.** This consists mostly of collagen and elastic fibers, and its elasticity is a factor in the lung's recoil after inhalation.

WORD	PRONUNCIATION		ELEMENTS	DEFINITION
diaphragm	**DIE**-ah-fram		Greek *diaphragm*	Musculoligamentous partition separating the abdominal and thoracic cavities
diaphragmatic (adj)	**DIE**-ah-frag-**MAT**-ic	S/ R/	-atic *pertaining to* diaphragm- *diaphragm*	Pertaining to the diaphragm
fissure fissures (pl)	**FISH**-ur	S/ R/	-ure *result of* fiss- *split*	Deep furrow or cleft
hilum hila (pl)	**HIGH**-lum **HIGH**-lah		Latin *small area*	The site where the nerves and blood vessels enter and leave an organ
lobe lobar (adj)	LOBE **LOH**-bar	S/ R/	Greek *lobe* -ar *pertaining to* lob- *lobe*	Subdivision of an organ or other part Pertaining to or part of a lobe
mediastinum	**MEE**-dee-ah-**STIE**-num	S/ P/ R/	-um *tissue, structure* media- *middle* -stin- *partition*	Area between the lungs containing the heart, aorta, venae cavae, esophagus, and trachea
mediastinal (adj)	**MEE**-dee-ah-**STIE**-nal	S/	-al *pertaining to*	Pertaining to or part of the mediastinum
parenchyma	pah-**RENG**-kih-mah		Greek *to pour in beside*	Characteristic functional cells of a gland or organ that are supported by the connective tissue framework
stroma	**STROH**-mah		Greek *bed*	Connective tissue framework that supports the parenchyma of an organ or gland
trachealis	tray-kee-**AY**-lis	S/ R/	-alis *pertaining to* trache- *trachea*	Pertaining to the trachea

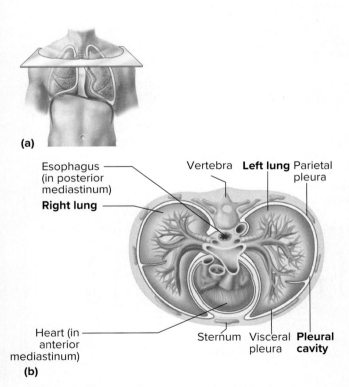

(a)

Esophagus (in posterior mediastinum)

Vertebra   **Left lung**   Parietal pleura

Right lung

Heart (in anterior mediastinum)

Sternum   Visceral pleura   **Pleural cavity**

(b)

▲ **Figure 13.9** **Pleural cavity and membranes.** (*a*) Site of cross-section of superior view. (*b*) Pleural cavity and membranes in the superior view.

Structure and Functions of Pleura

The surface of each lung is covered with a serous membrane called the **visceral pleura** (*Figure 13.9*). At the hilum, the visceral pleura turns back on itself to form the **parietal pleura,** which lines the rib cage. The space between the visceral and parietal pleurae is called the **pleural cavity,** which contains a thin film of lubricant called the **pleural fluid.**

The functions of the **pleurae** and pleural fluid are to:

1. **Reduce friction.** The lubricant quality of the pleural fluid enables the lungs to expand during inhalation (**inspiration**) and contract during **exhalation** (**expiration**) with minimal friction.

2. **Assist in inspiration.** The pressure in the pleural cavity is lower than the pressure of the atmospheric air in the lungs. This assists the **inflation** of the lungs on inspiration.

3. **Separation.** The **pleurae, mediastinum,** and **pericardium** protect the organs inside them to prevent infections from spreading easily from one organ to another.

Structure of Bronchi

As the inhaled air continues down the respiratory tract, the trachea divides and air flows into the right and left main (primary) bronchi, which enter each lung at the hilum.

In turn, the main bronchi divide into a secondary (lobar) bronchus for each lobe. There are three secondary bronchi in the right lung and two in the left lung. Each secondary bronchus divides into tertiary bronchi that supply segments of each lobe *(Figure 13.10)*.

Structure and Functions of Bronchioles and Alveoli

The tertiary bronchi divide into **bronchioles,** which in turn divide into **terminal bronchioles** and then smaller respiratory bronchioles *(Figure 13.11)*. None of these bronchioles has cartilage in the walls, but smooth muscle enables them to dilate or constrict. These bronchioles in turn divide into thin-walled alveoli.

Each alveolus is a thin-walled sac with its cells supported by a thin **respiratory membrane** that allows the exchange of gases with the surrounding **pulmonary** capillary network *(Figure 13.11)*. About 5% of the alveolar cells secrete a detergent-like substance called **surfactant** that keeps the alveolar sacs from collapsing. There are approximately 300 million alveoli in the two lungs.

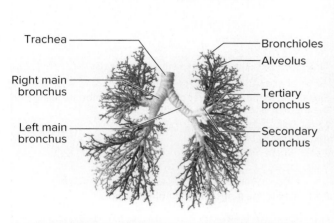

▲ **Figure 13.10** Latex cast of tracheobronchial tree.

Dave King/Dorling Kindersley/Science Source

▲ **Figure 13.11** Bronchioles and alveoli.

Mechanics of Respiration

A resting adult breathes 10 to 15 times per minute, **inhales** about 500 mL of air during inspiration *(Figure 13.12a)*, and **exhales** it during expiration *(Figure 13.12b)*. The mission is to get air into and out of the alveoli so that O_2 can get into the blood and CO_2 can get out of the blood.

The diaphragm does most of the work. In inspiration it drops down and flattens to expand the volume of the thoracic cavity and reduce the pressure in the airways *(Figure 13.12a)*. In addition, the external intercostal muscles lift the chest wall up and out to further expand the thoracic cavity.

Expiration is a passive process of letting go. The diaphragm and intercostal muscles relax, and the thoracic cavity springs back to its original volume *(Figure 13.12b)*.

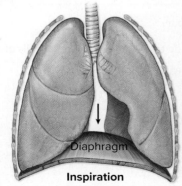

Inspiration

Diaphragm contracts; vertical dimensions of thoracic cavity increase.

(a)

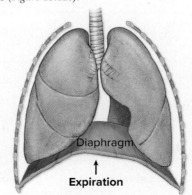

Expiration

Diaphragm relaxes; vertical dimensions of thoracic cavity decrease.

(b)

▲ **Figure 13.12** Inspiration and expiration.

Did you know...

- **Hiccups** are reflex spasms of the diaphragm, causing an involuntary inhalation followed by a sudden closure of the glottis that produces an audible sound—the "hic." The etiology is unknown, and there is no specific medical cure.

- **Yawning** is a reflex that originates in the brainstem in response to hypoxia, boredom, or sleepiness. The exact mechanisms are not known.

S = Suffix   P = Prefix   R = Root   R/CF = Combining Form

WORD	PRONUNCIATION		ELEMENTS	DEFINITION
exhale (verb)	EKS-hail		Latin *breathe out*	Breathe out
exhalation	EKS-huh-**LAY**-shun	P/	ex- *out*	The process of breathing out
		R/	-hale *breathe*	
		S/	-ation *process*	
expire	**EKS**-pire	P/	ex- *out*	
		R/	-(s)pire- *to breathe*	
expiration	EKS-puh-**RAY**-shun	S/	-ation *process*	
inflate (verb)	in-**FLAYT**		Latin *blow up*	Expand with air
inflation (noun)	in-**FLAY**-shun	S/	-ation *process*	Process of expanding with air
inhale (verb)	in-**HALE**		Latin *to breathe in*	Breathe in
inhalation	**IN**-huh-**LA**-shun	P/	in- *in*	Process of breathing in
		R/	-hale *breathe*	
		S/	-ation *process*	
inspire	in-**SPIRE**	P/	in- *in*	
		R/	-(s)pire- *to breathe*	
inspiration	**IN**-spih-**RAY**-shun	S/	-ation *process*	
membrane	**MEM**-brain		Latin *parchment*	Thin layer of tissue covering a structure or cavity
parietal	pah-**RYE**-eh-tal	S/	-al *pertaining to*	Pertaining to the outer layer of the serous membrane lining
		R/	pariet- *wall*	the thoracic and other body cavities
pleura	**PLOOR**-ah		Greek *rib, side*	Membrane covering the lungs and lining the ribs in the thoracic cavity
pleurae (pl)	**PLOOR**-ee			Pertaining to the pleura
pleural (adj)	**PLOOR**-al	S/	-al *pertaining to*	
		R/	pleur- *pleura*	
pulmonary	**PULL**-moh-**NAIR**-ee	S/	-ary *pertaining to*	Pertaining to the lungs and their blood supply
		R/	pulmon- *lung*	
surfactant	ser-**FAK**-tant		acronym for **SUR**face **ACT**ive age**NT**	A protein and fat compound that reduces surface tension to hold lung alveolar walls apart

Check Point Section 13.3

A. Precision in communication means using the correct form of the medical term, as well as the correct spelling. *Test your knowledge of plurals, adjectives, and spelling with this exercise. Select the correct choice.* **LO 13.1, 13.3**

1. The area between the lungs containing the heart, aorta, venae cavae, esophagus, and trachea is the

    a. mediastenum   **b.** medisternum   **c.** mediastinum   **d.** midiasternum

2. The patient was diagnosed with _____ pneumonia.

    a. lobe   **b.** lobular   **c.** lobar   **d.** lumbar

3. _____ is the term for the functional cells of an organ.

    a. Perenchyma   **b.** Parenchyma   **c.** Perinchkima   **d.** Perenkima

4. Because there is a hilum in each lung, collectively they are referred to as the

    a. hilla   **b.** hila   **c.** hilia   **d.** hilea

5. The muscle separating the abdominal and thoracic cavities is the

    a. diaphram   **b.** diaphragm   **c.** diahragm   **d.** diapragm

6. Removal of a lobe of a lung would be a

    a. lobotomy   **b.** lobectomy   **c.** lobarectomy   **d.** lobarotomy

B. Select the correct pronunciation of the following two terms. LO 13.4

1. stroma
   a. **STROM**-a
   b. **STRO**-mah
   c. **STROH**-mah
   d. **STROH**-ma
   e. **STROM**-ah

2. diaphragm
   a. **DIE**-a-fram
   b. **DI**-a-frame
   c. **DI**-ah-fram
   d. **DIE**-ah-fram
   e. **DE**-a-fram

C. Define structure and functions of the pleura, bronchi, bronchioles, and alveoli. *The structures are distinct and have a distinct purpose. It is important to be able to differentiate these structures and functions.* **LO 13.1**

1. The substance that lines the alveoli to help keep them open: _____

2. The smallest of the airways that do not participate in gas exchange: _____

3. The serous membrane that covers the lungs: _____ pleura

4. The fluid that reduces friction between the lungs and the thoracic cavity: _____ fluid

5. The large airway that enters each lung at the hilum: _____

D. These elements all appear in the language of pulmonology. *Challenge your knowledge of these elements, and make the correct match. Fill in the blanks.* **LO 13.1, 13.2**

_____ 1. *re-*	a. to narrow
_____ 2. *em*	b. process
_____ 3. *capn*	c. pull
_____ 4. *-ole*	d. dilation
_____ 5. *-osis*	e. back
_____ 6. *constrict*	f. CO_2
_____ 7. *-ation*	g. into
_____ 8. *tract*	h. bronchus
_____ 9. *-ectasis*	i. small
_____ 10. *bronchi*	j. condition

Section 13.4 Disorders of the Respiratory System

Disorders of the Upper Respiratory Tract

Disorders of the Nose

The **common cold** is a viral **upper respiratory infection (URI)**. It is contagious, being transmitted from person to person in airborne droplets from coughing and sneezing. There is no proven effective treatment.

   Rhinitis is an inflammation of the nasal mucosa, usually viral in origin. It is also called **coryza.**

   Allergic rhinitis affects 15% to 20% of the population. There is swelling of the mucous membranes of the nose, pharynx, and sinuses, with a clear watery discharge.

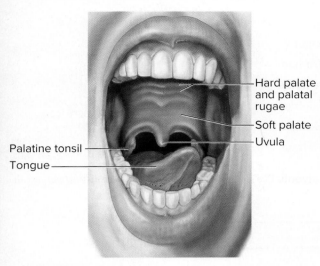

Hard palate and palatal rugae

Soft palate

Uvula

Palatine tonsil

Tongue

▲ **Figure 13.13** **Soft tissues at back of mouth.**

Sinusitis is an infection of the paranasal sinuses, often following a cold. The infection can be bacterial, producing a **mucopurulent** discharge from the nose. Treatment with **antibiotics** and **decongestants** may be indicated.

Epistaxis is bleeding from the septum of the nose, usually from trauma.

Disorders of the Pharynx

Twenty-five percent of normal adults are habitual snorers. The condition is most frequent in overweight males, and it becomes worse with age. The noises of **snoring** are made at the back of the mouth and nose where the tongue and upper pharynx meet the soft palate and uvula *(Figure 13.13).* When there is obstruction to the free flow of air, these structures hit each other, and the vibration produces the sounds of snoring.

Obstructive sleep apnea occurs when obstruction by the soft tissues at the back of the nose and mouth causes frequent episodes of gasping for breath followed by complete cessation of breathing **(apnea).** These episodes of apnea can last for 10 to 30 seconds and occur many times every hour of sleep. The episodes reduce the level of O_2 in the blood **(hypoxemia),** causing the heart to pump harder. After several years with this problem, hypertension and cardiac enlargement can occur.

Pharyngitis is an acute or chronic infection involving the pharynx, tonsils, and uvula. It is usually of viral origin in children.

Tonsillitis is an infection of the tonsils in the oropharynx by a virus or, in less than 20% of cases, a streptococcus.

Nasopharyngeal carcinoma is a rare form of cancer that occurs mostly in males between the ages of 50 and 60.

Disorders of the Larynx

Laryngitis is inflammation of the mucosal lining of the larynx, producing hoarseness and sometimes progressing to loss of voice **(aphonia).**

Epiglottitis is inflammation of the epiglottis. **Acute epiglottitis** is typically seen in children between ages 2 and 7 years and is caused by *Haemophilus influenzae type b* bacteria. Swelling in the epiglottis can cause acute airway obstruction. It is preventable with an available vaccine.

Laryngotracheobronchitis (LTB), commonly referred to as **croup,** is a viral respiratory infection in children aged 3 months to 5 years. It causes inflammation and obstruction of the upper airway. It produces a characteristic cough that sounds like a seal barking. In severe cases, the child makes a high-pitched, squeaky inspiratory noise called **stridor.**

Papillomas or laryngeal **polyps** are benign tumors of the larynx that result from overuse or irritation.

Carcinoma of the larynx produces a persistent hoarseness. Its incidence peaks in smokers in their fifties and sixties.

S = Suffix   P = Prefix   R = Root   R/CF = Combining Form

WORD	PRONUNCIATION	ELEMENTS		DEFINITION
apnea	**AP**-nee-ah	P/ R/	**a-** *without* **-pnea** *breathe*	Absence of spontaneous respiration
aphonia	ay-**FOH**-nee-ah	S/ P/ R/	**-ia** *condition* **a-** *without* **-phon-** *voice*	Loss of voice
hypoxemia	**HIGH**-pok-**SEE**-mee-ah	S/ P/ R/	**-emia** *blood condition* **hyp(o)-** *below* **-ox-** *oxygen*	Decreased levels of oxygen in the blood
anoxia	an-**OK**-see-ah	S/ P/	**-ia** *condition* **an-** *without*	Complete deprivation of oxygen supply
coryza *rhinitis* **(syn)**	koh-**RYE**-zah		Greek *catarrh*	Viral inflammation of the mucous membrane of the nose
epiglottitis	ep-ih-glot-**TIE**-tis	P/ R/ S/	**epi-** *above* **-glott-** *opening of larynx* **-itis** *inflammation*	Inflammation of the epiglottis
epistaxis	ep-ih-**STAK**-sis	S/ P/ R/	**-is** *condition* **epi-** *above, over* **-stax-** *fall in drops*	Nosebleed
laryngitis	lair-in-**JIE**-tis	S/ R/	**-itis** *inflammation* **laryng-** *larynx*	Inflammation of the larynx
laryngotracheobronchitis *croup* **(syn)**	lah-**RING**-oh-**TRAY**-kee-oh-brong-**KIE**-tis	R/CF R/CF R/	**laryng/o-** *larynx* **-trache/o-** *trachea* **-bronch-** *bronchus*	Inflammation of the larynx, trachea, and bronchi
mucopurulent	myu-koh-**PYUR**-you-lent	S/ R/CF R/	**-ent** *forming* **muc/o-** *mucus* **-purul-** *pus*	Mixture of pus and mucus
pharyngitis	fair-in-**JIE**-tis	S/ R/	**-itis** *inflammation* **pharyng-** *pharynx*	Inflammation of the pharynx
polysomnography	pol-ee-som-**NOG**-rah-fee	S/ P/ R/CF	**-graphy** *process of recording* **poly-** *many* **-somn/o-** *sleep*	Test to monitor brain waves, muscle tension, eye movement, and oxygen levels in the blood as the patient sleeps
rhinitis *coryza* **(syn)**	rye-**NIE**-tis	S/ R/	**-itis** *inflammation* **rhin-** *nose*	Inflammation of the nasal mucosa
sinusitis	sigh-nuh-**SIGH**-tis	S/ R/	**-itis** *inflammation* **sinus-** *sinus*	Inflammation of the lining of a sinus
snore	SNORE		Old English *snore*	Noise produced by vibrations in the structures of the nasopharynx
tonsillitis (note the double "ll")	ton-sih-**LIE**-tis	S/ R/	**-itis** *inflammation* **tonsill-** *tonsil*	Inflammation of the tonsils

Disorders of the Lower Respiratory Tract

Common Signs and Symptoms of Respiratory Disorders

1. **Coughing** is triggered by irritants in the respiratory tract. You close the glottis and contract the muscles of expiration to develop high pressure in the lower tract. Then you suddenly open the glottis to release an explosive blast of air.

   The irritants can be cigarette smoke, infection, or tumors (as in lung cancer). A productive cough produces sputum that can be swallowed or **expectorated**. Bloody sputum is called **hemoptysis.** Thick, yellow (purulent) sputum indicates infection. A nonproductive cough is dry and hacking. Abnormal amounts of expectorated clear mucus are called **phlegm.**

2. **Dyspnea,** or shortness of breath (SOB), can be on exertion or, in severe disorders, at rest when all the respiratory muscles can exchange only a small volume of air.

Dyspnea can result from airway obstruction. Wheezing associated with dyspnea is the sound of air being forced through constricted airways, as in asthma. Dyspnea also can be produced by fibrosis of lung tissues, when the lungs' **compliance** is reduced. Compliance is the ability of the lungs to expand on inspiration.

3. **Cyanosis** is seen when the blood has increased levels of **unoxygenated hemoglobin,** which has a characteristic dark gray–blue color. The color is best seen in the lips, mucous membranes, and nail beds where there is no skin pigmentation to mask it.

   • **Peripheral cyanosis** occurs when there is peripheral vasoconstriction. The reduced flow allows hemoglobin to yield more of its O_2, leading to increased unoxygenated hemoglobin.

   • **Central cyanosis** occurs with inadequate blood oxygenation in the lungs as a result of impaired airflow or impaired blood flow through the lungs. Central cyanosis is detected by examining the color of the lips, gums, and tongue.

4. **Changes in rate of breathing. Eupnea** is the normal, easy, automatic respiration—around 15 breaths per minute in a resting adult. Both **tachypnea** (rapid rate of breathing) and **hyperpnea** (breathing deeper and more rapidly than normal) are signs of respiratory difficulty, as is **bradypnea** (slow breathing).

5. **Sneezing** is caused by irritants in the nasal cavity. The glottis stays open while the soft palate and tongue block the flow of air from getting out. Then they suddenly release to let air burst out through the nose.

Word Analysis and Definition: Signs and Symptoms of Respiratory Disorders

S = Suffix   P = Prefix   R = Root   R/CF = Combining Form

WORD	PRONUNCIATION		ELEMENTS	DEFINITION
bradypnea (opposite of tachypnea)	brad-ip-**NEE**-ah	R/ P/	**-pnea** *breathe* **brady-** *slow*	Slow breathing
compliance	kom-**PLY**-ance	S/ R/	**-ance** *state of, condition* **compli-** *fulfill*	Measure of the capacity of a chamber or hollow viscus to expand, in this case, the lungs
cyanosis	sigh-ah-**NOH**-sis	S/ R/	**-osis** *condition* **cyan-** *blue*	Blue discoloration of the skin, lips, and nail beds due to low levels of oxygen in the blood
cyanotic (adj)	sigh-ah-**NOT**-ik	S/ R/CF	**-tic** *pertaining to* **cyan/o-** *blue*	Marked by cyanosis
dyspnea	disp-**NEE**-ah	R/ P/	**-pnea** *breathe* **dys-** *difficult*	Difficulty breathing
eupnea	yoop-**NEE**-ah	R/ P/	**-pnea** *breathe* **eup-** *normal*	Normal breathing
expectorate	ek-**SPEC**-toh-rate	S/ P/ R/	**-ate** *process* **ex-** *out* **-pector-** *chest*	Cough up and spit out mucus from the respiratory tract
hemoptysis	hee-**MOP**-tih-sis	R/CF R/	**hem/o-** *blood* **-ptysis** *spit*	Bloody sputum
hyperpnea	high-perp-**NEE**-ah	R/ P/	**-pnea** *breathe* **hyper-** *excessive*	Deeper and more rapid breathing than normal
phlegm	FLEM		Greek *flame*	Abnormal amounts of mucus expectorated from the respiratory tract
sputum	**SPYU**-tum		Latin to *spit*	Matter coughed up and spat out by individuals with respiratory disorders
tachypnea (opposite of bradypnea)	tak-ip-**NEE**-ah	R/ P/	**-pnea** *breathe* **tachy-** *rapid*	Rapid breathing

Disorders of the Lower Respiratory Tract

Acute bronchitis can be viral or bacterial, leading to the production of excess mucus with some obstruction of airflow. A single episode resolves without significant residual damage to the airway.

Chronic bronchitis is the most common obstructive disease, due to cigarette smoking or repeated episodes of acute bronchitis. In addition to excess mucus production, cilia are destroyed. A pattern develops, involving chronic cough, sputum production, dyspnea, and recurrent acute infections.

In advanced chronic bronchitis, **hypoxia** and **hypercapnia** develop, and heart failure follows.

Bronchiolitis, inflammation of the small airway bronchioles, occurs in the adult as the early and often unrecognized beginning of airway changes in cigarette smokers or those exposed to "secondhand smoke," inhaling the smoke produced by other peoples' cigarettes.

Bronchiolitis affects children under the age of 2 because their small airways become blocked very easily. The disease is viral and in severe cases can cause marked respiratory distress, with drawing in of the neck and intercostal spaces of the chest with each breath (known as **retractions**).

Pulmonary emphysema is a disease of the respiratory bronchioles and alveoli. These airways become enlarged, and the septa between the alveoli are destroyed, forming large sacs **(bullae).** There is a loss of surface area for gas exchange. Because the septa contain elastic tissue that assists the lungs' recoil in exhalation, recoil becomes more difficult, and air is trapped in the bullae. This leads to **hyperinflation** of the lungs and the enlarged "barrel chest" shown by many patients with emphysema.

Chronic airway obstruction (CAO) is also called **chronic obstructive pulmonary disease (COPD)** is a progressive disease. It involves both chronic bronchitis and emphysema. A history of heavy cigarette smoking, with chronic cough and sputum production, is followed by exertional dyspnea. By the time Mr. Jacobs' dyspnea was severe, irreversible lung damage *(Figure 13.14)* had led to emphysema, recurrent infections, and episodes of respiratory insufficiency. The insufficiency became permanent, and supplementary O_2 is now necessary round the clock. Right-sided heart failure **(cor pulmonale)** is the end-result of pulmonary hypertension and blood backing up into the right ventricle *(see Chapter 10).*

Bronchiectasis is the abnormal dilatation of the small bronchioles due to repeated infections. The damaged, dilated bronchi are unable to clear secretions, so additional infections and more damage can occur.

Bronchial asthma is a disorder with recurrent acute episodes of bronchial obstruction as a result of constriction of bronchioles **(bronchoconstriction), hypersecretion** of mucus, and inflammatory swelling of the bronchiolar lining. The airflow obstruction these produce is mainly during expiration, and the wheezing exhalation heard in asthma is the result of forcing air out of the lungs through constricted, swollen bronchioles. Between attacks, breathing can be normal. The **etiology** of asthma is an allergic response to substances such as pollen, animal dander, or the feces of house dust mites.

Cystic fibrosis (CF) is caused by an increased viscosity of secretions from the pancreas, salivary glands, liver, intestine, and lungs. In the lungs, a particularly thick mucus obstructs the airways and causes repeated infections. Respiratory failure is the cause of death, often before the age of 30. The disorder is genetic.

Pulmonary edema is the collection of fluid in the lung tissues and alveoli. It is most frequently the result of left ventricular failure or mitral valve disease with **congestive heart failure (CHF).** Noncardiogenic pulmonary edema can result from sepsis, renal failure, disseminated intravascular coagulation (DIC) *(see Chapter 11),* and opiate or barbiturate poisoning.

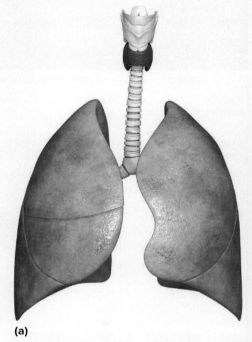

(a)

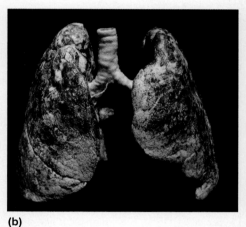

(b)

▲ **Figure 13.14** **Whole lungs.** (*a*) Nonsmoker's lungs. (*b*) Smoker's lungs. Pixologic Studio/Science Source imageBROKER/Alamy Stock Photo

WORD	PRONUNCIATION		ELEMENTS	DEFINITION
asthma asthmatic (adj)	**AZ**-mah az-**MAT**-ic	S/ R/	Greek *asthma* -tic *pertaining to* asthma- *asthma*	Episodes of breathing difficulty due to narrowed or obstructed airways Pertaining to, or suffering from, asthma
bronchiectasis	brong-kee-**EK**-tah-sis	S/ R/CF	-ectasis *dilation* bronch/i- *bronchus*	Chronic dilation of the bronchi following inflammatory disease and obstruction
bronchiolitis	brong-kee-oh-**LIE**-tis	S/ R/	-itis *inflammation* bronchiol- *small bronchus*	Inflammation of the small bronchioles
bronchoconstriction	**BRONG**-koh-kon-**STRIK**-shun	S/ R/CF R/	-ion *process* bronch/o- *bronchus* -constrict- *to narrow*	Reduction in diameter of a bronchus
bulla bullae (pl)	**BULL**-ah **BULL**-ee		Latin *bubble*	Bubble-like dilated structure
cor pulmonale	KOR pul-moh-**NAH**-lee	S/ R/	cor Latin *heart* -ale *pertaining to* pulmon- *lung*	Right-sided heart failure arising from chronic lung disease
cystic fibrosis (CF)	**SIS**-tik fie-**BROH**-sis	S/ R/ S/ R/	-ic *pertaining to* cyst- *cyst* -osis *condition* fibr- *fiber*	Genetic disease in which excessive viscid mucus obstructs passages, including bronchi
emphysema	em-fih-**SEE**-mah	P/ R/	em- *in, into* -physema *blowing*	Dilation of respiratory bronchioles and alveoli
hypercapnia	**HIGH**-per-**KAP**-nee-ah	S/ P/ R/	-ia *condition* hyper- *excessive* -capn- *carbon dioxide*	Abnormal increase of carbon dioxide in the arterial bloodstream
hyperinflation	**HIGH**-per-in-**FLAY**-shun	S/ P/ P/ R/	-ion *process* hyper- *excessive* -in- *in* -flat- *blow up*	Overdistension of pulmonary alveoli with air resulting from airway obstruction
hypersecretion	**HIGH**-per-seh-**KREE**-shun	S/ P/ R/	-ion *process* hyper- *excessive* -secret- *secrete*	Excessive secretion of mucus (or enzymes or waste products)
hypoxia hypoxic (adj)	high-**POK**-see-ah high-**POK**-sik	S/ P/ R/ S/	-ia *condition* hyp(o)- *deficient, below* -ox- *oxygen* -ic *pertaining to*	Decrease below normal levels of oxygen in tissues, gases, or blood Deficient in oxygen
retraction	ree-**TRAK**-shun	S/ P/ R/	-ion *process* re- *back* -tract- *pull*	A pulling back, as a pulling back of the intercostal spaces and the neck above the clavicle

Disorders of the Lower Respiratory Tract Continued

Pneumonia is an acute infection affecting the alveoli and lung parenchyma (*Figure 13.15*). Bacterial infections focus on the alveoli; viral infections, on the parenchyma. **Lobar pneumonia** is an infection limited to one lung lobe. **Bronchopneumonia** is used to describe an infection in the bronchioles that spreads to the alveoli.

When an area of the lung (segment) or a lobe becomes airless as a result of the infection, the lung is **consolidated.** When an area of the lung collapses as a result of bronchial obstruction, the condition is called **atelectasis.**

Pleurisy, an inflammation of the pleurae, can be a complication of pneumonia. This condition is very painful on breathing. The inflammation often leads to an exudate accumulating in the pleural cavity—a **pleural effusion.** If the pleural effusion contains pus, it is called **empyema (pyothorax).** If it contains blood, it is called **hemothorax.**

Lung abscess can be a complication of bacterial pneumonia or cancer. Long-term antibiotics are used, and surgical resection of the abscess may be required.

Pneumothorax is the entry of air into the pleural cavity (*Figure 13.16*). The cause can be unknown (**spontaneous pneumothorax**), but it often results from trauma when a fractured rib, knife blade, or bullet lacerates the parietal pleura.

Thromboembolism is caused by an embolus, usually arising in the deep vein of the calf and lodging in a branch of the pulmonary artery. The symptoms are chest pain, dyspnea, tachypnea (increased respiratory rate), and a reduction in blood O_2 levels.

Acute respiratory distress syndrome (ARDS) is sudden life-threatening lung failure caused by a variety of underlying conditions, from major trauma to sepsis. The alveoli fill with fluid and collapse, and gas exchange is shut down. Hypoxia results. Mechanical ventilation has to be provided. The mortality is from 35% to 50%.

Neonatal respiratory distress syndrome (NRDS) is seen in premature babies whose lungs have not matured enough to produce surfactant. The alveoli collapse, and mechanical ventilation is needed to keep them open.

Chronic infections of the lung parenchyma are the result of prolonged exposure to infection or to occupational irritant dusts or droplets. These disorders are called **pneumoconioses.** Levels of dust inhalation overwhelm the airways' particle-clearing abilities; the dust particles accumulate in the alveoli and parenchyma, leading to fibrosis. **Asbestosis** from inhaling asbestos particles can lead to a cancer (**mesothelioma**) in the pleura. **Silicosis** from inhaling silica particles is called *stone mason's lung.* **Anthracosis** from inhaling coal dust particles is called *coal miners' lung.* **Sarcoidosis** is an **idiopathic** fibrotic disorder of the lung parenchyma.

Pulmonary tuberculosis is a chronic, infectious disease of the lungs.

Lung cancer, related to tobacco use, used to be a male disease, but now fatalities in women from lung cancer exceed those from breast cancer. Ninety percent of lung cancers arise in the mucous membranes of the larger bronchi and are called **bronchogenic carcinomas.** The tumor obstructs the bronchus, spreads into the surrounding lung tissues, and metastasizes to lymph nodes, liver, brain, and bone.

Acute respiratory failure (ARF) is abnormal respiratory function resulting in inadequate tissue oxygenation or CO_2 elimination that is severe enough to impair vital organ functions. Causes of ARF include congestive heart failure (CHF), chronic obstructive pulmonary disease (COPD), chest trauma with resultant **flail chest,** spinal cord injury, and neuromuscular disorders in which the muscles of respiration are weak or paralyzed.

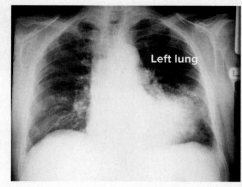

▲ **Figure 13.15** **Chest x-ray of patient with pneumonia in the left lung.** A normal lung appears as mostly black space but with some lung markings on an x-ray because its spongy structure is filled with air. In contrast, a pneumonic lung appears white or opaque on an x-ray as a result of accumulation of fluid and cells in the alveoli. Anthony Ricci/Shutterstock

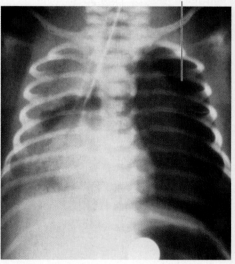

▲ **Figure 13.16** **Left pneumothorax.** There are no lung markings seen in the area of the pneumothorax. Wellcome Photo Library

S = Suffix   P = Prefix   R = Root   R/CF = Combining Form

WORD	PRONUNCIATION	ELEMENTS		DEFINITION
anthracosis	an-thra-**KOH**-sis	S/ R/	-osis *condition* anthrac- *coal*	Lung disease caused by the inhalation of coal dust
asbestosis	as-bes-**TOH**-sis	S/ R/	-osis *condition* asbest- *asbestos*	Lung disease caused by the inhalation of asbestos particles
abscess	**AB**-ses		Latin *a going away*	A collection of pus surrounded by infected tissue that is swollen and inflamed
atelectasis	at-el-**EK**-tah-sis	P/ R/	atel- *incomplete* -ectasis *dilation*	Collapse of part of a lung
bronchogenic	brong-koh-**JEN**-ik	S/ R/CF	-genic *creation* bronch/o- *bronchus*	Arising from a bronchus
bronchopneumonia	**BRONG**-koh-new-**MOH**-nee-ah	S/ R/CF R/	-ia *condition* bronch/o- *bronchus* -pneumon- *air, lung*	Acute inflammation of the walls of smaller bronchioles with spread to lung parenchyma
consolidate (v) consolidated (adj) consolidation	kon-**SOL**-i-date kon-**SOL**-i-day-tid kon-**SOL**-i-day-shun	S/ S/	Latin *to make solid* -ed *pertaining to* -ion *process*	Making firm or solid An aerated tissue that has become firm or solid Area of solid tissue that was once aerated
effusion	eh-**FYU**-shun		Latin *pouring out*	Collection of fluid that has escaped from blood vessels into a cavity or tissues
empyema pyothorax (syn)	**EM**-pie-**EE**-mah **PIE**-oh-**THOR**-aks	S/ P/ R/ S/ R/CF	-ema *result* em- *in* -py- *pus* -thorax *chest* py/o- *pus*	Pus in a body cavity, particularly in the pleural cavity Empyema in a pleural cavity
flail chest	FLAIL CHEST		**flail** Old English *flapping* **chest** Greek *basket, hamper*	Condition in which three or more consecutive ribs have been fractured, resulting in uncontrolled movement of that segment of the chest
hemothorax	hee-moh-**THOR**-aks	R/ R/	thorax *chest* hem/o- *blood*	Blood in the pleural cavity
idiopathic	**ID**-ih-oh-**PATH**-ik	S/ R/CF R/	-ic *pertaining to* idi/o- *personal, distinct, unknown* -path- *disease*	Pertaining to a disease of unknown etiology
mesothelioma	**MEEZ**-oh-thee-lee-**OH**-mah	S/ P/ R/CF	-oma *tumor, mass* meso- *middle* -thel/i- *lining*	Cancer arising from the cells lining the pleura or peritoneum
pleurisy	**PLOOR**-ih-see	S/ R/	-isy *inflammation* pleur- *pleura*	Inflammation of the pleura
pneumoconiosis	new-moh-koh-nee-**OH**-sis	S/ R/CF R/	-osis *condition* pneum/o- *air, lung* -coni- *dust*	Fibrotic lung disease caused by the inhalation of different dusts
pneumonia pneumonitis (syn)	new-**MOH**-nee-ah new-moh-**NIE**-tis	S/ R/ S/	-ia *condition* pneumon- *air, lung* -itis *inflammation*	Inflammation of the lung parenchyma
pneumothorax	new-moh-**THOR**-aks	S/ R/CF	-thorax *chest* pneum/o- *air, lung*	Air in the pleural cavity
sarcoidosis (*Note:* Two suffixes.)	sar-koy-**DOH**-sis	S/ S/ R/	-osis *condition* -oid- *resembling* sarc- *sarcoma*	Granulomatous lesions of lungs and other organs; cause is unknown
silicosis	sil-ih-**KOH**-sis	S/ R/	-osis *condition* silic- *silicon*	Fibrotic lung disease from inhaling silica particles
thromboembolism	**THROM**-boh-**EM**-boh-lizm	S/ R/CF R/	-ism *condition* thromb/o- *blood clot* -embol- *plug*	A piece of detached blood clot (embolus) blocking a distant blood vessel
tuberculosis	too-**BER**-kyu-**LOH**-sis	S/ R/	-osis *condition* tubercul- *nodule, tuberculosis*	Infectious disease that can infect any organ or tissue

Check Point Section 13.4

 Case Report (CR) 13.1

You are

. . . a sleep technologist in the Sleep Disorders Clinic at Fulwood Medical Center. You are about to position the electrodes on your patient for an overnight **polysomnography** (sleep study).

Your patient is

. . . Mr. Tye Gawlinski, a 29-year-old professional football player.

Mr. Gawlinski's wife states that he snores loudly and has 40 or 50 periods in the night when he stops breathing. The snoring is so loud that she cannot sleep even in the adjoining bedroom. Mr. Gawlinski complains of being tired all day and not having the energy he needs for his job. The sleep study is being performed to confirm a diagnosis of **obstructive sleep apnea.**

A. After reading Case Report 13.1, answer the following questions. LO 13.5, 13.6

1. What are Mr. Gawlinski's symptoms? (Choose all that apply)

   a. daytime sleepiness   **b.** sore throat   **c.** lack of energy   **d.** runny nose

2. Mr. Gawlinski underwent the diagnostic procedure of:

   a. tonsillectomy   **b.** endoscopy   **c.** polysomnography   **d.** sonogram

3. If left untreated, his chronic obstructive sleep apnea could cause:

   a. sinus infection   **b.** hypertension   **c.** cardiac arrest   **d.** lymphedema

4. What causes Mr. Gawlinski's obstructive sleep apnea to occur?

   a. smoking   **b.** carcinoma   **c.** increased neck tissue   **d.** hypoxemia

5. Why is polysomnography done overnight?

   a. The test requires at least 8 hours of monitoring.   **b.** The technicians are only hired for the night shift.

   c. Sleep apnea only occurs in the nighttime hours.   **d.** The test requires monitoring of a typical night's sleep.

B. Deconstruct. *For long or short medical terms, deconstruction into word elements is your key to solving the meaning of the term. If there is no particular element, leave the space blank.* **LO 13.2, 13.5, 13.6**

1. apnea

Rewrite this term, and slash all its elements:

_____ / _____ / _____
P   R/CF   S

2. epiglottitis

Rewrite this term, and slash all its elements:

_____ / _____ / _____
P   R/CF   S

3. aphonia

Rewrite this term, and slash all its elements:

_____ / _____ / _____
P   R/CF   S

C. Define disorders of the larynx. *It is important to discriminate between the different disorders of the larynx. Given the definition, write the condition it is describing.* **LO 13.6**

1. Viral infection of the larynx, trachea, and bronchi. Another term for the condition called croup: _____

2. Inflammation of the larynx: _____

3. Bacterial infection of the epiglottis: _____

D. Build terms. *Knowing just one element will enable you to build more terms with the addition of other elements. Practice building your pulmonology terms with the following root and various prefixes. Fill in the blanks.* **LO 13.2, 13.6**

1. The suffix *-pnea* means _____.

Add the following prefixes to *-pnea* to form new terms for questions 2 through 6.

tachy	brady	dys	eu	hyper

2. Difficult breathing _____pnea

3. Deeper breathing than normal _____pnea

4. Slow breathing _____pnea

5. Normal breathing _____pnea

6. Rapid breathing _____pnea

E. Differentiate between the types of conditions of the pleura. *Word elements indicate major differences in conditions and thus the approach to care of patients. Identify the meanings of the following terms as they relate to abnormal contents of the pleural cavity.* **LO 13.2, 13.6**

1. Abnormal contents of the pleural cavity often contain the suffix:

   a. *osis*   **b.** *pulmon/o*   **c.** *pleur*   **d.** *thorax*

2. An abnormal collection of blood in the pleural cavity contains the combining form:

   a. *hem/o*   **b.** *pleur/o*   **c.** *idi/o*   **d.** *purul/o*

Section 13.5 Procedures and Pharmacology

Pulmonary Diagnostic Procedures

Pulmonary Function Tests

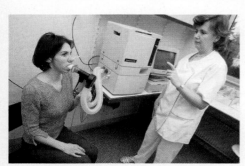

▲ **Figure 13.17** **Spirometer.** Philippe Garo/ Science Source

Many of the diagnostic and therapeutic procedures used in the diagnosis and treatment of respiratory disorders are performed by registered respiratory therapists (RRTs) or respiratory care practitioners under the orders of **pulmonologists** and physicians of other specialties. It is important to understand the medical language used to order, perform, and document these procedures. A **spirometer** is a device used to measure the **volume** of air that moves in and out of the respiratory system *(Figure 13.17)*. You ask the patient to breathe in as deeply as possible and then breathe out as rapidly and completely as possible through the spirometer. The volume of air expired at the end of this **pulmonary function test (PFT)** is the patient's **forced vital capacity (FVC).**

The spirometer also measures **flow rates.** The **forced expiratory volume in 1 second (FEV$_1$)** is the amount of air expired in the first second of the test.

In obstructive lung disorders such as asthma or COPD, the lumina of the airways are constricted and resistant to airflow. This will cause a reduction in the FEV$_1$.

In restrictive lung disorders in which the lung tissue is fibrotic or scarred and resists expansion, there will be a reduction in the FVC.

A **peak flow meter** records the greatest flow of air that can be sustained for 10 milliseconds **(msec)** on forced expiration, the **peak expiratory flow rate (PEFR).** It is of value in following the course of asthma.

Arterial blood gases (ABGs), the measurement of the levels of O_2 and CO_2 in the blood, are good indicators of respiratory function.

Auscultation

The stethoscope is used to detect normal (**vesicular**) and abnormal (**adventitious**) breath sounds. Abnormal breath sounds are categorized as:

- **Wheezes (rhonchi):** musical quality; associated with bronchoconstriction found with asthma. Wheezes are characteristic of asthma.
- **Crackles** (formally known as **rales**): nonmusical, explosive sounds; attributed to the popping opening of the airways with or without the movement of air through secretions in larger airways. Crackles can be auscultated with pneumonia, pulmonary edema, and atelectasis.
- **Pleural rub:** nonmusical sound, often described as a grating or creaking sound. It is caused by the inflamed visceral and parietal pleurae rubbing together, which can occur with pleurisy.
- **Stridor:** loud, high-pitched sound with a musical quality. Associated with constriction of the airways of the upper respiratory tract such as croup.

Word Analysis and Definition: Pulmonary Diagnostic Procedures

S = Suffix   P = Prefix   R = Root   R/CF = Combining Form

WORD	PRONUNCIATION	ELEMENTS		DEFINITION
crackle rale (syn) rales (pl)	**KRAK**-el RAHL RAHLS		*To crack* French *rattle*	Explosive popping sound due to the sudden opening of small airways or air moving through secretions
pleural rub	**PLOOR**-al RUB	S/ R/	**-al** *pertaining to* **pleur-** *pleura* **rub** East Frisian *to rub, scrape*	Grating sound due to pleural membranes rubbing against each other
pulmonary (adj)	**PULL**-moh-**NAIR**-ee	S/ R/	**-ary** *pertaining to* **pulmon-** *lung*	Pertaining to the lungs and their blood supply
pulmonology	**PULL**-moh-**NOL**-oh-jee	S/ R/CF	**-logy** *study of* **pulmon/o-** *lung*	Study of the lungs, or the medical speciality of disorders of the respiratory tract
pulmonologist	**PULL**-moh-**NOL**-oh-jist	S/	**-logist** *one who studies, specialist*	Medical specialist in pulmonary disorders
rhonchus rhonchi (pl) *wheeze* (syn)	**RONG**-kuss **RONG**-key		Greek *snoring*	Wheezing sound heard on auscultation of the lungs, made by air passing through a constricted lumen
spirometer	spy-**ROM**-eh-ter	R/CF R/	**spir/o-** *to breathe* **-meter** *measure*	An instrument used to measure respiratory volumes
stridor	**STRIE**-door		Latin *a harsh, creaking sound*	High-pitched noise made when there is respiratory obstruction in the larynx or trachea
wheeze wheezes (pl)	WEEZ		Old English *action of blowing*	Musical sound of the airways associated with asthma

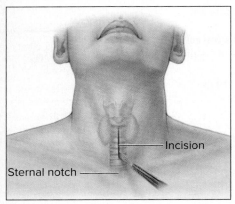

① Tracheotomy incision is made superior to sternal notch.

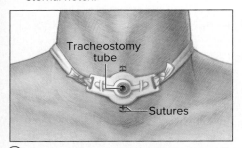

② A tracheostomy tube is inserted, and the remaining incision is sutured closed.

▲ **Figure 13.18** **Tracheostomy procedure.** Carolyn Cole/Los Angeles Times/ Getty Images

Diagnostic Procedures

Chest x-ray (CXR) is a radiograph image of the chest taken in **anteroposterior (AP)**, **posteroanterior (PA)**, lateral, and sometimes oblique and lateral decubitus positions.

Computed tomography (CT), **angiography** of the pulmonary circulation using contrast materials, **magnetic resonance angiography (MRA)** to define emboli in the pulmonary arteries, and **ultrasonography** of the pleural space are chest imaging techniques in current use. **Positron emission tomography (PET)** can sometimes distinguish benign from malignant lesions.

Bronchoscopy is the insertion of a fiber-optic endoscope (called a **bronchoscope**) into the bronchial tree to visually examine it, take a tissue biopsy, or take a wash for secretions.

Mediastinoscopy is used to stage lung cancer and diagnose mediastinal masses. The mediastinoscope is inserted through an incision in the sternal notch.

Tracheal aspiration uses a soft catheter that allows brushings and washings to be performed to remove cells and secretions from the trachea and main bronchi. It can be passed throuᵧh a tracheostomy, **endotracheal** tube, or the mouth or nose.

Thoracentesis is the insertion of a needle through an intercostal space to remove fluid from a pleural effusion for laboratory study or to relieve pressure. It is also called a **pleural tap.**

Thoracotomy is used to obtain an open biopsy of tissue from the lung, hilum, pleura, or mediastinum. It is performed through an intercostal incision under general anesthesia.

In many disorders of the lower respiratory tract, during auscultation of the chest, the air bubbling through abnormal fluid in the alveoli and small bronchioles (as in pulmonary edema) produces a noise called **rales**. When the bronchi are partly obstructed and air is being forced past an obstruction, a high-pitched noise called a rhonchus is heard.

Therapeutic Procedures

Rhinoplasty is a surgical procedure to alter the size and/or shape of the nose.

Cautery (burning and scarring) with silver nitrate or electrical cautery treats epistaxis if pinching the nose or packing the nostril with gauze does not stop the bleeding.

Pulmonary rehabilitation includes education, breathing retraining, exercises for the upper and lower extremities, and psychosocial support.

Nutritional support is critical for patients who have difficulty breathing or who lose a lot of weight.

Immunizations are available against influenza and the pneumococcus bacterium, the most common cause of bacterial pneumonia.

Postural drainage therapy (PDT) uses gravity to promote drainage of secretions from lung segments by positioning and tilting the patient. Chest percussion (tapping) can help loosen, mobilize, and drain the retained secretions.

Continuous positive airway pressure (CPAP) and **Bi-level positive airway pressure (BiPAP)** apply pressure to airways through a mask or nose piece. CPAP provides the one pressure during inhalation and exhalation; BiPAP provides different pressures during inhalation and exhalation.

CPAP and BiPAP is used at home for obstructive sleep apnea (OSA).

Noninvasive ventilation is the application of CPAP or BiPAP to avoid invasive mechanical ventilation in acute respiratory failure or COPD exacerbation. This application is performed by a health care professional.

Mechanical ventilation is a process by which gases are moved into and out of the lungs via a device that is set to meet the respiratory requirements of the patient. It requires that a tracheostomy tube or endotracheal tube be attached to the mechanical ventilator. It can augment or replace the patient's own ventilatory efforts.

Endotracheal intubation involves visualizing the larynx with a **laryngoscope** to aid in the placement of a tube into the trachea. This allows patients to be placed on a ventilator and their breathing controlled. Endotracheal intubation and mechanical ventilation are used when the patient is unable to adequately ventilate on his or her own, such as when the patient is paralyzed, has ARDS, has a significant lung infection, or has a COPD or asthma exacerbation.

Tracheotomy is an incision made into the trachea (windpipe) so that a temporary or permanent opening into the windpipe, called a **tracheostomy,** can be created *(Figure 13.18)*. A tracheostomy tube is placed into the opening to provide an airway. A tracheostomy is used to maintain an airway when there is obstruction or paralysis in the respiratory structures above it and for long-term ventilation.

Pulmonary resection is the surgical removal of lung tissue.

Wedge resection is the removal of a small localized area of diseased lung.

Segmentectomy is the removal of lung tissue attached to a bronchus.

Lobectomy is the removal of a lobe.

Pneumonectomy is the removal of an entire lung.

Word Analysis and Definition: Therapeutic Procedures

S = Suffix   P = Prefix   R = Root   R/CF = Combining Form

WORD	PRONUNCIATION		ELEMENTS	DEFINITION
bronchoscope	**BRONG**-koh-skope	S/	-scope *instrument for viewing*	Endoscope used for bronchoscopy
bronchoscopy	brong-**KOS**-koh-pee	R/CF S/	bronch/o- *bronchus* -scopy *to examine*	Examination of the interior of the tracheo-bronchial tree with an endoscope
cautery	**KAW**-ter-ee		Greek *a branding iron*	Agent or device used to burn or scar a tissue
endotracheal	en-doh-**TRAY**-kee-al	S/ P/ R/	-al *pertaining to* endo- *inside* -trache- *trachea*	Pertaining to being inside the trachea
laryngoscope	lah-**RING**-oh-skope	R/CF S/	laryng/o- *larynx* -scope *instrument for viewing*	Hollow tube with a light and camera used to visualize or operate on the larynx
lobectomy	loh-**BEK**-toh-mee	S/ R/	-ectomy *surgical excision* lob- *lobe*	Surgical removal of a lobe of the lungs
mediastinoscopy	**MEE**-dee-ass-tih-**NOS**-koh-pee	S/ P/ R/CF	-scopy *to examine* media- *middle* stin/o- *partition*	Examination of the mediastinum using an endoscope
pneumonectomy	**NEW**-moh-**NEK**-toh-mee	S/ R/	-ectomy *surgical excision* pneumon- *lung, air*	Surgical removal of a lung
resection resect (verb)	ree-**SEK**-shun ree-**SEKT**	S/ P/ R/	-ion *action* re- *back* -sect- *cut off*	Removal of a specific part of an organ or structure
rhinoplasty	**RYE**-noh-plas-tee	S/ R/CF	-plasty *surgical repair* rhin/o- *nose*	Surgical procedure to change the size or shape of the nose
segmentectomy	seg-men-**TEK**-toh-mee	S/ R/	-ectomy *surgical excision* segment- *a section*	Surgical excision of a segment of a tissue or organ
thoracentesis pleural tap (syn)	**THOR**-ah-sen-**TEE**-sis	S/ R/	-centesis *to puncture* thora- *chest*	Insertion of a needle into the pleural cavity to withdraw fluid or air
thoracotomy	thor-ah-**KOT**-oh-mee	S/ R/CF	-tomy *surgical incision* thorac/o- *chest*	Incision through the chest wall
tomography	toh-**MOG**-rah-fee	S/ R/CF	-graphy *process of recording* tom/o- *section*	Radiographic image of a selected slice or section of tissue
tracheostomy tracheotomy	tray-kee-**OST**-oh-mee tray-kee-**OT**-oh-mee	S/ R/CF S/	-stomy *new opening* trache/o- *trachea* -tomy *surgical incision*	Surgical opening into the windpipe, through which a tube can be inserted to assist breathing Incision made into the trachea to create a tracheostomy
ultrasonography	**UL**-trah-soh-**NOG**-rah-fee	S/ P/ R/CF	-graphy *process of recording* ultra- *beyond* -son/o- *sound*	Delineation of deep structures using sound waves

Respiratory Drugs

Respiratory infections are treated with antibiotics or nothing if viral.

Oxygen is used in hypoxia and can be given by nasal **cannula** or by mask. Patients with severe COPD can be attached to a portable oxygen cylinder.

Aerosol therapy is the administration of a mist to be breathed into the airway. Nasal pumps deliver aerosol to the nasal passages and sinuses. For inhalation into the lungs, aerosol can be delivered via DPI, MDI, or nebulizer. A DPI allows for the patient to inhale a dry medicated powder into the lungs. An MDI delivers a premeasured puff of medicated mist for oral inhalation. A nebulizer creates an aerosol mist via compressed air. The mist may contain medication or can be composed of sterile water, which can be administered to soothe the upper airway, as in the treatment of croup.

Decongestants via nasal pump oxymetazoline (*Afrin*) are used to relieve nasal congestion by producing local vasoconstriction. **Pseudoephedrine** (*Sudafed*) or **phenylephrine** (*Sudafed PE*) are tablets that are nasal decongestants.

Leukotriene receptor antagonists, such as montelukast (*Singulair*), reduces airway swelling and mucus production due to allergies.

Benralizumab (*Fasenra*) treats eosinophilic asthma.

Glucocorticosteroids These medications can be inhaled into the nose to decrease swelling due to allergies fluticasone (*Flonase*), or orally to reduce airway inflammation in asthma, providing improvement in symptoms. Examples are beclomethasone dipropionate (*QVAR*), budesonide DPI (*Pulmicort DPI*), and fluticasone propionate (*Flovent HFA, Flovent Diskus*).

Bronchodilators relax bronchial smooth muscles. This decreases resistance in the airway, increases airflow to the lungs, and increases the forced expiratory volume in one second (FEV_1).

COPD and asthma are treated with a combination of short-acting, long-acting, corticosteroids, immunotherapy. Choice of medication and delivery method is decided between the patient and health care provider.

β_2-receptor agonists and anticholinergics relax the smooth muscles of the airways by different mechanisms. Short-acting medications provide quick relief for 4–6 hours; long-acting medications provide relief for 12–24 hours.

Short acting β_2-receptor agonists (SABAs) include albuterol (*salbutamol, Proventil,* or *Ventolin*) and levalbuterol (*Xopenex*).

Long-acting β_2-receptor agonists (LABAs) include arformoterol (*Brovana*), formoterol (*Foradil, Perforomist*), and salmeterol (*Serevent*).

Short-acting anticholinergic (SAMA)—ipratropium bromide (*Atrovent*)

Long-acting anticholinergics (LAMAs) aclidinium (*Tudorza Pressair*), tiotropium (*Spiriva Handihaler DPI* or *Spiriva Respimat* as a mist).

Combination medications contain more than one classification of medication in one device. Examples are albuterol and ipratropium bromide (*Combivent Respimat*), fluticasone and salmeterol (*Advair Diskus*), beclomethasone, formoterol, and glycopyrronium (*Trimbow*).

Expectorants increase the amount of hydration of bronchial secretions and as a byproduct lubricate an irritated respiratory tract. **Guaifenesin** is an expectorant available in many cough syrups, tablets, and caplets.

Mucolytics break down the chemical structure of mucus molecules so that the mucus becomes thinner and can be removed more easily by coughing. There are several mucolytic agents: **erdosteine** (Erdostin, Mucotec), **acetylcysteine** (Mucomyst, Bronkyl, Fluimucil), and **carbocysteine** (Mucodyne). **Dornase alfa** (*Pulmozyme*) breaks down excess DNA in mucus that is only seen in patients with cystic fibrosis.

Word Analysis and Definition: Respiratory Drugs

S = Suffix   P = Prefix   R = Root   R/CF = Combining Form

WORD	PRONUNCIATION		ELEMENTS	DEFINITION
aerosol	**AIR**-oh-sol	S/ R/CF	-sol *solution* aer/o- *air*	Stable liquid suspension intended for use by inhalation
agonist	**AG**-on-ist		Greek *contest*	Agent that combines with receptors on cells to initiate drug actions
anticholinergic	**AN**-tee-kohl-ih-**NER**-jik	S/ P/ R/ R/	-ic *pertaining to* anti- *against* -cholin- *choline* -erg- *work*	Antagonistic to the action of parasympathetic nerve fibers
cannula cannulae (pl)	**KAN**-you-lah **KAN**-you-lee		Latin *reed*	Tube inserted into a cavity or blood vessel as a channel for fluid or gases
decongestant	dee-con-**JESS**-tant	S/ P/ R/	-ant *pertaining to* de- *take away* -congest- *accumulation of fluid*	Agent that reduces the swelling and fluid in the nose and sinuses
glucocorticosteroid	**GLU**-koh-**KOR**-tih-koh-**STER**-oyd	S/ R/CF R/CF R/	-oid *resemble* gluc/o- *sugar* -cortic/o- *cortex* -ster- *solid*	Hormone of the adrenal cortex that influences glycogen metabolism and exerts an anti-inflammatory effect
inhalation	in-hah-**LAY**-shun	S/ P/ R/	-ation *process* in- *in* -hal- *breathe*	The act of breathing in—inspiration
inhaler	in-**HALE**-er	S/	-er *agent*	Instrument for delivering medication by inhalation
mucolytic	**MYU**-koh-**LIT**-ik	S/ R/CF R/	-ic *pertaining to* muc/o- *mucus* -lyt- *dissolve*	Agent capable of dissolving or liquefying mucus
nebulizer	**NEB**-you-lize-er	S/ R/	-izer *line of action* nebul- *cloud*	Device used to deliver liquid medicine in a fine mist for inhalation

Check Point Section 13.5

A. Elements. *Work with elements to build your knowledge of the language of pulmonology.* **LO 13.1**

1. The root in the term **rhinitis** means:

   a. shell **b.** inflammation **c.** cavity **d.** nose

2. The suffix in the term **tracheotomy** means:

   a. new opening **b.** surgical incision **c.** windpipe **d.** voice box

3. The prefix in the term **paranasal** means:

   a. above **b.** nose **c.** adjacent to **d.** pertaining to

B. Define components of pulmonary function testing (PFT). *Given the description of the PFT result, choose the PFT that it used to help diagnose the respiratory disorder.* **LO 13.5**

1. The measurement used in the evaluation of asthma.

   a. forced vital capacity

   b. peak expiratory flow rate

   c. forced expiratory volume in 1 second

2. If this value is less than 70% of predicted, it indicates the presence of COPD.

   a. forced vital capacity

   b. peak expiratory flow rate

   c. forced expiratory volume in 1 second

3. If this value is less than 70% of predicted, it indicates the presence of restrictive lung disease.

   a. forced vital capacity

   b. peak expiratory flow rate

   c. forced expiratory volume in 1 second

C. Define adventitious breath sounds. *Breath sounds can be used to indicate the presence of disease. Match the adventitious breath sound with its correct description.* **LO 13.5**

_____ **1.** musical sound, indicating narrowing of the lower airways

_____ **2.** grating sound

_____ **3.** explosive, popping sound

_____ **4.** high-pitch sound associated with constricted upper airway

a. stridor

b. crackle

c. pleural rub

d. wheeze

D. Put the following elements into the right combinations to form medical terms for the definitions provided. *Some elements you will use more than once; some elements you will not use at all. Fill in the blanks.* **LO 13.2, 13.7**

endo-	-ectomy	trans-	bronch/o-	-trache/o-	-ion
lob-	-al	-ator	pharyng/e-	pneumon-	immuniz-
-ation	-son/o-	-tomy	-trache-	in-	-scopy
-sect-	ultra-	re-	thorac/o-	-stomy	ventil-
-graphy	-ic	-stomy	hyper-	tom/o	

1. Surgical removal of a lung _____
2. Examination of a bronchus _____
3. Radiographic image of a selected slice of tissue _____
4. Image of deep structures using sound waves _____
5. Pertaining to being inside the trachea _____
6. Removal of a specific part of an organ _____
7. Incision through the chest wall _____
8. New opening in the neck to the trachea _____

E. Medications used in the treatment of respiratory diseases have different mechanisms of action. *Respiratory medications act by increasing the internal size of the airway or by helping to clear mucus from the body. Identify the mechanism of action of the following medications. Some questions have more than one correct answer as indicated. Answers can be used more than once.* **LO 13.7**

decongestant   anticholinergic   β agonist   mucolytic   glucocorticosteroid

1. Thins the mucus. _____

2. Relaxes bronchial smooth muscles. (choose 2 answers) _____

3. Reduces swelling in the upper and lower airways. _____

4. Used to treat swelling in the nose and sinuses. (choose 2 answers) _____

F. Identify the devices that deliver medications to the respiratory airways. *Match the devices on the left with their correct description on the right.* **LO 13.7, 13.9**

1. nasal pump _____   a. delivers mist via compressed air

2. MDI _____   b. creates a dry powder for inhalation

3. nebulizer _____   c. generates a premeasured puff of wet aerosol for oral inhalation

4. DPI _____   d. used to administer aerosol to the nasal airways and sinuses

Table 13.1 Chapter 13 Abbreviations

ABG	arterial blood gas	**MDI**	metered dose inhaler
AP	anteroposterior	**MRA**	magnetic resonance angiography
ARDS	acute respiratory distress syndrome	**msec**	millisecond
ARF	acute respiratory failure	**NRDS**	neonatal respiratory distress syndrome
BP	blood pressure	**O$_2$**	oxygen
CAO	chronic airway obstruction	**OSA**	obstructive sleep apnea
CF	cystic fibrosis	**PA**	posteroanterior
CHF	congestive heart failure	**PDT**	postural drainage therapy
CO$_2$	carbon dioxide	**PEEP**	positive endexpiratory pressure
COPD	chronic obstructive pulmonary disease	**PEFR**	peak expiratory flow rate
CPAP	continuous positive airway pressure	**PET**	positron emission tomography
CXR	chest Xray	**PFT**	pulmonary function test
DPI	dry powder inhaler	**RRT**	registered respiratory therapists
FEV1	forced expiratory volume in 1 second	**SABA**	shortacting β2 receptor agonist
FVC	forced vital capacity	**SAMA**	Short-acting anticholinergic
LABA	longacting β2 receptor agonist	**SOB**	shortness of breath
LAMA	Long-acting anticholinergic	**URI**	upper respiratory infection
LTB	laryngotracheobronchitis	**VS**	vital signs

Table 13.2 Comparison of Selected Respiratory Disorders - Signs, Symptoms, and Treatments

Disorder or Disease	Signs and Symptoms	Diagnostic Tests	Treatment
Asthma	Dyspnea, short of breath, wheezing, cough	PFTs, peak flow meter, auscultation	Long acting bronchodilator, inhaled glucocorticoid, benralizumab, short-acting bronchodilators when needed
COPD	Dyspnea, shortness of breath, wheezing, difficulty exhaling	PFTS, auscultation	Long-acting anticholinergic, inhaled glucocorticoid, short-acting bronchodilators when needed
Pneumonia	Crackles, rhonchi	Chest x-ray, sputum sample for culture to determine type of infection.	Antibiotics, bronchodilators as needed, oxygen as needed
Obstructive sleep apnea	Snoring, periods of sleep apnea, not feeling rested	Sleeping test that can be administered at home or at sleep clinic	CPAP or BiPAP device
Papilloma of the larynx	hoarse voice	viewing with laryngoscope	Removal with laryngoscope

2014 Nucleus Medical Media

Respiratory System

Challenge Your Knowledge

A. **Plurals.** Refresh your memory for the rules of plurals with this exercise. Fill in the chart with the plural. **LO 13.3**

Medical Term	Plural
1. alveolus	
2. cilium	
3. bronchus	
4. concha	
5. naris	

B. **Spelling.** The following terms come directly from Latin and Greek. Choose the correct spelling based on the definition following the numbers. Select the best answer. **LO 13.3**

1. reed	**a.** cannula	**b.** canula	**c.** canulla
2. passage	**a.** miatus	**b.** meatis	**c.** meatus
3. shell	**a.** conca	**b.** conka	**c.** concha
4. branding iron	**a.** cautiry	**b.** cautery	**c.** cautary
5. lack of breath	**a.** apenea	**b.** apnea	**c.** apnia
6. throat	**a.** pharynix	**b.** parynix	**c.** pharynx
7. ring	**a.** cricoid	**b.** crickoid	**c.** crecoid
8. creaking sound	**a.** strideor	**b.** stridore	**c.** stridor
9. oblong shield	**a.** thyrhoid	**b.** thiroyd	**c.** thyroid
10. nerves enter and leave this area	**a.** hylum	**b.** hilum	**c.** hylim

C. **Pharmacology.** For any body system, it is important to know the various types of medications and when they might be prescribed. Demonstrate your knowledge of pharmacology for the respiratory system by assigning the correct drug category in the right column to the statements in the left column. *Answers may be used more than once.* The first one has been done for you. **LO 13.7**

___d___ 1. Example: penicillin   **a.** bronchodilators

_____ 2. Relax smooth muscles of the bronchioles   **b.** anti-inflammatories

_____ 3. Corticosteroids   **c.** mucolytics

_____ 4. Used in hypoxia   **d.** antibiotics

_____ 5. Used when a bacterial infection is present   **e.** O_2

_____ 6. Best given by inhalation

_____ 7. Administered by nasal cannula

_____ 8. Breaks up mucus

D. Language of pulmonology. You are a new student in the Respiratory Therapy program. The following questions contain terminology you will use every day on the job. Select the answer that correctly completes each statement. **LO 13.1, 13.6, 13.7**

1. **Cyanosis** signals deficient oxygenation of blood and will turn nail beds
   - **a.** yellow
   - **b.** red
   - **c.** black
   - **d.** white
   - **e.** blue

2. A shell-shaped bone in the nose is the
   - **a.** meatus
   - **b.** concha
   - **c.** nares
   - **d.** vestibule
   - **e.** choana

3. Which of the following medical terms can be associated with mucopurulent discharge?
   - **a.** pleurisy
   - **b.** sinusitis
   - **c.** epistaxis
   - **d.** pneumonia
   - **e.** nasal polyps

4. A segment of the chest wall separates from the rest of the thoracic cage in
   - **a.** pneumoconiosis
   - **b.** epiglottitis
   - **c.** flail chest
   - **d.** thoracentesis
   - **e.** ARF

5. Surgical repair of the nose is
   - **a.** rhinoplasty
   - **b.** thoracentesis
   - **c.** tracheostomy
   - **d.** lobectomy

E. Construct terms. The suffix -itis is one that you will meet over and over again in this book. Build the correct medical term to match its definition. Fill in the blanks. **LO 13.2, 13.6**

1. inflammation of the bronchus _____itis
2. inflammation of the organ of voice production _____itis
3. inflammation of the tonsils _____itis
4. inflammation of the throat _____itis
5. inflammation of the nose _____itis
6. inflammation of the epiglottis _____itis
7. croup _____itis
8. inflammation of the small bronchioles _____itis
9. inflammation of the lung parenchyma _____itis

F. Analyze. Knowledge of medical terms includes choosing the correct term for the meaning you want to convey either verbally or in documentation. Analyze the suffixes to help you choose the term. Use the following medical terms to fill in the statements, all relating to the bronchus. Fill in the blanks. **LO 13.1, 13.6**

bronchogenic	bronchi	bronchopneumonia	bronchioles	bronchiolitis
bronchus	bronchial asthma	bronchial	bronchitis	bronchiectasis

1. Greek word for *windpipe:* _____

2. Plural of the word bronchus: _____

3. Pertaining to the windpipe: _____

4. Tertiary bronchi divide into these: _____

5. Inflammation of the bronchus: _____

6. Abnormal dilation of bronchioles due to repeated infections: _____

7. Infection in the bronchioles that usually spreads to the alveoli: _____

8. Inflammation of the bronchioles: _____

9. Recurrent acute episodes of bronchial obstruction due to constriction: _____

10. Arising from a bronchus: _____

Now, using the word elements that follow, build new terms relating to the bronchus. Your root or combining form will still be bronch/o-.

	stenosis	plasty
scope	pathy	pulmonary
dilation	scopy	dilator
		gram

11. An instrument used to see into the bronchus: _____

12. Drug meant to open bronchial passages: _____

13. Surgical procedure for plastic repair on a bronchus: _____

14. Any disease of a bronchus: _____

15. Pertaining to the bronchus and the lung: _____

16. Widening the area of the bronchus: _____

17. The procedure of looking into the bronchus: _____

18. Constriction or narrowing of the bronchus: _____

19. The record obtained by bronchography: _____

G. Deconstruct the following terms, and then answer the following questions. **LO 13.2**

Medical Term	Prefix	Root/Combining Form	Suffix
empyema	1.	2.	3.
mesothelioma	4.	5.	6.
expectorate	7.	8.	9.

Choose the correct preceding terms to complete the following sentences. Use the terms that you deconstructed above.

10. Cancer arising from the cells lining the pleura _____.

11. Pleural effusion containing pus is also termed _____.

12. To cough up and spit out mucus _____.

H. **Trace the pathway.** The tracheobronchial tree begins with the trachea, which starts air on its pathway all the way down to the alveoli, where gas exchange can occur. Trace this path by sequentially lettering the following choices A through H. **LO 13.1**

1. Each secondary bronchus divides into tertiary bronchi.   _____

2. Terminal bronchioles divide into several alveoli.   _____

3. Bronchi enter the lung at the hilum.   _____

4. Bronchioles divide into terminal bronchioles.   _____

5. Main bronchi divide into a secondary bronchus for each lobe.   _____

6. Tertiary bronchi divide into bronchioles.   _____

7. At the carina, the trachea divides into right and left main bronchi.   _____

8. The trachea starts air on the pathway to the alveoli.   _____

I. **Test-taking skills.** Employ your test-taking skills when you answer multiple-choice questions. Start by reading the question and ALL the answers. Immediately eliminate answers you know to be incorrect. With the choices you have left, one answer will clearly be the *best* choice. Select the answer that correctly completes the statement or answers the question. **LO 13.1, 13.5**

1. The hairlike structures in the nasal cavity are called

    a. polyps

    b. cilia

    c. adenoids

    d. bullae

    e. trachealis

2. What is the total number of lobes in *both* lungs?

    a. 4

    b. 5

    c. 6

    d. 2

    e. 3

3. What exactly is a lobe?

   a. an opening into an organ

   b. an exit from an organ

   c. a subdivision of an organ

   d. a blood reservoir in an organ

   e. a pathway through an organ

4. An instrument used to measure breathing volume is called

   a. bronchoscope

   b. spirometer

   c. endoscope

   d. tonometer

   e. sphygmomanometer

5. What is surfactant?

   a. creates surface tension

   b. a mucous membrane

   c. keeps a muscle from collapsing

   d. a subcutaneous lesion

   e. a place where two bones meet to make a joint

J. **Use your knowledge of the language of respiration to answer the following questions.** Select the answer that correctly completes the statement or answers the question. **LO 13.1, 13.5, 13.6**

1. The measure of the capacity of a chamber or hollow viscus to expand is called

   a. expectorate   d. postural drainage

   b. idiopathic   e. consolidation

   c. compliance

2. Which of the following is another name for the nasal **conchae** on the lateral wall of each nasal cavity?

   a. meatus   d. turbinates

   b. choana   e. septum

   c. nares

3. A bubblelike structure is called a

   a. bronchiole   d. bronchus

   b. barbiturate   e. bradypnea

   c. bulla

4. The sense of smell is

    a. external respiration

    b. aspiration

    c. internal respiration

    d. exhalation

    e. olfaction

5. Which of the following is another term for heart failure?

    a. cyanosis

    b. conchae

    c. choana

    d. cor pulmonale

    e. chordae tendineae

6. Laryngeal polyps are

    a. benign tumors of the larynx

    b. localized infection of the larynx

    c. papillomas

    d. malignant tumors of the trachea

    e. verruca in the larynx

7. The medical term for the nostrils is

    a. nares

    b. adenoids

    c. polyps

    d. tonsils

    e. papillomas

K. **Define abbreviations that relate to the respiratory system.** Match the definition in the first column to the correct abbreviation in the second column **LO 13.9**

Disease	Abbreviation
_____ **1.** common cold	**a.** COPD
_____ **2.** dyspnea	**b.** CF
_____ **3.** CAO is also called	**c.** SOB
_____ **4.** condition is inherited	**d.** ARF
_____ **5.** sudden, life-threatening lung failure	**e.** URI

L. **Diagnostic and therapeutic procedures are performed for different reasons.** Use the language of pulmonology to identify their medical terminology. Select letter **a** if the term is a diagnostic procedure; letter **b** if the term is a therapeutic procedure. **LO 13.5, 13.7, 13.9**

1. intubation

   a. diagnostic

   b. therapeutic

2. PDT

   a. diagnostic

   b. therapeutic

3. tracheotomy

   a. diagnostic

   b. therapeutic

4. CXR

   a. diagnostic

   b. therapeutic

5. mediastinoscopy

   a. diagnostic

   b. therapeutic

6. CT

   a. diagnostic

   b. therapeutic

7. bronchoscopy

   a. diagnostic

   b. therapeutic

M. **Pronunciation is important whether you are saying the word or listening to a word from a coworker.** Identify the proper pronunciation of the following medical terms. Correctly spell the term. **LO 13.3, 13.4, 13.5, 13.6, 13.7**

1. The correct pronunciation for the inflammation of the pleura

   a. PLOOR-is-see

   b. PLOOR-it-is

   c. KOR-ee-zah

   d. koh-**RYE**-zah

      Correctly spell the term: _____

2. The correct pronunciation for the region of the pharynx below the epiglottis that

3. includes the larynx

   a. LAIR-ink-oh-**FAIR**-inks

   b. lah-**RING**-oh-**FAIR**-inks

   c. NAY-zoh-**FAIR**-inks

   d. NOH-zoh-**FAIR**-inks

      Correctly spell the term: _____

4. The correct pronunciation for the process of breathing out

    a. IN-spy-eh-**RAY**-shun

    b. in-spih-**RAY**-shun

    c. EKS-pie-er-**AY**-shun

    d. EKS-pih-**RAY**-shun

        Correctly spell the term: _____

5. The correct pronunciation explosive popping sound due to the suddenopening of small airways or air moving through secretions

    a. RAILS

    b. RAHLS

    c. RONG-key

    d. RONG-kih

        Correctly spell the term: _____

6. The correct pronunciation for the term that agent capable of dissolving or liquefying mucus

    a. MYU-koh-**LIT**-ik

    b. MYU-cool-**IT**-ik

    c. AG-on-ist

    d. AYG-on-ist

        Correctly spell the term: _____

Case Reports

A. Interpretation. Use your knowledge of the **language of pulmonology** to understand the Case Report and answer the following questions. **LO 13.4, 13.6, 13.7, 13.9, 13.10**

Case Report 13.2

You are

. . . an advanced-level RRT working in the Acute Respiratory Care Unit of Fulwood Medical Center with pulmonologist Tavis Senko, MD.

Your patient is

. . . Mr. Jude Jacobs, a 68-year-old white retired mail carrier, who is known to have COPD and is on continual oxygen by nasal prongs. He has smoked two packs a day for his adult life. Last night, he was unable to sleep because of increased shortness of breath and cough. His cough produced yellow sputum. He had to sit upright in bed to be able to breathe.

VS are T 101.6°F, P 98, R 36, BP 150/90. On examination, he is cyanotic and frightened and has nasal prongs in his nose. Air entry is diminished in both lungs, and there are crackles at both bases. You have been ordered to draw blood for ABGs and to measure the amount of air entering and leaving his lungs by using spirometry.

Mr. Jacobs' FEV_1 was only 40% of the predicted value for a man of his age, height, and weight. Mr. Jacobs' FVC also was reduced because of the fibrotic effects of repeated infections on his lung tissues reducing the volume in his airways. When he was off O_2, Mr. Jacobs' O_2 levels were below 50% of normal. Even with nasal prongs and the administration of O_2, his blood O_2 levels were only 75% of normal.

1. What is your profession?

   a. nurse

   b. physical therapist

   c. physician

   d. respiratory therapist

2. What is another name for nasal "prongs"?

   a. cannula

   b. ventilator

   c. respirator

   d. intubation

3. The medical term for "shortness of breath" is

   a. tachypnea

   b. apnea

   c. dyspnea

   d. eupnea

4. The yellow sputum is indicative of

   a. asthma

   b. bacterial infection

   c. atelectasis

   d. pleurisy

5. Cyanosis may indicate

   a. decreased oxygen in the blood

   b. he has a barrel chest

   c. increased heart rate

   d. increased carbon dioxide in the blood

6. An ABG comes from

   a. pleural fluid

   b. exhaled air

   c. arterial blood

   d. sputum analysis

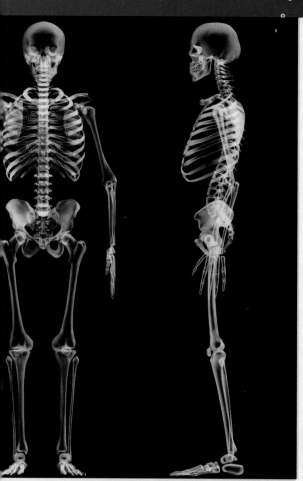

alengo/E+/Getty Images

Chapter Sections

14.1 Functions of the Skeletal System and Joints

14.2 The Axial and Appendicular Skeleton

14.3 Disorders and Injuries of Skeleton System

14.4 Procedures and Pharmacology

Skeletal System
Language of Orthopedics

Chapter Learning Outcomes

Upon completion of this chapter, you will be able to:

LO 14.1   Identify and describe the anatomy and physiology of the skeletal system.

LO 14.2   Use roots, combining forms, suffixes, and prefixes to construct and analyze medical terms related to the skeletal system.

LO 14.3   Spell medical terms related to the skeletal system.

LO 14.4   Pronounce medical terms related to the skeletal system.

LO 14.5   Describe diagnostic procedures utilized for injuries and disorders of the skeletal system.

LO 14.6   Identify and describe injuries, disorders, and pathological conditions related to the skeletal system.

LO 14.7   Describe the therapeutic procedures and pharmacologic agents used with the skeletal system.

LO 14.8   Apply knowledge of medical terms relating to the skeletal system to documentation, medical records, and communication.

LO 14.9   Identify and correctly use abbreviations of terms used that refer to the skeletal system.

LO 14.10   Identify health professionals involved in the care of patients with skeletal injuries and disorders.

Many health professionals that treat the skeletal system also treat the muscular system. Many of the professions below, you will see discussed in both *Chapters 14 and 15*. These professions include:

- **Orthopedic surgeons (orthopedists),** physicians who deal with the prevention, correction, disorders, and injuries of the skeletal system.
- **Osteopathic physicians,** who have earned a doctorate in **osteopathy** (**DO**) and receive additional training in the skeletal system and how it affects the whole body.
- **Physiatrists,** who are physicians specializing in physical medicine and rehabilitation.
- **Chiropractors (DCs),** who focus on the manual adjustments of joints—particularly the spine—to maintain and restore health.
- **Physical therapists (PT),** diagnose and treat injuries, disabilities, or other health conditions to improve a patient's ability to move, reduce pain, restore function, and prevent disability.
- **Physical therapist assistants (PTA),** assist physical therapists in the treatment of patients.
- **Orthopedic technologists** and **technicians,** who assist orthopedic surgeons in treating patients.
- **Podiatrists,** who are practitioners in the diagnosis and treatment of disorders and injuries of the foot.
- **Orthotists,** who make and fit orthopedic appliances (**orthotics**).

Section 14.1 Functions of the Skeletal System

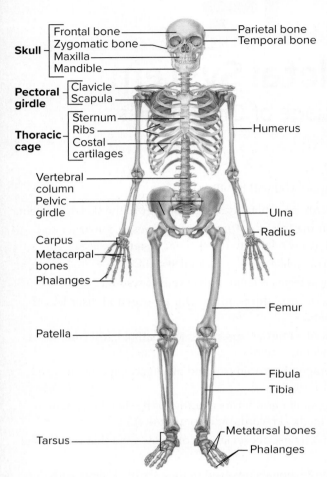

Skull —
Frontal bone
Zygomatic bone
Maxilla
Mandible

Parietal bone
Temporal bone

Pectoral girdle —
Clavicle
Scapula

Thoracic cage —
Sternum
Ribs
Costal cartilages

Humerus

Vertebral column
Pelvic girdle

Ulna
Radius

Carpus
Metacarpal bones
Phalanges

Femur

Patella

Fibula
Tibia

Tarsus

Metatarsal bones
Phalanges

▲ **Figure 14.1** Adult skeleton: Anterior view.

Did you know...

Bones are divided into four classes based on their shape: long, short, flat, and irregular.

Functions of the Skeletal System

If you didn't have a skeleton, you'd be like a rag doll, shapeless and unable to move. Your skeleton provides support, protects many organ systems, and is the landmark for much of medical terminology. For example, the radial artery you use for taking a pulse is so named because it travels beside the radial bone of the forearm. In addition, the surface anatomy of bones and their markings enable you to describe and document the sites of symptoms, signs, and clinical, diagnostic, and therapeutic procedures. The four components of the skeletal system (*Figure 14.1*) are

1. *Bones*
2. *Cartilage*
3. *Tendons*
4. *Ligaments*

The bones provide the following functions:

- **Support.** The bones of your vertebral column, pelvis, and legs hold up your body. The jawbone supports your teeth. **Cartilage** supports your nose, ears, and ribs. **Tendons** support and attach your muscles to bone. **Ligaments** support and hold your bones together.

- **Protection.** The skull protects your brain. The vertebral column protects your spinal cord. The rib cage protects your heart and lungs.

- **Movement. Muscles** could not function without their attachments to skeletal bones, and muscles are responsible for your movements (*see Chapter 15*).

- **Blood formation.** Bone marrow in many bones is the major producer of blood cells, including most of those in your immune system (*see Chapter 12*).

- **Mineral storage and balance.** The skeletal system stores calcium and phosphorus. These are released when your body needs them for other purposes. For example, calcium is needed for muscle contraction (*see Chapter 15*), communication between neurons (*see Chapter 9*), and blood clotting (*see Chapter 11*).

- **Detoxification.** Bones remove metals such as lead and radium from your blood, store them, and slowly release them for excretion.

Word Analysis and Definition: Functions of the Skeletal System

S = Suffix P = Prefix R = Root R/CF = Combining Form

WORD	PRONUNCIATION		ELEMENTS	DEFINITION
cartilage	**KAR**-tih-lij		Latin *gristle*	Nonvascular, firm connective tissue found mostly in joints
detoxification	dee-**TOKS**-ih-fih-**KAY**-shun	S/ P/ R/CF	**-fication** *remove* **de-** *from, out of* **tox/i-** *poison*	Removal of poison from a tissue or substance
ligament	**LIG**-ah-ment		Latin *band, sheet*	Band of fibrous tissue connecting two structures
muscle	**MUSS**-el		Latin *muscle*	Tissue consisting of contractile cells
tendon	**TEN**-dun		Latin *sinew*	Fibrous band that connects muscle to bone

Bone Growth and Structure

Bone Growth

Factors that affect bone growth include:

1. **Genes.** Genes determine the size and shape of bones and the ultimate adult height.
2. **Nutrition.** Calcium and phosphorus are needed to develop good bone density.
3. **Exercise.** Exercise increases bone density and total bone mass.
4. **Mineral deposition.** Calcium and phosphate are taken from plasma and deposited in bone.
5. **Mineral resorption.** Calcium and phosphate are released from bone back into the plasma when they are needed elsewhere. For example, calcium is needed for muscle contraction, communication between neurons, and blood clotting. Phosphate is a component of deoxyribonucleic acid (DNA) and ribonucleic acid (RNA).
6. **Vitamins.** Vitamin A activates **osteoblasts;** vitamin C is essential for collagen synthesis; vitamin D stimulates absorption of calcium and phosphate, its transport, and its deposition into bones.
7. **Hormones.** For example, growth hormone stimulates the epiphyseal plate to calcify, and estrogen and testosterone accelerate bone growth after puberty and maintain bone density *(see Chapter 17).*

Structure of Bones

Long bones are the most common type of bone in the body *(Figure 14.2a).*

The shaft of a long bone is called the **diaphysis.** Each end of the bone is called the **epiphysis** and is expanded to provide extra surface area for the attachment of ligaments and tendons.

Sandwiched between the diaphysis and epiphysis is a thin area called the **metaphysis.** Thin layers of cartilage cells in the **epiphyseal plate** enable the diaphysis (bone shaft) to grow in length. When growth stops, compact bone grows into the epiphyseal plate and forms the **epiphyseal line** *(Figure 14.2b).*

A tough connective tissue sheath called **periosteum** covers the outer surface of all bones and is attached to the compact or **cortical** bone by tough collagen fibers. The periosteum protects the bone and anchors blood vessels and nerves to the surface of the bone.

The hollow cylinder inside the diaphysis is called the **medullary cavity.** It contains bone **marrow** and is lined by a thin membrane called the **endosteum.** The marrow is a fatty tissue that contains blood cells in different stages of development *(see Chapter 11).*

The endosteum and periosteum contain **osteoblasts,** cells that produce the matrix of new bone tissue. This process is called **osteogenesis.** Bone **matrix** consists of cells, collagen fibers, a gel that supports and suspends the fibers, and calcium phosphate crystals that give bone its hardness.

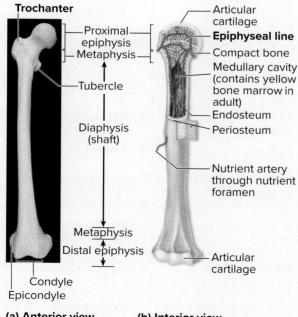

(a) **Anterior view**   (b) **Interior view**

▲ **Figure 14.2** Femur: Long bone of the thigh.

(a) Christine Eckel/McGraw Hill

When osteoblasts are incorporated into the new bone, they become **osteocytes**. These cells, which maintain the matrix, reside in small spaces in the matrix called **lacunae**.

Osteoclasts are produced by the bone marrow. They dissolve calcium, phosphorus, and the organic components of the bone matrix. There is a continual balancing act going on as osteoclasts remove matrix and osteoblasts produce matrix. If osteoclasts outperform the osteoblasts, then **osteoporosis** occurs.

Word Analysis and Definition: Bone Growth and Structure

S = Suffix   P = Prefix   R = Root   R/CF = Combining Form

WORD	PRONUNCIATION		ELEMENTS	DEFINITION
cortex cortical (adj)	**KOR**-teks **KOR**-tih-kal	S/ R/	Latin *bark* -al *pertaining to* cortic- *cortex*	Outer portion of an organ, such as bone Pertaining to the cortex
diaphysis	die-**AF**-ih-sis		Greek *growing between*	The shaft of a long bone
endosteum	en-**DOSS**-tee-um	S/ P/ R/	-um *tissue, structure* end- *within* -oste- *bone*	A membrane of tissue lining the inner (medullary) cavity of a long bone
epiphysis	eh-**PIF**-ih-sis	P/ R/	epi- *upon, above* -physis *growth*	Expanded area at the proximal and distal ends of a long bone that provides increased surface area for attachment of ligaments and tendons
epiphyseal plate	eh-pih-**FIZ**-ee-al PLATE	S/ R/	-eal *pertaining to* -phys- *growth* plate Greek *broad, flat*	Layer of cartilage between epiphysis and metaphysis where bone growth occurs
haversian canals (also called **central canals**)	hah-**VER**-shan ka-**NALS**		Clopton Havers, 1655–1702, English physician	Vascular canals in bone
lacuna lacunae (pl)	la-**KOO**-nah la-**KOO**-nee		Latin *a pit, lake*	Small space or cavity within the matrix of bone
marrow	**MAH**-roh		Old English *marrow*	Fatty, blood-forming tissue in the cavities of long bones
matrix	**MAY**-triks		Latin *mother, womb*	Substance that surrounds cells, is manufactured by cells, and holds them together
medulla medullary (adj)	meh-**DULL**-ah **MED**-ul-ah-ree	S/ R/	Latin *marrow* -ary *pertaining to* medull- *middle*	Central portion of a structure surrounded by cortex Pertaining to the medulla
metaphysis	meh-**TAF**-ih-sis	P/ R/	meta- *beyond, after, subsequent to* -physis *growth*	Region between the diaphysis and the epiphysis where bone growth occurs
osteoblast	**OS**-tee-oh-blast	S/ R/CF	-blast *germ cell* oste/o- *bone*	Bone-forming cell
osteoclast	**OS**-tee-oh-klast	S/ R/CF	-clast *break down* oste/o- *bone*	Bone-removing cell
osteocyte	**OS**-tee-oh-site	S/ R/CF	-cyte *cell* oste/o- *bone*	Bone-maintaining cell
osteogenesis	**OS**-tee-oh-**JEN**-eh-sis	S/ R/CF	-genesis *creation* oste/o- *bone*	Creation of new bone
osteogenic (adj)	**OS**-tee-oh-**JEN**-ik	S/	-genic *producing*	Relating to the creation of new bone
osteoporosis	**OS**-tee-oh-poh-**ROH**-sis	S/ R/CF R/	-osis *condition* oste/o- *bone* -por- *opening*	Condition in which the bones become more porous, brittle, and fragile, and are more likely to fracture
periosteum	**PER**-ee-**OSS**-tee-um	S/ P/ R/	-um *tissue, structure* peri- *around* -oste- *bone*	Strong membrane surrounding a bone
periosteal (adj)	**PER**-ee-**OSS**-tee-al	S/	-al *pertaining to*	Pertaining to the periosteum

All bones are well supplied with blood *(Figure 14.3)*. The blood vessels travel through the bone in a system of small **central (haversian) canals.** Because of its good blood supply, bone heals.

Joints

Classes of Joints

Joints allow you to move, but movable parts that rub together can wear out. Damage or disease in a joint can make movement very difficult and painful. The structure of any joint, or articulation, is directly related to its mobility and function. Joints are classified structurally into three types:

1. **Fibrous** joints are two bones tightly bound together by bands of fibrous tissue with no joint space. They come in three varieties:

   a. **Sutures** occur between the bones of the skull *(Figure 14.4)*; the two opposing bones have interlocking processes to add stability to the joint. The **periosteum** on each of the outer and inner surfaces of the two bones is continuous and holds the joint together.

   b. **Syndesmosis** is a joining of two bones with fibrous ligaments. Their movement is minimal. An example is the joint above the ankle where the tibia and fibula are attached.

   c. **Gomphoses** are pegs that fit into sockets and are held in place by fine collagen fibers. Examples are the joints between teeth and their sockets.

2. **Cartilaginous** joints join two bones with cartilage:

   a. **Synchondroses** join two bones with **hyaline** cartilage, which allows little or no movement between them, as between your ribs and costal cartilages.

   b. **Symphyses** join two bones with **fibrocartilage.** An example is the symphysis pubis, where your two pubic bones meet at the front of your pelvis.

3. **Synovial** joints contain synovial fluid as a lubricant and allow considerable movement *(Figure 14.5)*. Most joints in the legs and arms are synovial joints. The ends of the bones are covered with hyaline **articular** cartilage. In some joints, an additional plate of fibrocartilage is located between the two bones. In the knee, this plate is incomplete and is called a **meniscus.**

A **bursa** is an extension of the synovial joint that forms a cushion between structures that otherwise would rub against each other; for example, in the knee joint between the patellar tendon and the patellar and tibial bones *(Figure 14.5)*.

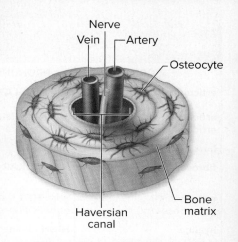

▲ **Figure 14.3** Blood supply to bone.

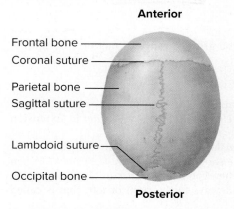

▲ **Figure 14.4** Sutures of skull: Superior view.

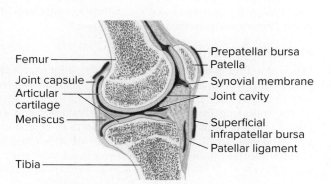

▲ **Figure 14.5** Synovial joint.

WORD	PRONUNCIATION	ELEMENTS		DEFINITION
articulation	ar-tik-you-**LAY**-shun	S/	-ation *process*	A joint
		R/	articul- *joint*	
articulate (verb)	ar-**TIK**-you-late	S/	-ate *pertaining to*	Joint movement
articular (adj)	ar-**TIK**-you-lar	S/	-ar *pertaining to*	Pertaining to a joint
bursa	**BURR**-sah		Latin *purse*	A closed sac containing synovial fluid
fibrocartilage	fie-broh-**KAR**-til-ij	R/CF	fibr/o- *fiber*	Cartilage containing collagen fibers
		R/CF	-cartilag/e *cartilage*	
gomphosis	gom-**FOH**-sis	S/	-osis *condition*	Joint formed by a peg and socket
gomphoses (pl)	gom-**FOH**-sees	R/	gomph- *bolt, nail*	
hyaline	**HIGH**-ah-line		Greek *glass*	Cartilage that looks like frosted glass and contains fine collagen fibers
meniscus	meh-**NISS**-kuss		Greek *crescent*	Disc of connective tissue cartilage between the bones of a joint; for example, in the knee joint
menisci (pl)	meh-**NISS**-kee			
suture	**SOO**-chur		Latin *a seam*	Place where two bones are joined together by a fibrous band continuous with their periosteum, as in the skull
sutures (pl)	**SOO**-churs			Also means to unite two surfaces by sewing; the material used in the sewing together; and the seam formed by the sewing together
symphysis	**SIM**-feh-sis		Greek *growing together*	Two bones joined by fibrocartilage
symphyses (pl)	**SIM**-feh-sees			
synchondrosis	sin-kon-**DROH**-sis	S/	-osis *condition*	A rigid articulation (joint) formed by cartilage
		P/	syn- *together*	
synchondroses (pl)	sin-kon-**DROH**-sees	R/	-chondr- *cartilage*	
syndesmosis	sin-dez-**MOH**-sis	S/	-osis *condition*	An articulation (joint) formed by ligaments
		P/	syn- *together*	
syndesmoses (pl)	sin-dez-**MOH**-sees	R/	-desm- *bind*	
synovial	sih-**NOH**-vee-al	S/	-al *pertaining to*	Pertaining to synovial fluid and synovial membrane
		P/	syn- *together*	
		R/CF	-ov/i- *egg*	

Joint Movement

Joints allow for variety of actions. Synovial joints provide the greatest range of motion through the body. These joint movements are as follows:

Flexion and Extension of Joints

When standing in anatomic position, every joint except the ankle is in extension. For most of the rest of the body, flexion is movement of a body part *anterior* to the **coronal plane** *(see Chapter 3)*. Extension is movement *posterior* to the coronal plane.

The following figures show **flexion** (bending) and **extension** (straightening) in the elbow joint *(Figure 14.6a and b)*, in the wrist joint *(Figure 14.6c–e)*, and in the shoulder joint *(Figure 14.6g and h)*. When you bend your trunk forward, that is flexion *(Figure 14.6f)*. When you bend your trunk backward, that is extension *(see Figure 14.6g)*. When you bend your trunk sideways to the right or left, that is called *lateral flexion.*

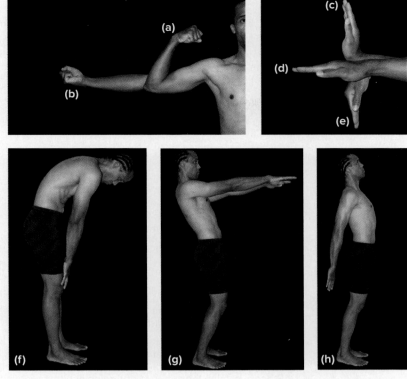

▲ **Figure 14.6 Joint flexion and extension.** (*a*) Flexion of the elbow. (*b*) Extension of the elbow. (*c*) Extension of the wrist. (*d*) Neutral position of the wrist. (*e*) Flexion of the wrist. (*f*) Flexion of the spine. (*g*) Flexion of the shoulder. (*h*) Extension of the shoulder. (a-h) Shaana Pritchard/McGraw Hill

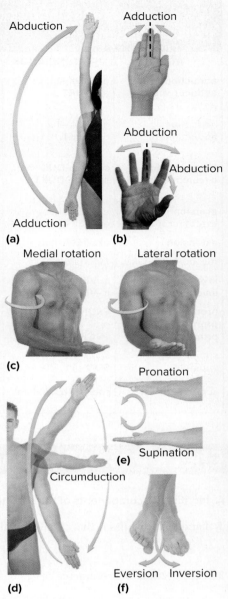

▲ **Figure 14.7 Movement of the limbs.** (*a*) Abduction and adduction of the upper limb. (*b*) Abduction and adduction of the fingers. (*c*) Medial and lateral rotation of the arm. (*d*) Circumduction. (*e*) Pronation and supination of the hand. (*f*) Eversion and inversion of the foot. (a-f) Eric Wise

Abduction and Adduction of Joints

Abduction is movement away from the midline. **Adduction** is movement toward the midline. Abduction of your arm is moving it sideways away from your trunk. Adduction is bringing it back to the side of your trunk *(Figure 14.7a)*. Abduction of your fingers is spreading them apart, away from the middle finger. Adduction is bringing them back together *(Figure 14.7b)*.

Rotation of Joints

Rotation is turning around an axis. Medial rotation of the upper arm bone, the humerus, with the elbow flexed brings the palm of the hand toward the body. Lateral rotation moves the palm away from the body *(Figure 14.7c)*.

Pronation and Supination

When you lie flat on the ground facedown on your belly with your palms touching the ground, you are **prone.** When you lie flat on your back with your spine on the floor and your palms facing up, you are **supine.**

When you rotate your forearm so that your palm faces the floor, that is **pronation.** When you rotate the forearm so that your palm is facing upward, that is **supination** *(Figure 14.7e)*.

Circumduction of Joints

Circumduction of the shoulder is moving it in a circular movement so that it forms a cone, with the shoulder joint as the apex of the cone *(Figure 14.7d)*.

Inversion and Eversion

When you turn your ankle so that the sole of your foot faces toward the opposite foot, that is supination or inversion. When you turn your ankle so that the sole of the foot faces laterally away from the other foot, that is pronation or **eversion** *(Figure 14.7f)*.

S = Suffix P = Prefix R = Root R/CF = Combining Form

WORD	PRONUNCIATION	ELEMENTS		DEFINITION
abduction abduct (verb)	ab-**DUK**-shun ab-**DUKT**	S/ P/ R/	**-ion** *process, action* **ab-** *away from* **-duct-** *lead*	Action of moving away from the midline
adduction adduct (verb)	ah-**DUK**-shun ah-**DUKT**	S/ P/ R/	**-ion** *process, action* **ad-** *toward* **-duct-** *lead*	Action of moving toward the midline
circumduction circumduct (verb)	ser-kum-**DUK**-shun ser-kum-**DUKT**	S/ P/ R/	**-ion** *process, action* **circum-** *around* **-duct-** *lead*	Movement of an extremity in a circular motion
eversion evert (verb)	ee-**VER**-shun ee-**VERT**		Latin *overturn*	A turning outward
extension	eks-**TEN**-shun		Latin *stretch out*	When a joint is straightened to increase its angle
flexion	**FLEK**-shun		Latin *to bend*	When a joint is bent to decrease its angle
inversion invert (verb)	in-**VER**-shun in-**VERT**		Latin *to turn about*	A turning inward
prone (adj) pronation pronate (verb)	PRONE proh-**NAY**-shun **PROH**-nate	 S/ R/	Latin *prone, lying down* **-ion** *process, action* **pronat-** *bend down*	Lying facedown, flat on your belly Process of lying facedown or of turning a hand or foot with the volar (palm or sole) surface down
supine (adj) supinate supination	soo-**PINE** **SOO**-pih-nate soo-pih-**NAY**-shun	 S/ R/	Latin *supine, lying face up* Latin *face up* **-ion** *process, action* **supinat-** *bend backward*	Lying face up, flat on your spine Rotate the forearm so that the surface of the palm faces anteriorly in the anatomical position Process of lying face upward or turning an arm or foot so that the palm or sole is facing up

Check Point Section 14.1

A. Identify the components of the skeletal system and the functions of the bones. *Choose the correct organ or tissue being described.* **LO 14.1**

1. Band of strong tissue that connects two structures (such as bone to bone).

   a. muscle   **b.** ligament   **c.** tendon   **d.** cartilage

2. Tissue containing contractile cells.

   a. muscle   **b.** ligament   **c.** tendon   **d.** cartilage

3. Firm connective tissue found mostly in joints.

   a. muscle   **b.** ligament   **c.** tendon   **d.** cartilage

4. Fibrous band that connects muscle to bone.

   a. muscle   **b.** ligament   **c.** tendon   **d.** cartilage

B. Identify the professionals related to the skeletal system. *Many professionals specialize in different aspects of the care of the skeletal system. It is important to understand their specialty. Refer to the Introduction section of this chapter to assist you in matching the specialty in the first column with its correct description in the second column.* **LO 14.10**

	Term		Meaning
_____	**1.** orthopedist		**a.** treats pain by physical therapeutic measures.
_____	**2.** chiropractor		**b.** treats mechanical disorders of the musculoskeletal system.
_____	**3.** podiatrist		**c.** makes and fits orthopedic devices.
_____	**4.** physical therapist		**d.** specialist in the treatment of the skeletal system.
_____	**5.** orthotist		**e.** specialist in the treatment of disorders and injuries of the feet.

C. The combining form oste/o means "bone" and is the main element in each of the following terms. *You choose the correct suffix to complete the term. Fill in the blanks.* **LO 14.1**

blast   cyte   genesis   clast   genic   porosis

The osteo_____ process begins with osteo_____, which produce the matrix of new bone tissue. Osteo_____ has begun. Once these cells incorporate into new bone, they are termed osteo _____. These cells maintain matrix. Osteo_____ are produced by bone marrow. A delicate balance must be maintained between cells that remove matrix and cells that produce matrix. If more matrix is removed than produced, osteo_____ will result.

D. Critical thinking: *Fill in the blanks.* **LO 14.1**

1. What organic element and vitamin are critical in bone health? _____ and vitamin _____ encourage bone health.

E. It is important to recognize the singular and plural versions of medical terms. *Identify the word as being singular or plural. Select the correct choice.* **LO 14.2, 14.3, 14.4**

1. syndesmoses

    a. singular   **b.** plural

2. suture

    a. singular   **b.** plural

3. gomphosis

    a. singular   **b.** plural

4. menisci

    a. singular   **b.** plural

F. Identify the word elements that compose medical terms. *Knowing the meaning of the word elements helps you to quickly define medical terms. Select the answer that correctly completes each sentence.* **LO 14.1, 14.2**

1. The root in the term *synchondroses* means:

    a. egg   **b.** joint   **c.** cartilage   **d.** seam

2. The prefix in the term *synchondroses* means:

    a. condition   **b.** together   **c.** crescent   **d.** pertaining to

3. The root in the term *syndesmoses* means:

    a. pertaining to   **b.** egg   **c.** bind   **d.** bolt

4. The root in the term *gomphosis* means:

    a. pertaining to   **b.** egg   **c.** bind together   **d.** bolt

G. Some medical terms can act as both a verb (action) and a noun (person, place, or thing). *The following pairs of terms are both verbs and nouns. Write the correct form of each term in the blank.* **LO 14.1, 14.3**

1. circumduct   circumduction

    The baseball pitcher was unable to _____ his arm to wind up his pitch.

2. invert   inversion

    A clubfoot would be an _____ of the foot.

3. abduct   abduction

    Moving away from the midline of the body is called _____.

4. evert   eversion

    The patient was unable to _____ her ankle due to great pain.

5. adduct   adduction

    The patient was asked to _____ his arms from a horizontal plane toward the center of his chest.

H. Translate the following statements that are in layman's terms into medical terminology. *Fill in the blanks.* **LO 14.3**

1. Moving your hand so the palm is facing upward: _____

2. Moving your foot so the sole of the foot is facing inward: _____

3. A patient is being prepared for back surgery. What would be his position on the operating room table? _____

Section 14.2 The Axial and Appendicular Skeleton

Structure of Axial Skeleton

The axial skeleton comprises the

1. Vertebral column   2. Skull   3. Rib cage

The axial skeleton is the upright axis of the body and protects the brain, **spinal** cord, heart, and lungs—most of the major centers of our physiology.

Components of the Vertebral Column

The **vertebral column** has 26 bones divided into five regions *(Figure 14.8)*:

1. **Cervical** region, with seven vertebrae, labeled C1 to C7 and curved anteriorly.
2. **Thoracic** region, with 12 vertebrae, labeled T1 to T12 and curved posteriorly.
3. **Lumbar** region, with five vertebrae, labeled L1 to L5 and curved anteriorly.
4. **Sacral** region, with one bone curved posteriorly.
5. **Coccyx** (tailbone), with one bone curved posteriorly.

The spinal cord lies protected in the vertebral canal. Spinal nerves leave the spinal cord through the **intervertebral foramina** to travel to other parts of the body.

Intervertebral discs consist of fibrocartilage and inhabit the intervertebral space between the bodies of adjacent vertebrae. They provide additional support and cushioning for the vertebral column. The center of the disc is a gelatinous nucleus pulposus.

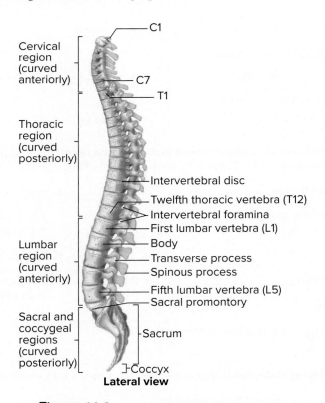

Lateral view

▲ **Figure 14.8** Vertebral column.

WORD	PRONUNCIATION		ELEMENTS	DEFINITION
cervical	SER-vih-kal	S/ R/	-al *pertaining to* cervic- *neck*	Pertaining to the neck region
coccyx	KOK-siks		Greek *coccyx*	Small tailbone at the lowest end of the vertebral column
disc	DISK		Latin or Greek *disk*	Flattened, round structure. In the skeletal system, a flattened round fibrocartilaginous structure between bones
foramen foramina (pl)	foh-RAY-men foh-RAM-in-ah		Latin *an aperture*	An opening through a structure
intervertebral	IN-ter-VER-teh-bral	S/ P/ R/	-al *pertaining to* inter- *between* -vertebr- *vertebra*	Located between two vertebrae
lumbar (adj)	LUM-bar		Latin *loin*	Relating to the region in the back and sides between the ribs and pelvis
sacrum sacral (adj)	SAY-krum SAY-kral	 S/ R/	Latin *sacred* -al *pertaining to* sacr- *sacrum*	Segment of the vertebral column that forms part of the pelvis Pertaining to the sacrum
spine spinal (adj)	SPINE SPY-nal	 S/ R/	Latin *spine* -al *pertaining to* spin- *spine*	Vertebral column, *or* a short projection from a bone Pertaining to the spine
thorax thoracic (adj)	THOR-aks thor-ASS-ik	 S/ R/	Greek *breastplate* -ic *pertaining to* thorac- *chest*	The part of the trunk between the abdomen and neck Pertaining to the chest (thorax)
vertebra vertebrae (pl) vertebral (adj)	VER-teh-brah VER-teh-bray VER-teh-bral	 S/ R/	Latin *spinal joint* -al *pertaining to* vertebr- *vertebra*	One of the bones of the spinal column Pertaining to the vertebrae

The Skull

The human skull has 22 bones, 8 of which make up the **cranium,** the upper part of the skull that encloses the **cranial cavity** and protects the brain *(Figure 14.9).* The bones of the cranium are:

1. **Frontal bone**—forms the forehead and the roofs of the orbits and contains a pair of right and left frontal sinuses above the orbits.

2. **Parietal bones** (2)—form the bulging sides and roof of the cranium.

3. **Occipital bone**—forms the back of and part of the base of the cranium.

4. **Temporal bones** (2)—form the sides and part of the base of the cranium.

5. **Sphenoid bone**—forms part of the base of the cranium and the orbits.

6. **Ethmoid bone**—forms parts of the nose and the orbits and is hollow, forming the ethmoid sinuses.

The bones of the cranium are joined together by sutures, joints that appear as seams, covered on the inside and outside by a thin layer of connective tissue.

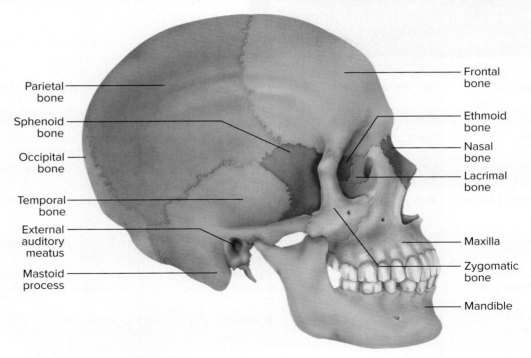

Parietal bone

Sphenoid bone

Occipital bone

Temporal bone

External auditory meatus

Mastoid process

Frontal bone

Ethmoid bone

Nasal bone

Lacrimal bone

Maxilla

Zygomatic bone

Mandible

▲ **Figure 14.9** Skull: Right lateral view.

The lower anterior part of the skull comprises the 14 bones of the facial skeleton *(Figure 14.10; see also Figure 14.9):*

1. **Maxillary** bones (2)—form the upper jaw, hold the upper teeth, and are hollow, forming the maxillary sinuses.
2. **Palatine** bones (2)—are located behind the maxilla.
3. **Zygomatic** bones (2)—form the prominences of the cheeks below the eyes.
4. **Lacrimal** bones (2)—form the medial wall of each eye orbit.
5. **Nasal** bones (2)—form the sides and bridge of the nose.
6. **Vomer** bone—separates the two nasal cavities *(Figure 14.10).*
7. Inferior nasal **conchae** (2)—are fragile bones in the lower nasal cavity.
8. **Mandible**—is the lower jawbone, which holds the lower teeth.

The third component of the axial skeleton, the rib cage, is discussed in *Chapter 13.*

Bones and Joints of Mastication

The **temporomandibular joint (TMJ)** connects the condyle of the mandible to a fossa in the temporal bone at the base of the skull. The joint acts like a hinge when you open and close your mouth.

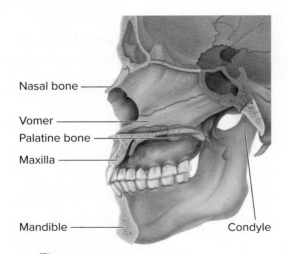

Nasal bone

Vomer

Palatine bone

Maxilla

Mandible

Condyle

▲ **Figure 14.10** Facial bones.

WORD	PRONUNCIATION		ELEMENTS	DEFINITION
concha conchae (pl)	**KON**-kah **KON**-kee		Latin *a shell*	Shell-shaped bone on medial wall of nasal cavity
cranium cranial (adj)	**KRAY**-nee-um **KRAY**-nee-al	 S/ R/	Greek *skull* -al *pertaining to* crani- *skull*	The upper part of the skull that encloses and protects the brain Pertaining to the skull
ethmoid bone	**ETH**-moyd BOHN	S/ R/	-oid *resemble* ethm- *sieve* **bone** Old English *bone*	Bone that forms the back of the nose and part of the orbits and encloses numerous air cells, forming the ethmoid sinuses
lacrimal	**LAK**-rim-al	S/ R/	-al *pertaining to* lacrim- *tears*	Pertaining to tears
mandible mandibular (adj)	**MAN**-di-bel man-**DIB**-you-lar	 S/ R/	Latin *jaw* -ar *pertaining to* mandibul- *the jaw*	Lower jawbone Pertaining to the mandible
maxilla maxillary (adj)	mak-**SILL**-ah **MAK**-sill-ah-ree	 S/ R/	Latin *jawbone* -ary *pertaining to* maxill- *maxilla*	Upper jawbone, containing right and left maxillary sinuses
occiput occipital bone	**OK**-si-put ok-**SIP**-it-al BOHN	 S/ R/	Latin *occiput* al- *pertaining to* occipit- *back of head* **bone** Old English *bone*	The back of the skull Bone that forms the back and part of the base of the cranium
palatine	**PAL**-ah-tine		Latin *palate*	Bone that forms the hard palate and parts of the nose and orbits
parietal bone	pah-**RYE**-eh-tal BOHN	S/ R/	-al *pertaining to* pariet- *wall* **bone** Old English *bone*	Bones that form the bulging sides and roof of the cranium
sphenoid bone	**SFEE**-noyd BOHN	S/ R/	-oid *resemble* sphen- *wedge* **bone** Old English *bone*	Wedge-shaped bone that forms part of the base of the cranium and the orbits
temporal bones	**TEM**-por-al BOHNZ	S/ R/	-al *pertaining to* tempor- *temple, side of head* **bone** Old English *bone*	Bones that form the sides and part of the base of the cranium
temporomandibular joint (TMJ)	**TEM**-por-oh-man-**DIB**-you-lar JOYNT	S/ R/CF R/ R/	-ar *pertaining to* tempor/o- *temple, side of head* -mandibul- *the jaw* **joint** Middle English *joint*	The joint between the temporal bone and the mandible
vomer	**VOH**-mer		Latin *ploughshare*	Lower nasal septum
zygoma zygomatic (adj)	zie-**GOH**-mah zie-goh-**MAT**-ik	 S/ R/	French *yoke* -ic *pertaining to* zygomat- *cheekbone*	Bone that forms the prominence of the cheek

Appendicular Skeleton
Shoulder Girdle and Upper Arm

The **pectoral** (shoulder) **girdle** connects the axial skeleton to the upper limbs and helps with movements of the upper limb.

The bones of the pectoral girdle are the **scapulae** (shoulder blades) and **clavicles** (*Figure 14.11*). The scapula extends over the top of the joint to form a roof called the **acromion**. The acromion is attached to the clavicle at the **acromioclavicular (AC)** joint. This also provides a connection between the axial skeleton, pectoral girdle, and upper arm. The clavicle acts as a strut to keep the scapula in place so that the arm hangs freely and can have maximum range of movement. It is commonly fractured by a fall on the shoulder tip or on the outstretched hand.

The joint that connects the pectoral girdle to the upper limb is the shoulder joint, located between the scapula and the **humerus** bone of the upper arm (see *Figure 14.11*).

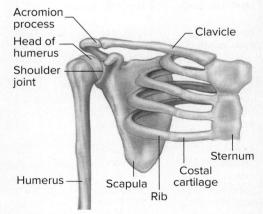

Acromion process
Clavicle
Head of humerus
Shoulder joint
Sternum
Humerus
Scapula
Costal cartilage
Rib

▲ **Figure 14.11** Pectoral girdle.

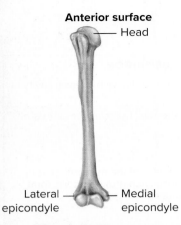

Anterior surface
— Head

Lateral
epicondyle

Medial
epicondyle

▲ **Figure 14.12** Humerus.

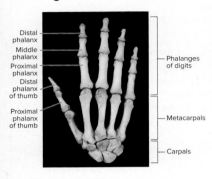

Distal phalanx
Middle phalanx
Proximal phalanx
Distal phalanx of thumb
Proximal phalanx of thumb

Phalanges of digits

Metacarpals

Carpals

▲ **Figure 14.13** The bones of the hand. Christine Eckel/ McGraw Hill.

This joint is a ball-and-socket joint in which the head of the humerus allows the greatest range of motion of any joint in the body. Several ligaments hold together the articulating surfaces of the humerus and scapula.

The **humerus** extends from the scapula to the elbow joint. The inferior end of the humerus has two **condyles** that articulate with the ulna to form the elbow joint *(Figure 14.12)*. A lateral projection on each condyle, the **epicondyle,** serves as an attachment for ligaments and tendons to allow for stabilization as well as movement of the joint.

The elbow joint has two **articulations:**

1. A hinge joint between the humerus and **ulna** bone of the forearm, which allows flexion and extension of the elbow.

2. A gliding joint between the humerus and **radius** bone of the forearm, which allows pronation and supination of the forearm and hand.

A joint capsule and ligaments hold the two articulations together.

Forearm, Wrist, and Hand

The hand and wrist have a complex structure comprised of 27 bones, and all the ligaments, joints, and muscles that allow for many complicated and delicate movements. The muscles of the forearm supinate and pronate the forearm, flex and extend the wrist joint and hand, and move the hand medially and laterally. The two bones of the forearm, the radius and ulna, attach distally to the carpal bones *(Figure 14.13)*. The carpal bones then articulate distally with five long bones called metacarpals, which form the palm of the hand. The **metacarpals** in turn articulate distally with the **phalanges** (finger bones). Your thumb has two phalanges, all the other fingers have three each.

Word Analysis and Definition: Shoulder Girdle, Arm, Elbow, and Hand

S = Suffix   P = Prefix   R = Root   R/CF = Combining Form

WORD	PRONUNCIATION	ELEMENTS		DEFINITION
acromion acromioclavicular (adj)	ah-**CROH**-mee-on ah-**CROH**-mee-oh-klah-**VIK**-you-lar	S/ R/ S/ R/CF R/	-ion *action* **acrom-** *acromion* -ar *pertaining to* **acromi/o-** *acromion* -**clavicul-** *clavicle*	Lateral end of the scapula, extending over the shoulder joint Pertaining to the joint between the acromion and the clavicle
carpus carpal (adj)	**KAR**-pus **KAR**-pal	 S/ R/	Greek *wrist* -al *pertaining to* **carp-** *bones of the wrist*	Collective term for the eight carpal bones of the wrist Pertaining to the wrist
clavicle clavicular (adj)	**KLAV**-ih-kul klah-**VIK**-you-lar	 S/ R/	Latin *collarbone* -ar *pertaining to* **clavicul-** *clavicle*	Curved bone that forms the anterior part of the pectoral girdle Pertaining to the clavicle
condyle epicondyle	**KON**-dile ep-ih-**KON**-dile	 P/ R/	Greek *knuckle* epi- *above* -**condyle** *knuckle*	Rounded bone surface that articulates with another bone Projection above the condyle for attachment of a ligament or tendon
humerus	**HYU**-mer-us		Latin *shoulder*	Single bone of the upper arm
metacarpal	**MET**-ah-**KAR**-pal	S/ P/ R/	-al *pertaining to* meta- *after* -**carp-** *bones of the wrist*	The five bones between the carpus and the fingers
pectoral	**PEK**-tor-al	S/ R/	-al *pertaining to* **pector-** *chest*	Pertaining to the chest
phalanx phalanges (pl)	**FAY**-lanks **FAY**-lan-jeez		Greek *line of soldiers*	A bone of a finger or toe
radius	**RAY**-dee-us		Latin *spoke of a wheel*	The forearm bone on the thumb side
scapula scapulae (pl) scapular (adj)	**SKAP**-you-lah **SKAP**-you-lee **SKAP**-you-lar	 S/ R/	Latin *shoulder blade* -ar *pertaining to* **scapul-** *scapula*	Shoulder blade Pertaining to the shoulder blade
ulna ulnar (adj)	**UL**-nah **UL**-nar	 S/ R/	Latin *elbow* -ar *pertaining to* **uln-** *forearm bone*	The medial and larger bone of the forearm Pertaining to the ulna or any of the structures (artery, vein, nerve) named after it

Pelvic Girdle

The pelvic girdle *(Figure 14.14)* is the two hip bones that articulate anteriorly with each other at the **symphysis pubis** and posteriorly with the **sacrum** to form the bowl-shaped **pelvis.** The two joints between the hip bones and the sacrum are the **sacroiliac (SI) joints.**

The pelvic girdle has the following functions:

1. Supports the axial skeleton.
2. Transmits the body's weight through to the lower limbs.
3. Provides attachments for the lower limbs.
4. Protects the internal reproductive organs, urinary bladder, and distal end of the large intestine.

Each hip bone is a fusion of three bones: the **ilium, ischium,** and **pubis** *(Figure 14.14a).* The fusion takes place in the region of the **acetabulum,** a cup-shaped cavity on the lateral surface of each hip bone that receives the **head** of the **femur** (thigh bone, *Figure 14.14b*).

The lower part of the pelvis is formed by the lower ilium, ischium, and **pubic** bones that surround a short canal-like cavity. This opening is larger in females than males to allow the infant to pass through during childbirth. The outlet from the cavity is spanned by strong muscular layers through which the rectum, vagina, and urethra pass.

Muscles anchor the pelvic girdle to the vertebrae and ribs of the axial skeleton *(Figure 14.14c).*

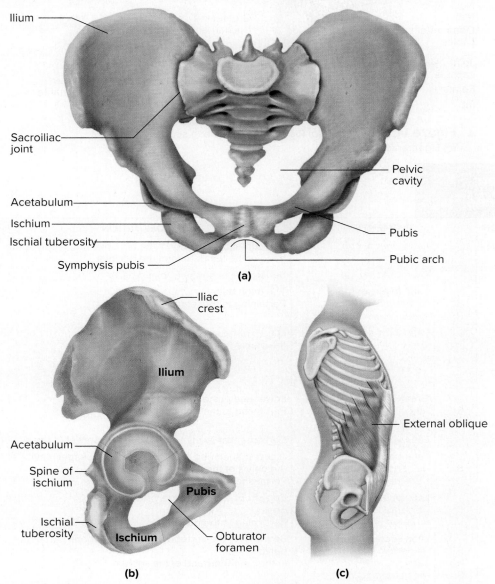

(a)

(b)

(c)

▲ **Figure 14.14** **Pelvic girdle.** (*a*) Front view. (*b*) Side view. (*c*) Abdominal muscles supporting the pelvic girdle.

Bones and Joints of the Hip and Thigh

The hip joint is a ball-and-socket synovial joint between the head of the femur and the cup-shaped **acetabulum** of the hip bone (*Figure 14.15a*). A ligament (ligamentum capitis) attached to the head of the femur from the lining of the acetabulum carries blood vessels to the head of the femur to nourish it.

The joint is held in place by a thick joint **capsule** reinforced by strong ligaments that connect the neck of the femur to the rim of the acetabulum (*Figure 14.15*).

The **labrum** is the cartilage that forms a rim around the socket of the joint; it cushions the joint and helps keep the head of the femur in place in the socket.

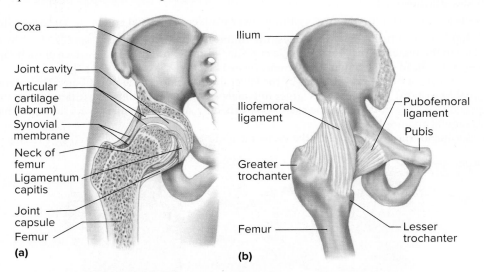

(a)

(b)

▲ **Figure 14.15** Hip joint. (*a*) Right frontal view of a section of hip joint. (*b*) Ligaments of hip joint.

Word Analysis and Definition: Bones and Joints of the Hip and Thigh

S = Suffix P = Prefix R = Root R/CF = Combining Form

WORD	PRONUNCIATION		ELEMENTS	DEFINITION
acetabulum	ass-eh-**TAB**-you-lum		Latin *vinegar cup*	The cup-shaped cavity of the hip bone that receives the head of the femur to form the hip joint
diastasis	die-**ASS**-tah-sis		Greek *separation*	Separation of normally joined parts
femur femoral (adj)	**FEE**-mur **FEM**-oh-ral	S/ R/	Latin *thigh* -al *pertaining to* femor- *femur*	The thigh bone Pertaining to the femur
ilium (***Note:*** The ileum is a section of the small intestine [Chapter 6].) ilia (pl)	**ILL**-ee-um **ILL**-ee-ah		Latin *to twist*	Large wing-shaped bone at the upper and posterior part of the pelvis
ischium ischia (pl) ischial (adj)	**ISS**-kee-um **ISS**-kee-ah **ISS**-kee-al	S/ R/CF	Greek *hip* -al *pertaining to* isch/i- *ischium*	Lower and posterior part of the hip bone Pertaining to the ischium
labrum	**LAY**-brum		Latin *lip-shaped*	Cartilage that forms a rim around the socket of the hip joint
pelvis pelvic (adj)	**PEL**-vis **PEL**-vic	S/ R/	Latin *basin* -ic *pertaining to* pelv- *pelvis*	A cup-shaped ring of bone; also a cup-shaped cavity, as in the pelvis of the kidney Pertaining to the pelvis
pubis pubic (adj)	**PYU**-bis **PYU**-bik	S/ R/	Latin *pubis* -ic *pertaining to* pub- *pubis*	Bony front arch of the pelvis of the hip; also called *pubic bone* Pertaining to the pubis
sacrum sacral (adj) sacroiliac joint	**SAY**-crum **SAY**-kral say-kroh-**ILL**-ih-ak JOYNT	S/ R/ S/ R/CF R/	Latin *sacred* -al *pertaining to* sacr- *sacrum* -ac *pertaining to* sacr/o- *sacrum* ili- *ilium* joint Middle English *joint*	Segment of the vertebral column that forms part of the pelvis In the neighborhood of the sacrum The joint between the sacrum and ilium

Bones and Joints of the Knee and Thigh

Knee Joint

The knee is a hinged joint formed with four bones:

1. The lower end of the **femur**, shaped like a horseshoe. The two ends of the horseshoe are the medial and lateral femoral **condyles** (*Figure 14.16b*).
2. The flat upper end of the **tibia.**
3. The **patella** (kneecap), a flat triangular bone embedded in the **patellar tendon.** The patella articulates with the femur between its two **condyles** (*Figure 14.16a*).
4. The **fibula,** which forms a separate joint by articulating with the tibia. This is called the **tibiofibular joint** (*see Figure 14.16b*).

Mechanically, the role of the patella is to provide an increase of about 30% in the strength of extension of the knee joint.

Within the knee joint, two crescent-shaped pads of cartilage lie on top of the tibia to articulate with the femoral condyles. They are the medial and lateral **menisci.** Their function is to distribute weight more evenly across the joint surface to minimize wear and tear. They play a crucial role in joint stability, lubrication, and transmission of force.

Bones and Joints of the Lower Leg, Ankle, and Foot

The two bones of the lower leg are the larger and medial **tibia** and the thinner and lateral **fibula.** The lower end of the tibia on its medial border forms a prominent process called the medial malleolus. The lower end of the fibula forms the lateral malleolus. You can **palpate** both these prominences at your own ankle.

The ankle has two joints:

1. One between the lateral malleolus of the fibula and the talus.
2. One between the medial malleolus of the tibia and the talus.

The **calcaneus** is the heelbone. The **talus** is the most superior of the seven **tarsal** bones of the ankle and proximal foot (*Figure 14.17*), and its surface articulates with the tibia. The tarsal bones help the ankle bear the body's weight. Strong ligaments on both sides of the ankle joint hold it together.

Attached to the tarsal bones are the five parallel **metatarsal** bones that form the instep and then fan out to form the ball of the foot, where they bear weight. Each of the toes has three phalanges, except for the big toe, which has only two. This is identical to the thumb and its relation to the hand. The tendons of the leg muscles are inserted into the phalanges.

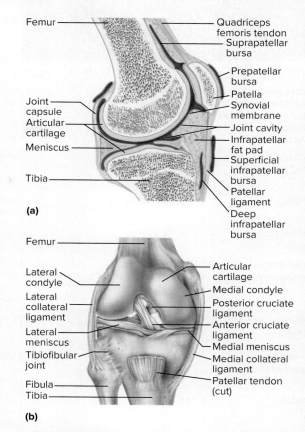

(a)

(b)

▲ **Figure 14.16** Knee joint. (*a*) Section of knee joint. (*b*) Right knee joint: anterior view.

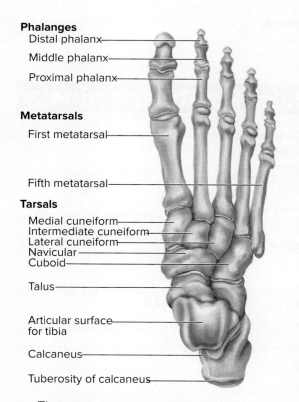

▲ **Figure 14.17** Twenty-six bones and 33 joints of right foot.

WORD	PRONUNCIATION		ELEMENTS	DEFINITION
calcaneus calcaneal tendon (same as Achilles tendon) Achilles	kal-**KAY**-nee-us kal-**KAY**-nee-al **TEN**-dun ah-**KIL**-eez	S/ R/	Latin *the heel* -al *pertaining to* calcane- *calcaneus* tendon Latin *sinew* **Achilles** mythical Greek warrior	The heel bone The tendon of the heel formed from gastrocnemius and soleus muscles and inserted into the calcaneus
fibula fibular (adj)	**FIB**-you-lah **FIB**-you-lar	S/ R/	Latin *clasp or buckle* -ar *pertaining to* fibul- *fibula*	The smaller of the two bones of the lower leg Pertaining to the fibula
hallux valgus	**HAL**-uks **VAL**-gus		**hallux** Latin *big toe* **valgus** Latin *turn out*	Deviation of the big toe toward the lateral side of the foot
meniscus menisci (pl)	meh-**NISS**-kuss meh-**NISS**-kee			Disc of connective tissue cartilage between the bones of a joint; for example, in the knee joint
metatarsus metatarsal (adj)	**MET**-ah-**TAR**-sus **MET**-ah-**TAR**-sal	S/ P/ R/ S/	-us *structure* meta- *behind* -tars- *ankle* -al *pertaining to*	A collective term referring to the five parallel bones of the foot between the tarsus and the phalanges Pertaining to the metatarsus
patella (kneecap [syn]) patellae (pl) patellar (adj) prepatellar	pah-**TELL**-ah pah-**TELL**-ee pah-**TELL**-ar pree-pah-**TELL**-ar	 S/ R/ P/	Latin *small plate* -ar *pertaining to* patell- *patella* pre- *before, in front of*	Thin, circular bone in front of the knee joint and embedded in the patellar tendon Pertaining to the patella (kneecap) In front of the patella
talus	**TAY**-luss		The tarsal bone that articulates with the tibia to form the ankle joint	The tarsal bone that articulates with the tibia to form the ankle joint
tarsus tarsal (adj)	**TAR**-sus **TAR**-sal	S/ R/	Latin *flat surface* -al *pertaining to* tars- *tarsus*	The collection of seven bones in the foot that form the ankle and instep Pertaining to the tarsus
tibia tibial (adj)	**TIB**-ee-ah **TIB**-ee-al	S/ R/	Latin *large shinbone* -al *pertaining to* tibi- *tibia*	The larger bone of the lower leg Pertaining to the tibia

Check Point Section 14.2

A. Deconstruct medical terms associated with the axial skeleton. *Breaking medical terms into their elements will make it easier to decipher their meaning. Fill in the blanks.* **LO 14.1**

1. intervertebral: _____ /_____ /_____
                   P   R/CF   S

2. cervical: _____ /_____
              R   S

3. thoracic: _____ /_____
              R   S

B. Construct medical terms related to the bones of the skull. *Given the definition, complete the medical term with the correct word element. Fill in the blank.* **LO 14.1, 14.2**

1. Wedge-shaped bone at the base of the skull. _____/oid

2. Bone that forms part of the base and sides of the skull. _____/al

3. Bone that forms the back of the nose and encloses numerous air cells. _____/oid

4. The two bones forming the sidewalls and roof of the cranium. _____/al

C. Not all bones are constructed with word elements. *Some bones are named for their shape. Given the description, enter the name of the bone. Fill in the blank.* **LO 14.2**

1. Bone that forms the hard palate and parts of the nose and orbits: _____

2. Shell-shaped bone on medial wall of nasal cavity: _____

3. Bone named because it resembled a *yoke:* _____

4. This bone has the shape of a *plow:* _____

5. The upper jawbone: _____

6. The lower jawbone: _____

D. Use your knowledge to complete the following medical terms. *Each blank represents a word element. If the term has a combining vowel, there is a blank for that as well. The first one has been done for you.* **LO 14.1, 14.2**

1. Lateral end of the scapula _____ acrom _____ / _____ ion _____

2. Joint between acromion and clavicle _____ / _____ / _____

3. Pertaining to the shoulder blade _____ / _____

E. Answer the following questions. *Write medical terms for the following layman's terms. Fill in the blanks.* **LO 14.1, 14.3**

1. the shoulder girdle (2 words) _____

2. shoulder blades _____

3. collarbones _____

F. Identify the bone structures of the upper arm. *From the provided definition, provide the term it is describing.* **LO 14.1, 14.3**

1. The forearm bone that is on the thumb side: _____

2. The structure of the humerus that articulates with the ulna: _____

3. The forearm bone that is on the medial side of the forearm: _____

4. The structure of the humerus that serves as an attachment for ligaments and tendons: _____

G. Terms related to the anatomy of the wrist. *Correctly identify the structures of the wrist.* **LO 14.1, 14.2**

1. The medical term that means *wrist:*

   a. carpal

   b. retinaculum

   c. radius

   d. ulna

H. Because the body has 206 bones, there is an extensive amount of orthopedic vocabulary. *Build your knowledge of hand terminology with this exercise. Select the answer that correctly completes each statement.* **LO 14.1**

1. The suffix *-al* means:

   a. pertaining to

   b. one who does

   c. study of

   d. condition

2. The prefix *meta-* means:

   a. before

   b. during

   c. after

   d. middle

3. The term **metacarpal** refers to the:

a. arm

b. elbow

c. forearm

d. hand

4. The bone of a finger *or* toe is called a(n):

a. carpus

b. fascia

c. eminence

d. phalanx

5. The nasal bone is _____ to the mandible.

a. inferior

b. posterior

c. superior

d. anterior

I. Match the language of the pelvic girdle to the correct definitions. *Match the definition in the first column with its correct term in the second column.* **LO 14.1**

_____ 1. receives head of femur

_____ 2. cup-shaped ring of bones

_____ 3. posterior part of hip bone

_____ 4. bony anterior arch of the pelvis

_____ 5. wing-shaped bone, upper part of pelvis

_____ 6. segment of vertebral column

_____ 7. thigh bone

a. sacrum

b. ilium

c. pubis

d. femur

e. pelvis

f. ischium

g. acetabulum

J. Continue working with the *language of orthopedics*. *Demonstrate your knowledge of the terms by selecting the best answer to each of the following statements* **LO 14.1**

1. The head of the femur fits into the _____ of the pelvis.

a. sacrum

b. acetabulum

c. labrum

d. foramen

2. The cartilage that forms a ring around the hip joint:

a. labrum

b. pubis

c. acetabulum

d. symphysis

K. Identify the structures that make up the knee joint. *Given the description, identify the structure that makes up the knee joint. Fill in the blanks.* **LO 14.1**

1. This cartilage is tough and functions to cushion and add stability to the joint._____

2. This bone protects the anterior portion of the knee joint. It is embedded in a tendon. _____

3. The femur articulates with this leg bone. _____

4. This lower leg bone is on the lateral side of the leg. _____

Section 14.3 Disorders and Injuries of Skeleton System

Diseases of Bone

Osteoporosis results from a loss of bone density (*Figure 14.18*) when the rate of bone **resorption** exceeds the rate of bone formation. It is more common in women than in men, and its incidence increases with age. Ten million people in the United States already have osteoporosis, and 18 million more have low bone density (**osteopenia**) and are at risk for developing osteoporosis.

In women, production of the hormone estrogen decreases after menopause, and its protection against osteoclast activity is lost. This leads to fragile, brittle bones. In men, reduction in testosterone has a similar but less marked effect.

Osteomyelitis is an inflammation of an area of bone due to bacterial infection, usually with a staphylococcus. Untreated tuberculosis can spread from its original infection in the lungs to bones via the bloodstream to produce tuberculous osteomyelitis.

Osteomalacia, known as **rickets** in children, is a disease caused by vitamin D deficiency. When bones lack calcium, they become soft and flexible. They are not strong enough to bear weight and become bowed. Osteomalacia occurs in some developing nations and occasionally in this country when children drink soft drinks instead of milk fortified with vitamin D.

Achondroplasia occurs when the long bones stop growing in childhood, but the bones of the axial skeleton are not affected (*Figure 14.19*). This leads to short-stature individuals who are about 4 feet tall. Intelligence and life span are normal. It is caused by a spontaneous gene mutation that then becomes a dominant gene for succeeding generations.

Osteogenic sarcoma is the most common malignant bone tumor. Peak incidence is between 10 and 15 years of age; the tumor often occurs around the knee joint.

Osteogenesis imperfecta is a rare genetic disorder, producing very brittle bones that are easily fractured, often in utero (while inside the uterus).

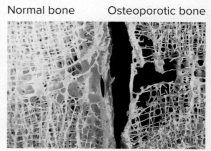

Normal bone   Osteoporotic bone

LM 5×

▲ **Figure 14.18** Normal bone and osteoporotic bone. Michael Klein/ Photolibrary/Getty Images

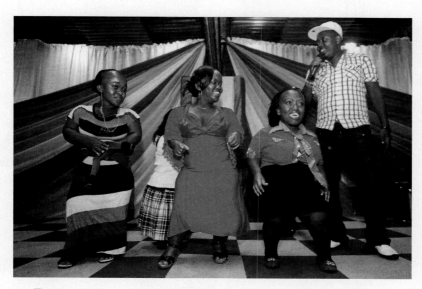

▲ **Figure 14.19** Achondroplastic dwarfs performing for friends. Daniel Irungu/EPA/Shutterstock

WORD	PRONUNCIATION	ELEMENTS		DEFINITION
achondroplasia	ay-kon-droh-**PLAY**-zee-ah	S/ P/ R/CF	-plasia *formation* a- *without* -chondr/o- *cartilage*	Condition with abnormal conversion of cartilage into bone, leading to dwarfism
osteogenesis imperfecta	**OS**-tee-oh-**JEN**-eh-sis im-per-**FEK**-tah	S/ R/CF	-genesis *creation* oste/o- *bone* **imperfecta** Latin *unfinished*	Inherited condition in which bone formation is incomplete, leading to fragile, easily broken bones
osteomalacia	**OS**-tee-oh-mah-**LAY**-shee-ah	S/ R/CF	-malacia *abnormal softness* oste/o- *bone*	Soft, flexible bones lacking in calcium
osteomyelitis	**OS**-tee-oh-my-eh-**LIE**-tis	S/ R/CF R/	-itis *inflammation* oste/o- *bone* -myel- *bone marrow*	Inflammation of bone tissue
osteopenia	**OS**-tee-oh-**PEE**-nee-ah	S/ R/CF	-penia *deficient* oste/o- *bone*	Decreased calcification of bone
resorption	ree-**SORP**-shun		Latin *to suck back*	Loss of substance, such as bone
rickets	**RIK**-ets		Old English *to twist*	Disease in children due to vitamin D deficiency, producing soft, flexible bones
sarcoma	sar-**KOH**-mah	S/ R/	-oma *tumor, mass* sarc- *flesh*	A malignant tumor originating in connective tissue
osteogenic sarcoma	**OS**-tee-oh-**JEN**-ik sar-**KOH**-mah	S/ R/CF	-genic *creation* oste/o- *bone*	Malignant tumor originating in bone-producing cells

Bone Fractures

A fracture is a break of a bone and can have a traumatic or pathological reason for occurring. The types of bone fractures are shown in *Figure 14.20*.

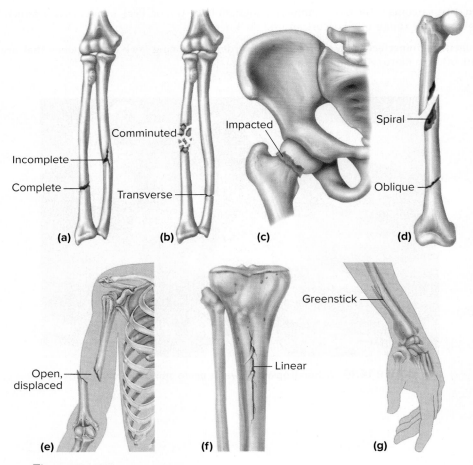

▲ **Figure 14.20** Bone fractures.

Healing of Fractures

Uncomplicated fractures take 8 to 12 weeks to heal.

Step 1: When a bone is fractured, blood vessels bleed into the fracture site, forming a **hematoma** (*Figure 14.21a*).

Step 2: A few days after the fracture (**Fx**), osteoblasts move into the hematoma and start to produce new bone. This is called a **callus** (*Figure 14.21b*).

Step 3: Osteoblasts produce immature, lacy, **cancellous** (spongy) bone that replaces the callus (*Figure 14.21c*).

Step 4: Osteoblasts continue to produce bone cells. They produce compact bone and fuse the bone segments together (*Figure 14.21d*).

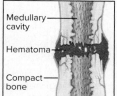

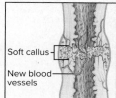

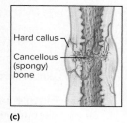

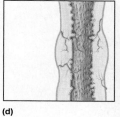

(a)   (b)   (c)   (d)

▲ **Figure 14.21** Healing of bone fracture.

Word Analysis and Definition: Fractures

S = Suffix   P = Prefix   R = Root   R/CF = Combining Form

WORD	PRONUNCIATION		ELEMENTS	DEFINITION
callus (*Note: Callous* is a nonmedical word meaning *insensitive*.)	**KAL**-us		Latin *hard skin*	The mass of fibrous connective tissue that forms at a fracture site and becomes the foundation for the formation of new bone
cancellous	**KAN**-sell-us		Latin *lattice*	Bone that has a spongy or lattice-like structure
closed fracture (opposite of open)	KLOHZD **FRAK**-chur	S/ R/	**closed** Latin *intact* -**ure** *result of* **fract-** *break*	A bone is broken but the skin over it is intact
comminuted fracture	**KOM**-ih-nyu-ted	S/ R/	-**ed** *pertaining to* **comminut-** *break into small pieces*	A fracture in which the bone is broken into pieces
complete fracture	kom-**PLEET**		Latin *fill up*	A bone is fractured into two separate pieces
compression fracture	kom-**PRESH**-un	S/ R/	-**ion** *condition, action* **compress-** *press together*	Fracture of a vertebra causing loss of height of the vertebra
displaced fracture	dis-**PLAYSD**	P/ R/	**dis-** *apart, away from* -**placed** *in an area*	A fracture in which the fragments are separated and are not in alignment
greenstick fracture	**GREEN**-stik	R/ R/	**green-** *green* -**stick** *branch, twig*	A fracture in which one side of the bone is partially broken and the other side is bent. Occurs mostly in children
hairline fracture	**HAIR**-line		**hair** Old English *hair* **line** Latin *a mark*	A fracture without separation of the fragments
hematoma	hee-mah-**TOH**-mah	S/ R/	-**oma** *tumor, mass* **hemat-** *blood*	Collection of blood that has escaped from the blood vessels into tissue
impacted fracture	im-**PAK**-ted	S/ P/ R/	-**ed** *pertaining to* **im-** *in* -**pact-** *driven in*	A fracture in which one bone fragment is driven into the other
incomplete fracture	in-kom-**PLEET**	P/ R/	**in-** *not* -**complete** *fill in*	A fracture that does not extend across the bone, as in a hairline fracture
linear fracture	**LIN**-ee-ar	S/ R/	-**ar** *pertaining to* **line-** *a mark*	A fracture running parallel to the length of the bone
oblique fracture	ob-**LEEK**		Latin *slanting*	A diagonal fracture across the long axis of the bone
open fracture	**OH**-pen		Old English *not enclosed*	The skin over the fracture is broken
pathologic fracture	path-oh-**LOJ**-ik	S/ R/CF R/	-**ic** *pertaining to* **path/o-** *disease* -**log-** *to study*	Fracture occurring at a site already weakened by a disease process, such as cancer. Also called stress fracture
spiral fracture	**SPY**-ral	S/ R/	-**al** *pertaining to* **spir-** *a coil*	A fracture in the shape of a coil
transverse fracture	trans-**VERS**	P/ R/	**trans-** *across* -**verse** *travel*	A fracture perpendicular to the long axis of the bone

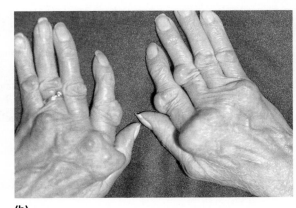

	Spinal cord
Compressed vertebrae	
Degenerative changes	Narrowed intervertebral disc space

(a) Lumbar vertebrae

(b)

▲ **Figure 14.22** **Arthritis.** (*a*) Magnetic resonance imaging (MRI) scan of lumbar vertebrae showing degenerative changes due to osteoarthritis. (*b*) Rheumatoid arthritis of the hands. [a] Du Cane Medical Imaging Ltd./Science Source [b] Image appears with permission from VisualDx

Diseases of Joints

Osteoarthritis (OA) is caused by the breakdown and eventual destruction of cartilage in a joint. It develops as the result of wear and tear and is common in the weight-bearing joints: the knee, hip, and lower back (*Figure 14.22a*). OA is often referred to **degenerative joint disease (DJD).** The degenerative process begins in the articular cartilage, which cracks and frays, eventually exposing the underlying bone. In addition, OA is common in the hands. As a finger joint deteriorates, small bony spurs called **Heberden nodes** can form.

Rheumatoid arthritis (RA), with destruction of joint surfaces, joint capsule, and ligaments, leads to marked deformity and joint instability (*Figure 14.22b*). It occurs mostly in women, with onset between ages 20 and 50. The great majority of patients have RA in the joints of their hands, wrists, and knees. The disease affects the synovial membrane that lines joints and tendons. The abnormal synovial membrane can invade the smooth, gliding joint surfaces and destroy them, or it can invade the surrounding joint capsule and ligaments and cause deformity and joint instability and pain. Lumps known as **rheumatic nodules** can form over or near joints with RA. Typically, rheumatoid nodules are near areas of repeated trauma or pressure and occur adjacent to joints on extensor surfaces, such as the elbow, fingers and forearms and knees. This occurs in one out of 4 patients with RA.

Juvenile rheumatoid arthritis (JRA) affects children under the age of 17 with inflammation and stiffness of joints. Many children grow out of it.

Bursitis is inflammation of a **bursa** that can result from overuse of a joint, repeated trauma, or diseases such as RA.

Word Analysis and Definition: Joint Disease

S = Suffix P = Prefix R = Root R/CF = Combining Form

WORD	PRONUNCIATION	ELEMENTS		DEFINITION
bursa bursitis	**BURR**-sah burr-**SIGH**-tis	S/ R/	Latin *purse* -itis *inflammation* burs- *bursa*	A closed sac containing synovial fluid Inflammation of a bursa
degenerative	dee-**JEN**-er-a-tiv	S/ R/	-ive *quality of* degenerat- *deteriorate*	Relating to the deterioration of a structure
Heberden node	**HEH**-ber-den NOHD		William Heberden, 1710–1801, English physician **node** Latin *a knot*	Bony lump on the terminal phalanx of the fingers in osteoarthritis
nodule	**NOD**-yule	S/ R/	-ule *little, small* nod- *node*	Small node or knotlike swelling
osteoarthritis	**OS**-tee-oh-ar-**THRIE**-tis	S/ R/CF R/	-itis *inflammation* oste/o- *bone* -arthr- *joint*	Chronic inflammatory disease of the joints with pain and loss of function
rheumatism rheumatic (adj) rheumatoid arthritis	**RHU**-mat-izm rhu-**MAT**-ik **RHU**-mah-toyd ar-**THRIE**-tis	S/ R/ S/ S/ S/ R/	-ism *condition* rheumat- *a flow* -ic *pertaining to* -oid *resembling* -itis *inflammation* arthr- *joint*	Pain in various parts of the musculoskeletal system Relating to or characterized by rheumatism Disease of connective tissue, with arthritis as a major manifestation

Common Disorders of the Vertebral Column

Abnormal spinal curvatures can result from disease, poor posture, or congenital defects in the vertebrae. The defect that is most common is called **scoliosis**, an abnormal lateral curve in the thoracic region (*Figure 14.23a*). In older people, particularly those with osteoporosis, an exaggerated thoracic curvature is called **kyphosis** (*Figure 14.23b*). An exaggerated lumbar curve is called **lordosis** (*Figure 14.23c*).

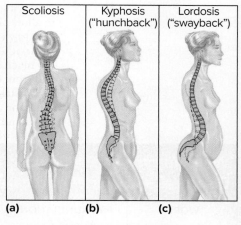

▲ **Figure 14.23** Abnormal spinal curvatures. Zephyr/Science Source

S = Suffix P = Prefix R = Root R/CF = Combining Form

Word Analysis and Definition: Abnormal Spinal Curvatures

WORD	PRONUNCIATION	ELEMENTS		DEFINITION
kyphosis	kie-**FOH**-sis	S/	-osis *condition*	A normal posterior curve of the thoracic spine that can be exaggerated in disease
		R/	kyph- *humpback*	
kyphotic (adj)	ki-**FOT**-ik	S/	-tic *pertaining to*	Pertaining to kyphosis
		R/CF	kyph/o- *humpback*	
lordosis	lore-**DOH**-sis	S/	-osis *condition*	An exaggerated forward curvature of the lumbar spine
		R/	lord- *bend backward*	
lordotic (adj)	lore-**DOT**-ik	S/	-tic *pertaining to*	Pertaining to lordosis
		R/CF	lord/o- *bend backward*	
scoliosis	skoh-lee-**OH**-sis	S/	-osis *condition*	An abnormal lateral curvature of the vertebral column
		R/	scoli- *crooked*	
scoliotic (adj)	**SKOH**-lee-**OT**-ik	S/	-tic *pertaining to*	Pertaining to scoliosis
		R/CF	scoli/o- *crooked*	

Common Disorders of the Shoulder

As the result of the increased range of motion of this joint, the shoulder joint also is the most unstable joint and is liable to **dislocation.** Shoulder dislocation occurs when the ball of the humerus slips out of the socket of the scapula, usually anteriorly. Shoulder **subluxation** occurs when the ball of the humerus slips partially out of position and then moves back in.

Shoulder **separation** is a dislocation of the acromioclavicular joint, usually due to a fall on the point of the shoulder. The other common injury caused by falling on the point of the shoulder is a fractured clavicle.

Common Disorders of the Wrist

Colles fracture is a common fracture of the radius just above the wrist joint. It occurs when a person tries to break a fall with an outstretched hand. The distal radius just proximal to the wrist is broken. In some cases, the distal ulna is also fractured and the wrist joint dislocated. The fracture is diagnosed with an x-ray (*Figure 14.24*).

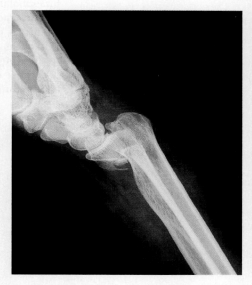

▲ **Figure 14.24** X-ray of Colles fracture with radius and ulna involved. ZephyrScience Source

Disorders of the Pelvic Girdle

Low back pain can be caused by a variety of problems with the interconnected network of bones, muscles, nerves, and discs in the lumbar spine. In adults 30 to 60 years old, the pain often can arise from disc degeneration or herniation in the lumbar spine or from muscle or other tissue strain. Adults over 60 years can suffer from lumbar joint degeneration and spinal stenosis. In February 2017, the American College of Physicians issued guidelines for the initial treatment of low back pain, recommending nondrug therapies such as superficial heat, massage, acupuncture, or spinal manipulation. If drugs are necessary, nonsteroidal anti-inflammatory drugs (NSAIDs) or skeletal muscle relaxants are recommended.

SI joint strain is a common cause of lower-back pain. Unlike most joints, the sacroiliac joint is only designed to move ¼ inch (approximately 6 mm) during weight bearing and forward flexion. Its main function is to provide shock absorption for the spine.

During pregnancy, hormones enable connective tissue to relax so that the pelvis can expand enough to allow birth. The stretching in the sacroiliac joint ligaments makes it excessively mobile and susceptible to wear-and-tear painful arthritis.

Another cause of pain in the sacroiliac joint is trauma, with tearing of the joint ligaments generating too much motion and pain. The pain is felt in the low back, in the buttock, and sometimes in the back and front of the thigh.

Diastasis symphysis pubis is another result of the stretching of pelvic ligaments during pregnancy. The softening and stretching of the ligaments of the symphysis pubis stretch the joint between the two pubic bones and lead to pain over the joint and difficulty in walking, climbing stairs, and turning over in bed.

Word Analysis and Definition: Disorders and Injuries of the Skeleton

WORD	PRONUNCIATION	ELEMENTS		DEFINITION
Colles fracture	**KOL**-ez **FRAK**-chur		Abraham Colles, 1773–1843, Irish surgeon	Fracture of the distal radius at the wrist
diastasis	die-**ASS**-tah-sis		Greek *separation*	Separation of normally joined parts
dislocation	dis-loh-**KAY**-shun	S/ P/ R/	**-ion** *action* **dis-** *apart* **-locat-** *a place*	The state of being completely out of joint
separation	sep-ah-**RAY**-shun	S/ R/	**-ion** *action* **separate** *move apart*	A shoulder separation is a dislocation of the acromioclavicular joint
subluxation	sub-luk-**SAY**-shun	S/ P/ R/	**-ion** *action* **sub-** *under, slightly* **-luxat-** *dislocate*	An incomplete dislocation in which some contact between the joint surfaces remains

Disorders of the Ankle and Foot

Podiatry is a health care specialty concerned with the diagnosis and treatment of disorders and injuries of the foot.

Bunions occur usually at the base of the big toe and are swellings of the bones that cause the metatarsophalangeal joint to be misaligned and stick out medially. This deformity is called **hallux valgus.**

Pott fracture is a term applied to a variety of fractures in which there is a fracture of the fibula near the ankle, often accompanied by a fracture of the medial malleolus of the tibia.

Gout is an extremely painful arthritis of the big toe and other joints caused by a buildup of uric acid in the blood, which forms needlelike crystals that accumulate in the joints.

Talipes equinovarus is a congenital deformity of the foot. The foot is turned inwardly at the ankle and is commonly referred to as "clubfoot."

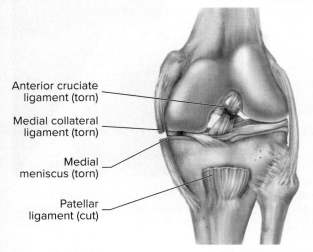

Anterior cruciate ligament (torn)

Medial collateral ligament (torn)

Medial meniscus (torn)

Patellar ligament (cut)

▲ **Figure 14.25** Complete tear of the medial collateral ligament, a complete tear of the anterior cruciate ligament (ACL), and a partial tear (avulsion) of the medial meniscus.

Common Disorders of the Knee

The anterior cruciate ligament (ACL) is the most commonly injured ligament in the knee (*Figure 14.25*), particularly in female athletes. The injury is often caused by a sudden **hyperextension** of the knee joint when landing awkwardly on flat ground. Because of its poor vascular supply, a torn ligament does not heal. The knee becomes unstable, risking further joint damage and arthritis.

Other major ligaments that are commonly injured are the medial and lateral collateral ligaments and the posterior cruciate ligament.

Meniscus injuries result from a twist to the knee. Pain and locking are the result of the torn meniscus flipping in and out of the joint as it moves. Loss of a meniscus leads to arthritic changes.

Patellar problems produce pain that is noticed particularly when descending stairs. The force on the patella when descending stairs is about seven times body weight, compared to about two times body weight when ascending stairs.

Chondromalacia patellae (runner's knee) is caused by irritation of the undersurface of the patella.

Patellar subluxation or **dislocation** produces an unstable, painful kneecap.

Prepatellar bursitis (housemaid's knee) produces painful swelling over the bursa at the front of the knee and is seen in people who kneel for extended periods of time, such as carpet layers.

WORD	PRONUNCIATION	ELEMENTS		DEFINITION
bunion	**BUN**-yun		French *bump*	A swelling at the base of the big toe
chondromalacia	**KON**-droh-mah-**LAY**-shee-ah	S/ R/CF	**-malacia** *abnormal softness* **chondr/o-** *cartilage*	Softening and degeneration of cartilage
gout	GOWT	Latin *drop*	Latin *drop*	Painful arthritis of the big toe and other joints
hyperflexion	high-per-**FLEK**-shun	S/ R/ P/	**-ion** *action, condition* **hyper-** *excess* **-flex-** *bend*	Flexion of a limb or part beyond the normal limits
meniscus menisci (pl)	meh-**NISS**-kuss meh-**NISS**-kee		Greek *crescent*	Disc of connective tissue cartilage between the bones of a joint; for example, in the knee joint
patella (kneecap (syn)) patellae (pl) patellar (adj) prepatellar	pah-**TELL**-ah pah-**TELL**-ee pah-**TELL**-ar pree-pah-**TELL**-ar	 S/ R/ P/	 Latin *small plate* **-ar** *pertaining to* **patell-** *patella* **pre-** *before, in front of*	Thin, circular bone in front of the knee joint and embedded in the patellar tendon Pertaining to the patella (kneecap) In front of the patella
pes planus	PES **PLAY**-nuss		**pes** Latin *foot* **planus** Latin *flat surface*	A flat foot with no plantar arch
Pott fracture	POT **FRAK**-chur	 S/ R/	Percival Pott, 1714–1788, London surgeon **-ure** *result of* **fract-** *break*	Fracture of lower end of fibula, often with fracture of tibial malleolus
podiatry podiatrist	poh-**DIE**-ah-tree poh-**DIE**-ah-trist	S/ R/ S/	**-iatry** *treatment* **pod-** *foot* **-iatrist** *practitioner*	Specialty concerned with the diagnosis and treatment of disorders and injuries of the foot Practitioner of podiatry
talipes equinovarus	**TAL**-ip-eez ee-kwie-noh-**VAY**-rus	R/ R/ R/CF S/	**-pes** *foot* **tali-** *ankle bone* **equin/o-** *horse* **-varus** *bent inward, bow-legged*	Deformity of the foot involving the talus

Check Point Section 14.3

A. Bone diseases can strike at any age. *Refer to the text regarding diseases of the bone for the correct terminology to identify each disease. Fill in the blanks.* **LO 14.6**

1. Inflammation of an area of bone, usually due to staph infection _____

2. Bone disease in children caused by vitamin D deficiency _____

3. Leads to short stature (height) _____

4. Rare, genetic disorder causing brittle bones _____

5. Decreased calcification of bone _____

6. Most common malignant bone tumor _____

7. Also known as *rickets* in children _____

8. When bone resorption exceeds bone formation, _____ results.

B. Fractures. You are working as the new radiology technician in the Radiology Department at the hospital. *You are attempting to identify the types of fractures with the pictures you see on the film. Match the description of the fracture on the left to its correct fracture on the right.* **LO 14.6**

Fracture Seen on the Film	Type of Fracture
_____ 1. Fracture at a right angle to the long axis of the radius	**a.** open fracture
_____ 2. Femur broken into two clean pieces	**b.** oblique fracture
_____ 3. Cancer patient with vertebral fracture	**c.** closed fracture
_____ 4. Broken ankle but no broken skin	**d.** transverse fracture
_____ 5. Diagonal fracture across the long axis of the femur	**e.** pathologic fracture
_____ 6. Fractured hand with bone fragments sticking out of the skin	**f.** displaced fracture

C. Use the appropriate abbreviation. *From the given list, choose the abbreviation that best fits the given description. Fill in the blanks.* **LO 14.6**

RA   DJD

1. Osteoarthritis is also known as _____

2. The arthritis in the joints was due to an autoimmune disease that caused the body to attack its own tissue. This type of arthritis is termed as _____

D. Deconstruct medical terms. *Deconstruct medical terms into their word elements. Fill in the blanks.* **LO 14.2, 14.6**

1. osteoarthritis: _____ / _____ / _____

2. degenerative: _____ / _____ / _____

E. Terms related to disorders of the wrist. *Correctly identify disorders of the wrist.* **LO 14.6**

1. A Colles fracture occurs at the:

   a. proximal radius

   b. distal radius

   c. proximal carpals

   d. distals carpals

2. The proper pronunciation for Colles is:

   a. cool ease   **c.** call ease

   b. cool ess   **d.** call ess

3. In a Colles fracture, the radius is displaced:

   a. medially   **c.** anteriorly

   b. laterally   **d.** posteriorly

F. Complete your knowledge of the skeleton by matching the statement in the left column to the appropriate term in the right column. LO 14.1, 14.6

_____ 1. forms ankle joint	**a.** hallux valgus
_____ 2. forms ankle and instep	**b.** gout
_____ 3. heel bone	**c.** tarsus
_____ 4. arthritis of big toe	**d.** talipes
_____ 5. deviation of big toe	**e.** metatarsus
_____ 6. swelling at base of big toe	**f.** talus
_____ 7. five parallel bones in the foot	**g.** calcaneus
_____ 8. foot deformity involving talus	**h.** bunion

Section 14.4 Procedures and Pharmacology

Diagnostic Procedures for Skeletal Disorders

Because bones are readily visible using x-rays, radiology is a common method to evaluate bone disorders. Radiography, CT scans, and MRI are frequently used to determine the presence of fractures or growths, such as tumors.

Arthrography is an x-ray of a joint taken after the injection of a contrast medium into the joint. A contrast medium makes the inside details of the joint visible.

Diagnostic arthroscopy is an exploratory procedure performed using an **arthroscope** to examine the internal compartments of a joint.

Women at risk for osteoporosis should have **bone mineral density (BMD)** screening using a **dual-energy x-ray absorptiometry (DEXA)** scan.

Therapeutic Procedures for the Skeletal System

Surgical Procedures

Arthrocentesis removes excess fluid from a joint, improving joint movement and relieving pain. Performed frequently for osteoarthritis.

Arthroscopy, performed through an **arthroscope,** allows for visual examination of a joint.

- **Ligament** reconstruction using **allograft, autograft,** or synthetic materials.
- **Cartilage** repair shoulder, knee, shoulder, ankle.
- **Meniscus** debridement, suturing, partial and total **meniscectomy** of the knee.

Arthroplasty repairs a joint by removing the diseased parts and replacing them with artificial parts made of titanium, other metals, and ceramics.

- **Total hip replacement (THP)** consists of replacing the femoral head and the hip socket (acetabulum) with a metal **prosthesis** (*Figure 14.26*).
- **Total knee arthroplasty (TKA)** (*Figure 14.27*) The lower end of the femur is replaced with a metal shell. The upper end of the tibia is replaced with a metal trough lined with plastic, and the back of the patella can be replaced with a plastic button.
- **Metacarpophalangeal arthroplasty** replaces osteoarthritic damaged finger joint with an artificial joint made of silicone rubber.

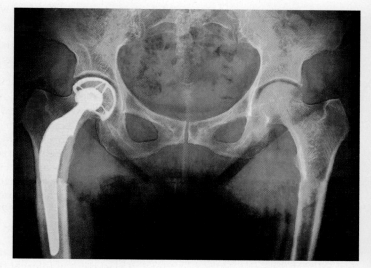

▲ **Figure 14.26** **Total hip replacement.** Colored x-ray of prosthetic hip. AJPhoto/Science Source

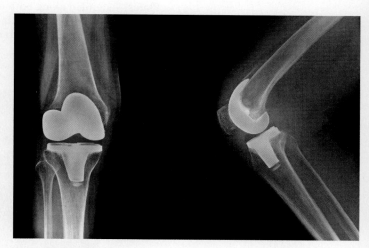

▲ **Figure 14.27** **Total knee replacement.** Colored x-ray of total knee replacement of left knee. ChooChin/Shutterstock

Treatment for SI Joint Pain

Fluoroscopic injection of local anesthetic into the joint can relieve the pain temporarily. Treatment is usually **stabilization** of the joint with a **brace** and physical therapy to strengthen the low-back muscles. Occasionally, **arthrodesis** of the joint is necessary.

Bone Fractures

The initial goal of fracture treatment is to bring the ends of the bone at the break opposite each other so that they fit together as they did in the original bone. This is called **alignment** and is necessary to ensure the bone heals

External devices are frequently used to keep bones into alignment and include:

- **Slings** hold the arm in place while allowing some movement.
- **Splints** and **braces** immobilize the bone and allow for a small amount of movement.
- **Casts** immobilize the bone and prevent movement of the muscles that move the joint. They are made of plaster and fiberglass.

Reduction moves a bone back to its correct place. Closed reduction pulls the bones from the distal end back into alignment.

Traction uses weights, pulley, and a metal frame to pull a bone into alignment.

Arthrodesis is the surgical fixation of a joint to prevent motion. Bone graft, wires, screws, or a plate can be used to stabilize the joint.

Fixation devices are plates, screws, and rods used to reassemble bones with multiple fractures or bone fragments. They can be made of stainless steel, titanium, or composites; certain types of composites can dissolve in the bone over time. These devices allow the patient to return to function quicker and reduces the incidence of **nonunion** and **malunion** (improper healing).

External fixation (*Figure 14.28*) uses fixation devices with one end inserted into the bone and the other attached to a metal frame or rod. These devices are removed when the bone has healed, around 6 to 8 weeks.

Open reduction internal fixation (**ORIF**) (*Figure 14.29*) surgery involves an incision to view the fracture and placement of internal fixation devices.

Fixation devices include:

Wires—used as sutures to "sew" the bone fragments together during ORIF.

Rods—can be inserted through the medullary cavity of both fragments to align the bones.

Plates—extended along both or all fragments of bone and held in place by screws.

Screws—can be used on their own as well as with plates.

Pins—a long, thick metal pin can be driven down the shaft of a bone from one end.

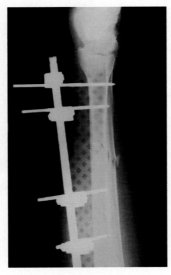

▲ **Figure 14.28**
External fixation devices.
Rod and pins
Stockbyte/Getty Images

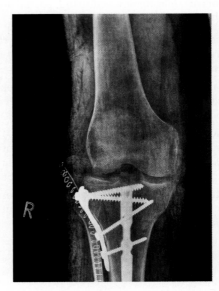

▲ **Figure 14.29** **Internal fixation devices.** Screws, rod, and plate
Stockbyte/Getty Images

Word Analysis and Definition: Diagnostic and Therapeutic Procedures

S = Suffix P = Prefix R = Root R/CF = Combining Form

WORD	PRONUNCIATION	ELEMENTS		DEFINITION
arthrocentesis	**AR**-throh-sen-**TEE**-sis	S/ R/CF	**-centesis** *to puncture* **arthr/o** - *joint*	Withdrawal of fluid from a joint with a needle
arthrodesis	**AR**-throh-**DEE**-sis	S/	**-desis** *bind together*	Fixation or stiffening of a joint by surgery
arthrography	ar-**THROG**-rah-fee	S/	**-graphy** *process of recording*	X-ray of a joint taken after injection of a contrast medium in the joint
arthroplasty	**AR**-throh-plas-tee	S/	**-plasty** *surgical repair*	Surgery to restore as far as possible the function of a joint
arthroscope	**AR**-throh-skope	S/	**-scope** *instrument for viewing*	Endoscope used to view the interior of a joint
arthroscopy	ar-**THROS**-koh-pee	S/	**-scopy** *to view*	Visual examination of the interior of a joint
cast	CAST		Old English *to create a mold*	Rigid encasement of a fractured bone to immobilize a fractured bone
sling	SLING		Middle English *sling*	Cloth tied behind the neck to support an arm
splint	SPLINT		Middle English *splint*	Device to prevent movement
fix			Old French *to fasten, fix*	Fix
fixation	fik-**SAY**-shun	S/	**-ation** *process*	Process of repairing
reduction	ree-**DUCK**-shun	S/ P/ R/	**-ion** *action condition, process* **re-** *backward* **-duct-** *lead*	Movement to place a structure back into anatomic position
traction	**TRAK**-shun		Latin *to pull*	A pulling or dragging force
malunion	mal-**YOU**-nee-un	S/ P/	**-ion** *action, condition, process* **mal-** *bad*	Condition in which the two bony ends of a fracture fail to heal together correctly
nonunion	non-**YOU**-nee-un	R/ P/	**-un-** *one* **non-** *not*	Total failure of healing of a fracture

Pharmacology

For osteoporosis, calcium (1,200 mg daily) and vitamin D (800 IU daily) are both the accepted baseline prevention and treatment.

For patients at risk of fractures, several medications approved by the U.S. **Food and Drug Administration (FDA)** are available for the treatment of osteoporosis. Most inhibit osteoclast activity to reduce the rate of loss of bone **(resorption)**, but some produce a direct increase in bone mass. As the turnover of bone is very slow, the time needed for assessing the effects of medications takes several years. Drugs that reduce the rate of bone resorption include estrogen, bisphosphonates, and calcitonin. **Bisphosphonates** (*Alendronate, Risedronate,* and others) are poorly absorbed from the gastrointestinal tract and can be given intravenously. **Calcitonin** also decreases osteoclast activity and is available as a subcutaneous injection or nasal spray. Several other drugs are available in other countries and/or are undergoing clinical trials in the United States.

Medications for osteoarthritis are numerous. **Acetaminophen** reduces mild pain but does not affect inflammation or swelling. It is used in combination with aspirin and/or caffeine (*Excedrin*) as an **OTC** medicine, and with codeine, or the narcotics hydrocodone (*Vicodin*) or oxycodone (*Percocet*) as prescription medications. Nonsteroidal anti-inflammatory drugs **(NSAIDs)** such as ibuprofen (*Advil*) and naproxen (*Aleve*) work well for pain but cause gastrointestinal problems and an increased risk of heart attacks and strokes.

Corticosteroids such as cortisone, prednisone, triamcinolone, and betamethasone, are used to reduce the pain and inflammation of severe osteoarthritis and are given orally or injected directly into the joint **(intra-articular)**. Corticosteroids are also used to reduce inflammation in rheumatoid arthritis **(RA)** but do not slow the progression of the disease. **Disease modifying anti-rheumatic drugs (DMARDs)** such as methotrexate (*Trexall*) are effective in reducing the signs and symptoms of RA, and other DMARDs such as hydrochloroquine (*Plaquenil*) and sulfasalazine (*Azulfidine*) can be added to methotrexate to enhance its effects. **Tumor necrosis factor (TNF)** is produced in RA joints by synovial macrophages and lymphocytes to attack the joint tissues and TNF **inhibitors** such as abatacept (*Orencia*) and rituximab (*Rituxan*) slow or halt the destruction.

Viscosupplementation is the intra-articular injection of a gel-like hyaluronic acid liquid, acting like synovial fluid by lubricating the joint and reducing the pain caused by osteoarthritis. Treatment for knee osteoarthritis requires multiple injections, given one week apart. It can take 8 to 12 weeks to feel pain reduction.

Did you know...

Viscosupplementation is given once all other treatments have failed.

S = Suffix P = Prefix R = Root R/CF = Combining Form

WORD	PRONUNCIATION	ELEMENTS		DEFINITION
acetaminophen	ah-seat-ah-**MIN**-oh-fen		Generic drug name	Medication that modifies or relieves pain
bisphosphonate	bis-**FOSS**-foh-nate	S/ P/ R/ R/	-ate *composed of* bi- *two* -phos- *light* -phon- *sound*	Drug that delays the rate of bone resorption
calcitonin	kal-sih-**TONE**-in	S/ R/CF R/	-in *chemical compound* calci- *calcium* -ton- *tension, pressure*	Hormone that moves calcium from blood to bones
corticosteroid	**KOR**-tih-koh-**STEHR**-oyd	S/ R/CF R/	-oid *resembling* cortic/o- *cortisone* -ster- *steroid*	A hormone produced by the adrenal cortex
inhibit (verb) inhibitor (noun)	in-**HIB**-it in-**HIB**-it-or		Latin *to keep back*	To curb or restrain Agent that curbs or restrains
intra-articular	**IN**-trah-ar-**TIK**-you-lar	S/ P/ R/	-ar *pertaining to* intra- *inside* -articul- *joint*	Pertaining to the inside of a joint

Check Point Section 14.4

A. There are several procedures that are specific to the joint. *Use the medical terms below to correctly complete each sentence. Not all terms will be used. Fill in the blanks.* **14.5, 14.6, 14.7**

arthrocentesis   arthrodesis   arthroplasty   arthroscope   arthroscopy

Mr. Johansen is a 54-year-old-man complaining of chronic, intense wrist pain and swelling. Dr. Lee believes that the pain is due to over-use and joint instability as a consequence of Mr. Johansen's years of college cheerleading due to repeated lifting of female cheerleaders.

In order to relieve the swelling, (**1**) _____ of the wrist was performed. In order to visualize the joint, an (**2**) _____ was ordered. During the surgery, Dr. Lee utilized the (**3**) _____ to determine that the best course of action was to fuse the bones of the wrist. Therefore, an (**4**) _____ was performed.

B. Construct medical terms related to therapeutic procedures. *You are given definitions of medical terms along with a few word elements. Fill in the blanks with the missing word elements to create the medical term.* **LO 14.7**

1. Movement to place a structure back into anatomic position   re /_____ /_____

2. Excision of a part of a mensicus: menisc /_____

3. Removal of necrotic tissue: _____ /_____/ment

4. Surgical fixation of a joint: _____ /o/_____

C. Use terms related to pharmacology. *Use terms and abbreviations to complete the following paragraph. Use the terms provided. Not all terms will be used. Fill in the blanks.* **LO 14.7**

DNARD   podiatrist   RA   OTC   chiropractor   acetaminophen   calcitonin   corticosteroid

Ms. Walker made an appointment with a _____ for pain in her shoulder. She participates in high-intensity weightlifting and fitness training. She has been taking _____ medication to treat the pain; specifically, the medication _____. She denies a personal or family history of _____.

D. Construct medical terms related to the pharmacology of the skeletal system. *Insert the correct word element that completes each term.* *Fill in the blanks.* **LO 14.2, 14.7**

1. Hormone that moves calcium from the blood to the bone: calc/i/_____/in

2. Hormone produced by the adrenal cortex: _____/_____/ster/oid

3. Pertaining to the inside of a joint: intra-_____/ar

Table 14. 2 Chapter 14 Abbreviations

Abbreviations	Meaning
AC	acromioclavicular
BMD	bone mineral density
DC	Doctor of Chiropractic
DEXA	dual-energy x-ray absorptiometry
DJD	degenerative joint disease
DMARD	disease modifying anti-rheumatic drug
DO	Doctor of osteopathy
FDA	Food and Drug Administration
Fx	fracture
JRA	juvenile rheumatoid arthritis
MD	Doctor of Medicine
NSAIDs	nonsteroidal anti-inflammatory drugs
OA	osteoarthritis
OTC	over the counter
MCL	medial collateral ligament
RA	rheumatoid arthritis
SI	sacroiliac
THR	total-hip replacement
TMJ	temporomandibular joint
TNF	tumor necrosis factor

Table 14. 2 Comparison of Selected Skeletal Disorders—Signs, Symptoms, and Treatments

Disorder or Disease	Signs and Symptoms	Diagnostic Tests	Treatment
Osteomalacia (rickets)	Pain in bones, joints, muscles.	X-ray, blood tests to measure amount of vitamin D and calcium levels.	Increase vitamin D and calcium intake through diet. Vitamin D and calcium supplements as needed.
Osteomyelitis	Can occur without signs or symptoms. Pain, warmth, redness in affected area. Fever and fatigue.	X-rays, MRI, CT scan. Blood tests for signs of infection—increased leukocytes.	Surgical removal of the infected bone followed by IV antibiotics.
Closed humerus fracture	Pain and redness of the arm. Patient supports arm by holding the elbow.	X-ray, CT scan.	Closed reduction, followed by splint, then brace after swelling has gone down. Depends on severity of break.
Torn anterior cruciate ligament (ACL)	Noncontact injury occurs with sudden stopping of leg motion, patient hears a sudden "pop" and then knee "gives out."	Manipulation of the joint, MRI.	Arthroscopic surgical reconstruction of ligament with tissue graft.

Challenge Your Knowledge

A. **Knowing the exact number of certain body parts, and their relative positions, will ensure precision in your medical documentation.** Match the correct number to the correct term. Use one answer twice. **LO 14.1**

_____ **1.** Number of lumbar vertebrae: _____

_____ **2.** Number of bones in the vertebral column: _____

_____ **3.** Number of cervical vertebrae: _____

_____ **4.** Number of components in the skeletal system: _____

_____ **5.** Number of regions in the vertebral column: _____

_____ **6.** Number of thoracic vertebrae: _____

a. 7

b. 5

c. 4

d. 12

e. 26

B. **Match the health professional in the second column with his or her job description in the first column. LO 14.10**

_____ **1.** Practitioner in the diagnosis and treatment of disorders and injuries of the foot

_____ **2.** Practitioner who evaluates and treats pain, disease, or injury by measures other than medical or surgical

_____ **3.** Practitioner who makes and fits orthopedic appliances

_____ **4.** Physician who specializes in physical medicine and rehabilitation

_____ **5.** Practitioner who focuses on manual adjustment of joints to maintain and restore health

a. orthotist

b. physiatrist

c. podiatrist

d. chiropractor

e. physical therapist

C. **Correct spelling and formation of plurals are important in medical documentation.** Improve your skill with this exercise. Fill in the blanks the correct spelling of the singular term, and then form the plural. The plural form is not provided for you. **LO 14.3**

1. epiphysis   epipisis   ephysis   epyisis

Correct spelling of the term: _____

Plural form of the term: _____

2. laccuna   lacuna   lecuna   lacunna

Correct spelling of the term: _____

Plural form of the term: _____

3. thoraax   torax   thorax   thoraxx

Correct spelling of the term: _____

Plural form of the term: _____

4. palanx   phalanx   phalynx   palanyx

Correct spelling of the term: _____

Plural form of the term: _____

D. The following prefixes have all appeared in this chapter. The meaning of the prefix is given to you—identify the prefix. Fill in the chart. **LO 14.2**

Prefix	Meaning of Prefix
1.	*from, out of*
2.	*beyond, making change*
3.	*two*
4.	*without*
5.	*between*
6.	*inside*
7.	*together*
8.	*away from*
9.	*toward*
10.	*around*

E. Demonstrate your knowledge of the upper-body bones and joints by selecting the correct answer to these questions. LO 14.6, 14.7

1. What is the long bone of the upper arm called?

   a. radius

   b. ulna

   c. humerus

   d. carpal

   e. scapula

2. What is a likely shoulder injury?

   a. separation

   b. lateral epicondylitis

   c. Colles fracture

   d. Carpal tunnel syndrome

3. What structures hold an articulation together?

   a. ligaments

   b. tendons

   c. joint capsule

   d. all of these

4. The injury that describes the condition of the humerus no longer touching the scapular surface

   a. subluxation

   b. separation

   c. arthrodesis

   d. avulsion

   e. dislocation

5. Where does a Colles fracture occur?

   a. shoulder

   b. hip

   c. shoulder

   d. elbow

   e. wrist

alengo/E+/Getty Images

F. **Many medical terms come directly from Greek or Latin.** Match the term on the left with its correct Greek or Latin meaning on the right. **LO 14.1**

Medical Term

Greek or Latin Meaning

_____ 1. bursa

a. mother, womb

_____ 2. callus

b. bark

_____ 3. cartilage

c. purse

_____ 4. condyle

d. hard skin

_____ 5. cortex

e. band, sheet

_____ 6. lacuna

f. knuckle

_____ 7. ligament

g. pit, lake

_____ 8. matrix

h. gristle

G. **Read the description and then enter the abnormal spinal curvature that it is describing.** Some conditions are used more than once. **LO 14.6**

1. An abnormal lateral curvature of the spine: _____

2. An abnormal posterior curvature of the thoracic vertebrae: _____

3. An abnormal anterior curvature of the lumbar vertebrae: _____

4. Osteoporosis can lead to this abnormal spinal curvature: _____

5. Of the three types of abnormal curvatures, this one occurs most frequently: _____

H. **Physical therapists instruct patients in range-of-motion (ROM) exercises to improve mobility.** The exercises are described for you—determine the correct medical term. Use the provided word bank to fill in the blanks with the correct action being described. **LO 14.1**

abduction	lateral rotation	rotation	pronation	supination
inversion	circumduction	medial rotation	adduction	eversion

1. Rotating the humerus with the elbow flexed while bringing the palm of the hand toward the body: _____

2. Elbow flexed at 90 degrees, rotating forearm so that palm is facing the floor: _____

3. Sole of the foot facing toward the opposite foot: _____. This is also called _____.

4. Action of moving toward the midline: _____

5. Turning a joint on its axis: _____

6. Sole of the foot facing laterally away from the other foot: _____ or _____

7. Moving the shoulder so that it forms a cone with the shoulder joint as the apex of the cone: _____

8. Spreading fingers apart, away from the middle finger: _____

9. Moving the palm away from the body: _____

10. Lying flat on your back, palms facing up: _____

I. Choose the correct medical term(s) from the list to complete the sentence. You will not use all the terms. Use the provided word bank to fill in the blanks with the correct action being described. **LO 14.1, 14.6, 14.7**

arthrodesis	symphysis	detoxification	intervertebral discs
cancellous	circumduction	pelvis	retinaculum
shoulder girdle	cortex	acetabulum	Colles
arthrocentesis	Pott	labrum	

1. Removal of excess fluid from a joint: _____.

2. A transverse, fibrous band on the wrist is called a _____.

3. _____ support and cushion the vertebral column.

4. A fracture of the fibula near the ankle is called a _____ fracture.

5. Moving the arms in a circular motion is termed _____.

6. Cartilaginous joint between two bones is called _____.

7. A _____ is a cartilage rim along a ball and socket joint.

8. Dr. Stannard performed a(n) _____ to remove the excess fluid from the knee.

9. The _____ is the hard outer bone shell.

J. Many professional certification exams are given in multiple-choice format. Decide on the answer by quickly eliminating the answers you know to be incorrect. Then select the remaining answer that correctly completes each statement. **LO 14.1, 14.6**

1. Bone growth occurs at the
   - a. origin
   - b. epiphyseal plate
   - c. diaphysis
   - d. epicondyle
   - e. lacuna

2. An inherited condition in which bone formation is incomplete is
   - a. osteoarthritis
   - b. osteomalacia
   - c. osteomyelitis
   - d. osteogenesis imperfecta
   - e. osteopenia

3. Lubricant for joint movement is
   - a. mucin
   - b. mucus
   - c. mucous
   - d. synovial
   - e. meniscus

4. The following is where two bones come together at a joint:
   - a. articulation
   - b. reduction
   - c. mastication
   - d. striation
   - e. herniation

5. An extension of synovial membrane that forms a cushion to prevent structures from rubbing together is
   - a. tendon
   - b. periosteum
   - c. ligament
   - d. bursa
   - e. muscle

6. Pulling a bone from the distal end back into alignment is
   - a. subluxation
   - b. dislocation
   - c. reduction
   - d. resorption
   - e. external fixation

7. The process of lying face upward, flat on your spine, is
   - a. pronation
   - b. abduction
   - c. adduction
   - d. supination
   - e. inversion

8. Joints between the teeth and their sockets are called
   - a. symphyses
   - b. gomphoses
   - c. sutures
   - d. syndesmoses
   - e. synchondroses

alengo/E+/Getty Images

K. **Build your orthopedic terminology by completing the medical terms defined here.** After you fill in the element on the line, write the type of element (prefix, root, combining form, suffix) you have used below the lines. Fill in the blanks. **LO 14.1, 14.2, 14.6, 14.7**

1. Bone softening   osteo/_____

2. Projection above the condyle   _____ /condyle

3. Membrane surrounding a bone   peri/ _____ / _____

4. Region between diaphysis and epiphysis   _____ /physis

5. Decreased calcification of bone   osteo/ _____

6. Bone cell that lives in a lacuna   osteo/ _____

7. Malignant tumor of connective tissue   _____ /oma

8. Moving toward the midline   _____ / _____ /ion

9. Fixation of a joint with surgery   arthro/ _____

L. **Identify the elements in each medical term and unlock the meaning of the word.** Fill in the chart. If the word does not have a particular word element, write n/a. **LO 14.2**

Medical Term	Meaning of Prefix	Meaning of Root/ Combining Form	Meaning of Suffix	Meaning of the Term
syndesmosis	1.	2.	3.	4.
osteogenesis	5.	6.	7.	8.
subluxation	9.	10.	11.	12.
periosteal	13.	14.	15.	16.
pectoral	17.	18.	19.	20.

M. **Write the correctly spelled terms for each of the following definitions.** **LO 14.1, 14.3**

1. Tailbone   _____

2. Joint formed by ligaments   _____

3. Lower/posterior part of the hip bone   _____

4. Compact bone grows in and forms this line   _____

5. Shoulder blades   _____

6. Posterior spinal curve   _____

N. **Pronunciation is important whether you are saying the word or listening to a word from a coworker.** Identify the proper pronunciation of the following medical terms. The correctly spell the term. **LO 14.1, 14.3, 14.5**

1. The correct pronunciation for a fracture that is broken into pieces

     a. IN-kom-plate   **c.** KOM-ih-nyu-ted

     b. in-kom-**PLEET**   **d.** kom-you-**TATE**-ed

     Correctly spell the term: _____

2. The correct pronunciation for multiple bones joined by fibrocartilage

    a. SIM-feh-sees

    b. sim-**FEE**-sis

    c. gom-**FOHS**-ees

    d. gom-**FOH**-sis

    Correctly spell the term: _____

3. The correct pronunciation for the inflammation of a closed sac containing synovial fluid

    a. burr-**SIGH**-tis

    b. by-**YOUR**-sigh-tis

    c. ar-**THRIE**-tis

    d. **ARTH**-right-us

    Correctly spell the term: _____

4. The correct pronunciation for multiple openings through a structure

    a. foh-**RAM**-in-ah

    b. for-**AY**-men-ah

    c. **KON**-dile

    d. kon-**DILE**

    Correctly spell the term: _____

5. The correct pronunciation for the bones that form the bulging sides and roof of the cranium

    a. pah-**RYE**-eh-tal

    b. **PAIR**-ee-**EYE**-tal

    c. ox-**IP**-it-al

    d. ok-**SIP**-it-al

    Correctly spell the term: _____

Case Reports

A. **After reading the following Case Report, correctly answer the following questions.** The answers to the questions may not be in the Case Report itself but can be found in the chapter content. **LO 14.1, 14.6, 14.7, 14.8, 14.9, 14.10**

Case Report (CR) 14.1

You are

. . . an **orthopedic technologist** working with Kevin Stannard, MD, an **orthopedist** in the Fulwood Medical Group.

Your patient is

. . . Mrs. Amy Vargas, a 70-year-old housewife, who tripped going down the front steps from her house. She has severe pain in her right hip and is unable to stand. Dr. Stannard examined her in the Emergency Department, and after reading her x-ray, admitted her for surgery.

For you to work with Dr. Stannard to give optimal care to Mrs. Vargas and help her and her family understand the significance of her bone disorder and injury, you will need to be familiar with the terminology of bone structure and function and bone disorders.

---

1. You are collecting Mrs. Vargas's medical history. She states that she the only exercise she does is walking 25 yards to get the mail and has smoked for over 30 years. Based on these facts and the facts in the Case Report, Mrs. Vargas like has the pre-existing condition:

    a. chondromalacia.

    b. bunions.

    c. osteoporosis.

    d. pes planus.

2. The health professional that will help Mrs. Vargas gain strength in her affected joint will be a:

    a. physical therapist.

    b. orthotist.

    c. chiropractor.

    d. podiatrist.

3. Based on the location of pain described by Mrs. Vargas, she has likely fractured her:

    a. tibia

    b. pelvis

    c. clavicle

    d. ulna

4. Which surgery do you predict Mrs. Vargas will have?

    a. DEXA

    b. THR

    c. MCP

    d. ACL

B. **After reading the following Case Report, correctly answer the following questions.** The answers to the questions may not be in the Case Report itself but can be found in the chapter content. **LO 14.6, 14.7, 14.8, 14.9, 14.10**

Case Report (CR) 14.2

You are

. . . an emergency technician working in the Emergency Department at Fulwood Medical Center.

Your patient is

. . . Mr. Luke Johnson, a 20-year-old university student.

Mr. Johnson presents with severe pain in his right shoulder area. At rugby practice, Mr. Johnson jumped to catch a pass, was tackled while in the air, and landed on the tip of his left shoulder. He is now complaining of pain in his upper chest near the shoulder, has his left arm held close to his chest, and is supporting it with his right hand. Examination shows swelling and tenderness over the midclavicular region and inability to abduct his left humerus.

The emergency physician sends Mr. Johnson for an x-ray, which shows a midshaft fracture of his clavicle.

---

1. Which device would probably provide Mr. Johnson immediate pain relief?

    a. Cast

    b. Plate

    c. Sling

    d. Splint

2. Based on the case report, Mr. Johnson is unable to move his:

    a. arm anteriorly.

    b. arm away from his side.

    c. forearm anteriorly.

    d. forearm away from his side.

3. Which type of specialist should be consulted to care for Mr. Johnson's injury?

    a. Orthopedic technologist

    b. Osteopathic physician

    c. Orthopedic surgeon

    d. Orthotist

4. The surgical correction for this condition would be an:

    a. open reduction with a plate.

    b. external reduction and a cast.

    c. arthrodesis and a sling.

    d. arthroplasty with a brace.

C. After reading the following Case Report, correctly answer the following questions. The answers to the questions may not be in the Case Report itself but can be found in the chapter content. **LO 14.6, 14.8**

 Case Report (CR) 14.3

You are

. . . an orthopedic technologist working with Kenneth Stannard, MD, at Fulwood Medical Center.

Your patient is

. . . James Fox, a 17-year-old male who complains of severe pain in his right wrist. While playing soccer a few hours earlier, he fell. James pushed his hand out to break his fall and heard his wrist snap. The wrist is now swollen and deformed.

VS are T 98.2, P 92, R 15, BP 110/76. On examination, his right wrist is swollen and tender and has a dinner-fork deformity. An IV has been started, and he has been given 3 mg of morphine IV. An x-ray of the wrist was ordered and reveals a closed Colles Fx.

1. What type of physician is Dr. Stannard?

a. podiatrist

b. orthotist

c. orthopedist

d. chiropractor

2. The fracture has been described as *closed:*

a. bones are out of placement

b. the skin is unbroken

c. bones are shifted laterally

d. it is complex and requires surgery

3. The abbreviation *Fx* means:

a. fracture

b. fixation

c. flexion

d. febrile

4. Why was James given morphine?

a. reduce swelling

b. decrease the respiratory rate

c. reduce the elevated blood pressure

d. treat the pain

5. In a Colles Fx, a bone that is likely affected is:

a. ulna

b. humerus

c. radius

d. phalange

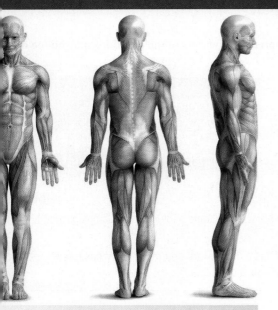
Adike/Shutterstock

CHAPTER
15

Muscles and Tendons, Physical Medicine and Rehabilitation (PM&R)
The Languages of Orthopedics and Rehabilitation

Chapter Sections

Chapter Learning Outcomes

Upon completion of this chapter, you will be able to:

LO 15.1 Identify and describe the anatomy and physiology of the muscular system.

LO 15.2 Use roots, combining forms, suffixes, and prefixes to construct and analyze medical terms related to the muscular system.

LO 15.3 Spell medical terms related to the muscular system.

LO 15.4 Pronounce medical terms related to the muscular system.

LO 15.5 Describe diagnostic procedures utilized for disorders of the muscular system.

LO 15.6 Identify and describe disorders and pathological conditions related to the muscular system.

LO 15.7 Describe rehabilitation procedures and pharmacologic agents used with the muscular system.

LO 15.8 Apply knowledge of medical terms relating to the muscular system to documentation, medical records, and communication.

LO 15.9 Identify and correctly use abbreviations of terms used that refer to the muscular system.

LO 15.10 Identify health professionals involved in the care of patients with muscular disorders.

The health professionals involved in the diagnosis and treatment of problems of the musculoskeletal system include:

- **Physiatrists,** who are physicians specializing in physical medicine and rehabilitation.
- **Physical therapists,** diagnose and treat injuries, disabilities, or other health conditions to improve a patient's ability to move, reduce pain, restore function, and prevent disability.
- **Physical therapist assistants,** assist physical therapists in the treatment of patients.
- **Occupational therapists,** who practice occupational therapy (OT) to help patients improve their activities of daily living (ADLs) and adapt to visual and other perceptual deficits.
- **Occupational therapy assistants** (COTAs), who assist occupational therapists.
- **Orthopedic technologists and technicians,** who assist orthopedic surgeons in treating patients.
- **Orthotists,** who make and fit orthopedic appliances (**orthotics**).

Section 15.1 Muscles and Tendons

Types of Muscle

Bones of the skeleton support the body and joints provide mobility. Neither of these functions can occur without muscles and their tendons to provide both. The three types of muscle are:

- **skeletal**
- **cardiac**
- **smooth**

Skeletal muscle contracts on demand to provide posture and movement.

Cardiac and smooth muscle contract and relax without conscious thought, cardiac muscle to power the heart contractions and smooth muscle to power the movement of food through the gastrointestinal tract (*see Chapter 5*), the process called **peristalsis.**

Functions and Structure of Skeletal Muscle

Functions of Skeletal Muscle

Skeletal muscle is attached to one or more bones. It is also called **voluntary muscle** because it is under conscious control. Because of their length, muscle cells are usually called muscle **fibers.** Each skeletal muscle consists of bundles of muscle fibers, blood vessels, and nerves, with connective tissue sheets that hold the fibers together and connect the muscle to bone.

Skeletal muscle has the following functions:

1. **Movement.** All skeletal muscles are attached to bones, and when a muscle **contracts,** it causes movement of the bones to which it is attached (*Figure 15.1*). This enables you to walk, run, and work with your hands.

2. **Posture.** The **tone** of skeletal muscles holds you straight when sitting, standing, or moving.

3. **Body heat.** When skeletal muscles contract, heat is produced as a by-product of the energy reaction. This heat is essential to maintain your body temperature.

4. **Respiration.** Skeletal muscles move the chest wall as you breathe.

5. **Communication.** Skeletal muscles enable you to speak, write, type, gesture, and grimace.

Structure of Skeletal Muscle

Skeletal muscle **fibers** (*Figure 15.2*) are narrow and long, up to 1½ inches (approximately 3.7 cm) in length. Each muscle fiber has a thin layer of connective tissue around it. Bundles of muscle fibers are grouped together into **fascicles** that are also surrounded by a layer of connective tissue. Skeletal muscle fibers contain alternating dark and light bands (**striations**) created by the pattern of protein filaments responsible for muscle contraction. Skeletal muscle can be referred to as **striated muscle.**

Bundles of fascicles form a muscle that is separated from adjacent muscles and kept in position by a dense layer of connective tissue called **fascia.** Fascia extends beyond the muscle to form a tendon. The tendon attaches to the periosteum of a bone at the **origin** and **insertion** of the muscle.

As an adult, you have the same number of muscle fibers as you had in late childhood. When you exercise and/or lift weights and your muscles enlarge or **hypertrophy,** you have increased the thickness of each muscle fiber. If you do not use your muscles, the reverse happens, and the muscles **atrophy.**

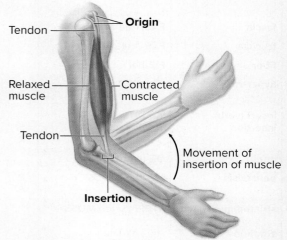

▲ **Figure 15.1** Muscle contraction.

Did you know...

- The **origin** of a muscle is its attachment to a more fixed part of the skeleton.
- The **insertion** of a muscle is its attachment to a more movable part of the skeleton.

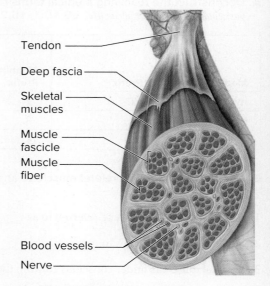

▲ **Figure 15.2** Structure of skeletal muscle.

S = Suffix P = Prefix R = Root R/CF = Combining Form

WORD	PRONUNCIATION	ELEMENTS		DEFINITION
atrophy	**AT**-roh-fee	P/ R/	a- *without* -trophy *nourishment*	The wasting away or diminished volume of tissue, an organ, or a body part
contract	kon-**TRAKT**	P/ R/	con- *with, together* -tract *draw*	Draw together or shorten
fascia	**FASH**-ee-ah		Latin *a band*	Sheet of fibrous connective tissue
fascicle	**FAS**-ih-kull		Latin *small bundle*	Bundle of muscle fibers
fiber	**FIE**-ber		Latin *fiber*	A strand or filament
hypertrophy	high-**PER**-troh-fee	P/ R/	hyper- *excessive* -trophy *nourishment*	Increase in size, but not in number, of an individual tissue element
insert (verb) insertion	in-**SIRT** in-**SIR**-shun	 S/ R/	Latin *to join* -ion *action, condition* insert- *put together*	The insertion of a muscle is the attachment of a muscle to a more movable part of the skeleton, as distinct from the origin
origin	**OR**-ih-gin		Latin *source of*	Fixed source of a muscle at its attachment to bone
peristalsis	per-ih-**STAL**-sis	P/ R/	peri- *around* -stalsis *constrict*	Waves of alternate contraction and relaxation of the alimentary canal wall to move food along the digestive tract
striated muscle	**STRIE**-ay-ted **MUSS**-el		striated Latin *stripe* muscle Latin *muscle*	Another term for skeletal muscle
striation	strie-**AY**-shun	S/ R/	-ion *action, condition* striat- *stripe*	Stripes
tone	TONE		Greek *tone*	Tension present in resting muscles
voluntary muscle	**VOL**-un-tare-ee **MUSS**-el	 S/ R/	-ary *pertaining to* volunt- *free will* muscle Latin *muscle*	Another term for skeletal muscle. It is under the control of the will

Check Point Section 15.1

A. Deconstruct the following medical terms related to muscles into their basic elements. *Fill in the chart. If the word does not have a particular word element, write n/a.* **LO 15.1, 15.2**

Medical Term	Prefix	Meaning of Prefix	Root/ Combining Form	Meaning of Root/ Combining Form	Suffix	Meaning of Suffix
hypertrophy	1.	2.	3.	4.	5.	6.
contract	7.	8.	9.	10.	11.	12.
atrophy	13.	14.	15.	16.	17.	18.

B. Use terms related to skeletal muscle to answer the following questions. *Fill in the blank to complete each statement correctly.* **LO 15.1, 15.3**

1. Skeletal muscle also can be referred to as _____ muscle.

2. Skeletal muscle attaches to _____.

3. Skeletal muscle is under conscious control; therefore, it is considered a _____ muscle.

4. Skeletal muscle must be used, or _____ (condition) occurs.

Section 15.2 Muscles and Tendons of the Upper and Lower Extremities

Shoulder Girdle

Your **shoulder girdle** connects your axial skeleton to your upper limbs and helps you to move these limbs. Without your shoulder girdle, you wouldn't be able to throw a ball, drive a car, or reach that top shelf of your closet or kitchen cabinet. In fact, you wouldn't be able to move your upper limbs.

The muscles and tendons in your shoulder girdle get plenty of use. Four muscles originate on your scapula, wrap around the shoulder joint, and fuse together. This fusion forms one large tendon (the **rotator cuff**), which is inserted into the humerus (*Figure 15.3*). Your rotator cuff keeps the ball of the humerus tightly in the scapula's socket and provides stability of the shoulder joint and the kind of strength needed by baseball pitchers.

The rotator cuff muscles are

1. Subscapularis
2. Supraspinatus
3. Infraspinatus
4. Teres minor

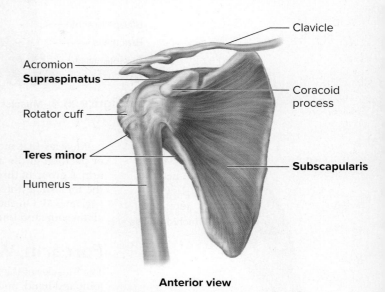

▲ **Figure 15.3** Rotator cuff muscles (anterior view).

Word Analysis and Definition: Shoulder Girdle				
				S = Suffix P = Prefix R = Root R/CF = Combining Form
WORD	**PRONUNCIATION**	**ELEMENTS**		**DEFINITION**
infraspinatus	IN-frah-spy-NAY-tuss	S/ P/ R/	-us *pertaining to* infra- *below, beneath* -spinat- *having spines*	Pertaining to beneath the spine (of the scapula)
rotator cuff	roh-TAY-tor CUFF	S/ R/	-or *one who does* rotat- *rotate* cuff Old English *band*	Part of the capsule of the shoulder joint
subscapularis	SUB-skap-you-LA-ris	S/ P/ R/	-is *pertaining to* sub- *below* -scapular- *scapula*	Pertaining to below the scapula
supraspinatus	sue-prah-spy-NAY-tuss	S/ P/ R/	-us *pertaining to* supra- *above* -spinat- *having spines*	Pertaining to above the spine (of the scapula)
teres major	TER-eze MAY-jor		teres Latin *long and round* major Latin *large*	One of the muscles that make up the rotator cuff

Upper Arm and Elbow Joint

Muscles connect the humerus (upper arm bone) to the shoulder girdle, vertebral column, and ribs. These muscles enable the arm to move freely at the shoulder joint. The major anterior muscles (those at the front of the body) are the **deltoid** (shoulder muscle) and **pectoralis major** (chest muscle) (*Figure 15.4a*). Among the major posterior muscles is the **latissimus dorsi,** found in the back (*Figure 15.4b*).

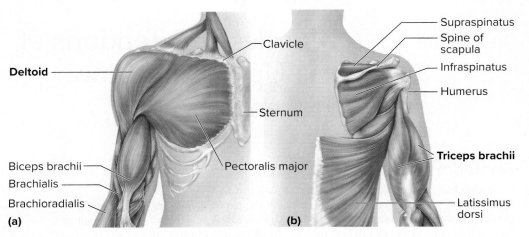

▲ **Figure 15.4** Muscles join arm to body. (a) Anterior view. (b) Posterior view.

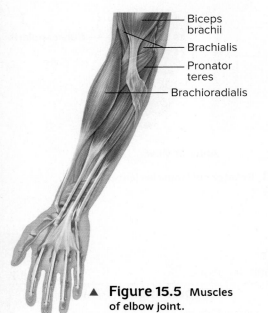

▲ **Figure 15.5** Muscles of elbow joint.

Muscles that move the elbow joint and forearm have their origins on the humerus or pectoral girdle and are inserted into the bones of the forearm. On the front of the arm, a group of three muscles (the **biceps brachii, brachialis,** and **brachioradialis**) flexes the forearm at the elbow joint and rotates the forearm and hand laterally (supination) *(Figure 15.5).* On the back of the arm, a single muscle, the **triceps brachii,** extends the elbow joint and forearm.

Forearm, Wrist, and Hand

The muscles of the forearm supinate and pronate the forearm, flex and extend the wrist joint and hand, and move the hand medially and laterally.

As the tendons pass over the wrist, they are surrounded by sheaths of synovial membrane and held in place on the wrist by a transverse, thick fibrous band called a **retinaculum** *(Figure 15.7).*

The Hand

When you look at the palm of your hand, you'll see a prominent pad of muscles (the **thenar eminence**) at the base of your thumb *(Figure 15.7).* A smaller pad of muscles (the **hypothenar eminence**) is located at the base of your little finger. The back of your hand is called the **dorsum.**

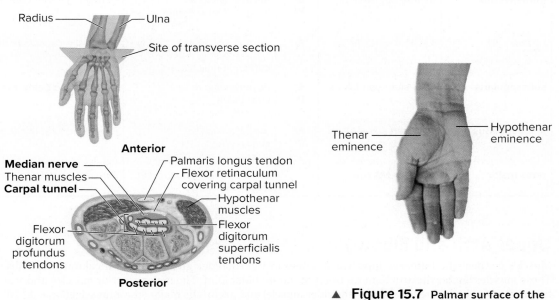

▲ **Figure 15.6** Carpal tunnel: Transverse section.

▲ **Figure 15.7** Palmar surface of the hand. Eric Wise

WORD	PRONUNCIATION	ELEMENTS		DEFINITION
biceps brachii	**BIE**-sepz **BRAY**-kee-eye	R/ P/ R/CF	**-ceps** *head* **bi-** *two* **brachi/i** *of the arm*	A muscle of the arm that has two heads or points of origin on the scapula
brachialis	**BRAY**-kee-al-is	S/ R/	**-alis** *pertaining to* **brachi-** *arm*	Muscle that lies underneath the biceps and is the strongest flexor of the forearm
brachioradialis	**BRAY**-kee-oh-**RAY**-dee-al-is	S/ R/CF R/	**-alis** *pertaining to* **brachi/o-** *arm* **-radi-** *radius*	Muscle that helps flex the forearm
deltoid	**DEL**-toyd	S/ R/	**-oid** *resembling* **delt-** *triangle*	Large, fan-shaped muscle connecting the scapula and clavicle to the humerus
dorsum dorsal (adj)	**DOR**-sum **DOR**-sal	S/ R/	Latin *back* **-al** *pertaining to* **dors-** *back*	The back of any part of the body, including the hand Pertaining to the back of any part of the body
latissimus dorsi	lah-**TISS**-ih-muss **DOR**-sigh	S/ R/ R/	**-imus** *most* **latiss-** *wide* **dorsi** *of the back*	The widest (broadest) muscle in the back
retinaculum	ret-ih-**NAK**-you-lum	S/ R/	**-um** *structure* **retinacul-** *hold back*	Fibrous ligament that keeps the tendons in place on the wrist so that they do not "bowstring" when the forearm muscles contract
thenar eminence	**THAY**-nar **EM**-in-ens	R/	**thenar** *palm* **eminence** Latin *stand out*	The fleshy mass at the base of the thumb
hypothenar eminence	high-poh-**THAY**-nar **EM**-in-ens	P/	**hypo-** *below, smaller*	The fleshy mass at the base of the little finger
triceps brachii	**TRY**-sepz **BRAY**-kee-eye	R/ P/ R/CF	**-ceps** *head* **tri-** *three* **brachi/i** *of the arm*	Muscle of the arm that has three heads or points of origin

Muscles of Pelvic Girdle and Lower Limb

Powerful muscles that support the hip joint and move the thigh have their origins on the pelvic girdle and their insertions into the femur. Prominent among them are the three **gluteus** muscles—**maximus, medius,** and **minimus** (*Figure 15.8*)—and the **adductor** muscles that run down the inner thigh.

Thigh Muscles

The thigh muscles move the knee joint and lower leg. The anterior thigh (the front of the thigh) contains the large **quadriceps femoris** muscle. This muscle has four heads: the rectus femoris, vastus lateralis, vastus medialis, and the vastus intermedius (which lies beneath the rectus femoris). These four muscle heads join into the **quadriceps tendon** (which contains the patella) and continue as the patellar tendon to be inserted into the tibia (*Figure 15.9*). The quadriceps muscle extends (straightens) the knee joint and, because of the lower leg's weight, it has to be a very strong muscle.

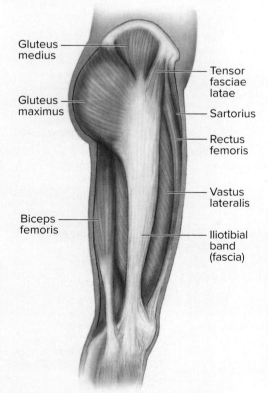

Gluteus medius
Gluteus maximus
Biceps femoris
Tensor fasciae latae
Sartorius
Rectus femoris
Vastus lateralis
Iliotibial band (fascia)

▲ **Figure 15.8** Muscles of the hip and thigh [lateral view].

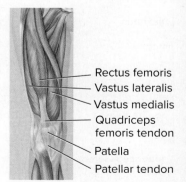

Rectus femoris
Vastus lateralis
Vastus medialis
Quadriceps femoris tendon
Patella
Patellar tendon

▲ **Figure 15.9** Anterior muscles of the thigh.

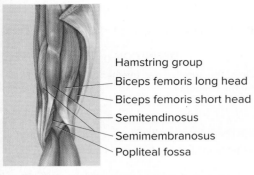

- Hamstring group
- Biceps femoris long head
- Biceps femoris short head
- Semitendinosus
- Semimembranosus
- Popliteal fossa

▲ **Figure 15.10** Posterior thigh muscles.

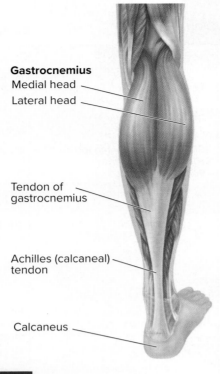

Gastrocnemius
- Medial head
- Lateral head

- Tendon of gastrocnemius

- Achilles (calcaneal) tendon

- Calcaneus

▶ **Figure 15.11** Muscles of the right lower leg [posterior view].

The posterior (rear) thigh is composed mostly of the three **hamstring muscles:** the **biceps femoris, semimembranosus,** and **semitendinosus** (*Figure 15.10*). These muscles flex (bend) the knee joint and rotate the lower leg. The hollow area at the back of the knee joint between the hamstring tendons is the **popliteal fossa.**

Muscles of the Lower Leg

The muscles of the lower leg move the ankle, foot, and toes. Those on the front of the leg are in a compartment between the tibia and fibula. They dorsiflex the foot at the ankle and extend the toes. Those on the lateral side of the leg evert the foot.

Those on the back of the leg plantar flex the foot at the ankle, flex the toes, and invert the foot (*Figure 15.11*). The **gastrocnemius** muscle forms a large part of the calf. The distal end of it joins with the tendon of the **soleus** muscle to form the **calcaneal (Achilles) tendon,** which is attached to the **calcaneus** (heel bone). The gastrocnemius muscle and the calcaneal tendon enable you to "push off" and start running or jumping.

Word Analysis and Definition: Muscles of Pelvic Girdle and Lower Limb

S = Suffix P = Prefix R = Root R/CF = Combining Form

WORD	PRONUNCIATION		ELEMENTS	DEFINITION
adductor	ah-**DUK**-tor	S/	**-or** *that which does something*	Muscle that moves the thigh toward the midline
		P/	**ad-** *toward*	
adduction	ah-**DUK**-shun	R/	**-duct-** *lead*	Action of moving toward the midline
		S/	**-ion** *action, condition*	
calcaneus	cal-**KAY**-nee-us		Latin *the heel*	The heel bone
calcaneal tendon	kal-**KAY**-knee-al **TEN**-dun	S/	**-al** *pertaining to*	The tendon of the heel formed from gastrocnemius and soleus muscles and inserted into the calcaneus
(*same as* **Achilles** tendon)		R/	**calcane-** *calcaneus*	
			tendon Latin *sinew*	
Achilles	ah-**KIL**-eez		**Achilles** mythical Greek warrior	
gastrocnemius	gas-trok-**NEE**-mee-us	S/	**-ius** *pertaining to*	Major muscle in back of the lower leg (the calf)
		R/	**gastrocnem-** *calf of leg*	
gluteus	**GLUE**-tee-us		Greek *buttocks*	Refers to one of three muscles in the buttocks
gluteal (adj)	**GLUE**-tee-al	S/	**-eal** *pertaining to*	Pertaining to the buttocks
		R/	**glut-** *buttocks*	
maximus	**MAKS**-ih-mus		Latin *the biggest*	The gluteus maximus muscle is the largest muscle in the body, covering a large part of each buttock
medius	**MEE**-dee-us		Latin *middle*	The gluteus medius muscle is partly covered by the gluteus maximus
minimus	**MIN**-ih-mus		Latin *smallest*	The gluteus minimus is the smallest of the gluteal muscles and lies under the gluteus medius
popliteal fossa	pop-**LIT**-ee-al **FOSS**-ah	S/	**-al** *pertaining to*	The hollow at the back of the knee
		R/CF	**poplit/e-** *ham, back of knee*	
			fossa Latin *trench, ditch*	
quadriceps femoris	**KWAD**-rih-seps **FEM**-or-is	S/	**-ceps** *head*	An anterior thigh muscle with four heads (origins)
		P/	**quadri-** *four*	
		S/	**-is** *belonging to, pertaining to*	
		R/	**femor-** *femur*	

Check Point Section 15.2

A. Deconstruct the names of the muscles that make up the rotator cuff. *The prefix and root elements explain the location of each muscle. Select the answer that correctly completes each statement.* **LO 15.1**

1. The muscle that is located *above the spine of the scapula:*

   a. supraspinatus

   b. subscapularis

   c. infraspinatus

   d. teres major

2. The muscle that is described as *large, long, and round:*

   a. supraspinatus

   b. subscapularis

   c. infraspinatus

   d. teres major

3. This muscle has a root element that means the *shoulder blade:*

   a. supraspinatus

   b. subscapularis

   c. infraspinatus

   d. teres major

B. Name the muscles of the upper arm and elbow joint. *Match the name of the muscle in the first column with its correct description listed in the second column.* **LO 15.4**

_____ 1. biceps brachii

_____ 2. deltoid

_____ 3. latissimus dorsi

_____ 4. triceps brachii

_____ 5. pectoralis major

a. the largest back muscle

b. located on the chest; moves the arm at the shoulder joint

c. flexes the forearm at the elbow joint

d. moves the arm at the shoulder joint

e. extends the forearm at the elbow joint

C. Deconstruct the term to decipher its meaning. *Defining the word element provides a clue to its meaning. Choose the correct answer for each statement.* **LO 15.1**

1. The prefix that means *four:*

   a. *ad-*   b. *quadri-*   c. *ab-*

2. The root that means *lead:*

   a. *calcan-*   b. *femor-*   c. *glut-*   d. *duct-*

3. The suffix that means *that which does something:*

   a. *-is*   b. *-ion*   c. *-al*   d. *-or*

4. The suffix *-ceps* means:

   a. trench, ditch   b. muscle   c. head   d. belong to

D. Identify medical terms that come from Latin. *Given the Latin meaning, write the medical term that it is defining. Fill in the blanks.* **LO 15.1, 15.3**

1. buttocks: _____

2. smallest: _____

3. the heel: _____

4. middle: _____

5. biggest: _____

Section 15.3 Disorders and Injuries of Muscles and Tendons

Disorders of Skeletal Muscles

Muscle disease and disorders are typically characterized by pain and muscle weakness.

Fibromyalgia affects muscles and tendons all over the body, causing chronic pain associated with fatigue and depression. Its etiology is unknown. There are no laboratory tests for it and no specific treatment except pain management, physiotherapy, and stress reduction.

Polymyalgia rheumatica is an inflammatory disease of muscles that causes pain and stiffness on both sides of the body, particularly in the shoulders, neck, upper arms, buttocks, and thighs with a general feeling of not being well. Most people who develop this disorder are older than 65.

Myasthenia gravis is a chronic autoimmune disease (*see Chapter 12*) characterized by varying degrees of weakness of the skeletal muscles. The weakness increases with activity and decreases with rest. Facial muscles are often involved, causing problems with eye and eyelid movements, chewing, and talking. Antibodies produced by the body's own immune system block the passage of **neurotransmitters** from motor nerves to muscles.

Muscular dystrophy is a general term for a group of hereditary, progressive disorders affecting skeletal muscles. **Duchenne muscular dystrophy (DMD)** is the most common, occurring in boys, who begin to have difficulty walking around the age of 3. Generalized muscle weakness and atrophy progress, and few live beyond 20 years. There is no effective treatment.

Injuries of Skeletal Muscles

Muscle injury is very common and usually results from athletics or vocation.

Muscle soreness may be a result of vigorous exercise, particularly if your muscles are not used to it. Exercise causes buildup of lactic acid in muscle fibers, and the resulting inflammation of them and their surrounding connective tissue produces soreness.

Muscle cramps are sudden, painful contractions of a muscle or group of muscles. They are usually of short duration. The etiology of cramps is unknown, but low blood potassium, calcium, and magnesium levels; use of caffeine and tobacco; and diminished blood supply are possible causes. There are no effective medications available. The cramp is usually self-limiting.

Muscle strains range from a simple stretch in the muscle or **tendon** to a partial or complete tear in the muscle or muscle-tendon combination. A **sprain** is a stretching or tearing of a ligament.

Rhabdomyolysis is the breakdown of muscle fibers. This releases a protein pigment called **myoglobin** into the bloodstream. Myoglobin breaks down into toxic compounds that cause kidney failure. Rhabdomyolysis can be caused by muscle trauma; severe exertion (marathon running); alcoholism; and use of cocaine, heroin, amphetamines, or phencyclidine (**PCP**).

Tenosynovitis is inflammation of the sheath that surrounds a **tendon.** It is usually related to repetitive use, occurs commonly in the wrist and hands in computer users, and is beginning to be seen in the thumbs of frequent texters. It produces pain, tenderness in the tendon, and difficulty in movement of a joint. Treatment is rest, immobilization, nonsteroidal anti-inflammatory drugs (**NSAIDs**), local corticosteroid injections, and, occasionally, surgery.

Achilles tendinitis results from a small stretch injury that causes the tendon to become swollen and painful. A larger partial or complete tear leads to loss of function with difficulty in walking and no ability to "push off."

Common Disorders of the Shoulder Girdle

Rotator cuff tears (a frequent injury to the shoulder girdle) are caused by wear and tear from overuse in work situations or in certain sports, such as baseball, football, and golf. These tears can be partial or complete (*Figure 15.3*).

Tendinitis of the shoulder joint is caused when the rotator cuff and/or biceps tendon becomes inflamed from overuse.

Bursitis, inflammation of the lubricating sac of the rotator cuff, also can be produced by overuse.

Common Disorders of the Elbow

Lateral epicondylitis (also known as Tennis elbow) is caused by overuse of the elbow joint or poor techniques in playing tennis or golf. Tendons of upper-arm and forearm muscles are inserted into the medial and lateral **epicondyles** of the humerus just above the elbow joint (*Figure 14.19*). Small tears in the tendons at their attachments occur with overuse, and eventually enough tears accumulate to cause pain and restrict elbow movement. The pain occurs when straightening the elbow or opening and closing the fingers.

Ligament strains and **bone fractures** due to a heavy fall or a blow to the elbow are also common injuries.

Common Disorders of the Wrist and Hand

Your wrists and hand are under constant use; therefore, they are prone to disorders and injuries.

Ganglion cysts are fluid-filled cysts arising when the synovial tendon sheaths that run over the back of the wrist are irritated or inflamed. They often disappear spontaneously.

Stenosing tenosynovitis is a painful inflammation of the synovial sheaths on the back of the wrist.

Carpal tunnel syndrome (CTS) develops on the front of the wrist and results from inflammation and swelling of overused tendon sheaths (*Figure 15.6*). Repetitive movements, like typing on a computer keyboard, can lead to CTS. A feeling of "pins and needles" or pain and loss of muscle power in the thumb side of the hand are common.

In the hand, flexor tendon injuries occur as a result of lacerations. Because the flexor tendons lie just beneath the skin on the palmar surfaces of the fingers, they are very susceptible to injury even with a shallow laceration. Even after repair, there can be residual stiffness and limited motion of the fingers.

Word Analysis and Definition: Disorders and Injuries of Muscle

S = Suffix P = Prefix R = Root R/CF = Combining Form

WORD	PRONUNCIATION		ELEMENTS	DEFINITION
cyst	SIST		Greek *fluid-filled sac*	An abnormal, fluid-containing sac
Duchenne muscular dystrophy	**DOO**-shen **MUSS**-kyu-lar **DISS**-troh-fee	S/ R/ P/ R/	Guillaume Benjamin Duchenne, 1806–1875, French neurologist -ar *pertaining to* muscul- *muscle* dys- *bad, difficult* -trophy *nourishment*	A condition with symmetrical weakness and wasting of pelvic, shoulder, and proximal limb muscles
fibromyalgia	fie-broh-my-**AL**-jee-ah	S/ R/CF R/	-algia *pain* fibr/o- *fiber* -my- *muscle*	Pain in the muscle fibers
ganglion	**GANG**-lee-on		Greek *swelling*	Fluid-containing swelling attached to the synovial sheath of a tendon
neurotransmitter (**Note:** *Transmitter* is a word in itself and begins with a prefix.)	**NYUR**-oh-trans-**MIT**-er	S/ R/CF P/ R/	-er *agent* neur/o- *nerve* -trans- *across* -mitt- *to send*	Chemical agent that relays messages from one nerve cell to the next
rhabdomyolysis	**RAB**-doh-my-**OL**-eye-sis	S/ R/CF R/CF	-lysis *destruction* rhabd/o- *rod shaped* -my/o- *muscle*	Destruction of muscle to produce myoglobin
stenosis	steh-**NOH**-sis	S/ R/CF	-sis *abnormal condition* sten/o- *narrow*	Narrowing of a passage
strain	STRAIN		Latin *to bind*	Overstretch or tear in a muscle or tendon
sprain	SPRAIN		Old English *tear*	A stretching or tearing of ligaments
tendon tendinitis (also spelled **tendonitis**)	**TEN**-dun ten-dih-**NIE**-tis	S/ R/	Latin *sinew* -itis *inflammation* tendin- *tendon*	Fibrous band that connects muscle to bone Inflammation of a tendon
tenosynovitis	**TEN**-oh-sin-oh-**VIE**-tis	S/ R/CF R/	-itis *inflammation* ten/o- *tendon* -synov- *synovial membrane*	Inflammation of a tendon and its surrounding synovial sheath

A. The following elements are all contained in the section tables. *Choose the best answer.* **LO 15.1, 15.2**

1. *Dys* is a

    a. suffix   b. prefix   c. root

2. *Fibro* is a

    a. combining form   b. root   c. suffix

B. Interpret definitions of medical terms. *Read the following sentences and determine the condition the patient is likely suffering from. Fill in each blank.* **LO 15.3, 15.6, 15.8**

1. The patient made an appointment with the nurse practitioner. She was complaining of chronic pain and fatigue, and had symptoms of depression. The probable diagnosis is _____.

2. Jon just completed his second marathon. He is now feeling quite ill and visits the emergency department. The note states that he is in acute kidney failure. The physician determines that the patient likely has the muscular condition _____.

3. After five years of no routine exercise, Analisa has decided to begin an aggressive weight-lifting program. The next day she is very sore and it is painful to move from a sitting to a standing position. After consulting a physician assistant, she is diagnosed with severe muscle _____.

4. Over the weekend, Marcus painted his mother's kitchen and living room. On Monday, his hands were achy and painful. He is likely suffering from _____ of the hands.

C. Identify disorders of the elbow and wrist joints. *Given the description, identify the condition. Fill in the blank to correctly complete each statement.* **LO 15.6**

1. A painful wrist condition caused by repetitive movements. Write the abbreviation for this condition: _____

2. Fluid-filled sacs located on the back of the wrist: _____ cysts

3. Painful inflammation of the synovial sheaths on the back of the wrist: stenosing _____

Section 15.4 Procedures and Pharmacology

Diagnostic Procedures for Disorders of Muscles and Tendons

A medical history and physical examination are essential components of a diagnostic examination. Additional diagnostic tests include:

- **Blood tests.** Damaged muscles release **enzymes** such as **creatine kinase (CK)** and aldolase into the blood, and their levels can be measured. An **erythrocyte sedimentation rate (ESR)** is not specific for any disease process, but it indicates the presence of **inflammation,** and serial readings can be used to measure changes in an inflammatory process.

- **Electromyography (EMG),** in which an **electrode** needle is inserted into the muscle to be tested to measure and record the electrical activity in that muscle as the muscle is contracted and relaxed.

- **Nerve conduction studies** are used to measure the speed at which motor or sensory nerves conduct impulses and also can show problems at the neuromuscular junction; for example, in myasthenia gravis.

- **Magnetic resonance imaging (MRI)** and **computed tomography scan (CT scan)** show detailed images of damage or disease in muscles.
- **Ultrasonography** can identify tears and inflammation of tendons and involves no exposure to radiation, unlike MRI and CT scan.
- **Muscle biopsy (Bx)** is performed by removing a small piece of the abnormal muscle through a hollow needle or a small incision to be sent to the laboratory for examination and analysis.
- **Genetic testing** of blood or tissues can show the mutations in some of the genes that cause the different types of muscular dystrophy.
- **Myositis specific antibodies (MSA)** can confirm a diagnosis of **dermatomyositis** or polymyositis. Dozens of these antibodies have been identified and research is ongoing to define their significance.

Word Analysis and Definition: Diagnostic Procedures

S = Suffix P = Prefix R = Root R/CF = Combining Form

WORD	PRONUNCIATION	ELEMENTS		DEFINITION
antibody	**AN**-tih-bod-ee	P/ R/	anti- *against* -**body** *substance*	Protein produced in response to an antigen
biopsy	**BIE**-op-see	S/ R/	-opsy *to view* **bi-** *life*	Removal of a tissue from a living person for laboratory examination
creatine kinase	**KREE**-ah-teen **KI**-nase	S/ R/ S/ R/	-ine pertaining to **creat-** *flesh* -ase enzyme **kin-** *motion*	Enzyme elevated in the plasma following heart muscle damage
electrode	ee-**LEK**-trode	S/ R/	-ode way, road **electr-** *electricity*	A device for conducting electricity
electromyography	ee-**LEK**-troh-my-**OG**-rah-fee	S/ R/CF R/CF	-graphy *process of recording* **electr/o-** *electricity* -**my/o-** *muscle*	Recording of electrical activity in a muscle
enzyme	**EN**-zime	P/ R/	en- *in* -**zyme** *fermenting*	Protein that induces change in other substances
erythrocyte sedimentation rate (ESR)	eh-**RITH**-roh-site **SED**-i-men-**TAY**-shun RATE	S/ R/CF S/ R/	-cyte cell **erythr/o-** *red* -ation *process* **sediment-** *settling* Latin *according to a fixed part*	The speed at which red blood cells sink from drawn blood
inflammation	in-flah-**MAY**-shun	S/ P/ R/	-ation *process* in- *in* -**flamm-** *flame*	A basic complex of reactions in blood vessels and adjacent tissues in response to injury or abnormal stimulation
ultrasonography	**UL**-trah-soh-**NOG**-rah-fee	S/ P/ R/CF	-graphy *process of recording* ultra- *beyond* -**son/o-** *sound*	Delineation of deep structures using sound waves

Therapeutic Procedures

Physical therapy is a profession dedicated to the treatment of functional impairments, decreased mobility, and pain. Physical therapy is widely utilized and supported by research as a successful course of treatment and rehabilitation for individuals of all ages. Physical therapy utilizes a wide variety of interventions to help patients.

Therapeutic Exercise

Therapeutic exercise is a systematic, progressive set of exercises, that a PT designs for each individual's needs. These exercises are designed to foster rehabilitation, maintain, or increase range of motion (ROM) and decrease pain. Therapeutic exercises are classified according to the purpose of the exercise being utilized. Primarily, these classifications are ROM, strengthening, postural, balance and coordination, and flexibility.

Manual Therapy

Dry Needling

Dry needling is a treatment performed by a PT certified in the procedure. Also referred to as intramuscular therapy, a thin monofilament needle penetrates the skin to treat a specific muscle. Dry needling can reduce pain, inactivate trigger points, and target tissues that are not manually palpable. Typically, dry needling is one component of a broader treatment plan incorporating other physical therapy interventions. It is important to note that dry needling is not acupuncture. Acupuncture is a practice based on traditional Chinese medicine and performed by licensed acupuncturists. Dry needling is an evidence-based intervention using modern western principles of medicine.

Cupping

Cupping therapy is a modality sometimes used by PTs for treating painful musculoskeletal issues. It uses a pulling effect on the fascia and underlying muscles to improve tissue extensibility, decrease fascial restrictions, treat muscular trigger points, and temporarily increase circulation.

Soft Tissue Mobilization and Myofascial Release

Fascia is the connective tissue that surrounds all the organs and muscles in the body holding them in place. **Myofascial release** is a therapy used to release tension in the fascia and improve the mobility between the different fascial planes in the body. **Soft tissue mobilization,** is an intervention PT's use to treat areas of increased tension in muscles and tendons. It can be used to treat trigger points, areas of pain, scar tissue, and reduced mobility. Both myofascial release and soft tissue mobilization are typically performed using manual pressure provided by the therapist's hands or fingers.

Instrument Assisted

Sometimes tools can be used to assist a therapist in soft tissue mobilization or myofascial release. These tools are used to work on soft tissues such as muscles, tendons, and ligaments to promote healing and tissue regeneration. Instruments are often utilized when soft tissues have significant scarring, injured or dysfunctional, or when mobility is restricted. Muscles are comprised of thousands of fibers which, in healthy and normal muscles, run parallel to each other. Sometimes when there is injury, damage, or dysfunction in a muscle, the muscle fibers will no longer run in the same direction throughout the entirety of the muscle. The use of tools on a dysfunctional muscle can help to straighten those muscle fibers back out to restore normal movement and function of that muscle. Instrument assisted soft tissue mobilization can be practiced by any PT, but there are also special certifications including ASTYM, and Graston technique requiring continuing education.

Physical Therapy Modalities

Physical therapy modalities refer to the use of electrical, thermal, or mechanical energy as a treatment technique.

Electrical Stimulation

Electrical stimulation (e-stim) is a common modality used to address pain. Electrodes are placed on the targeted area and electrical pulses are sent through the skin. These electrical pulses can interrupt the normal transmission of nociceptors in the area providing some pain relief. **Interferential current therapy (IFC)** is one type of e-stim which uses a frequency sweep pattern to prevent the body from accommodating to the stimulation and therefore extending its effectiveness. Occasionally, electrical stimulation is used to cause muscle contractions intended to preserve or increase muscular function. These treatments are typically used in patients with a significantly impaired ability to contract the muscle independently. If a patient can actively contract a muscle, this is almost always a superior method of strengthening to electrical stimulation.

Thermal Modalities

Thermal modalities use heat or cold to produce an effect in the targeted tissue. The use of heat can increase blood flow and extensibility of the targeted area. This can be particularly useful for areas that are avascular (very limited blood supply) to increase healing and repair.

Cold can be used to limit swelling by reducing blood flow to an area and slowing the inflammatory response. Inflammation is needed for injury repair, but also increases pain due to the release of certain cellular messengers known as **cytokines** that can trigger nociceptors. Inflammation can also impact surrounding healthy tissue which is why cold therapy is important.

Ultrasound

An **ultrasound** machine in the physical therapy setting utilizes a sound wave to mechanically cavitate the cells in a targeted area creating a deep heating effect. Typically, this is not felt by the patient as the sound waves have little impact on the cutaneous nerves as they pass through to heat the underlying tissue. Occasionally, if the ultrasound wand is left too long over a bony area, then the buildup of sound waves along the periosteum can produce a sharp spike of pain. This pain dissipates as soon as the wand is removed from the area.

Musculoskeletal Drugs

NSAIDs inhibit the two cyclooxygenase (**COX**) enzymes that are involved in producing the inflammatory process. They have **analgesic** and **antipyretic** effects and are used for treatment of tissue injury, pyrexia, rheumatoid arthritis, osteoarthritis, gout, and nonspecific joint and tissue pains. The three major NSAIDs, each of which is available OTC, are:

1. **Acetylsalicylic acid** (aspirin), which, in addition to the above effects and uses, also has an antiplatelet effect due to its inhibition of one of the COX enzymes; thus, it is often used in the prevention of heart attacks.

2. **Ibuprofen** (*Advil, Motrin,* and several other trade names), which acts by inhibiting both the COX enzymes, essential elements in the enzyme pathways involved in pain, inflammation, and fever. It is taken orally, but in 2009 an injectable form of ibuprofen (*Caldolor*) was approved for use. In some studies, ibuprofen has been associated with the prevention of Alzheimer and Parkinson diseases, but further studies are needed.

3. **Naproxen** (*Aleve* and many other trade names), which is taken orally once a day and also inhibits both the COX enzymes.

Indomethacin, an NSAID that inhibits both COX enzymes, is a potent drug with many serious side effects. It is not used as an analgesic for minor aches and pains or for fever.

Paracetamol (acetaminophen), an active **metabolite** of phenacetin (not an NSAID), is a widely used OTC analgesic and antipyretic. It is used for the relief of minor aches and pains and is an **ingredient** in many cold and flu remedies.

Skeletal muscle relaxants are FDA-approved for spasticity (baclofen, dantrolene, tizanidine) or for muscular conditions like multiple sclerosis (carisoprodol, chlorzoxazone, cyclobenzaprine, metaxalone, methocarbamol, orphenadrine). The only drug with available evidence of efficacy in spasticity is tizanidine (*Zanaflex, Sirdalud*), but cyclobenzaprine (*Amrix*) appears to be somewhat effective.

Anabolic steroids are related to testosterone but have been altered so that their main effect is to cause skeletal muscle to hypertrophy. They are used illegally in many sports to increase muscle strength. They have marked, often irreversible, side effects, including stunting the height of growing adolescents, shrinking testes and sperm counts, masculinizing women, and causing delusions and paranoid jealousy. In the long term, there are increased risks of heart attacks and strokes, kidney failure, and liver tumors.

Did you know...

Spasticity is a state of increased muscular tone with exaggeration of the tendon reflexes.

Word Analysis and Definition: Therapeutic Terms and Musculoskeletal Drugs

S = Suffix P = Prefix R = Root R/CF = Combining Form

WORD	PRONUNCIATION	ELEMENTS		DEFINITION
anabolic steroid	an-ah-**BOL**-ik **STER**-oyd	S/ R/ S/ R/	-ic *pertaining to* anabol- *to raise up* -oid *resembling* ster- *solid*	Prescription drug used by some athletes to increase muscle mass
analgesia	an-al-**JEE**-zee-ah	S/ P/	-ia *condition* an- *without*	State in which pain is reduced
analgesic		R/ S/	-alges- *sensation of pain* -ic *pertaining to*	Agent that produces analgesia
antipyretic	**AN**-tee-pie-**RET**-ik	S/ P/ R/	-ic *pertaining to* anti- *against* -pyret- *fever*	Agent that reduces fever
cytokine	**SIGH**-toh-kine	S/ R/CF	-kine *movement* cyt/o- *cell*	A hormone like protein that regulates the intensity of an immune response
ingredient	in-**GREE**-dee-ent	S/ P/ R/	-ent *end result, ertaining to* in- *in, into* -gredi- *to go*	An element in a mixture
metabolism	meh-**TAB**-oh-lizm	S/ R/	-ism *condition* metabol- *change*	The constantly changing physical and chemical processes in the cell
metabolite	meh-**TAB**-oh-lite	S/	-ite *associated with*	Any product of metabolism
ultrasound	**UL**-trah-sownd	P/ R/	ultra-*higher* -sound *noise*	Very high-frequency sound waves

Check Point Section 15.4

A. Determine the appropriate diagnostic test. *Read each scenario and determine which diagnostic test is indicated to support the diagnosis. Fill in the blanks. Not all answers will be used.* **LO 15.5, 15.9**

ESR   EMG   CK   Bx   MSA

1. The physician ordered a(n) _____ to determine the strength of muscular contraction in the patient with polio.

2. In order to support the diagnosis of myositis, a(n) _____ of the muscle tissue was ordered.

3. Dr. Novak sent a blood sample to the lab to have the medical technologist measure the _____ to determine if the patient had rhabdomyolysis.

4. The patient's blood was sent to the lab with an order for the medical technologist to measure the _____ in order to determine if the patient had a chronic inflammatory condition.

B. Select the correct medical term to complete the following questions. *Choose the correct answer.* **LO 15.7**

1. NSAIDS inhibit enzymes that are involved in the _____ process.

    a. respiratory   d. pulmonary

    b. digestive   e. inflammatory

    c. urinary

2. The class of medication that treats muscle spasticity:

    a. COX inhibitor   c. muscle relaxant

    b. analgesic   d. antipyretic

3. The analgesic listed that is NOT an NSAID:

    a. naproxen   c. aspirin

    b. ibuprofen   d. paracetamol

4. An NSAID that is described as a potent pain reliever but is not used for minor aches and pains due to its serious side effects:

    a. orphenadrine   c. indomethacin

    b. naproxen   d. cyclobenzaprine

5. A medication that lowers a fever is termed a(n):

    a. metabolite   c. ingredient

    b. antipyretic   d. anti-inflammatory

Section 15.5 Physical Medicine and Rehabilitation (PM&R)

Physical Medicine and Rehabilitation

Physical medicine and rehabilitation (PM&R) health professionals are listed and defined at the beginning of this chapter.

Physical medicine and rehabilitation is also called **physiatry.** Its goal is to develop a comprehensive program to put together the different pieces of a person's life—medical, social, emotional, and **vocational**—after injury or disease. PM&R programs cover a wide spectrum, from prevention of injury in athletes to treating sports-related injuries in sports medicine to coping with complicated multiple trauma.

Rehabilitation Definitions

The following definitions of terms or phrases specific to rehabilitation will help you to understand more precisely the different kinds of rehabilitation in which you may be involved as a health professional.

Rehabilitation medicine focuses on function. Being able to function is essential to an individual's independence and ability to have a good quality of life (*Figure 15.12*).

Restorative rehabilitation restores a function that has been lost, such as after a hip fracture, hip replacement, or stroke. This process can be intense, but it's also usually short term.

Maintenance rehabilitation strengthens and maintains a function that is gradually being lost. It is less intense than restorative rehabilitation but often long term. Problems of senescence (old age), like difficulty with balance or flexibility, require this long-term approach.

Rehabilitation medicine is also involved with the **prevention** of function loss and the prevention of injury. In sports medicine, an example is the prevention of shoulder and elbow injuries often experienced by baseball pitchers.

Activities of daily living (ADLs) are the routine activities of personal care. The six basic ADLs are eating, bathing, dressing, grooming, toileting, and transferring. Assistive devices are designed to make ADLs easier to perform and help maintain the patient's independence. Examples of these devices include reachers and grabbers, easy-pull sock aids, long shoehorns, jar openers, and eating aids. ADLs are also a measurement to assess therapy needs and monitor its effectiveness.

Instrumental activities of daily living (IADLs) relate to independent living. These activities include managing money, using a telephone, cooking, driving, shopping for groceries and personal items, and doing housework.

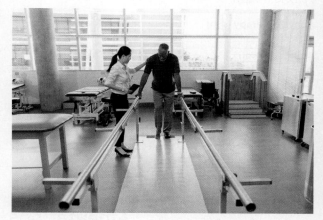

▲ **Figure 15.12** **Assistive device for walking.**
SDI Productions/E+/Getty Images

WORD	PRONUNCIATION	ELEMENTS		DEFINITION
occupational therapy	**OK**-you-**PAY**-shun-al **THAIR**-ah-pee	S/ R/	-al *pertaining to* **occupation-** *work* **therapy** Greek *medical treatment*	Use of work and recreational activities to increase independent function
orthotic	or-**THOT**-ik	S/ R/	-ic *pertaining to* **orthot-** *correct*	Orthopedic appliance to correct an abnormality
orthotist	or-**THOT**-ist	S/	-ist *specialist*	Specialist who makes and fits orthopedic appliances
physiatry (*Note:* The "i" in the root is dropped because "iatry" also begins with "i")	fih-**ZIE**-ah-tree	S/ R/	-iatry *treatment, field of medicine* **phys-** *body*	Physical medicine
physiatrist	fih-**ZIE**-ah-trist	S/ R/	-ist *specialist* -iatr- *treatment*	Specialist in physical medicine
physical medicine	**FIZ**-ih-cal **MED**-ih-sin	S/ R/ S/ R/	-al *pertaining to* **physic-** *body* -ine *pertaining to, substance* **medic-** *medicine*	Diagnosis and treatment by means of remedial agents, such as exercises, manipulation, heat, etc.
physical therapy (also known as physiotherapy)	**FIZ**-ih-cal **THAIR**-ah-pee	S/ R/	-al *pertaining to* **physic-** *body* **therapy** Greek *medical treatment*	Use of remedial processes to overcome a physical defect
physiotherapy (syn)	**FIZ**-ee-oh-**THAIR**-ah-pee	S/ R/CF	-therapy *treatment* **physi/o-** *body*	Another term for physical therapy
rehabilitation	**REE**-hah-bil-ih-**TAY**-shun	S/ P/ R/	-ion *action, condition* **re-** *again* **-habilitat-** *restore*	Therapeutic restoration of an ability to function as before
therapy	**THAIR**-ah-pee		Greek *medical treatment*	Systematic treatment of a disease, dysfunction, or disorder
therapist	**THAIR**-ah-pist	S/ R/	-ist *specialist* **therap-** *treatment*	Professional trained in the practice of a particular therapy
therapeutic (adj)	**THAIR**-ah-**PYU**-tik	S/ R/	-ic *pertaining to* **therapeut-** *treatment*	Relating to the treatment of a disease or disorder

Amputations

Seventy-five percent of all **amputations** are performed on people over 65 years of age with **peripheral vascular disease (PVD).** This includes complications from arteriosclerosis and diabetes. Most of these cases involve **below-the-knee amputations (BKAs).**

Recently, the wars in Iraq and Afghanistan have led to soldiers losing their arms or legs due to the detonation of explosive devices. In some of these cases, amputations are also required, depending on the level of damage an explosion has caused to the soldier's body.

Rehabilitation after amputation (*Figure 15.12*) is an increasingly important component in rehabilitation programs. Immediately after surgery, the objectives of the rehabilitation team are to:

- Promote healing of the stump;
- Strengthen the muscles above the site of the amputation;
- Strengthen arm muscles to assist in ambulation or help with walking using a cane, crutches, or other assistive devices;
- Prevent **contractures** or tightening of the joints above the amputation (knee and hip for BKAs);
- Shrink the post-amputation stump with elastic cuffs or bandages to fit the socket of a temporary **prosthesis** (*Figure 15.13 and 15.4*); and
- Provide emotional, psychological, and family support.

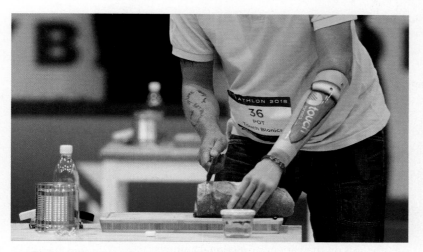

▲ **Figure 15.13** Teenager doing ADL after amputation. REUTERS/ Arnd Wiegmann/Alamy

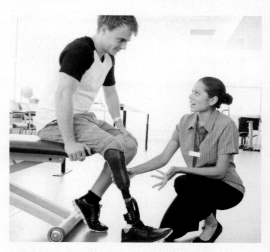

▲ **Figure 15.14** Young man being fitted with a prosthesis. JohnnyGreig/Getty Images

Word Analysis and Definition: Amputations

S = Suffix P = Prefix R = Root R/CF = Combining Form

WORD	PRONUNCIATION	ELEMENTS		DEFINITION
amputation	am-pyu-**TAY**-shun	S/ R/	-ation *process* amput- *prune*	Removal of a limb, part of a limb, or other projecting body part
contracture	kon-**TRAK**-chur	S/ R/	-ure *result of* contract- *pull together*	Muscle shortening due to spasm or fibrosis
prevention	pree-**VEN**-shun	S/ R/	-ion *action, condition* prevent- *prevent*	Process to prevent occurrence of a disease or health problem
prosthesis	**PROS**-thee-sis		Greek *an addition*	An artificial part to remedy a defect in the body
restorative rehabilitation	ree-**STOR**-ah-tiv **REE**-hah-bil-ih-**TAY**-shun	S/ R/ S/ P/ R/	-ative *quality of* restor- *renew* -ion *action, process* re- *begin again* -habilitat- *restore*	Therapy that promotes renewal of health and strength

Check Point Section 15.5

A. Use the correct term to complete each sentence. *Use the terms provided to complete each sentence.* **LO 15.10**

therapist   therapy   therapeutic   orthotic   orthotist

1. The physician prescribes two shoe inserts as _____ devices to relieve the patient's foot pain.

2. After breaking her fingers, the patient was prescribed occupational _____ to regain strength and function in her hand.

3. The physiatrist used warm, moist heat as a _____ measure to relieve the muscle strain.

4. The _____ created an ankle brace for the child.

5. After having surgery to repair a rotator cuff tear, the physical _____ created a strengthening plan for the patient.

B. Describe the treatment of amputations. *Choose the correct answer for each statement.* **LO 15.7**

1. When employing the use of physical therapy for strengthening muscles, the area for strengthening the muscles is _____ the amputation site.

   a. above

   b. below

   c. lateral to

   d. medial to

2. In order to prepare patients for walking with crutches, which muscles should be strengthened?

a. back

c. arm

b. chest

d. leg

3. Family support is an important part of rehabilitation therapy for patients with amputation.

a. True

b. False

C. Define terms associated with rehabilitation. *Match the term in the first column with its correct definition in the second column.* **LO 15.7**

_____ 1. maintenance rehabilitation

a. activities specific to independent living

_____ 2. restorative rehabilitation

b. short-term therapy, aimed at returning the patient to prior function

_____ 3. rehabilitation medicine

c. routine activities of personal care

_____ 4. instrumental activities of daily living

d. long-term therapy; helps to prevent loss of current strength

_____ 5. activities of daily living

e. focuses on the patient's functional abilities

D. Matching: Match the therapeutic procedure to the definitions provided LO 15.7

1. Cupping

a. Purposeful exercise is used to foster rehabilitation

2. Therapeutic exercise

b. Uses a pulling effect on the facia and underling muscles

3. Myofascial release

c. The use of electrical impulses to provide pain relief

4. Dry needling

d. Utilized to release tension in the facia

5. ASTYM

e. A monofilament needle is used in the course of treatment

6. e-stim

f. A form of instrument assisted therapy

Table 15.1 Chapter 15 Abbreviations

Abbreviations	Meaning
ADLs	activities of daily living
BKA	below-the-knee amputation
Bx	biopsy
CK	creatine kinase
CT	computed tomography
CTS	carpal tunnel syndrome
COTA	certified occupational therapist assistant
COX	Cyclooxy genase enzymes
DMD	Duchenne muscular dystrophy
EMG	electromyography

Abbreviations	Meaning
e-stim	electrical stimulation
IDALs	instrumental activities of daily living
MRI	magnetic resonance imaging
MSA	myositis specific antibodies
SI	sacroiliac
PCP	phencyclidine
PM&R	physical medicine and rehabilitation
PVD	peripheral vascular disease
ROM	range of motion

Table 15.2 Comparison of Selected Muscular Disorders – Signs, Symptoms, and Treatments

Disorder or Disease	Signs and Symptoms	Diagnostic Tests	Treatment
Fibromyalgia	Chronic pain, fatigue	None. Diagnosis is by elimination of other diseases and disorders.	Physiotherapy and pain management. NSAIDs, acetaminophen, cyclobenzaprine relieves pain and may help sleep. Antidepressants and anti-seizure drugs may ease pain.
Muscle pain and strain	Acute pain in area of muscle		Physiotherapy. Treatment modalities include Gaston technique, cupping, and myofascial release.
Myasthenia gravis	Progressive weakness starting at the upper extremities, moving downward. Weakness increases with activity	Physical examination. Typically presents with drooping eyelid.	Cannot be cured. Corticosteroids and immunosuppressants treat symptoms.
Tennis elbow (lateral epicondylitis)	Pain on the outside of the elbow. Gripping increases pain.	Physical examination. Touching outside of elbow may produce pain	NSAIDs, elbow brace, physiotherapy, ultrasound.

Adike/Shutterstock

Challenge Your Knowledge

A. **Match the health professional in the second column with his or her job description in the first column.** **LO 15.7**

_____ **1.** Practitioner who evaluates and treats pain, disease, or injury by measures other than medical or surgical

_____ **2.** Practitioner who makes and fits orthopedic appliances

_____ **3.** Physician who specializes in physical medicine and rehabilitation

_____ **4.** Practitioner who focuses on helping patients with activities of daily living

a. orthotist

b. physiatrist

c. occupational therapist

d. physical therapist

B. **Describe the function of skeletal muscle.** From the given example, identify the function being described. Use the provided terms to fill in the blank. **LO 15.1**

movement   posture   heat   respiration   communication

1. The function of skeletal muscles that Mr. Schwartz uses when he greets patients when they arrive to the clinic: _____

2. The children were cold, so they ran around the house to warm up. The function of warming up: _____

3. The occupational therapy assistant helped his patient to bring the spoon to her mouth. Bringing the spoon to the mouth is an example of: _____

4. Skeletal muscles contract to keep the back straight: _____

5. Breathing to bring oxygen into the body and move carbon dioxide out: _____

C. **Demonstrate your knowledge of the muscular system anatomy and disorders by choosing the correct answer to complete each statement.** **LO 15.1, 15.6**

1. The type of muscle only found in the heart:

a. smooth   **b.** skeletal   **c.** cardiac

2. Due to their long size, skeletal muscle cells are also known as muscle:

a. strings

b. fascicles

c. fibers

d. junction

3. The stripes seen in a microscopic view of skeletal muscle are called:

a. striations

b. fascia

c. interneurons

d. osteoclasts

4. Muscle that has decreased in size is said to have the condition of:

a. edema

b. hypertrophy

c. atrophy

d. paralysis

5. Lifting heavy objects over a long period of time can result in muscle:

   a. polymyalgia

   b. tenosynovitis

   c. atrophy

   d. hypertrophy

6. The location where a skeletal muscle attaches to the bone that is moved with muscle contraction is termed the:

   a. origin

   b. insertion

   c. fascicle

   d. fascia

7. The broadest muscle in the back is the:

   a. biceps

   b. triceps

   c. brachii

   d. latissimus dorsi

   e. deltoid

8. Ganglion cysts are fluid-filled cysts arising from the:

   a. muscles

   b. joints

   c. synovial tendon sheaths

   d. articulations

   e. bursa

9. Four muscles that originate on the scapula, wrap around the joint, and fuse to form one large tendon are called the:

   a. articulation

   b. rotator cuff

   c. brachialis

   d. scapulae

   e. pectoral

10. An overstretch or tear in a muscle is termed a:

   a. strain

   b. fasciotomy

   c. sprain

   d. tenosynovitis

   e. cyst

D. **Common disorders of skeletal muscle.** Match the skeletal muscle disorder in the first column with its correct description in the second column. **LO 15.6**

_____ 1. rhabdomyolysis

_____ 2. tenosynovitis

_____ 3. Duchenne muscular dystrophy

_____ 4. tendonitis

_____ 5. fibromyalgia

_____ 6. strain

   a. symmetrical weakness and wasting of pelvic, shoulder, and proximal limb muscles

   b. overstretch of a muscle or tendon

   c. inflammation of tendon and its surrounding synovial sheath

   d. destruction of muscle to produce myoglobin

   e. inflammation of a tendon

   f. pain in the muscle fibers

E. Skeletal muscles that move the arms, legs, and feet. Select the answer that correctly completes each statement. **LO 15.1**

    1. The smallest gluteal muscle is the gluteus:

        a. maximus   **b.** medius   **c.** minimus

    2. The group of muscles located on the anterior side of the femur:

        a. hamstrings   **c.** rotator cuff

        b. quadriceps   **d.** gluteals

    3. A muscle located directly below the spine of the scapula:

        a. vastus lateralis   **c.** brachioradialis

        b. subscapularis   **d.** infraspinatus

    4. The pad of muscle located on the thumb side of your hand:

        a. dorsum   **c.** thenar eminence

        b. bursa   **d.** hypothenar eminence

    5. The origin of all muscles that make up the rotator cuff:

        a. scapula   **c.** clavicle

        b. humerus   **d.** radius

    6. The meaning of the muscle *teres major*:

        a. above the acromion   **c.** pertaining to the earth

        b. wide and broad   **d.** big, long, and round

    7. The muscle that extends the arm at the elbow joint:

        a. triceps brachii   **c.** deltoid

        b. biceps brachii   **d.** subscapularis

    8. The largest muscle that makes up the buttocks is the:

        a. gluteus minimus   **d.** vastus lateralis

        b. gluteus medius   **e.** vastus medialis

        c. gluteus maximus

F. Disorders of the muscles of the arm, thigh, leg, and foot. Given the description, identify the likely disorder related to the muscular system. Match the description in the first column with its matching term in the second column. **LO 15.6**

_____ **1.** Pain and tingling in the hand due to repetitive wrist movements   **a.** bursitis

_____ **2.** Injury due to overuse of the shoulder joint   **b.** lateral epicondylitis

_____ **3.** Painful condition caused by overuse of the elbow joint   **c.** rotator cuff tear

_____ **4.** Inflammation of the lubricating sac found near a joint   **d.** carpal tunnel syndrome

Adike/Shutterstock

G. Deconstructing words related to physical medicine and rehabilitation. Identify the meaning of the element in each medical term. Select the answer that correctly completes each statement. **LO 15.2, 15.10**

1. The suffix in the term **physiatry** means:

    a. pertaining to

    b. nature

    c. treatment

    d. specialist

2. The root in the term **therapeutic** means:

    a. specialist

    b. treatment

    c. body

    d. pertaining to

3. The word element in the term **rehabilitation** that means *again:*

    a. prefix   **b.** root   **c.** suffix

4. The root in the term **occupational** means:

    a. work

    b. aid, help

    c. body

    d. treatment

5. The suffix in **kinase** means:

    a. restore

    b. enzyme

    c. nature of

    d. pertaining to

H. Use medical terms to complete professional documentation. Read the following case study and replace the words in italics with the medical term it is describing. **LO 15.8**

Mr. Vernon has arrived to the clinic today to see Dr. Cho, **(1)** *a specialist in the treatment of bone and muscle disorders.* He states that he experienced a constant pain in his shoulder that he thinks may be due to an **(2)** *inflamed tendon.* He was an avid tennis player for over 15 years, which may be related to his condition.

Dr. Cho examines Mr. Vernon and notes that he is limited in his ability to move his arm away from his body. Dr. Cho diagnoses the patient with a tear in the **(3)** *muscles that support the shoulder joint.* He recommends that Mr. Vernon see a **(4)** *specialist in the strengthening of muscles* for five weeks followed by surgery to repair the tear.

1. _____

2. _____

3. _____

4. _____

I. Prefixes: Match the correct medical term in the first column with the meaning of its prefix in the second column. LO 15.2

Medical Term	Meaning of the Prefix
_____ 1. hypothenar	**a.** two
_____ 2. triceps	**b.** together
_____ 3. adductor	**c.** toward
_____ 4. quadriceps	**d.** above
_____ 5. contract	**e.** three
_____ 6. supra	**f.** four
_____ 7. biceps	**g.** below, deficient

J. Identify abbreviations that describe medical terms. Match the abbreviation in the first column to its correct description in the second column. **LO 15.9**

_____ **1.** COTA   **a.** examples include toileting, brushing one's hair, brushing one's teeth

_____ **2.** NSAID   **b.** removal of the lower leg and foot

_____ **3.** CTS   **c.** a professional that assists people in improving their activities of daily living

_____ **4.** BKA   **d.** hereditary muscular condition with general muscle weakness and atrophy

_____ **5.** ADLs   **e.** repetitive movements that cause a feeling of "pins and needles" in the hand

_____ **6.** DMD   **f.** a type of medication used to treat muscle pain

K. Identify the elements in each medical term and unlock the meaning of the word. _Fill in the chart. If the word does not have a particular word element, write n/a. The first one has been done for you._ **LO 15.2**

Medical Term	Prefix	Meaning of Prefix	Root/ Combining Form	Meaning of Root/ Combining Form	Suffix	Meaning of Suffix	Meaning of Term
dorsal	1. n/a	2. n/a	3. *dors-*	4. back	5. *-al*	6. pertaining to	7. pertaining to the back
analgesia	8.	9.	10.	11.	12.	13.	14.
deltoid	15.	16.	17.	18.	19.	20.	21.
hypertrophy	22.	23.	24.	25.	26.	27.	28.
infraspinatus	29.	30.	31.	32.	33.	34.	35.

L. Pronunciation is important whether you are saying the word or listening to a word from a coworker. Identify the proper pronunciation of the following medical terms. The correctly spell the term. **LO 15.1, 15.6, 15.7**

1. The correct pronunciation for a breakdown of muscle fibers

     a. rab-**DOH**-my-oh-**LIE**-sis   **c.** **RAB**-doh-my-**OL**-eye-sis

     b. **RAB**-doh-**MY**-oh-lie-sis   **d.** rab-doh-**MY**-oh-**LIE**-sis

     Correctly spell the term: _____

2. The correct pronunciation for inflammation of a tendon and surrounding synovial sheath

     a. **TEN**-oh-sine-oh-**VIE**-tis   **c.** **TEN**-oh-**SINE**-oh-vie-tis

     b. ten-**OH**-sine-oh-**VIE**-tis   **d.** **TEN**-oh-**SINE**-oh-**VIE**-tis

     Correctly spell the term: _____

3. The correct pronunciation for recording of electrical activity in a muscle

     a. **EE**-lek-troh-my-og-**RAH**-fee   **c.** **UL**-trah-soh- **NOG**-rah-fee

     b. ee-**LEK**-troh-my-**OG**-rah-fee   **d.** ul-**TRAH**-soh-nog-**RAFEE**

     Correctly spell the term: _____

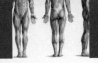
4. The correct pronunciation for the fibrous tissue that surrounds muscle and organs

    a. FIE-ber

    b. fie-**BER**

    c. fash-**EE**-ah

    d. FASH-ee-ah

    Correctly spell the term: _____

5. The correct pronunciation for the fibrous ligament that keeps the tendons in place on the wrist

    a. ret-ih-**NAK**-you-lum

    b. RET-ih-nak-you-lum

    c. FAS-ih-kull

    d. fa-**SIH**-kull

    Correctly spell the term: _____

Case Report

A. **Read the Case Report presented below.** Choose the correct answer to each question. **LO 15.8, 15.9, 15.10**

Case Report (CR) 15.1

You are

. . . a certified occupational therapist assistant working in the Rehabilitation Unit at Fulwood Medical Center.

Your patient is

. . . Mr. Hank Johnson, a 65-year-old print shop owner.

One year ago, Mr. Johnson had an elective left total-hip replacement for osteoarthritis. Four months later, he had a myocardial infarction. Two weeks ago, while on his exercise bike, he had a stroke. His right arm and leg were paralyzed, he lost his speech, and he had difficulty swallowing. He arrived in the Emergency Department within 3 hours of the stroke and received thrombolytic therapy (*see Chapter 9*). Mr. Johnson is now receiving physical therapy, occupational therapy, and speech therapy in the inpatient Rehabilitation Unit. He is able to say some simple words and has begun to have voluntary movements in the arm and leg. Your roles are to help him regain function in his arm and leg and to monitor and record his progress.

---

1. When completing required patient documentation, you would likely abbreviate your job title. Which abbreviation would you use?

    a. PTA

    b. COTA

    c. OT

    d. PT

2. The fact that his movements in his arm and leg are **voluntary** means that:

    a. his arm and leg muscles have atrophied

    b. he has no control over the movement of his arm and leg

    c. his arm and leg are weak

    d. he can choose to move his arm and leg

3. Which of the following may be an occupational therapy goal in regards to his arm?

    a. use a cane for walking

    b. ride a bicycle

    c. chew and swallow solid food

    d. brush his hair and teeth

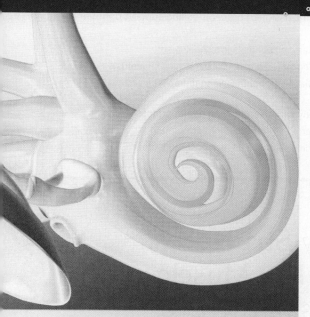

2014 Nucleus Medical Media

CHAPTER 16

Special Senses of the Eye and Ear

The Languages of Ophthalmology and Otology

Chapter Sections

16.1 Accessory Structures and Functions of the Eye

16.2 Disorders of the Eye

16.3 Procedures and Pharmacology-The Eye

16.4 The Ear and Hearing

16.5 Disorders of the Ear

16.6 Procedures and Pharmacology-The Ear

Chapter Learning Outcomes

Upon completion of this chapter, you will be able to:

LO 16.1 Identify and describe the anatomy and physiology of the eyes and ears.

LO 16.2 Use roots, combining forms, suffixes, and prefixes to construct and analyze medical terms related to the eyes and ears.

LO 16.3 Spell medical terms related to the eyes and ears.

LO 16.4 Pronounce medical terms related to the eyes and ears.

LO 16.5 Describe diagnostic procedures utilized for injuries and disorders of the eyes and ears.

LO 16.6 Identify and describe injuries, disorders, and pathological conditions related to the eyes and ears.

LO 16.7 Describe the therapeutic procedures and pharmacologic agents used with the ophthalmology and otology systems.

LO 16.8 Apply knowledge of medical terms relating to ophthalmology and otology to documentation, medical records, and communication.

LO 16.9 Identify and correctly use abbreviations of terms used in ophthalmology and otology.

LO 16.10 Identify health professionals involved in the care of patients with eye and ear disorders.

Note: The sense of smell is discussed as an integral part of the respiratory system *(Chapter 13)*, the sense of taste as an integral part of the digestive system *(Chapter 5)*, and the sense of touch as an integral part of the nervous system *(Chapter 9)*.

In your future career, you may work directly and/or indirectly with the following health professionals in the area of ophthalmology:

- **Ophthalmologists,** who are medical specialists (MDs) in the diagnosis and treatment of diseases of the eye.
- **Optometrists** (ODs), who are doctors of optometry and are skilled in the measurement of vision. They are not medical doctors and cannot prescribe medication.
- **Opticians,** who are licensed to make corrective lenses, adjust and repair spectacles, and fit contact lenses.

Continued

The health professionals in the following list perform specific assigned procedures and support ophthal-mologists according to the depth of their training:

- Certified ophthalmic medical technicians
- Certified ophthalmic assistants
- Certified ophthalmic technicians
- Certified ophthalmic technologists
- Registered ophthalmic ultrasound biometrists
- Diagnostic ophthalmic sonographers

In the area of otology, you may work directly and/or indirectly with the following health professionals:

- **Otologists,** who are medical specialists in diseases of the ear.
- **Otorhinolaryngologists,** who are medical specialists (MDs) in diseases of the ear, nose, and throat (ENT).
- **Audiologists,** who evaluate hearing function.

Section 16.1 Accessory Structures, Extrinsic Eye Muscles and Functions of the Eye

Accessory Structures, Extrinsic Muscles and Their Functions

The components of the eye work together so we can see. The function of the eye is to receive and bend light rays, convert them to electric energy, send it to the brain which creates the images we see.

Accessory Structures

Accessory structures serve as assistants to the eye so that it can receive the light rays.

- **Eyebrows** keep sweat from running into the eye and function in nonverbal communication.
- **Eyelids** consist mostly of muscle that fans out from each eyelid onto the forehead and cheek to open and close the eyelids. They are covered in the body's thinnest layer of skin.
  Functions of eyelids are to close to protect the eye from foreign objects; blink to move tears across the surface of the eye and sweep debris away; close in sleep to keep out visual stimuli.
- The **tarsus** is a flat, fibrous connective tissue layer in the eyelid, whose ducts open along the edge of the eyelid.
- **Tarsal glands** are found within the tarsus, with ducts open along the edge of the eyelid. They secrete an oily fluid that keeps the eyelids from sticking together.
- **Eyelashes** are strong hairs that help keep debris out of the eyes. They arise on the edge of the lids from hair follicles (*see Chapter 4*).
- **Canthi** (singular, **canthus**) are the two corners where the upper and lower eyelids meet.
- **Conjunctiva** is a transparent mucous membrane that lines the inside of both eyelids and covers the front of the eye except the central portion, the cornea. The conjunctiva is freely moveable, has numerous small blood vessels, and is richly supplied with nerve endings that make it very sensitive to pain. Numerous goblet cells within the conjunctiva secrete a thin film of mucin that prevents the surface of the eyeball from dehydrating.
  The **lacrimal apparatus** (*Figure 16.1*) consists of four structures.

1. The **lacrimal (tear) gland,** located in the upper, lateral corner of the orbit, secretes tears.
2. Short **lacrimal ducts** carry the tears to the surface of the conjunctiva. Tears wash across the conjunctiva.
3. The **lacrimal sac** collects the tears at the medial corner of the eye.
4. The **nasolacrimal duct** carries the tears into the nose, from where they are swallowed.

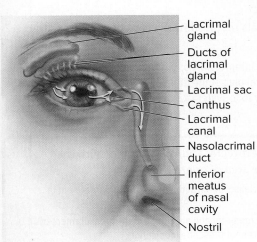

Lacrimal gland
Ducts of lacrimal gland
Lacrimal sac
Canthus
Lacrimal canal
Nasolacrimal duct
Inferior meatus of nasal cavity
Nostril

▲ **Figure 16.1** Lacrimal apparatus and accessory structures.

The functions of tears are to:
- Clean and lubricate the surface of the eye.
- Deliver nutrients and oxygen to the conjunctiva.
- Prevent infection through a bactericidal enzyme called **lysozyme.**

Extrinsic Muscles of the Eye

Humans, with their two eyes working closely together, have developed very good three-dimensional perception (**stereopsis**) and hand-eye coordination. Stereopsis depends on an accurate alignment of the two eyes.

This alignment is held in place by the coordination of six **extrinsic eye muscles** (also called **extraocular muscles**) for each eye that are attached to the inner wall of the orbit and to the outer surface of the eyeball (*Figure 16.2*). The function of these muscles is to move the eye in all directions.

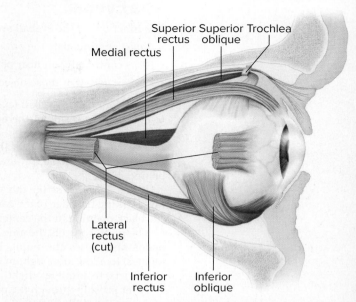

▲ **Figure 16.2** Extrinsic muscles of the right eye (lateral view).

Word Analysis and Definition: The Eye

S = Suffix P = Prefix R = Root R/CF = Combining Form

WORD	PRONUNCIATION		ELEMENTS	DEFINITION
canthus canthi (pl)	**KAN**-thus **KAN**-thee		Greek *corner of the eye*	Corner of the eye where upper and lower lids meet
conjunctiva conjunctival (adj)	kon-junk-**TIE**-vah kon-junk-**TIE**-val	S/ R/	Latin *inner lining of eyelids* **-al** *pertaining to* **conjunctiv-** *conjunctiva*	Inner lining of the eyelids Pertaining to the conjunctiva
extrinsic	eks-**TRIN**-sik		Latin *on the outer side*	Muscles that are located on the outside of the eye
intrinsic	in-**TRIN**-sik		Latin *on the inner side*	Muscles that are located inside the eye
lacrimal	**LAK**-rim-al	S/ R/	**-al** *pertaining to* **lacrim-** *tears*	Pertaining to tears
lacrimal duct lacrimal sac nasolacrimal duct	**LAK**-rim-al DUKT **LAK**-rim-al SAK **NAY**-zoh-**LAK**-rim-al DUKT	R/ R/CF	**duct** *to lead* **sac** Latin *bag, pocket* **nas/o-** *nose*	Carries tears to the conjunctiva Where tears leave the eye at the medial corner Passage from the lacrimal sac to the nose
lysozyme	**LIE**-soh-zime	S/ R/CF	**-zyme** *enzyme* **lys/o-** *decomposition*	Enzyme that dissolves the cell walls of bacteria
orbit	**OR**-bit		Latin *circle*	The bony socket that holds the eyeball Pertaining to the orbit
orbital (adj)	**OR**-bit-al	S/ R/	**-al** *pertaining to* **orbit-** *orbit*	
periorbital	per-ee-**OR**-bit-al	S/ P/ R/	**-al** *pertaining to* **peri-** *around* **-orbit-** *orbit*	Pertaining to tissues around the orbit
stereopsis	ster-ee-**OP**-sis	S/ R/	**-opsis** *vision* **stere-** *three-dimensional*	Three-dimensional vision
tarsus (**Note:** *Tarsus* also is used to refer to the seven bones in the instep of the foot.)	**TAR**-sus		Greek *flat*	The flat fibrous plate that gives shape to the outer edges of the eyelids
tarsal (adj)	**TAR**-sal	S/ R/	**-al** *pertaining to* **tars-** *tarsus*	Pertaining to the tarsus

The Eyeball

The functions of the eyeball are to:

- *Adjust* continuously the amount of light it lets in to reach the retina.
- *Focus* continually on near or distant objects.
- *Produce images* of those objects and instantly transmit them to the brain.

The front of the eyeball (except for the cornea) is covered by the conjunctiva, a thin layer of tissue that covers the inside of the eyelids and curves over the eyeball to meet the **sclera,** the tough, white outer layer of the eye.

The center of the front of the eye is a transparent, dome-shaped membrane called the **cornea.** The cornea has no blood supply and obtains its nutrients from tears and from fluid in the **anterior chamber** behind it.

When light rays strike the eye, they pass through the cornea. Because of its domed curvature, those rays striking the edge of the cornea are bent toward its center. The light rays then go through the **pupil,** the black opening in the center of the colored area (the **iris**) in the front of the eye.

The pupil controls the amount of light entering the eye. The **sphincter pupillae muscle** *(Figure 16.3)* opens and closes the pupil. When you are in a dark place, the sphincter pupillae muscle opens (dilates) to allow more light to enter. When you are in bright light, the sphincter pupillae muscle closes (constricts) to admit less light.

After passing through the pupil, the light rays pass through the transparent **lens.** The ciliary muscle of the **ciliary body** makes the lens thicker and thinner, enabling it to bend the light rays and focus them on the **retina** at the back of the eye. This process of changing focus is called accommodation. The process of bending the light rays by the cornea and lens is called **refraction.**

The lens has no supply of blood vessels or nerves. With increasing age, the lens loses its elasticity.

Did you know...

- The cornea protects the eye and, by changing shape, provides about 60% of the eye's focusing power.
- The pupil controls the amount of light entering the eye.
- The lens changes its shape to focus rays of light onto the retina.
- Both the cornea and the lens refract light rays. Neither has a blood supply, which compromises healing from injury or disease.

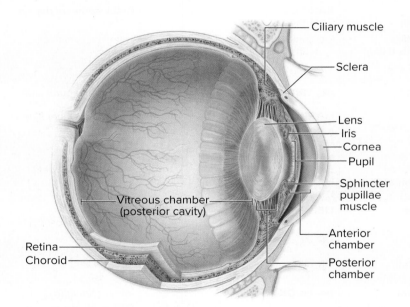

▲ **Figure 16.3** Anatomy of the eyeball.

WORD	PRONUNCIATION	ELEMENTS		DEFINITION
ciliary body	**SILL**-ee-air-ee **BOD**-ee	S/ R/ R/	-ary *pertaining to* cili- *eyelid* body *mass*	Muscles that make the lens of the eye thicker and thinner
cornea	**KOR**-nee-ah		Latin *web, tunic*	The central, transparent part of the outer coat of the eye covering the iris and pupil
iris	**EYE**-ris		Greek *diaphragm of the eye*	Colored portion of the eye with the pupil in its center
lens	LENZ		Latin *lentil shape*	Transparent refractive structure behind the iris
pupil pupillae (pl) pupillary (adj)	**PYU**-pill pyu-**PILL**-ee **PYU**-pill-**AH**-ree	 S/ R/	Latin *pupil* -ary *pertaining to* pupill- *pupil*	The opening in the center of the iris that allows light to reach the lens Pertaining to the pupil
refract (verb) refraction (noun)	ree-**FRAKT** ree-**FRAK**-shun	 S/ R/	Latin *break up* -ion *action, condition, process* refract- *break up*	Make a change in direction of, or bend, a ray of light The change in direction of a ray of light when it passes from one optic medium to another
retina retinal (adj)	**RET**-ih-nah **RET**-ih-nal	 S/ R/	Latin *net* -al *pertaining to* retin- *retina*	Light-sensitive innermost layer of eyeball Pertaining to the retina
sclera scleral (adj)	**SKLAIR**-ah **SKLAIR**-al	 S/ R/	Greek *hard* -al *pertaining to* scler- *hard, white of eye*	Fibrous outer covering of the eyeball and the white of the eye Pertaining to the sclera
sphincter	**SFINK**-ter		Greek *band*	Band of muscle that encircles an opening; when it contracts, the opening squeezes closed

The Retina

The final destination of the light rays is the **retina,** the thin lining at the back of your eye *(Figure 16.4a).* It's an area the size of a small postage stamp that has 10 layers of cells. The retina has 130 million **rods** *(Figure 16.4b),* which perceive only light, not color, and function mostly when the light is dim. There are 6.5 million **cones** *(see Figure 16.4b),* which are activated by light and color and have precise **visual acuity.** Different cones respond to red, blue, and green light. The perception of color is based on the intensity of different mixtures of colors from the three types of cones.

Rods and cones are called **photoreceptor** cells. The rods and cones convert the energy of the light rays into electrical impulses, and the **optic nerve,** a bundle of more than a million nerve fibers, transmits these impulses to the visual cortex at the back of the brain. The area where the optic nerve leaves the retina is called the **optic disc.** Because it has no rods and cones, the optic disc cannot form images and is called the **blind spot.**

Just lateral to the optic disc at the back of the retina is a circular, yellowish region called the **macula lutea** *(see Figure 16.4a).* In the center of the macula is a small pit called the **fovea centralis,** which has 4,000 tiny cones and no rods. Each cone has its own nerve fiber, and this makes the fovea the area of sharpest vision. As you read this text, the words are precisely focused on your fovea centralis. The rods and cones outside of the macula provide **peripheral vision.**

Behind the photoreceptor layer of the retina is a very **vascular** layer called the **choroid.** This layer, together with the iris and ciliary body, is called the **uvea.**

Segments of the Eye

The eyeball is divided into two fluid-filled segments separated by the lens and the ciliary muscle. The fluids maintain the shape of the eyeball. In the back, the **posterior cavity** extends from the back of the lens to the retina and contains a transparent jelly called the **vitreous humor,** which helps maintain the shape of the eyeball.

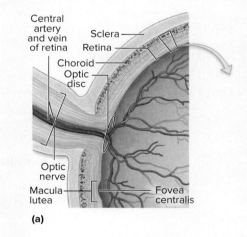

(a)

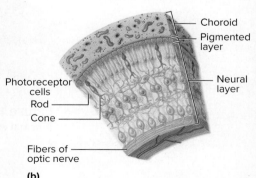

(b)

▲ **Figure 16.4** Structure of the retina.

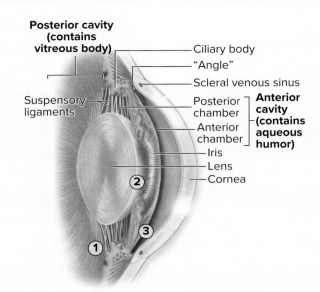

Ciliary body
"Angle"
Scleral venous sinus
Posterior chamber
Anterior cavity (contains aqueous humor)
Suspensory ligaments
Anterior chamber
Iris
Lens
Cornea

▲ Figure 16.5 Circulation of aqueous humor.

In front, the **anterior cavity** extends from the cornea to the lens and is divided into two chambers. The **anterior chamber** extends from the cornea to the iris, and the **posterior chamber** extends from the iris to the lens (*Figure 16.5*). **Aqueous humor** is produced in the posterior chamber as a filtrate from plasma (Step 1). It passes through the pupil into the anterior chamber (Step 2) where it is continually reabsorbed into a vascular space called the **scleral venous sinus** (Step 3) and taken into the venous bloodstream. The aqueous humor also removes waste products and helps maintain the internal chemical environment of the eye.

Visual Pathway

After the optic nerves leave the back of the retina and eyeball, they leave each orbit through the **optic foramen.** They converge into an "X" called the **optic chiasm** (*Figure 16.6*). Here, the fibers from the medial half of each retina cross to the opposite side of the brain.

After leaving the chiasm, the fibers form the **optic tract** and then the **optic radiation** to take the nerve impulses to the **visual cortex** in the **occipital lobes** at the back of the brain. Here the incoming visual stimuli are interpreted.

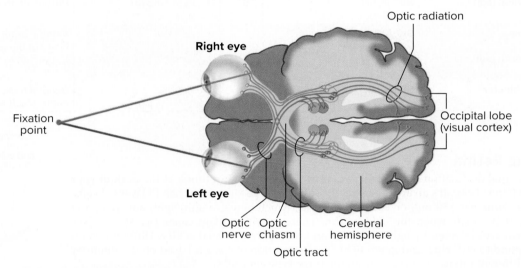

Optic radiation

Right eye

Fixation point

Occipital lobe (visual cortex)

Left eye

Optic nerve   Optic chiasm   Cerebral hemisphere

Optic tract

▲ Figure 16.6 Visual pathway.

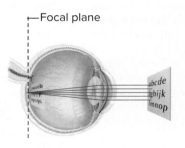

Focal plane

abcde
fghijk
lmnop

▲ Figure 16.7 Emmetropia (normal vision).

Refraction

Light is traveling at a speed of 186,000 miles per second when it hits the eye. Light rays that hit the center of the cornea pass straight through, but because of the curvature of the cornea, rays that hit away from center are bent toward the center. The light rays then hit the lens, are bent again, and, in normal vision, the image is focused sharply on the retina (*Figure 16.7*). This normal vision is called **emmetropia.**

Word Analysis and Definition: The Retina and Segments of the Eye

S = Suffix P = Prefix R = Root R/CF = Combining Form

WORD	PRONUNCIATION		ELEMENTS	DEFINITION
aqueous humor	AYK-wee-us HEW-mor	S/ R/CF	-ous *pertaining to* aqu/e- *watery* humor Greek *liquid*	Watery liquid in the anterior and posterior chambers of the eye
chiasm chiasma (alternative term)	KIE-asm kie-AZ-mah		Greek *cross*	X-shaped crossing of the two optic nerves at the base of the brain
choroid	KOR-oid		Greek *membrane*	Region of the retina and uvea
fovea centralis	FOH-vee-ah sen-TRAH-lis		fovea Latin *a pit* centralis Latin *central, in the center*	Small pit in the center of the macula that has the highest visual acuity
macula lutea	MAK-you-lah LOO-tee-ah		macula Latin *small spot* lutea Latin *yellow*	Yellowish spot on the back of the retina; contains the fovea centralis
optic	OP-tik	S/ R/	-ic *pertaining to* opt- *vision, eye*	Pertaining to vision or the eye
optical (adj)	OP-tih-kal	S/	-ical *pertaining to*	Pertaining to vision or the eye
photoreceptor	foh-toh-ree-SEP-tor	S/ R/CF R/	-or *that which does something* phot/o- *light* -recept- *receive*	A photoreceptor cell receives light and converts it into electrical impulses
tract	TRAKT		Latin *path*	Bundle of nerve fibers with a common origin and destination
uvea	YOU-vee-ah		Greek *layer of eyeball*	Middle coat of eyeball; includes iris, ciliary body, and choroid
visual acuity	VIH-zhoo-wal ah-KYU-ih-tee	S/ R/	-al *pertaining to* visu- *sight* acuity Latin *sharpen*	Sharpness and clearness of vision
vitreous humor	VIT-ree-us HEW-mor	S/ R/	-ous *pertaining to* vitre- *glassy* humor Greek *liquid*	A gelatinous liquid in the posterior cavity of the eyeball with the appearance of glass

Check Point Section 16.1

A. Define the accessory structures of the eye. *Match the accessory structure of the eye with its correct definition.* **LO 16.1**

_____ 1. lysozyme

_____ 2. canthus

_____ 3. tarsus

_____ 4. eyelash

_____ 5. eyebrow

_____ 6. lacrimal gland

_____ 7. conjunctiva

_____ 8. tarsal gland

a. corner of the eye where eyelids meet

b. strong hairs that keep debris out of the eye

c. secretes tears

d. secretes an oily substance to keep eyelids from sticking together

e. enzyme that destroys bacteria

f. hair that keeps sweat out of the eyes

g. transparent mucous membrane that lines the eyelids and the front of the eye (except for the cornea)

h. fibrous connective tissue that gives structure to the eyelids

B. Notice in this exercise that not every medical term needs a prefix and/or a suffix. *However, every medical term does contain one or more roots and/or combining forms.* **Deconstruct** *the following medical terms into their elements. Fill in the chart.* **LO 16.1, 16.2, 16.6**

Medical Term	Prefix	Root(s)/Combining Form	Suffix
conjunctival		1.	2.
periorbital	3.	4.	5.
aqueous		6.	7.
refraction		8.	9.
stereopsis		10.	11.

C. Recognize the definitions of structures of the eye with two roots/combining forms that are being described. *Fill in the blanks.* **LO 16.1, 16.2**

1. muscles that make the lens of the eye thicker and thinner _____

2. a cell that receives light and converts into electrical impulses _____

3. passage from the lacrimal sac to the nose _____

4. carries tears to the conjunctiva _____

D. Components of the eyeball: Enhance your knowledge of the components of the eyeball and their functions. *This will help you to understand the vision process. Match the phrase in the left column with the appropriate medical term in the right column.* **LO 16.1**

_____ **1.** Colored portion of the eye   **a.** lens

_____ **2.** Change direction of a ray of light   **b.** retina

_____ **3.** Opening in the iris   **c.** sphincter

_____ **4.** Band of muscle that encircles an opening   **d.** pupil

_____ **5.** Transparent, refractive structure   **e.** ciliary body

_____ **6.** Innermost layer of eyeball   **f.** refract

_____ **7.** White of the eye   **g.** iris

_____ **8.** Operates the lens   **h.** sclera

E. Identify the structures of the eyeball. *Select the best answer.* **LO 16.1**

1. Sharpness and clearness of vision is called
  a. optical
  b. acuity
  c. vascular
  d. aqueous
  e. choroid

2. The term **photoreceptor** has
  a. two combining forms and a suffix
  b. a prefix, root, and suffix
  c. a root, a combining form, and a suffix
  d. two roots and a suffix
  e. a suffix and a root

3. The choroid, iris, and ciliary body make up the
  a. optic disc
  b. blind spot
  c. uvea
  d. visual cortex
  e. optic nerve

4. The gel contained in the posterior cavity is called
  a. vitreous humor
  b. ciliary body
  c. visual cortex
  d. aqueous humor
  e. macula lutea

5. This helps maintain the shape of the eyeball:

    a. vitreous humor

    b. rods

    c. fovea centralis

    d. cones

    e. macula lutea

6. The area of sharpest vision is the

    a. cornea

    b. rods

    c. macula lutea

    d. fovea centralis

    e. choroid

Section 16.2 Disorders of the Eye

Disorders of the Accessory Structures and Extrinsic Eye Muscles

Disorders of the accessory structures of the eye occur separately, but often are a result of another accessory structure disorder.

Eyelid edema can be a result of eyelid disorders (e.g., stye and chalazion), or is often produced by an allergic reaction due to cosmetics, pollen in the air, or stings and bites from insects. It can also be caused by conjunctivitis or dacryostenosis.

Ptosis occurs when the upper eyelid is constantly drooped over the eye due to **paresis** (partial paralysis) of the muscle that raises the upper lid *(Figure 16.11)*. It can be associated with diabetes, myasthenia gravis, brain tumor, and muscular dystrophy, all of which are described in previous subsequent chapters. The term **blepharoptosis** is used for sagging of the eyelids due to excess skin.

Blepharitis occurs when multiple eyelash follicles and tarsal glands become infected. The margin of the eyelid shows persistent redness and crusting and may become ulcerated. The infection is usually staphylococcal.

A **chalazion** is a small, painless, localized, whitish swelling inside the lid when a tarsal gland becomes blocked *(Figure 16.12)*. It usually disappears spontaneously.

A **stye**, or **hordeolum,** is an infection of an eyelash follicle producing an abscess *(Figure 16.13)*, with localized pain, swelling, redness, and pus formation at the edge of the eyelid.

Conjunctivitis *(Figure 16.14)* has several causes. Viral and bacterial conjunctivitis are contagious.

- **Viral** is commonly caused by viruses that cause the common cold.

- **Bacterial** is frequently due to staphylococcal or streptococcal bacteria; may be caused by rubbing eyes, sharing makeup that is not your own.

- **Allergic conjunctivitis** can be part of seasonal hay fever or be produced by year-round allergens such as animal dander and dust mites *(see Chapter 12)*.

- **Irritant conjunctivitis** can be caused by air pollutants (smoke and fumes) and by chemicals such as chlorine and those found in soaps and cosmetics.

- **Neonatal conjunctivitis (ophthalmia neonatorum)** can be caused by a blocked tear duct in the baby, by the antibiotic eyedrops given routinely at birth, or by sexually transmitted bacteria in an infected mother's birth canal.

- **Dry eyes** are a common and chronic condition which over 75 million Americans suffer from. It is due to the tears losing water and becoming too salty so that the eyes sting and burn and vision becomes blurry.

Dacryostenosis is a blockage of the drainage of tears, usually due to narrowing of the nasolacrimal ducts. Approximately 6% of newborns have this condition, but it may not be noticeable at birth because infants do not produce

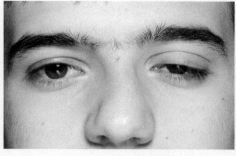

▲ **Figure 16.11** **Ptosis of right eyelid.**
Mediscan/Alamy Stock Photo

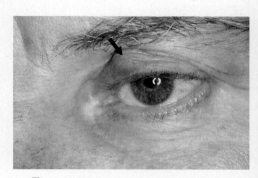

▲ **Figure 16.12** **Chalazion in upper eyelid.** SPL/Science Source

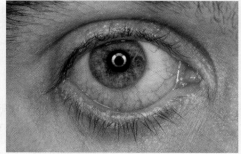

▲ **Figure 16.14** **Conjunctivitis.** Pavel L Photo and Video/Shutterstock

Stye

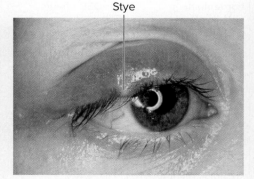

▲ **Figure 16.13** **Stye showing pus-filled cyst.** Western Opthamolic Hospital/Science Source

tears until they are several weeks old. Fortunately, nearly all blocked ducts open by the age of one year and do not require surgical opening.

Dacryocystitis is an infection of the lacrimal sac, with swelling and pus at the medial corner of the eye.

Disorders of Extrinsic Eye Muscles

Strabismus, "squinting," is the loss of alignment of the eyes due to muscle control. Types of strabismus:

Exotropia, an outward turning of one eye.

Esotropia, "crossed eyes," is the eye turned in toward the nose *(Figure 16.10)*. In congenital or infantile esotropia, both eyes look in toward the nose—the right eye looks to the left, and the left eye looks to the right.

Accommodative esotropia is caused by uncorrected hyperopia (a refractive disorder). An eye will cross when attempting to keep a distant object in focus.

Word Analysis and Definition: Disorders of the Accessory Glands

S = Suffix P = Prefix R = Root R/CF = Combining Form

WORD	PRONUNCIATION	ELEMENTS		DEFINITION
accommodate (verb)	ah-**KOM**-oh-date		Latin *to adjust*	To adjust something to make it fit its needs
accommodation (noun)	ah-kom-oh-**DAY**-shun	S/ R/	-ion *action* accommodat- *adjust*	The act of adjusting something to make it fit the needs
accommodative (adj)	ah- **KOM** -oh-day-tiv	S/ R/	-ive *pertaining to, quality of* accommodat- *adjust*	Willing to adjust to create agreement
blepharitis	blef-ah-**RIE**-tis	S/ R/	-itis *inflammation* blephar- *eyelid*	Inflammation of the eyelid
blepharoptosis	**BLEF**-ah-rop-**TOH**-sis	S/ R/CF	-ptosis *drooping* blephar/o- *eyelid*	Drooping of the upper eyelid
chalazion	kah-**LAY**-zee-on		Greek *lump*	Cyst on the outer edge of an eyelid caused by a blocked tarsal gland
conjunctivitis	kon-junk-tih-**VIE**-tis	S/ R/	-itis *inflammation* conjunctiv- *conjunctiva*	Inflammation of the conjunctiva
contagious	kon-**TAY**-jus	S/ R/	-ous *pertaining to* contagi- *transmissible by contact*	Able to be transmitted, as infections transmitted from person to person, from person to air, or from surface to person
dacryocystitis	**DAK**-ree-oh-sis-**TIE**-tis	S/ R/CF R/	-itis *inflammation* dacry/o- *tears* -cyst- *sac*	Inflammation of the lacrimal sac
dacryostenosis	**DAK**-ree-oh-steh-**NOH**-sis	S/ R/CF	-sis *abnormal condition* -sten/o- *narrowing*	Narrowing of the nasolacrimal duct
esotropia	es-oh-**TROH**-pee-ah	S/ P/ R/	-ia *condition* eso- *inward* -trop- *turn*	A turning of the eye inward toward the nose
exotropia	ek-soh-**TROH**-pee-ah	S/ P/ R/	-ia *condition* exo- *outward* -trop- *turn*	A turning of the eye outward away from the nose
hordeolum stye (syn)	hor-**DEE**-oh-lum STY		Latin *stye in the eye*	Abscess in an eyelash follicle
infectious	in-**FEK**-shus	S/ R/CF	-ous *pertaining to* infect/i- *internal invasion*	Capable of being transmitted, or caused by infection by a microorganism
ophthalmia neonatorum	off-**THAL**-mee-ah nee-oh-nay-**TOR**-um	S/ R/ S/ P/ R/	-ia *condition* ophthalm- *eye* -orum *function of* neo- *new* -nat- *born*	Conjunctivitis of the newborn
paresis	par-**EE**-sis		Greek *paralysis*	Partial paralysis
ptosis (*Note:* The first consonant is silent.**)**	**TOH**-sis		Greek *drooping*	Sinking down of an eyelid or an organ
strabismus	strah-**BIZ**-mus	S/ R/	-ismus *take action* strab- *squint*	A turning of an eye away from its normal position

Disorders of the Anterior Eyeball

Corneal abrasions can be caused by foreign bodies, direct trauma (such as being poked by a fingernail), or badly fitting contact lenses. The abrasion can grow into an ulcer *(see Figure 16.15).*

Scleritis, inflammation of the sclera (the white outer covering of the eyeball), can affect one or both eyes. It causes dull pain and intense redness, and is often associated with rheumatoid arthritis *(see Chapter 14)* and the digestive disorder Crohn's disease *(see Chapter 5).*

Uveitis, inflammation of the iris, ciliary body, and choroid, produces pain, intense **photophobia,** blurred vision, and constriction of the pupil. There is usually an underlying disease, such as rheumatoid arthritis.

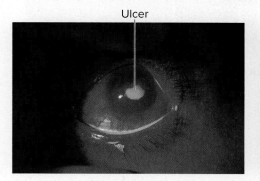

▲ **Figure 16.15** Fluorescein-stained corneal ulcer. Shutterstock/ARZTSAMUI

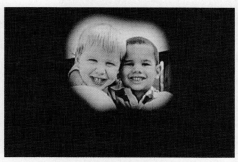

▲ **Figure 16.16** Vision with glaucoma. National Eye Institute

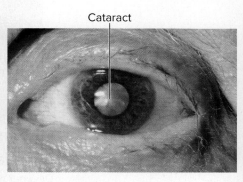

▲ **Figure 16.17** Cataract. Dr. P. Marazzi/ Science Source

Glaucoma

The circulation of aqueous humor was described earlier in this chapter. If the aqueous humor cannot escape from the eye into the bloodstream, the fluid continues to be produced and pressure builds up inside the eye. The increased **intraocular** pressure interferes with the blood supply to the retina, causing death of retinal cells. Eventually the optic nerve fibers are damaged. This condition is called **glaucoma** and is a major cause of blindness *(Figure 16.16).*

Cataracts

A **cataract** is a cloudy or opaque area in the lens *(Figure 16.17).* It is typically caused by deterioration of the lens due to aging and may be associated with diabetes and with cigarette smoke. It presents with blurring of vision and **photosensitivity** or may be discovered on routine eye examination. It is another major cause of blindness.

The majority of cataracts occur in the center of the lens, but those associated with diabetes can be cortical (around the outside of the lens). Cortical cataracts can cause diminished **peripheral vision** and photosensitivity. The blurred vision obtained when a cataract is present is shown in *Figure 16.18.*

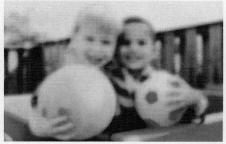

▲ **Figure 16.18** Vision with cataract. National Eye Institute

Word Analysis and Definition: Disorders of the Anterior Eyeball

S = Suffix P = Prefix R = Root R/CF = Combining Form

WORD	PRONUNCIATION		ELEMENTS	DEFINITION
abrasion	ah-**BRAY**-shun	S/ R/	-ion *action, condition, process* abras- *scrape off*	Area of skin or mucous membrane that has been scraped off
cataract	**KAT**-ah-rakt		Greek *waterfall*	Complete or partial opacity of the lens
glaucoma	glaw-**KOH**-mah	S/ R/	-oma *mass, tumor* glauc- *lens opacity*	Increased intraocular pressure
intraocular	in-trah-**OK**-you-lar	S/ P/ R/	-ar *pertaining to* intra- *inside* -ocul- *eye*	Pertaining to the inside of the eye
photophobia	foh-toh-**FOH**-bee-ah	S/ R/CF	-phobia *fear* phot/o- *light*	Fear of the light because it hurts the eyes
photophobic (adj)	foh-toh-**FOH**-bik	S/ R/	-ic *pertaining to* -phob- *light*	Relating to or suffering from photophobia
photosensitive (adj)	foh-toh-**SEN**-sih-tiv	R/CF R/CF	phot/o- *light* -sensitiv/e *sensitive*	An eye in which light induces pain
photosensitivity	foh-toh-sen-sih-**TIV**-ih-tee	S/ R/	-ity *condition* -sensitiv- *sensitive*	Condition in which light produces pain in the eye

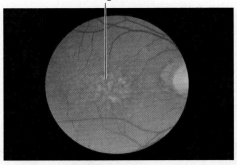

Macular degeneration

▲ **Figure 16.19** Ophthalmoscopic view of macular degeneration. Paul Parker/Science Source

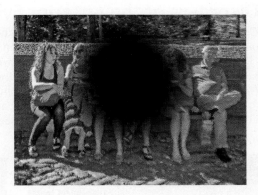

▲ **Figure 16.20** Vision with macular degeneration. Spencer Grant/Science Source

Diseases of the Retina

Macular Degeneration

Degeneration of the central macula results in loss of visual acuity, with a dark blurry area of vision loss in the center of the visual field *(Figures 16.19 and 16.20).*

There is photoreceptor cell loss and bleeding, with capillary proliferation and scar formation. The condition can progress to blindness. Most cases occur in people over age 55.

Retinal Detachment

Separation of the retina from its underlying choroid layer may be partial or complete and produces a retinal tear or hole. The detachment can happen suddenly, without pain. The patient sees a dark shadow invading his or her peripheral vision. The detachment can be seen on ophthalmoscopic examination.

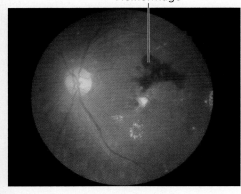

Hemorrhage

▲ **Figure 16.21** Ophthalmoscopic view of diabetic retinopathy. memorisz/iStock/Getty Images

Diabetic Retinopathy

This disease occurs most frequently in diabetics whose blood sugar levels are not controlled. Some 50% of diabetics have **retinopathy.**

In the early stages, **microaneurysms** of the small retinal blood vessels form. There are usually no symptoms. Later, hemorrhages can occur, leading to destruction of the photoreceptor cells (rods and cones) and visual difficulties *(Figure 16.21).*

Symptoms of diabetic retinopathy include blurred vision, dark areas in vision *(Figure 16.22)* and vision loss.

Papilledema

Papilledema is swelling of the optic disc due to increased **intracranial** pressure. It is not a diagnosis; it is a sign of some underlying pathology. It is seen on ophthalmoscopic examination.

Cancer of the Eye

Tumors of the skin of the eyelids include the **squamous cell** and **basal cell carcinomas** and **melanoma,** described in *Chapter 4.*

Retinoblastoma is typically diagnosed at two years of age, rarely after 6 years of age. It is curable if diagnosed early and if it has not metastized to other parts of the body. It has a 5-year survival rate of 96%. The condition can be hereditary.

The first symptom is a white appearance of the pupil (**leukocoria).** With early detection and aggressive treatment based on chemotherapy and laser surgery, 90% of cases are cured.

In adults, the most common cancers are **metastases** to the eye from cancer of the lung in men and the breast in women.

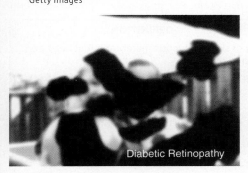

Diabetic Retinopathy

▲ **Figure 16.22** Vision with diabetic retinopathy. National Institutes of Health/National Eye Institute

Color Blindness

Some people have a hereditary lack of response by one or more of the three types of cones and show **color blindness.** The most common form is red-green color blindness, in which these colors and related shades cannot be distinguished from each other.

Night blindness is the inability to see in poor light. It is a symptom of an underlying problem that can be

- Uncorrected nearsightedness.
- Cataracts.
- Retinitis pigmentosa.
- Vitamin A deficiency.
- Glaucoma medications (such as pilocarpine) that constrict the pupil.

Word Analysis and Definition: Diseases of the Retina

S = Suffix P = Prefix R = Root R/CF = Combining Form

WORD	PRONUNCIATION	ELEMENTS		DEFINITION
leukocoria	loo-koh-**KOH**-ree-ah	S/ R/CF R/	-ia *condition* leuk/o- *white* -cor- *pupil*	Reflection in pupil of white mass in the eye
metastasis metastases (pl)	meh-**TAS**-tah-sis meh-**TAS**-tah-sees	P/ R/	meta- *beyond* -stasis *stay in one place*	Spread of disease from one part of the body to another
microaneurysm	my-kroh-**AN**-yu-rizm	P/ R/	micro- *small* -aneurysm *dilation*	Focal dilation of retinal capillaries
papilledema	pah-pill-eh-**DEE**-mah	R/ S/	papill- *pimple* -edema *swelling*	Swelling of the optic disc in the retina
retinoblastoma	**RET**-in-oh-blas-**TOH**-mah	S/ S/ R/CF	-oma *tumor, mass* -blast- *germ cell* retin/o- *retina*	Malignant neoplasm of primitive retinal cells
retinopathy	ret-ih-**NOP**-ah-thee	S/	-pathy *disease*	Degenerative disease of the retina

Disorders of Refraction

Farsighted people are said to have **hyperopia** *(Figure 16.8)* in which only distant objects can be seen clearly. Because the eyeball is shortened, objects close to the eye are focused behind the retina and vision is blurred. Convex lenses are needed to correct the problem.

Nearsighted people are said to have **myopia** *(Figure 16.9)*, in which only close objects can be clearly seen. Because the eyeball is elongated, faraway objects are focused in front of the retina.

In **presbyopia,** the lens loses its flexibility, so there is difficulty focusing for near vision. This happens when you reach your forties.

In **astigmatism,** unequal curvatures of the cornea cause unequal focusing and blurred images.

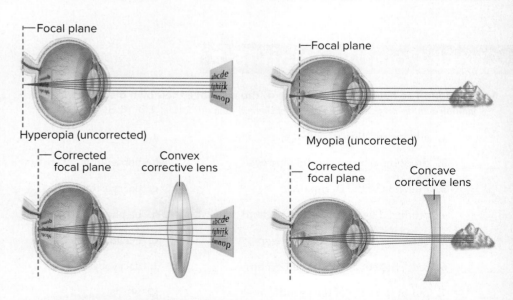

▲ **Figure 16.8** Hyperopia (farsightedness).　　▲ **Figure 16.9** Myopia (nearsightedness).

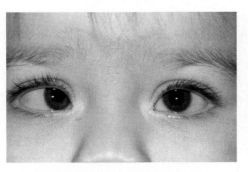

Accommodative esotropia is an inward eye turn, usually noticed around 2 years of age (*Figure 16.10*). It can be caused by underlying conditions, such as uncorrected hyperopia.

Amblyopia, or "lazy eye," occurs in children when vision in one eye has not developed as well as in the other. Amblyopia can be caused by disorders of refraction, family history, prematurity, or muscle imbalance (strabismus amblyopia).

▲ **Figure 16.10** **Strabismus with right eye turned inward.** BioPhoto Associates/ Science Source

Word Analysis and Definition: Disorders of Refraction

S = Suffix P = Prefix R = Root R/CF = Combining Form

WORD	PRONUNCIATION	ELEMENTS		DEFINITION
amblyopia	am-blee-OH-pee-ah	P/ R/	ambly- *dull* -opia *sight*	Failure or incomplete development of the pathways of vision to the brain
astigmatism	ah-**STIG**-mah-tism	S/ P/ R/	-ism *action* a- *without* -stigmat- *focus*	Inability to focus light rays that enter the eye in different planes
emmetropia	em-eh-**TROH**-pee-ah	P/ R/	emmetr- *measure* -opia *sight*	Normal refractive condition of the eye
hyperopia	high-per-**OH**-pee-ah	P/ R/	hyper- *beyond* -opia *sight*	Able to see distant objects but unable to see close objects
myopia (*Note:* An "o" is removed from the elements.)	my-**OH**-pee-ah	P/ R/	myo- *to blink* -opia *sight*	Able to see close objects but unable to see distant objects
presbyopia tract	prez-bee-**OH**-pee-ah TRAKT	R/ R/	presby- *old person* -opia *sight* Latin *path*	Difficulty in nearsighted vision occurring in middle and old age in both sexes Bundle of nerve fibers with a common origin and destination

Check Point Section 16.2

A. Disorders: The accessory structures of the eye have their own disorders. *The patient conditions are described in the left column; match the condition with the correct medical term (right column) from this lesson.* **LO 16.6**

_____ 1. allergic reaction to pollen

_____ 2. drooping of upper eyelid over eye

_____ 3. infection of the lacrimal sac

_____ 4. produced by a blocked tarsal gland

_____ 5. blockage of the drainage of tears

_____ 6. red, crusted, and ulcerated eyelid

_____ 7. pus at the edge of the eyelid

a. chalazion

b. hordeolum

c. dacryostenosis

d. blepharitis

e. eyelid edema

f. dacryocystitis

g. ptosis

B. Create new medical terms by applying different prefixes to the root *-opia*. *The definition of each term is provided; you construct the medical term. Fill in the blanks.* **LO 16.1, 16.6**

1. Meaning of *-opia*: _____

2. Difficulty in nearsighted vision occurring in middle and old age: _____ /opia

3. Normal refractive condition of the eye: _____ /opia

4. Able to see close objects but unable to see distant ones: _____ /opia

5. Able to see distant objects but unable to see close objects: _____ /opia

6. *Challenge question:* If *dipl/o* means *double* and *two,* what then is **diplopia?** _____

C. Choose the correct answer, using the *language of ophthalmology*. **LO 16.1**

1. Which eye condition has unequal curvatures of the lens?

   a. astigmatism   **d.** emmetropia

   b. myopia   **e.** presbyopia

   c. hyperopia

D. Review the medical terms. *Use the language of ophthalmology to complete the sentences. Use each term only once. Fill in the blanks.* **LO 16.6**

1. _____ is a result of increased intraocular pressure.

2. Sensitivity to light that produces eye pain is _____.

3. Avoiding the light because you know it will hurt your eyes is _____.

4. Inflammation of the iris, ciliary body, and choroid is termed _____.

E. Deconstruct medical terms into their word elements. **LO 16.2, 16.6**

1. abrasion: _____ / _____
                      R   S

2. glaucoma: _____ / _____
                     R   S

3. intraocular: _____ / _____ / _____
                   P   R   S

F. Identify the disorders of the eye. *Given the description, identify the disease being described. Fill in the blanks.* **LO 16.6**

1. This is a cancer of the eye. It is the most common cancer occurring in children: _____.

2. Increased intracranial pressure can lead to swelling of the optic disc, correctly termed as _____.

3. This condition can occur in diabetics and can lead to blindness. This condition is diabetic _____.

4. A loss of central vision due to the degeneration of the retina lateral to the optic disc: _____ degeneration.

G. Define the word elements to decipher the meaning of medical terms. *Word elements provide clues to the meanings of medical terms.*
Choose the correct answer to complete the following statements. **LO 16.2, 16.6**

1. In the term **leukocoria,** the root element *cor-* means:

   a. cornea

   b. vessel

   c. white

   d. pupil

   e. condition

2. In the term **retinopathy,** the suffix means:

   a. choroid

   b. disease

   c. uvea

   d. retina

   e. cancer

3. In the term **retinoblastoma,** the word element that means *germ cell* is:

   a. *retin/o*

   b. *-blast*

   c. *-oma*

4. In the term **papilledema,** the root *papill-* means:

   a. pimple

   b. cancer

   c. pupil

   d. swelling

Section 16.3 Procedures and Pharmacology for the Eye

Ophthalmic Diagnostic Procedures

Ophthalmologists and optometrists are both skilled to perform diagnostic procedures of the eye; optometrists refer patients to ophthalmologists for certain eye disorders needing further diagnostic tests. The difference between their professions is discussed in the Therapeutic Procedures section of this chapter. Examination of the eye includes evaluation of pupillary reaction. Medical shorthand for this quick normal eye examination can be **PERRLA,** which means *p*upils *e*qual, *r*ound, *r*eactive to *l*ight and *a*ccommodation.

Visual acuity, the sharpness and clearness of vision, is tested for each eye with the opposite eye covered with a solid object. For **distance vision,** patients look at a **Snellen letter chart** *(Figure 16.23a)* 20 feet away and vision is recorded as the smallest line in which the patient can read half of the letters. For **near vision,** the patient reads a standard **Jaeger reading card** *(Figure 16.23b)* at a distance of 14 inches.

Color vision is tested using the **Ishihara color system.** In the example shown in *Figure 16.24,* people with red-green color blindness would not be able to detect the number 74 among the colored dots.

Refractive error, the nature and degree to which light is bent by the eye, is measured with a **refractometer.**

Visual fields can be impaired by lesions anywhere in the neural visual pathway and in glaucoma, and can be assessed grossly by **direct confrontation.** The patient maintains a fixed gaze at the examiner's nose and a small object or finger is brought into the patient's visual periphery (peripheral vision) in each of the four visual quadrants. The patient indicates when the object is first seen. Each eye is tested separately.

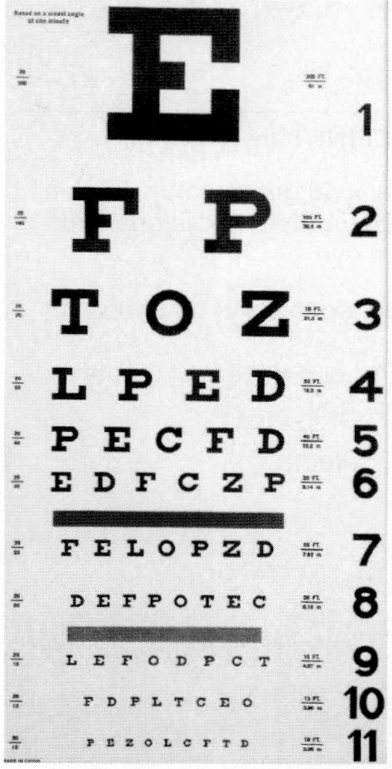

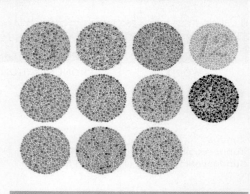

Figure 16.23 (a) on the left shows an eye chart with lines numbered 1-11:

E
F P
T O Z
L P E D
P E C F D
E D F C Z P
F E L O P Z D
D E F P O T E C
L E F O D P C T
F D P L T C E O
P E Z O L C F T D

(a)

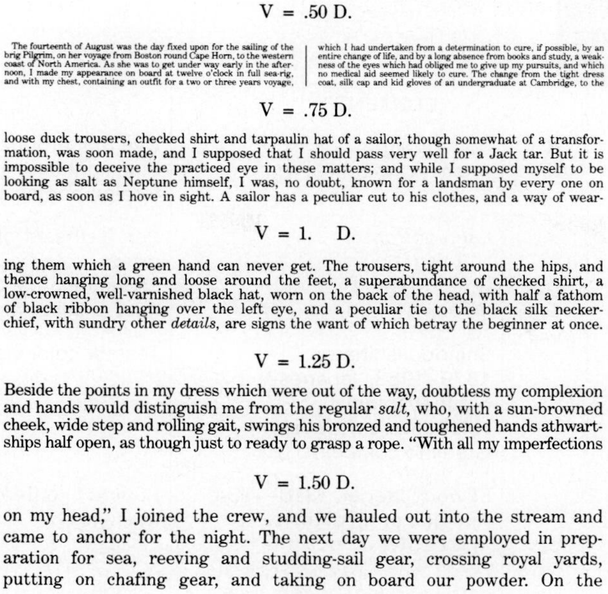

V = .50 D.

The fourteenth of August was the day fixed upon for the sailing of the brig Pilgrim, on her voyage from Boston round Cape Horn, to the western coast of North America. As she was to get under way early in the afternoon, I made my appearance on board at twelve o'clock in full sea-rig, and with my chest, containing an outfit for a two or three years voyage, which I had undertaken from a determination to cure, if possible, by an entire change of life, and by a long absence from books and study, a weakness of the eyes which had obliged me to give up my pursuits, and which no medical aid seemed likely to cure. The change from the tight dress coat, silk cap and kid gloves of an undergraduate at Cambridge, to the

V = .75 D.

loose duck trousers, checked shirt and tarpaulin hat of a sailor, though somewhat of a transformation, was soon made, and I supposed that I should pass very well for a Jack tar. But it is impossible to deceive the practiced eye in these matters; and while I supposed myself to be looking as salt as Neptune himself, I was, no doubt, known for a landsman by every one on board, as soon as I hove in sight. A sailor has a peculiar cut to his clothes, and a way of wear-

V = 1.   D.

ing them which a green hand can never get. The trousers, tight around the hips, and thence hanging long and loose around the feet, a superabundance of checked shirt, a low-crowned, well-varnished black hat, worn on the back of the head, with half a fathom of black ribbon hanging over the left eye, and a peculiar tie to the black silk neckerchief, with sundry other *details*, are signs the want of which betray the beginner at once.

V = 1.25 D.

Beside the points in my dress which were out of the way, doubtless my complexion and hands would distinguish me from the regular *salt*, who, with a sun-browned cheek, wide step and rolling gait, swings his bronzed and toughened hands athwartships half open, as though just to ready to grasp a rope. "With all my imperfections

V = 1.50 D.

on my head," I joined the crew, and we hauled out into the stream and came to anchor for the night. The next day we were employed in preparation for sea, reeving and studding-sail gear, crossing royal yards, putting on chafing gear, and taking on board our powder. On the

(b)

▲ **Figure 16.23** **Visual acuity tests.** (a) Rick Brady/McGraw Hill. (b) Courtesy Good-Lite Company.

Complete **Ishihara** color test plates

▲ **Figure 16.24** **Test for color blindness.** Reproduced with permission from *Ishihara's Tests for Color Deficiency*, published by Kanehara Trading Inc., Tokyo, Japan. Tests for color deficiency cannot be conducted with this figure. For accurate testing, the original plates should be used. Alexander Kaludov/Alamy Stock Photo

Corneal examination uses **fluorescein** staining to reveal abrasions and ulcers.

Pupillary reaction to light is tested in each eye with a penlight as the patient looks into the distance.

Extrinsic muscles of the eyeball are tested by guiding the patient to look in 8 directions (up, up and right, right, down and right, down, down and left, left, left and up) with a moving finger or penlight.

Fundoscopy using an **ophthalmoscope** *(Figure 16.25)* can detect lens opacities, retinal changes, and retinal vascular changes. The vascular changes can be areas of hemorrhage or changes in the retinal arteries indicating hypertension or arteriosclerosis. The retinal changes can show age-related macular degeneration, retinoblastoma, retinal detachment, signs of diabetes, signs of glaucoma, or signs of raised intracranial pressure (**papilledema**).

Slit-lamp examination focuses the height and width of a beam of light to give a **stereoscopic** view of the interior structures of the eyeball. It is used for identifying corneal foreign bodies and abrasions, and identifying retinal diseases.

Intraocular pressure is measured with a **tonometer,** which determines the eyeball's resistance to tension or indentation. There are several methods of **tonometry,** which include pneumatonometry and Goldmann tonometry.

Optic disc

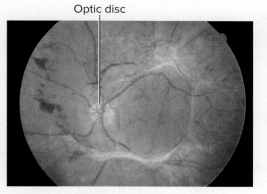

▲ **Figure 16.25** **Ophthalmoscopic examination of the eye.** Lisa R. Klancher

Did you know...

- Glaucoma contributed 8.5% of world bindness.

- The number of glaucoma patients is expected to increase due increase in aging population

WORD	PRONUNCIATION	ELEMENTS		DEFINITION
fluorescein	flor-**ESS**-ee-in	P/	**fluo-** *fluorine*	Dye that produces a vivid green color under a blue light to diagnose corneal abrasions and foreign bodies in the eye
		R/	**-rescein** *resin*	
fundus fundoscopy fundoscopic (adj)	**FUN**-dus fun-**DOS**-koh-pee fun-doh-**SKOP**-ik	S/ R/CF S/	Latin *bottom* **-scopy** *to examine* **fund/o-** *fundus* **-ic** *pertaining to*	Part farthest from the opening of a hollow organ Examination of the fundus (retina) of the eye As a result of fundoscopy
Ishihara color system	ish-ee-**HAR**-ah **KUH**-ler **SIS**-tem		Shinobu Ishihara, 1879–1963, Japanese ophthalmologist **color** Latin *color* **system** Greek *to combine*	Test for color vision defects
Jaeger reading cards	**YAY**-ger **REED**-ing CARDS	 S/ R/	Edward Jaeger, 1818–1884, Austrian ophthalmologist **-ing** *quality of, doing* **read-** *advise, interpret, read* **card** Latin *leaf of papyrus*	Printed in different sizes of print for testing near vision
ophthalmology ophthalmologist ophthalmic (adj)	off-thal-**MALL**-oh-jee off-thal-**MALL**-oh-jist off-**THAL**-mik	S/ R/CF S/ S/ R/	**-logy** *study of* **ophthalm/o-** *eye* **-logist** *one who studies, specialist* **-ic** *pertaining to* **ophthalm-** *eye*	Medical specialty that diagnoses and treats diseases of the eye Medical specialist in ophthalmology Pertaining to the eye
ophthalmoscope ophthalmoscopy ophthalmoscopic (adj)	off-**THAL**-moh-skope **OFF**-thal-**MOS**-koh-pee **OFF**-thal-moh-**SKOP**-ik	S/ R/CF S/ S/	**-scope** *instrument for viewing* **ophthalm/o-** *eye* **-scopy** *to examine, to view* **-ic** *pertaining to*	Instrument for viewing the retina The process of viewing the retina Pertaining to the use of an ophthalmoscope
optician	op-**TIH**-shun	S/ R/CF	**-cian** *having a skill or art* **opt/i-** *vision*	Someone who is licensed to make corrective lenses, adjust and repair spectacles, and fit contact lenses
optometrist	op-**TOM**-eh-trist	S/ R/CF	**-metrist** *skilled in measurement* **opt/o-** *vision*	Someone who is skilled in the measurement of vision but cannot treat eye diseases or prescribe medication
refractometer	ree-frak-**TAH**-meh-tur	S/ R/CF	**-meter** *measure, instrument to measure* **refract/o-** *to bend (light)*	Device that measures refractive errors of the cornea
Snellen letter chart	**SNEL**-en **LET**-er CHART		Hermann Snellen, 1834–1908, Dutch ophthalmologist **letter** Latin *letter of the alphabet* **chart** Latin *piece of papyrus, document*	Test for acuity of distance vision
tonometer tonometry	toh-**NOM**-eh-ter toh-**NOM**-eh-tree	S/ R/CF S/	**-meter** *measure, instrument to measure* **ton/o-** *pressure, tension* **-metry** *process of measuring*	Instrument for determining intraocular pressure The measurement of intraocular pressure

Therapeutic Procedures for Diseases and Disorders of the Eye

Photocoagulation therapy is used to reattach a torn or detached portion of the retina and to prevent further growth of abnormal blood vessels that can cause a detachment. A high-intensity, narrowly focused beam of light from the **argon laser** is absorbed by pigment in the retinal cells and converted into heat, which welds the edge of the retinal detachment against the underlying choroid. **Retinal cryopexy (cryotherapy)** uses intense cold to have the same effects as the heat of photocoagulation.

Photocoagulation therapy is also used to heal bleeding **microaneurysms** of small blood vessels in the early stages of **diabetic retinopathy,** and is used with **chemotherapy** in the treatment of **retinoblastoma.** It also can be used for wet age-related macular degeneration to destroy or seal off new blood vessels to prevent leakage, but the many small retinal scars it creates cause blind spots in the patient's visual field.

When a **cataract** is interfering with vision, the opaque lens is removed by **phacoemulsification** in which ultrasonic waves fragment the cataract to make its removal much easier. The lens is then replaced with an artificial **intraocular** lens, which becomes a permanent part of the eye.

Laser corneal surgery is a procedure that uses a laser to reshape the surface of the eye to change the curvature of the cornea. The surgical procedure **radial keratotomy** is used to treat myopia. Radial cuts, like the spokes of a wheel, flatten the cornea and enable it to refract the light rays to focus on the retina. In flattening the cornea, it can correct myopia (nearsightedness) and astigmatism (uneven curvature of the cornea) and alter the outer edges of the cornea to correct hyperopia/hypermetropia (farsightedness). These procedures are also called **refractive surgery** and **laser-assisted in situ keratomileusis (LASIK).** An alternative to LASIK is **photorefractive keratectomy (PRK),** in which spoke-like incisions are cut into the cornea to flatten its surface and correct nearsightedness.

Glaucoma is treated with a combination of eye drops *(see next section on ocular pharmacology)*, pills, laser surgery, and traditional surgery with the goal of preventing loss of vision. The most commonly used laser procedure is **trabeculoplasty,** in which the eye's drainage system is changed by the laser beam to enable the aqueous humor fluid to drain out more easily into the blood stream. **Trabeculectomy** is the most common traditional surgical procedure, in which a passage is created in the sclera to allow excess fluid to drain out of the eye. More recently, a small silicone tube has been placed from the surface of the eye into the anterior chamber to allow drainage of the excess fluid. Future research is investigating gene therapy for congenital glaucoma. The placement of a plug in the lacrimal apparatus that provides sustained release of glaucoma medication is being evaluated.

Corrective Lenses

Corrective lenses correct disorders of refraction. They bend light rays before they meet the eye's lens.

Concave lens corrects myopia.

Convex lens corrects hyperopia.

Convex bifocal or **progressive** lens corrects presbyopia.

Cylindrical lens corrects this astigmatism.

Exotropia and esotropia treatments depend on the severity of the problem. One treatment is patching the good eye so that the affected eye is required to focus. Surgical treatment of extrinsic eye muscle is an option with large deviation or if previous management is unsuccessful.

Amblyopia treatments include patching the good eye. Treatment is necessary to strengthen the neural connections from the affected eye to the brain. Lifetime poor vision results if amblyopia is not treated.

(Continued)

WORD	PRONUNCIATION		ELEMENTS	DEFINITION
argon laser	AR-gon LAY-zer		**argon** Greek *lazy* **laser** acronym for **L**ight **A**mplification by **S**timulated **E**mission of **R**adiation	Laser used for ophthalmic procedures consisting of photons in the blue and/or green spectrum
bifocal	bi-FOH-cal	S/ P/ R/	**-al** *pertaining to* **bi-** *two* **-foc-** *focus*	Two powers on lens
concave (*Note:* concave is used as a noun or adjective.)	con-CAVE or CON-cave		Latin *arched, vaulted*	Curve outward
convex (*Note:* concave is used as a noun or adjective.)	CON-vecks or con-VECKS		Latin *arched, vaulted*	Curved outward
cryotherapy	CRY-oh- THAIR-ah-pee	S/	**-therapy** *treatment*	The use of cold in the treatment of disease
cryopexy	CRY-oh-PEK-see	R/CF S/	**cry/o-** *cold* **-pexy** *fixation*	Repair of a detached retina by freezing it to surrounding tissue
cylindrical	sih- LIN-drih-kul	S/	Greek *a roll* **-al** *pertaining to*	Surface shape having long straight sides and two round ends
in situ	IN SIGH-tyu		Latin *in its original place*	In the correct place
keratectomy	KAIR-ah-TEK-toh-mee	S/ R/	**-ectomy** *excision* **kerat-** *cornea*	Surgery to remove corneal tissue
keratomileusis	KAIR-ah-toh-mie-LOO-sis	R/CF R/	**kerat/o-** *cornea* **-mileusis** *lathe*	A surgical procedure that involves cutting and shaping the cornea
keratotomy	KAIR-ah-TOT-oh-mee	S/	**-tomy** *surgical incision*	Incision in the cornea
phacoemulsification	FACK-oh-ee-mul-sih-fih-KAY-shun	S/ R/CF R/	**-ation** *process* **phac/o-** *lens* **-emulsific-** *to milk out*	Technique used to fragment the center of the lens into very tiny pieces and suck them out of the eye
photocoagulation	foh-toh-koh-ag-you-LAY-shun	S/ R/CF R/	**-ation** *process* **phot/o-** *light* **-coagul-** *clot*	The use of light (laser beam) to form a clot
photoreactive	foh-toh-ree-AK-tiv	P/ R/	**-re-** *again* **-active** *movement*	Initiation by light of a process previously inactive
progressive	pro-GRESS-iv	S/	Latin *going forward* **-ive** *nature of, quality of, pertaining to*	Lens power gradually changes form point to point
trabeculectomy	trah-BEK-you-LEK-toh-mee	S/ R/	**-ectomy** *excision* **trabecul-** *eye's fluid drainage system*	Surgical creation of passage in sclera to allow fluid to drain out of the eye
trabeculoplasty	trah-BEK-you-loh-plas-tee	S/ R/CF	**-plasty** *surgical repair* **trabecul/o-** *eye's fluid drainage system*	Laser repair of eye's fluid drainage system

Ocular Pharmacology

There are a wide variety and number of medications placed directly into the conjunctival sac to treat different eye disorders or to help the clinician examine the eye more thoroughly and more easily.

- **Mydriatics** are drugs that cause the pupil to dilate and are mainly used to examine the eye fundus. **Mydriacil** (*Tropicamide*) takes 15 minutes for the eye to fully dilate and can last for 3 to 6 hours with blurred vision. Other dilating drops, for example, **atropine** and **homatropine,** are long acting, lasting 7 to 10 days.
- **Miotics** are drugs that constrict the pupil (**miosis**); for example, **pilocarpine,** which can be part of a regimen for treating glaucoma.
- **Ocular topical anesthetics** temporarily block nerve conduction in the conjunctiva and cornea. They have a quick onset of 10 to 20 seconds and last for 10 to 20 minutes. They are used to assist with eye examinations and visual **acuity** testing and to help treat chemical burns, welding flash, and foreign bodies. Examples are **amethocaine,** 0.5% and 1%, and **oxybupricaine,** 0.4%.

- **Ocular diagnostic drops** stain conjunctival cells to improve diagnostic capabilities; for example, the presence of a foreign body or a corneal abrasion. Examples are **fluorescein** and **Lissamine Green.** The drops do not interfere with vision but are taken up by soft contact lenses, which should be removed prior to instillation of the drops.
- **Ocular lubricant drops** are used to replace tears, treat dry eyes, moisten hard contact lenses, protect the eye during eye surgical procedures, and help treat keratitis. Examples are *Visine, Refresh Optive,* and *Retaine.*
- **Anti-infective eye medications,** both drops and ointments, can be **antibacterial,** for example, **glatifloxacin** (*Zymaxid*) and **sulfacetamide** (*Klaron, Ovace*); **antifungal,** such as **natamycin** (*Natacyn*); and **antiviral,** for example, **idoxuridine** (*Herplex*) and **trifluridine** (*Viroptic*).
- **Anti-inflammatory eye medications** are used in allergic disorders, to prevent scarring and visual loss in inflammation of the eye, and to decrease postoperative eye inflammation and scarring. Examples are **corticosteroids** such as **dexamethasone** (*Decadron*) and nonsteroidal antiinflammatory agents such as **flurbiprofen** (*Ocufen*) and **suprofen** (*Profenal*).
- In **glaucoma,** numerous eye medications are available and are used individually, in combinations, and/or with surgery (*see previous section on eye therapeutic procedures*). **Miotics** decrease the size of the pupil and widen the trabecular network to enable fluid to escape more easily. **Beta-adrenergic blockers** decrease production of aqueous humor; examples are **timolol maleate** (*Timoptic*) and **betaxolol** (*Betoptic*). **Carbonic anhydrase inhibitors** reduce production of aqueous humor; examples are **acetazolamide sodium** (*Diamox*) and **dichlorphenamide** (*Daranide*); **alpha-adrenergic agents** increase the outflow of aqueous humor by unknown mechanisms; examples are **epinephrine** (*Epifrin*) and **phenylephrine** (*Neo-synephrine*).

Word Analysis and Definition: Ocular Pharmacology

S = Suffix P = Prefix R = Root R/CF = Combining Form

WORD	PRONUNCIATION	ELEMENTS		DEFINITION
antibacterial	**AN**-teh-bak-**TEER**-ee-al	S/ P/ R/CF	-al *pertaining to* anti- *against* -bacter/i- *bacteria*	Destructive of or preventing the growth of bacteria
antifungal	**AN**-teh-**FUN**-gal	R/	-fung- *fungus*	Destructive of or preventing the growth of fungi
anti-infective	**AN**-teh-in-**FEK**-tiv	S/ R/	-ive *nature of* -infect- *taint*	Made incapable of transmitting an infection
anti-inflammatory	**AN**-teh-in-**FLAM**-ah-toh-ree	S/ P/ R/	-ory *having the function of* -in- *in* -flammat- *inflammation*	Reducing, removing, or preventing inflammation
antiviral	an-teh-**VIE**-ral	R/	-vir- *virus*	To weaken or abolish the action or replication of a virus
atropine	**AT**-roh-peen		Greek *belladonna*	Pharmacologic agent used to dilate pupils
inhibitor	in-**HIB**-ih-tor	S/ P/ R/	-or *one who does* in- *in* -hibit- *keep back*	An agent that restrains or retards physiologic, chemical, or enzymatic action
miosis	my-**OH**-sis		Greek *lessening*	Contraction of the pupil
miotic	my-**OT**-ik	S/ R/CF	-tic *pertaining to* mi/o- *less*	An agent that causes the pupil to contract
mydriasis	mih-**DRY**-ah-sis		Greek *dilation of the pupil*	Dilation of the pupil
mydriatic	mid-ree-**AT**-ik	S/ R/	-atic *pertaining to* mydri- *dilation of the pupil*	Pertaining to or an agent that causes dilation of the pupil

Check Point Section 16.3

A. The ophthalmic technician in Dr. Chun's office needs to be familiar with all these terms in order to communicate with Dr. Chun and her patients. *Show your understanding of the terms by choosing the correct answers.* **LO 16.5**

1. The test used to measure color blindness is
   - **a.** Snellen
   - **b.** Jaeger
   - **c.** Ishihara
   - **d.** visual fields
   - **e.** otoscope

2. Peripheral vision measures the outer edge of the
   - **a.** anterior segment
   - **b.** vitreous body
   - **c.** aqueous humor
   - **d.** posterior segment
   - **e.** visual field

3. A test for near vision is the
   - **a.** Snellen chart
   - **b.** ophthalmoscope
   - **c.** Jaeger card
   - **d.** Ishihara
   - **e.** visual fields

4. This is used to detect corneal abrasions or ulcers
   - **a.** ophthalmoscope
   - **b.** refractometer
   - **c.** tonometer
   - **d.** fluorescein

B. Identify the meaning of the word elements related to ophthalmology. *Match the element in the first column with its correct meaning in the second column.* **LO 16.2, 16.5, 16.7**

Word Element	Meaning
_____ 1. *kerat-*	a. cold
_____ 2. *cry/o-*	b. light
_____ 3. *-ectomy*	c. surgical repair
_____ 4. *-plasty*	d. eye's fluid drainage system
_____ 5. *phot/o-*	e. cornea
_____ 6. *trabecul-*	f. excision

C. Identify the medication that would treat each condition. *Match the medication on the left with its correct indicated use.* **LO 16.7**

_____ 1. antibacterial	a. a treatment for glaucoma
_____ 2. mydriatic	b. dry eyes
_____ 3. anti-inflammatory	c. bacterial infection of the eye
_____ 4. miotic	d. allergic disorder of the eye
_____ 5. ocular topical anesthetic	e. dilate the pupil in order to view the eye fundus
_____ 6. lubricant	f. chemical burn to the eyes

Section 16.4 The Ear and Hearing

Your ear has three major sections *(Figure 16.26):* the external ear, the middle ear, and the inner ear.

External Ear

The **auricle,** or **pinna,** is a wing-shaped structure that directs sound waves coming through the air into the **external auditory meatus** and **external auditory canal.** This in turn ends at the **tympanic membrane.** The external auditory canal not only protects the middle and inner ears but also acts as a resonator to augment the transmission of sound to the middle and inner ears.

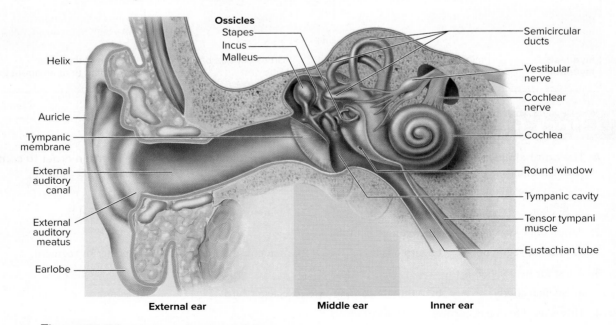

▲ **Figure 16.26** Anatomical regions of the ear.

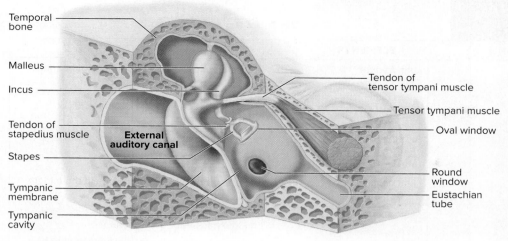

▲ **Figure 16.27** Middle ear.

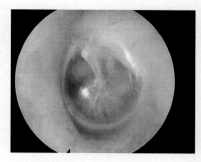

▲ **Figure 16.28**
Otoscopic view of normal tympanic membrane. Professor Tony Wright, Institute of Laryngology & Otology/Science Source

The external auditory canal is the only skin-lined cul-de-sac in the body. Its interior is dark, warm, and prone to become moist. These are ideal conditions for bacterial and fungal growth.

The meatus and canal are lined with skin that contains many modified sweat glands called ceruminous glands, which secrete **cerumen.** The cerumen and hairs growing in the meatus help to keep out foreign objects. Cerumen combines with dead skin cells to form **earwax.**

Middle Ear

The middle ear has four components: the tympanic membrane, the tympanic cavity, the **eustachian tube (auditory) tube,** and the ossicles *(Figure 16.27)*.

1. The **tympanic membrane (eardrum)** is located at the inner end of the external auditory canal. It is suspended in a bony groove, is concave on its outer surface, and vibrates freely as sound waves hit it. It has a good nerve supply and is very sensitive to pain. The tympanic membrane is transparent and reflects light *(Figure 16.28)*.

2. The **tympanic cavity** *(Figure 16.27)* is immediately behind the tympanic membrane. It is filled with air that enters through the eustachian (auditory) tube, and the cavity is continuous with the **mastoid** air cells in the bone behind it. The presence of air in the cavity maintains equal air pressure on both sides of the tympanic membrane, which is essential for normal hearing. The cavity contains the **ossicles.**

3. The eustachian (auditory) tube *(Figure 16.27)* connects the middle ear with the **nasopharynx** (throat), into which it opens close to the pharyngeal **tonsil (adenoid)** *(Figure 16.29)*. In children under 5 years, the tube is not fully developed. It is short and horizontal, and the valvelike flaps in the throat that protect it are not developed. When you are landing in an airplane and moving from a high altitude to a lower one, the air pressure in the external auditory canal increases and pushes the tympanic membrane inward. If your eustachian (auditory) tube is blocked, no air can get into the middle ear to equalize the pressure, and your eardrum is painful. If you can force some air up the eustachian (auditory) tube by chewing or swallowing, then your ear "pops" as the tympanic membrane moves back to its normal position.

4. The three **ossicles**—the **malleus, incus,** and **stapes** *(Figure 16.27)*—are attached to the wall of the tympanic cavity by tiny ligaments that are covered by a mucous membrane. The malleus is attached to the tympanic membrane and vibrates with the membrane when sound waves hit it. The malleus is also attached to the incus, which also vibrates and passes the vibrations onto the stapes. The stapes is attached to the oval window, an opening that transmits the vibrations to the inner ear. The stapes is the smallest bone in the body.

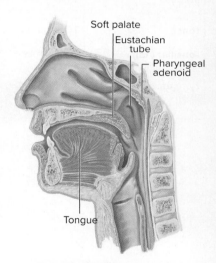

▲ **Figure 16.29** Nasopharynx (throat).

Word Analysis and Definition: External and Middle Ear

S = Suffix P = Prefix R = Root R/CF = Combining Form

WORD	PRONUNCIATION		ELEMENTS	DEFINITION
auditory	AW-dih-tor-ee		Latin *hearing*	Pertaining to the sense or organs of hearing
auricle	AW-ri-kul		Latin *ear*	The shell-like external ear
cerumen	seh-ROO-men		Latin *wax*	Waxy secretion of ceruminous glands of external ear canal
eustachian tube auditory tube (syn)	you-STAY-shun TYUB		Bartolommeo Eustachio, 1524–1574, Italian anatomist **tube** Latin *trumpet*	Tube that connects the middle ear to the nasopharynx
incus	IN-cuss		Latin *anvil*	Middle one of the three ossicles in the middle ear; shaped like an anvil
malleus	MAL-ee-us		Latin *hammer*	Outer (lateral) one of the three ossicles in the middle ear; shaped like a hammer
mastoid	MASS-toyd	S/ R/	**-oid** *resembling* **mast-** *breast*	Small bony protrusion immediately behind the ear
meatus	mee-AY-tus		Latin *passage*	Passage or channel; also used to denote the external opening of a passage
meatal (adj)	mee-AY-tal	S/ R/	**-al** *pertaining to* **meat-** *passage or channel*	Pertaining to a meatus
nasopharynx	NAY-zoh-FAIR-inks	R/CF R/	**nas/o-** *nose* **-pharynx** *throat*	Region of the pharynx at the back of the nose and above the soft palate
ossicle	OS-ih-kel	S/ R/	**-icle** *small* **oss-** *bone*	A small bone, particularly relating to the three bones in the middle ear
pinna pinnae (pl)	PIN-ah PIN-ee		Latin *wing*	Another name for auricle
stapes	STAY-pees		Latin *stirrup*	Inner (medial) one of the three ossicles of the middle ear; shaped like a stirrup
tonsil	TON-sill		Latin *tonsil*	Mass of lymphoid tissue on either side of the throat at the back of the tongue
tonsillar (adj)	TON-sih-lar	S/ R/	**-ar** *pertaining to* **tonsill-** *tonsil*	Pertaining to the tonsils
tympanic	tim-PAN-ik	S/ R/	**-ic** *pertaining to* **tympan-** *eardrum, tympanic membrane*	Pertaining to the tympanic membrane or tympanic cavity

Inner Ear for Hearing

The inner ear is a **labyrinth** *(Figure 16.30)* of complex, intricate systems of passages. The passages in the **cochlea,** a part of the labyrinth, contain receptors to translate vibrations into nerve impulses so that the brain can interpret them as different sounds.

The membrane of the oval window separates the middle ear from the **vestibule** of the inner ear. From the tympanic membrane (① *in Figure 16.31*), the stapes ② moves the oval membrane to generate pressure waves in the fluid inside the cochlea ③. The pressure waves cause **vestibular** and **basilar membranes** inside the cochlea to vibrate ④ and sway fine hair cells attached to the basilar membrane ⑤. The hair cells convert this motion into nerve impulses, which travel via the **cochlear nerve** to the brain. The excess pressure waves in the cochlea escape the inner ear via the round window ⑥.

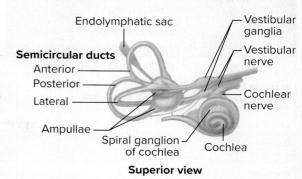

▲ **Figure 16.30** Inner ear.

Inner Ear for Equilibrium and Balance

The **vestibule** and the three **semicircular canals** *(Figure 16.32)* are the organs of balance.

Inside the fluid-filled vestibule are two raised, flat areas (**maculae**) covered with hair cells and a gelatinous material. This gelatinous material contains crystals of calcium and protein called **otoliths.** The position of the head alters the pressure applied to the hair cells by the gelatinous mass. The hair cells respond to horizontal and vertical changes and send impulses to the brain indicating the position to which the head has tilted.

Each of the three fluid-filled semicircular canals has a dilated end called an **ampulla** that contains a mound of hair cells embedded in a gelatinous material that together are called a **crista ampullaris** *(Figure 16.33)*. They detect rotational movements of the head that distort the hair cells and lead to stimulation of connected nerve cells. The nerve impulses travel via the vestibular nerve and go to the brain. From the brain, nerve impulses travel to the muscles to maintain **equilibrium** and balance.

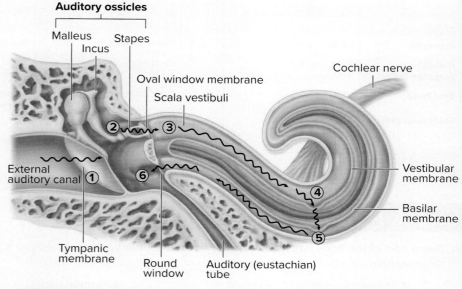

▲ **Figure 16.31** Hearing process in the inner ear.

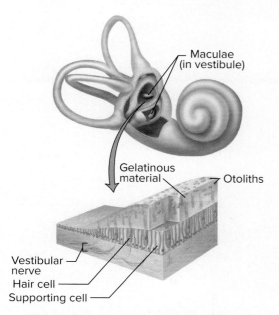

▲ **Figure 16.32** Vestibule and maculae.

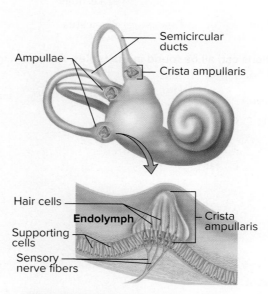

▲ **Figure 16.33** Semicircular ducts.

WORD	PRONUNCIATION	ELEMENTS		DEFINITION
ampulla crista ampullaris	am-**PULL**-ah **KRIS**-tah am-pull-**AIR**-is	R/ S/ R/	Latin *two-handled bottle* crista *crest* -aris *pertaining to* ampull- *bottle-shaped*	Dilated portion of canal or duct Mound of hair cells and gelatinous material in the ampulla of a semicircular canal
basilar	**BAS**-ih-lar	S/ R/	-ar *pertaining to* basil- *base, support*	Pertaining to the base of a structure
cochlea	**KOK**-lee-ah		Latin *snail shell*	An intricate combination of passages; used to describe the part of the inner ear used in hearing
cochlear (adj)	**KOK**-lee-ar	S/ R/	-ar *pertaining to* cochle- *cochlea*	Pertaining to the cochlea
equilibrium	ee-kwih-**LIB**-ree-um	P/ R/	equi- *equal* -librium *balance*	Being evenly balanced
labyrinth	**LAB**-ih-rinth		Greek *labyrinth*	The inner ear
macula maculae (pl)	**MAK**-you-lah **MAK**-you-lee		Latin *small spot*	Small area of special function; in the ear, a sensory receptor
vestibule	**VES**-tih-byul		Latin *entrance*	Space at the entrance to a canal Pertaining to the vestibule of the inner ear
vestibular (adj)	ves-**TIB**-you-lar	S/ R/	-ar *pertaining to* vestibul- *vestibule of the inner ear*	

Check Point Section 16.4

A. Every part of the body has its own specialized vocabulary. *Test your knowledge of the language of otology by matching correct answers. Match the phrase in the left column with the appropriate medical term in the right column.* **LO 16.1**

_____ 1. External opening of a passage   **a.** pinna

_____ 2. Shell-like external ear   **b.** auditory

_____ 3. Another name for auricle   **c.** auricle

_____ 4. Pertaining to the sense or organs of hearing   **d.** tympanic

_____ 5. Earwax   **e.** cerumen

_____ 6. Pertaining to the eardrum   **f.** meatus

B. Answers to the following questions can all be found in the tables. *Review the terms before you start this exercise. Pay special attention to the spelling. Select the best choice.* **LO 16.1, 16.2**

1. In the term **mastoid,** the suffix means
   a. condition   **b.** resembling   **c.** inflammation

2. The element *mast-* means
   a. throat   **b.** breast   **c.** ear

3. The **stapes** is a(n)
   a. gland   **b.** ossicle   **c.** mastoid

4. The element *pharynx-* means
   a. throat   **b.** nose   **c.** gland

5. The term *nasopharynx* is composed of
   a. prefix + suffix   **b.** root + root   **c.** combining form + root

6. The _____ is shaped like a hammer.

    a. malleus   **b.** malleolus   **c.** maleus

7. One of the names for the tube that connects the middle ear to the nasopharynx is the _____ tube.

    a. eusstachian   **b.** eustashian   **c.** eustachian

8. The _____ is shaped like an anvil.

    a. incus   **b.** stapes   **c.** adenoid

C. This exercise pertains to the ossicles. *Use the language of otology for your answers.* **LO 16.1**

1. How many bones make up the ossicles? _____

2. Which of the ossicles is the smallest bone in the body? _____

3. Which bone is attached to the tympanic membrane and the incus? _____

4. Are the ossicles in the external ear, the middle ear, or the inner ear? _____

D. Choose the correct answer to each statement. LO 16.2

1. The term **nasopharynx**, -pharynx is the

    a. suffix   **b.** prefix   **c.** root   **d.** Latin term

2. In the term **crista ampullaris,** the word element that means *pertaining to* is:

    a. -ta   **b.** -aris   **c.** ampull-

3. In the term **equilibrium,** the word element *-librium* means:

    a. pertaining to   **b.** equal   **c.** passage for hearing   **d.** balance

E. Increase your knowledge of the language of otology by correctly answering the following questions. *Review the material regarding the middle ear structures and their disorders; then choose the best answer.* **LO 16.2**

1. In the term **basilar,** *basil-* is a

    a. prefix   **b.** root   **c.** combining form

2. The **entrance to the inner ear** is the

    a. vestibule   **b.** labyrinth   **c.** cochlea   **d.** aqueous   **e.** choroid

3. The element *neur-* means

    a. never   **b.** nerve   **c.** nose

4. An **intricate combination of passages** in the ear is the

    a. cochlea   **b.** vestibule   **c.** labyrinth

5. The suffix meaning *pertaining to* is found in the term

    a. vestibular   **b.** labyrinthitis   **c.** audiometer

F. Challenge your knowledge of the ear by filling in the correct terms for the following definitions. *Fill in the blanks.* **LO 16.1**

Definition	Medical Term
1. Evenly balanced	_____
2. Dilated portion of a canal or duct	_____
3. Small area of special function	_____
4. Calcium particle in the vestibule	_____
5. Mound of hair cells found in ampulla	_____

Section 16.5 Disorders of the Ear

Disorders of External Ear

Otitis externa is an infection of the lining of the external auditory canal *(Figure 16.34)*. It produces a painful, red, swollen ear canal, sometimes with purulent drainage. The infection can be bacterial or fungal. Fungal infections are responsible for 10% of otitis externa cases and are called **otomycoses.**

Conditions helping to cause otitis externa include trauma to the canal during attempts to self-clean it; use of unclean earplugs, earphones, or hearing aids; and the presence of other skin diseases, such as seborrhea and psoriasis *(see Chapter 4)*.

Swimmer's ear is a form of otitis externa that comes after swimming, particularly if the water is polluted.

Overproduction of cerumen can completely block the external canal (**cerumen impaction**), causing hearing loss and preventing examination of the tympanic membrane with an **otoscope.**

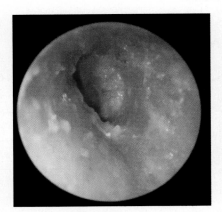

▲ **Figure 16.34** **Anatomical regions of the ear.** Otoscopic view of otitis externa with purulent exudate (shown in yellow). Dr. Michael Hawke

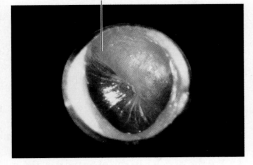

Inflamed membrane

▲ **Figure 16.35** Otoscopic view of otitis media (acute), showing inflamed tympanic membrane. Lester V. Bergman/ Corbis NX/Getty Images

Disorders of Middle Ear

Acute otitis media (AOM) is the presence of pus in the middle ear with pain in the ear, fever, and redness of the tympanic membrane. This occurs most often in the first 2 to 4 years of age because:

- Eustachian tubes in children are shorter and more horizontal than in adults, making it easier for bacteria and viruses to find their way into the middle ear from the nasopharynx.
- Adenoids at the back of the nasopharynx near the eustachian tubes can block the opening of the eustachian tubes.
- Children's immune systems are not fully developed until 7 years of age, and they have difficulty fighting infections.

If the infections are viral, they will go away on their own. If bacterial, oral antibiotics may be necessary.

Chronic otitis media (COM) occurs when the acute infection subsides but the eustachian tube is still blocked. The **effusion** (fluid) in the middle ear cannot drain out and gradually becomes stickier. This is called **chronic otitis media with effusion (OME)** and produces hearing loss because the sticky fluid prevents the ossicles from vibrating. You can see the fluid through the otoscope *(Figure 16.35)*.

A **perforated tympanic membrane** can occur in acute otitis media when pus in the middle ear cannot escape down the eustachian tube. It builds up pressure and perforates the eardrum *(Figures 16.36 and 16.37)*. Other causes of perforation include a puncture by a cotton swab, an open-handed slap to the ear, or large pressure changes (as may be induced in scuba diving). Most perforations will heal spontaneously in a month, leaving a small scar.

Cholesteatoma is a complication of chronic otitis media with effusion or of poor eustachian tube function. Chronically inflamed cells in the middle ear multiply and collect into a tumor. They damage the ossicles and can spread to the inner ear. Surgical removal is required.

Otosclerosis is a middle-ear disease that usually affects people between 18 and 35 years of age. It can affect one ear or both and produces a gradual hearing loss for low and soft sounds. Its etiology is unknown. Spongy bone forms around the junction of the oval window and stapes, preventing the stapes from conducting the sound vibrations to the inner ear. The only treatment is to replace the stapes with a metal or plastic **prosthesis.**

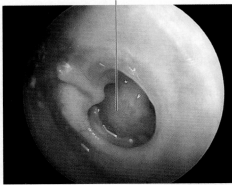

Perforation

▲ **Figure 16.36** Otoscopic view of otitis media (chronic) with perforated tympanic membrane. Professor Tony Wright, Institute of Laryngology & Otology/Science Source

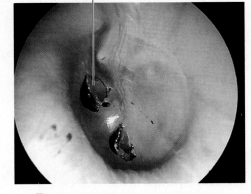

Perforation

▲ **Figure 16.37** Perforated tympanic membrane. Professor Tony Wright, Institute of Laryngology & Otology/Science Source

S = Suffix P = Prefix R = Root R/CF = Combining Form

WORD	PRONUNCIATION	ELEMENTS		DEFINITION
cholesteatoma	koh-less-tee-ah-**TOH**-mah	S/ R/CF R/	-oma *tumor, mass* chol/e- *bile* -steat- *fat*	Yellow, waxy tumor arising in the middle ear
effusion	eh-**FYU**-shun		Latin *pouring out*	Collection of fluid that has escaped from blood vessels into a cavity or tissues
impacted	im-**PAK**-ted		Latin *driven in*	Immovably wedged, as with earwax blocking the external ear canal
otomycosis	**OH**-toh-my-**KOH**-sis	S/ R/CF R/CF	-sis *abnormal condition* ot/o- *ear* -myc/o- *fungus*	Fungal infection of the external ear canal
otosclerosis	oh-toh-skler-**OH**-sis	S/ R/CF R/CF	-sis *abnormal condition* ot/o- *ear* -scler/o- *hardening*	Hardening at the junction of the stapes and oval window that causes loss of hearing
otitis media	oh-**TIE**-tis **MEE**-dee-ah	S/ R/ R/	-itis *inflammation* ot- *ear* media *middle*	Inflammation of the middle ear
perforated	**PER**-foh-ray-ted		Latin *to bore through*	Punctured with one or more holes
tympanic	tim-**PAN**-ik	S/ R/	-ic *pertaining to* tympan- *eardrum, tympanic membrane*	Pertaining to the tympanic membrane or tympanic cavity

Disorders of the Inner Ear

Hearing

Today, the most common cause of hearing loss is damage to the fine hairs in the cochlea by exposure to repeated loud noise, related either to work (for example, jackhammers, leaf blowers) or to leisure activities (such as amplified music at concerts, personal listening devices, and motorcycles). This is a **sensorineural hearing loss.** A **conductive hearing loss** occurs when sound is not conducted efficiently through the external auditory canal to the tympanic membrane and the ossicles. Causes include:

- Middle ear pathology, such as acute otitis media, otitis media with effusion, or a perforated eardrum.
- Impacted cerumen.
- An infected external auditory canal.
- A foreign body in the external canal.

Balance

The sensation of spinning or whirling is called **vertigo,** often described by patients as dizziness. The ringing in his ears is called **tinnitus.** Both sensations arise in the inner ear.

Acute labyrinthitis is an acute viral infection of the labyrinth, producing extreme vertigo, nausea, and vomiting. It usually lasts 1 to 2 weeks.

Benign paroxysmal positional vertigo (BPPV) presents with short (less than 60 seconds) episodes of vertigo occurring with certain head positions due to displacement of otoliths. It is diagnosed clinically and treated with otolith repositioning maneuvers.

Word Analysis and Definition: Disorders of the Inner Ear

WORD	PRONUNCIATION		ELEMENTS	DEFINITION
conductive hearing loss	kon-**DUK**-tiv **HEER**-ing LOSS	S/ R/	**conductive** Latin *to lead* **-ing** *quality of* **hear-** *to perceive sounds* **loss** Middle English *to lose*	Hearing loss caused by lesions in the outer ear or middle ear
labyrinthitis	**LAB**-ih-rin-**THIE**-tis	S/ R/	**-itis** *inflammation* **labyrinth-** *inner ear*	Inflammation of the inner ear
Ménière disease	men-**YEAR** diz-**EEZ**	 P/ R/	Prosper Ménière, 1799–1862, French physician **dis-** *apart* **-ease** *normal function*	Disorder of inner ear with cluster of symptoms of acute attacks of tinnitus, vertigo, and hearing loss
paroxysmal	par-ok-**SIZ**-mal	S/ R/	**-al** *pertaining to* **paroxysm-** *irritation*	Occurring in sharp, spasmodic episodes
recurrent	ree-**KUR**-ent	S/ P/ R/	**-ent** *pertaining to* **re-** *back* **-curr-** *to run*	Symptoms or lesions returning after an intermission
sensorineural hearing loss	**SEN**-sor-ih-**NYUR**-al **HEER**-ing LOSS	S/ R/CF R/ S/ R/	**-al** *pertaining to* **sensor/i-** *sensory* **-neur-** *nerve* **-ing** *quality of* **hear-** *to perceive sounds* **loss** Middle English *to lose*	Hearing loss caused by lesions of the inner ear or the auditory nerve
tinnitus	**TIN**-ih-tus		Latin *jingle*	Persistent ringing, whistling, clicking, or booming noise in the ears
vertigo	**VER**-tih-go		Latin *dizziness*	Sensation of spinning or whirling

Check Point Section 16.5

A. Challenge your knowledge of the ear by filling in the correct terms for the following definitions. *Fill in the blanks.* **LO 16.6**

Definition	Medical Term
1. Persistent ringing in the ears	_____
2. Sensation of spinning or whirling	_____
3. Occurring in sharp, spasmodic episodes	_____

B. Build medical terms. *Fill in the blanks with the correct element to complete the terms.* **LO 16.2, 16.6**

1. Pertaining to the eardrum: _____ /ic

2. Hardening at the junction of the stapes and oval window:

ot/o/_____ /sis

3. Yellow, waxy tumor in the middle ear:

_____ / _____ / _____ /oma

C. Increase your knowledge of the language of otology by correctly answering the following questions. *Review the material regarding the middle ear structures and their disorders; then choose the best answer.* **LO 16.6**

1. **Labyrinthitis** is a(n)

   a. procedure

   b. symptom

   c. inflammation

2. **Hearing loss** caused by lesions of the outer ear or middle ear is

   a. auditory

   b. basilar

   c. sensorineural

   d. aqueous

3. The suffix meaning of inflammation can be found in the word

   a. vestibule

   b. labyrinthitis

   c. otology

4. **Hearing loss** caused by lesions of the inner ear is called hearing loss.

   a. auditory

   b. basilar

   c. sensorineural

Section 16.6 Procedures and Pharmacology for the Ear

Diagnostic Procedures for Diseases of the Ear

Basic hearing test procedures that can be performed in an office include:

- **Whispered speech testing,** which is a simple screening method in which one ear of the patient is covered and the patient is asked to identify whispered sounds.
- **Tuning fork screening tests,** which can identify on which side a hearing loss is located **(Weber test)** and whether the hearing loss is due to loss of bone or air conduction **(Rinne test).**

An **audiometer** is an electronic device that generates sounds in different frequencies and intensities and prints out a graph (**audiogram**) of the patient's responses (*Figure 16.38*). **Audiometry** measures hearing function and is often performed by an **audiologist**. An audiologist is a specialist in **audiology**. **Tympanometry** helps detect problems between the tympanic membrane and the inner ear by using a small earpiece that generates pressure and sound in the ear canal to gather information (**tympanography**) about changes of pressure inside the ear.

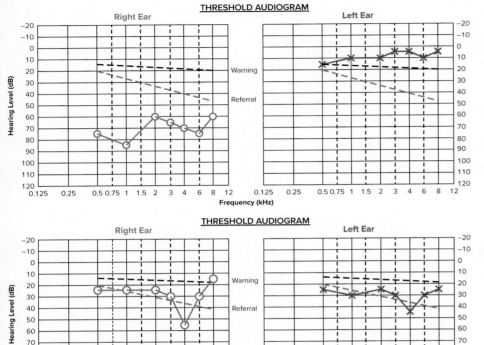

▲ **Figure 16.38** Examples of audiometry results.

When recording the results of hearing testing, **A.D.** is shorthand for the right ear, **A.S.** for the left ear, and **A.U.** for both ears.

The pinna (auricle) is examined visually and by touch. The external ear and the middle ear are examined via **otoscopy** with an **otoscope** (*Figure 16.39*). The pinna (auricle) of the ear is gently manipulated in order for a health care provider to obtain an **otoscopic** view of the external and middle ear. The otoscopic view enables the tympanic membrane and the ossicles behind it to be visualized.

A **pneumatic otoscope** pushes air into the ear and enables the examiner to see if the eardrum moves freely.

Electrocochleography (ECOG) measures the response to sound by the nervous system. A soft electrode is placed deeply in the external ear canal and other electrodes are placed on the forehead to measure responses to sound.

Auditory brainstem response test (ABR) also measures the nervous system response to sound with a setup and procedure similar to ECOG.

Magnetic resonance imaging (MRI) of structures in the inner ear can be helpful in the diagnosis of some vestibular disorders. **Computerized axial tomography (CAT scan)** can help diagnose problems in and around the inner ear.

Balance

Electronystagmography (ENG) and **videonystagmography (VNG)** evaluate the movement of the eyes as they follow different visual targets to evaluate vestibular dysfunction, ENG uses small electrodes placed on the skin around the eyes and VNG uses goggles with video cameras to monitor the eye movements.

Rotation tests, such as head rotation or a computerized rotary chair, also measure associated eye movements using electrodes or goggles to determine how well the balance organs are functioning.

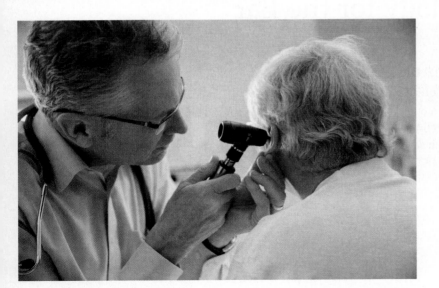

▲ **Figure 16.39** Physician using an otoscope to examine patient's ear.
Hero Images Inc./Alamy Stock Photo

WORD	PRONUNCIATION	ELEMENTS		DEFINITION
audiology	aw-dee-**OL**-oh-jee	S/ R/CF/ S/	-logy *study of* audi/o- *hearing* -logist *specialist*	Study of hearing disorders Specialist in evaluation of hearing function
audiologist	aw-dee-**OL**-oh-jist			
audiometer	aw-dee-**OM**-eh-ter	R/CF/ S/ S/ R/ S/	audi/o- *hearing* -meter *measure* -ic *pertaining to* -metr- *measure* -metry *process of measuring*	Instrument to measure hearing Pertaining to the measurement of hearing The measurement of hearing
audiometric (adj)	**AW**-dee-oh-**MET**-rik			
audiometry	aw-dee-**OM**-eh-tree			
auditory	**AW**-dih-tor-ee	S/ R/	-ory *having the function of* audit- *hearing*	Pertaining to the sense of hearing or to the organs of hearing
electrocochleography	ee-**LEK**-troh-kok-lee-**OG**-rah-fee	S/ R/CF R/CF	-graphy *process of recording* electr/o- *electric* -cochle/o- *cochlea*	Measurement of the electric potentials generated in the inner ear by sounds
electronystagmography	ee-**LEK**-troh-nys-tag-**MOG**-rah-fee	S/ R/CF R/CF R/CF	-graphy *process of recording* electr/o- *electric* -nystagm/o- *nystagmus* vide/o- *visual*	Test using electrodes to measure eye movements to evaluate vestibular dysfunction Test using goggles with video cameras to measure eye movements to evaluate vestibular dysfunction
videonystagmography	**VID**-ee-oh-nys-tag-**MOG**-rah-fee			
otoscope	**OH**-toh-scope	S/ R/CF S/ S/	-scope *instrument for viewing* ot/o- *ear* -ic *pertaining to* -scopy *to examine*	Instrument for examining the external and middle ears Pertaining to examination with an otoscope Examination of the ear
otoscopic (adj) otoscopy	oh-toh-**SKOP**-ik oh-**TOS**-koh-pee			
pneumatic	new-**MAT**-ik	S/ R/	-ic *pertaining to* pneumat- *structure filled with air*	Pertaining to a structure filled with air
Rinne test	**RIN**-eh TEST		Friedrich Rinne, 1819–1868, German otologist **test** Latin *earthen vessel*	Test for conductive hearing loss
tympanography	**TIM**-pan-**OG**-rah-fee	S/ R/CF	-graphy *process of recording* tympan/o- *eardrum, tympanic membrane* -metry *process of measuring*	Recording pressure changes inside the ear Measurement of pressure changes between the middle and inner ears
tympanometry	**TIM**-pan-**OM**-eh-tree	S/		
Weber test	**VAY**-ber TEST		Ernst Weber, 1794–1878, German physiologist **test** Latin *earthen vessel*	Test for sensorineural hearing loss

Therapeutic Procedures for the Ear

Hearing

Ear clearing to equalize the pressure in the middle ear with the outside air pressure by making the ear(s) "pop" can be performed by yawning, swallowing, or using a method like a **Valsalva maneuver,** in which the nose is pinched, the mouth is closed, and attempts are made to breathe out through the nose.

Ear wax blockage is removed by loosening it with oil, and then flushing, **curetting,** or suctioning out the softened wax.

Debridement is the removal of **necrotic** tissue and debris from the external ear canal in **otitis externa** using dry cotton wipes and/or suction. Mild otitis externa can then be treated with 2% acetic acid and hydrocortisone drops. Moderate infections require the addition of a **topical antibacterial suspension,** and severe infections require the insertion of an ear wick into the canal, wetted four times a day with a topical antibiotic or 5% aluminum acetate solution. Very severe infections may need systemic antibiotics. **Swimmer's ear** is a form of otitis externa and can be prevented by applying a few drops of a 1:1 mixture of rubbing alcohol and vinegar immediately after swimming.

Acute otitis media responds to an antibiotic such as amoxicillin, though some infections may subside spontaneously.

In **chronic otitis media with effusion,** when the sticky fluid persists in the middle ear, a **myringotomy** can be performed and a small, hollow plastic tube inserted through the tympanic membrane to allow

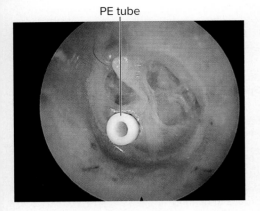

PE tube

Figure 16.40 Pressure equalization (PE) tube in tympanic membrane.
Professor Tony Wright, Institute of Laryngology & Otology/Science Source

the effusion to drain out. These tubes are called **tympanostomy tubes,** or **pressure equalization tubes (PE tubes)** (*Figure 16.40*). Surgical removal is required for a **cholesteatoma.**

Hearing aids can help a sensorineural hearing loss and an **audiologist** will recommend the type of device for each patient.

Cochlear implants can be used for a severe hearing loss. Unlike a hearing aid that amplifies sound and directs it through the ear canal, a cochlear implant compensates for damaged or nonworking elements in the cochlea. The devices pick up sound and **digitize** it, convert the digitized sound into electrical signals, and transmit those signals to electrodes embedded in the cochlea. The electrodes stimulate the cochlear nerve, sending signals to the brain.

Balance

Otolith repositioning procedures, performed by physical therapists with specialized training, are employed to return the tiny otolith granules to their correct resting place to resolve positional vertigo.

Exercises taught in a physical therapy setting can help with dizziness and vertigo to improve balance in different positions and activities.

Medications for the Ear

In the external ear canal, buildup of wax can be loosened with oil or with carbamide peroxide solution (*Debrox*). Otitis externa can be treated with acetic acid drops to change the pH of the external canal or with drops containing an antibiotic or an antibiotic and steroid such as ciprofloxacin and dexamethazone (*Ciprodex*) or neomycin, polymycin, and hydrocortisone (*Corticosporin*).

For infections of the middle ear, antibiotics such as penicillin, amoxicillin, and erythromycin are used.

For inner ear disorders, the antihistamine meclizine and the anti-anxiety medication diazepam (*Valium*) are used to diminish the vertigo of BPPV. The treatment of Ménière's disease has been revolutionized with the use of a single transtympanic injection of a low dose of gentamycin.

Word Analysis and Definition: Therapeutic Procedures and Medications

S = Suffix P = Prefix R = Root R/CF = Combining Form

WORD	PRONUNCIATION	ELEMENTS		DEFINITION
curette **curettage** (***Note:*** the final "e" of curette is dropped because the suffix "–age" begins with a vowel.)	kyu-**RET** kyu-reh-**TAHZH**	S/ S/ R/	French *cleanse* -age *related to* currett- *cleanse*	Scoop-shaped instrument for scraping the interior of a cavity or removing new growths Scraping the interior of a cavity or removing a new growth
debridement	day-**BREED**-mon	S/ P/ R/	-ment *resulting state* de- *take away* -bride- *rubbish*	The removal of necrotic or injured tissue
digitize	**DIJ**-ih-tize	S/ R/	-ize *affect in a specific way* digit- *finger, toe, number*	To change analog information into a numerical format to facilitate computer processing
maneuver	mah-**NYU**-ver		French *to work by hand*	A planned movement or procedure
myringotomy	mir-in-**GOT**-oh-mee	S/ R/CF	-tomy *surgical incision* myring/o- *tympanic membrane*	Incision in the tympanic membrane
necrosis	neh-**KROH**-sis	S/ R/	-osis *condition* necr- *death*	Pathologic death of one or more cells
necrotic (adj)	neh-**KROT**-ik	S/ R/CF	-tic *pertaining to* necr/o- *death*	Affected by necrosis
topical	**TOP**-ih-kal	S/ R/	-al *pertaining to* topic- *local*	Medication applied directly to obtain a local effect
tympanostomy	tim-pan-**OS**-toh-mee	S/ R/CF	-stomy *new opening* tympan/o- *eardrum, tympanic membrane*	Surgically created new opening in the tympanic membrane to allow fluid to drain from the middle ear
Valsalva	val-**SAL**-vah		Antonio Valsalva, 1666–1723, Italian physician	Any forced expiratory effort against a closed airway

Check Point Section 16.6

A. Define the different auditory diagnostic tests. *The different auditory tests are indicated for different disorders of the ear. Knowing what they test for gives clues to the patient's condition. Match the test on the left with its correct description on the right.* **LO 16.5**

_____ **1.** tympanometry

_____ **2.** Rinne test

_____ **3.** otoscopy

_____ **4.** Weber test

a. used to view the external ear and tympanic membrane

b. test for conductive hearing loss

c. test for sensorineural hearing loss

d. measures pressure changes between the middle and inner ears

B. Deconstruct medical terms relating to the diagnostic tests of the ear. *Deconstruct the terms in order to decipher their meanings.* **LO 16.2, 16.5**

1. tympanometry: _____ / _____
CF   S

2. audiometry: _____ / _____
CF   S

3. audiologist: _____ / _____
CF   S

C. Use the following table *to list all the combining forms in the terms given and give their meaning:* **LO 16.2, 16.5**

Terms	Combining Forms	Meaning of Combining Forms
otoscope		
electrocochleography		
electronystagmography		
videonystagmography		

D. Identify the therapeutic procedure indicated for each disorder. *Select the correct answer for each question.* **LO 16.7**

1. Chronic otitis media is treated with:

  a. Valsalva maneuver

  b. tympanostomy tubes

  c. rubbing alcohol drops

  d. physical therapy

2. An acute otitis media is treated with:

  a. myringotomy

  b. tympanostomy tubes

  c. oral antibiotics

  d. antihistamines

3. Positional vertigo can be treated with:

  a. physical therapy

  b. anti-anxiety medications

  c. cochlear implants

  d. myringotomy

4. Excessive cerumen in the auditory canal is treated with:

  a. alcohol and vinegar drops

  b. antibiotic drops

  c. myringotomy

  d. curettage

5. Cholesteatoma is treated with:

  a. debridement

  b. excision

  c. acetic acid drops

  d. oral antibiotics

Table 16.1 Chapter 16 Abbreviations

Abbreviations	Meaning
ABR	auditory brainstem response
AD	Latin is auris dexter right ear
AOM	acute otitis media
AS	Latin is auris sinistra left ear
AU	Latin is aures unitas or auris uterque both ears
BOM	bilateral otitis media
BPPV	benign paroxysmal positional vertigo
CAT	computed axial tomography
COM	chronic otitis media
ECOG	electrocochleography
ENG	electronystagmography
LASIK	laser-assisted in situ keratomileusis
mg	milligram
MRI	magnetic resonance imaging
PERRLA	pupils equal, round, reactive to light and accommodation
PE	pressure equalization (tubes)
PRK	photorefractive keratectomy
p.r.n	when necessary
OD	Doctor of Optometry
OME	otitis media with effusion
OT	ophthalmic technician
q.4.h	every four hours
q.i.d	four times each day
URI	upper respiratory infection
VNG	videonystagmography

Table 16.2 Comparison of Selected Eye and Ear Disorders—Signs, Symptoms, and Treatments

Eye Disorder or Disease	Signs and Symptoms	Diagnostic Tests	Treatment
Blepharitis	Redness, irritation, burning, tearing, crusting of eyelashes. Symptoms typically worse in the morning.	Eye evaluation Slit-lamp biomicroscopy Cultures	Warm compress Eyelid cleansing Antibiotics if due to bacterial infection.
Amblyopia "Lazy Eye"	Squinting Shutting one eye Tilting head	Eye exam	Treatment causes the affected eye to be the source of vision. This strengthens the nerve connection between the affected eye and the brain. Eye patch—patch the good eye Atropine eye drops in the good eye—temporarily blurs the vision in the good eye
Cholesteatoma	History of middle ear infections Ear discharge Gradual loss of hearing	Otoscopy CT scan MRI	Surgical removal of the cholesteatoma. Access by transcanal (going through ear canal) or transauricular (incision behind the ear, then moving the external ear forward). Mastoidectomy to remove infected bone and tympanoplasty to repair the eardrum
Sensorineural hearing loss	Ask people to repeat what they are saying Turn up the volume of TV louder than others in the room need it to be Trouble hearing with background noise	Weber's Test Rinne Test Audiogram	Hearing aids This type of hearing loss is permanent
Ear wax impaction	Difficulty hearing Feeling of ear fullness Tinnitus Cough	Otoscopy	Irrigation Oils to soften Curettage

Special Senses of the Eye and Ear

Challenge Your Knowledge

A.   Suffixes. The following terms all have a suffix with a common meaning. Write the suffix for each term. Write it with the hyphen, for example, -itis. Fill in the blanks. **LO 16.2**

     1. periorbital   _____

     2. lacrimal   _____

     3. necrotic   _____

     4. intraocular   _____

     5. neural   _____

     6. optic   _____

     7. tarsal   _____

     8. pupillary   _____

     9. retinal   _____

     10. recurrent   _____

     These suffixes all mean _____.

B.   Prefixes. Use your knowledge of prefixes to deconstruct the following terms; write the prefix for each term. **LO 16.2**

Term	Prefix
periorbital	**1.**
esotropia	**2.**
astigmatism	**3.**
emmetropia	**4.**
intraocular	**5.**
exotropia	**6.**
bilateral	**7.**
equilateral	**8.**

C.   Diagnosis. You are preparing to code the claim forms for various patients seen in the clinic today. The doctor has given each diagnosis in general terms on the charge slip. Write the correct medical term for each general term. **LO 16.6**

     1. Pink eye   _____

     2. Sensitivity to light   _____

     3. Nearsighted   _____

     4. Scratched cornea (2 words)   _____

     5. Inflammation of the iris   _____

     6. "Lazy eye"   _____

     7. Farsighted   _____

     8. Inflamed eyelash and tarsal gland   _____

     9. Droopy eyelid   _____

     10. Cross-eyed   _____

D. **Match the Latin and Greek terms in the left column to their meanings in the right column.** LO 16.1, 16.6

_____ 1. orbit   a. flat

_____ 2. extrinsic   b. drooping

_____ 3. chalazion   c. on the outer side

_____ 4. cornea   d. paralysis

_____ 5. cortex   e. lump

_____ 6. ptosis   f. corner of the eye

_____ 7. canthus   g. web

_____ 8. contagious   h. circle

_____ 9. tarsus   i. outer shell

_____ 10. paresis   j. touch closely

E. **Identify the meaning of the medical term below. Terms can be from the eye or the ear section of this chapter.** Fill in the blanks. LO 16.1, 16.3, 16.6

1. Persistent ringing in the ears _____

2. Sensation of spinning or whirling _____

3. Occurring in sharp, spasmodic episodes _____

4. Eye turning away from its normal position _____

5. Partial paralysis _____

6. Sinking down of an eyelid or organ _____

7. Collection of fluid that has escaped from blood vessels into a cavity or tissues _____

8. Punctured with one or more holes _____

9. The structure that carries tears to the conjunctiva _____

F. **Master your documentation—it is a legal record.** Select the most appropriate choice, and insert the correct abbreviation where indicated on the line. LO 16.3, 16.6, 16.7, 16.9

1. Patient complains of sticky eyelids with (purulent/perulent) discharge, prescription eye drops prescribed to be given every four

   hours (_____ [abbreviation]). Diagnosis: (scleritis/conjunctivitis)

2. The optometrist (_____ [abbreviation]) determined with the patient's vision now 20/40 in the right eye,

   with correction.

3. The (diagnosis/prognosis) for Mr. Baker is continued decreasing vision in his right eye if his diabetes remains uncontrolled and

   his (retinopathy/retinoblastoma) worsens.

4. (Opthalmoscopic/Ophthalmoscopic) examination of the left eye reveals (microaneurisms/microaneurysms) forming.

   The (Fluoreseen/Fluorescein) angiography is ordered for more details.

5. The (ophthalmologist/ophthalamologist) determined that the patient's pupils are equal, round, and reactive to light and accom-

   modation (_____ [abbreviation]).

G. Terminology challenge. The following medical terms are associated with either an eye specialist or an ear specialist. Check (✓) the appropriate specialist for the term. **LO 16.10**

Term	Otologist	Ophthalmologist
1. uveitis		
2. otolith		
3. vertigo		
4. cholesteatoma		
5. conjunctivitis		
6. glaucoma		
7. labyrinthitis		
8. papilledema		
9. canthus		
10. audiologist		
11. hordeolum		
12. dacryostenosis		
13. LASIK		
14. ptosis		

H. Word elements. Learning word elements is your most valuable tool for increasing your medical vocabulary. Use your knowledge of word elements to answer the following questions. Select the correct answer. **LO 16.1, 16.2, 16.5, 16.6**

1. The root for *tear* is

   a. blephar

   b. tamin

   c. commodat

   d. strab

   e. lacrim

2. This word means partial paralysis:

   a. parietal

   b. periorbital

   c. paresis

   d. ptosis

   e. presbyopia

3. On the basis of its suffix, you can tell that a **keratotomy** is a

   a. body part

   b. procedure

   c. diagnosis

   d. medication

   e. infection

4. The prefix in **microaneurysm** tells you that this aneurysm is

   a. large

   b. black

   c. small

   d. painful

   e. red

5. In the term **amblyopia,** *-opia* means

   a. sound

   b. light

   c. sight

   d. movement

   e. pain

6. **In situ** is a Latin phrase that means *(Be precise!)*

    a. in this place   **d.** in the place

    b. in another place   **e.** in place of

    c. in its original place

7. In the terms **retinoblastoma** and **retinopathy,** the combining form tells you that both these terms concern the

    a. cornea   **d.** vitreous body

    b. iris   **e.** retina

    c. lens

8. **Tonometry** is a diagnostic test for

    a. intraocular pressure   **d.** distance vision

    b. refractive errors   **e.** gland

    c. blood vessel

9. In the term **periorbital,** *peri-* is a prefix that means

    a. within   **d.** against

    b. outside   **e.** around

    c. on top of

I.   **Abbreviations.** The following abbreviations are all part of the *language of otology.* Match the abbreviation in the left column with its meaning in the right column. **LO 16.9**

_____ **1.** PE		**a.**	ear infection with fluid collection
_____ **2.** BPPV		**b.**	both ears
_____ **3.** A.S.		**c.**	four times each day
_____ **4.** p.r.n.		**d.**	right ear
_____ **5.** q.i.d.		**e.**	common cold
_____ **6.** OME		**f.**	sensation of spinning or whirling
_____ **7.** A.U.		**g.**	chronic otitis media
_____ **8.** COM		**h.**	pressure equalization tubes
_____ **9.** URI		**i.**	left ear
_____ **10.** A.D.		**j.**	when necessary

J. Identify the elements in each medical term and unlock the meaning of the word. *Fill in the chart. If the word does not have a particular word element, write n/a. The first one has been done for you.* **LO 16.2**

Medical Term	Prefix	Meaning of Prefix	Root/Combining Form	Meaning of Root/Combing Form	Suffix	Meaning of Suffix	Meaning of the Term
mydriatic	1. n/a	2. n/a	3. *mydri-*	4. dilation of the pupil	5. *-atic*	6. pertaining to	7. Pertaining to the dilation of the pupil
tympanic	8.	9.	10.	11.	12.	13.	14.
debridement	15.	16.	17.	18.	19.	20.	21.
myringotomy	22.	23.	24.	25.	26.	27.	28.
otoscope	29.	30.	31.	32.	33.	34.	35.

K. Match the term in the left column with its meaning in the right column. LO 16.1, 16.6

_____ 1. humor   a. pouring out

_____ 2. impacted   b. wing

_____ 3. auricle   c. jingle

_____ 4. vertigo   d. stirrup

_____ 5. meatus   e. driven in

_____ 6. effusion   f. liquid

_____ 7. cerumen   g. dizziness

_____ 8. pinna   h. ear

_____ 9. stapes   i. wax

_____ 10. tinnitus   j. go through

L. Schedule your patients. The following doctors and ancillary personnel are seeing patients in the clinic today. Based on the patient's needs, schedule the patient for the correct physician or technician. **16.10**

ophthalmologist   **ophthalmic technician**

otologist   **otorhinolaryngologist**

Patient Needs/Has	Schedule with
refraction	1.
PE tubes	2.
phacoemulsification	3.
instruction in using eyedrops	4.
cholesteatoma	5.
patient hit in eye with tree branch	6.
removal of tonsils and adenoids	7.
LASIK surgery	8.
child has bubblegum in nose	9.
runny nose, stopped-up ears, sore throat	10.
broken eyeglasses	11.

M. **Apply what you know about the middle ear to choose the answer.** Select the best choice. **LO 16.1, 16.6**

1. Which of these is NOT a component of the middle ear?

   a. tympanic membrane

   b. eustachian (auditory) tube

   c. malleus, incus, stapes

   d. nasopharynx

   e. tympanic cavity

2. The eustachian (auditory) tube connects the

   a. tonsils and nasopharynx

   b. middle ear and nasopharynx

   c. nasopharynx and ossicles

   d. nasopharynx and tympanic membrane

   e. tympanic cavity and tympanic membrane

3. Identify the three ossicles:

   a. pinna, auricle, stapes

   b. eustachian (auditory) tube, mastoid cells, tonsils

   c. nasopharynx, tonsils, middle ear

   d. malleus, incus, stapes

   e. tonsils, stapes, incus

4. What is a complication of chronic otitis media with effusion?

   a. vertigo

   b. acute infection

   c. cholesteatoma

   d. dizziness

   e. nausea

5. Which of these would NOT cause a perforated eardrum?

   a. puncture by a cotton swab

   b. open-handed slap to the ear

   c. scuba diving

   d. pus from acute otitis media

   e. sinusitis

N. **Pronunciation is important whether you are saying the word or listening to a word from a coworker. Identify the proper pronunciation of the following medical terms.** **LO 16.1, 16.3, 16.4, 16.6**

1. The correct pronunciation for the last name of the French physician that describes an inner ear disorder that have cluster attacks of tinnitus, vertigo, and hearing loss.

   a. val-sale-**VAH**

   b. val-**SAL**-vah

   c. men-**YEAR**

   d. man-**YARE**

   Correctly spell the term: _____

2. The correct pronunciation for a fungal infection in an ear

   a. ves-**TIB**-you-lar

   b. **VES**-tih-byul-ar

   c. **OH**-toh-migh-**KEY**-oh-sis

   d. **OH**-toh-my-**KOH**-sis

   Correctly spell the term: _____

3. The correct pronunciation for another name for auricle

   a. **PIN**-ee

   b. **PIN**-ah

   c. **PIN**-ay

   d. **PIN**-ahs

   Correctly spell the term: _____

4. The correct pronunciation for pertaining to tears

   a. pair-ee-**OR**-bit-al

   b. **PER**-ih-or-bit-al

   c. Lak-**RIME**-al

   d. **LAK**-rim-al

   Correctly spell the term: _____

5. The correct pronunciation for the ability to see close objects but unable to see distant objects

   a. me-**OH**-pee-ah

   b. my-**OH**-pee-ah

   c. em-eh-**TOH**-pee-ah

   d. em-eh-try-**OH**-pee-ah

   Correctly spell the term: _____

Case Reports

A. **After reading Case Report (CR) 16.1, answer the following questions.** *For multiple choice questions, select the correct answer.* **LO 16.5, 16.6, 16.7, 16.8**

 Case Report (CR) 16.1

Mrs. Jenny Hughes's "pink eye" is called acute **contagious** conjunctivitis. It responds well to **antibiotic** eyedrops. Her hands were **contaminated** from the keyboard of the employee who had left work and gone home with "pink eye." Mrs. Hughes transmitted the infection from her fingers to her eyes by touching or rubbing.

Your documentation of Mrs. Hughes's office visit could read:

Progress Note 04/10/21

Mrs. Jenny Hughes was brought directly into the clinical area at 1030 hrs. with what appeared to be conjunctivitis, "pink eye." Both eyelids were red and swollen with a purulent discharge. She complained of headache and photophobia. Dr. Chun prescribed Neosporin eyedrops, 1–2 drops every four hours (**q.4.h**) for 7 days. A swab was sent to the laboratory. I instructed and watched Mrs. Hughes wash her hands and use an alcohol-based hand gel. I then had her sign in and sign our Notice of Privacy Practices. I instructed her in the use of the drops and emphasized home care and hand care measures to prevent the infection from spreading to her family. She was given a return appointment in 1 week and told to call the office if the drops did not help. Daphne Butras, OT. 1055 hrs.

1. Which of the following statements correctly describes Mrs. Hughes's condition?

    a. Inflammation of the inner lining of the eyelid

    b. Partial paralysis of the eyelid

    c. Infection of the tear duct

    d. Abscess in an eyelash follicle

2. Her condition can:

    a. can cause a fever

    b. can lead to paralysis of the eye

    c. is an infection that can be given to other people

    d. remains in your body for up to one year

3. You can tell Mrs. Hughes that the medication in the eye drops:

    a. relieves your dry eyes

    b. fights off allergens

    c. dilates your pupils

    d. kills the bacterial infection

B. After reading Case Report (CR) 16.2, then select the correct answer for each question. LO 16.5, 16.7, 16.8, 16.10

 Case Report (CR) 16.2

You are

. . . an ophthalmic technician working with Angela Chun, MD, an ophthalmologist at Fulwood Medical Center.

Your patient is

. . . Sam Hughes, a 2-year-old boy, who has been referred by his pediatrician to Dr. Chun.

His mother, Mrs. Jenny Hughes, states that she has noticed for the past couple of months that his right eye has turned in. The only visual difficulty she has noticed is that he sometimes misses a Cheerio when he tries to grab it. Otherwise, he is healthy.

You are responsible for documenting Sam's diagnostic and therapeutic procedures and explaining the significance of these to his mother.

1. What is the medical term for eye turned in toward the nose:

    a. Astigmatism

    b. Glaucoma

    c. Esotropia

    d. Amblyopia

2. Which of the following diagnostic tests might Dr. Chun use to determine Sam's eye condition?

    a. Slit lamp to evaluate his eye muscles

    b. Have Sam follow a moving penlight

    c. CT scan of eye and optic nerve

    d. Determine Sam's visual acuity

3. According to the Case Report, how did Mrs. Hughes decide to seek Dr. Chun's medical opinion?

    a. performed an Internet search

    b. a friend suggested she see Dr. Chun

    c. she was referred by her son's doctor

    d. Dr. Chun was called to see Sam in the ER

4. Which of the following might be a therapeutic method to treat Sam's eye condition?

    a. Eyeglasses with a concave lens

    b. LASIK to the good eye

    c. Patch the good eye

    d. Occasional use of prism

Chapter 16 Review

2014 Nucleus Medical Media

C. After reading Case Report (CR), correctly answer the following questions. LO 16.2, 16.5, 16.7, 16.8, 16.9, 16.10

 Case Report (CR) 16.3

You are

. . . a medical assistant working with **primary care** physician Susan Lee, MD, of the Fulwood Medical Group on March 16, 2021.

Your patients are

. . . 3-year-old Eddie Cardenas and his mother, Mrs. Carmen Cardenas.

Mrs. Cardenas has brought in her son, Eddie. She tells you that he has had a cold for a couple of days. Early this morning he woke up screaming, felt hot, and was tugging his ears. She gave him **acetaminophen** with some orange juice, and he threw up. This is the third similar episode in the past year. Since the last time, she is concerned that he is not hearing normally. You see a worried mother and a very unhappy, restless toddler with a green nasal discharge. His oral temperature taken with an electronic digital thermometer is 102.4°F, pulse 100. Dr. Lee examines Eddie and finds that he has an **(URI)** with **(BOM).** She prescribes amoxicillin 250 mg (q.i.d). for 10 days, and acetaminophen 160 mg (p.r.n.) for pain, after which she will see Eddie again. After the acute infection subsides, if there remains an **effusion** in the middle ear, she will refer Eddie to an **otologist.** Luisa Guittierez, CMA. 1115 hrs. 3/16/17.

1. Dr. Lee has recommended the use of acetaminophen as an:

    a. analgesic

    b. antibiotic

    c. antihistamine

2. What type of medication is the amoxicillin?

    a. antipyretic

    b. analgesic

    c. antibiotic

3. Which diagnostic tool will Dr. Lee use to determine if there is an effusion in the middle ear?

    a. tonometer

    b. otoscope

    c. ophthalmoscope

    d. curette

    Dr. Chun asks that you explain the prescriptions and how often they are given to Eddie. Also, explain the medical plan to Mrs. Hughes if Eddie needs to see an otologist.

4. Provide the three words that URI stands for:

    _____ _____ tract _____

5. How often is Mrs. Hughes to give the antibiotic?

    a. three times a day

    b. four times a day

    c. when he has a fever

    d. when he has pain

6. If Eddie is not better in time for his next appointment, Dr. Chun will:

    a. refer him to an ear specialist

    b. prescribe another antibiotic

    c. use a curette to remove the infection

    d. refer him to a throat specialist

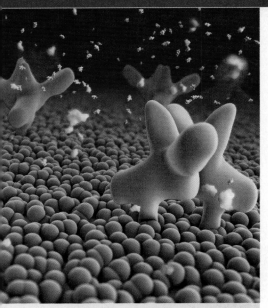

2014 Nucleus Medical Media

Chapter Sections

CHAPTER

17

Endocrine System
The Language of Endocrinology

Chapter Learning Outcomes

Upon completion of this chapter, you will be able to:

LO 17.1 Identify and describe the anatomy and physiology of the endocrine system.

LO 17.2 Use roots, combining forms, suffixes, and prefixes to construct and analyze medical terms related to the endocrine system.

LO 17.3 Spell medical terms related to the endocrine system.

LO 17.4 Pronounce medical terms related to the endocrine system.

LO 17.5 Describe diagnostic procedures utilized for disorders of the endocrine system.

LO 17.6 Identify and describe disorders and pathological conditions related to the endocrine system.

LO 17.7 Describe the therapeutic procedures and pharmacologic agents used with the endocrine systems.

LO 17.8 Apply knowledge of medical terms relating to endocrinology to documentation, medical records, and communication.

LO 17.9 Identify and correctly use abbreviations of terms used in endocrinology.

LO 17.10 Identify health professionals involved in the care of patients with endocrine disorders.

Health professionals involved in the treatment of patients with **endocrinological** problems include:

- **Endocrinologists,** who are medical specialists concerned with the endocrine glands that produce hormonal secretions.
- **Pediatric endocrinologists,** who are medical specialists concerned with the diagnosis and management of children with endocrine disorders and diabetes.
- **Diabetologists,** who are physicians and endocrinologists whose practice and research are concentrated in diabetes care. **Diabetology** is not a recognized medical specialty.
- **Endocrine physician assistants,** who work as a team with endocrinologists to provide care and education to endocrine and diabetes patients.
- **Endocrine nurse practitioners,** who also work as a team with endocrinologists to provide care and education to endocrine and diabetes patients.
- **Certified diabetic educators,** licensed health care professionals including registered nurses, registered dietitians, and pharmacists, who are certified to possess distinct and specialized knowledge in diabetes self-management education and monitoring.

Section 17.1 Endocrine System Overview

Endocrine System

The endocrine system is composed of 14 major **glands** (*Figure 17.1*)

- **Pituitary** gland and the nearby hypothalamus
- **Pineal** gland
- Thyroid gland
- **Parathyroid** glands (4)
- Thymus gland
- Adrenal glands (2)
- Pancreas
- Gonads: testes (2) in the male; ovaries (2) in the female

In addition, endocrine cells found in tissues all over the body secrete hormones. Examples are:

- **Cells in the upper GI tract** that secrete the hormone **gastrin,** which stimulates gastric secretions, and the hormone **cholecystokinin,** which contracts the gallbladder *(see Chapter 5).*
- **Cells in the kidney** that secrete **erythropoietin,** which stimulates erythrocyte production *(see Chapter 6).*
- **Fat cells** that secrete **leptin,** which helps suppress appetite. Lack of it can lead to overeating and obesity.
- **Cells in tissues throughout the body** that secrete **prostaglandins,** which act locally to dilate blood vessels, relax airways, stimulate uterine contractions in menstrual cramps or labor, and lower acid secretion in the stomach. When tissues are injured, prostaglandins promote an inflammatory response.

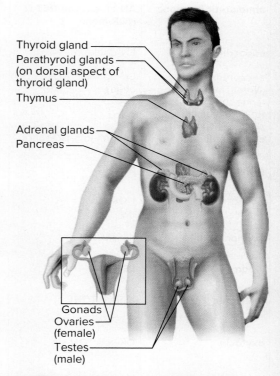

Thyroid gland
Parathyroid glands (on dorsal aspect of thyroid gland)
Thymus
Adrenal glands
Pancreas
Gonads
Ovaries (female)
Testes (male)

▲ **Figure 17.1** Major endocrine glands.

Hypothalamus

The hypothalamus (*Figure 17.2*) forms the floor and walls of the brain's third ventricle *(see Chapter 9)* and produces eight hormones. Six of them are local hormones that regulate the production of hormones by the anterior pituitary gland *(see page 592)*. Two of them, **oxytocin** and **antidiuretic hormone (ADH),** are transported to the posterior pituitary, where they are stored until they are needed elsewhere in the body.

Pineal Gland

The pineal gland is located on the roof of the third ventricle of the brain, posterior to the hypothalamus (*Figure 17.2*). It secretes **serotonin** by day and converts it to **melatonin** at night. The gland reaches its maximum size in childhood and may regulate the timing of puberty. It also may play a role in **seasonal affective disorder (SAD),** in which people are depressed in the dark days of winter.

Did you know...

- A hormone is secreted by an organ and carried by the bloodstream to act at distant target sites.
- The medical specialty concerned with the hormonal secretions of the endocrine glands, their physiology, and pathology is called **endocrinology.**

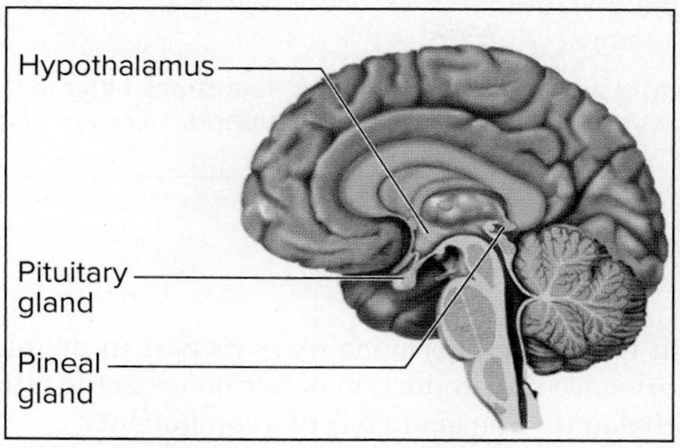

Hypothalamus
Pituitary gland
Pineal gland

▲ **Figure 17.2** Hypothalamus, pituitary gland, and pineal gland.

WORD	PRONUNCIATION		ELEMENTS	DEFINITION
antidiuretic (*Note:* This term has two prefixes.)	AN-tih-die-you-RET-ik	S/ P/ P/ R/	-ic *pertaining to* anti- *against* -di- *complete* -uret- *urination*	An agent that decreases urine production
antidiuretic hormone	AN-tih-die-you-RET-ik HOR-mohn		hormone Greek *to set in motion*	Posterior pituitary hormone that decreases urine output by acting on the kidney; also called *vasopressin*
endocrine	EN-doh-krin	S/ P/	-crine *secrete* endo- *within*	Pertaining to a gland that produces an internal or hormonal secretion
endocrinology (*Note:* The "e" in -*crine* changes to "o" for easier pronunciation.)	EN-doh-krih-NOL-oh-jee	S/ R/CF	-logy *study of* -crin/o- *secrete*	Medical specialty concerned with the production and effects of hormones
endocrinologist	EN-doh-krih-NOL-oh-jist	S/	-logist *one who studies, specialist*	A medical specialist in endocrinology
gland	GLAND		Latin *glans, acorn*	A collection of cells functioning as a secretory or excretory organ
hormone	HOR-mohn		Greek *to set in motion*	Chemical formed in one tissue or organ and carried by the blood to stimulate or inhibit a function of another tissue or organ
hormonal (adj)	hor-MOHN-al	S/ R/	-al *pertaining to* hormon- *chemical messenger*	Pertaining to a hormone(s) or the endocrine system
leptin	LEP-tin	S/ R/	-in *chemical compound* lept- *thin, small*	Hormone secreted by adipose tissue
melatonin	mel-ah-TONE-in	S/ R/ R/	-in *chemical compound* mela- *black* -ton- *tension, pressure*	Hormone formed by the pineal gland
oxytocin	OK-see-TOH-sin	S/ P/ R/	-in *chemical compound* oxy- *quick* -toc- *labor, birth*	Hypothalamic hormone, stored in the posterior pituitary, that stimulates the uterus to contract
parathyroid	pair-ah-THIGH-royd	P/ S/ R/	para- *beside* -oid *resembling* -thyr- *an oblong shield*	Endocrine glands embedded in the back of the thyroid gland
pineal	PIN-ee-al		Latin *like a pine cone*	Pertaining to the pineal gland
pituitary	pih-TOO-ih-tair-ee	S/ R/	-ary *pertaining to* pituit- *pituitary*	Pertaining to the pituitary gland
prostaglandin	PROS-tah-GLAN-din	S/ R/CF R/	-in *chemical compound* prost/a- *prostate* -gland- *gland*	Hormone present in many tissues, but first isolated from prostate gland
seasonal affective disorder (*Note:* The abbreviation for this is SAD, which is how you feel with this disorder.)	SEE-zon-al af-FEK-tiv dis-OR-der	S/ R/ S/ R/ P/ R/	-al *pertaining to* season- *period of the year* -ive *pertaining to* affect- *mood* dis- *apart, away from* -order *arrange*	Depression that occurs at the same time every year, often in winter
serotonin	ser-oh-TOH-nin	S/ R/CF R/	-in *substance* ser/o- *serum* -ton- *tension, pressure*	A neurotransmitter in the central and peripheral nervous systems

Pituitary Gland

While there is no single conductor of the endocrine orchestra in which each hormone plays its part in maintaining **homeostasis,** the pituitary gland and the hypothalamus work together and often influence the production of hormones in the other endocrine glands.

The pituitary gland (**hypophysis**) is suspended from the hypothalamus. The gland has two components:

1. A large anterior lobe called the **adenohypophysis.**
2. A smaller posterior lobe called the **neurohypophysis.**

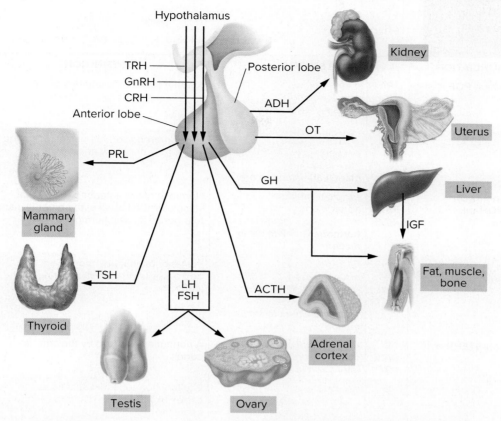

▲ **Figure 17.3** Hormones of the pituitary gland and their target organs.

Anterior lobe hormones are six in number *(Figure 17.3):*

- **Follicle-stimulating hormone (FSH)** stimulates target cells in the ovaries to develop eggs and stimulates sperm production in the testes.
- **Luteinizing hormone (LH)** stimulates ovulation and the formation of a corpus luteum in the ovary *(see Chapter 8)* to secrete estrogen and progesterone. In the male, LH stimulates production of testosterone *(see Chapter 7).*

(FSH and LH are gonadotropins and are released under the control of gonadotropin-releasing hormone [**GnRH**] of the hypothalamus.)

- **Thyroid-stimulating hormone (TSH),** or **thyrotropin,** stimulates the growth of the thyroid gland and the production of **thyroxine.**
- **Adrenocorticotropic hormone (ACTH),** or **corticotropin,** stimulates the **adrenal glands** to produce hormones called **corticosteroids.**
- **Prolactin (PRL)** stimulates the mammary glands after pregnancy to produce milk.
- **Growth hormone (GH),** or **somatotropin,** is produced in quantities at least a thousand times as great as any other pituitary hormone. It stimulates cells to enlarge and divide to produce growth, particularly in childhood and adolescence.

Tropic (also spelled **trophic**) **hormones** are hormones that stimulate other endocrine glands to produce their hormones. All of the anterior lobe hormones except PRL and GH are tropic hormones.

Posterior lobe hormones, which are produced by nuclei in the hypothalamus and then stored in and released by the pituitary posterior lobe, are of two types *(Figure 17.4):*

- **Oxytocin (OT)** in childbirth stimulates uterine contractions and in lactation forces milk to flow down ducts to the nipple. In both sexes, its production increases during sexual intercourse to help give the feelings of satisfaction and emotional bonding.
- **Antidiuretic hormone (ADH)** reduces the volume of urine produced by the kidneys. It is also called **vasopressin.**

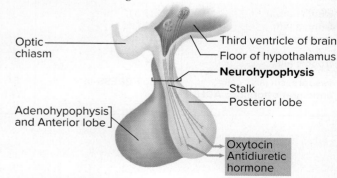

▲ **Figure 17.4** Hormones of the posterior lobe of the pituitary gland.

Word Analysis and Definition: Pituitary Gland

WORD	PRONUNCIATION	ELEMENTS		DEFINITION
adenohypophysis (*Note:* The prefix *hypo-* is part of **hypophysis,** which is a term in itself.)	**AD**-en-oh-high-**POF**-ih-sis	P/ R/CF R/	**-hypo-** *below* **aden/o-** *gland* **-physis** *growth*	Anterior lobe of the pituitary gland
adrenal gland	ah-**DREE**-nal GLAND	S/ P/ R/	**-al** *pertaining to* **ad-** *near, toward* **-ren-** *kidney* **gland** Latin *glans, acorn*	The suprarenal, or adrenal, gland on the upper pole of each kidney
adrenocorticotropic hormone	ah-**DREE**-noh-**KOR**-tih-koh-**TROH**-pik **HOR**-mohn	S/ R/CF R/CF	**-tropic** *stimulator* **adren/o-** *adrenal gland* **-cortic/o-** *cortisone, cortex* **hormone** Greek *to set in motion*	Hormone of the anterior pituitary that stimulates the cortex of the adrenal gland to produce its own hormones
antidiuretic hormone (ADH) (also called **vasopressin**)	**AN**-tih-die-you-**RET**-ik **HOR**-mohn	S/ P/ P/ R/CF	**-ic** *pertaining to* **anti-** *against* **-di-** *complete* **-uret-** *urinary system* **hormone** Greek *to set in motion*	Posterior pituitary hormone that decreases urine output by acting on the kidney
corticosteroid	**KOR**-tih-koh-**STEHR**-oyd	S/ R/CF R/	**-oid** *resembling* **cortic/o-** *cortisone* **-ster-** *steroid*	A hormone produced by the adrenal cortex
corticotropin	**KOR**-tih-koh-**TROH**-pin	S/ R/CF	**-tropin** *stimulation* **cortic/o-** *cortisone, cortex*	Pituitary hormone that stimulates the cortex of the adrenal gland to secrete cortisone
hypophysis	high-**POF**-ih-sis	P/ R/	**hypo-** *below* **-physis** *growth*	Another name for the pituitary gland
neurohypophysis	**NYUR**-oh-high-**POF**-ih-sis	P/ R/CF R/	**-hypo-** *below* **neur/o-** *nervous tissue* **-physis** *growth*	Posterior lobe of the pituitary gland
prolactin	proh-**LAK**-tin	S/ P/ R/	**-in** *chemical compound* **pro-** *before* **-lact-** *milk*	Pituitary hormone that stimulates the production of milk
somatotropin (also called **growth hormone**)	**SOH**-mah-toh-**TROH**-pin	S/ R/CF	**-tropin** *stimulation* **somat/o-** *the body*	Hormone of the anterior pituitary that stimulates growth of body tissues
thyroid	**THIGH**-royd	S/ R/	**-oid** *resembling* **thyr-** *an oblong shield*	Endocrine gland in the neck, or a cartilage of the larynx
thyrotropin	thigh-roh-**TROH**-pin	S/ R/CF	**-tropin** *stimulation* **thyr/o-** *thyroid*	Hormone from the anterior pituitary gland that stimulates function of the thyroid gland
thyroxine	thigh-**ROK**-seen	S/ R/ R/	**-ine** *pertaining to* **thyr-** *an oblong shield* **-ox-** *oxygen*	Thyroid hormone T$_4$, tetraiodothyronine
tropin (noun) **trophin** (alt) **tropic** (adj) **trophic** (alt)	**TROH**-pin **TROH**-fin **TROH**-pik **TROH**-fic	S/ R/ R/	Greek *a turning* Greek *nourishment* **-ic** *pertaining to* **trop-** *turning* **troph-** *nourishment*	Hormone Hormone Tropic hormones stimulate other endocrine glands to produce hormones
vasopressin (also called **antidiuretic hormone ADH**)	vay-soh-**PRESS**-in	S/ R/CF R/	**-in** *chemical compound* **vas/o-** *blood vessel* **-press-** *press, close*	Pituitary hormone that constricts blood vessels and decreases urine output

Thyroid Gland

The thyroid gland lies just beneath the skin of the neck and below the thyroid cartilage (Adam's apple). It is about 2 inches (5 cm) across and shaped like a bow tie. Two lobes extend up on either side of the trachea and are joined by an isthmus (*Figure 17.5*).

The thyroid is a soft, very vascular organ composed mostly of small follicles lined with epithelial cells. These cells secrete the two thyroid hormones: **triiodothyronine** **(T_3)** and **thyroxine** **(T_4)**. The term **thyroid hormone** refers to T_3 and T_4 collectively.

Thyroid hormone acts in three interrelated ways:

- **Stimulates** almost every tissue in the body to produce proteins.
- **Increases** the amount of oxygen that cells use.
- **Controls** the speed at which the body's chemical functions proceed (metabolic rate).

The thyroid gland extracts **iodine** from the blood to produce T_3 and T_4. The hormones are produced in response to **thyroid-stimulating hormone (TSH)** from the anterior pituitary gland. The pituitary gland, in turn, increases or slows the release of TSH in response to the level of thyroid hormone in the blood.

The thyroid also produces the hormone **calcitonin** from the **C cells** found between the follicles. Calcitonin stimulates osteoblastic activity (*see Chapter 14*) to promote calcium deposition and bone formation.

Parathyroid Glands

The **parathyroid glands** are usually four in number and are partially embedded in the posterior surface of the thyroid gland (*Figure 17.6*). They secrete **parathyroid hormone (PTH)** in response to hypocalcemia. Calcitonin and PTH are **antagonistic:** PTH stimulates osteoclasts to reabsorb bone and bring calcium back into the blood while calcitonin takes calcium from the blood and stimulates osteoblasts to lay down bone (*see Chapter 14*).

Thymus Gland

The thymus **gland** is located in the mediastinum behind the sternum between the lungs and above the heart (*Figure 17.7*). It is large in children and decreases in size until, in the elderly, it is mostly fibrous tissue. It secretes a group of hormones that stimulate the production of T lymphocytes (*see Chapter 12*).

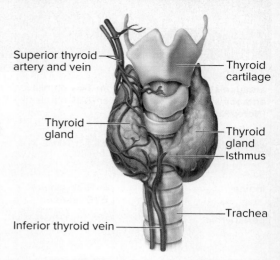

▲ **Figure 17.5** Anatomy of the thyroid gland.

Superior thyroid artery and vein
Thyroid cartilage
Thyroid gland
Thyroid gland
Isthmus
Inferior thyroid vein
Trachea

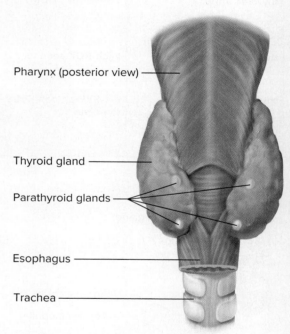

▲ **Figure 17.6** Site of parathyroid glands: Posterior view.

Pharynx (posterior view)
Thyroid gland
Parathyroid glands
Esophagus
Trachea

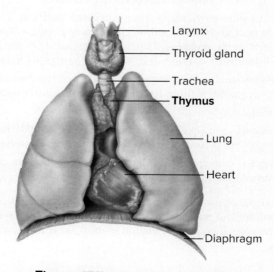

Larynx
Thyroid gland
Trachea
Thymus
Lung
Heart
Diaphragm

▲ **Figure 17.7** Position of thymus gland in the mediastinum.

WORD	PRONUNCIATION	ELEMENTS		DEFINITION
antagonist antagonistic (adj) (*Note:* Two suffixes.)	an-**TAG**-oh-nist an-**TAG**-oh-nis-tik	S/ P/ R/ S/	-ist *agent* ant- *against* -agon- *to fight* -ic *pertaining to*	An opposing structure, agent, disease, or process Having an opposite function
calcitonin	kal-sih-**TONE**-in	S/ R/CF R/	-in *chemical compound* calc/i- *calcium* -ton- *pressure, tension*	Thyroid hormone that moves calcium from blood to bones
iodine	**EYE**-oh-dine or **EYE**-oh-deen	S/ R/	-ine *pertaining to* iod- *violet, iodine*	Chemical element, the lack of which causes thyroid disease
parathyroid	pair-ah-**THIGH**-royd	S/ P/ R/	-oid *resembling* para- *adjacent* -thyr- *an oblong shield*	Endocrine glands embedded in the back of the thyroid gland
thymus	**THIGH**-mus		Greek *sweetbread*	Endocrine gland located in the mediastinum
thyroid hormone	**THIGH**-royd **HOR**-mohn	S/ R/	-oid *resembling* thyr- *an oblong shield* **hormone** Greek *to set in motion*	Collective term for the two thyroid hormones, T_3 and T_4
thyroxine	thigh-**ROK**-seen	S/ R/ R/	-ine *pertaining to* thyr- *an oblong shield* -ox- *oxygen*	Thyroid hormone T_4, tetraiodothyronine
triiodothyronine	trie-**EYE**-oh-doh- **THIE**-roh-neen	S/ P/ R/CF R/CF R/	-ine *pertaining to* tri- *three* -iod/o- *violet, iodine* -thyr- *an oblong shield* -on *chemical substance*	Thyroid hormone T_3

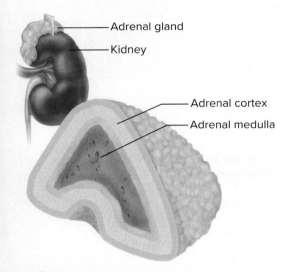

- Adrenal gland
- Kidney
- Adrenal cortex
- Adrenal medulla

▲ **Figure 17.8** Adrenal gland.

Adrenal Glands and Hormones

An **adrenal (suprarenal) gland** is anchored like a cap on the upper pole of each kidney (*Figure 17.8*).

The outer layer of the gland, the **adrenal cortex,** synthesizes more than 25 steroid hormones known collectively as **adrenocortical hormones, corticosteroids,** or **corticoids.** There are three groups of corticosteroids:

1. **Glucocorticoids**—particularly **hydrocortisone (cortisol).** These hormones stimulate fat and protein catabolism and help regulate blood glucose levels, particularly as the body resists stress (*see Lesson 17.4*). Hydrocortisone also has an anti-inflammatory effect and is used in ointments to relieve inflammation.

2. **Mineralocorticoids**—the principal one of which is called **aldosterone.** This hormone promotes sodium retention and potassium excretion by the kidneys.

3. **Sex steroids:**

   a. **Androgens**—principally **dehydroepiandrosterone (DHEA),** which is a weak androgen but is converted by other tissues into testosterone (*see Chapter 7*).

   b. **Estrogens**—principally estradiol, which is produced in much smaller quantities than in the ovaries (*see Chapter 8*).

The inner layer of the adrenal gland, the **adrenal medulla,** secretes hormones called **catecholamines,** principally **epinephrine (adrenaline)** and **norepinephrine.** These hormones prepare the body for physical activity. They raise blood pressure, increase circulation to muscles, increase pulmonary blood flow, and stimulate gluconeogenesis.

Word Analysis and Definition: Adrenal Glands and Hormones

S = Suffix P = Prefix R = Root R/CF = Combining Form

WORD	PRONUNCIATION	ELEMENTS		DEFINITION
adrenal gland	ah-**DREE**-nal GLAND	S/ R/	-al *pertaining to* adren- *adrenal gland* gland Latin *glans, acorn*	The suprarenal, or adrenal, gland on the upper pole of each kidney
adrenaline epinephrine (syn)	ah-**DREN**-ah-lin ep-ih-**NEF**-rin	S/	-ine *pertaining to*	One of the catecholamines
adrenocortical	ah-**DREE**-noh-**KOR**-tih-kal	S/ R/CF R/	-al *pertaining to* adren/o- *adrenal gland* -cortic- *cortex, cortisone*	Pertaining to the cortex of the adrenal gland
aldosterone	al-**DOS**-ter-ohn	S/ R/CF R/	-one *hormone* ald/o- *organic compound* -ster- *steroid*	Mineralocorticoid hormone of the adrenal cortex
catecholamine	kat-eh-**KOHL**-ah-meen	S/ R/	-amine *nitrogen-containing* catechol- *benzene derivative*	Any major hormones in stress response; includes epinephrine and norepinephrine
corticoid corticosteroid (syn)	**KOR**-tih-koyd **KOR**-tih-koh-**STEHR**-oyd	S/ R/ R/CF R/	-oid *resemble* cortic- *cortex, cortisone* cortic/o- *cortex, cortisone* -ster- *steroid*	One of the steroid hormones produced by the adrenal cortex A hormone produced by the adrenal cortex
cortisol hydrocortisone (syn)	**KOR**-tih-sol	S/ R/	-ol *chemical substance* cortis- *cortisone*	One of the glucocorticoids produced by the adrenal cortex; has anti-inflammatory effects
dehydroepian-drosterone (DHEA)	dee-**HIGH**-droh-eh-pee-an-**DROS**-ter-ohn	S/ P/ R/CF P/ R/CF R/	-one *hormone* de- *without, change of* -hydr/o- *water* -epi- *above* -andr/o- *male, masculine* -ster- *steroid*	Precursor to testosterone; produced in the adrenal cortex
epinephrine adrenaline (syn)	ep-ih-**NEF**-rin	S/ P/ R/	-ine *pertaining to* epi- *above* -nephr- *kidney*	Main catecholamine produced by the adrenal medulla
glucocorticoid	glue-koh-**KOR**-tih-koyd	S/ R/CF R/	-oid *resemble* gluc/o- *glucose* -cortic- *cortex, cortisone*	Hormone of the adrenal cortex that helps regulate glucose metabolism
hydrocortisone cortisol (syn)	high-droh-**KOR**-tih-sohn	S/ R/CF R/	-one *hormone* hydr/o- *water* -cortis- *cortisone*	Potent glucocorticoid with anti-inflammatory properties
mineralocorticoid	**MIN**-er-al-oh-**KOR**-tih-koyd	S/ R/CF R/	-oid *resemble* mineral/o- *inorganic materials* -cortic- *cortex, cortisone*	Hormone of the adrenal cortex that influences sodium and potassium metabolism
norepinephrine noradrenaline (syn)	**NOR**-ep-ih-**NEF**-rin	S/ P/ P/ R/	-ine *pertaining to* nor- *normal* -epi- *above* -nephr- *kidney*	Parasympathetic neurotransmitter that is a catecholamine hormone of the adrenal gland

Pancreas

The location and structure of the **pancreas** are detailed in *Chapter 5*. Most of the pancreas is an exocrine gland that secretes digestive juices into the duodenum through a duct (*Figure 17.9*). Scattered throughout the pancreas are clusters of endocrine cells grouped around blood vessels. These clusters are called **pancreatic islets** (**islets of Langerhans**). Within the islets are three distinct cell types:

1. **Alpha cells,** which secrete the hormone **glucagon** in response to a low blood glucose. Glucagon's actions are:

   a. In the liver, to stimulate **gluconeogenesis, glycogenolysis,** and the release of glucose into the bloodstream.

   b. In adipose tissue, to stimulate fat catabolism and the release of free fatty acids.

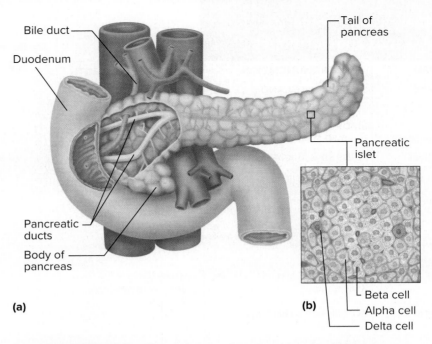

▲ **Figure 17.9** **Pancreas.** (*a*) General anatomy. (*b*) Alpha, beta, and delta cells.

2. **Beta cells,** which secrete **insulin** in response to a high blood glucose. Insulin has the opposite effects of glucagon:

   a. In muscle and fat cells, to encourage absorption of glucose and to store glycogen and fat.

   b. In the liver, to stimulate the conversion of glucose to glycogen and to inhibit the conversion of noncarbohydrates to glucose.

3. **Delta cells,** which secrete **somatostatin,** which acts within the pancreas to inhibit the secretion of glucagon and insulin.

   These three types of cell secrete their hormones directly into the bloodstream.

Word Analysis and Definition: Pancreas

S = Suffix P = Prefix R = Root R/CF = Combining Form

WORD	PRONUNCIATION		ELEMENTS	DEFINITION
glucagon	**GLUE**-kah-gon	S/ R/	**-agon** *contest* **gluc-** *glucose*	Pancreatic hormone that supports blood glucose levels
gluconeogenesis	**GLUE**-koh-nee-oh-**JEN**-eh-sis	S/ P/ R/CF	**-genesis** *creation* **-neo-** *new* **gluc/o-** *glucose*	Formation of glucose from noncarbohydrate sources
glycogenolysis	**GLIE**-koh-jeh-**NOL**-ih-sis	S/ R/CF R/CF	**-lysis** *break down* **glyc/o-** *glycogen* **-gen/o-** *to create*	Conversion of glycogen to glucose
insulin	**IN**-syu-lin	S/ R/	**-in** *chemical compound* **insul-** *island*	A hormone secreted by the islet cells of the pancreas
pancreas	**PAN**-kree-ass		Greek *sweetbread*	Lobulated gland, the head of which is tucked into the curve of the duodenum
pancreatic (adj)	pan-kree-**AT**-ik	S/ R/	**-ic** *pertaining to* **pancreat-** *pancreas*	Pertaining to the pancreas
pancreatic islets	pan-kree-**AT**-ik **EYE**-lets	S/ R/ S/ R/	**-ic** *pertaining to* **pancreat-** *pancreas* **-et** *little* **isl-** *island*	Areas of pancreatic cells that produce insulin and glucagon
islets of Langerhans (syn)	**EYE**-lets of **LAHNG**-er-hahnz		Paul Langerhans, 1847–1888, German anatomist	
somatostatin	**SOH**-mah-toh-**STAT**-in	S/ R/CF	**-statin** *inhibit* **somat/o-** *body*	Hormone that inhibits release of growth hormone and insulin

Check Point Section 17.1

A. Elements are listed in the left column. *In the first blank, write P for prefix, R/CF for root/combining form, or S for suffix. Finish the exercise by writing the meaning of the element in the right column.* **LO 17.1, 17.2**

Element	P, R/CF, or S	Meaning of Element
1. *di*	_____	_____
2. *anti*	_____	_____
3. *endo*	_____	_____
4. *mela*	_____	_____

B. Many hormones are known by their abbreviation. *Match the description in the left column to the correct abbreviation in the right column.* **LO 17.1, 17.9**

_____ 1. Stimulates formation of corpus luteum   **a.** OT

_____ 2. Stimulates production of corticosteroids   **b.** LH

_____ 3. Stimulates uterine contractions   **c.** FSH

_____ 4. Stimulates ovaries to develop eggs   **d.** ACTH

C. Describe the location and function of the parathyroid glands and the thymus gland. *Choose the correct answer for each of the following statements.* **LO 17.1**

1. There are normally _____ parathyroid glands.

    a. two   **b.** three   **c.** four   **d.** five

2. The parathyroid glands are located on the _____ surface of the thyroid gland.

    a. lateral   **b.** medial   **c.** anterior   **d.** posterior

3. The thymus gland is located _____ to the heart.

    a. anterior   **b.** posterior   **c.** inferior   **d.** superior

4. This hormone is released when blood calcium levels are low.

    a. parathyroid hormone   **b.** calcitonin   **c.** thyroxine   **d.** somatostatin

5. The function of the thymus gland is to:

    a. increase calcium levels in the blood.   **b.** decrease the body's metabolic rate.

    c. stimulate the production of T lymphocytes.   **d.** secrete testosterone.

D. Word elements are the building blocks that enable you to define the meaning of unknown words. *Match the elements in 1–10 to their correct meanings in a–j.* **LO 17.1, 17.2**

_____ 1. *hydro*	**a.** normal		_____ 6. *andr/o*	**f.** steroid
_____ 2. *adren/o*	**b.** resemble		_____ 7. *gluc/o*	**g.** kidney
_____ 3. *oid*	**c.** hormone		_____ 8. *nor*	**h.** adrenal
_____ 4. *epi*	**d.** glucose		_____ 9. *one*	**i.** above
_____ 5. *ster*	**e.** water		_____ 10. *nephr*	**j.** male

E. Describe the functions of the pancreas. *Choose the correct answer for each of the following statements.* **LO 17.1**

1. The effect of glucagon is:

   a. decrease blood sugar levels   b. increase blood sugar levels

2. Glucagon is secreted by the _____ cells.

   a. alpha   b. beta   c. delta

3. Clusters of alpha, beta, and delta cells in the pancreas are called:

   a. pancreatic clusters   b. pancreatic islets   c. pancreatitis   d. gluconeogenesis

4. The process of gluconeogenesis will cause blood sugar levels to:

   a. increase   b. decrease   c. stay the same

5. Storage of glycogen is stimulated by the hormone:

   a. somatostatin   b. glucagon   c. insulin

F. Identify the meaning of word elements. *Recognizing the meaning of the word elements makes short work of knowing the meaning of the entire medical term. Choose the correct answer.* **LO 17.2**

1. The suffix in the term **glycogenolysis** means:

   a. creation   b. contest   c. break down   d. store

2. The root in the term **glucagon** means:

   a. chemical compound   b. create   c. sugar   d. contest

3. The suffix in the term **somatostatin** means:

   a. inhibit   b. pertaining to   c. creation   d. body

4. The prefix in the term **gluconeogenesis** means:

   a. sugar   b. new   c. creation   d. pertaining to

Section 17.2 Disorders of the Endocrine System

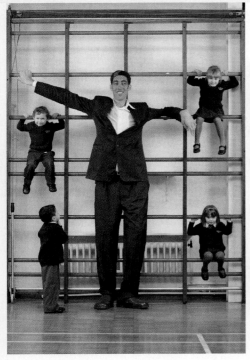

▲ **Figure 17.10** Pituitary gigantism.
Solent News/Shutterstock

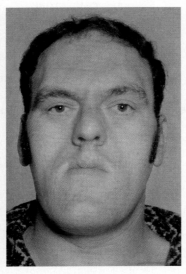

▲ **Figure 17.11** Man with acromegaly, Age 52. Clinical Photography, Central Manchester University Hospitals NHS Foundation Trust, UK/Science Source

Disorders of Pituitary Hormones

Overproduction of Pituitary Hormones

Overproduction of growth hormone stimulates excessive growth of bones and muscles. It is almost always caused by a benign pituitary **adenoma.**

In children, the excessive production starts before the growth plates of the long bones have closed. The long bones grow enormously, producing **gigantism** *(Figure 17.10).* Puberty can be delayed, genitalia may not develop fully, and diabetes can be a problem.

In adults, excessive growth hormone produces **acromegaly** *(Figure 17.11).* Signs include enlarged hands and feet, protruding jaw (**prognathism**), coarse hair, and sweating.

Treatment of acromegaly is difficult.

A **prolactinoma** is a benign prolactin-secreting tumor of the pituitary gland in both men and women. It can lead to breast milk production in women who are not breast-feeding and produce scanty menstrual periods. In men it leads to breast milk production and impotence. The abnormal production of breast milk is called **galactorrhea** *(see Chapter 13).*

Underproduction of Pituitary Hormones

Underproduction of growth hormone can be present at birth and leads to **pituitary dwarfism** (*Figure 17.12*). The short stature becomes evident at around 1 year of age and is associated with episodes of hypoglycemia.

Hypopituitarism is uncommon. It can be caused by a pituitary tumor and cause a decline in the production of several hormones at the same time, a condition called **panhypopituitarism.**

Diabetes insipidus (DI) results from a decreased production of ADH, which helps regulate the amount of water in the body. (Diabetes mellitus is an entirely different disorder; *see* Disorders of Pancreatic Hormones: Diabetes Mellitus.) Antidiuretic hormone is produced in the hypothalamus and stored in the posterior pituitary lobe. Diabetes insipidus can result from insufficient production of ADH in the hypothalamus or failure of the pituitary gland to release it.

Symptoms begin with excessive urine production (**polyuria**) by day and by night. This leads to thirst and the need to drink up to 40 quarts of fluid per day. Urine in diabetes insipidus is dilute and does not contain sugar.

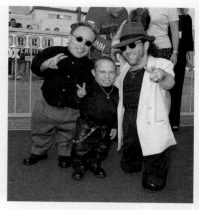

▲ **Figure 17.12** **Pituitary dwarfism.** Frank Trapper/Getty Images

Word Analysis and Definition: Disorders of Pituitary Hormones

S = Suffix   P = Prefix   R = Root   R/CF = Combining Form

WORD	PRONUNCIATION		ELEMENTS	DEFINITION
acromegaly	ak-roh-**MEG**-ah-lee	P/ R/	acro- *highest point, extremity* -megaly *enlargement*	Enlargement of the head, face, hands, and feet due to excess growth hormone in an adult
adenoma	**AD**-eh-**NOH**-mah	S/ R/	-oma *tumor* aden- *gland*	A benign neoplasm of epithelial tissue
diabetes insipidus	die-ah-**BEE**-teez in-**SIP**-ih-dus	S/ P/ R/	**diabetes** Greek *siphon* -us *pertaining to* in- *not, without* -sipid- *flavor*	Excretion of large amounts of dilute urine as a result of inadequate ADH production
dwarfism	**DWORF**-izm	S/ R/	-ism *condition* dwarf- *miniature*	Short stature due to underproduction of growth hormone
gigantism	jie-**GAN**-tizm	S/ R/	-ism *condition* gigant- *giant*	Abnormal height and size of entire body
hypopituitarism	**HIGH**-poh-pih-**TYU**-ih-tah-rizm	S/ P/ R/	-ism *condition* hypo- *deficient* -pituitar- *pituitary*	Condition of one or more deficient pituitary hormones
panhypopituitarism	pan-**HIGH**-poh-pih-**TYU**-ih-tah-rizm	S/ P/ P/ R/	-ism *condition* pan- *all* -hypo- *deficient* -pituitar- *pituitary*	Deficiency of all the pituitary hormones
polyuria	pol-ee-**YOU**-ree-ah	S/ P/ R/	-ia *condition* poly- *excessive* -ur- *urine*	Excessive production of urine
prognathism	**PROG**-nah-thizm	S/ P/ R/	-ism *condition* pro- *before, in front* -gnath- *jaw*	Condition of a forward-projecting jaw
prolactinoma	proh-lak-tih-**NOH**-mah	S/ S/ P/ R/	-oma *tumor* -in- *chemical compound* pro- *before, in front* -lact- *milk*	Prolactin-producing tumor

Disorders of the Thyroid Gland

Hyperthyroidism (Thyrotoxicosis)

Whatever the cause of **hyperthyroidism (thyrotoxicosis)**, the symptoms are those of increased body metabolism. These include tachycardia, hypertension, sweating, shakiness, anxiety, weight loss despite increased appetite, and diarrhea. Weight loss may be severe causing **emaciation.**

Graves disease is an autoimmune disorder (*see Chapter 12*) in which an antibody stimulates the thyroid to produce and secrete excessive quantities of thyroid hormones into the blood. It is associated with one or more symptoms of **goiter** (enlarged thyroid gland), **exophthalmos,** and pretibial **myxedema.**

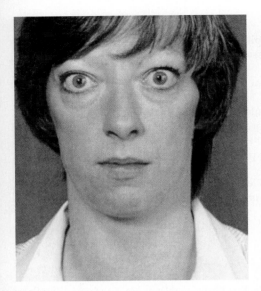

▲ **Figure 17.13** **Hyperthyroidism may cause the eyes to protrude (exophthalmos).** Biophoto Associates/Science Source

Exophthalmos, in which the eyes bulge outward *(Figure 17.13),* is caused by a substance that builds up behind the eyes. The same substance is occasionally deposited in the skin over the shins and called *pretibial myxedema.*

Thyroiditis is an inflammation of the thyroid gland. It presents in three forms:

- **Silent lymphocytic thyroiditis** is characterized by some thyroid enlargement and a self-limiting hyperthyroid phase of a few weeks, followed by recovery to the normal **euthyroid** state.

- **Subacute thyroiditis** has a history of an antecedent viral upper respiratory infection (URI) followed by signs of hyperthyroidism with a diffusely enlarged thyroid gland. It is self-limiting.

- **Hashimoto disease** is an autoimmune disease with lymphocytic infiltration of the thyroid gland. Hypothyroidism results, necessitating lifelong synthetic thyroid hormone replacement therapy.

Toxic thyroid adenoma is a nodule in the gland that produces thyroid hormones without stimulation by the pituitary's TSH. The nodule can be removed surgically.

Goiter *(Figure 17.14)* is an enlargement of the thyroid gland that, as it enlarges, can cause difficulty in swallowing and breathing. A goiter is most often the result of an iodine deficiency. They can also be caused by the above diseases, and in some cases; goiters can develop during pregnancy.

Thyroid storm is a medical emergency. It occurs when the thyroid gland releases large amounts of thyroid hormone in a short amount of time. It can be brought on when an illness or stressful event occurs in patients with untreated Grave's disease.

Hypothyroidism

Hypothyroidism results from an inadequate production of thyroid hormone, leading to a slowing of the body's metabolism. Primary hypothyroidism, in which no specific cause is found, affects 10% of older women. Severe hypothyroidism is called *myxedema.* In developing countries, a common cause is lack of iodine in the diet. In the United States, iodine is added to table salt to prevent hypothyroidism, and iodine is also found in dairy products and seafood.

Hypothyroidism causes the body to function slowly. Symptoms develop gradually. They include loss of hair; dry, scaly skin; puffy face and eyes; slow, hoarse speech; weight gain; constipation; and inability to tolerate cold *(Figure 17.15).*

Diagnosis of primary hypothyroidism is confirmed with a TSH blood level that is high. Treatment is to replace the thyroid hormone with synthetic T_4 (L-thyroxine), which is started in small doses.

Cretinism *(Figure 17.16)* is a congenital form of thyroid deficiency that severely retards mental and physical growth. If it is diagnosed and treated early with thyroid hormones, significant improvement can be achieved.

Thyroid cancer usually presents as a symptomless **nodule** in the thyroid gland.

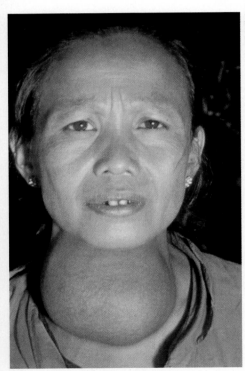

▲ **Figure 17.14** **Woman with goiter.** Lester V. Bergman/Getty Images

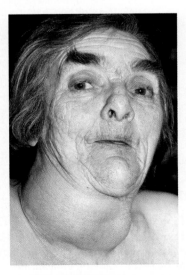

▲ **Figure 17.15** **Elderly woman with hypothyroidism.** Dr. P. Marazzi/SPL/Science Source

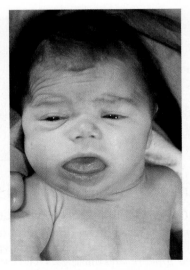

▲ **Figure 17.16** **Infant with cretinism.** Mediscan/Alamy Stock Photo

WORD	PRONUNCIATION		ELEMENTS	DEFINITION
cretin cretinism	**KREH**-tin **KREH**-tin-ism	S/ R/	French *cretin* -ism *condition, process* cretin- *cretin*	A person with severe congenital hypothyroidism Condition of severe congenital hypothyroidism
emaciation emaciated (adj)	ee-**MAY**-see-**AY**-shun ee-**MAY**-see-**ATE**-ed	S/ R/CF S/	-ation *process* emac/i- *make thin* -ated *composed of*	Abnormal thinness Abnormally thin and wasted
euthyroid	you-**THIGH**-royd	S/ P/ R/	-oid- *resembling* eu- *good, normal* -thyr- *an oblong shield*	Normal thyroid function
exophthalmos	ek-sof-**THAL**-mos	P/ R/	ex- *out, out of* -ophthalmos *eye*	Protrusion of the eyeball
goiter	**GOY**-ter		Latin *throat*	Enlargement of the thyroid gland
Graves disease	GRAYVZ diz-**EEZ**	 P/ R/	Robert Graves, 1796–1853, Irish physician dis- *apart* -ease *normal function*	Hyperthyroidism with toxic goiter
Hashimoto disease Hashimoto thyroiditis (syn)	hah-shee-**MOH**-toh diz-**EEZ**	 P/ R/	Hakaru Hashimoto, 1881–1934, Japanese surgeon dis- *apart* -ease *normal function*	Autoimmune disease of the thyroid gland
hypercalcemia	**HIGH**-per-kal-**SEE**-mee-ah	S/ P/ R/	-emia *condition of the blood* hyper- *above, excessive* -calc- *calcium*	Excessive level of calcium in the blood
hyperthyroidism	high-per-**THIGH**-royd-ism	S/ S/ P/ R/	-ism *condition, process* -oid- *resembling* hyper- *excessive* -thyr- *an oblong shield*	Excessive production of thyroid hormones
hypothyroidism	high-poh-**THIGH**-royd-ism	S/ S/ P/ R/	-ism *condition, process* -oid- *resembling* hypo- *deficient* -thyr- *an oblong shield*	Deficient production of thyroid hormones
myxedema	mik-seh-**DEE**-mah	P/ S/	myx- *mucus* -edema *swelling*	Waxy, nonpitting edema of the skin
nodule	**NOD**-yule		Latin *small knot*	Small node or knotlike swelling
thyroid storm	**THIGH**-royd STORM	S/ R/	-oid *resembling* thyr- *an oblong shield* storm Old High German *storm, crisis*	Medical crisis and emergency due to excess thyroid hormones
thyroiditis	thigh-roy-**DIE**-tis	S/ S/ R/	-itis *inflammation* -oid- *resembling* thyr- *an oblong shield*	Inflammation of the thyroid gland
thyrotoxicosis	**THIGH**-roh-tok-sih-**KOH**-sis	S/ R/CF R/CF	-sis *abnormal condition* thyr/o- *an oblong shield* -toxic/o- *poison*	Disorder caused by excessive thyroid hormone production

Disorders of the Parathyroid and Thymus Glands

Disorders of Parathyroid Glands

Hypoparathyroidism is a deficiency of parathyroid hormone that lowers levels of blood calcium (**hypocalcemias**). Most symptoms are neuromuscular, ranging from tingling in the fingers to muscle cramps and the painful muscle spasms of **tetany** (not tetanus).

Hyperparathyroidism is an excess of parathyroid hormone. It is seen more often than hypoparathyroidism and is usually caused by one of the four glands enlarging and secreting excess parathyroid hormone in an unregulated manner. It leads to four major abnormalities:

1. Bones are depleted of calcium (osteopenia) (*see Chapter* 14) and become brittle.
2. High blood calcium levels (**hypercalcemia**) lead to decreased bowel motility and constipation and to increased gastric acidity and heartburn.
3. Extra excretion of calcium in the urine leads to kidney stones (nephrolithiasis) (*see Chapter 6).*
4. High blood calcium leads to mental symptoms such as depression and fatigue and can lead to coma.

Disorders of Thymus Gland

DiGeorge syndrome is a genetic immunodeficiency disorder (*see Chapter 12*) in which the thymus is underdeveloped or absent at birth. Abnormalities of the thymus and parathyroid glands, heart, and facial structure are present, with few or no T lymphocytes. Transplantation of stem cells or thymus tissue can cure the immunodeficiency.

Thymomas, benign tumors, and **thymic carcinomas** are rare tumors that can be associated with myasthenia gravis (*see Chapter 9*) and other autoimmune syndromes, such as lupus erythematosus and rheumatoid arthritis.

Word Analysis and Definition: Disorders of the Parathyroid and Thymus Glands

S = Suffix P = Prefix R = Root R/CF = Combining Form

WORD	PRONUNCIATION		ELEMENTS	DEFINITION
DiGeorge syndrome	dee-**JORJ SIN**-drome	 P/ R/	Angelo M. DiGeorge, 1921–2009, U.S. pediatrician, described syndrome in 1968 **syn-** *together* **-drome** *course*	Congenital absence of the thymus gland
hypercalcemia hypocalcemia	**HIGH**-per-kal-**SEE**-mee-ah **HIGH**-poh-kal-**SEE**-mee-ah	S/ R/ P/ P/	**-emia** *condition of the blood* **calc-** *calcium* **hyper-** *above, excessive* **hypo-** *deficient*	Excessive level of calcium in the blood Deficient levels of calcium in the blood
hyperparathyroidism hypoparathyroidism	**HIGH**-per-pair-ah-**THIGH**-royd-ism **HIGH**-poh-pair-ah-**THIGH**-royd-ism	S/ R/ P/ P/	**-ism** *condition, process* **-thyr-** *an oblong shield* **hyper-** *excessive* **hypo-** *deficient*	Excessive levels of parathyroid hormone Deficient levels of parathyroid hormone
tetany tetanic (adj)	**TET**-ah-nee teh-**TAN**-ik	 S/ R/	Greek *convulsive tension* **-ic** *pertaining to* **tetan-** *tetany, tetanus*	Severe muscle twitches, cramps, and spasms Pertaining to tetany or tetanus
thymoma	thigh-**MOH**-mah	S/ R/	**-oma** *tumor, mass* **thym-** *thymus gland*	Benign tumor of the thymus gland

Disorders of Adrenal Glands

Adrenal cortical hypofunction can be primary when the disorder is in the adrenal cortex (Addison disease) or secondary when there is a lack of ACTH from the pituitary gland.

Addison disease is caused mostly by idiopathic atrophy of the adrenal cortex. Production of the three groups of adrenocortical steroids is diminished or absent:

- **Decreased cortisol production** leads to weakness, fatigue, diminished resistance to stress, increased susceptibility to infection, and weight loss.
- **Decreased aldosterone production** leads to dehydration, decreased circulatory volume, hypotension, and circulatory collapse.

Acute adrenocortical insufficiency in patients with Addison disease is called an **adrenal crisis.** It can be precipitated by an infection or trauma and leads to peripheral vascular collapse and kidney failure.

Adrenal cortical hyperfunction is due to excessive production of the groups of the corticosteroids.

Hypersecretion of glucocorticoids produces **Cushing syndrome** *(Figure 17.18)*. Clinical manifestations include "moon" **facies,** obesity of the trunk, muscle wasting and weakness, osteoporosis, kidney stones, and reduced resistance to infection. Most cases of Cushing syndrome are due to a pituitary tumor secreting too much ACTH, thereby causing the normal adrenal glands to produce too much cortisol.

Often, the symptoms of Cushing syndrome can result from therapeutic administration of excess cortisol medications.

Hypersecretion of aldosterone (aldosteronism, or **Conn syndrome)** leads to sodium retention and potassium loss with increased blood volume, hypertension, excessive thirst, and excessive urination. A benign adenoma (**aldosteronoma**) is the most common cause and can be removed by laparoscopic **adrenalectomy.**

Hypersecretion of androgens is called **adrenal virilism** or **adrenogenital syndrome.** In adult women, manifestations include **hirsutism,** baldness, acne, deepened voice, decreased breast size, and other signs of masculinization. If a tumor is found by CT or MRI scan, it can be removed surgically.

Pheochromocytoma is a tumor of the adrenal medulla that overproduces the catecholamines epinephrine and norepinephrine. It produces marked hypertension that is difficult to control, with severe headaches, tachycardia, palpitations, and feelings of impending death.

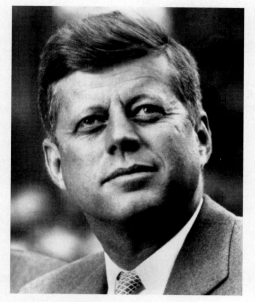

▲ **Figure 17.17** **John F. Kennedy.** Historical/Corbis Historical/Getty Images

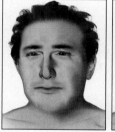 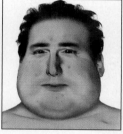

▶ **Figure 17.18** **Cushing syndrome.** (a) Patient before onset of the syndrome. (b) The same person, only 4 months later, showing the "moon face" characteristic of Cushing syndrome. Mikkel Juul Jensen/Science Source

(a)　　**(b)**

Stress Syndrome

There are two types of stress, eustress and distress. Examples of eustress would be getting married or starting a new job. Examples of distress are your financial insecurity, job pressure, etc. Did you know that our body responds to eustress and distress the same way it would if you were under attack from a bear or in a car accident? This is called *"fight or flight"* and it is your body becoming physically prepared for the stress. Regardless of whether the perceived stressor is considered positive, negative, acute fear, or just life pressure; your body responds the same way.

The *general adaptation syndrome (GAS),* developed by Hans Selye, explains the pattern of physiological responses that the body goes through after being exposed to a stressor. There are three stages: alarm, resistance, and exhaustion.

Alarm—This occurs when we first perceive something as stressful, and then the body initiates the fight-or-flight response.

Resistance—If the stress persists, the body stays activated at a higher metabolic level. Our body cannot maintain this level for a long period of time and our resources deplete.

Exhaustion—Prolonged exposure to the stressor will result in the depletion of the body's resources. This will result in suppression of the immune system and cause bodily functions to deteriorate. This can lead to a multiple health issues including heart disease, digestive problems, depression, and diabetes.

WORD	PRONUNCIATION		ELEMENTS	DEFINITION
Addison disease	ADD-ih-son diz-EEZ Thomas Addison, 1793–1860, English physician	P/ R/	dis- *apart* -ease *normal function*	An autoimmune disease leading to decreased production of adrenocortical steroids
adrenalectomy	ah-DREE-nal-EK-toh-mee	S/ S/ P/ R/	-ectomy *surgical excision* -al- *pertaining to* ad- *near, toward* -ren- *kidney* gland *Latin glans, acorn*	Removal of part or all of an adrenal gland
adrenogenital syndrome	ah-DREE-noh-JEN-it-al SIN-drome	S/ R/CF R/ P/ R/	-al *pertaining to* adren/o- *adrenal gland* -genit- *primary male or female sex organs* syn- *together* -drome *course*	Hypersecretion of androgens from the adrenal gland
aldosteronism	al-DOS-ter-ohn-izm	S/ R/CF R/	-ism *condition, process* ald/o- *organic compound* -steron- *steroid*	Condition caused by excessive secretion of aldosterone
aldosteronoma	al-DOS-ter-oh-NOH-mah	S/	-oma *tumor, mass*	Benign adenoma of the adrenal cortex
Conn syndrome (syn)	KON SIN-drome	 P/ R/	Jerome W. Conn, 1907–1981, American endocrinologist syn- *together* -drome *course*	
Cushing syndrome	KUSH-ing SIN-drome	 P/ R/	Harvey Cushing, 1869–1939, American neurosurgeon syn- *together* -drome *course*	Hypersecretion of cortisol (hydrocortisone) by the adrenal cortex
facies	FASH-eez		Latin *appearance*	Facial expression and features characteristic of a specific disease
hirsutism	HER-sue-tizm		Latin *shaggy*	Excessive body and facial hair
pheochromocytoma	fee-oh-KROH-moh-sigh-TOH-mah	S/ P/ R/CF R/	-oma *tumor* pheo- *gray* -chrom/o- *color* -cyt- *cell*	Adenoma of the adrenal medulla secreting excessive catecholamines
virilism	VIR-ih-lizm	S/ R/	-ism *condition, process* viril- *masculine*	Development of masculine characteristics by a woman or girl

Disorders of Pancreatic Hormones: Diabetes Mellitus

Diabetes mellitus (DM) is a syndrome characterized by hyperglycemia resulting from an absolute or relative impairment of insulin secretion and/or insulin action. This leads to a disruption of carbohydrate, fat, and protein metabolism. It is the world's most prevalent metabolic disease and the leading cause of blindness, renal failure, and gangrene. There are four categories of diabetes mellitus:

1. **Type 1 diabetes,** also called **insulin-dependent diabetes mellitus (IDDM),** accounts for 10% to 15% of all cases of DM but is the predominant type of DM under the age of 30. When symptoms become apparent, 90% of the pancreatic insulin-producing cells have been destroyed by **autoantibodies.** The incidence of type 1 diabetes is increased in patients with Graves disease, Hashimoto disease, and Addison disease.

2. **Type 2 diabetes,** also called **non-insulin-dependent diabetes mellitus (NIDDM),** accounts for 90% to 95% of all cases of DM. Almost 7% of U.S. residents are diagnosed with type 2 diabetes, and the incidence is increasing rapidly. Not only is there some impairment of insulin response, but there is decreased insulin effectiveness in stimulating glucose uptake by tissues and in restraining

hepatic glucose production. This is called **insulin resistance.** In addition to type 2 diabetes, insulin resistance leads to other common disorders such as obesity, hypertension, hyperlipidemia, and coronary artery disease. Type 2 diabetes can be secondary to Cushing syndrome, acromegaly, pheochromocytoma, and aldosteronism.

3. **Gestational diabetes** is seen in the latter half of 5% of pregnancies. While most cases of gestational diabetes resolve after the pregnancy, a woman who has this complication of pregnancy has a 30% chance of developing type 2 diabetes within 10 years.

4. **Mature-onset diabetes of youth (MODY)** is genetically inherited, occurs in thin individuals who are in their teens and twenties, and is comparable to type 2 diabetes in its severity.

Hypoglycemia is present when blood glucose is below 70 mg/dL. Hormonal defense mechanisms (glucagon and adrenaline) are activated as the blood glucose drops below 55 mg/dL. Because brain metabolism depends primarily on glucose, the brain is the first organ affected by hypoglycemia. Impaired mental efficiency starts to be seen when the blood glucose falls below 65 mg/dL. It becomes very obvious (shakiness, anxiety, confusion, tremor) around 40 mg/dL, and below that figure seizures can occur. If the blood glucose falls below 10 mg/dL, the neurons become electrically silent, resulting in diabetic **coma.** Symptomatic hypoglycemia is sometimes called **insulin shock.**

Low blood glucose can be raised to normal in minutes by taking 3 to 4 ounces of orange, apple, or grape juice. Symptoms should begin to improve in 5 minutes, with full recovery in 10 to 15 minutes. In an emergency, if the patient is not able to take oral sugar, treatment is begun with a rapid IV **bolus** of 25 mL of 50% glucose solution, followed by an intravenous infusion of glucose.

Word Analysis and Definition: Diabetes Mellitus

S = Suffix P = Prefix R = Root R/CF = Combining Form

WORD	PRONUNCIATION	ELEMENTS		DEFINITION
autoantibody	aw-toh-**AN**-tee-bod-ee	P/ P/ R/	**auto-** *self, same* **-anti-** *against* **-body** *body*	Antibody produced in response to an antigen from the host's own tissue
bolus	**BOH**-lus		Greek *a lump*	Single mass of a substance
coma	**KOH**-mah		Greek *deep sleep*	State of deep unconsciousness
diabetes mellitus	die-ah-**BEE**-teez **MEL**-ih-tus		**diabetes** Greek *a siphon* **mellitus** Latin *sweetened with honey*	Metabolic syndrome caused by absolute or relative insulin deficiency and/or insulin ineffectiveness
diabetic (adj)	die-ah-**BET**-ik	S/ R/	**-ic** *pertaining to* **diabet-** *diabetes*	Pertaining to or suffering from diabetes
hypoglycemia	**HIGH**-poh-glie-**SEE**-mee-ah	S/ P/ R/	**-emia** *blood condition* **hypo-** *below, deficient* **-glyc-** *glucose*	Low level of glucose (sugar) in the blood
hypoglycemic (adj)	**HIGH**-poh-glie-**SEE**-mik	S/	**-emic** *in the blood*	Pertaining to or suffering from hypoglycemia

Diabetes Mellitus—Hyperglycemia

The classic symptoms of **hyperglycemia** are polyuria (excessive urination), **polydipsia** (excessive thirst), and **polyphagia** (excessive hunger), with unexplained weight loss.

Symptomatic hyperglycemia is how type 1 diabetes usually presents. Type 2 diabetes can be symptomatic or asymptomatic and is often found during a routine health examination.

Because of high glucose levels, hyperglycemia damages capillary endothelial cells in the retina and renal glomerulus and neurons and neurolemmocytes in peripheral nerves. Of all diabetics, 85% develop some degree of diabetic retinopathy, while 30% develop diabetic nephropathy, which can progress to end-stage renal disease *(see Chapter 6).* Diabetic neuropathy causes sensory defects with numbness, tingling, and **paresthesias** in the stocking-glove (feet-hands) distribution.

In larger blood vessels, the hyperglycemia contributes to endothelial cell lining damage and atherosclerosis. Coronary artery disease and peripheral vascular disease with claudication *(see Chapter 10)* are complications. Hyperglycemia is the most common cause of foot ulcers followed by gangrene of the lower extremity, sometimes necessitating amputation. The risk of infection is increased by the cellular hyperglycemia and the circulatory deficits.

The complications of hyperglycemia can be kept at bay by strict control of blood glucose levels.

Diabetic ketoacidosis (DKA) is a state of marked hyperglycemia with dehydration, **metabolic acidosis,** and **ketone formation.** It is seen mostly in type 1 diabetes and is usually the result of a lapse in insulin treatment, acute infection, or trauma that renders the usual insulin treatment inadequate.

DKA presents with polyuria, vomiting, and lethargy and can progress to coma. **Acetone** (a ketone) can be smelled on the breath. Diabetic ketoacidosis is a medical emergency and requires rapid fluid volume expansion, correction of hyperglycemia, prevention of hypokalemia, and treatment of any infection. There is a 2% to 5% mortality from circulatory collapse.

Diabetic coma, a severe medical emergency, has three causes, which have been described earlier:

- **Diabetic ketoacidosis (DKA).**
- **Hyperglycemia** with dehydration, but not the ketosis and acidosis of DKA. This condition is called **hyperosmolar coma.**
- **Hypoglycemic coma.** A blood glucose test will differentiate hypoglycemia from the other two causes.

Word Analysis and Definition: Diabetes Mellitus—Hyperglycemia

S = Suffix P = Prefix R = Root R/CF = Combining Form

WORD	PRONUNCIATION	ELEMENTS		DEFINITION
acetone	**ASS**-eh-tone		Latin *vinegar*	Ketone that is found in blood, urine, and breath when diabetes mellitus is out of control
hyperglycemia	**HIGH**-per-glie-**SEE**-mee-ah	S/ P/ R/	-emia *blood condition* hyper- *above* -glyc- *glucose*	High level of glucose (sugar) in blood
hyperglycemic (adj)	**HIGH**-per-glie-**SEE**-mik	S/	-emic *in the blood*	Pertaining to high blood sugar
hyperosmolar	**HIGH**-per-os-**MOH**-lar	S/ P/ R/	-ar *pertaining to* hyper- *above* -osmol- *concentration*	Marked hyperglycemia without ketoacidosis
ketoacidosis	**KEY**-toh-ass-ih-**DOH**-sis	S/ R/CF R/	-osis *condition* ket/o- *ketone* -acid- *acid*	Excessive production of ketones, making the blood acid
ketone	**KEY**-tone		Greek *acetone*	Chemical formed in uncontrolled diabetes or in starvation
ketosis (**Note:** With the "o" in ket/o- preceding the "o" in -osis, one "o" drops out for simpler pronunciation.)	key-**TOH**-sis	S/ R/	-osis *condition* ket- *ketone*	Excessive production of ketones
metabolic acidosis	met-ah-**BOL**-ik ass-ih-**DOH**-sis	S/ R/ S/ R/	-ic *pertaining to* metabol- *change* -osis *condition* acid- *acid*	Decreased pH in blood and body tissues as a result of an upset in metabolism
paresthesia paresthesias (pl)	par-es-**THEE**-zee-ah par-es-**THEE**-zee-as	S/ P/ R/	-ia *condition* par- *abnormal* -esthes- *sensation*	An abnormal sensation; for example, tingling, burning, pricking
polydipsia	pol-ee-**DIP**-see-ah	S/ P/ R/	-ia *condition* poly- *many, much* -dips- *thirst*	Excessive thirst
polyphagia	pol-ee-**FAY**-jee-ah	S/ P/ R/	-ia *condition* poly- *many, much* -phag- *to eat*	Excessive eating

A. After reading Case Report (CR) 17.1, answer the following questions. *Fill in the blanks with the correct answer or choose the correct letter(s) for the multiple-choice questions.* **LO 17.5, 17.6, 17.7**

 ## Case Report (CR) 17.1

You are

. . . a registered nurse (**RN**) working with endocrinologist Sabina Khalid, MD, in the Endocrinology Clinic at Fulwood Medical Center.

Your patient is

. . . Mrs. Gina Tacher, a 33-year-old schoolteacher. She complains of coarsening of her facial features and enlargement of the bones of her hands. Over the past 10 years, her nose and jaw have increased in size, and her voice has become husky. She brought photos of herself at ages 9 and 16. She has no other health problems.

Dr. Khalid's examination of Mrs. Gina Tacher showed a protruding mandible (**prognathism**) and an enlarged, deeply grooved tongue. Her feet and hands were enlarged. She had noticed an increase in her shoe size and an inability to remove her wedding band. Her ribs were thickened, her heart was enlarged, and her blood pressure (**BP**) was 140/90. Her body hair was dark and coarse, and she was sweating freely.

X-rays showed a thickened skull with enlarged nasal sinuses and thickened terminal phalanges of her hands. A diagnosis of **acromegaly** was made.

Computed tomography (**CT**) and magnetic resonance imaging (**MRI**) scans showed a tumor in the pituitary that occupies most of the sella turcica *(see Chapter 5)*.

Blood tests showed high levels of growth hormone and **insulin-like growth factor (IGF)**.

---

1. What is the medical term for *protruding mandible*? _____

2. Which of the following are the signs (observable on the outside) that Mrs. Tacher is exhibiting? (Choose all that apply.)
   a. protruding mandible
   b. observed sweating
   c. increase in shoe size
   d. enlarged heart
   e. change in voice

3. Which of the following are the symptoms (felt by the patient)? (Choose all that apply.)
   a. protruding mandible
   b. observed sweating
   c. increase in shoe size
   d. enlarged heart
   e. change in voice

4. Was her blood pressure elevated?
   a. Yes
   b. No

5. Which of the following are the diagnostic tests used by her physician to determine a disorder? (Choose all that apply.)
   a. change in shoe size
   b. CT scan
   c. tongue appearance
   d. blood tests
   e. MRI

6. In the diagnosis **acromegaly,** which element means *enlargement*? _____

_____

7. Why wasn't her condition considered to be gigantism?
   a. Gigantism is caused by another hormone.
   b. People with gigantism do not have enlarged feet.
   c. Her disorder occurred after puberty.
   d. Acromegaly only occurs in females.

8. Mrs. Tacher's acromegaly was caused by:
   a. cancer of her hypothalamus
   b. inappropriate diet
   c. decreased production of ADH
   d. tumor of her anterior pituitary gland

B. After reading Case Report (CR) 17.2, answer the following questions. LO 17.6, 17.8

 Case Report (CR) 17.2

You are

. . . an emergency medical technician (**EMT**) working in the Emergency Room at Fulwood Medical Center at 0200 hours.

Your patient is

. . . Ms. Norma Leary, a 22-year-old college student living with her parents for the summer.

Ms. Leary is **emaciated,** extremely agitated, restless, and at times disoriented and confused. Her parents tell you that, in the past 3 or 4 days, she has been coughing and not feeling well. In the past 12 hours, she has become feverish and been complaining of a left-sided chest pain. With questioning, the parents reveal that prior to this acute illness, she had lost about 20 pounds in weight, although she was eating voraciously. Her vital signs (VS) are T 105.2°F, P 180 and irregular, R 24, BP 160/85.

You call for Dr. Hilinski **STAT** (immediately). On his initial examination, he believes that the patient is in **thyroid storm.** This is a medical emergency. There are no immediate laboratory tests that can confirm this diagnosis.

1. Someone who appears **emaciated** is:

   a. obese

   b. sleepy

   c. rude

   d. thin

2. Which of the following are *signs* that a disorder is present? (choose all that apply)

   a. agitation

   b. not feeling well

   c. pain

   d. increased body temperature

   e. rapid respirations

3. Which of the following are *symptoms* felt by Ms. Leary?

   a. agitation

   b. not feeling well

   c. pain

   d. increased body temperature

   e. rapid respirations

4. What is her diagnosed condition? (choose all that apply)

   a. diabetes insipidus

   b. thyroid storm

   c. dyspnea

   d. bradycardia

   e. osteoporosis

5. Which of the following terms in the Case Report means *immediately*:

   a. feverish

   b. voraciously

   c. disoriented

   d. irregular

   e. STAT

6. *Thyroid storm* is due to:

   a. excessive thyroid hormones

   b. increased somatostatin

   c. shrinking isthmus

   d. decreased blood iodine

C. Elements: One word or phrase in each of the descriptions in the following questions is in bold. *This is your clue to finding the correct medical term in the word bank. Fill in the blanks with the language of endocrinology.* **LO 17.6**

thyroiditis	euthyroid	antithyroid	exophthalmos
thyrotoxicosis	hyperthyroidism	myxedema	

1. **Excessive production** of thyroid hormones: _____

2. **Swelling** with a waxy substance: _____

3. **Inhibition** of production of thyroid hormone: _____

4. **Normal** thyroid function: _____

5. **Inflammation** of the thyroid gland: _____

6. **Protrusion** of the eyeball: _____

D. Language of endocrinology: The meaning of a word element never changes, regardless of the term that contains it. *Demonstrate your knowledge of word elements by making the correct choice in the following multiple-choice questions.* **LO 17.6**

1. On the basis of its suffix, an **aldosteronoma** is a
   - **a.** condition
   - **b.** facial hair
   - **c.** tumor
   - **d.** facial expression
   - **e.** gland

2. In the term **pheochromocytoma,** the prefix is one of
   - **a.** size
   - **b.** shape
   - **c.** direction
   - **d.** color
   - **e.** gender

3. Select the term with a root that means *masculine:*
   - **a.** hirsutism
   - **b.** aldosteronism
   - **c.** facies
   - **d.** virilism
   - **e.** aldosteronoma

4. The suffix in this term means *surgical excision:*
   - **a.** adrenalectomy
   - **b.** virilism
   - **c.** aldosteronoma
   - **d.** facies
   - **e.** pheochromocytoma

E. Discuss the stress response. *Place the events of the stress response in the correct order starting with A for the first stage and C for the last stage.* **LO 17.1**

_____ **1.** body uses alternative metabolic pathways to produce glucose

_____ **2.** fight or flight response is initiated and glucose is released

_____ **3.** glycogen and fat stores are depleted

F. Diabetes is the world's most prevalent metabolic disease. *Many patients have diabetes as a concurrent condition with other health problems— which always makes it a consideration in treatment and prescribing medications. Test your knowledge of this disease by answering the following questions. Choose the correct answer.* **LO 17.6**

1. Diabetes mellitus is the leading cause of
   - **a.** blindness
   - **b.** hypotension
   - **c.** hemorrhage
   - **d.** kidney stones
   - **e.** reflux disease

2. The first organ affected by hypoglycemia is the
   - **a.** kidney
   - **b.** heart
   - **c.** pancreas
   - **d.** brain
   - **e.** liver

3. The predominant type of diabetes mellitus in patients under the age of 30 is
   - **a.** type 1
   - **b.** type 2
   - **c.** non-insulin-dependent DM
   - **d.** gestational diabetes type 3

4. Impairment of insulin response and decreased insulin effectiveness are termed insulin
   - **a.** production
   - **b.** resistance
   - **c.** autoantibodies
   - **d.** control
   - **e.** conversion

5. Most cases of gestational diabetes resolve after
   - **a.** medication
   - **b.** treatment
   - **c.** testing
   - **d.** delivery
   - **e.** surgery

6. Symptomatic hypoglycemia is sometimes called
   - **a.** insulin resistance
   - **b.** coma
   - **c.** insulin shock
   - **d.** glucolysis
   - **e.** bolus

7. Type 1 diabetes is also known as

    a. IDDM   **b.** NIDDM   **c.** hypoglycemia   **d.** hyperglycemia   **e.** coma

8. Insulin resistance can lead to

    a. obesity   **b.** aldosteronoma   **c.** hirsutism   **d.** myxedema   **e.** virilism

9. Low blood glucose can be raised to normal with a

    a. vitamin   **b.** hormone   **c.** enzyme   **d.** carbohydrate   **e.** electrolyte

10. What can raise blood glucose levels in type 2 diabetes?

    a. stress   **b.** dehydration   **c.** nausea   **d.** coughing   **e.** vomiting

G. Answer the following questions. *Fill in the blanks.* **LO 17.6**

1. **Hyperglycemic** means that the level of _____ is too high in the patient's blood.

2. **Hyperosmolar coma** is the same thing as _____.

H. Translate the explanation of a condition into the medical term it is describing. *As a health care provider, you will need to be able to correctly interpret conditions into a medical term. You will need to be able to correctly spell the term. Fill in the blanks.* **LO 17.3, 17.6**

1. The abbreviation for the condition that has the signs of ketone formation, metabolic acidosis, and marked hyperglycemia: _____

2. Excessive thirst: _____

3. Excessive urination: _____

4. Pertaining to high sugar in the blood: _____

5. Condition of excess ketones: _____

6. Excessive eating: _____ .

7. Condition of excess ketones causing the blood to be acidic: _____

Section 17.3 Procedures and Pharmacology

Diagnostic and Therapeutic Procedures for Disorders of the Pituitary Gland

Diagnostic Procedures

Visual field tests can show the presence of a **pituitary tumor** as the tumor presses on the **optic chiasma** (*see Figure 16.11*), causing loss of vision in the peripheral visual fields.

Levels of pituitary hormones in the blood and/or urine can be measured directly to show the presence of a hormone-producing pituitary **adenoma.**

Examples are the levels of **growth hormone** and **insulin-like growth factor-1** (IGF-1). When growth hormone levels are high, they cause the liver to produce more IGF-1. When both levels are very high, a pituitary tumor is the diagnosis. If the levels are only slightly increased, a **glucose suppression test** is performed. Ingestion of a large amount of sugar normally leads to a drop in growth hormone levels. If growth hormones remain high, a pituitary adenoma is the cause. High levels of growth hormone are found in gigantism, beginning in children, and acromegaly, beginning in adults.

Blood **prolactin** levels can be measured to check for a prolactinoma; **ACTH (corticotropin)** levels help distinguish ACTH-secreting pituitary tumors from adrenal gland tumors: **TSH (thyrotropin)** levels usually identify thyrotropin-secreting adenomas.

Diabetes insipidus, caused by failure in production of **ADH (antidiuretic hormone)** by the hypothalamus or by failure of the posterior pituitary to release it due to an adenoma, is diagnosed primarily by measurement of the amount of urine and its **osmolality.**

Magnetic resonance imaging (MRI) can show pituitary tumors greater than 3 mm across.

Biopsy of the tumor is sometimes needed to make a firm diagnosis. When pituitary tumors are removed surgically, they are always examined under a microscope to confirm the exact diagnosis.

Therapeutic Procedures

Surgical removal of a pituitary tumor is necessary if the tumor is pressing on the optic nerves or if it is overproducing hormones. In 99% of cases, this is performed by an **endoscopic transnasal transsphenoidal approach** in which the surgery is performed through the nose and sphenoid sinus using an **endoscope. Craniotomy,** in which a very large tumor is removed through the upper part of the skull, is occasionally necessary. The surgery can be made more efficient by using **image-guided stereotactic surgery** in which advanced computers create a three-dimensional image of the tumor to guide the surgeon.

Radiation therapy can be used alone, after surgery, or if the tumor persists or returns after surgery. Methods of radiation therapy include:

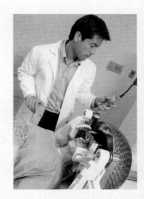

▲ **Figure 17.19** Gamma **knife.** Cathy Yeulet/123RF

- **Gamma Knife stereotactic radiosurgery** *(Figure 17.19),* which delivers a single high-dose radiation beam the size and shape of the tumor using special brain-imaging techniques.

- **Proton beam therapy,** which delivers positively charged ions (protons) rather than x-rays in beams that are finely controlled with minimal risk to surrounding healthy tissues.

- **External beam radiation,** which delivers x-rays in small increments, usually five times a week over a four- to six-week period. It may damage surrounding healthy pituitary and brain tissues.

Medications and Hormone Replacement Therapy

Medications can help to block excessive hormone secretion and sometimes reduce pituitary tumor size:

- **Growth hormone-secreting tumors** have two types of drugs used if surgery has been unsuccessful in normalizing growth hormone production. **Somatostatin analogs** *(Sandostatin, Somatuline Depot)* cause a decrease in growth hormone production and are given by injection every four weeks. The second type, **pegvisomant** *(Somavert),* blocks the effect of excess growth hormone, is given by daily injection, and may cause liver damage.

- **Prolactin-secreting tumors (prolactinomas)** are treated with two drugs, **cabergoline** *(Dostinex)* and **bromocriptine** *(Parlodel),* that decrease prolactin secretion, but they can have serious side effects, including developing compulsive behaviors.

Pituitary hormone replacement therapy is needed after surgery or radiation therapy to maintain normal hormone levels. The medication taken depends on the hormones that need to be replaced, which include adrenocorticotropic hormone (ACTH), thyroxine, estrogen and progesterone, testosterone, antidiuretic hormone (ADH), and synthetic growth hormones. Treatment of diabetes insipidus is with vasopressin or desmopressin, synthetic modified forms of ADH. They are taken as a nasal spray several times daily, the dose being adjusted to maintain a normal urine output.

WORD	PRONUNCIATION		ELEMENTS	DEFINITION
adenoma	AD-eh-NOH-mah	S/ R/	-oma *tumor* aden- *gland*	A benign neoplasm of epithelial tissue
analog	AN-ah-log		Greek *proportionate*	A compound that resembles another in structure but not in function; analog is a means of the transmission of continuous information to our senses, in contrast with the digital transmission of only zeros and ones
biopsy (*Note:* the extra "o" is dropped.)	BIE-op-see	S/ R/	-opsy *to view* bi- *life*	Process of removing tissue from living patients for microscopic examination
chiasm chiasma (alt)	KIE-asm kie-AZ-mah		Greek *cross*	X-shaped crossing of the two optic nerves at the base of the brain
craniotomy	kray-nee-OT-oh-mee	S/ R/	-tomy *incision* crani/o- *cranium*	Incision of the skull
endoscope endoscopic (adj)	EN-doh-skope EN-doh-SKOP-ik	P/ R/ S/	endo- *inside* -scope *instrument for viewing* -ic *pertaining to*	Instrument for viewing the inside of a tubular or hollow organ Pertaining to an endoscope.
gamma knife	GAM-ah NIFE		**gamma** *third letter in Greek alphabet* **knife** Old English *knife*	A minimally invasive radiosurgical system
optic	OP-tik	S/ R/	-ic *pertaining to* opt- *vision*	Pertaining to the eye
osmolality	OZ-moh-LAL-ih-tee	S/ S/ R/	-ity *state* -al- *pertaining to* osmol- *concentration*	The concentration of a solution
proton	PROH-ton		Greek *first*	The positively charged unit of the nuclear mass
stereotactic	STER-ee-oh-TAK-tik	S/ R/CF R/	-ic *pertaining to* stere/o *three-dimensional* -tact- *orderly arrangement*	Pertaining to a precise three-dimensional method to locate a lesion or a tumor
transnasal	trans-NAY-zal	S/ P/ R/	-al *pertaining to* trans- *across, through* -nas- *nose*	Through the nose
transsphenoid	trans-SFEE-noyd	S/ P/ R/	-oid *resembling* trans- *through* -sphen- *wedge*	Through the sphenoid sinus
tumor	TOO-mer		Latin *swelling*	Any abnormal swelling

Diagnostic and Therapeutic Procedures for Disorders of the Thyroid Gland

Diagnostic Procedures

Thyroid-stimulating hormone (TSH) levels in the blood are low if the gland is overactive.

Thyroid hormone levels in the blood detail the activity of the gland; the levels are high if the gland is overactive.

Antithyroid antibodies are associated with autoimmune inflammatory diseases of the thyroid.

Isotopic thyroid scans detail the nature of the thyroid enlargement and the function of the gland.

Serum calcitonin level is elevated in medullary carcinoma.

Fine needle aspiration biopsy distinguishes benign from malignant nodules.

Ultrasonography reveals the size of the gland and the presence of nodules.

Therapeutic Procedures

Radioactive iodine (I-131) therapy uses the **isotope** of iodine that emits radiation to treat hyperthyroidism and thyroid cancer. When a small dose of the isotope is swallowed, it is absorbed into the bloodstream, taken up from the blood, and concentrated by the cells of the thyroid gland, where it begins destroying the gland's cells.

Hypothyroidism, in most cases, can be treated adequately with a constant daily dose of **levothyroxine (LT4).** For hypothyroidism due to destruction of thyroid cells, **TSH** levels are monitored. For central (pituitary or hypothalamic) hypothyroidism, **T** levels are used for monitoring.

Thyroid surgery is indicated for a variety of conditions including **cancerous** and **benign nodules, goiters,** and **overactive thyroid glands.** The types of surgery that can be performed include:

- **Excisional biopsy:** removal of a small part of the gland.
- **Hemilobectomy:** removal of half of the thyroid gland.
- **Total thyroidectomy:** removal of all thyroid tissue.
- **Near-total thyroidectomy:** removal of all but a very small part of the gland.
- **Endoscopic thyroidectomy:** performed through a single small incision using a flexible lighted tube and video monitor to guide the surgical procedure.
- **Laser ablation:** a minimally invasive procedure used to remove benign thyroid nodules using ultrasound guidance without affecting the surrounding organ.

Thyroid Pharmacology

Antithyroid medications prevent formation of thyroid hormones in the gland's cells.

Propylthiouracil and **methimazole** both decrease the amount of thyroid hormone produced by the gland's cells and can be used to treat hyperthyroidism. Unfortunately, they both have the major and frequent side effects of agranulocytosis and aplastic anemia and are no longer recognized as a front-line medication.

Thyroid replacements are:

- L-thyroxine. This synthetic T_4 is a preferred replacement.
- Liothyronine sodium. This synthetic T_3 has a rapid turnover and must be monitored frequently.

Word Analysis and Definition: Diagnostic and Therapeutic Procedures for Disorders of the Thyroid Gland

S = Suffix P = Prefix R = Root R/CF = Combining Form

WORD	PRONUNCIATION		ELEMENTS	DEFINITION
ablation	ab-**LAY**-shun	S/ R/	-ion *process* ablat- *take away*	Removal of tissue to destroy its function
aspiration	**AS**-pih-**RAY**-shun	S/ R/	-ion *process* aspirat- *breathe in*	Removal by suction of fluid or gas from a body cavity
isotope isotopic (adj)	**EYE**-so-tope	P/ R/ S/ R/	iso- *equal* -tope *part* -ic *pertaining to* -top- *part*	Radioactive element; some of these elements are used in diagnostic procedures Of identical chemical composition
lobectomy	loh-**BEK**-toh-mee	S/ R/	-ectomy *surgical excision* lob- *lobe*	Surgical removal of a lobe of the lungs or the thyroid gland
lymphadenectomy	lim-**FAD**-eh-**NEK**-toh-mee	S/ R/	-ectomy *surgical excision* lymphaden- *lymph node*	Surgical excision of a lymph node
radioactive iodine	**RAY**-dee-oh-**AK**-tiv **EYE**-oh-dine	S/ R/CF R/	-ive *pertaining to* radi/o- *radiation* -act- *performance* iodine *nonmetallic element*	Any of the various tracers that emit alpha, beta, or gamma rays
ultrasonography	**UL**-trah-soh-**NOG**-rah-fee	S/ P/ R/CF	-graphy *recording* ultra- *beyond* son/o- *sound*	Delineation of deep structures using sound waves

Therapeutic Procedures for the Parathyroid and Thymus Glands

Parathyroid Glands

Parathyroid gland disorders are diagnosed by blood tests calcium and vitamin D levels.

Hyperparathyroidism

Watchful waiting, surgery to remove enlarged parathyroid glands Surgical removal of the enlarged gland is **curative.**

- **Calcimimetics** such as cinacalcet (*Sensipar*) trick the parathyroid gland into thinking there is more calcium in the blood than there actually is, decreasing secretion of PTH.
- **Vitamin D supplements** if blood levels of vitamin D are low.

Hypoparathyroidism

- high-dose calcium and vitamin D supplements.
- A genetically engineered recombinant form of PTH

Thymus

DiGeorge syndrome—Transplantation of stem cells or thymus tissue is curative.
Thymectomy—Thymomas or thymic carcinomas followed by **adjuvant** radiotherapy.

Word Analysis and Definition: Therapeutic Procedures for Disorders of the Parathyroid and Thymus Glands

S = Suffix P = Prefix R = Root R/CF = Combining Form

WORD	PRONUNCIATION	ELEMENTS		DEFINITION
adjuvant	**AD**-joo-vant	S/ R/	-ant *pertaining to* adjuv- *give help*	Additional treatment after a primary treatment has been used
curative	**KYUR**-ah-tiv	S/ R/	-ive *quality of* curat- *to care for*	That which heals or cures
mimetic calcimimetic	mi-**MET**-ick kal-sih-mi-**MET**-ick	S/ R/ R/	Greek *imitate* -tic *pertaining to* calc/i- *calcium* -mime- *imitate*	Imitate Substance that imitates calcium
thymectomy	thigh-**MEK**-toh-mee	S/ R/	-ectomy *surgical excision* thym- *thymus gland*	Surgical removal of the thymus gland

Diagnostic and Therapeutic Procedures for Disorders of the Adrenal Glands

Diagnostic Procedures

Congenital adrenal hyperplasia can be diagnosed in the fetus using amniocentesis and chorionic villus sampling (*see Chapter 8*) and in the newborn through a heel stick to obtain a blood sample. The test detects elevated levels of 17-hydroxy-progesterone (17-HP) and, as with all screening tests, a confirmatory test(s) has to be performed. Treatment can then be started in the womb or immediately after birth.

   Cushing syndrome can be confirmed with three tests: elevated cortisol levels in saliva, elevated cortisol levels in 24-hour urine, and suppression of cortisol production by the synthetic steroid dexamethasone.

Addison disease can be diagnosed based on routine blood tests showing hypercalcemia, hypoglycemia, hyponatremia, and hyperkalemia; the diagnosis is confirmed by the ACTH stimulation test, in which the synthetic pituitary ACTH hormone **tetracosactide** fails to stimulate the production of cortisol.

Pheochromocytoma is diagnosed by measuring **catecholamines** and **metanephrines** in plasma or by 24-hour urinary collection. CT scan or MRI can localize the tumor.

Hyperaldosteronism (Conn syndrome) is diagnosed by high levels of aldosterone and low levels of potassium in blood or urine tests. CT scan or MRI can locate the tumor in the adrenal gland.

Therapeutic Procedures

Congenital adrenal hyperplasia, when diagnosed in a female fetus, can require the pregnant mother to take a **corticosteroid** drug such as **dexamethasone** during pregnancy. This drug crosses the placenta to reduce the secretion of the fetal male hormones and allow the female genitals to develop normally. When diagnosed in childhood, dexamethasone or hydrocortisone are needed daily, and in some infant girls who have **ambiguous external genitalia,** reconstructive surgery to correct the appearance and function of the **genitals** is performed.

Addison disease is daily hydrocortisone **by mouth (PO).** Additionally, fluorocortisone is given PO to replace aldosterone. **Intercurrent** infections require that the hydrocortisone dose be doubled.

Pheochromocytoma is treated with surgery to remove the adrenal tumor, usually by **laparoscopic** surgery.

Adrenal cortical carcinomas or benign adenomas are usually treated with surgery.

Medications and Hormone Replacement Therapy

The **adrenal medulla** secretes **epinephrine (adrenaline).** The **adrenal cortex** synthesizes **steroids** from cholesterol. The outer zona glomerulosa secretes **mineralocorticoids,** which regulate salt and water metabolism (aldosterone) by affecting excretory organs such as the kidney, colon, salivary glands, sweat glands, and brain. The middle zona fasciculate synthesizes **glucocorticoids,** which regulate normal metabolism and resistance to stress (cortisol) by affecting every organ in the body including the brain. The inner zona reticularis secretes adrenal **androgens** that control the development and activity of the male sex organs and male secondary sex characteristics. Androgens are the precursor of all **estrogens.** The primary androgen is testosterone, present in males and females.

Word Analysis and Definition: Adrenal Procedures and Pharmacology				
				S = Suffix P = Prefix R = Root R/CF = Combining Form
WORD	**PRONUNCIATION**		**ELEMENTS**	**DEFINITION**
ambiguous	am-**BIG**-you-us		Latin *to wander*	Uncertain
androgen	**AN**-droh-jen	S/ R/CF	-gen *to produce* andr/o- *male*	Hormone that produces masculine characteristics
cortex	**KOR**-teks		Latin *outer covering*	Outer portion of an organ
genital	**JEN**-ih-tal	S/ R/	-al *pertaining to* genit- *primary male or female sex organs*	Relating to the primary male or female sex organs
hyperplasia	high-per-**PLAY**-zee-ah	S/ P/ R/	-ia *condition* hyper- *excessive* -plas- *formation*	Increase in the number of cells in a tissue or organ
intercurrent	**IN**-ter-**KUR**-ent	S/ P/ R/	-ent *end result, pertaining to* inter- *among, between* -curr- *to run*	A disease attacking a person who already has another disease
medulla	meh-**DULL**-ah		Latin *marrow*	Central part of a structure surrounded by cortex
steroid	**STER**-oyd	S/ R/	-oid *resemble* ster- *solid*	Large family of chemical substances found in hormones, body components, and drugs

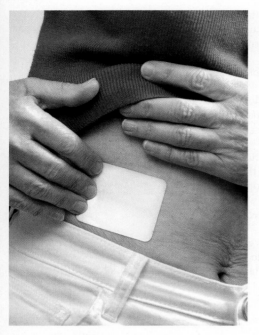

Hormone replacement therapy (HRT) (also called hormone therapy or HT) uses estrogen and progestin to treat symptoms of menopause *(see Chapter 8).* HRT comes as a tablet, patch *(Figure 17.20),* injection, vaginal cream, or vaginal ring; protects against osteoporosis *(see Chapter 14);* and reduces the risk for uterine cancer, but it may increase the risk for blood clots, breast cancer, heart disease, stroke, and gallstones. At this time, short-term (up to 5 years) use of HRT given in the lowest possible dose to treat the symptoms of menopause appears to be safe for many women.

Estrogen makes hormone-receptor-positive breast cancers *(see Chapter 8)* grow. HRT medications treat hormone-receptor-positive breast cancers by lowering the amount of estrogen in the body and/or blocking the action of estrogen on breast cancer cells. They are used after surgery to help slow the growth of advanced-stage or metastatic hormone-receptor-positive breast cancers. There are three main types of HRT agents:

- **Aromatase inhibitors (AIs),** which stop the production of estrogen from androgen in post-menopausal women. These medications are anastrozole *(Arimidex),* exemestane *(Aromasin),* and letrozole *(Femara).* Each is given in a pill form taken once a day. Anastrozole and letrozole are available in generic form.

- **Selective estrogen receptor modulators (SERMs),** which block estrogen in the estrogen receptors of breast cells so that the cells can't grow and multiply. The SERMs are tamoxifen *(Nolvadex),* raloxifene *(Evista),* and toremifene *(Fareston).*

- **Estrogen-receptor downregulators (ERDs)** act just like SERMs, sitting in the receptors of breast cells to block estrogen. Fulvestrant *(Faslodex)* is the only approved ERD at this time.

▲ **Figure 17.20** Hormone replacement patch (HRT). AJ Photo/Science Source

Word Analysis and Definition: Adrenal Procedures and Pharmacology

S = Suffix P = Prefix R = Root R/CF = Combining Form

WORD	PRONUNCIATION	ELEMENTS		DEFINITION
aromatase	ah-**ROH**-mah-taze	S/	-ase *enzyme*	An enzyme responsible for a key step in the production of estrogens from androgens
		R/	aromat- *spice*	
aromatase inhibitor	ah-**ROH**-mah-taze in-**HIB**-ih-tor	S/	-or *a doer*	An agent that stops the production of estrogen in post-menopausal women
		R/	inhibit- *repress*	
estrogen	**ES**-troh-jen	S/	-gen *produce, create*	Generic term for hormones that stimulate female secondary sex characteristics
		R/CF	estr/o- *woman*	
modulator	mod-you-**LAY**-tor		Latin *to measure off properly*	An agent that regulates or adjusts

Diagnosis and Treatment of Diabetes Mellitus

Criteria for the Diagnosis of Diabetes Mellitus

The accepted **criteria** for the diagnosis of diabetes mellitus (DM) include either a fasting (8 hours) plasma glucose of 126 mg/dL or greater; or symptoms (polyuria, polydipsia, polyphagia, unexplained weight loss) and a random plasma glucose of 200 mg/dL or higher.

Treatment of Diabetes Mellitus

The basic principle of diabetes treatment is to avoid hyperglycemia and hypoglycemia. The following are the areas of treatment:

- **Diet and exercise.** To achieve weight reduction of 2 pounds per week in overweight type 2 patients is essential. For insulin-treated diabetics, detailed diet management restricts variations in timing, size, and content of meals.

- **Patient education.** Patients are taught to understand the disease process, to recognize the indications for seeking immediate medical care, and to follow a regimen of foot care.
- **Plasma glucose monitoring.** This is an essential skill that all diabetics must learn. Patients on insulin must learn to adjust their insulin doses. Home glucose analyzers use a drop of blood obtained by a spring-powered lancet from the fingertip or forearm. The frequency of testing is varied individually. As a rule, insulin-treated patients should test their plasma glucose before meals, 2 hours after meals, and at bedtime.
- **Continuous glucose monitor (CGM)** *(Figure 17.21)*. The device measures glucose levels through the skin. A transmitter worn over the skin sends a signal to an app that displays glucose levels.
- **Routine physician visits.** The patient is assessed for symptoms or signs of complications. Skin condition, pulses, and sensation in feet are tested. Urine is tested for **microalbuminuria** by using **immunoassays.** This detects smaller increases in urinary albumin than does conventional urine testing.
- **Periodic laboratory evaluation.** This includes **blood urea nitrogen (BUN)** and serum creatinine (kidney function), lipid profile, electrocardiogram (**ECG**), and an annual complete ophthalmologic evaluation.

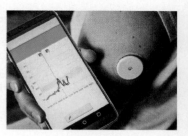

▲ **Figure 17.21** Continuous glucose monitor.
dzikamrowka/123RF

   Glycosylated hemoglobin (Hb A1c) is used to monitor plasma glucose control during the preceding 1 to 3 months. It is formed at rates that increase with plasma glucose levels. Normal Hb A1c is less than 6%. In poor control, the value is 9% to 12%. It is also part of a periodic laboratory evaluation.

   Fructosamine is formed by glucose combining with plasma protein and reflects plasma glucose control over the preceding 1 to 3 weeks. A standard reference range for this test is not available.

   Insulin preparations routinely contain 100 units (U/mL) (**U-100 insulin**). The insulin is injected subcutaneously by using disposable syringes that hold 0.5 mL. In addition, already prepared mixtures of intermediate and regular insulins in different ratios are available. An **insulin pen** is an injection device that holds several days' dosage.

   Continuous subcutaneous insulin infusion is given by a battery-powered, programmable pump that provides continuous insulin through a small needle in the abdominal wall.

Pharmacology of Diabetes Mellitus

Oral antidiabetic drugs are used for type 2 but not type 1 diabetes. These drugs include:

- **Metformin,** which acts by decreasing hepatic glucose production. It also promotes weight loss and decreases lipid levels. It is **synergistic** in combination with sulfonylureas.
- **Sulfonylureas,** which act by stimulating the beta cells to secrete insulin.

Word Analysis and Definition: Diabetes Mellitus Procedures and Pharmacology

S = Suffix P = Prefix R = Root R/CF = Combining Form

WORD	PRONUNCIATION		ELEMENTS	DEFINITION
criterion criteria (pl)	kri-**TEER**-ee-on kri-**TEER**-ee-ah		Greek *a standard*	Standard or rule for judging
fructosamine	**FRUK**-toh-sah-meen	S/ R/	-amine *nitrogen-containing* fructos- *fruit sugar*	Organic compound with fructose as its base
glycosylated hemoglobin (Hb A1c)	**GLIE**-koh-sih-lay-ted **HEE**-moh-**GLOH**-bin	S/ R/CF R/CF R/	-sylated *linked* glyc/o- *glucose* -hem/o- *blood* -globin *protein*	Hemoglobin A fraction linked to glucose; used as index of glucose control
immunoassay	**IM**-you-noh-**ASS**-ay	R/CF R	immun/o- *immune response* -assay *evaluate*	Biochemical test that uses the reaction of an antibody to its antigen to measure the amount of a substance in a liquid
microalbuminuria	**MY**-kroh-al-byu-min-**YOU**-ree-ah	S/ P/ R/ R/	-ia *condition* micro- *small* -albumin- *albumin* -ur- *urine*	Presence of very small quantities of albumin in urine that cannot be detected by conventional urine testing
synergist	**SIN**-er-jist	S/ P/ R/	-ist *specialist* syn- *together* -erg- *work*	Agent or process that aids the action of another
synergistic (adj)		S/	-ic *pertaining to*	Working together

Check Point Section 17.3

A. Use abbreviations to describe the condition. *Health care professionals often use abbreviations in documentation; therefore, it is important to know the meanings of abbreviations. Given the description, write the abbreviation for the hormone. Fill in the blank.* **LO 17.1, 17.5, 17.9**

1. Lack of this hormone would increase urine production. _____

2. This hormone will be increased with thyrotropin-secreting adenomas. _____

3. Helps distinguish corticotropin pituitary tumors from adrenal gland tumors. _____

B. Define the word elements to quickly decipher the meaning of the medical term. *Knowing the meaning of the word elements makes short work of defining medical terms. Identify the meaning of the element on the left with its correct meaning on the right.* **LO 17.2**

_____	1. *osmol-*	**a.**	tumor
_____	2. *-oma*	**b.**	gland
_____	3. *bio-*	**c.**	to view
_____	4. *-opsy*	**d.**	concentration
_____	5. *aden-*	**e.**	life

C. Explain the therapeutic procedures for disorders of the pituitary gland. *Choose the correct answer to complete the sentence or answer the question.* **LO 17.7**

1. Treatment of pituitary tumors is aimed at:

    a. shrinking or removing the tumor   **c.** increasing pituitary hormone levels

    b. removing the entire pituitary gland   **d.** suppressing adrenal gland secretion

2. Large pituitary tumors may require a:

    a. MRI   **b.** craniotomy   **c.** lithotripsy   **d.** lobectomy

3. After treatment of pituitary tumors, what type of therapy is often begun?

    a. physical   **b.** occupational   **c.** radiation   **d.** hormone-replacement

D. Deconstruct the terms relating to therapeutic procedures to treat disorders of the pituitary gland. *Identifying the word elements will help you understand the purpose of the procedure. Choose the correct answer.* **LO 17.2, 17.7**

1. The suffix of the term **endoscopic** means

    a. process of viewing   **b.** use of a microscope   **c.** across   **d.** pertaining to

2. The suffix in the term **transsphenoid** means:

    a. pertaining to   **b.** bony projection   **c.** resembling   **d.** across   **e.** butterfly

3. The suffix in the term **craniotomy** means:

    a. incision into   **b.** removal of   **c.** skull   **d.** treatment of   **e.** covering

E. Certain kinds of tests are performed for the purpose of arriving at the correct diagnosis for treatment. *Select the correct diagnostic test for each described condition.* **LO 17.5, 17.7**

1. Is associated with autoimmune inflammatory disease of the thyroid:

    a. serum calcitonin levels   **c.** antithyroid hormone levels

    b. thyroid-stimulating hormone levels   **d.** fine needle aspiration biopsy

2. Blood test to measure activity of the thyroid gland:

    a. serum calcitonin levels   **c.** antithyroid hormone levels

    b. thyroid hormone levels   **d.** fine needle aspiration biopsy

3. Level becomes elevated in medullary carcinoma:

    a. serum calcitonin levels   **c.** antithyroid hormone levels

    b. thyroid-stimulating hormone levels   **d.** fine needle aspiration biopsy

4. Reveals the size of the gland and the presence of nodules:

    a. radioactive iodine therapy   **c.** ultrasonography

    b. fine needle aspiration biopsy   **d.** serum calcitonin levels

5. Distinguishes benign from malignant nodules:

    a. radioactive iodine therapy   **c.** ultrasonography

    b. fine needle aspiration biopsy   **d.** isotopic thyroid scans

6. Details the nature of the thyroid enlargement and the function of the gland:

    a. isotopic thyroid scans   **c.** ultrasonography

    b. fine needle aspiration biopsy   **d.** serum calcitonin levels

F. Deconstruct medical terms into their component parts. *Using the terms in the chapter, place the correct element on each blank.* **LO 17.2, 17.5, 17.7**

1. Increase in the number of cells in a tissue: _____ / _____ / _____

2. Hormone that produces masculine characteristics: _____ / _____ / _____

3. Large family of chemical substances found in hormones: _____ / _____

G. Explain the therapeutic procedures for disorders of the adrenal glands. *Choose the correct answer for each statement.* **LO 17.7**

1. Treatment for this condition requires lifelong hormone replacement with hydrocortisone:

    a. pheochromocytoma   **c.** Cushing syndrome

    b. Addison disease   **d.** adrenal cortex carcinoma

2. In this condition, it is the mother who takes medication to treat the fetal condition:

    a. congenital adrenal hyperplasia   **c.** Addison disease

    b. pheochromocytoma   **d.** Cushing syndrome

3. A condition that is often treated with laparoscopic surgery and removal of the adrenal tumor:

    a. Cushing syndrome   **c.** pheochromocytoma

    b. Addison disease   **d.** congenital adrenal hyperplasia

H. Answer the questions employing the medical language of pharmacology. *Match the abbreviation to its correct description.* **LO 17.7, 17.9**

Description		Abbreviation
_____ **1.** block estrogen receptor cells; tamoxifen		**a.** ERD
_____ **2.** stop production of estrogen from androgen		**b.** SERMs
_____ **3.** used to relieve symptoms of menopause		**c.** AI
_____ **4.** block estrogen receptors; fulvestrant		**d.** HRT

I. Medications: Diabetics will deal with medications for the rest of their lives. *Choose the correct medication that is being described. Select the one drug that is the correct answer for each statement.* **LO 17.7**

1. Act(s) by stimulating the beta cells to secrete insulin

    a. metformin   **b.** sulfonylureas   **c.** thiazolidinedione

2. Suppress(es) hepatic glucose production

    a. metformin   **b.** sulfonylureas   **c.** cinacalcet

3. Improve(s) insulin sensitivity in skeletal muscle

    a. metformin   **b.** sulfonylureas   **c.** cinacalcet

J. Treatment of diabetes mellitus. *Health care providers involved with the care of patients with diabetes mellitus must constantly educate them regarding the proper treatment and self-care. Test your knowledge of the treatment of patients with diabetes mellitus by identifying statements as T for true and F for false.* **LO 17.7**

    1. All patients with diabetes mellitus follow the same plasma glucose monitoring schedule.   **T**   **F**

    2. An important part of the daily routine is foot care.   **T**   **F**

    3. The standard reference for fructosamine levels is 0.5 U/dl.   **T**   **F**

    4. The HbA1c is a record of blood sugar control over the preceding 1 to 3 months.   **T**   **F**

    5. An option for some patients is a continuous infusion of insulin via a programmable pump.   **T**   **F**

Table 17.1 Chapter 17 Abbreviations

Abbreviations	Meaning	Abbreviations	Meaning
ACTH	adrenocorticotropic hormone	IGF-1	insulin-like growth factor-1
ADH	antidiuretic hormone	LH	luteinizing hormone
AI	aromatase inhibitor	MRI	magnetic resonance imaging
BP	blood pressure	MODY	mature-onset diabetes of youth
BUN	blood urea nitrogen	NIDDM	non-insulin-dependent diabetes mellitus
CT	computed tomography	OGTT	oral glucose tolerance test
DKA	diabetic ketoacidosis	OT	oxytocin
DM	diabetes mellitus	PRL	prolactin
DI	diabetes insipidus	PTH	parathyroid hormone
ECG	electrocardiogram	PO	by mouth
EMT	emergency medical technician	RN	registered nurse
ERD	estrogen-receptor downregulator	SAD	seasonal affective disorder
FSH	follicle-stimulating hormone	SERM	selective estrogen receptor modulator
GAS	general adaptation syndrome	SGLT2	sodium-glucose cotransporter-2
GH	growth hormone	STAT	Immediately
GnRH	gonadotropin-releasing hormone	TSH	thyroid-stimulating hormone
Hb A1c	glycosylated hemoglobin (hemoglobin A one-C)	T_3	triiodothyronine
HRT	hormone replacement therapy	T	thyroxine (tetraiodothyronine
HT	hormone therapy	U	unit
IDDM	insulin-dependent diabetes mellitus		

Table 17.2 Comparison of Selected Endocrine Disorders—Signs, Symptoms, and Treatments

Disorder or Disease	Signs and Symptoms	Diagnostic Tests	Treatment
Diabetes insipidus	Polyuria, nocturia, polydipsia	24-hour urine collection, used to measure osmolality, Plasma ADH level.	Desmopressin nasal spray
Addison Disease	Fatigue, weight loss, decreased appetite. Symptoms are gradual and often unnoticed.	Blood tests—electrolyte levels low cortisol and aldosterone levels.	Glucocorticoid replacement with prednisone. Mineralcorticoid replacement with fludrocortisone.
Pheochromocytoma	Hypertension, severe headaches, tachycardia, palpitations, fear of impending death. May have bruising and unintentional weight loss or gain.	Blood tests—catecholamines and metanephrines. CT scan to locate adrenal tumor.	Adrenalectomy
Cushing Syndrome	Obesity of the trunk, round face, kidney stones.	Tests to determine elevated cortisol levels—saliva and 24-hour urine collection.	spirinolacone (*Aldactone*)

Challenge Your Knowledge

A.   Diseases and disorders. Identify the diseases and disorders of the endocrine system as described in the following statements. Special attention to the prefixes will aid you in matching your correct choice. **LO 17.6**

_____ 1. Autoimmune disease with lymphocytic infiltration manifesting with hypothyroidism

_____ 2. Congenital form of thyroid deficiency

_____ 3. Excess of parathyroid hormone

_____ 4. Severe hypothyroidism

_____ 5. Presents as symptomless thyroid nodule

_____ 6. Inflammation of the thyroid gland

_____ 7. Hyperthyroidism associated with a goiter

_____ 8. Deficiency of parathyroid hormone

_____ 9. Enlargement of the thyroid gland

_____ 10. Eyes bulging outward

a. Graves disease

b. thyroid cancer

c. hypoparathyroidism

d. thyroiditis

e. Hashimoto disease

f. goiter

g. exophthalmos

h. hyperparathyroidism

i. myxedema

j. cretinism

B.   Latin and Greek terms. Latin and Greek terms cannot be further deconstructed into prefix, root, or suffix. You must know them for what they are. Test your knowledge of these terms with the following exercise. Match the meaning in the left column with the correct medical term in the right column. **LO 17.1**

_____ 1. Outer covering

_____ 2. Cross

_____ 3. Deep sleep

_____ 4. Stimulation, change

_____ 5. Sweet bread

_____ 6. A lump

_____ 7. Convulsive tension

_____ 8. Appearance

_____ 9. Shaggy or hairy

_____ 10. To set in motion

a. tetany

b. coma

c. tropin

d. cortex

e. chiasm

f. facies

g. hirsutism

h. bolus

i. hormone

j. thymus

C.   Language of endocrinology. Knowing the endocrine system will aid you in understanding the overall body process of _homeostasis_. Apply the _language of endocrinology_ to the following questions about the anatomy and physiology of the endocrine system; choose the correct answer. **LO 17.1**

1. Which of the following is **not** a part of the endocrine system?

a. pancreas

b. pituitary

c. pineal

d. parathyroid

e. palatine

2. The abnormal production of breast milk is called

   a. dysmenorrhea

   b. polydipsia

   c. galactorrhea

   d. dysphagia

   e. menorrhagia

3. The speed at which the body's chemical functions proceed is called

   a. cardiac rate

   b. vasoconstriction

   c. metabolic rate

   d. blood pressure

   e. homeostasis

4. The only hormone that lowers blood glucose is

   a. glucagon

   b. cortisol

   c. aldosterone

   d. corticosterone

   e. insulin

D. **Language of endocrinology.** Apply the *language of endocrinology* to the following questions about the anatomy and physiology of the endocrine system; choose the correct answer. **LO 17.1, 17.6**

   1. A congenital form of thyroid deficiency that severely retards mental and physical growth is

      a. goiter

      b. thyroid adenoma

      c. cretinism

      d. pretibial myxedema

      e. hyperthyroidism

   2. **Tetany** is

      a. lockjaw

      b. painful muscle spasm

      c. protrusion of the eyeball

      d. enlargement of the thyroid gland

      e. excessive production of thyroid hormones

   3. A condition produced by a pituitary tumor that causes a decline in the production of several hormones at the same time is called

      a. hypopituitarism

      b. hyperpituitarism

      c. panhypopituitarism

      d. prolactinoma

      e. diabetes mellitus

   4. Another name for **epinephrine** is

      a. corticosteroid

      b. corticosterone

      c. adrenalin

      d. hydrocortisone

      e. cortisol

   5. The pineal gland secretes **serotonin** by day and converts it to _____ at night.

      a. melatonin

      b. a vasodilator

      c. vasopressin

      d. prolactin

      e. an enzyme

E. **Hormones.** Hormones are bloodborne messengers secreted by endocrine glands. Each has a specific purpose. Correctly use the following terms or abbreviations to fill in the blanks after each definition. **LO 17.1**

ACTH	FSH	somatotropin	PRL	tropic
insulin	glucocorticoid	melatonin	LH	thyrotropin

1. Hormone that stimulates the growth of the thyroid gland: _____

2. Hormones that stimulate other endocrine glands to produce hormones: _____

3. Hormone that stimulates ovulation and testosterone production: _____

4. Hormone of the adrenal cortex that helps regulate glucose metabolism: _____

5. Hormone that stimulates cells to enlarge and divide: _____

6. Hormone that regulates blood sugar: _____

7. Hormone of the anterior pituitary that stimulates cortex of adrenal gland to produce its own hormones: _____

8. Hormone that stimulates target cells in the ovaries and testes: _____

9. Hormone that replaces serotonin at night: _____

10. Hormone that stimulates the mammary glands after pregnancy to produce milk: _____

F. **Plurals.** Enhance your command of plurals in medical terminology by completing this exercise. Select the best choice for the correct form of the plural in the sentence. Fill in the blank. **LO 17.3**

1. Patient complains of multiple _____ (paresthesiae/paresthesias) on her left side.

2. There are several _____ (criterion/criteria) by which to judge this patient's recovery.

3. _____ (Catecholamines/Catecholamina) are major elements in stress response.

G. **Terminology construction.** Construct the *language of endocrinology.* Build the term for the definition provided. Fill in the blanks. **LO 17.2**

1. Hormone formed by the pineal gland _____ /tonin

2. Protrusion of the eyeball ex/ _____

3. Hormone produced by the adrenal cortex _____ /o/steroid

4. Deficiency of all the pituitary hormones _____ /hypo/pituitar/ism

5. Another name for the pituitary gland _____ /physis

6. Hormone that stimulates the uterus to contract oxy/ _____ /in

7. Removal of part or all of the adrenal gland adrenal/_____

8. Prolactin-producing tumor prolactin/ _____

9. Waxy, nonpitting edema of skin _____ /edema

10. Excess of growth hormone that produces enlarged hands and feet _____ /megaly

H. **Elements.** Use your knowledge of word elements to answer the following questions about hormones in other body systems. Fill in the blanks. **LO 17.1, 17.2**

1. Based on its root, the hormone gastrin would have a connection with which body organ? _____

2. Based on its root, the hormone cholecystokinin has an effect on which body organ? _____

3. Both of the above organs are part of which body system that you have already studied? _____ (answer is one word)

4. Based on its root, the hormone erythropoietin stimulates production of _____.

I. Deconstruction. Deconstruct these medical terms into the meanings of their basic elements. Fill in the chart. If the term does not have an element, write n/a. **LO 17.1, 17.2**

Medical Term	Meaning of Prefix	Meaning of Root/ Combining Form	Meaning of Suffix	Meaning of Medical Term
polyuria	1.	2.	3.	4.
parathyroid	5.	6.	7.	8.
thyrotropin	9.	10.	11.	12.
oxytocin	13.	14.	15.	16.
prognathism	17.	18.	19.	20.

J. Abbreviations. This exercise contains all the letters you need to form the correct abbreviations for the terms described. Fill in the blanks. **LO 17.9**

A   D   G   H   I   K   M   N   O   P   S   T

1. Stored in the posterior pituitary: _____

2. Type 2 diabetes: _____

3. Thyrotropin: _____

4. Somatotropin: _____

5. Secreted in response to hypocalcemia: _____

6. Type 1 diabetes: _____

7. Winter depression: _____

8. Marked hyperglycemia with dehydration: _____

9. Used occasionally to diagnose type 2 diabetes: _____

10. Disorder caused by insulin deficiency: _____

K. Terminology challenge. An element may have more than one meaning. For example, *hypo-* can mean either *below* (location) or *deficient* (less in quantity or number). The following five terms all start with *hypo-*. Choose the meaning of the prefix in the following section. **LO 17.2**

1. hypoglycemia

    a. below   **b.** deficient

2. adenohypophysis

    a. below   **b.** deficient

3. neurohypophysis

    a. below   **b.** deficient

4. hypopituitarism

    a. below   **b.** deficient

5. hypophysis

    a. below   **b.** deficient

2014 Nucleus Medical Media

Now match the term to its correct definition. **LO 17.6**

_____ **6.** hypoglycemia

_____ **7.** adenohypophysis

_____ **8.** hypothalamus

_____ **9.** hypopituitarism

_____ **10.** hypophysis

a. another name for the pituitary gland

b. produces eight hormones

c. anterior lobe of the pituitary gland

d. condition of one or more deficient pituitary hormones

e. pertaining to low blood sugar

L. **Pronunciation is important whether you are saying the word or listening to a word from a coworker.** Identify the proper pronunciation of the following medical terms. Correctly spell the term. **LO 17.1, 17.3, 17.4, 17.6**

1. The correct pronunciation for the condition of a forward-projecting jaw

    a. prog-**NAH**-thizm

    b. **PROG**-nah-thizm

    c. ak-roh-**MEG**-ah-lee

    d. ak-roh-mega-**AH**-LEE

    Correctly spell the term: _____

2. The correct pronunciation for thyroid hormone T4, tetraiodothyronine

    a. thigh-**ROK**-seen

    b. **THIGH**-rok-sin

    c. kal-sih-**TONE**-in

    d. kal-**SIH**-toh-nine

    Correctly spell the term: _____

3. The correct pronunciation for one of the catecholamines

    a. kor-**tik**-oyd

    b. **KOR**-tih-koyd

    c. ep-**EE**-nefr-in

    d. ep-ih-**NEF**-rin

    Correctly spell the term: _____

4. The correct pronunciation for inflammation of the thyroid gland

    a. thigh-roy-**DIE**-tis

    b. thigh-ro-id-**EYE**-tis

    c. ant-**EE**-thigh-royd

    d. an-tee-**THIGH**-royd

    Correctly spell the term: _____

5. The correct pronunciation for excessive body and facial hair

    a. hair-**SUIT**-izm

    b. **HER**-sue-tizm

    c. **VIR**-ih-lizm

    d. vire-**LYE**-izm

    Correctly spell the term: _____

Case Report

A. **After reading the following Case Report, correctly answer the following questions.** The answers to the questions may not be in the Case Report itself but can be found in the chapter content. **LO 17.3, 17.6, 17.8, 17.9**

 Case Report (CR) 17.3

You are

. . . a medical assistant working with Susan Lee, MD, In her primary care clinic at Fulwood Medical Center.

Your patient is

. . . Mrs. Martha Jones, who is here for her monthly checkup.

Mrs. Martha Jones is a 53-year-old type 2 diabetic on insulin, with diabetic retinopathy and diabetic neuropathy of her feet. Bariatric surgery has enabled her to reduce her weight from 275 to 156 pounds. The time is 0930 hrs. She is complaining of having a cold and cough for the past few days. Now she is feeling drowsy and nauseous and has a dry mouth. As you talk with her, you notice that her speech is slurred. She cannot remember if she gave herself her morning insulin. Examination of her lungs reveals rales at her right base. Her vital signs are T 97.8°F, P120, R 20, BP 100/50. You perform her blood glucose measurement. The reading is 525 mg/dL.

1. You would document Mrs. Jones's blood sugar level with the term _____.

2. Which of her symptoms suggests that she is dehydrated?

   a. Cough

   b. Slurred speech

   c. Dry mouth

   d. Nausea

3. Why are respiratory symptoms of a cold, cough, and rales in her lungs important information?

   a. They contributed to her blood sugar of 525 mg/dL.

   b. Left untreated, these symptoms will cause permanent lung damage.

   c. These symptoms indicate that her bariatric surgery is failing.

   d. Diabetes causes these symptoms.

4. Dr. Lee immediately transfers Mrs. Jones to the hospital because she is in:

   a. IDDM

   b. PTH

   c. DKA

   d. IGF

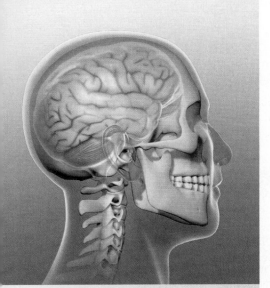

2014 Nucleus Medical Media

Mental Health

The Languages of Psychology and Psychiatry

Chapter Sections

18.1 Mental Health and Affective Disorders

18.2 Anxiety Disorders

18.3 Schizophrenia and Personality Disorders

18.4 Procedures and Pharmacology

Chapter Learning Outcomes

Upon completion of this chapter, you will be able to:

LO 18.1   Define key medical terms in psychiatry and psychology for classifying and describing mental disorders.

LO 18.2   Spell medical terms related to mental health.

LO 18.3   Pronounce medical terms related to mental health.

LO 18.4   Describe diagnostic procedures utilized for mental health disorders.

LO 18.5   Identify and describe mental health disorders.

LO 18.6   Describe the therapeutic procedures and pharmacologic agents used in the treatment of mental health disorders.

LO 18.7   Apply knowledge of medical terms relating to mental health to documentation, medical records, and communication.

LO 18.8   Identify and correctly use abbreviations of terms used in mental health.

LO 18.9   Identify health professionals involved in the care of patients with mental health disorders.

The health professionals involved in the diagnosis and treatment of patients with mental health disorders include:

- **Psychiatrists,** who are medical doctors licensed in the diagnosis and treatment of mental disorders.

- **Clinical psychologists,** who are professionals licensed in the science concerned with the behavior of the human mind.

- **Psychiatric and mental health nurses or nurse practitioners,** who evaluate and provide care for patients with psychiatric disorders, medical mental conditions, and substance abuse problems.

- **Psychiatric social workers,** who assess, develop treatment plans, and provide case management and rights advocacy to patients with mental health problems.

- **Psychiatric technicians,** who provide front-line care to patients with mental illnesses and/or developmental disabilities and who carry out doctors' orders and serve as the eyes and ears of the diagnosing professional.

Section 18.1 Mental Health and Affective Disorders

Definitions in Mental Health

Mental health is defined as emotional, behavioral, and social well-being such that an individual can cope with internal and external events.

Psychology is defined as the scientific study of behavior and mental processes. **Behavior** is anything you do—talking, sleeping, reading, interacting with others. **Mental processes** are your private, internal experiences—thinking, feeling, remembering, dreaming.

A licensed specialist in psychology is called a **psychologist.** Psychologists can have a master's degree or a doctorate in philosophy **(PhD)** or a doctorate in psychology **(PsyD).** They can practice in many different career specialties, including being a **psychotherapist** or a **psychoanalyst.** Psychologists are not licensed to prescribe medications.

Psychiatry is the medical specialty concerned with the origin, diagnosis, prevention, and treatment of mental, emotional, and behavioral disorders. **Psychiatrists** have an MD or a DO degree and a minimum of 4 years of residency training in the specialty. As physicians, psychiatrists are licensed to prescribe medications.

Many psychiatrists and psychologists work together in a team approach to therapy. Other health professionals in the mental health team include **clinical social workers, psychiatric nurses,** and **psychiatric technicians.**

Mental disorder can be defined as any behavior or emotional state that:
- Causes a person to suffer emotional distress (e.g., depression, anxiety).
- Is harmful to the individual sufferer (impairs the individual's ability to work, take care of personal needs, or get along with others).
- Is self-destructive (e.g., substance abuse, gambling and other addictions, self-injury).
- Endangers others or the community (antisocial behaviors, **homicidal** intent, **pyromania** [setting fires]).

Insanity is a *legal* term for a severe mental illness, present at the time a crime was committed, that impaired the defendant's capacity to understand the moral wrong of the act. *It is not a medical diagnosis.*

Did you know...

- The *Diagnostic and Statistical Manual of Mental Disorders*, fifth edition (DSM-5) classifies and describes psychiatric disorders.
- The DSM-5 contains over 200 diagnoses grouped into 17 major categories.

Word Analysis and Definition: Mental Health

S = Suffix   P = Prefix   R = Root   R/CF = Combining Form

WORD	PRONUNCIATION		ELEMENTS	DEFINITION
behavior	be-**HAYV**-yur	S/ R/	**-ior-** *pertaining to* **behav-** *mental activity*	Mental or motor activity
behavioral (adj)	be-**HAYV**-yur-al	S/	**-al** *pertaining to*	Pertaining to any mental or motor activity
homicide	**HOM**-ih-side	S/ R/CF	**-cide** *to kill* **hom/i-** *man*	Killing of one human by another
homicidal (adj)	hom-ih-**SIDE**-al	S/	**-cidal** *pertaining to killing*	Having a tendency to commit homicide
insanity	in-**SAN**-ih-tee	S/ P/ R/	**-ity** *condition* **in-** *not* **-san-** *sound, healthy*	Nonmedical term for person unable to be responsible for actions
mental	**MENT**-al	S/ R/	**-al** *pertaining to* **-ment-** *mind*	Pertaining to the mind
psychiatry	sigh-**KIE**-ah-tree	S/ R/	**-iatry** *treatment* **psych-** *mind*	Diagnosis and treatment of mental disorders
psychiatric (adj)	sigh-kee-**AH**-trik	S/	**-ic** *pertaining to*	Pertaining to psychiatry
psychiatrist	sigh-**KIE**-ah-trist	S/	**-iatrist** *one who treats, practitioner*	Licensed medical specialist in psychiatry
psychology	sigh-**KOL**-oh-jee	S/ R/CF	**-logy** *study of* **psych/o-** *mind*	Scientific study of the human mind and behavior
psychological (adj)	sigh-koh-**LOJ**-ik-al	S/	**-ical** *pertaining to*	Pertaining to psychology
psychologist	sigh-**KOL**-oh-jist	S/	**-logist** *specialist*	Licensed specialist in psychology
psychoanalysis	sigh-koh-ah-**NAL**-ih-sis	R/	**-analysis** *process to define*	Method of psychotherapy
psychoanalyst	sigh-koh-**AN**-ah-list	R/	**-analyst** *one who defines*	Practitioner of psychoanalysis
psychotherapy	sigh-koh-**THAIR**-ah-pee	S/	**-therapy** *treatment*	Treatment of mental disorders through communication
psychotherapist	sigh-koh-**THAIR**-ah-pist	R/	**-therapist** *one who treats*	Practitioner of psychotherapy
pyromania	pie-roh-**MAY**-nee-ah	S/ R/CF	**-mania** *frenzy* **pyr/o-** *fire*	Morbid impulse to set fires

Affective disorders are not a clearly delineated group of disorders. Included are the **mood disorders** of **unipolar** and **bipolar depression.**

Mood Disorders

You will feel sad and blue and down in the dumps from time to time and occasionally feel the grief of the death of a loved one and the tragedy of injury or severe emotional hurt. Everyone does. But people with **major depression** are so deeply sad for at least 2 weeks that they feel despairing and hopeless, see nothing but sorrow in the future, and may not want to live anymore (*Figure 18.1*). They see themselves as worthless and unlovable. They have difficulty getting up and going to school or work.

Physical symptoms occur. These may include difficulty concentrating, difficulty falling asleep, feeling tired all the time, and losing weight. Thoughts of harming oneself, thoughts of suicide or attempting suicide are serious symptoms requiring immediate intervention. There is more than one type of depression. Forms of depression include:

- **Seasonal affective disorder (SAD)** is a mood disorder associated with episodes of depression during the fall and winter months, subsiding during spring and summer. It appears to be related to a lack of sunshine causing increased melatonin production by the pineal gland (*see Chapter 14*).
- **Perinatal depression** can occur during pregnancy (*see Chapter 8*).
- **Postnatal depression** can occur after pregnancy (*see Chapter 8*).

Bipolar disorder is alternating episodes of depression with **mania.** Mania is the opposite of depression, described as an excessive state of overexcitement and impulsive behavior. It used to be called **manic-depressive disorder.**

In the **manic** phase, the person is **hyperactive** and **distractible** and may not sleep for days yet shows no fatigue. Thinking and speech are rapid and disjointed and cannot be interrupted. The person may give away possessions or go on a spending spree. Untreated pure manic episodes usually last 6 weeks. Untreated mixed (manic and depressive) episodes usually last 17 weeks.

Dysphoric mania, a form of bipolar disorder, combines the frenetic energy of mania with dark thoughts and paranoid delusions.

Did you know...

- Approximately 6 million Americans suffer from bipolar disorder.
- A study published in 2017 from the University of Texas at Houston linked a volume decrease in specific parts of the brain's hippocampus (*see Chapter 9*).
- Studies are finding signs of neuroinflammation in the remaining hippocampal tissue of people with bipolar disorder.

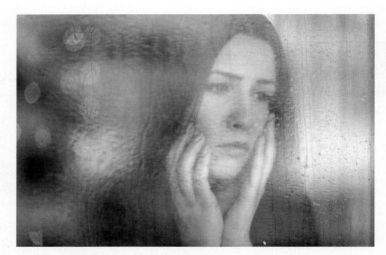

▲ **Figure 18.1** **Depressed woman at window.** Bojan Kontrec/iStock/ Getty Images

WORD	PRONUNCIATION	ELEMENTS		DEFINITION
affect affective (adj)	AF-fekt af-FEK-tiv	S/ R/	Latin *state of mind* -ive *pertaining to* affect- *mood*	External display of feelings, thoughts, and emotions Expressing emotion
bipolar disorder	bi-POH-lar dis-OR-der	S/ P/ R/ P/ R/	-ar *pertaining to* bi- *two* -pol- *pole* dis- *apart, away from* -order *arrange*	A mood disorder with alternating episodes of depression and mania, the two poles of the disorder
depression	de-PRESH-un	S/ R/	-ion *condition, process* depress- *press down*	Mental disorder with feelings of deep sadness and despair
distract (verb) distractibility	dis-TRAKT dis-TRAK-ti-BILL-ih-tee	S/	Latin *pull in different directions* -ibility *being able*	To turn the mind away Inability to keep the mind one topic
dysphoria dysphoric (adj)	dis-FOR-ee-ah	S/ P/ R/ S/	-ia *condition* dys- *bad, difficult* -phor- *carry, bear* -ic *pertaining to*	A condition of severe depression, agitation, and paranoid delusions Pertaining to dysphoria
hyperactive (adj) hyperactivity	HIGH-per-ac-TIV HIGH-per-ac-TIV-ih-tee	P/ R/ S/ R/	hyper- *excessive* -active- *movement* -ity *state, condition* -activ- *movement*	Excessive restlessness and movement Condition of being hyperactive
mania manic (adj) manic-depressive disorder	MAY-nee-ah MAN-ik MAN-ik dee-PRESS-iv dis-OR-der	 S/ R/ S/ R/ P/ R/	Greek *frenzy* -ic *pertaining to* man- *affected by frenzy* -ive *quality of* depress- *press down* dis- *apart, away from* -order *arrange*	Mood disorder with hyperactivity, irritability, and rapid speech Pertaining to or characterized by mania An outdated name for bipolar disorder
suicide suicidal (adj)	SOO-ih-side SOO-ih-SIGH-dal	S/ R/CF S/	-cide *to kill* su/i- *self* -cidal *pertaining to killing*	The act of killing oneself Wanting to kill oneself
unipolar disorder	you-nih-POLE-ar dis-OR-der	S/ P/ R/ P/ R/	-ar *pertaining to* uni- *one* -pol- *pole (at the pole of depression)* dis- *apart, away from* -order *arrange*	Depression

Check Point Section 18.1

A. Reinforce your learning of the *languages of psychology and psychiatry* by providing the term that is being defined. *Fill in the blank.* **LO 18.1, 18.10**

1. A medical doctor who specializes in the origin, diagnosis, prevention, and treatment of mental, emotional, and behavioral

    disorders: _____

2. A front-line worker who directly cares for those with mental illnesses and/or developmental disabilities: _____ technician.

3. The general term for a licensed specialist in psychology: _____

B. Choose the correct answer for the question. LO 18.1

1. Which of the following choices cannot be classified under the term *behavior*?

    a. talking

    b. sleeping

    c. reading

    d. depression

    e. interacting with others

2. Which of the following statements *best* describes a mental process?

    a. your private, internal experiences

    b. thinking

    c. feeling

    d. remembering

    e. dreaming

3. Which of the following terms contains a prefix, root, and suffix?

   a. psychology

   b. hallucination

   c. insanity

   d. homicidal

   e. psychiatry

C. Differentiate between the conditions and signs of bipolar and unipolar disorders. *Use the words below to fill in the blanks in the following sentences.* **LO 18.6**

bipolar	unipolar	mania	manic	depression

1. A patient who experiences episodes of mania with episodes of depression is diagnosed with _____ disorder.

2. While experiencing the periods of hyperactivity, irritability, and paranoid delusions, the patient is said to be in a _____ state.

3. A patient whose symptoms are limited to deep sadness suffers from _____.

4. Clinical depression is the same as _____ disorder.

5. A person with bipolar disorder is experiencing _____ when he speaks very rapidly, is irritable, and is hyperactive.

Section 18.2 Anxiety Disorders

Anxiety Disorders

Anxiety disorders are the most common category of mental disorders found in the United States. They are characterized by an **unreasonable anxiety** or **fear** that is inappropriate to the circumstances and so intense and chronic that it disrupts the person's life.

There are five major categories of anxiety disorder:

1. **Generalized anxiety disorder (GAD)** consists of persistent, excessive worrying, and uncontrollable anxiety that is not focused on one particular situation and has lasted for at least 6 months. People with this disorder are frightened of something but are unable to articulate a specific fear. They develop physical fear reactions including palpitations, **insomnia,** difficulty concentrating, and irritability.

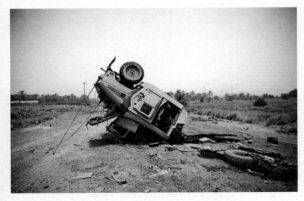

▲ **Figure 18.2** **The remains of an American Humvee, one of four that were disabled by massive IEDs, lies on a dirt road on August 4, 2007, in Hawr Rajab, Iraq.** Benjamin Lowy/Getty Images

2. **Posttraumatic** stress disorder (PTSD) occurs when a person who has gone through a significant trauma shows stress symptoms that last for longer than a month and impair the person's ability to function. The trauma can be a life-threatening accident, a natural disaster, loss of a loved one, torture or abuse, or combat (*Figure 18.2*) and its related incidents.

3. **Panic disorder** is characterized by sudden, brief attacks of **intense fear** that cause physical symptoms. The fear rises abruptly, often for no reason, and peaks in 10 minutes or less. The frequency of the attacks varies widely over many years. The disorder runs in families, but whether it is due to genetics or a shared environment is not clear.

4. **Phobias** differ from generalized anxiety and panic attacks in that a specific situation or object brings on the strong fear response. The danger is small, and the person realizes the fear is irrational, but there is still overwhelming anxiety. There are two categories of phobia:

   • **Situational phobias** involve a fear of specific situations. Examples include **agoraphobia** (fear of crowded places, buses, and elevators), **acrophobia** (fear of heights), fear of flying or driving in tunnels, and fear of specific animals (snakes, mice). The basic fear of being trapped in a confined space is called **claustrophobia.**

   • **Social phobias** involve fear of being embarrassed in social situations. The most common are fear of public speaking (stage fright) and of eating in public. In many, the fear is so strong that it makes normal life impossible.

5. In **obsessive-compulsive disorder (OCD),** a majority of patients have both **obsessions** and **compulsions.** The obsessions are recurrent thoughts, fears, doubts, images, or impulses. The compulsions are recurrent, irresistible impulses to perform actions such as counting, hand washing, checking, and systematically arranging things. The recurrent thoughts can be violent or sexual.

Most patients recognize the senselessness of their behaviors, but if they resist doing them, the fear and anxiety become intolerable.

Psychosomatic and Somatoform Disorders

Psychosomatic disorder is a real, physical disorder that, at least in part, has a psychologic cause. Tension headaches have real pain caused by muscle spasm, but stress and anxiety play a role in causing the symptoms.

Somatoform disorder occurs when there is no identifiable physical cause to explain physical symptoms. The symptoms are real to the patient and are not under voluntary control.

In **conversion disorder,** symptoms progress to involve loss of feeling, paralysis, deafness, or blindness.

Somatic symptom disorder (SSD) is a condition in which the patient has distressing physical (somatic) symptoms together with abnormal thoughts, feelings, and behaviors in response to these symptoms.

Did you know...

- The DSM-5 has replaced the disorder **hypochondriasis** with the diagnosis of **somatic symptom disorder** and **illness anxiety disorder.**

Word Analysis and Definition: Anxiety Disorders

S = Suffix P = Prefix R = Root R/CF = Combining Form

WORD	PRONUNCIATION	ELEMENTS		DEFINITION
acrophobia	ak-roh-**FOH**-bee-ah	S/ R/CF	**-phobia** *fear* **acr/o-** *peak, highest point*	Pathologic fear of heights
agoraphobia	ah-gor-ah-**FOH**-bee-ah	S/ R/CF	**-phobia** *fear* **agor/a-** *marketplace*	Pathologic fear of being trapped in a public place
anxiety	ang-**ZIE**-eh-tee		Greek *distress, anxiety*	Distress caused by fear
claustrophobia	klaw-stroh-**FOH**-bee-ah	S/ R/CF	**-phobia** *fear* **claustr/o-** *confined space*	Pathologic fear of being trapped in a confined space
compulsion	kom-**PUL**-shun	S/ R/	**-ion** *action, condition* **compuls-** *drive, compel*	Uncontrollable impulses to perform an act repetitively
compulsive (adj)	kom-**PUL**-siv	S/	**-ive** *nature of, quality of*	Possessing uncontrollable impulses to perform an act repetitively
conversion disorder	kon-**VER**-shun dis-**OR**-der	S/ P/ R/ P/ R/	**-ion** *action, condition* **con-** *with, together* **-vers-** *turned* **dis-** *apart, away from* **-order** *arrange*	An unconscious emotional conflict is expressed as physical symptoms with no organic basis
insomnia	in-**SOM**-nee-ah	S/ P/ R/	**-ia** *condition* **in-** *not* **-somn-** *sleep*	Inability to sleep
obsession	ob-**SESH**-un	S/ R/	**-ion** *action, condition* **obsess-** *besieged by thoughts*	Persistent, recurrent, uncontrollable thoughts or impulses
obsessive (adj)	ob-**SES**-iv	S/	**-ive** *nature of, quality of*	Possessing persistent, recurrent, uncontrollable thoughts or impulses
phobia	**FOH**-bee-ah		Greek *fear*	Pathologic fear or dread
posttraumatic	post-traw-**MAT**-ik	S/ P/ R/	**-ic** *pertaining to* **post-** *after* **-traumat-** *wound*	Occurring after and caused by trauma
psychosomatic	sigh-koh-soh-**MAT**-ik	S/ R/CF R/	**-ic** *pertaining to* **psych/o-** *mind* **-somat-** *body*	Pertaining to disorders of the body usually resulting from disturbances of the mind
somatic symptom disorder	soh-**MAT**-ik **SIMP**-tum dis-**OR**-der	S/ R/ P/ R/	**-ic** *pertaining to* **somat-** *body* **symptom** Greek *sign* **dis-** *apart, away from* **-order** *arrange*	Distressing physical symptoms occur, causing abnormal thoughts, feelings, and behaviors
somatoform	soh-**MAT**-oh-form	S/ R/CF	**-form** *appearance of* **somat/o-** *body*	Physical symptoms occurring without identifiable physical cause

A. Identify the word elements in each medical term. *Choose the correct answer for each question below.* **LO 18.2**

1. Which of the following terms has a word element that means *not*?

   a. insomnia

   b. posttraumatic

   c. anxiety

2. Which of the following terms has a word element that means *wound*?

   a. insomnia

   b. posttraumatic

   c. anxiety

3. Which of the following terms has a word element that means *condition*?

   a. insomnia

   b. posttraumatic

   c. anxiety

B. Match the term to its correct definition. *Pay close attention to the word elements to assist you in choosing the correct definition for each term.*
LO 18.6

_____	**1.** psychosomatic	**a.** Fear of being trapped in a public space
_____	**2.** acrophobia	**b.** Fear of heights
_____	**3.** obsessive	**c.** Physical symptoms occurring without a physical cause
_____	**4.** hypochondriasis	**d.** Disorder of body due to disturbance of the mind
_____	**5.** somatoform	**e.** Belief that a minor symptom indicates a severe disease
_____	**6.** agoraphobia	**f.** Uncontrollable impulses to perform act repetitively
_____	**7.** compulsion	**g.** Persistent, recurrent, uncontrollable thoughts

Section 18.3 Schizophrenia and Personality Disorders

Schizophrenia

Schizophrenia is a form of **psychosis** in which there is a loss of contact with reality. Symptoms of schizophrenia typically come on in the late teens and twenties and people do not get it after their 40's. People with schizophrenia do *not* have a split personality, but their words can be separated from the meaning, their perceptions separated from reality, and behaviors separated from their thought processes *(Figure 18.3)*. Typically, people with schizophrenia are not violent toward others but may harm themselves.

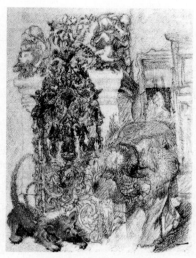

▲ **Figure 18.3** **Artwork by schizophrenic patient.** Wellcome Images/Science Source

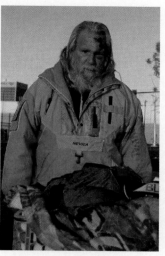

▲ **Figure 18.4** **Homeless schizophrenic man on the street.** George Rose/Getty Images

Sometimes their speech is disorganized and can be incoherent. Their behaviors are often totally inappropriate. People with schizophrenia have their sensory perceptions jumbled and distorted, have difficulty concentrating, and perceive things without a stimulation—**hallucinations.** Hallucinations can occur in any of the senses but are most often auditory. They also suffer from **delusions,** mistaken beliefs that are contrary to facts. The delusions can be **paranoid,** with pervasive distrust and suspicion of others.

People with schizophrenia can withdraw from society, become homeless, and refuse to communicate *(Figure 18.4)*. In extreme cases, their blunted emotions and withdrawal can progress to **catatonia,** and possibly become **mute.**

Word Analysis and Definition: Schizophrenia

S = Suffix P = Prefix R = Root R/CF = Combining Form

WORD	PRONUNCIATION		ELEMENTS	DEFINITION
catatonia	kat-ah-**TOH**-nee-ah	S/ P/ R/	-ia *condition* cata- *down* -ton- *pressure, tension*	Syndrome characterized by physical immobility and mental stupor
catatonic (adj)	kat-ah-**TON**-ik	S/	-ic *pertaining to*	Pertaining to or characterized by catatonia
delusion	dee-**LOO**-shun	S/ R/	-ion *condition, process* delus- *deceive*	Fixed, unyielding, false belief or judgment held despite strong evidence to the contrary
delusional (adj)	dee-**LOO**-shun-al	S/	-al *pertaining to*	Pertaining to having delusions
hallucination	hah-loo-sih-**NAY**-shun	S/ R/	-ation *process* hallucin- *imagination*	Perception of an object or event when there is no such thing present
mute mutism	MYUT **MYU**-tizm	 S/ R/	Latin *silent* -ism *condition, process* mut- *silent*	Unable or unwilling to speak Absence of speech
paranoia	pair-ah-**NOY**-ah	P/ R/	para- *abnormal, beside* -noia *to think*	Mental disorder with persecutory delusions
paranoid (adj)	**PAIR**-ah-noyd	R/	-noid *abnormal thinking*	Having delusions of persecution
psychosis	sigh-**KOH**-sis	S/ R/	-osis *condition* psych- *mind*	Disorder causing mental disruption and loss of contact with reality
schizophrenia	skitz-oh-**FREE**-nee-ah	S/ R/CF R/	-ia *condition* schiz/o- *to split, cleave* -phren- *mind*	Disorder of perception, thought, emotion, and behavior
schizophrenic (adj)	skitz-oh-**FREN**-ik	S/	-ic *pertaining to*	Relating to, or suffering from, schizophrenia

Personality Disorders

Personality is defined as an individual's unique and stable patterns of thoughts, feelings, and behaviors. When these patterns become rigid and inflexible in response to different situations, they can cause impairment of the individual's ability to deal with other people (i.e., to function socially).

Borderline personality disorder (BPD) is a frequent diagnosis in people who are impulsive, unstable in mood, and manipulative. They can be exciting, charming, and friendly one moment and angry, irritable, and sarcastic the next. Their identity is fragile and insecure, their self-worth low. They can be promiscuous and self-destructive; for example, committing **self-mutilation (self-injury)** *(Figure 18.5)* or suicide. People with **narcissistic personality disorder** have an exaggerated sense of self-importance, seek constant attention, and lack **empathy.**

Antisocial personality disorder, used interchangeably with the terms **sociopath** and **psychopath,** describes people who lie, cheat, steal, make trouble for others, and have no sense of responsibility and no anxiety or guilt about their behavior. The psychopaths have these characteristics but tend to be more violent and anger more easily than sociopaths.

Schizoid and **paranoid personality disorders** describe people who are absorbed with themselves, untrusting, and fearful of closeness with others.

Treatment for personality disorders may not successful.

Dissociative Disorders

Dissociative disorders involve a disassociation (splitting apart) of past experiences from present memory or consciousness. Being unable to recall identity is called **dissociative amnesia.** The development of distinctly separate personalities is called **dissociative identity disorder (DID).** It was formerly called **multiple personality disorder (MPD).**

The basic origin of all these disorders is the need to escape, usually from extreme trauma, and most often from sexual, emotional, or physical abuse in childhood.

The most severe of this group of disorders is DID. Two or more distinct personalities, each with their own memories and behaviors, inhabit the same person at the same time *(Figure 18.6)*. Treatment is with psychotherapy.

Impulse Control Disorders

Impulse control disorders are an inability to resist an impulse to perform an action that is harmful to the individual or to others. These disorders include:

- **Intermittent explosive disorder,** which is characterized by recurrent episodes of unrestrained aggression toward people, furniture, or property, with violent resistance to attempts to restrain. The etiology is thought to be epileptic-like activity in the brain.

- **Kleptomania,** which is characterized by stealing—not for gain, but to satisfy an irresistible urge to steal.

- **Trichotillomania (TTM),** which is characterized by the repeated urge to pull out scalp, beard, pubic, and other body hair.

- **Substance abuse** and **chemical dependence,** which involve a person's continued use of drugs or alcohol despite having had significant problems or distress related to their use. This **addiction** affects the brain and behavior, and develops an increased need for the substance and an inability to stop using it.

- **Pyromania,** which is repeated fire setting with no motive other than a fascination with fire and fire engines. Some pyromaniacs end up as volunteer firefighters. Treatment with behavioral therapy is sometimes successful.

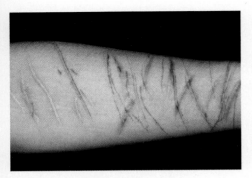

▲ **Figure 18.5** Self-mutilated arm.
Dr. P. Marazzi/SPL/Science Source

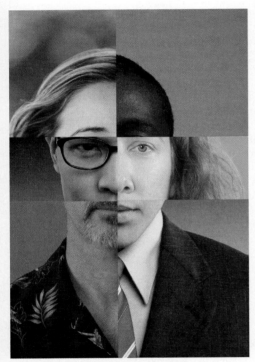

▲ **Figure 18.6** Dissociative identity disorder (multiple personality disorder).
John Lund/Blend Images/Getty Images

Did you know...

- **Empathy** is understanding another person's feelings.
- **Sympathy** is to feel sorry about a person's problem.

Word Analysis and Definition: Personality Disorders

WORD	PRONUNCIATION	ELEMENTS		DEFINITION
addict addiction	**AD**-ikt ah-**DIK**-shun	P/ R/ S/	**ad-** *toward* **-dict** *surrender* **-ion** *condition, action*	Person with a psychologic or physical dependence on a substance or practice Habitual psychologic and physiologic dependence on a substance or practice
amnesia	am-**NEE**-zee-ah		Greek *forgetfulness*	Total or partial inability to remember past experiences
antisocial personality disorder	**AN**-tee-**SOH**-shal person-**AL**-ih-tee dis-**OR**-der	S/ P/ R/ S/ S/ R/ P/ R/	**-al** *pertaining to* **anti-** *against* **-soci-** *partner, ally, community* **-ity** *condition, state* **-al** *pertaining to* **person-** *person* **dis-** *apart, away from* **-order** *arrange*	Disorder of people who lie, cheat, steal, and have no guilt about their behavior
dissociative identity disorder	di-**SO**-see-ah-tiv eye-**DEN**-tih-tee dis-**OR**-der	S/ P/ R/ P/ R/	**-ative** *quality of* **dis-** *apart, away from* **-soci-** *partner, ally, community* **identity** Latin *repeatedly, again and again* **dis-** *apart, away from* **-order** *arrange*	Mental disorder in which part of an individual's personality is separated from the rest, leading to multiple personalities
empathy	**EM**-pah-thee	P/ R/CF	**em-** *into* **-pathy** *disease*	Ability to place yourself into the feelings, emotions, and reactions of another person
kleptomania	klep-toh-**MAY**-nee-ah	S/ R/CF	**-mania** *frenzy* **klept/o-** *to steal*	Uncontrollable need to steal
narcissism narcissistic (adj)	**NAR**-sih-sizm **NAR**-sih-**SIS**-tik	 S/ R/ S/	**Narcissus,** Greek mythical character who was in love with his own reflection in water **-ism** *a process* **narciss-** *self-love* **-istic** *pertaining to*	Self-love; person interprets everything purely in relation to himself or herself Relating everything to oneself; pertaining to, or suffering from, narcissism
psychopath	**SIGH**-koh-path	S/ R/CF	**-path** *disease* **psych/o-** *mind*	Person with antisocial personality disorder who is prone to anger and violence
pyromania	pie-roh-**MAY**-nee-ah	S/ R/CF	**-mania** *frenzy* **pyr/o-** *fire*	Morbid impulse to set fires
schizoid	**SKITZ**-oyd	S/ R/	**-oid** *resemble* **schiz-** *split*	Withdrawn, socially isolated
self-mutilation	self-myu-tih-**LAY**-shun	S/ R/ R/	**-ation** *process* **self-** *own individual* **-mutil-** *to maim*	Injury or disfigurement made to one's own body
sociopath	**SOH**-see-oh-path	S/ R/CF	**-path** *disease* **soci/o-** *partner, ally, community*	Person with antisocial personality disorder
sympathy	**SIM**-pa-thee	P/ R/CF	**sym-** *together* **-pathy** *disease*	Appreciation and concern for another person's mental and emotional state

Check Point Section 18.3

A. After reading Case Report (CR) 18.3, *choose the correct answer to complete each statement.* **LO 18.6, 18.8**

Case Report (CR) 18.3

You are

. . . an emergency medical technician (EMT) working in the Emergency Department at Fulwood Medical Center.

Your patient is

. . . Mr. Dante Costello, a 21-year-old homeless man brought in by the police after he was found sitting in the middle of a main street.

Mr. Costello's explanation is "the voices told me to do it." He has heard voices telling him to do things for the past year. The voices often comment on his behavior. He has isolated himself from other people because "they are not who they say they are, and they are trying to get me." He is taking no drugs or medications and denies any **suicidal** or homicidal intent. Mr. Costello is dirty and disheveled, with poor hygiene. He can give no home or family address. His **affect** is **congruent,** though expressionless. His speech is slow, and his thoughts are disorganized and confused. The most probable diagnosis is **schizophrenia.** He needs to be admitted to the hospital because he is a danger to himself and other people.

Mr. Costello stated he was hearing voices of people who were not there speaking to him (hallucination). Mr. Costello was also paranoid, believing that people were "out to get him." He withdrew from society and became homeless. His behavior of sitting immobile in the middle of the street for long periods is inappropriate and is **catatonic.**

1. The term that means *wanting to kill oneself:*

   a. homicidal

   b. schizophrenic

   c. suicidal

   d. psychotic

2. Mr. Costello's inappropriate behavior is due to:

   a. homicidal thoughts

   b. poor hygiene

   c. hearing voices

   d. homelessness

3. His behavior of sitting in the street for long periods of time describes which condition?

   a. paranoia

   b. mutism

   c. homicidal

   d. catatonia

B. Use the correct abbreviation for personality disorders. *Read the description of the personality disorder and give the correct abbreviation for which it is describing.* **LO 18.6, 18.9**

1. A person who pulls the hairs from the eyebrows and eyelids: _____

2. The current title for a condition in which a person states that he or she has two separate and distinct personalities: _____

3. The older abbreviation for a person with two separate and distinct personalities: _____

4. This person is known to be manipulative, yet charming. His or her moods are unstable and behavior is impulsive: _____

Section 18.4 Procedures and Pharmacology

Diagnostic Methods for Mental Disorders

While mental illness is common (about one in five adults has a mental illness in any given year) and is a leading cause of disability, diagnostic tests and treatment procedures are limited, and medications do not cure the illness but can significantly improve symptoms. At this time, there are no tests (examination of blood or body fluids) for mental illnesses as is the case with a physical health condition, though research to identify markers for schizophrenia and depression is ongoing. To define a mental health diagnosis, the following steps can be taken:

- A **physical examination** by a primary care physician to rule out physical problems that could be causing the symptoms.
- **Lab tests** to rule out physical causes of the symptoms; for example, tests of thyroid function and screening for alcohol and drugs.
- A **psychological evaluation** by a psychiatrist or psychologist to determine the patient's symptoms, thoughts, feelings, mood **congruence**, and behavior patterns by talking to the patient and using questionnaires. The defining symptoms of each mental illness are detailed in the *Diagnostic and Statistical Manual of Mental Disorders,* **fifth edition (DSM-5),** compiled by the American Psychiatric Association, which is used by mental health providers to make the diagnosis of mental health disorders and by insurance companies to set reimbursements for treatment.

Brain imaging scans (neuroimaging scans) are being used to help detect and diagnose medical disorders, but their use for mental disorders is in research to try to learn more about the mental disorders.

The diagnosis of mental disorders is even more challenging in children, where the U.S. Surgeon General estimates that one in five children has a diagnosable mental illness. Children are developing mentally as well as physically and actions such as anger, anxiety, or shyness can be a temporary condition as part of developmental growth rather than an illness. When troubling behaviors occur over a period of time or in a way that disrupts daily life, they can then be considered symptoms of a disorder.

Therapeutic Methods for Mental Disorders

Mental disorders are characterized by changes in mood, thought, and/or behavior that interfere with the daily activities of living and impair the ability to work and interact with family and the community. The National Survey on Drug Use and Health Data for 2019 shows that 51.5 million adults aged 18 and older experienced some form of mental illness in that year, about 20.6% of the population.

Bright light therapy stimulates the pineal gland to treat seasonal affective disorder. This is one of the few mental health disorders that has a treatment outside of psychotherapy. **Psychotherapy,** also called talk therapy, explores with a trained mental health professional thoughts, feelings, and behaviors on the assumption that the cure for a person's suffering lies within that person. The therapist's roles are to generate emotional awareness and insight to help the person identify the source of the problems and consider alternatives for dealing with them. There are six types of psychotherapy:

1. **Supportive psychotherapy,** in which the expression of feelings is encouraged and the therapist provides help with problem solving.
2. **Psychoanalysis,** which is the oldest form of psychotherapy, developed by Sigmund Freud in the early 20th century. It encourages the person to say whatever comes to mind and helps the person develop an understanding of how the past affects the present, enabling the person to develop new and more adaptive ways of functioning.
3. **Psychodynamic psychotherapy,** which is similar to psychoanalysis and focuses on identifying unconscious patterns in current thoughts, feelings, and behaviors.
4. **Cognitive therapy,** which helps people identify distortions in interpreting experiences and learn to think in different ways about the experiences, which leads to an improvement in behavior and feelings.
5. **Behavioral therapy,** which is similar to cognitive therapy. A combination of the two—**cognitive behavioral therapy (CBT)**—is often used. Behavioral therapy believes that abnormal behaviors are due to faulty learning, and these maladaptive behaviors can be unlearned and corrected.
6. **Interpersonal therapy** involves treatment for depression and focuses on unresolved grief and conflicts that arise when people have to fill roles that differ from their expectations both at work and in the family.

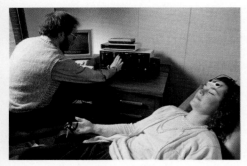

▲ **Figure 18.7** Patient receiving biofeedback therapy. Will & Deni McIntyre/ Science Source

Phototherapy, also called bright light therapy, uses bright fluorescent lights to stimulate the pineal gland to treat seasonal affective disorder.

Eye movement desensitization and reprocessing (EMDR) is an eight-phase treatment found to be as effective as CBT for patients suffering from PTSD and for patients who have experienced traumatic situations. The process involves the patient recalling painful memories while the clinician provides sensory input for the patient, such as side-to-side eye movements.

Biofeedback *(Figure 18.7)* and relaxation techniques can be helpful in reducing the tension and spasm associated with psychosomatic disorders.

Brain stimulation treatment, in the form of **electroconvulsive therapy (ECT),** is an effective treatment for severe depression that is unresponsive to other treatments. Electrodes are attached to the head and a series of electrical shocks are delivered to the brain to induce a brief seizure. The effect of this on the brain cells is not fully understood. Other brain stimulation therapies such as **repetitive transcranial magnetic stimulation** and **deep brain stimulation** are experimental.

The treatment of **posttraumatic stress disorder** is **multimodal,** involving **psychotherapy,** social interventions, and family and patient education. Forms of psychotherapy are **cognitive behavioral therapy (CBT)** and **cognitive processing therapy (CPT),** in which thoughts and beliefs generated by the trauma are reframed.

Care in a **psychiatric hospital** may be necessary for severe mental illness and can take the form of 24-hour inpatient care, partial or day hospitalization, or residential treatment to provide a temporary supportive place to live.

Word Analysis and Definition: Therapeutic Methods

S = Suffix P = Prefix R = Root R/CF = Combining Form

WORD	PRONUNCIATION	ELEMENTS		DEFINITION
biofeedback (**Note:** This term has no prefix or suffix.)	bye-oh-**FEED**-back	S/ R/ R/	**-back** *back, return* **bio-** *life* **-feed-** *to nourish*	Training techniques to achieve voluntary control of responses to stimuli
cognitive behavioral therapy (**Note:** Behavioral has two suffixes.)	**KOG**-nih-tiv be-**HAYV**-yur-al **THAIR**-ah-pee	S/ R/ S/ S/ R/	**-ive** *quality of* **cognit-** *thinking* **-al** *pertaining to* **-ior-** *pertaining to* **behav-** *mental activity* **therapy** Greek *medical treatment*	Psychotherapy that emphasizes thoughts and attitudes in one's behavior
cognitive processing therapy	**KOG**-nih-tiv **PROSS**-es-ing **THAIR**-ah-pee	S/ R/ S/ P/ R/	**-ive** *quality of* **cognit-** *thinking* **-ing** *doing* **pro-** *before* **cess-** *going forward* **therapy** Greek *medical treatment*	Psychotherapy to build skills to deal with the effects of trauma in other areas of life
electroconvulsive	ee-**LEK**-troh-**KON-VUL**-siv	S/ R/CF P/ R/	**-ive** *quality of* **electr/o-** *electricity* **-con-** *with* **-vuls-** *tear, pull*	Use of electrical current to produce convulsions
multimodal	mul-tee-**MOH**-dal	S/ P/ R/	**-al** *pertaining to* **multi-** *many* **-mod-** *method*	Using many methods
psychoanalysis	sigh-koh-ah-**NAL**-ih-sis	R/CF R/	**psych/o-** *mind* **-analysis** *process to define*	Method of psychotherapy
psychodynamic	sigh-koh-die-**NAM**-ik	S/ R/CF R/	**-ic** *pertaining to* **psych/o-** *mind* **-dynam-** *power*	The interplay between motivation and emotion
transcranial	trans-**KRAY**-nee-al	S/ P/ R/CF	**-al** *pertaining to* **trans-** *through* **-crani-** *skull*	Through the skull

Pharmacologic Agents Used for Mental Disorders

Psychiatric medications do not cure mental disorders, but they can significantly improve symptoms and help to make other treatments such as psychotherapy more effective. Commonly used classes of prescription medications are discussed below. Two examples of psychiatric medications and their effect on anxiety disorder are listed in in *Table 18.1*.

- **Selective serotonin reuptake inhibitors (SSRIs),** with generic and brand names fluoxetine (*Prozac*), fluoxamine (*Luvox*), paroxeline (*Paxil*), and sertraline (*Zoloft*); depression, bipolar disorder, anxiety disorders.

- **Serotonin and norepinephrine reuptake inhibitors (SNRIs),** with generic and brand names venlafaxine (*Effexor*), milnacipran (*Dalcipran*), and duloxetine (*Cymbalta*); depression, bipolar disorder.

- **Affect mainly dopamine and norepinephrine**—bupropion (*Wellbutrin*); depression.

- **Novel serotonergic drugs** such as vortioxetine (*Trintellix*—formerly called *Brintellix*) or vilazodone (*Viibryd*); major depressive disorder.

- **Tricyclic antidepressants (TCAs),** with generic names amitriptyline, protriptyline, clomipramine, imipramine, and trimipramine; depression.

- **Monoamine oxidase inhibitors (MAOIs),** with generic and brand names isocarboxazid (*Marplan*), phenelzine (*Nardil*), selegiline (*Ensam*), and tranylcypromine (*Parnate*); depression.

- **Mood stabilizers** to control manic or hypomanic episodes are lithium (*Lithobid*), valproic acid (*Depakene*), divalproex (*Depakote*), carbamazepine (*Tegretol*), and lamotrigine (*Lamictal*); bipolar disorder.

- **Antipsychotics** to help persistent symptoms of depression or mania are the newer, second-generation aripiprazole psychotics olanzapine (*Zyprexa*), risperidone (*Risperdal*), quetiapine (*Seroquel*), and aripiprazole (*Abilify*). These medications are also used to treat schizophrenia, often in combination with **benzodiazepine.**

- **Antidepressant-psychotic**—the medication *Symbyax* is a combination of the antidepressant fluoxetine and the antipsychotic olanzapine and is approved for the treatment of depressive disorders in bipolar disorder.

- **Benzodiazepines** such as diazepam (*Valium*), alprazolam (*Xanax*), clonazepam (*Klonopin*), and lorazepam (*Ativan*); anxiety disorders.

- **Stimulants** such as dextroamphetamine (*Adderal, Dexedrene*) and methylphenidate (*Ritalin, Metylin*) are used to treat attention-deficit/hyperactivity disorder (ADHD) and are also available in long-acting formats.

- **Hypnotics** such as zolpidem (*Ambien*), zaleplon (*Sonata*), and eszopiclone (*Lunesta*) also are used to treat insomnia.

- **Tranquilizers** such as chlorpromazine (*Thorazine*), haloperidol (*Aloperidin*), and the benzodiazepines calm like sedatives but without a sleep-inducing effect.

Table 18.1 Pharmacotherapy of panic disorder

Type of Drug	Effect
Benzodiazepines:	Effective prophylaxis
alprazolam *(Xanax)*	Reduce anticipatory anxiety
clonazepam *(Klonopin)*	Rapid onset of action
lorazepam *(Ativan)*	
diazepam *(Valium)*	
Selective Serotonin Reuptake Inhibitors (SSRIs):	Reduce frequency of attacks
sertraline *(Zoloft)*	Reduce intensity of panic
paroxetine *(Paxil)*	Take 2 weeks to produce effect
fluvoxamine *(Luvox)*	

Word Analysis and Definition: Pharmacologic Agents

S = Suffix P = Prefix R = Root R/CF = Combining Form

WORD	PRONUNCIATION	ELEMENTS		DEFINITION
antidepressant	**AN**-tih-dee-**PRESS**-ant	S/ P/ R/	-ant *agent* anti- *against* -depress- *press down*	An agent to suppress the symptoms of depression
antipsychotic	**AN**-tih-sigh-**KOT**-ik	S/ P/ R/CF	-tic *pertaining to* anti- *against* -psych/o- *mind*	An agent helpful in the treatment of psychosis
barbiturate	bar-**BIT**-chu-rat	S/ R/	-urate *salt of uric acid* barbit- *barbituric acid*	Central nervous system depressant used as a hyp-notic, anxiolytic, or anticonvulsant
benzodiazepine	ben-zoh-die-**AZ**-ah-peen	S/ P/ R/CF	-pine *pine* -diaze- *organic compound* benz/o- *benzene*	Central nervous system depressant used as a hyp-notic, anxiolytic, or anticonvulsant, or to produce amnesia
hypnotic	hip-**NOT**-ik	S/ R/CF	-tic *pertaining to* hypn/o- *sleep*	An agent that promotes sleep
sedative	**SED**-ah-tiv	S/ R/	-tive *quality of* sedat- *to calm*	Agent that calms nervous excitement
stabilizer	**STAY**-bill-ize-er	S/ S/ R/	-er *agent* -ize- *action* stabil- *fixed, steady*	Agent that helps create a steady state
stimulant	**STIM**-you-lant	S/ R/	-ant *forming* stimul- *excite*	Agent that excites functional activity
tranquilizer	**TRANG**-kwih-lie-zer	S/ R/	-izer *affects in a particular way* tranquil- *calm, serene*	Agent that calms without sedating or depressing

Did you know...

Dependence on drugs can be both psychological and physical.

Psychoactive Drugs

Psychoactive drugs are chemicals that change consciousness, awareness, or perception (*Table 18.2*). The most commonly used drugs are caffeine, tobacco, and alcohol.

Table 18.2 Psychoactive drugs

Type/Mode of Action	Name	Common Effects	Effects of Abuse
Stimulants ("uppers")	caffeine	Wakefulness, shorter reaction time, alertness	Restlessness, insomnia, heartbeat irregularities
Speed up activity in the central nervous system (CNS)	nicotine	Varies from alertness to calm-ness, appetite for carbohydrates decreases	Heart disease; high blood pressure; vaso-constriction; bronchitis; emphysema; lung, throat, mouth cancer
	amphetamines	Wakefulness, alertness, increased metabolism, decreased appetite	Nervousness, high blood pressure, delu-sions, psychosis, convulsions, death
	cocaine	**Euphoria,** high energy, illusions of power	Excitability, paranoia, anxiety, panic, depression, heart failure, death
Depressants ("downers")	alcohol	**1–2 drinks**—reduced inhibitions and anxiety	Blackouts, mental and neurologic impair-ment, psychosis, cirrhosis of liver, death
Slow down activity in the CNS		**Many drinks**—slow reaction time, poor coordination and memory	Impaired motor and sensory functions, amnesia, loss of consciousness, death
	barbiturates and tranquilizers	Reduced anxiety and tension, sedation	
Narcotics	codeine, opium, morphine, heroin	Euphoria, pleasure, relief of pain	High tolerance of pain, nausea, vomiting, constipation, convulsions, coma, death
Mimic the actions of natu-ral **endorphins**			
Psychedelics	marijuana **(THC)**	Relaxation, euphoria, increased appetite, pain relief	Sensory distortion, hallucinations, paranoia, throat and lung damage
Disrupt normal thought processes	**LSD,** mescaline, **MDMA** (ecstasy), **PCP** (angel dust)	Exhilaration, euphoria, hallucina-tions, insightful experiences	Panic, extreme delusions, bad trips, paranoia, psychosis

Drug abuse refers to the use of drugs that cause emotional or physical harm to an individual as consumption becomes frequent and compulsive.

Addiction occurs when a person feels compelled to use a drug or perform a certain activity and cannot control the use.

Psychological dependence is the mental desire or **craving** for the effects produced by a drug.

Physical dependence is the changes in the body processes that make the drug necessary for daily functioning. If the drug is stopped, the withdrawal symptoms include physical pain as well as intense cravings.

Tolerance occurs when the body adjusts to the effects of the drug, and higher and higher doses produce less and less effect. The brain, liver, heart, and other organs can be damaged.

Comorbidity is the presence of a combination of disorders. It is very common. Alcohol dependence and abuse overlap with almost all other mental disorders, including anxiety disorders, mood disorders, and personality disorders. In such cases, stopping drinking alcohol is only the first step in solving the problem.

Word Analysis and Definition: Psychoactive Drugs

S = Suffix P = Prefix R = Root R/CF = Combining Form

WORD	PRONUNCIATION	ELEMENTS		DEFINITION
comorbidity	koh-mor-**BID**-ih-tee	S/ P/ R/	-ity *condition, state* co- *with, together* -morbid- *disease*	Presence of two or more diseases at the same time
craving	**KRAY**-ving		Latin *desire*	Deep longing or desire
dependence	dee-**PEN**-dense	S/ R/	-ence *forming, quality of* depend- *relying on*	State of needing someone or something
depressant	dee-**PRESS**-ant	S/ P/ R/	-ant *agent* de- *away from* -press- *press down*	Substance that diminishes activity, sensation, or tone
endorphin	en-**DOR**-fin	P/ R/	end- *within* -orphin *morphine*	Natural substance in the brain that has same effect as opium
euphoria	yoo-**FOR**-ee-ah	S/ P/ R/	-ia *condition* eu- *normal* -phor- *bear, carry*	Exaggerated feeling of well-being
narcotic	nar-**KOT**-ik	S/ R/CF	-tic *pertaining to* narc/o- *sleep, stupor*	Drug derived from opium or a synthetic drug with similar effects
psychedelic	sigh-keh-**DEL**-ik	S/ R/CF R/	-ic *pertaining to* psych/e- *mind, soul* -del- *manifest, visible*	Agent that intensifies sensory perception
psychoactive	sigh-koh-**AK**-tiv	S/ R/CF R/	-ive *quality of, nature of* psych/o- *mind, soul* -act- *performance*	Able to alter mood, behavior, and/or cognition
stimulant	**STIM**-you-lant	S/ R/	-ant *agent* stimul- *excite*	Agent that excites or strengthens functional activity
tolerance	**TOL**-er-ants	S/ R/	-ance *condition, state of* toler- *endure*	The capacity to become accustomed to a stimulus or drug

Check Point Section 18.4

A. Identify the meaning of the word element to help you determine the meaning of the medical term. *One word element can change the entire meaning of the word. Match the term on the left with its correct definition on the right.* **LO 18.1, 18.7**

1. _____ psychotherapy

2. _____ psychoanalysis

3. _____ psychodynamic

a. method of psychotherapy

b. interplay between motivation and emotion

c. treatment of mental disorders through talking

B. Elements remain your best clue to the meaning of a medical term. *Match the element in the left column with its correct meaning in the right column.* **LO 18.2**

_____	**1.** *electr/o*	**a.**	mental activity
_____	**2.** *cognit*	**b.**	before
_____	**3.** *bio*	**c.**	nourish
_____	**4.** *pro-*	**d.**	pertaining to
_____	**5.** *vuls*	**e.**	tear
_____	**6.** *behav*	**f.**	life
_____	**7.** *con-*	**g.**	quality of
_____	**8.** *-ior*	**h.**	electricity
_____	**9.** *-ive*	**i.**	with
_____	**10.** *feed*	**j.**	thinking

C. Apply the elements of the language of medical terminology to answer the following questions. *Fill in the blanks.* **LO 18.7**

1. What are the differences between *behavioral, processing,* and *feedback* therapies?

a. Behavioral therapy _____

_____

b. Processing therapy _____

_____

c. Biofeedback therapy _____

_____

D. Define the types of medications used to treat mental disorders. *Choose the correct definition for the given medication.* **LO 18.7**

1. The action of a **sedative** is to:
   a. suppress the symptoms of depression   **b.** calm without depressing
   c. promote wakefulness   **d.** calm nervous excitement

2. The action of a **stabilizer** is to:
   a. create a steady state in mood   **b.** excite functional activity
   c. treat psychosis   **d.** promote sleep

3. The difference between a **tranquilizer** and a **sedative** is:
   a. tranquilizers treat psychosis and sedatives treat mania   **b.** sedatives treat depression and tranquilizers treat mania
   c. tranquilizers are used for inducing sleep and a sedative does not   **d.** sedatives induce sleep and tranquilizers do not

4. A patient may be prescribed a **hypnotic** to:
   a. promote sleep   **b.** reduce anxiety   **c.** prevent hallucinations   **d.** improve psychotherapy

5. A reason why a physician would prescribe a **benzodiazepine** would be due to its ability to induce:
   a. seizures   **b.** muscle spasms   **c.** memory loss   **d.** insomnia

E. Identify the action of medications and provide the abbreviation. *Read the description of the medications and treatments for mental disorders. Write the correct abbreviation for what is being described.* **LO 18.7, 18.9**

1. This medication affects the neurotransmitters serotonin and norepinephrine: _____

2. This medication is old and works by inhibiting an enzyme that breaks down neurotransmitters: _____

3. This medication prevents the reuptake of only serotonin: _____

F. Review all the new terms you have learned. *From the provided terms below, choose the correct medical term to insert into each of the following sentences. Fill in the blanks.* **LO 18.7**

| craving | endorphins | narcotic | psychoactive | psychedelic | stimulant | tolerance |

1. After repeated use of a drug, a person can build up a _____, which would cause the person to need a higher dose of the drug to get the same effect.

2. Marathon runners can experience the natural stimulatory effect from _____.

3. A(n) _____ mimics the effect of the naturally occurring substance endorphin.

4. A broad category of drugs that can alter mood, behavior, and/or cognition is _____.

5. A(n) _____ is an agent that can create feelings of euphoria along with pain relief and increased appetite.

6. Deep longing or desire is a(n) _____.

7. Nicotine is classified as a(n) _____.

Table 18.3 Chapter 18 Abbreviations

Abbreviations	Meaning
ADHD	attention-deficit/ hyperactivity disorder
BPD	borderline personality disorder
CBT	cognitive behavioral therapy
CPT	cognitive processing therapy
DID	dissociative identity disorder
DSM-5	Diagnostic and Statistical Manual of Mental Disorders, fifth edition
ECT	Electroconvulsive therapy
EMDR	eye movement desensitization and reprocessing
GAD	generalized anxiety disorder
LSD	lysergic acid diethylamide
MAOI	monoamine oxidase inhibitor
MDMA	methylenedioxymethamphetamine
MPD	multiple personality disorder
OCD	obsessive-compulsive disorder
PCP	phencyclidine
PhD	doctorate in philosophy
PsyD	doctorate in psychology
PTSD	posttraumatic stress disorder
SAD	seasonal affective disorder
SNRI	serotonin and norepinephrine reuptake inhibitor
SSD	somatic symptom disorder
SSRI	selective serotonin reuptake inhibitor
TCA	tricyclic antidepressant
THC	tetrahydrocannabinol
TTM	trichotillomania

Table 18.4 Comparison of Selected Mental Disorders—Signs, Symptoms, and Treatments

Disorder or Disease	Signs and Symptoms	Diagnostic Tests	Treatment
Schizophrenia	Hallucinations, delusions, disorganized speech	Complete and thorough physical examination to rule out other causes or illnesses.	Medications—*Seroquel, Risperdal.* psychotherapy
Bipolar disorder	Cycle of mania and depression. Mania may include high level of energy, no sleeping, reckless decisions. Depression with symptoms slow speaking, change in appetite, thoughts of suicide	Complete and thorough physical examination to rule out other causes or illnesses. Diagnosis is made by psychiatrist or other mental health professional.	Mood stabilizer medications—*Lamictal, Lithium, Tegretol*
Generalized anxiety disorder (GAD)	Frequent days of: Excessive worry, difficulty in controlling the worry, irritability	Complete and thorough physical examination to rule out other causes or illnesses. Anxiety disrupts normal functioning in work or social functions.	Exercise, SSRI's (*Lexapro, Prozac, Zoloft*), SRNI's (*Cymbalta*)
Obsessive–compulsive disorder	Fear of dirt and contamination, wanting things to be in perfect order, creating ritual behaviors	Complete and thorough physical examination to rule out other causes or illnesses. Attempt to ignore obsessive thoughts, uses compulsive behavior as a way to stop obsessive thoughts.	Medications—*Paxil, Prozac, Zoloft* Cognitive-behavioral therapy
ADHD in adults	Trouble multitasking, poor planning, trouble completing tasks, difficulty in coping with stress, hot temper	Complete and thorough physical examination to rule out other causes or illnesses ADHD rating test	Stimulants—dextroamphetamine (*Adderal*), bupropion (*Wellbutrin*) Cognitive behavioral therapy
Borderline personality disorder	Fear of abandonment, risky behavior, impulsiveness, suicidal threats, intense anger	Complete and thorough physical examination to rule out other causes or illnesses Can have a family history of BPD, usually occurs with other mental health disorders such as depression, eating disorders, and substance abuse disorder	Psychotherapy Medication may be indicated to treat the mental health disorders that are occurring with BPD.

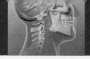
Challenge Your Knowledge

A. **Abbreviations.** Apply your knowledge of abbreviations to complete the following patient documentation. Choose from the following abbreviations to correctly fill in the blanks. You will have more answers than questions. **LO 18.9**

ECT   CNS   PTSD   BPD   DID   CBT   SSRI   STAT

  1. Patient now has developed three distinct, separate personalities. Her _____ is rapidly progressing.

  2. Patient is suffering from unipolar depression, and a(n) _____ medication will be prescribed.

  3. Patient's nightmares are increasing and are always the same replay of his automobile accident. I am sending him

      for _____ in the hopes this can alleviate some of his _____ and help him sleep better. Sleep medication is also prescribed.

  4. Patient exhibits frequent mood changes and has become manipulative in her relationship with her parents.

      Her _____ is escalating her insecurity.

  5. _____ will be prescribed for this patient as a last resort for treatment of his mania.

B. **Prefixes.** Test your recall of word element meanings by answering the following questions about prefixes. The medical term is given; fill in the blank with the word element that is the prefix, then select the best answer. **LO 18.2**

  1. *bipolar:* Prefix is _____ and means

     a. one

     b. two

     c. three

     d. four

     e. five

  2. *hypochondriasis:* Prefix is _____ and means

     a. after

     b. around

     c. deficient

     d. next to

     e. excessive

  3. *depressant:* Prefix is _____ and means

     a. toward

     b. forming

     c. within

     d. away from

     e. around

  4. *catatonia:* Prefix is _____ and means

     a. up

     b. around

     c. through

     d. down

     e. beside

  5. *addiction:* Prefix is _____ and means

     a. toward

     b. from

     c. for

     d. with

     e. up

  6. *euphoria:* Prefix is _____ and means

     a. marketplace

     b. mind

     c. normal

     d. madness

     e. wound

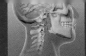

7. *paranoia:* Prefix is _____ and means

   a. above

   b. excessive

   c. abnormal

   d. condition

   e. study of

8. *unipolar:* Prefix is _____ and means

   a. one

   b. four

   c. many

   d. few

   e. none

9. *dissociative:* Prefix is _____ and means

   a. painful

   b. apart

   c. abnormal

   d. irregular

   e. together

10. *convulsive:* Prefix is _____ and means

   a. in front of

   b. with

   c. next to

   d. yellow

   e. small

C. **Language of psychology and psychiatry.** Employ your knowledge of the *language of mental health* to match the statement in the left column with the correct medical vocabulary in the right column. **LO 18.1, 18.5, 18.6**

_____ **1.** lack of contact with reality

_____ **2.** symptoms with no physical cause

_____ **3.** refusal or inability to speak

_____ **4.** legal term, not a diagnosis

_____ **5.** motor immobility for hours

_____ **6.** deep sadness and despair

_____ **7.** mistaken belief, contrary to fact

_____ **8.** individual's unique pattern of thought

_____ **9.** unable to recall identity

_____ **10.** emotional state that is self-destructive

   a. delusion

   b. mutism

   c. dissociative amnesia

   d. personality

   e. mental disorder

   f. catatonia

   g. somatoform

   h. psychosis

   i. depression

   j. insanity

D. **Define terms that are unique to psychiatry and psychology.** Match the terms on the left with their correct description on the right. **LO 18.6, 18.8, 18.10**

_____ **1.** psychologist

_____ **2.** psychiatrist

_____ **3.** psychotherapist

_____ **4.** insanity

_____ **5.** homicidal

_____ **6.** delusion

_____ **7.** suicidal

   a. wanting to kill oneself

   b. fixed false belief held despite strong evidence to the contrary

   c. condition in which person is unable to be responsible for his actions

   d. licensed specialist in treatment of human mind and behavior

   e. wanting to kill another human being

   f. medical doctor who diagnoses and treats mental disorders

   g. practitioner who uses communication to treat mental disorders

Using the terms above in the left column, write the term that best defines the following sentences.

Mr. Robinson has a mental disorder that he and a female celebrity have a romantic relationship. The celebrity does not know Mr. Robinson. His family recommends that he talk to a professional to talk about this belief. He would benefit from speaking with a **(8.)** _____.

A patient comes to a hospital's emergency department because she feels like taking her life. She is **(9.)** _____. The emergency department contacts a **(10.)** _____, who can effectively diagnose and treat her current condition.

The police have been called to a residence because the adult male in the home has been threatening to kill the other people in the home. He is being suspected of having **(11.)** _____ thoughts. His family has reported that he talks to people that are not in the room and behaves oddly, leading them to think he may be suffering from **(12.)** _____.

E. **Latin and Greek terms cannot be further deconstructed into prefix, root, or suffix.** You must know them for what they are. Test your knowledge of these terms with this exercise. Match the meaning in the first column with the correct medical term in the second column. **LO 18.1**

_____ 1. silent   **a.** mania

_____ 2. medical treatment   **b.** affect

_____ 3. knowledge   **c.** mute

_____ 4. frenzy   **d.** phobia

_____ 5. desire   **e.** craving

_____ 6. forgetfulness   **f.** anxiety

_____ 7. fear   **g.** amnesia

_____ 8. distress   **h.** cognitive

_____ 9. state of mind   **i.** therapy

F. **Deconstruction.** Deconstruct these medical terms into the meanings of their basic elements. Fill in the chart. If the term does not have an element, write n/a. **LO 18.2**

Medical Term	Prefix	Meaning of Prefix	Root/ Combining Form	Meaning of Root/ Combining Form	Suffix	Meaning of Suffix	Meaning of Term
antipsychotic	1.	2.	3.	4.	5.	6.	7.
pyromania	8.	9.	10.	11.	12.	13.	14.
insomnia	15.	16.	17.	18.	19.	20.	21.
comorbidity	22.	23.	24.	25.	26.	27.	28.
endorphin	29.	30.	31.	32.	33.	34.	35.

2014 Nucleus Medical Media

G. **Use your knowledge of the language of psychology and psychiatry.** Choose the correct answer to the following questions. *Remember:* There is only one *best* answer. **LO 18.7, 18.9**

1. A personality disorder in which a person pulls out his or her body hairs:

   a. PTSD

   b. SAD

   c. TTM

   d. OCD

   e. MPD

2. Manic-depressive disorder is now known as

   a. borderline personality

   b. unipolar disorder

   c. generalized anxiety disorder

   d. mania

   e. bipolar disorder

3. A TCA used to treat depression is

   a. *Prozac*

   b. *Paxil*

   c. amitriptyline

   d. *Zoloft*

   e. duloxetine

4. Significant trauma can lead to

   a. OCD

   b. TTM

   c. SAD

   d. DID

   e. PTSD

5. Select the drug NOT prescribed for a panic disorder:

   a. *Tegretol*

   b. *Paxil*

   c. *Xanax*

   d. *Zoloft*

   e. *Klonopin*

H. **Apply your knowledge of the language of psychology and psychiatry.** Choose the correct answer to the following questions. *Remember:* There is only one *best* answer. **LO 18.6, 18.9**

1. A combination of CBT and EMDR would be treatment for

   a. MPD

   b. DID

   c. OCD

   d. PTSD

   e. TTM

2. No identifiable physical cause to explain physical symptoms characterizes

   a. hypochondriasis

   b. acrophobia

   c. conversion disorder

   d. agoraphobia

   e. somatoform disorder

3. Perceiving things without a stimulation is a(n)

   a. compulsion

   b. delusion

   c. hallucination

   d. obsession

   e. tangent

4. Higher doses of a drug produce less effect:

    a. psychological dependence   **d.** physical dependence

    b. addiction   **e.** comorbidity

    c. tolerance

5. Schizophrenia is a form of

    a. delusion   **d.** mood disorder

    b. phobia   **e.** obsession

    c. psychosis

I. Suffixes. Mental health practitioners can be either *psycho*logists or *psychi*atrists. The root/combining form *psych/o-* is present in all the following terms. The suffix is what makes the difference. Challenge your knowledge of the language of mental health by applying the correct term to the following statements. Fill in the blanks, using the choices below. **LO 18.10**

psychopath	**psychiatry**	**psychiatric**	**psychotherapy**
psychotic	**psychoactive**	**psychoanalysis**	**psychology**
psychiatrist	**psychoanalyst**	**psychologist**	**psychological**
psychosomatic	**psychotherapist**	**psychosis**	

1. An agent able to alter mood, behavior, or cognition is _____.

2. Treatment of mental disorders through communication is called _____.

3. _____ is the science concerned with the behavior of humans.

4. A licensed specialist in psychology is known as a _____.

5. The patient's _____ state was starting to affect his physical well-being.

6. A method of psychotherapy is _____.

7. What type of technician is the health care worker in the first CR at the beginning of this chapter? _____ *technician*

8. A medical specialist in psychiatry is a _____.

9. A practitioner of psychoanalysis is called a _____.

10. Disorder causing mental disruption and loss of contact with reality is _____.

11. _____ is the medical specialty dealing with the diagnosis and treatment of mental disorders.

12. A practitioner of psychotherapy is a _____.

13. A real, physical disorder that, at least in part, has a psychological cause is _____.

14. Pertaining to or affected by psychosis is _____.

15. A serial killer can be termed a _____.

J. **Pronunciation is important whether you are saying the word or listening to a word from a coworker.** Identify the proper pronunciation of the following medical terms. **LO 18.4**

1. The correct pronunciation for the inability to sleep

    a. dis-**FOR**-ee-ah

    b. dis-for-**EE**-ah

    c. in-**SOM**-nee-ah

    d. in-som-**NEE**-ah

    Correctly spell the term: _____

2. The correct pronunciation for disorder of perception, thought, emotion, and behavior

    a. skitz-oh-**FREE**-nee-ah

    b. skitz-oh-free-**NEE**-ah

    c. kat-ah-**TOH**-nee-ah

    d. **KAT**-ah-toh-nee-ah

    Correctly spell the term: _____

3. The correct pronunciation for physical symptoms occurring without identifiable physical cause

    a. soh-**MAT**-oh-form

    b. **SOH**-mat-oh-form

    c. sigh-koh-soh-**MAT**-ik

    d. sigh-**KOH**-soh-**MAT**-ik

    Correctly spell the term: _____

4. The correct pronunciation for expressing emotion

    a. ay-FEK-**TIV**

    b. af-**FEK**-tiv

    c. **AY**-fect-iv

    d. af-**FEK**-tiev

    Correctly spell the term: _____

5. The correct pronunciation for a central nervous system depressant used as a hypnotic, anxiolytic, or anticonvulsant

    a. bar-**BIT**-chu-rat

    b. bar-bit-**CHU**-rat

    c. trang-**KWIH**-lie-zer

    d. **TRANG**-kwih-lie-zer

    Correctly spell the term: _____

Case Reports

A. After reading the following Case Report, correctly answer the following questions. The answers to the questions may not be in the Case Report itself but can be found in the chapter content. **LO 18.1, 18.3, 18.5, 18.6, 18.8, 18.10**

 Case Report (CR) 18.1

You are

. . . a **psychiatric technician** employed in the Psychiatric Department of Fulwood Medical Center. Your patient has been referred from the Emergency Department where he was seen earlier this morning.

Your patient Is

. . . Mr. Harlan Diment, a 40-year-old construction worker. He was brought to the Emergency Department by his roommate, who says that Mr. Diment has slept only a couple of hours each night for the past 3 weeks. He stays up most of the night, cleaning their apartment and drinking beer. He has bought a new home entertainment set, including a big-screen TV, that he cannot afford. He is very irritable and explosive when challenged about his behavior. His roommate has seen no signs of drugs and is not aware of any medical problems. Mr. Diment is usually very quiet, thoughtful, and introverted.

A mental status examination shows Mr. Diment to be alternately irritable and excited. His speech is rapid and loud, and it is difficult to interrupt him. He paces the room, claims to feel "great," and is angry with his roommate for insisting that he come to the hospital. He says he has no suicidal thoughts, **hallucinations,** or **delusions.**

---

1. You are assessing the patient for causes of his behavior. Which method would help you quickly rule out drugs as a cause of his behavior?

   a. MRI
   b. urinalysis

   c. psychological analysis
   d. biofeedback

2. The medical term that could be substituted for his sleeping pattern is:

   a. insomnia
   b. apathy

   c. obstructive
   d. dysphoric

3. Which of the following questions would determine if Mr. Diment has delusions?

   a. "Do you feel like hurting yourself?"
   b. "Does buying expensive things make you feel better?"

   c. "Do you see objects that you know don't truly exist?"
   d. "Do you think that you have abilities that no other people have?"

4. Based on the presented symptoms, which mental health disorder do you suspect Mr. Diment has?

   a. manic phase
   b. narcissism

   c. social phobia
   d. anxiety

5. The type of physician with the specialty in mental health disorders that will be called to evaluate Mr. Diment would be a:

_____

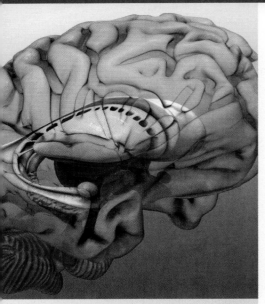

2014 Nucleus Medical Media

Chapter Sections

Chapter Learning Outcomes

Upon completion of this chapter, you will be able to:

LO 19.1 Describe the aging and the process, senescence, and death.

LO 19.2 Use roots, combining forms, suffixes, and prefixes to construct and analyze medical terms related to geriatrics.

LO 19.3 Spell medical terms related to geriatrics.

LO 19.4 Pronounce medical terms related to geriatrics.

LO 19.5 Describe diagnostic procedures utilized in geriatrics.

LO 19.6 Identify and describe disorders of aging.

LO 19.7 Describe the therapeutic procedures and pharmacologic agents used in geriatrics.

LO 19.8 Apply knowledge of medical terms relating to geriatrics to documentation, medical records, and communication.

LO 19.9 Identify and correctly use abbreviations of terms used in geriatrics.

LO 19.10 Identify health professionals involved in the care of geriatric patients.

In many situations, a team of health professionals can work together to meet the different needs of older patients. The team can include:

- **Geriatricians,** who are physicians who specialize in the care of elderly people.
- **Gerontologists,** who are professionals who study the aging process.
- **Geriatric nurse practitioners (NP),** who are nurses with special training in the care of the elderly.
- **Social workers, nutritionists, and physical and occupational therapists,** who are also members of the geriatric care team as needs for their services arise.

Section 19.1 Aging and Senescence

Aging

Aging is the gradual, spontaneous changes resulting in maturation through childhood, adolescence, and young adulthood and causing a decline in function (rather than maturation) through late adulthood and old age.

Senile is a term used to refer to the characteristics of old age, and **senility** is the general term used in referring to a person who demonstrates a variety of conditions of mental disorders occurring in old age.

Gerontology is the study of the social, mental, and physical aspects of aging. Professionals from diverse fields call themselves **gerontologists**. The medical field that involves the study, care, and treatment of the elderly *(Figure 19.1)* is called **geriatrics**, and a medical specialist in geriatrics is called a **geriatrician**.

- **Life span** is the age to which individual humans aspire to live and the process of getting there.
- **Life expectancy** is the average length of life for any given population.
- **Longevity** is living beyond the normal life expectancy.
- **Senescence** is the loss over time of the ability of cells to divide, grow, and function, a process that terminates in death. It is sometimes used interchangeably with the term aging.

Profile of Older Americans

According to the latest statistics published by the Administration on Aging (AoA) of the U.S. Department of Health and Human Services in 2019:

- The population aged 65 and older numbered 52.4 million in 2018, compared to 38.8 million in 2018, and is projected to be 94.7 million in 2060.
- About one in every seven, or 14.9% of the population, is 65 or older.
- Persons reaching age 65 have an average life expectancy of an additional 19.4 years (20.6 years for females and 18 years for males).
- Older women outnumber older men at 29.1 million older women to 23.3 million older men.
- In 2018, 23% of persons 65+ were members of racial or ethnic minority populations: 9% were African American, 5% were Asian, and 8% were Hispanic.
- As of 2019, about 28% (14.7 million) of noninstitutionalized older persons live alone (9.7 million women, 5 million men).
- The 85+ population is projected to increase from 6.5 million to 14.6 million in 2040.
- Over 5.1 million adults (9.7%) were below the poverty level in 2018.
- Most older people have at least one chronic medical condition, and many have multiple conditions.
- The most frequently occurring conditions among the elderly are:
  - Arthritis (54%)
  - Hypertension (67% of men and 79% of women)
  - All types of heart disease (28%)
  - Any cancer (19%)
  - Diabetes (28%)

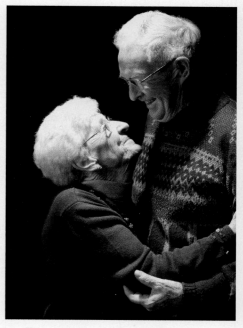

▲ **Figure 19.1 Elderly couple.** Darren Greenwood/Design Pics

Did you know...

- Future estimates of Americans with Alzheimer's disease will increase due to changes in how it is diagnosed.

WORD	PRONUNCIATION	ELEMENTS		DEFINITION
aging	**AY**-jing		Latin *aging*	The process of human maturation and decline
aged	**AY**-jid		Latin *being old*	Having lived to an advanced age
geriatrics (*Note:* This term contains two roots.)	jer-ee-**AT**-riks	S/ R/ R/	-ics *knowledge of* ger- *old age* -iatr- *medical treatment*	Medical specialty that deals with the problems of old age
geriatrician	jer-ee-ah-**TRISH**-an	S/	-ician *expert*	Medical specialist in geriatrics
gerontology	jer-on-**TOL**-oh-jee	S/ R/CF	-logy *study of* geront/o- *process of aging*	Study of the process and problems of aging
gerontologist	jer-on-**TOL**-oh-jist	S/	-logist *specialist*	Specialist in the process and general problems of aging
life expectancy	LIFE ek-**SPEK**-tan-see	S/ R/	-ancy *state of* expect- *await* life Old English *life*	Statistical determination of the number of years an individual is expected to live
life span	LIFE SPAN		span Old English *reach* or *stretch*	The age that a person reaches
longevity	lon-**JEV**-ih-tee	S/ R/	-ity *condition, state* longev- *long life*	Duration of life beyond the normal expectation
senescence	seh-**NES**-ens	S/ R/	-ence *state of, quality of* senesc- *growing old*	The state of being old
senescent (adj)		S/	-ent *end result, state of*	Growing old
senile	**SEE**-nile	S/ R/	-ile *capability* sen- *old age*	Characteristic of old age
senility	seh-**NIL**-ih-tee	S/ R/	-ity *condition, state* senil- *characteristic of old age*	Mental disorders occurring in old age

Senescence of Organ Systems

Organ systems begin to show signs of senescence at very different ages and do not degenerate at the same speed. Most physiologic studies show general peak physical performance occurs during a person's twenties, but surprisingly, **autopsies (postmortems)** in children will often reveal atherosclerosis in the arteries supplying the heart. Autopsies are usually performed by a **pathologist** or a medical examiner.

Integumentary system (*see Chapter 4*) changes begin in a person's forties. Melanocytes die, and hair becomes gray and thinner. The skin becomes paper thin, loses elasticity, and hangs loose, and wrinkles appear (*Figure 19.2*). Flat brown-black spots called **senile lentigines** (age spots) appear on the back of the hands and areas exposed to sunlight.

Special senses start to decline in the twenties. Visual acuity declines at that time. In the forties, presbyopia (*see Chapter 16*) begins, and many people develop cataracts later, in old age. Hearing loss occurs as the ossicles become stiffer and the number of cochlear hair cells (*see Chapter 16*) declines. Taste and smell also are blunted late in life, as taste cells and olfactory buds decline in number.

Skeletal system (*see Chapter 14*) changes appear during a person's thirties, as osteoblasts become less active than osteoclasts. The result is osteopenia, which later develops into osteoporosis—particularly in postmenopausal women. The joints of people in their later years have less synovial fluid and thinner articular cartilage, and often, osteoarthritis results.

Muscular system (*see Chapter 15*) changes occur with age as muscle mass is lost (**sarcopenia**) and replaced with fat. As muscle **atrophies**, there are fewer muscle fibers to do the work; as a result, the available blood supply decreases. Tasks that used to be easy become difficult, such as buttoning shirts and tying shoelaces.

Nervous system (*see Chapter 9*) changes begin around age 30, when the brain weighs twice as much as it does at age 75. Motor coordination, intellectual function, and short-term memory decline more quickly than long-term memory and language skills.

Cardiovascular systems (*see Chapter 10*) always have coronary artery atherosclerosis, even at a very early age. As a result, when aging myocardial cells die, the heart wall gets thinner and weaker, and cardiac output declines. This causes the decline in physical capabilities with aging. Atherosclerotic plaques narrow arteries and trigger thrombosis, leading to strokes and heart attacks. In veins, valves become weaker, and blood flows back and pools in the legs, leading to poor venous return to the heart and heart failure.

Respiratory system *(see Chapter 13)* changes are noticeable in the thirties, as pulmonary ventilation declines. This decline is a factor in the gradual loss of stamina that occurs as people age. The rib cage becomes less flexible, and the lungs become less elastic and have fewer alveoli. Respiratory function declines. As respiratory health declines, hypoxic degenerative changes occur in all the other organ systems.

Urinary system *(see Chapter 6)* changes begin in a person's twenties, when the number of nephrons starts to decline. Later in life, many of the remaining glomeruli become atherosclerotic. The body's glomerular filtration rate (GFR) decreases, and the kidneys become less efficient. For example, drug doses in the elderly are generally lower than those for younger people because drugs cannot be cleared from the elderly's blood as rapidly.

Immune system *(see Chapter 12)* function declines in the elderly, as the amounts of lymphatic tissue and red bone marrow in their bodies decrease with age. This leads to a reduction in both cellular and humoral (antibody) immunity. As a result, the elderly have lower levels of protection against infectious diseases and cancer.

Specific **disorders of senescence** and their terminology are described in each of the body system chapters in this book.

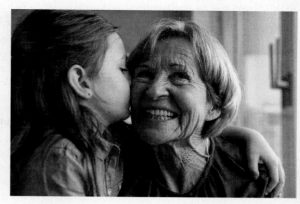

▲ **Figure 19.2** Senescence of the skin. Elderly Tibetan woman with her granddaughter. Westend61/ Getty Images

Word Analysis and Definition: Senescence

S = Suffix P = Prefix R = Root R/CF = Combining Form

WORD	PRONUNCIATION	ELEMENTS		DEFINITION
atrophy atrophies (verb)	**AT**-roh-fee **AT**-roh-feez	P/ R/	a- *without* -trophy *development, nourishment*	Wasting or diminished volume of a tissue or organ
autopsy postmortem (syn)	**AWE**-top-see post-**MOR**-tem	S/ P/ P/ R/	-opsy *to view* aut- *self, same* post- *after* mortem Latin *death*	Examination of the body and organs of a dead person to determine the cause of death
lentigo lentigines (pl)	len-**TIE**-go len-**TIHJ**-ih-neez		Greek *lentil*	Age spot; small, flat, brown-black spot in the skin of older people
pathologist	pa-**THOL**-oh-jist	S/ R/CF	-logist *one who studies, specialist* path/o- *disease*	A specialist in pathology (study of disease or characteristics of a particular disease)
sarcopenia	sar-koh-**PEE**-nee-ah	S/ R/CF	-penia *deficiency* sarc/o- *flesh*	Progressive loss of muscle mass and strength in aging

Theories of Senescence

The causes of **senescence** are unknown. **Heredity** plays a role because longevity or early death tends to run in families. Theories of senescence include:

- **Protein abnormalities.** One-quarter of the body's protein is collagen. With age, collagen and other proteins show abnormal structures in their cells and tissues, and become less soluble and more rigid. The cells accumulate more of these dysfunctional proteins as they age, and their functions are impaired, leading to **senescent** changes.

- **Free radicals.** These are chemical particles with an extra electron. For example, the stable oxygen molecule (O_2) has two atoms with many electrons. If it picks up an extra electron through some metabolic reaction, by radiation, or by chemical action, it becomes a free radical. The free radical's life is short because it combines quickly with other molecules that, in turn, become free radicals with the addition of the extra electron. A chain reaction occurs as more and more molecules become free radicals. Among the damage they cause are cancer, myocardial infarction, and perhaps senescence. They can be neutralized by **antioxidants**.

- **Autoimmune-altered molecules** *(see Chapter 12)*. These molecules may be recognized as foreign antigens, and an immune response may be generated against the body's own tissues. This theory is helped by the fact that autoimmune diseases such as rheumatoid arthritis are more common in old age.

Complex Effects of Aging

Decline in physiologic reserve can produce complications from mild problems. The appearance of symptoms of aging depends on the remaining healthy reserves of organs as they decline with age. For example, renal **impairment** can be part of aging, but renal **failure** is not. Most drugs are excreted by the liver or kidneys, either of which can be impaired in the elderly. As a result, the dosage of medications may need to be adjusted to avoid excessive levels in the blood and undesirable side effects.

Vague and **nonspecific symptoms** require health care providers to take time and care to discover their root cause. For example, pneumonia can present with low-grade fever, confusion, or falls rather than with the high fever and cough seen in younger adults. Something as simple as constipation can cause **delirium** in the elderly. Some older adults may have difficulty describing their symptoms, particularly if they have cognitive impairment.

Polypharmacy can result in **adverse** drug interactions. Polypharmacy includes prescription medications, over-the-counter (OTC) medications, and herbal supplements. It is important that the primary care health provider or gerontologist work with the patient to **deprescribe** unnecessary drugs.

Technologies assist patients in taking the right drug at the right time to avoid adverse effects of polypharmacy. Pill organizers (*Figure 19.3*) sort pills by day and times; calendars and notebooks can document times when drugs were taken; mobile apps can provide reminders to take the correct medication at the right time.

Aging has some benefits and advantages for many people. These include:

- Increased knowledge of life (wisdom).
- Freedom from many of the day-to-day responsibilities that working adults face.
- Freedom to be gentle and grow with oneself.
- Time to enjoy family.
- Freedom to choose to participate in childrearing for grandchildren or other relatives.
- Increased participation in volunteer organizations.

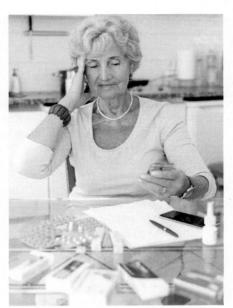

▲ **Figure 19.3** Elderly woman confused about her medications.
Iakov Filimonov/Shutterstock

Did you know...

- Polypharmacy is frequently described as the use of five or more prescribed drugs at one time.
- An estimated 28% of older people in America are receiving polypharmacy.
- When a physician or a nurse practitioner or a pharmacist oversees an elderly patient's medication regimen, drug-related problems are less likely to occur.
- The elderly patient should bring all of his/her medications to every hospital or office visit, including prescription drugs, over-the-counter (**OTC**) drugs, and all supplements.

Word Analysis and Definition: Effects of Aging

S = Suffix   P = Prefix   R = Root   R/CF = Combining Form

WORD	PRONUNCIATION		ELEMENTS	DEFINITION
adverse	**AD**-vers	P/ R/	**ad-** *toward* **-verse** *turned*	Noxious, unintended, undesired
antioxidant	an-tee-**OKS**-ih-dant	S/ P/ R/	**-ant** forming **anti-** *against* **-oxid-** *oxidize*	Substance that can prevent cell damage by neutralizing free radicals
delirium	deh-**LIR**-ee-um	S/ R/	**-um** structure **deliri-** *confusion, disorientation*	Acute altered state of consciousness with agitation and disorientation
deprescribe	dee-**PREE**-skribe	P/ P/ R/	**de-** *take away* **-pre-** *before* **-scribe** *write*	Process of stopping drugs that are no longer needed or may be causing harm
failure	**FAIL**-yer		Old French *to fail*	Unable to perform a normal function
free radical	FREE **RAD**-ih-kal	 S/ R/	**free** Old English *free* **-al** pertaining to **radic-** *root*	Short-lived product of oxidation in a cell that can be damaging to the cell
heredity	heh-**RED**-ih-tee	S/ R/	**-ity** condition, state **hered-** *inherited through genes*	Transmission of characteristics from parents to offspring through genes
impairment	im-**PAIR**-ment	S/ R/	**-ment** *action, state* **impair-** *worsen*	Diminishing of normal function
polypharmacy	pol-ee-**FAR**-mah-see	P/ R/	**poly-** *many* **-pharmacy** *drug*	The administration of many drugs at the same time

Check Point Section 19.1

A. Choose the correct definition for each of the following medical terms from the *languages of geriatrics and gerontology*. *Match the medical term in the first column with its correct meaning in the second column.* **LO 19.1**

_____ 1. senile

_____ 2. longevity

_____ 3. senility

_____ 4. geriatrics

_____ 5. gerontology

_____ 6. life expectancy

_____ 7. life span

a. mental disorders that occur in old age

b. new field that involves study, care, and treatment of the elderly

c. characteristic of old age

d. duration of life beyond the normal expected time

e. the age a person reaches

f. study of the process and problems of aging

g. the number of years a person is expected to live

B. Proper pronunciation of medical terms. *Identify the proper pronunciation of the bolded area of each medical term.* **LO 19.6**

1. sarco**pe**nia

   a. pie   **b.** pay   **c.** pee   **d.** peh

2. len**ti**go

   a. tie   **b.** tay   **c.** tee   **d.** the

3. lentig**ines**

   a. nighs   **b.** nays   **c.** knees   **d.** nose

C. Choose the correct answer for the following questions. **LO 19.6**

1. What does the medical term **lentigo** identify?

   a. skin lesion   **b.** skin tumor   **c.** skin type   **d.** skin spots   **e.** skin wrinkles

2. What is the correct plural of **lentigo**?

   a. lentigos   **b.** lentigoes   **c.** lentigones   **d.** lentigines   **e.** lentigons

3. Another medical term used for **autopsy** is

   a. senescence   **b.** senility   **c.** geriatrics   **d.** atrophy   **e.** postmortem

4. What is the correct element that means *after*?

   a. *post*   **b.** *em*   **c.** *mort*   **d.** *auto*   **e.** *patho*

5. What is the purpose of a *postmortem*?

   a. to discover the patient's blood type

   b. to discover the cause of death

   c. to discover the weight of the body organs

   d. to discover the body's final blood volume

   e. to discover the presence of foreign bodies

D. Complete the sentences with the correct medical term. *Fill in the blanks.* **LO 19.1**

1. Elderly persons often need care from several health care providers. Often, the specialists prescribe medications without knowing all of the other medications a patient may be taking. It is possible for patients to suffer from the interaction *multiple medications* (1) _____.

2. A person's life span can be affected by *inherited traits* (2) _____. The effect of *products that can damage cells* (3) _____ can also play a role. A healthy diet rich in *substances that neutralize free radicals* (4) _____ can be helpful.

E. Use the appropriate abbreviation to complete the sentence. *Fill in the blanks.* **LO 19.9**

1. Medications that do not require a prescription: _____

2. Chronic obstructive pulmonary diseases: _____

Section 19.2 Disorders of Aging

Disorders of Aging

The major categories of impairment in elderly people as they begin to fail (the so-called **Geriatric Giants**) include:

- immobility
- instability
- incontinence
- impaired intellect/memory

Immobility is a common pathway produced by many diseases and problems, particularly those that involve prolonged bed rest, immobilization, or inactivity. It can also occur when it is self-imposed—when elderly patients do not exercise to keep limbs flexible, promote circulation, and improve well-being. Many factors influencing the elderly's state of immobility are **iatrogenic**, or arising from medical regimens, institutional policies, and resident and staff characteristics in nursing homes. The negative consequences of immobility often can be avoided with careful and vigilant medical and nursing management.

Instability, or difficulty in balance *(Figure 19.4)*, is often the first problem that the elderly person encounters. The instability and associated falls can result from a single disease process or the accumulated effects of multiple diseases. It is essential to take a careful, detailed history and examination to define all the factors contributing to the instability and to develop the appropriate interventions to prevent future falls. Instability and falling are not inevitable in aging but are problems that arise from identifiable disabilities that are often treatable.

Incontinence is the inability to prevent the discharge of urine or feces. It is a common, but never normal, part of aging. Urinary incontinence can cause a decrease in quality of life and an increase in the need for care. There are five main types of urinary incontinence:

- **Urge incontinence,** the loss of urine before one can get to the toilet, is the most common form in the elderly. It can be caused by strokes, multiple sclerosis, dementia, and pelvic floor atrophy in women or prostate enlargement in men.
- **Stress incontinence** is caused by weak bladder muscles. It occurs when the abdominal pressure when you cough, sneeze, laugh, or climb stairs overcomes the closing pressure of the bladder.
- **Overflow incontinence** is rare. It occurs when the bladder never completely empties and leaks small amounts of urine.
- **Functional incontinence** is an inability to reach the toilet in time; for example, due to arthritis, stroke, or dementia.
- **Mixed incontinence** is usually a combination of stress and urge incontinence.

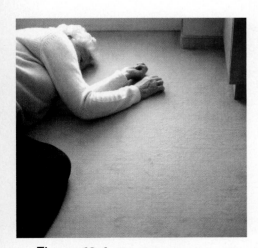

▲ **Figure 19.4** **Elderly woman injured in a fall.** Cristina Pedrazzini/Science Source

Fecal incontinence occurs in about one-third of the elderly in institutional care, and is the second most common reason for committing the elderly to a nursing home. It can be produced by local causes such as chronic laxative abuse or muscle damage to the sphincter muscles in surgery or childbirth. It also is seen in dementia, multiple sclerosis, and diabetes.

Impaired intellect/memory that is present for at least six months is called **dementia**. The **cognitive** functions that are affected include decision making, judgment, memory, thinking, reasoning, and verbal communication. Dementia is not a normal part of aging, but advancing age is the greatest risk factor. More than 5 million people aged 65 and older have dementia and more than 500,000 people under 65 have early-onset dementia.

Dementia

Dementia is an overall term for diseases characterized by a decline in memory and **cognitive** (thinking) skills. In mild dementia, there is evidence of cognitive decline and recent memory loss that do not interfere with **activities of daily living (ADLs)**. Then dementia progresses to cause significant cognitive decline in memory, language, and learning, sufficient to interfere with independence in ADLs. Ultimately confusion; disorientation; and difficulty speaking, swallowing, and walking take away independent living. All dementias are caused by damage inside and around the brain's neurons with different pathological changes. There is no cure.

Alzheimer disease (AD) accounts for 60% to 80% of dementias and is a slowly progressive dementia that begins well before clinical symptoms arise. **Vascular dementia** arises from infarcts (strokes) or bleeding into the brain and accounts for about 10% of dementia cases. In older individuals, pathologic changes of both Alzheimer and vascular dementia are found; this is called **mixed dementia**.

Dementia with Lewy bodies (DLB), **frontotemporal lobar degeneration (FTLD)**, and **Parkinson disease (PD)** are other causes of dementia.

Diagnosis of dementia is often difficult in the early stages, particularly as there is no one simple test for it. Initial assessment involves a detailed history from the patient and a close family member; physical examination and blood tests to identify other conditions present; and tests of mental abilities using both pen-and-paper tests and questions. These will test memory, language, and **visuospatial** skills, and can provide a baseline to measure future changes. Computerized tomography (CT) and magnetic resonance imaging (MRI) scans can show structural brain changes (*Figure 19.5*). If the diagnosis of the type of dementia is still unclear, single photon emission computerized tomography **(SPECT)** and positron emission tomography **(PET)** scans showing changes in brain activity may help clarify the diagnosis.

Treatment options, as there is no cure, aim to maximize the patient's quality of life and ability to communicate. **Environmental modifications** such as reducing visual and auditory clutter, providing cues (simple signs), and displaying personal items can improve memory, awareness, and orientation. External memory aids such as personal digital assistants **(PDAs)**, message boards, and pictures can help with memory difficulties.

Reminiscence therapy (RT) uses photographs, familiar items, past activities and experiences to improve the patient's memory to reinforce understanding and awareness of the environment. Other similar programs attempt to achieve similar goals.

Medications cannot stop dementia from progressing, but they may lessen symptoms of memory loss and confusion for a limited time. For treating Alzheimer disease, the FDA has approved two types of medications: **cholinesterase inhibitors** donepezil *(Aricept)*, rivastigmine *(Exelon)*, and galantamine *(Razadyne)*, as well as **memantine** *(Namenda)*, which has benefits similar to those induced by cholinesterase inhibitors.

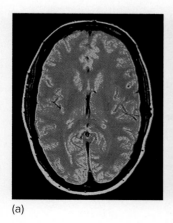
(a)

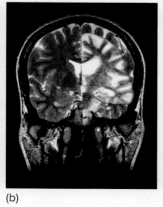
(b)

◄ **Figure 19.5** MRI scans. (a) Normal brain; (b) brain scan of individual with Alzheimer disease showing cerebral atrophy (green). Jessica Wilson/Medical Body Scans/Science Source

Word Analysis and Definition: Disorders of Aging

S = Suffix P = Prefix R = Root R/CF = Combining Form

WORD	PRONUNCIATION	ELEMENTS		DEFINITION
Alzheimer disease	AWLZ-high-mer diz-EEZ	P/ R/	Alois Alzheimer, 1894–1915, German neurologist dis- *apart* -ease *normal function*	Most common form of dementia
cognition cognitive (adj)	kog-NIH-shun KOG-nih-tiv	S/ R/ S/	-ion *process* cognit- *thinking* -ive *quality of*	Process of acquiring knowledge through thinking and learning Pertaining to the mental activities of thinking and learning
dementia	dee-MEN-she-ah	S/ P/ R/	-ia *condition* de- *without* -ment- *mind*	Chronic, progressive, and irreversible loss of the mind's cognitive and intellectual functions
hallucination	hah-loo-sih-NAY-shun	S/ R/	-ation *process* hallucin- *imagination*	Perception of an object or event when there is no such thing present
iatrogenic	eye-at-roh-JEN-ik	S/ P/ R/	-ic *pertaining to* iatro- *medical treatment* -gen- *producing*	An unfavorable response to medical or surgical treatment, caused by the treatment itself
incontinence incontinent	in-KON-tin-ence in-KON-tin-ent	S/ P/ R/ S/	-ence *state of* in- *not* -contin- *hold together* -ent *pertaining to*	Inability to prevent discharge of urine or feces Denoting incontinence
Lewy body	LOO-ee BOD-ee		Frederic Lewy, 1895–1950, German neurologist body Old English *body*	Abnormal cell found in brain in this form of dementia
visuospatial	VIZ-you-oh-SPAY-shall	S/ R/CF R/	-ial *pertaining to* visu/o- *vision* -spat- *space*	Denoting the ability to conceptualize visual representations and spatial relationships in learning

Check Point Section 19.2

A. Medical terms related to geriatrics. *Select the correct answer as it relates to terms and elements related to geriatrics.* **LO 19.6**

1. The patient does not have the strength to walk because he is confined to a bed. The inability to walk has a(n) _____ cause.

   a. cognitive   **b.** iatrogenic   **c.** dementia   **d.** skeletal

2. The general term that relates to a progressive, irreversible loss of cognitive and intellectual functions:

   a. senility   **b.** incontinence   **c.** dementia   **d.** Alzheimer disease

3. The medical term that contains the root meaning **thinking:**

   a. iatrogenic   **b.** dementia   **c.** hallucination   **d.** cognition

4. The root in the term **hallucination** means:

   a. recognition   **b.** mind   **c.** imagination   **d.** physician

5. The suffix -*ia* means:

   a. condition   **b.** pertaining to   **c.** producing   **d.** without

B. Use the new medical terminology you have learned in this chapter to select the correct answer for each question. LO 19.6

1. What is incontinence? (Read carefully and choose the BEST answer.)

   a. inability to prevent the discharge of urine

   b. inability to prevent the discharge of feces

   c. inability to prevent the discharge of flatus

   d. inability to prevent the discharge of urine or feces

   e. inability to prevent diarrhea

2. Coughing can cause a specific type of urinary incontinence. What is the medical term for this condition?

    a. stress incontinence

    b. urge incontinence

    c. overflow incontinence

    d. functional incontinence

    e. mixed incontinence

C. Use abbreviations within medical documentation. *Read the descriptions of the conditions and diagnosis related to dementia. Use the appropriate abbreviation to complete the sentence. Fill in the blanks.* **LO 19.9**

1. Cholinesterase inhibitors can be used to treat _____.

2. People with dementia may not be able to perform _____, such as brushing their hair, cooking meals, and routine cleaning tasks.

3. If all other diagnostic methods are unable to confirm the diagnosis of dementia, a(n) _____ scan may show changes in brain activity to clarify the diagnosis.

D. Diagnosis and treatment for dementia. *Choose the correct answer for each statement.* **LO 19.5, 19.6, 19.7**

1. Use of past activities and experiences to help patient with dementia with understanding of current environment:

    a. Namenda medication

    b. physical therapy

    c. environmental modifications

    d. reminiscence therapy

2. There is no definitive diagnostic test for dementia.

    a. True

    b. False

3. Medications such as rivastigmine *(Exelon)* will cure Alzheimer disease.

    a. True

    b. False

Section 19.3 Dying and Death

Death

In the past century in the United States, life expectancy has risen from age 47 to 84 and individuals over 90 are now the most rapidly growing portion of the population. While death can occur without warning in assaults and trauma, and sudden death can occur in certain illnesses, death usually comes at the end of a chronic illness or the frailty of old age. As a result, more and more health professionals of different disciplines are becoming involved in the care of dying elderly patients. Dying is inevitable. Just as fetal life in the womb is a preparation for birth, living and aging are a preparation for **death**. Death is a deeply personal, yet highly subjective experience. You can prepare for death in different ways, most of which are done with your family's involvement and many of which require legal assistance.

Legal Issues in Dying and Death

Medical issues are clearly significant in the process of dying. Your views on the types and extent of medical treatment you wish to have during the process of dying should be clearly stated. This is done through an **advance medical directive**, which consists of two documents:

1. Medical (durable) power of attorney, in which you appoint someone you know and trust as your agent and authorize that person to make medical decisions for you when you cannot.

2. Living will, in which you provide a set of instructions detailing what treatment you do and do not want in a terminal illness, including **hospice** treatment. If there are special instructions, such as **do not resuscitate (DNR)**, these must be stated clearly. It should also include a Health Insurance Portability and Accountability Act **(HIPAA) authorization** that enables your agent to receive the medical information about you that is necessary for making decisions about treatment. This is needed because HIPAA imposes tough privacy-of-medical-information rules on doctors and hospitals.

> **Did you know...**
>
> - Both PVS and MCS differ from **coma**, in which the individual is unresponsive and keeps his/her eyes closed.

Your primary care doctor should have a copy of your advance medical directive and read the document with you. This document should be part of your medical record. In some states, a document known as **Physician's Orders for Life-Sustaining Treatment (POLST)** is now available. This formal document is effectively a physician's order statement that is based on the patient's current medical condition and wishes. It has specific sections that list the patient's wishes for cardiopulmonary resuscitation (CPR), medical interventions, and artificially administered nutrition. It becomes a valid, durable component of the patient's medical record that health professionals must obey.

The process of dying, rather than death itself, is of concern to most elderly people. Dying should be free from physical and emotional pain and dignified, and occurring in the place most acceptable, usually the home. Death with Dignity state laws allow terminally ill adults to voluntarily request and receive a prescription medication from their physician to enable them to die in a peaceful, humane, and dignified manner. As of May 2021, these laws have been passed in 10 states, with an additional state, Montana, with Death with Dignity being made legal by court decision. Thirteen states introduced Death with Dignity bills between January and May 2021. Thirteen states have introduced similar laws 2021.

A **hospice** provides **palliative care** and provides for the emotional and spiritual needs of terminally ill patients and their loved ones at an inpatient facility or in the patient's home. Palliative care is designed to provide pain and symptom management to maintain the highest quality of life for as long as life remains.

Legal Definition of Death

In most states in the United States, death is now defined in terms of **brain death (BD),** when there is no cerebral or brainstem activity and the electroencephalogram (EEG) is flat for a specific length of time. Two other conditions involving brain damage and loss of brain function cause medical difficulty and should be addressed in your living will:

1. **Persistent vegetative state (PVS)** occurs in people who suffer enough brain damage that they are unaware of themselves or their surroundings, even though their eyes are open. Yet they still have certain reflexes and can breathe and pump blood because the brainstem still functions. Even reflex events like crying and smiling and the sleep–wake cycle can be seen. With medical care and artificial feeding, patients can survive for decades.

2. **Minimally conscious state (MCS)** is a condition of severely altered consciousness in which minimal evidence of awareness of self or surroundings is demonstrated. There is inconsistent communication or command following. However, positron emission tomography (PET) scans of MCS patients show cortical function when their loved ones speak to them. They are more likely to improve than are PVS patients.

Diagnostic and Therapeutic Procedures and Medications

The procedures used in geriatrics are identical to the procedures used for other patients and have been described in previous chapters on body systems. However, history taking and observing the elderly patient to determine his or her ability to live independently are of great importance. A Katz Activities of Daily Living Scale uses history taking to score patients in the areas of eating, dressing, bathing, transferring (e.g., moving in and out of bed), toileting, and continence.

Word Analysis and Definition: Death

S = Suffix P = Prefix R = Root R/CF = Combining Form

WORD	PRONUNCIATION		ELEMENTS	DEFINITION
advance medical directive	ad-**VANTS MED**-ih-kal die-**REK**-tiv	S/ R/ S/ R/	**advance** Latin *in front* -**al** *pertaining to* **medic-** *medicine* -**ive** *nature of, pertaining to* **direct-** *straight*	Legal document signed by the patient dealing with issues of prolonging or ending life in the event of life-threatening illness
death	DETH		Old English *to die*	Total and permanent cessation of all vital functions
hospice	**HOS**-pis		Latin *lodging*	Facility or program that provides care to the dying and their families
palliative care	**PAL**-ee-ah-tiv KAIR	S/ R/ R/	-**ive** *nature of, pertaining to* **palliat-** *reduce suffering* **care** *be responsible for*	Care that relieves symptoms and pain without curing
vegetative	**VEJ**-eh-tay-tiv	S/ R/	-**ive** *nature of, pertaining to* **vegetat-** *growth*	Functioning unconsciously as plant life is assumed to do

A. Use abbreviations that are commonly part of verbal and written communication. *Choose the correct abbreviation for the described medical term.* **LO 19.8, 19.9**

1. Document that allows the release of a patient's private medical information.

   a. DNR   b. POLST   c. ADL   d. HIPAA

2. This document provides instructions for a patient's care in a specific condition, such as which medical interventions should be administered:

   a. POLST   b. HIPAA   c. DNR   d. BD

B. List the documents that form a complete Advance Medical Directive. LO 19.1

_____

_____

_____

C. What is the single critical difference between an Advance Medical Directive and a POLST document? LO 19.1

_____

_____

D. Differentiate between medical terms associated with death and dying. *Match the term on the left with its correct definition on the right.* **LO 19.7**

_____ 1. hospice

_____ 2. minimally conscious state

_____ 3. palliative care

_____ 4. vegetative state

_____ 5. death

a. cessation of life

b. patient is completely unaware of surroundings

c. facility to provide care for dying patients and their families

d. patient that does not demonstrate awareness of self or surroundings

e. care that treats but does not cure

Table 19.1 Chapter 19 Abbreviations

Abbreviations	Meaning
AD	Alzheimer disease
ADE	adverse drug effect
ADLs	activities of daily living
BD	brain death
DLB	dementia with Lewy bodies
DNR	do not resuscitate
FTLD	frontotemporal lobar degeneration
HIPAA	Health Insurance Portability and Accountability Act
MCS	minimally conscious state
OTC	over the counter
PD	Parkinson disease
PDA	personal digital assistant
PET	positron emission tomography
POLST	Physician's Orders for Life-Sustaining Treatment
PVS	persistent vegetative state
RT	reminiscence therapy
SPECT	single photon emission computerized tomography

Challenge Your Knowledge

A. Abbreviations. Regardless of whether you are an administrative or clinical health care worker, you will be reading patient documentation with abbreviations, which can mean a diagnosis, procedure, disease, and so on. To interpret this documentation correctly and safely, you must know the meanings of the abbreviations. Challenge yourself to *define* each of the following abbreviations correctly. Fill in the chart. **LO 19.9**

Abbreviation	Meaning of Abbreviation
BD	1.
MCS	2.
PVS	3.

B. Elements. Even though these elements do not appear here in the context of a medical term, you should be able to recognize their meaning out of context. Match the correct element in the left column with its meaning in the right column. Fill in the blanks. **LO 19.2**

_____ 1. *-ician*   a. after

_____ 2. *-ity*   b. old age

_____ 3. *-trophy*   c. against

_____ 4. *sarc/o*   d. without

_____ 5. *-ile*   e. confusion

_____ 6. *post-*   f. expert

_____ 7. *anti-*   g. capability

_____ 8. *a* or *an*   h. condition, state

_____ 9. *deliri-*   i. many

_____ 10. *poly-*   j. flesh

_____ 11. *geront/o*   k. development

C. Latin and Greek terms cannot be further deconstructed into prefix, root, or suffix. You must know them for what they are. Test your knowledge of these terms with this exercise. Match the meaning in the left column with the correct medical term in the right column. **LO 19.1**

_____ 1. death   a. hospice

_____ 2. age spots   b. mortem

_____ 3. lodging   c. lentigo

D. Medical language. Employ the *languages of geriatrics and gerontology* to answer the following multiple-choice questions. Select the correct answer. **LO 19.1, 19.6**

1. Impaired intellect or memory that is present for at least six months is called

   a. dementia
   b. delirium
   c. hallucinations
   d. senescence
   e. cognition

2. In most U.S. states, *death* is described in terms of

   a. lack of breathing
   b. lack of blood flow to the body
   c. brain death
   d. lack of muscle response
   e. lack of speech and hearing

3. It is highly likely that senescence has more than one

   a. result

   b. free radical

   c. cause

   d. antioxidant

   e. autoimmune reaction

4. This condition is not a normal part of aging:

   a. renal failure

   b. renal impairment

   c. cataracts

   d. arthritis

   e. osteoporosis

5. A document that appoints someone you trust to make medical decisions for you is called a

   a. living will

   b. medical power of attorney

   c. DNR order

   d. consent form

   e. HIPAA authorization

6. The term meaning an unfavorable response to medical or surgical treatment, caused by the treatment itself, is

   a. polypharmacy

   b. iatrogenic

   c. senescence

   d. heredity

   e. dementia

7. The condition sarcopenia affects the _____ system.

   a. skeletal

   b. integumentary

   c. nervous

   d. muscular

   e. urinary

8. Free radicals can be neutralized by

   a. T lymphocytes (T cells)

   b. organ systems

   c. antioxidants

   d. enzymes

   e. hormones

9. What medical term describes an acute, altered state of consciousness with agitation and disorientation?

   a. delirium

   b. dementia

   c. hallucination

   d. persistent vegetative state

   e. migraine

10. Which of the following is NOT one of the so-called geriatric giants?

   a. immobility

   b. impaired intellect/memory

   c. instability

   d. incontinence

   e. loss of hearing

11. Which type of incontinence is caused by weak bladder muscles?

   a. overflow incontinence

   b. urge incontinence

   c. stress incontinence

   d. mixed incontinence

   e. functional incontinence

12. What disease accounts for 60–80% of all dementias?

   a. delirium

   b. Alzheimer disease

   c. fecal incontinence

   d. Lewy bodies

   e. impaired memory

13. Exercise and good nutrition are helpful in preventing

    a. wrinkles

    b. hair loss

    c. freckles

    d. osteopenia

    e. COPD

14. Which of the following statements is NOT true about hospice and the palliative care it provides?

    a. Hospice care can be provided in a hospital or in your home.

    b. Palliative care cannot cure anything.

    c. The main purpose of hospice is to alleviate pain and make you comfortable until you die.

    d. Hospice care does not charge the patient any fees.

    e. Hospice provides emotional support to the patient's family as well.

15. Which of the following statements applies to brain death?

    a. You have no cerebral or brainstem activity, and your EEG is flat for a specific length of time.

    b. You lose your sense of smell.

    c. You cannot hear anything around you.

    d. You cannot speak.

    e. You cannot walk.

E. **Use one of the following words to fill in the appropriate spaces with the *language of gerontology.*** Use each term only once; some terms will not be used. **LO 19.1, 19.6, 19.10**

sarcopenia	pathologist	postmortem	hospice
polypharmacy	adverse	incontinence	cognitive
dementia	iatrogenic	gerontologist	

  1. Because of her _____, the patient needs to wear diapers.

  2. The _____ will perform the autopsy tomorrow morning.

  3. The patient is suffering from _____ and needs physical therapy to strengthen his weakened muscles.

  4. A(n) _____ drug reaction is not beneficial to the patient.

  5. The family decided that _____ would be appropriate for their dying father.

F. **Prefixes and suffixes are good clues to the meaning of a medical term.** Analyze each medical term for the meaning of its prefix and suffix. Then give the complete meaning of the medical term in the last column. Every term may not have both a prefix and a suffix. If it does not have a particular word element, write n/a. Fill in the blanks. **LO 19.2**

Medical Term	Meaning of Prefix	Meaning of Root/ Combining Form	Meaning of Suffix	Meaning of Term
palliative	1.	2.	3.	4.
iatrogenic	5.	6.	7.	8.
dementia	9.	10.	11.	12.
atrophy	13.	14.	15.	16.

G. **Pronunciation is important whether you are saying the word or listening to a word from a coworker.** Identify the proper pronunciation of the following medical terms. Correctly spell the term. **LO 19.1, 19.3, 19.6, 19.7**

1. The correct pronunciation for multiple small, flat, brown-black spots in the skin of older people

    a. LOW-ee **BOD**-ee

    b. LOO-ee **BOD**-ee

    c. lent-ih-**JIHN**-ez

    d. len-**TIHJ**-ih-neez

    Correctly spell the term: _____

2. The correct pronunciation for the process of stopping drugs that are no longer needed or may be causing harm

    a. pol-ee-**FAR**-mah-see

    b. POL-ee-farm-**MAH**-see

    c. dee-**PREE**-skribe

    d. duh-**PREH**-skribe

    Correctly spell the term: _____

3. The correct pronunciation for an unfavorable response to medical or surgical treatment, caused by the treatment itself

    a. eye-a-**TROH**-jen-ik

    b. eye-at-roh-**JEN**-ik

    c. PAL-ee-ah-tiv KAIR

    d. PAIL-ih-ah-tiv KAIR

    Correctly spell the term: _____

4. The correct pronunciation for an acute altered state of consciousness with agitation and disorientation; condition is reversible

    a. dee-**MEN**-she-ah

    b. duh-men-**SHE**-ah

    c. deh-**LIR**-ee-um

    d. duh-**LEER**-ee-um

    Correctly spell the term: _____

5. The correct pronunciation for the state of being old

    a. seh-**NES-**ens

    b. sigh-**NES-**ens

    c. SEE-nile

    d. SIGHN-ile

    Correctly spell the term: _____

Case Reports

A. **After reading the following Case Report, correctly answer the following questions.** The answers to the questions may not be in the Case Report itself but can be found in the chapter content. **LO 19.6, 19.8**

Case Report (CR) 19.1

You are

. . . a family physician in a small group practice.

Your patient is

. . . Mrs. Virtanen, who is an 85-year-old female who is seeing you today for her annual well visit. Mrs. Virtanen is accompanied by her two daughters. They communicate to you that their mother is beginning to forget routine facts and she also has a decreased appetite. Two months ago, Mrs. Virtanen was involved in a minor traffic accident. She entered traffic in front of a car and misjudged the distance and speed of the oncoming car. The daughters are concerned that their mother should perhaps not drive. Mrs. Virtanen becomes very upset, as she does not want to lose her ability to come and go as she wants.

You perform a checkup and note the following: VS P 82, RR 18, BP 115/72, T 98.4 F. Her weight is down 15 pounds from last year's visit.

1. Mrs. Virtanen fears:

    a. loss of independence   **b.** incontinence   **c.** placement in assisted living

2. What is the likely explanation for her decreased appetite?

    a. dementia   **c.** probable malignancy

    b. decreased sensation of taste   **d.** abnormally low body temperature

3. Her inability to judge the speed and distance of the car may represent:

    a. early onset Alzheimer disease   **c.** low oxygen delivery to the brain

    b. a decline in her visuospatial skills   **d.** presence of lentigines

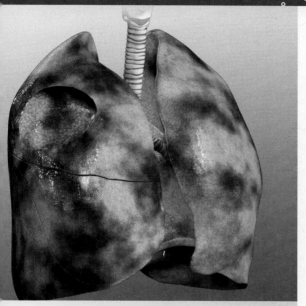

2014 Nucleus Medical Media

CHAPTER
20
Cancer
The Language of Oncology

Chapter Learning Outcomes

Upon completion of this chapter, you will be able to:

LO 20.1   Describe the different types of cancer.

LO 20.2   Identify and describe carcinogens and different environmental pollutants.

LO 20.3   Use roots, combining forms, suffixes, and prefixes to construct and analyze medical terms related to oncology.

LO 20.4   Spell medical terms related to oncology.

LO 20.5   Pronounce medical terms related to oncology.

LO 20.6   Describe screening for and detecting cancer.

LO 20.7   Describe the therapeutic procedures and pharmacologic agents used in oncology.

LO 20.8   Apply knowledge of medical terms relating to oncology to documentation, medical records, and communication.

LO 20.9   Identify and correctly use abbreviations of terms used in oncology.

LO 20.10 Identify health professionals involved in the care of cancer patients.

Note: In previous chapters on individual body systems, the terminology of cancers specific to each body system has been detailed. In this chapter, the terminology that relates to cancer in general will be explored.

Health professionals involved in the diagnosis and treatment of cancer include:

- **Oncologists,** who are physicians who specialize in the diagnosis and treatment of patients with cancer. There are many subspecialties of oncologists, including medical oncologists, surgical oncologists, pediatric oncologists, and radiation oncologists; their titles are self-explanatory.

- **Oncology clinical nurse specialists,** who are registered nurses with advanced clinical practice in the care of cancer patients.

- **Oncology social workers,** who have master's degrees in medical social work and provide for the social and emotional needs of cancer patients and their families.

Section 20.1 Types of Cancer

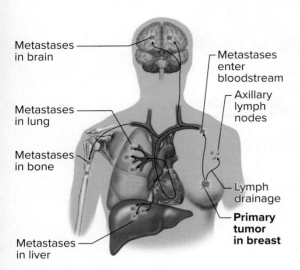

Metastases in brain

Metastases enter bloodstream

Axillary lymph nodes

Metastases in lung

Metastases in bone

Lymph drainage

Primary tumor in breast

Metastases in liver

▲ **Figure 20.1** **Metastases from primary breast cancer.** Metastases may be via lymph drainage to the axillary lymph nodes or via the bloodstream to the brain, lung, liver, and bone.

Did you know...

- The American Cancer Society estimates 1,800,000 new cases of cancer in 2020 with 606,520 cancer deaths.
- In females, 30% of new cancers are in the breast, 12% in the lungs, and 8% in the colon and rectum.
- In males, 20% are in the prostate, 13% in the lungs, and 9% in the colon and rectum.
- Between 2017 and 2018, the most recent years for which data are available, overall death rates for cancer decreased by 2.2% in the United States.
- The decline in cancer death rates is due to a decrease in smoking, better prevention efforts, new screening methods, and more effective treatments.

Types of Cancer

Normal tissue development is a balance between cell growth and cell death. If cells multiply more quickly than cells die, tumors (**neoplasms**) are formed. Neoplasms whose cells proliferate rapidly and spread to distant sites (metastasize) are called malignant. Neoplasms that grow slowly, stay localized, do not invade surrounding tissues, and do not metastasize are called benign. The study of tumors is called **oncology,** and medical specialists in this field are called **oncologists. Cancer (CA)** is a class of malignant diseases characterized by uncontrolled cell division. The basic cause of this uncontrolled growth is damage to the cells' DNA. This damage produces **mutations** to the genes that control cell division. These mutations, which can be inherited or acquired, lead to the uncontrolled cell division and malignant tumor formation. Thus, all cancer is genetic; that is, it develops because something in a cell's genes has changed (mutated).

Less than 10% of all cancers are inherited; that is, the genetic change is passed from parent to child. Almost 90% of cancers are acquired—something has caused the gene mutation in specific cells in a particular individual. A few genes mutated within a cell nucleus are enough to cause cancer. These gene mutations give the cells a superpower to proliferate in an uncontrolled way.

The Cells of Malignant Tumors

- Have unlimited, unregulated growth potential.
- Grow directly into adjacent tissues (invasion or **infiltration**).
- Invade the lymphatic system and are carried to local and distant lymph nodes (*Figure 20.1*).
- Invade the bloodstream and are carried to other distant organs and tissues (**metastasis;** *Figure 20.1*).

In contrast, **benign** tumors do not show such unregulated, invasive growth.

The Cells of Benign Tumors

- Grow slowly.
- Are surrounded by a connective tissue capsule.
- Do not invade or infiltrate adjacent tissues.
- Do not spread to other organs (metastasize) or to lymph nodes.
- Can compress surrounding tissues, causing functional problems.

Causes of Death

In 2017, the three most common causes of death in the United States were:

1. Cardiovascular disease (23.1% of all deaths).
2. Cancer (21.8% of all deaths).
3. Accidents (unintentional injuries) (5.9% of all deaths).

Environmental factors, particularly cigarette smoke, are associated with many forms of cancer. In this chapter, we will use a case of lung cancer to illustrate the characteristics of an acquired cancer and to discuss methods of detection and treatment.

Word Analysis and Definition: Cancer

WORD	PRONUNCIATION	ELEMENTS		DEFINITION
benign (adj)	bee-**NINE**		Latin *kind*	Denoting the nonmalignant character of a neoplasm or illness
cancer cancerous (adj)	**KAN**-ser **KAN**-ser-us	S/ R/	Latin *crab* -ous *pertaining to* cancer- *cancer*	General term for a malignant neoplasm Pertaining to a malignant neoplasm
infiltrate (verb) infiltration	**IN**-fil-trate in-fil-**TRAY**-shun	S/ P/ R/ S/	-ate *composed of, pertaining to* in- *in* -filtr- *strain through* -ation *process*	To penetrate and invade a tissue or cell The invasion into a tissue or cell
malignant (adj) malignancy (noun)	mah-**LIG**-nant mah-**LIG**-nan-see	 S/ R/	Latin *hurtful* -ancy *state of* malign- *cancer*	Capable of invading surrounding tissues and metastasizing to distant organs Tumor that invades surrounding tissues and metastasizes to distant organs
metastasis (noun) metastases (pl) metastatic (adj)	meh-**TAS**-tah-sis meh-**TAS**-tah-seez meh-tah-**STAT**-ik	P/ R/ S/ R/	meta- *after, beyond* -stasis *stay in one place* -ic *pertaining to* -stat- *stand still*	Spread of disease from one part of the body to another Able to metastasize
mutation mutagen	myu-**TAY**-shun **MYU**-tah-jen	S/ R/ S/	-tion *process* muta- *genetic change* -gen *produce*	A change in the chemistry of a gene that is continued in subsequent divisions of the cell Agent that produces a mutation in a gene
neoplasm (noun) neoplastic (adj) (**Note:** The "m" in -*plasm* is removed to allow the elements to flow.) neoplasia	**NEE**-oh-plazm **NEE**-oh-**PLAS**-tic **NEE**-oh-**PLAY**-zee-ah	P/ R/ S/ R/ S/	neo- *new* -plasm *to form* -tic *pertaining to* -plas- *molding, formation* -ia *growth*	A new growth, either a benign or a malignant tumor Pertaining to a neoplasm Process that results in formation of a tumor
oncology oncologist	on-**KOL**-oh-jee on-**KOL**-oh-jist	S/ R/CF S/	-logy *study of* onc/o- *tumor* -logist *one who studies, specialist*	The science dealing with cancer Medical specialist in oncology
proliferate	proh-**LIF**-eh-rate	S/ R/CF R/	-ate *composed of, pertaining to* prol/i- *bear offspring* -fer- *to bear*	To increase in number through reproduction
tumor	**TOO**-mor		Latin *swelling*	Any abnormal swelling

Within the broad classes of cancer *(Table 20.1)* are many subgroups, depending on the type of cells in the cancer. The term **carcinoma in situ (CIS)** describes an early form of carcinoma in which there is no invasion of surrounding tissues. In many instances, it is a precursor that will transform into an invasive or malignant cancer.

Table 20.1 Types of cancer

Class of Cancer	Cells of Origin	Examples
carcinoma	Epithelial	Cervical cancer, stomach cancer, squamous cell skin cancer, lung cancer
sarcoma	Connective tissue, bone, cartilage, muscle	**Osteosarcoma, chondrosarcoma, rhabdomyosarcoma**
leukemia	Blood-forming tissues	Acute lymphocytic leukemia, chronic myelogenous leukemia
lymphoma	Lymph nodes	Hodgkin disease, non-Hodgkin lymphoma
melanoma	Melanocytes (pigment-producing skin cells)	Malignant melanoma

Lung Cancer

Lung cancer has three main subgroups:

1. **Non–small cell lung cancer** accounts for 85% of cases, and 80% of patients die within 5 years of diagnosis. Included in this type are:

   a. **Squamous cell carcinoma,** arising from *round cells* that have replaced damaged cells in the epithelial lining cells of a major bronchus. It accounts for 25% to 40% of lung cancers.

   b. **Adenocarcinoma,** arising from the *mucus-producing cells* in the bronchi. It accounts for between 30% and 50% of lung cancers. It is the most common lung cancer in women, and its incidence is increasing.

   c. **Large cell carcinoma,** which includes cancers that cannot be identified under the microscope as squamous cell or adenocarcinoma. It accounts for 10% to 20% of lung cancers.

2. **Small cell lung cancer,** like squamous cell carcinoma, is derived from the epithelial cells of the bronchi but replicates at a faster rate, producing smaller cells. It accounts for 14% of all lung cancers; most patients die within 18 months of diagnosis.

3. **Mesothelioma** is a rare tumor arising from the cells lining the pleura and is associated with asbestosis.

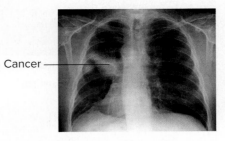

▲ **Figure 2O.2** **X-ray of small cell cancer of right upper lung.** Scott Camazine/Callista Images/Image Source

Did you know...

- The three most common cancers in men and the three leading causes of cancer death are prostate cancer, lung cancer, and colorectal cancer.
- The three most common cancers in women are breast cancer, lung cancer, and colorectal cancer.

Word Analysis and Definition: Types of Cancer

S = Suffix P = Prefix R = Root R/CF = Combining Form

WORD	PRONUNCIATION	ELEMENTS		DEFINITION
adenocarcinoma	AD-eh-noh-kar-sih-NOH-mah	S/ R/CF R/	-oma *tumor* aden/o- *gland* -carcin- *cancer*	A cancer arising from glandular epithelial cells
carcinoma	kar-sih-NOH-mah	S/ R/	-oma *tumor* carcin- *cancer*	A malignant and invasive epithelial tumor
carcinoma in situ (CIS)	kar-sih-NOH-mah IN SIGH-tyu		in situ Latin *in its place*	Carcinoma that has not invaded surrounding tissues
chondrosarcoma	KON-droh-sar-KOH-mah	S/ R/CF R/	-oma *tumor* chondr/o- *cartilage* -sarc- *flesh*	Cancer arising from cartilage cells
leukemia	loo-KEE-mee-ah	S/ R/	-emia *blood condition* leuk- *white*	Disease in which the blood is taken over by white blood cells and their precursors
lymphoma	lim-FOH-mah	S/ R/	-oma *tumor* lymph- *lymph*	Any neoplasm of lymphatic tissue
melanoma	MEL-ah-NOH-mah	S/ R/	-oma *tumor, mass* melan- *black*	Malignant neoplasm formed from cells that produce melanin
mesothelioma	MEEZ-oh-thee-lee-OH-mah	S/ P/ R/	-oma *tumor* meso- *middle* -theli- *lining*	Cancer arising from the cells lining the pleura or peritoneum
osteosarcoma	OS-tee-oh-sar-KOH-mah	S/ R/CF R/	-oma *tumor* oste/o- *bone* -sarc- *flesh*	Cancer arising in bone-forming cells
rhabdomyosarcoma	RAB-doh-MY-oh-sar-KOH-mah	S/ R/CF R/CF R/	-oma *tumor* rhabd/o- *rod-shaped, striated* -my/o- *muscle* -sarc- *flesh*	Cancer derived from skeletal muscle
sarcoma	sar-KOH-mah	S/ R/	-oma *tumor* sarc- *flesh*	A malignant tumor originating in connective tissue

Carcinogenesis

Carcinogenesis, literally the creation of cancer, is the abnormal rate of cell division as a result of damaged DNA causing gene mutation. Normally, the balance between cell division and proliferation and cell death **(apoptosis,** or **programmed cell death [PCD])** is tightly controlled to maintain the integrity of organs and tissues. Gene mutations that cause cancer disrupt this orderly process. Mutation in a single gene is usually not enough to cause cancer, and carcinogenesis requires multiple mutations in many genes.

Most normal cells cannot divide unless a **growth factor** binds to a receptor on the cell's surface. This growth factor then stimulates the cell to undergo mitosis *(see Chapter 3)* and **differentiate** into mature, functional cells *(Figure 20.3)*.

Two types of genes have been identified that play a part in the abnormal cell division and proliferation of cancer cells:

1. **Protooncogenes** are healthy genes that promote normal cell growth. Mutated **oncogenes** cause malfunctions in the normal growth mechanisms. For example, an oncogene called *SIS* stimulates blood vessels to grow into a tumor and provide the rich blood supply it needs to proliferate rapidly. An oncogene called *RAS* generates abnormal growth-factor receptors that switch on constant cell division signals. An oncogene called *HER-2* causes many cases of breast and ovarian cancer. The drug *Herceptin* is an antibody that targets the *HER-2* receptors on the cancer cells. This cuts off the chemical signals that the cell needs to keep proliferating. It also marks the abnormal cells for destruction by the immune system.

2. **Tumor suppressor (TS) genes** normally suppress mitosis and are activated by DNA damage. Their function is to stop cell division so that the abnormal genetic structure cannot be passed on to daughter cells. **Mutated TS genes** cannot do this, so the abnormal cells can divide and proliferate. A mutated TS gene called *p53* is present in half of all cancers and is associated with a poor prognosis and resistance to chemotherapy.

Mutations in both types of genes are usually required for cancer to develop. The oncogenes turn on the abnormal cell growth, and the mutated TS genes cannot stop it.

Cancer is due to the accumulation of genetic injury and mutations. Agents that cause these mutations are called **mutagens,** and mutagens that cause cancer are called **carcinogens.** Particular carcinogens are linked to specific types of cancer. Examples are inhalation of asbestos fibers with mesothelioma, prolonged exposure to radiation and ultraviolet radiation with melanoma and other skin malignancies, and tobacco smoking with lung cancer. Although the link between cigarette smoking and lung cancer is well established, only 15% to 20% of smokers develop lung cancer. In addition, about 10% of the population carries a gene that protects against lung cancer.

Studies in 2004 and 2005 of the epithelial cells in the large bronchi found a large number of genes altered by cigarette smoking. The studies defined genes whose alteration correlated with cumulative pack-years of smoking, and they identified 13 genes whose alterations do not return to normal after smoking is stopped. This could explain the persistent risk of lung cancer in former smokers. In addition, a subset of smokers was identified whose gene alterations have a different profile from that of other smokers. It is possible that this subset is the group who develop lung cancer.

Secondhand smoke, called **environmental tobacco smoke (ETS),** contains the same chemicals and carcinogens as those inhaled by smokers. It is responsible for 3,000 lung cancer cases each year in America. The genetic mutations caused by the carcinogens are probably similar to those in the subset of smokers discussed earlier, even though exposure to the carcinogens is much less than that for smokers.

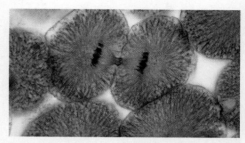
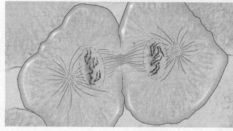

▲ **Figure 20.3** **End stage of mitosis.** For simplicity, the schematic drawing of the cell *(bottom)* is shown with only two chromosome pairs. Ed Reschke/Getty Images

Did you know...

- A pack-year equals the number of packs of cigarettes smoked per day multiplied by the number of years the person has smoked.

- Cigarette smoke contains over 60 known carcinogens.

- Several countries and states in the United States ban cigarette smoking in a car with minors to protect them from ETS

Word Analysis and Definition: Carcinogenesis

S = Suffix P = Prefix R = Root R/CF = Combining Form

WORD	PRONUNCIATION	ELEMENTS		DEFINITION
apoptosis	**AP**-op-**TOH**-sis	S/ P/	-ptosis *drooping* apo- *separation from*	Programmed normal cell death
carcinogen	kar-**SIN**-oh-jen	S/ R/CF	-gen *produce* carcin/o- *cancer*	Cancer-producing agent
carcinogenic (adj) carcinogenesis	**KAR**-sin-oh-**JEN**-ik **KAR**-sin-oh-**JEN**-eh-sis	S/ S/	-ic *pertaining to* -genesis *creation*	Causing cancer Origin and development of cancer
different (adj) differentiate (verb)	**DIF**-er-ent **DIH**-feh-**REN**-she-ate	S/ R/CF	Latin *difference* -ate *pertaining to, process* different/i- *different*	Not alike To change from generalized to specialized
oncogene	**ONG**-koh-jeen	S/ R/CF	-gene *producer, give birth* onc/o- *tumor*	One of a family of genes involved in cell growth that work in concert to cause cancer
oncogenic (adj)	**ONG**-koh-**JEN**-ik	S/	-genic *creation, producing*	Capable of producing a neoplasm
protooncogene	pro-toh-**ONG**-koh-jeen	S/ P/ R/CF	-gene *producer, give birth* proto- *first* -onc/o- *tumor*	A normal gene involved in normal cell growth

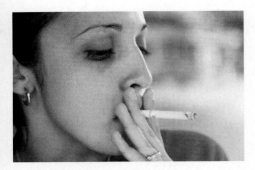

▲ **Figure 20.4** **Woman smoking.** Gary He/McGraw Hill

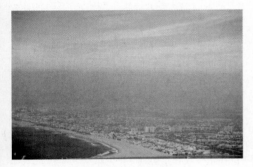

▲ **Figure 20.5** **Air pollution over a large city.** Patrick Clark/Photodisc/Getty Images

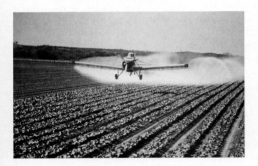

▲ **Figure 20.6** **Pesticide spraying of field of vegetables.** Garry D. McMichael/ Science Source

▲ **Figure 20.7** **No smoking sign.** Stockbyte/Photodisc Collection/Getty Images

Environmental Pollution

Pollution is a trigger of many cancers. For example, cigarette smoke *(Figure 20.4)* causes 87% of all lung cancers and acts in the following way: In the smoke are approximately 4,000 chemicals, some 60 of which are known to be carcinogenic and trigger genetic mutations that lead to cancer. Among the inhaled chemicals are cyanide, benzene, formaldehyde, acetylene, tar, arsenic, and ammonia, all of which can increase the risk for cancer.

Radon, a radioactive gas that you cannot see or smell, is the second leading cause of lung cancer (after smoking). It is produced by decaying **uranium** and is found in nearly all soils. In underground miners, it increases the risk of cancer to 40%. It gets into homes through cracks in the foundations or construction joints and is a problem in 1 out of 15 homes. Cigarette smoking on top of radon significantly increases the risk of lung cancer. Testing for radon is cheap and easy.

Air pollution may be the cause of the 10% to 40% increase in lung cancer mortality between urban and rural areas *(Figure 20.5)*. **Particulate matter,** especially very small **particles,** includes soot; organic material such as hydrocarbons; and metals such as arsenic, chromium, and nickel—all of which are known mutagens and carcinogens. A new analysis shows that premature death from cardiovascular ailments is increased by 24% among people exposed to tiny soot particles.

Chemical toxins are estimated to cause more than 75% of all cancers. Some 77,000 chemicals are used in this country. Over 3,000 are added to our food, and most Americans have between 400 and 800 chemicals stored in their bodies, mostly in fat cells. The toxins known to cause cancer include:

- **Chlorine.** Used in drinking water, chlorine produces carcinogenic compounds. Cancer risk among people drinking chlorinated water is 93% higher than that of people not drinking chlorinated water.
- **Lead.** Found in lead-based paint and contaminated air, water, and soil, lead poisoning can severely affect mental and physical development, particularly in children younger than 6. In 2014, over 100,000 residents of Flint, Michigan, including 12,000 children, were exposed to high levels of lead in their drinking water. The lead came from the polluted river source of water and from lead pipes used to supply the water.
- **Polychlorinated biphenyls (PCBs).** These were banned years ago but still persist in the environment, and are found in farmed salmon.
- **Pesticides.** According to the **Environmental Protection Agency (EPA),** 60% of herbicides, 90% of fungicides, and 30% of insecticides are known to be carcinogenic *(Figure 20.6)*. Farmers using pesticides have a 14% greater risk for developing prostate cancer than do organic farmers.
- **Dioxins.** These are chemical compounds produced by combustion processes from waste incineration and from burning fuels like wood, coal, and oil.
- **Asbestos.** This insulating material was used in the 1950s to 1970s on floors, ceilings, water pipes, and heating ducts. When the material becomes old and crumbly, it releases fibers into the air. Inhalation of the fibers is the cause of mesothelioma.
- **Arsenic.** This is used by insecticide and herbicide sprayers and oil refinery workers.

Occupational Safety and Health Administration **(OSHA)** regulations are designed to protect workers from these environmental hazards.

Prevention of Cancer

More than 50% of cancers could be prevented by **changes in lifestyle and environment.** The same carcinogens that affect the lining of the respiratory tract cause cancer of the oral cavity, pharynx, larynx, and esophagus. They also are absorbed into the bloodstream and disseminated, thereby becoming factors that can cause cancer in the pancreas, stomach, kidney, bladder, prostate, and cervix. **Stopping smoking** alone would reduce most of the 30% of all deaths due to lung cancer and reduce the incidence of many of the other cancers related to smoking *(Figure 20.7)*.

Clean air measures that are being implemented to reduce the more than 2 billion pounds of toxic air pollutants emitted into the atmosphere annually in this country can reduce the incidence of cancer.

Obesity is said to be linked to about 10% of breast and colorectal cancers and up to 40% of kidney, esophageal, and endometrial cancers. The mechanisms of obesity linked to these cancers are not understood.

Word Analysis and Definition: Environmental Pollution

S = Suffix P = Prefix R = Root R/CF = Combining Form

WORD	PRONUNCIATION	ELEMENTS		DEFINITION
chlorine	**KLOR**-een		Greek *greenish-yellow*	A toxic agent used as a disinfectant and bleaching agent
dioxin	die-**OK**-sin	S/ P/ R/	-in *chemical compound* di- *two* -ox- *oxygen*	Carcinogenic contaminant in pesticides
environment	en-**VIE**-ron-ment	S/ R/	-ment *resulting state* environ- *surroundings*	All the external conditions affecting the life of an organism
environmental (adj)	en-**VIE**-ron-**MEN**-tal	S/	-al *pertaining to*	Pertaining to the environment
particle	**PAR**-tih-kul		Latin *little piece*	A small piece of matter
particulate (adj)	par-**TIK**-you-let	S/ R/	-ate *composed of, pertaining to* particul- *little piece*	Relating to a fine particle
pesticide	**PES**-tih-side	S/ R/CF	-cide *to kill* pest/i- *pest*	Agent for destroying flies, mosquitoes, and other pests
pollution	poh-**LOO**-shun		Latin *dirty*	Condition that is unclean, impure, and a danger to health
radon	**RAY**-don		German *radium*	Colorless, tasteless, and odorless gas that can cause lung cancer
uranium	you-**RAY**-nee-um		Greek mythological character, Uranus	Radioactive metallic element

Check Point Section 20.1

A. Demonstrate that you can use various forms of the same term correctly. *Insert the appropriate medical term in the following blanks.*
LO 20.1, 20.4

neoplasm   neoplastic   neoplasia

1. The process of _____ results in the formation of a tumor, which can be either malignant or benign.

2. Another name for a tumor is a _____.

3. The tumor exhibited _____ behavior and was immediately biopsied.

metastases   metastatic   metastasis

4. A _____ carcinoma is cancer that has spread to a different site than the primary tumor.

5. The patient has _____ in his brain and kidneys.

6. Finding a primary tumor before _____ has occurred increases the chances for a cure.

B. Deconstruct the following language of oncology into elements. *These elements will form the basis for many additional oncologic terms. Give the one-word definition for the following word elements. Fill in the blank.* **LO 20.3**

1. *sarc/o* _____

2. *oste/o* _____

3. *-oma* _____

4. *my/o* _____

5. *chondr/o* _____

6. *aden/o* _____

7. *carcin-* _____

8. *mes/o* _____

9. *leuk-* _____

10. *melan-* _____

SECTION 20.1 Types of Cancer   663

C. Use the language of oncology to answer questions. *The following questions can be either true or false. Choose T if the statement is true. Choose F if the answer is false.* **LO 20.2**

1. Carcinogenesis is the creation of cancer.   T   F

2. Damaged blood cells cause gene mutation.   T   F

3. Programmed cell death is another term for apoptosis.   T   F

4. Mutagens that cause cancer are called carcinogens.   T   F

5. It is not possible to get cancer from secondhand smoke.   T   F

D. Many medical terms can be deconstructed into their word elements. *Choose the correct meaning of the word elements.* **LO 20.2, 20.3**

1. In the medical term **protooncogene,** the root means:

   a. produce   **b.** pertaining to   **c.** first   **d.** tumor

2. The prefix in the medical term **apoptosis** means:

   a. separation from   **b.** source   **c.** without   **d.** tumor

3. The root/combining form in the medical term **carcinogenic** means:

   a. produce   **b.** cancer   **c.** genetic change   **d.** tumor

4. The suffix in the medical term **oncogene** means:

   a. tumor   **b.** cancer   **c.** producer   **d.** first

E. Demonstrate your knowledge of the following terminology by deconstructing the terms into their elements. *Fill in the blanks. If the term does not a particular word element, leave the blank empty.* **LO 20.2, 20.3**

1. particulate   _____/_____/_____
                              P   R/CF   S

2. environment   _____/_____/_____
                              P   R/CF   S

3. pesticide   _____/_____/_____
                              P   R/CF   S

4. dioxin   _____/_____/_____
                              P   R/CF   S

F. Use the medical terms in context. *Use terms related to Environment Pollution to complete the following sentences. Fill in the blanks.* **LO 20.1**

1. Decaying _____ causes the release of radon, which can lead to lung cancer.

2. Consumption of water treated with _____ can increase the incidence of cancer.

3. Burning fuels such as coal releases the toxin _____, which can cause cancer.

4. Small bits of material are called _____.

5. A farmer may spray a chemical _____ on his produce to prevent insects from destroying the crops.

Screening for and Detecting Cancers

One genetic mutation in one cell, the mother or **progenitor** cell, can produce cancer, and the daughter cells can reproduce rapidly. But clinical detection is rare for a tumor mass less than 1 cm in diameter, which can include 1 billion cancer cells. The earlier and the more localized the tumor is detected, the better the chance of a cure. For the four major types of cancer (lung, breast, prostate, colorectal) combined, the National Cancer Institute estimates that in 2001–2016 there will be 772,000 new cases and 133,470 deaths in the United States alone. The ability to find cancers before they cause symptoms (like a lump that can be felt) and have spread would greatly improve the **prognosis** for people with this disease. The goal of **screening** tests is to achieve this outcome.

Breast Cancer Screening

The medical procedures used in screening for breast cancer include:

Examination and **palpation.**

Self-examination of the breast following a period.

Mammograms to record images of the breast on x-ray film.

Digital mammography to record images in computer code.

Computer-aided mammography using a laser beam to produce a digital signal that can be processed by a computer to highlight suspicious areas.

Ultrasound using sound waves to make a computer image of the inside of the breast, particularly to see changes in women with dense breast tissue and to tell the difference between benign fluid-filled cysts and a possibly malignant solid mass.

Magnetic resonance imaging (MRI) creating detailed images of the breast in different planes.

Ductal lavage using saline solution introduced through a fine catheter inserted into a milk duct through its opening on the surface of the nipple. The solution is **aspirated** out and examined microscopically to check for abnormal cells.

Biopsy of a suspicious lesion can detect the type of lung cancer (*see Chapter 13*). X-rays or ultrasound are used to guide accurate insertion of a needle into the suspicious lesion.

Several national organizations have developed guidelines for the age when screening for breast cancer should be started and how often procedures should be performed. Unfortunately, they are all slightly different, making it confusing for patients.

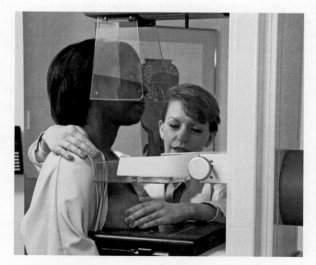

▲ **Figure 20.8** **Mammography.** Keith Brofsky/Photodisc/Getty Images

WORD	PRONUNCIATION	ELEMENTS		DEFINITION
biopsy (**Note:** The "o" in the root *bio* is dropped from the spelling.)	**BIE**-op-see	S/ R/CF	-opsy *to view* bi/o- *life*	Removal of living tissue for laboratory examination
duct	DUKT		Latin *to lead*	A tubular structure allowing any fluid to flow through it
ductal (adj)	**DUCK**-tal	S/ R/	-al *pertaining to* duct- *to lead*	Pertaining to a duct
lavage	lah-**VAHZH**		Latin *to wash*	Washing out of a hollow tube, cavity, or organ
mammogram	**MAM**-oh-gram	S/ R/CF	-gram *a record* mamm/o- *breast*	The record produced by x-ray imaging of the breast
mammography	mah-**MOG**-rah-fee	S/	-graphy *process of recording*	Process of x-ray examination of the breast
palpate (verb) palpation (noun)	**PAL**-pate pal-**PAY**-shun	S/ R/	Latin *to touch* -ion *action* palpat- *touch, stroke*	Examination with the fingers and hand To examine using the fingers and hands
progenitor	pro-**JEN**-ih-tor	P/ R/	pro- *before* -genitor *offspring*	Founder; beginning of an ancestry
prognosis	prog-**NO**-sis	P/ R/	pro- *before* -gnosis *knowledge*	Forecasting of the probable course of a disease
screen (verb) screening (noun)	SKREEN **SKREEN**-ing		French *examine*	To evaluate a group The evaluation of a group
self-examination	**SELF**-ek-zam-ih-**NAY**-shun	S/ R/ R/	-ation *process* examin- *test* self- *me*	To examine part of one's own body

The medical terms used in screening for and detecting lung cancer are:

Chest x-rays are thought of as **the** screening method for lung cancer. Frequently when lung cancer is detectable on chest x-ray it has spread beyond the lungs.

Computed tomography (CT) scans are more effective at identifying early lung cancers than are chest x-rays.

Magnetic resonance imaging (MRI) is being used to screen for lung cancer in high-risk patients.

Sputum analysis of coughed up sputum can be a useful and cost-effective method of identifying cancer cells arising from the lining of the airways.

Biomarkers are substances released by specific cancers and can be found in blood, sputum, and tissue samples. The blood test **anti-malignin antibody screen** can detect the presence of any kind of cancer and is non-specific.

More specific tests for detecting the presence of lung cancer cells include:

Positron emission tomography (PET) scans are expensive and not widely available. They are the most accurate non-invasive test for identifying if the cancer has spread outside lung tissue.

Scintigraphy *(Figure 20.9)* uses low-level **radioactive** agents that bind to cancer cells and can be tracked by special cameras to reveal the exact locations of cancer cells.

Bronchoscopy can locate cancers in the linings of the major airways. Biopsy specimens are obtained by cutting tissue, by brushings, or by a washing process called **bronchoalveolar lavage (BAL).**

Mediastinoscopy uses a fiber-optic tube with a camera and is inserted into the mediastinum via the suprasternal notch to locate affected mediastinal lymph nodes for biopsy.

Needle biopsy of tumors in the periphery of the lungs is performed by inserting a needle between the ribs and guiding it to the tumor with **fluoroscopy** or CT scan.

Brain metastases are identified by MRI and bone metastases by technetium-99m radionuclide bone scans.

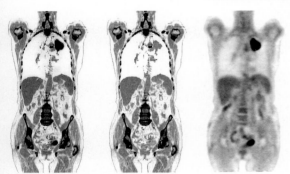

▲ **Figure 20.9 Diagnostic images.** (a) and (b) MRI scans and (b) scintigram of the same individual with lung cancer and a tumor in the abdomen.

SIMON FRASER/Science Source

Staging Lung Cancer

The **tumor-node-metastasis (TNM) system** is used to stage cancer:

- **T** stands for *tumor* and describes its size and its spread within the lung and to nearby tissues such as the pleura, diaphragm, and pericardium.
- **N** stands for spread to lymph *nodes* around the affected lung.
- **M** stands for *metastasis* to distant sites such as brain liver and bones.
- **O**nce the TNM categories have been assigned, the information is combined and given an overall stage of O, I, II, III, or IV.

Word Analysis and Definition: Cancer Screening

S = Suffix P = Prefix R = Root R/CF = Combining Form

WORD	PRONUNCIATION		ELEMENTS	DEFINITION
biomarker	**BI**-oh-**MARK**-er	R/CF R/	**bi/o**- *life* **-marker** *sign*	A biological marker or product by which a cell can be identified
bronchoalveolar	**BRONG**-koh-al-**VEE**-oh-lar	S/ R/CF R/	**-ar** *pertaining to* **bronch/o**- *bronchus* **-alveol**- *alveolus*	Pertaining to the bronchi and alveoli
bronchoscope bronchoscopy	**BRONG**-koh-scope brong-**KOS**-koh-pee	S/ R/CF S/	**-scope** *instrument for viewing* **bronch/o**- *bronchus* **-scopy** *to examine*	Endoscope used for bronchoscopy Examination of the interior of the tracheobronchial tree with an endoscope
fluoroscopy	flor-**OS**-koh-pee	S/ R/CF	**-scopy** *to examine* **fluor/o**- *x-ray beam*	Examination of the structure of the body by x-rays
mediastinoscopy	**ME**-dee-ass-tih-**NOS**-koh-pee	S/ R/CF	**-scopy** *to examine* **mediastin/o**- *mediastinum*	Examination of the mediastinum using an endoscope
scintigraphy	sin-**TIG**-rah-fee	S/ R/CF	**-graphy** *process of recording* **scint/i**- *spark*	Recording of radioactivity using a special camera
stage staging	STAYJ **STAY**-jing		Latin *to stand*	Definition of extent and dissemination of a malignant neoplasm Process of determination of the extent of the distribution of a neoplasm

Check Point Section 20.2

A. Learning word elements are the key to quickly knowing the medical term. *Match the element in the left column with its correct meaning in the right column.* **LO 20.3, 20.6**

_____ **1.** *ion*   **a.** before

_____ **2.** *opsy*   **b.** to lead

_____ **3.** *gram*   **c.** process

_____ **4.** *ation*   **d.** life

_____ **5.** *pro*   **e.** action

_____ **6.** *bi*   **f.** to view

_____ **7.** *duct*   **g.** a record

B. Language of Oncology: Test your knowledge of the language of oncology with this exercise. *Select the best answer(s).* **LO 20.6**

1. Which of the following terms contains a prefix?

   a. biomarker   **c.** prognosis

   b. bronchoscopy   **d.** scintigraphy

2. Which term contains the suffix meaning *to examine*?

   a. bronchoscope

   b. fluoroscopy

   c. scintigraphy

   d. staging

3. Which term would mean a recording with a special camera?

   a. biomarker

   b. fluoroscopy

   c. scintigraphy

   d. bronchoscope

4. Which of the following terms is a procedure on the chest?

   a. mediastinoscopy

   b. scintigraphy

   c. bronchoalveolar

   d. biomarker

Section 20.3 Treating Cancer

Treatment of any cancer depends on its location, its size, its localization or spread to surrounding tissues and lymph nodes, the presence of metastases, and the cancer's aggressiveness (as determined by pathologic findings on biopsy or surgical removal).

If the cancer is still localized, it can be removed and cure is possible. Unfortunately, few patients are diagnosed at such an early stage, particularly with lung cancer. Even if the original tumor is removed, cancer recurrence rates are high. Additional treatments with **radiation** and **chemotherapy** are used and can produce unpleasant side effects. A patient will have to balance a diminished quality of life against a chance for a modestly prolonged survival.

In the elderly, studies have shown that survival rates are the same for therapies aimed at relieving pain as they are for aggressive, unpleasant treatment **regimens** with their diminished quality of life.

Surgical Procedures

Surgical procedures for specific body system cancers are discussed in the relevant chapters. For example, surgery for breast cancer is covered in *Chapter 8* and for prostate cancer in *Chapter 7*.

The type of surgery for lung cancer depends on the amount of lung tissue that has to be removed.

Wedge resection (segmentectomy) removes only a small part of the lung. It is used for carcinoma in situ, small tumors, frailer patients who cannot tolerate lobectomy, or patients with lung disease.

Lobectomy is removal of one lobe of the lung and is used if the cancer has not spread beyond the lobe or into lymph nodes.

Pneumonectomy removes an entire lung and has a mortality of 5% to 8%.

Radiation Procedures (Radiotherapy)

Radiotherapy does not remove the lesion but distorts the DNA of the cancer cells so that they lose their ability to reproduce and to retain fluids; the cells shrink over time. Side effects of radiotherapy depend on the type of therapy used, and occur when healthy cells are damaged during the treatment. Tiredness, nausea, loss of appetite, and sore skin in the treatment area can be short-term effects.

External-beam radiation focuses a beam of radiation directly on the tumor. It is generally used for metastasized cancer.

Brachytherapy implants radioactive seeds through thin tubes directly into the tumor to give high doses of radiation to the tumor while reducing radiation exposure to the surrounding tissues (*Figure 20.10*). It can be used for inoperable cancers.

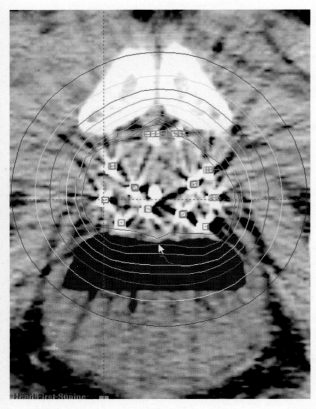

▲ **Figure 20.10** Radioactive seeds implanted in a tumor. Courtesy Varian Medical Systems

Continuous hyperfractionated accelerated radiotherapy (CHART) administers standard doses of radiation multiple times per day. It allows the total dose of radiation to be administered in a shorter period of time than the standard 6 weeks.

Stereotactic radiosurgery (SRS) uses three-dimensional computer programming to deliver a precise, single high dose of radiation in a one-day session. The most common form of SRS used in the United States is a cobalt-60–based machine called the gamma knife. Though this technique is labeled and implied as "surgery," there is no actual surgery involved.

Word Analysis and Definition: Treating Cancer

S = Suffix P = Prefix R = Root R/CF = Combining Form

WORD	PRONUNCIATION	ELEMENTS		DEFINITION
brachytherapy	brah-kee-**THAIR**-ah-pee	P/ R/	brachy- *short* -therapy *medical treatment*	Radiation therapy in which the source of irradiation is implanted in the tissue to be treated
chemotherapy	**KEE**-moh-**THAIR**-ah-pee	R/CF R/	chem/o- *chemical* -therapy *medical treatment*	Treatment using chemical agents
hyperfractionated (adj)	high-per-**FRAK**-shun-ay-ted	S/ P/ R/	-ated *process* hyper- *excessive* -fraction- *small amount*	Given in smaller amounts and more frequently
lobectomy	loh-**BEK**-toh-mee	S/ R/	-ectomy *surgical excision* lob- *lobe*	Surgical removal of a lobe of the lungs
pneumonectomy	**NEW**-moh-**NEK**-toh-mee	S/ R/	-ectomy *surgical excision* pneumon- *lung*	Surgical removal of a whole lung
radiation	ray-dee-**AY**-shun	S/ R/	-ation *process* radi- *x-ray, radiation*	Treatment with x-rays
radiotherapy	**RAY**-dee-oh-**THAIR**-ah-pee	R/CF R/	radi/o- *x-ray, radiation* -therapy *medical treatment*	Treatment using radiation
regimen	**REJ**-ih-men		Latin *direction*	Program of treatment
segmentectomy	seg-men-**TEK**-toh-mee	S/ R/	-ectomy *surgical excision* segment- *section*	Surgical excision of a segment of a tissue or organ

Medications

Chemotherapy (chemo) is the use of any drug to treat any disease, but the term is mostly used for drugs that treat cancer. Chemotherapy drugs target cells at different phases of the process of forming new cells. Cancer cells form new cells more quickly than normal cells and this makes them a better target for chemotherapy. But chemotherapy drugs cannot tell the difference between healthy cells and cancer cells. This means that normal cells are damaged along with cancer cells, and this causes **side effects.** Fatigue, nausea, vomiting, and hair loss are common side effects. Anemia and blood-clotting problems can arise from side effects on the bone marrow.

Sometimes cancer can be treated solely with chemotherapy, either as a single drug or with several drugs commonly given at regular intervals, called cycles. A cycle can be a dose of chemotherapy followed by several days or weeks without therapy. This gives normal cells time to recover from the effects of the chemotherapy.

More often, chemotherapy is used with surgery or radiation therapy, or both:

- Chemotherapy can be used to shrink a tumor before surgery or radiation therapy.
- Chemotherapy can be used after surgery or radiation therapy to help kill any remaining cancer cells.

In many cases, with treatment the cancer does not go away but can be controlled and managed as a chronic disease. In other cases, the cancer may seem to have gone away but returns. Chemotherapy can then be given again.

When the cancer is at an advanced stage, is not under control, and has metastasized to other parts of the body, chemotherapy can help shrink a tumor that is causing pain or pressure to improve the quality of life for the patient. This is called **palliation.**

There are more than 100 chemotherapy drugs of a dozen different types.

Did you know...

- As well as affecting cancer cells, chemotherapy alters the function of normal cells, causing side effects.
- Gene therapy is an experimental treatment that can target healthy cells to enhance their ability to fight cancer or can target cancer cells to destroy them.

Biologic Therapies (Immunotherapy)

Biologic therapies use the body's immune system, directly or indirectly, to attack cancer cells or to lessen the side effects that can be caused by radiation and chemotherapy. **Biologic response modifiers** alter the immune system's response to cancer cells and include interferons, interleukins, monoclonal antibodies, vaccines, and gene therapy.

Monoclonal antibodies (MOABs) are antibodies produced by a single type of cell and are specific for a single antigen. Examples of MOABs are rituximab (*Rituxan*), used for non-Hodgkin lymphoma, and trastuzumab (*Herceptin*), used in breast cancer for tumors that produce a protein called *HER-2*.

Cytostatics inhibit cell division. Examples include cyclophosphamide (*Cytoxan*) which is a potent agent; methotrexate (*Amethopterin*); cyclosporine (*Cyclosporin A*); mechlorethamine (*Nitrogen mustard*).

Antiangiogenesis therapy interferes with the genetic mechanisms that increase blood supply for the active growth of cancer cells. The drug *Avastin* has led to a great increase in the survival of patients with colon cancer and also is being used in lung and breast cancer.

Gene therapy is now a focus of cancer therapy. In 2005, the **National Cancer Institute (NCI)** and the **National Human Genome Research Institute (NHGRI)** announced a 3-year pilot project to map the genetic alterations in cancer cells. New technologies called **microarrays** or **gene chips** (small slivers of glass or nylon that can be coated with genes) enable every gene that is active in a cancer cell to be identified.

Gene therapy involves introducing a normal gene into a person's cells to replace an abnormal disease-producing gene (*see Chapter 21*). Numerous trials are under way to define gene therapy's applications in the biologic treatment of cancer.

Immune therapy is a recent focus of cancer therapy research. **Vaccines** against lymphoma, prostate cancer, breast cancer, and pancreatic cancer have shown promise in stimulating the immune system to attack cancer cells and extend survival rates. In 2010, the **FDA** approved the first-ever tumor vaccine, called *Provenge,* to treat prostate cancer. Another FDA-approved immunotherapy, *Yervoy,* is used in metastatic melanoma, but it only extends average survival by a few months.

Targeted immune modulators are new drugs used for diseases such as rheumatoid arthritis and psoriatic arthritis. Evidence of their effectiveness is evolving.

Many types of biological therapy are still in clinical trials, and biological therapy for cancer is a very active area of cancer research. In 2016, the FDA approved the immunotherapy drug pembrolizumab (*Keytruda*) as a first-line treatment for non–small cell lung cancer prior to chemotherapy and also to treat people who had already received chemotherapy.

Word Analysis and Definition: Pharmacological and Biologic Therapies

S = Suffix   P = Prefix   R = Root   R/CF = Combining Form

WORD	PRONUNCIATION	ELEMENTS		DEFINITION
angiogenesis	**AN**-jee-oh-**JEN**-eh-sis	S/	**-genesis** *origin, creation, formation*	Creation of new blood vessels
		R/CF	**angi/o-** *blood vessel*	
antiangiogenesis	**AN**-tee-**AN**-jee-oh-**JEN**-eh-sis	P/	**anti-** *against*	The prevention of growth of new blood vessels
biology	bie-**OL**-oh-jee	S/	**-logy** *study of*	Science concerned with life and living organisms
		R/CF	**bi/o-** *life*	
biologic (adj)	**BI**-oh-**LOJ**-ik	S/	**-ic** *pertaining to*	
				Pertaining to life and living organisms
clone	KLOHN		Greek *cutting used for propagation*	A colony of organisms or cells all having identical genetic constitutions
monoclonal (adj)	**MON**-oh-**KLOH**-nal	S/	**-al** *pertaining to*	Derived from a protein from a single clone of cells, all molecules of which are the same
		P/	**mono-** *one*	
		R/	**-clon-** *cutting used for propagation*	
microarray (also called gene chips)	**MY**-kroh-ah-**RAY**	P/	**micro-** *small*	Technique for studying one gene in one experiment
		R/	**-array** *place in order*	

Check Point Section 20.3

A. Match the word element in the first column with its correct meaning found in the second column. *Some of these elements have appeared in earlier chapters as well.* **LO 20.3, 20.7**

_____ 1. *chem/o*   a. small amount

_____ 2. *pneumon*   b. lobe

_____ 3. *brachy*   c. excessive

_____ 4. *hyper*   d. treatment

_____ 5. *ectomy*   e. lung

_____ 6. *lob*   f. short

_____ 7. *therapy*   g. chemical

_____ 8. *fraction*   h. surgical excision

B. Review the content related to the pharmacologic treatment of cancer to find the answers to the following questions. *Choose the best answer.* **LO 20.3**

1. The term containing a combining form that means *blood vessel* is

   a. hemolysis   **b.** angiogenesis   **c.** environmental

2. The prefix in this term means *one*:

   a. biologic   **b.** dioxin   **c.** monoclonal

3. The suffix in this term means *study of*:

   a. microarray   **b.** biology   **c.** brachytherapy

4. The suffix in this term means *origin*:

   a. biologic   **b.** antiangiogenesis   **c.** microarray

5. The term containing a word element that means *small* is

   a. lobectomy   **b.** stereotactic   **c.** microarray

6. The term that does NOT contain a prefix is

   a. biology   **b.** monoclonal   **c.** microarray

C. Medications used to treat cancer. *From the provided terms, complete the statements regarding medications that are used to treat cancer. Fill in the blank.* **LO 20.7**

palliation   chemotherapy   tumor   nausea   cycles

1. The use of drugs to treat cancer is termed _____.

2. Medication can shrink a _____ prior to its surgical removal.

3. Doses of medication are given at scheduled _____ to allow the patient to recover from its side effects.

4. Side effects of chemotherapy include fatigue, hair loss, and _____.

5. Chemotherapy that relieves symptoms but does not cure would be _____ therapy.

Abbreviations	Meaning
AMAS	anti-malignin antibody screen
BAL	bronchoalveolar lavage
BSE	breast self-examination
CA	cancer
CEA	carcinoembryonic antigen
CHART	continuous hyperfractionated accelerated radiotherapy
CIS	carcinoma in situ
CT	computed tomography
DRE	digital rectal examination
EPA	Environmental Protection Agency
ETS	environmental tobacco smoke
FDA	Federal Drug Administration
FOBT	fecal occult blood test
MOAB	monoclonal antibody
MRI	magnetic resonance imaging
NCI	National Cancer Institute
NHGRI	National Human Genome Research Institute
OSHA	Occupational Safety and Health Administration
Pap	papanicolaou cervical smear test
PCA3	prostate cancer antigen 3
PCBs	polychlorinated biphenyls
PCD	programmed cell death
PET	positron emission tomography
PSA	prostate-specific antigen
SRS	stereotactic radiosurgery
TNM	tumor-node-metastasis
TS	tumor suppressor
1°	primary
2°	secondary

2014 Nucleus Medical Media

Challenge Your Knowledge

A. Prefixes. Not every medical term will have a prefix, but when they do, it is an extra clue for you in determining the meaning of the term. Given the definition, identify the correct prefix it is describing. Fill in the blank. **LO 20.1, 20.2, 20.3, 20.6**

1. Programmed normal cell death: _____ ptosis

2. Carcinogenic released from burning wood: _____ oxin

3. Given in smaller amounts, more often: _____ fractionated

4. Cancer arising from the cells lining the pleural cavity or peritoneum: _____ thelioma

5. Spread of disease to another body part: _____ stasis

6. Technique for studying one gene in one experiment: _____ array

7. Derived from a single protein from a single clone of cells: _____ clonal

8. New growth, benign or malignant: _____ plasm

9. Founder, beginning of an ancestry: _____ genitor

10. A normal gene, in normal cell growth: _____ oncogene

B. Roots. Identify the meaning of the root/combining form in each term below. **LO 20.3**

_____ 1. mediastinoscopy
_____ 2. neoplastic
_____ 3. antiangiogenesis
_____ 4. palpation
_____ 5. monoclonal
_____ 6. apoptosis
_____ 7. lobectomy
_____ 8. progenitor

a. to form
b. offspring
c. cutting used for propagation
d. mediastinum
e. touch
f. lobe
g. blood vessel
h. falling

C. Complete the sentence with the correct term. From the words provided, complete the sentences with the best answer. Fill in the blanks. **LO 20.6, 20.7**

lavage   neoplasm   infiltrate   carcinogen   metastasis

pneumonectomy   digital   fluoroscopy   oncologist   chemotherapy

1. The family practice physician referred the patient to a(n) _____ for the proper treatment of her cancer.

2. The annual mammogram revealed a _____ in the right breast.

3. The physician ordered a ductal _____ to determine the presence of abnormal breast cells.

4. Because the tumor invaded the entire lung, a _____ was performed.

5. The tumor in the breast began to _____ healthy tissue.

6. The osteosarcoma is a result of the _____ of the liver cancer.

7. Modern radiography utilizes _____ imaging.

8. The radiologist utilized _____ to guide the needle to the tumor.

9. After removing the small cancerous growth, the oncologist recommended five weeks of _____.

10. Radon gas is a known _____.

D. **Suffixes can provide additional information about a medical term.** Analyze the suffix in each of the following terms, and use it to provide a clue about the term. Fill in the blanks. The first one has been done for you. **LO 20.1, 20.3, 20.6, 20.7**

Medical Term	Suffix	Meaning of Suffix	Meaning of Term
angiogenesis	1. -*genesis*	2. origin, creation, production	3. Creation of new blood vessels
neoplasia	4.	5.	6.
oncology	7.	8.	9.
oncologist	10.	11.	12.
pneumonectomy	13.	14.	15.
chondrosarcoma	16.	17.	18.
proliferate	19.	20.	21.
scintigraphy	22.	23.	24.
malignancy	25.	26.	27.
mammogram	28.	29.	30.

E. **Compare and contrast benign and malignant tumors to meet a lesson objective.** You are given a statement about a tumor. Indicate whether it refers to a benign or malignant tumor by writing B for benign and M for malignant. **LO 20.1**

1. Grows slowly: _____

2. Invades the lymph system: _____

3. Does not metastasize to other organs: _____

4. Invades the bloodstream and travels to other organs: _____

5. Lipoma: _____

6. Surrounded by connective tissue capsule: _____

7. Can compress surrounding tissues and cause functional problems: _____

8. Does not invade or infiltrate adjacent tissues: _____

9. Unlimited, unregulated growth potential: _____

10. Invades or infiltrates adjacent tissues: _____

11. Does not spread to lymph nodes: _____

12. Mesothelioma: _____

F. Correct usage. Demonstrate your knowledge of the *language of oncology*. These are similar medical terms, but each has only one correct use in the paragraph. Fill in the blanks. **LO 20.2**

carcinogen   carcinoma   carcinogenic   carcinogenesis

1. Raquel Sacco was unknowingly exposed to a _____ in the form of secondhand smoke. This _____ substance brought about the _____ of her tumors. Her primary _____ has already metastasized; her prognosis is poor.

metastasis   metastasized   metastases   metastatic

2. The _____ of Raquel's primary cancer to a secondary site was discovered after diagnostic study. The _____ in her brain were not the site of her current surgery. Her _____ lesions may require radiation therapy if they are inoperable. Because her cancer has already _____, her chances of survival are poor.

G. Cancer quiz. Assess your knowledge of this chapter by correctly answering the following questions on cancer. The *language of oncology* will aid your understanding of the questions and possible answers. Choose the correct choice, and remember there is only one *best* answer. **LO 20.1, 20.2, 20.7, 20.9**

1. Second-leading cause of lung cancer (after smoking):
   a. air pollution
   b. radon
   c. chemical toxins
   d. polychlorinated biphenyls
   e. particulate matter

2. Used to vacuum out suspicious breast tissue through a needle:
   a. gamma knife
   b. lavage
   c. bronchoscopy
   d. mammotome
   e. mammogram

3. In the TNM staging system for cancer, the "N" stands for
   a. nothing
   b. normal
   c. neoplasm
   d. node
   e. noninvasive

4. A medication that halts cell division:
   a. oncogene
   b. cytostatic
   c. antineoplastic
   d. protooncogene

5. A tumor that has invaded or infiltrated has
   a. grown into adjacent tissue
   b. died
   c. become weaker
   d. mutated
   e. necrotized

6. Healthy genes that promote normal cell growth are called
   a. tumor suppressor genes
   b. mutated tumor suppressor genes
   c. protooncogenes
   d. mutated genes
   e. receptor genes

7. A benign tumor is
   a. surrounded by a capsule
   b. cytostatic
   c. metastatic
   d. necrotic
   e. invasive

8. An early form of carcinoma in which there is no invasion of surrounding tissues is
   a. large cell carcinoma
   b. small cell carcinoma
   c. adenocarcinoma
   d. carcinoma in situ
   e. squamous cell carcinoma

9. The abbreviation PCD means the same as

   a. protooncogene

   b. apoptosis

   c. oncogene

   d. polychlorinated biphenyls

   e. progenitor

10. Detecting an abnormal growth by touch is defined as:

    a. palpation

    b. lavage

    c. curettage

    d. aspiration

    e. ultrasound

H. **Abbreviations.** Use with care to ensure you are conveying precise information. Demonstrate your knowledge of this chapter's abbreviations by correctly matching the definition in the first column to the abbreviation in the second column. **LO 20.9**

   _____ 1. genes normally suppress mitosis

   _____ 2. chemical toxin banned years ago

   _____ 3. general test for detecting cancer

   _____ 4. tests for blood in stool

   _____ 5. washing process with a scope

   _____ 6. apoptosis

   _____ 7. detailed images in planes

   a. PCD

   b. FOBT

   c. AMAS

   d. MRI

   e. TS

   f. PCB

   g. BAL

I. **Procedures.** There are many different procedures associated with cancer diagnosis and treatment. Can you correctly identify these procedures used for cancer patients? Choose the best answer. **LO 20.6**

1. Removal of the entire lung:

   a. pneumonectomy   b. bronchoscopy   c. lobectomy

2. The most accurate non-invasive test for identifying if the cancer has metastasized:

   a. thoracoscopy   b. cystoscopy   c. positron emission tomography

3. Treatment aimed at decreasing pain or discomfort; not curative

   a. brachytherapy   b. chemotherapy   c. palliation

4. Fiber-optic tube with a camera is inserted into the space between the lungs:

   a. computed tomography   b. mediastinoscopy   c. fluoroscopy

5. Implants radioactive seeds into the tumor for direct radiation:

   a. brachytherapy   b. stereotactic radiosurgery   c. scintigraphy

6. Removal of only a small part of the lung; used for carcinoma in situ:

   a. SRS   b. segmentectomy   c. pneumonectomy

7. Creates three-dimensional images of a lesion for accurate insertion of a needle:

   a. positron emission tomography   b. stereotactic-guided biopsy   c. ductal lavage

8. A program of therapy:

   a. aspiration   b. prognosis   c. regimen

9. Employed for cutting tissue, collecting brushings, and performing washings in the lung:

    a. bronchoscopy   **b.** scintigraphy   **c.** chest x-ray

10. More effective than chest x-rays at identifying early tumors:

    a. CT   **b.** PET   **c.** MRI

J. **Build your knowledge of elements with this exercise in the language of oncology.** The element is given to you in the left column; fill in the meaning of the element in the middle column and identify the type of element (prefix, root, combining form, or suffix) in the right column. Fill in the blanks. **LO 20.3**

Element	Meaning of Element	Type of Element (P, R, CF, S)
proto	**1.** _____	**2.** _____
apo	**3.** _____	**4.** _____
muta	**5.** _____	**6.** _____
genesis	**7.** _____	**8.** _____
gen	**9.** _____	**10.** _____
onco	**11.** _____	**12.** _____
carcino	**13.** _____	**14.** _____
ptosis	**15.** _____	**16.** _____
gene	**17.** _____	**18.** _____

K. **Elements.** You are given the meaning of the element. Choose the term in which it appears. **LO 20.2**

    1. The root meaning *surroundings* is in the term

        a. environment   **b.** dioxin   **c.** pollution

    2. The suffix meaning *produce* is in the term

        a. carcinogen   **b.** pesticide   **c.** particle

    3. The prefix meaning *new* is in the term

        a. proliferate   **b.** neoplastic   **c.** dioxin

    4. The suffix meaning *to kill* is in the term

        a. cytostatic   **b.** pesticide   **c.** pollution

    5. The suffix meaning *pertaining to* is in the term

        a. pollution   **b.** environmental   **c.** prognosis

    6. The prefix meaning *two* is in the term

        a. pesticide   **b.** dioxin   **c.** monoclonal

    7. The combining form meaning *spark* is in the term

        a. fluoroscopy   **b.** osteosarcoma   **c.** scintigraphy

    8. The root meaning *flesh* is in the term

        a. sarcoma   **b.** leukemia   **c.** carcinoma

L. Elements can provide a clue to the origin of a tumor. Analyze the medical terms in the left column and match them to the cancer source in the right column. **LO 20.1**

Medical Term

_____ 1. mesothelioma

_____ 2. sarcoma

_____ 3. adenocarcinoma

_____ 4. osteosarcoma

_____ 5. melanoma

_____ 6. chondrosarcoma

_____ 7. carcinoma

_____ 8. lymphoma

_____ 9. rhabdomyosarcoma

Cancer Arises from

a. epithelial cells

b. lymph nodes

c. cells lining pleural cavity

d. connective tissue cells

e. glandular epithelial cells

f. skeletal muscle

g. bone-forming cells

h. pigment-producing skin cells

i. cartilage cells

M. Commonalities. Analyze the following medical terms and discover what they all have in common. Choose the correct answer. **LO 20.6, 20.7, 20.9**

1. Lobectomy, segmentectomy, and mastectomy are all

a. diagnoses   b. procedures   c. diagnostic tests

2. Chondrosarcoma, adenocarcinoma, and osteosarcoma are all

a. neoplasms   b. genes   c. flavonoids

3. PET, MRI, and CT are all

a. blood tests   b. diagnostic tests   c. surgeries

4. Bronchoscopy, and mediastinoscopy are

a. chest procedures   b. pelvic procedures   c. abdominal procedures

5. Pathologist, oncologist, and histologist are all

a. diseases   b. specialists   c. conditions

N. Procedures. An important distinction to learn about procedures is understanding which ones are diagnostic (used to determine a diagnosis) and which ones are therapeutic (carry out treatment). Analyze the following list of medical terms and abbreviations to determine whether they are diagnostic or therapeutic procedures. Write the letter D if it is a diagnostic term and the letter T if it is therapeutic. **LO 20.8**

1. segmentectomy: _____

2. BAL: _____

3. brachytherapy: _____

4. DRE: _____

5. stereotactic biopsy: _____

6. pneumonectomy: _____

7. ductal lavage: _____

8. mediastinoscopy: _____

9. CHART: _____

O. Pronunciation is important whether you are saying the word or listening to a word from a coworker. Identify the proper pronunciation of the following medical terms. The correctly spell the term. **LO 20.1, 20.4, 20.5**

1. The correct pronunciation for able to metastasize

   a. meh-**TAS**-tas-tik

   b. meh-**TAS**-tah-tik

   c. **MET**-tah-**STAT**-ik

   d. meh-tah-**STAT**-ik

   Correctly spell the term: _____

2. The correct pronunciation for cancer arising from the cells lining the pleura or peritoneum

   a. **MEZ**-oh-thay-lee-**OH**-mah

   b. **MEEZ**-oh-thee-lee-**OH**-mah

   c. sar-**KOH**-mah

   d. sark-**OH**-mah

   Correctly spell the term: _____

3. The correct pronunciation for a malignant tumor originating in connective tissue

   a. sar-**KOH**-mah

   b. sark-oh-**MOH**

   c. kar-**SIN**-oh-jeen-ik

   d. **KAR**-sin-oh-**JEN**-ik

   Correctly spell the term: _____

4. The correct pronunciation for programmed normal cell death

   a. **AP**-op-**TOH**-sis

   b. ape-oh-**TOH**-sis

   c. **NEE**-oh-plazm

   d. nee-**OP**-lazm

   Correctly spell the term: _____

5. The correct pronunciation for the term that means a growth that is not cancerous

   a. **MAL**-ig-nant

   b. mah-**LIG**-nant

   c. ben-**IH**-jen

   d. bee-**NINE**

   Correctly spell the term: _____

Chapter 20 Review

2014 Nucleus Medical Media

Case Report

A. **After reading the following Case Report, correctly answer the following questions.** The answers to the questions may not be in the Case Report itself but can be found in the chapter content. **LO 20.4, 20.8, 20.9**

 ### Case Report (CR) 20.1

You are

. . . an advanced-level **respiratory therapist** employed by Fulwood Medical Center working with Tavis Senko, MD, a **pulmonologist.**

Your patient is

. . . Raquel Sacco, a 44-year-old mother of two teenage boys, who is the owner of a quilting fabrics store. She is 2 days postop from a lung surgery for non–small cell lung cancer. From her records, you see that she has two **secondary metastases** in her brain. She has been a nonsmoker all her life. Her 70-year-old father is a two-pack-a-day smoker, as is her husband. They both show no evidence of cancer on chest x-rays. Before Raquel is discharged, as part of her **postoperative** respiratory care plan, you are using **incentive spirometry**—also called **sustained maximal inspiration (SMI)**—to increase her **inspiratory** volume and improve her inspiratory muscle performance. You also will be taking an arterial blood sample to check her **arterial** oxygen pressure (PaO_2).

Adenocarcinoma was found in Raquel Sacco. It was **diagnosed** because she had a **seizure,** and **neurologic** tests revealed the presence of two metastases in her brain, leading to a search for the **primary** tumor, which was found in her lung. Raquel Sacco probably developed her lung cancer as a result of inhaling **secondhand** smoke all her life (from her father and husband). Because Raquel Sacco's cancer has **metastasized** to her brain, she is placed in stage IV. The outlook for Mrs. Sacco is bleak.

Non–Small Cell Lung Cancer Survival

Stage	5-Year Relative Survival Rate
I	47%
II	26%
III	8%
IV	2%

1. Which term means *after surgery?* _____

2. Does Mrs. Sacco have a personal history of smoking? _____

3. Is there anyone in her immediate family with a history of cancer? (yes or no) _____

4. Did her cancer spread? (yes or no) _____

5. Where did the metastases appear? _____

6. Are the metastases the 1° or 2° cancer? _____

7. Where does her 1° cancer originate? _____

8. What specific type of cancer is the 1° cancer? _____

9. What problem first brought Mrs. Sacco to the doctor? _____

10. What stage of cancer has Mrs. Sacco been diagnosed with? _____

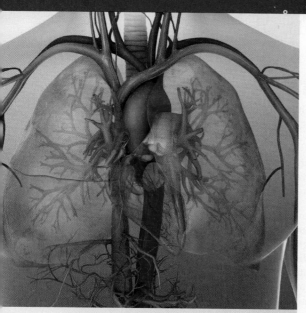

2014 Nucleus Medical Media

Radiology and Nuclear Medicine
The Language of Medical Imaging

Chapter Sections

Chapter Learning Outcomes

Upon completion of this chapter, you will be able to:

LO 21.1 Describe the characteristics of x-rays and the different techniques used for acquiring radiologic images.

LO 21.2 Describe the characteristics of radioactive materials used in medical imaging.

LO 21.3 Use roots, combining forms, suffixes, and prefixes to construct and analyze medical terms related to medical imaging.

LO 21.4 Spell medical terms related to medical imaging.

LO 21.5 Pronounce medical terms related to medical imaging.

LO 21.6 Explain the use of medical imaging in diagnosing disease.

LO 21.7 Describe the different nuclear medicine therapies and radiologic techniques used in the treatment of disease.

LO 21.8 Apply knowledge of medical terms relating to medical imaging to documentation, medical records, and communication.

LO 21.9 Identify and correctly use abbreviations of terms used in medical imaging.

LO 21.10 Identify health professionals involved in medical imaging.

The health professionals involved in radiology and nuclear medicine include:

- **Radiologists,** who are physicians with specialized training in obtaining and interpreting medical images.
- **Radiographers, radiologic technologists, radiologic technicians,** and **radiologic assistants,** who provide radiologists with the images they need to diagnose and treat medical conditions.
- **Sonographers,** who operate ultrasound imaging devices to produce diagnostic images.
- **Nuclear medicine specialists,** who are radiologists with specialized training in the use of **radiopharmaceuticals** for the purpose of diagnosis, treatment, and research.
- **Nuclear medicine technologists,** who administer radiopharmaceuticals to patients and operate cameras to detect and map the radioactive drug in the patient's body to create diagnostic images.
- **Radiotherapists,** who are physicians who specialize in the treatment of disease using x-rays and radioactive materials.

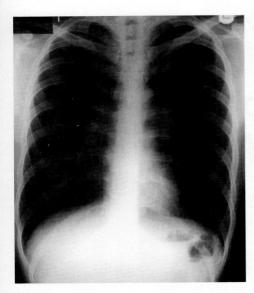

▲ **Figure 21.1** **X-ray image of a female chest.** UIG/Getty Images

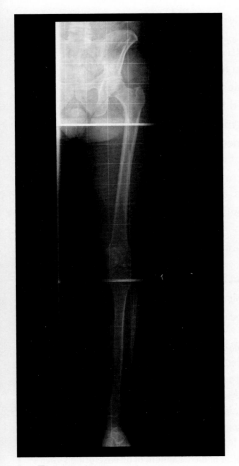

▲ **Figure 21.2** **X-ray image of a femur.** Warrick G./Science Source

X-ray Characteristics and Effects

X-rays were first discovered in 1895 by Wilhelm Conrad Röntgen. These x-rays, like light and radio waves, are a form of electromagnetic radiation. The characteristics of x-rays include:

- **Velocity.** Because they are **electromagnetic,** x-rays in a vacuum travel at the speed of light, 186,000 miles per second. This velocity is reduced as x-rays penetrate the different substances of the body according to their density.

- **Wavelength.** X-rays have a very short wavelength compared with other electromagnetic waveforms. Only gamma rays from an atomic explosion have a shorter wavelength. This short wavelength is a major factor in enabling x-rays to pass through many materials and tissues to different degrees. Air is the most **radiolucent** and allows the greatest penetration (photographic plates show black, *Figure 21.1*). Fat is denser than air, water is more dense, and bone is the most dense (**radiopaque**) (photographic plates show white, *Figure 21.2*).

- **Invisibility.** X-rays cannot be detected by sight, sound, or touch, so health professionals working in radiology wear a film badge to detect and record radiation to which they are exposed *(Figure 21.3)*.

- **Ionization.** An **ion** is an atom or group of atoms carrying an electric charge by having gained or lost one or more electrons. When x-rays **ionize** matter, they can both kill cancerous cells and damage normal cells to produce the side effects of radiation as well as genetic mutations that cause malignant changes. Radiation also can cause damage to a fetus, so the use of x-rays in pregnancy is kept to a minimum.

Recording of X-ray Images

A special type of photographic film is used to record x-ray pictures. The x-rays are converted into light, and the more energy that passes through body tissues to reach the photographic film or plate, the darker that region of film will be. Lungs will be dark; bones that prevent the passage of energy will be white. X-rays can now also be detected electronically using a recorder similar to that used in a digital camera. This means that they can be read immediately and stored more easily.

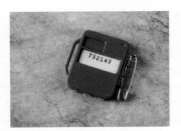

▲ **Figure 21.3** **Radiation monitor.** Film badge used to determine a person's exposure to radiation. The badge is worn on a person's clothing and contains a piece of photographic film. Radiation affects the film in a similar way to light. Martyn F. Chillmaid/Science Source

S = Suffix P = Prefix R = Root R/CF = Combining Form

WORD	PRONUNCIATION	ELEMENTS		DEFINITION
electromagnetic	ee-**LEK**-troh-mag-**NET**-ik	S/ R/CF R/	-ic *pertaining to* electr/o- *electricity* -magnet- *magnet*	Pertaining to energy propagated through matter and space
ion	**EYE**-on		Greek *going*	An atom or group of atoms having gained or lost one or more electrons
ionization (noun)	**EYE**-on-ih-**ZA**-shun	S/ R/	-ization *process of affecting in a specific way* ion- *atom or group of atoms carrying an electric charge*	The process of causing an atom or group of atoms to gain or lose one or more electrons
ionize (verb)		S/	-ize *to affect in a specific way*	To cause the process of ionization
radiolucent	ray-dee-oh-**LOO**-sent	S/ R/CF	-lucent *open* radi/o- *radiation*	Penetrable by x-rays or other forms of radiation
radiopaque	ray-dee-oh-**PAKE**	S/	-paque *shady*	Impenetrable to x-rays or other forms of radiation

Patient Alignment

In many situations where x-ray images are taken, the x-ray tube that produces the radiation, the patient, and the photographic film must be aligned to direct the x-ray beam to the lesion being examined in the best possible way. **Radiologic technicians** place patients are responsible for placing patients in the proper position as ordered by a health care provider. Terms describing the direction of the projection of x-ray beams are of importance in chest x-rays and are:

- **Posteroanterior (PA),** in which x-rays travel from a posterior source to an anteriorly placed image receiver. This is the most common chest x-ray view.

- **Anteroposterior (AP),** in which x-rays travel from an anterior source to a posteriorly placed image receiver.

- **Lateral view.** In a left lateral view, x-rays travel from a source located to the right of a patient and travel to an image recorder to the left of the patient. This is reversed in a right lateral view.

- **Mediolateral oblique (MLO),** which is commonly used in **mammography.**

- **Craniocaudal (CC)**—head-to-foot, commonly used in mammography.

- **Oblique,** in which x-rays travel at an angle from the perpendicular plane and pass behind the heart and lung hilum to show structures normally hidden in PA and AP views.
  The terms *anterior, posterior,* and other directional terms are described in *Chapter 3.*

Acquisition of Radiologic Images

Radiologists are physicians with specialized training in obtaining and interpreting medical images. Radiologist further specialize in acquisition of images, interventional radiology, nuclear medicine, or radiation therapy.

Plain (Projectional) Radiography

Plain radiography was the only modality available in the first 50 years of radiology. The x-rays that pass through a patient strike an undeveloped film held in a light-tight cassette. The film is then developed chemically to produce an image on the film. Now, **digital radiography (DR)** is replacing film screen radiography; x-rays strike a plate of sensors that convert the signals generated into digital information and an image on a computer screen. Because of its lower cost and availability, plain radiography is the first-line examination of choice in radiologic diagnosis *(Figure 21.4).* Lead aprons can be used to protect patients and technicians from receiving unwanted radiation.

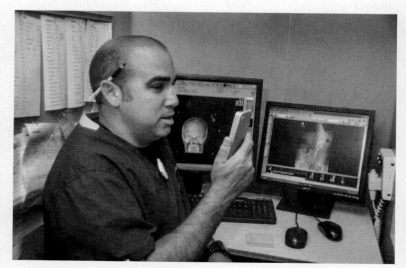

▲ **Figure 21.4** **Radiologist dictates a report.** Marmaduke St. John/Alamy Stock Photo

Fluoroscopy

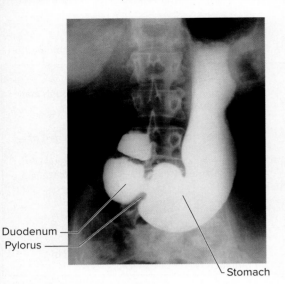

In **fluoroscopy,** a continuous x-ray image is shown on a monitor like an x-ray movie. This allows real-time imaging of structures in motion; for example, blood vessels or the gastrointestinal **(GI)** tract. **Radiocontrast** agents, such as barium sulfate and iodine, are administered orally, rectally, intravenously, or into an artery and enhance the real-time imaging of dynamic processes such as blood flow in arteries and veins (**angiography**) or peristalsis in the GI tract. Iodine contrast also may be concentrated in tumors, cysts, or inflamed areas to make them more **opaque** and conspicuous in imaging. A barium meal *(Figure 21.5)*, also known as an upper gastrointestinal series, enables radiographs of the esophagus, stomach, and duodenum to be taken after barium sulfate is ingested. However, the diagnostic use of a barium meal has declined with the increasing use of esophagogastroduodenoscopy **(EGD)**, which allows direct visual inspection of suspicious areas in the esophagus, stomach, and duodenum.

Duodenum —
Pylorus —

└ Stomach

▲ **Figure 21.5** **Barium meal showing stomach, pylorus, and duodenum.** Biophoto Associates/ Science Source

Word Analysis and Definition: Radiologic Images

S = Suffix P = Prefix R = Root R/CF = Combining Form

WORD	PRONUNCIATION	ELEMENTS		DEFINITION
angiography	an-jee-**OG**-rah-fee	S/ R/CF	-graphy *process of recording* angi/o- *blood vessel*	Radiography of blood vessels after injection of contrast material
angiogram	**AN**-jee-oh-gram	S/	-gram *a record*	The radiograph obtained by angiography
angioplasty	**AN**-jee-oh-**PLAS**-tee	S/	-plasty *surgical repair*	Recanalization of a blood vessel by surgery
anteroposterior	**AN**-teh-roh-pos-**TEER**-ee-or	S/ R/CF R/	-ior *pertaining to* anter/o- *coming before* -poster- *coming behind*	The direction the x-ray beam passes through the patient: from front to back (AP)
fluoroscopy	flor-**OS**-koh-pee	S/ R/CF	-scopy *to examine* fluor/o- *x-ray beam*	Examination of the structures of the body by x-rays
oblique	ob-**LEEK**		Latin *slanting*	Slanting; in radiology, a projection that is neither frontal nor lateral
mediolateral oblique	**MEE**-dee-oh-**LAT**-er-al ob-**LEEK**	S/ P/ R/	-al *pertaining to* medio- *middle* -later- *side*	An angled side view of a structure
opaque	oh-**PAKE**		Latin *shady*	Impervious to light; impenetrable by x-rays or other forms of radiation
posteroanterior	**POS**-ter-oh-an-**TEER**-ee-or	S/ R/CF R/	-ior *pertaining to* poster/o- *coming behind* -anter- *coming before*	The direction the x-ray beam passes through the patient: from back to front (PA)
radiocontrast	**RAY**-dee-oh-**CON**-trast	S/ R/CF	-contrast *against* radi/o- *radiation*	Agents that make structures stand out in x-ray imaging
craniocaudal	**KRAY**-nee-oh-**KAW**-dal	S/ R/CF R/	-al *pertaining to* crani/o- *skull* -caud- *tail*	A view of a structure from head to foot
mammography	mah-**MOG**-rah-fee	S/ R/CF	-graphy *process of recording* mamm/o- *breast*	X-ray imaging of the breast
mammogram	**MAM**-oh-gram	S/	-gram *a record*	The x-ray record produced by mammography
radiograph	**RAY**-dee-oh-graf	S/ R/CF	-graph *record* radi/o- *radiation*	Image made by exposure to x-rays
radiographer	ray-dee-**OG**-rah-fer	S/	-er *one who records*	Technologist who performs x-ray procedures
radiographic (adj)	ray-dee-oh-**GRAF**-ik	S/	-ic *pertaining to*	Pertaining to x-rays
radiology	ray-dee-**OL**-oh-jee	S/ R/CF	-logy *study of* radi/o- *radiation*	The study of medical imaging
radiologic (adj)	ray-dee-oh-**LOJ**-ik	S/	-ic *pertaining to*	Pertaining to radiology
radiologist	ray-dee-**OL**-oh-jist	S/	-logist *specialist*	Specialist in radiology

Interventional Radiology

Interventional radiology (IR) uses minimally invasive procedures both for diagnostic purposes (e.g., angiogram) and for treatment (e.g., **angioplasty**). X-ray images are used for guidance, and the basic instruments used are needles and catheters. The images provide a road map to enable the instruments to be guided to the areas containing disease for diagnosis and for treatment. Benefits from these procedures include short recovery time, shortened hospital stays, reduced infection rates, and reduced costs.

Computed Tomography

The first commercially viable **computed tomography (CT)** scanner was produced at EMI Labs in England in 1972. EMI owned the rights to the Beatles music, and their profits funded the research. CT scans use x-rays in conjunction with computer **algorithms** to produce a computer-generated cross-sectional image (**tomogram**) in the **axial** plane. From these images, the computer can reconstruct **coronal** and **sagittal** images. Radiocontrast agents can be used with CT to enhance the delineation of anatomy. CT scans have become the test of choice in diagnosing some emergency conditions such as cerebral hemorrhage *(Figure 21.6)*, pulmonary embolism *(see Chapter 13)*, aortic dissection *(see Chapter 10)*, and kidney stones *(see Chapter 6)* and in identifying small lung cancers *(see Chapter 13)*. Unfortunately, CT scans expose the patient to much more ionizing radiation than does an x-ray.

Ultrasound

Medical **ultrasonography** uses **ultrasound (US)** (high-frequency sound waves) functioning in real time to visualize soft tissue structures in the body. No ionizing radiation is involved. Because of this, it plays a vital role in obstetrics, enabling early diagnosis of fetal abnormalities and multiple gestations *(Figure 21.7)*. Ultrasound measures the severity of peripheral vascular disease and evaluates the dynamic function of the heart, heart valves, and major blood vessels. In trauma victims, it also can assess the integrity of the major viscera (including liver, spleen, and kidneys) and the presence of bleeding into the peritoneum.

Magnetic Resonance Imaging

Magnetic resonance imaging (MRI) uses strong magnetic fields to align atomic nuclei in tissues, then it uses a radio signal to disrupt the nuclei and observes the radio frequency signal as the nuclei return to their baseline states. MRI can produce images in axial, coronal, sagittal, and oblique planes and also can give the best soft tissue contrast of all imaging modalities. It is an important tool in musculoskeletal radiology and neuroradiology *(Figure 21.8)*. Its disadvantages are that the patient has to lie in a noisy, confined space (tube) for long periods of time, and it cannot be used for patients with pacemakers or any metallic implant such as artificial joints or implanted surgical hardware (plates, rods). For patients with **claustrophobia,** anti-anxiety medication can be prescribed to be taken before entering the scanner.

Teleradiology involves the transmission of radiographic digital images from one location to another for interpretation by a radiologist. It can provide real-time emergency radiology services and expert consultation around the clock.

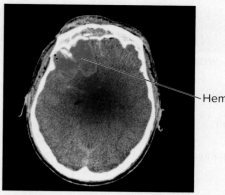

▲ **Figure 21.6** **Brain hemorrhage, colored computed tomography (CT) Scan.** The front of the brain is at top, and a large mass of blood (hematoma, purple) is seen at upper left in the frontal lobe. Bleeding (hemorrhage) in the brain occurs when a blood vessel, such as an artery, ruptures. It may be caused by a head injury, high blood pressure, or vascular disease. In this case, a tree fell on the patient's head. The area of the brain supplied by the ruptured artery may die due to lack of oxygenated blood, leading to a stroke. Du Cane Medical Imaging Ltd./Science Source

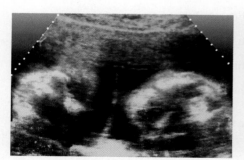

▲ **Figure 21.7** **Twins, ultrasound biometry.** VEM/Science Source

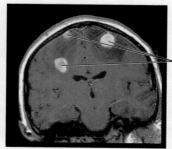

▲ **Figure 21.8** **MRI of brain showing Metastases.** BSIP/Science Source

Word Analysis and Definition: Radiologic Images

S = Suffix   P = Prefix   R = Root   R/CF = Combining Form

WORD	PRONUNCIATION	ELEMENTS		DEFINITION
axis axial (adj)	AK-sis AK-see-al	S/ R/	Greek central support -ial pertaining to ax- central support	A line of central support Pertaining to an axis
coronal	KOR-oh-nal	S/ R/	-al pertaining to coron- crown	Vertical plane dividing the body into anterior and posterior portions
fibroglandular	fie-broh-GLAN-dyu-lar	S/ R/CF R/	-ar pertaining to fibr/o- fiber -glandul- little gland	A mixture of fibrous and glandular tissue
interventional	IN-ter-VEN-shun-al	S/ S/ R/	-al pertaining to -ion- action, process intervent- to come between	Pertaining to an overt act to change an event or outcome
sagittal	SAJ-ih-tal	S/ R/	-al pertaining to sagitt- arrow	Pertaining to the vertical plane dividing the body into right and left portions
teleradiology	TEL-eh-ray-dee-OL-oh-jee	S/ P/ R/CF	-logy study of tele- distant -radi/o- radiation, x-ray	The interpretation of digitized diagnostic images transmitted from a distance
tomogram tomography	TOH-moh-gram toh-MOG-rah-fee	S/ R/CF S/	-gram a record tom/o- section -graphy process of recording	Radiographic image of a selected section or slice of tissue Process of taking a tomogram
ultrasound ultrasonography	UL-trah-sownd UL-trah-soh-NOG-rah-fee	P/ R/ S/ R/CF	ultra- higher, beyond -sound noise -graphy process of recording -son/o- sound	Very-high-frequency sound waves Delineation of dynamic structures using sound waves

Check Point Section 21.1

A. Answer the following questions about the characteristics of x-rays. *Select the correct answer.* **LO 21.1**

1. Which of the following is NOT a characteristic of an x-ray?

    a. velocity   **b.** wavelength   **c.** ionization   **d.** invisibility   **e.** weight

2. Which of the following characteristics of x-rays is most damaging to a fetus?

    a. velocity   **b.** radiation   **c.** wavelength   **d.** ionization   **e.** speed

3. X-rays in a vacuum travel at the speed of light. This is called

    a. wavelength   **b.** radiolucent   **c.** velocity   **d.** radiopaque   **e.** invisibility

B. Define the views used in radiography. *Match the term in the first column with its correct description in the second column.* **LO 21.1**

_____   **1.** posteroanterior   **a** x-ray beam passes through the body at an angle

_____   **2.** anteroposterior   **b.** x-ray beam passes through the structure from the middle to the side

_____   **3.** oblique   **c.** x-ray beam passes through the patient from back to front

_____   **4.** mediolateral   **d.** x-ray beam passes through the patient from front to back

C. Using the three medical terms below, insert the appropriate medical terms into the paragraph. LO 21.1, 21.6

    angioplasty   **angiogram**   **angiography**

1. The doctor is using _____ as a diagnostic tool.

2. After seeing the _____, he has decided to schedule the patient for a surgical procedure.

3. He has asked you to schedule the patient's _____ for tomorrow morning.

D. Analyze the continuation of the Case Report for Mrs. Coffrey, and then answer the following questions. LO 20.1, 20.8

 Case Report (CR) 21.1

You are

. . . Anita Scherraga, a radiologic technologist working in the radiology department at Fulwood Medical Center.

Your patient is

. . . Mrs. Carole Coffrey, a 46-year-old health information technologist with two children who is complaining of pain in her breasts. You are to perform a **mammogram** on Mrs. Coffrey using parallel-plate compression in a **full-field digital mammography** (FFDM) unit. You will be taking two views of Mrs. Coffrey's breasts: a head-to-foot (**craniocaudal [CC]**) and an angled side view (**mediolateral oblique [MLO]**).

Mrs. Coffrey's mammogram report was sent to her in writing. It reads, "There are scattered **fibroglandular** densities bilaterally. There is a benign-appearing area of glandular tissue in the right lower inner breast. There are a few faint calcifications in the lower inner and central left breast. There is no associated mass or distortion."

1. The type of image that the radiologist read:

   a. mammography   **b.** mammogram   **c.** angiography   **d.** angiogram

2. Were there any malignancies found in Mrs. Coffrey's report?

   a. yes   **b.** no

3. Associated mass would be another term for _____.

4. The medical term in the Case Report that mean both sides: _____

5. From the information in the mammogram report, does Mrs. Coffrey have breast cancer?

   a. Yes

               b. No

6. What term in the report led you to this conclusion? (fill in the blank) _____

7. In which breast(s) is/are the fibroglandular densities located?

   a. left only

   b. right only

   c. left and right

8. Which medical professional created the mammogram report?

   a. gerontologist

               c. sonographer

   b. podiatrist

               d. radiologist

E. Improve your knowledge of diagnostic procedures by matching the definition to the appropriate abbreviation. LO 21.9

_____ **1.** This uses minimally invasive procedures for diagnosis and treatment.   **a.** MRI

_____ **2.** This is the test of choice for diagnosing some emergency conditions.   **b.** IR

_____ **3.** This uses high-frequency sound waves to visualize soft tissue.   **c.** CT

_____ **4.** Patients with pacemakers are unable to use this modality.   **d.** US

Section 21.2 Nuclear Medicine

Radiopharmaceuticals

In nuclear medicine, **radionuclides** can be combined with pharmaceutical compounds to form **radiopharmaceuticals,** which are labeled with a radioactive **tracer.** When administered to a patient orally, injected intravenously, or inhaled as a gas, these compounds can localize to a specific organ or cells. Then, external detectors (gamma cameras) capture and form images from the radiation emitted by the tracers. This two-dimensional imaging is called **scintigraphy.** With computer processing, the information can be displayed as axial, coronal, and sagittal images *(see Chapter 3),* known as single-**photon** emission computed tomography **(SPECT)** images, to produce an image of a "slice" of a patient in a particular plane. A collection of parallel slices form a slice-stack, a three-dimensional representation of how the radionuclide is distributed in the patient.

The most commonly used tracers include:

- **Technetium-99m,** used in 85% of all nuclear medicine imaging including for bone scans, liver scans, renal function studies, labeling of red blood cells, and use as a gas/aerosol.
- **Iodine-123,** used mainly for thyroid scans.
- **Iodine-131,** used mainly for the destruction of thyroid tissues.
- **Gallium-67,** used in **positron emission tomography (PET)** scans *(see the following)* and for localizing infections.
- **Indium-111,** used to label and identify the movements of white blood cells.
- **Thallium-201,** used for myocardial perfusion scans in stress tests.
- **18F-FDG** (fludeoxyglucose), used in the diagnosis and staging of cancer and most commonly in PET scans.

Positron emission tomography (PET) scanning produces two opposite traveling gamma rays to be detected concurrently to improve resolution. 18F-FDG is injected intravenously into the patient, and the radiation emitted is detected to produce multiplanar images of the body. Tissues, such as cancer, that are most metabolically active concentrate the 18F-FDG more than normal tissues. PET images can be fused with an anatomical CT image to improve diagnostic accuracy. In academic and research settings, PET images are now being fused with MRI images.

Radiation Dose

The radiation doses delivered to a patient in a nuclear medicine procedure present a very small risk of inducing cancer. The radiopharmaceuticals are inside the body and emit ionizing radiation that travels a short distance, thus minimizing unwanted side effects and damage to noninvolved nearby structures. The radiopharmaceuticals decay and are excreted from the body through normal bodily functions.

Word Analysis and Definition: Nuclear Medicine

S = Suffix P = Prefix R = Root R/CF = Combining Form

WORD	PRONUNCIATION		ELEMENTS	DEFINITION
photon	FOH-ton		Greek *light*	A particle of light or other electromagnetic radiation
positron	POZ-ih-tron		Greek *positive element*	A subatomic particle equal in mass to an electron but with the opposite (positive) charge
radionuclide	RAY-dee-oh-NYU-klide	S/ R/CF R/	-ide *having a particular quality* radi/o- *radiation* -nucl- *nucleus*	Radioactive agent used in nuclear medicine
radiopharmaceutical	RAY-dee-oh-far-mah-SOO-tik-al	S/ S/ R/CF R/CF	-ical *pertaining to* -ceut- *relating to* radi/o- *radiation* -pharm/a- *drug industry*	Radioactive drugs
scintigraphy	sin-TIG-rah-fee	S/ R/CF	-graphy *process of recording* scint/i- *spark*	Recording of radioactivity with gamma cameras
tracer	TRAY-ser		Latin *track*	Radioactive agent used to trace metabolic processes

Radiation Therapy

Radiation therapy (**radiotherapy**) is defined as treatment with x-rays or radionuclides. **Radiotherapists** follow the physician's order for radiation treatment by applying radiation to the precise location of area needing treatment.

X-ray Therapy

Ionizing radiation works by damaging the DNA of tissues exposed to it. However, the x-rays often have to pass through skin and other organs to reach a target tumor. To spare normal tissues from the harmful side effects of x-rays, narrow radiation beams are aimed from several angles to intersect at the target tumor. This provides a much larger local dose to the tumor than to the surrounding healthy tissues. It is also common to combine x-ray therapy with surgery, chemotherapy, hormone therapy, immunotherapy, or any combination.

There are five types of x-ray therapy:

- **Conventional external-beam radiation therapy** consists of a single beam of radiation delivered to the tumor from several directions. The concern is the effect of the radiation on the healthy tissues close to the tumor being irradiated. For complex reasons, large tumors respond less well to radiation than small tumors. Strategies to overcome this include surgical resection prior to chemotherapy (as in the treatment of breast cancer), chemotherapy to shrink the tumor prior to radiation therapy, and the administration of radiosensitizing drugs during radiation therapy. Examples are cisplatin *(Platinol)* and cetuximab *(Erbitux).*

- **Stereotactic radiation** is a specialized form of external-beam radiation therapy. It focuses radiation beams by using detailed imaging scans. In **stereotactic radiosurgery (SRS),** radiation is applied to the tumor with multiple (as many as 200), separate narrow beams, so that the tumor receives a very high dose of radiation in one treatment, yet the surrounding tissues are minimally irradiated. In areas of the body where there is motion by breathing or blood flow, a combination of continuous imaging, motion detection, and robotic guidance enable the beams to remain focused on the tumor. **Stereotactic body radiation treatment (SBRT)** refers to the use of these techniques in such areas as the lungs. A technique called **hypofractionation** is the giving of a much higher dose of radiation per session with greater accuracy and the sparing of normal surrounding tissue. Brand names for these stereotactic radiation therapies include Gamma Knife, Cyberknife, Tomotherapy, and Truebeam.

- **3-Dimensional conformal radiation therapy (3DCRT)** is the result of being able to delineate tumors and surrounding normal tissues in three dimensions using CT or MRI scanners and planning software. The profile of each radiation beam and the treatment volume conform to the shape of the tumor, allowing a higher dose of radiation to be delivered to the tumor with a reduced toxicity to the surrounding normal tissues.

- **Intensity-modulated radiation therapy (IMRT)** is the next generation of 3DCRT in which, if the tumor is wrapped around a vulnerable structure such as a blood vessel or major organ, the pattern of radiation delivery can avoid the normal structure.

- **Proton beam therapy** has the advantage that the proton only gives up its energy when it hits the tumor and does not continue on through the tumor to hit normal tissue on the far side. Very high doses of radiation can be given without adjacent normal tissue damage. Prostate cancer is the most common cancer to be treated by proton beam therapy.

Nuclear Medicine Therapy

In **radioactive iodine (I-131) therapy,** the I-131 is taken orally and absorbed into the bloodstream from the GI tract. From the blood, it is concentrated by the thyroid gland, where it destroys cells in that organ and is used to treat thyroid cancer, thyroid nodules, and hyperthyroidism. Common nuclear medicine therapies treat lymphoma, neuroendocrine tumors, and palliative bone pain. Implanted capsules of isotopes **(brachytherapy)** are used for such cancers as prostate and breast cancer.

Radioimmunotherapy (RIT) combines radiation therapy and immunotherapy. In immunotherapy, a laboratory-produced molecule called a **monoclonal antibody** is designed to recognize and bind to the surface of cancer cells; this mimics the body's naturally produced antibodies. In RIT, a monoclonal antibody is fused with a radioactive material and injected into the patient's bloodstream. The antibody travels to and binds to the cancer cells, delivering a high dose of radiation directly to the cells in the cancer.

Word Analysis and Definition: Radiation Therapy

S = Suffix P = Prefix R = Root R/CF = Combining Form

WORD	PRONUNCIATION	ELEMENTS		DEFINITION
brachytherapy	brah-kee-**THAIR**-ah-pee	P/ R/	**brachy-** *short* **-therapy** *medical treatment*	Internal radiation therapy delivered by placing radiation sources into the tumor
hypofractionation	**HIGH**-poh-frak-shun-**AY**-shun	S/ S/ P/ R/	**-ation** *process* **-ion-** *action, process* **hypo-** *below* **-fract-** *small amount*	Larger measures of a dose of radiation given less frequently
monoclonal	**MON**-oh-**KLOH**-nal	S/ P/ R/	**-al** *pertaining to* **mono-** *one, single* **-clon-** *cutting*	Pertaining to protein from a single clone of cells
proton	**PROH**-ton		Greek *first*	The positively charged unit of the nuclear mass
radioimmunotherapy	**RAY**-dee-oh-**IM**-you-noh-**THAIR**-ah-pee	R/CF R/CF R/	**radi/o-** *radiation* **-immun/o-** *immune response* **-therapy** *medical treatment*	The combination of radiotherapy and the use of antibodies, e.g., monoclonal antibodies
radiotherapy	**RAY**-dee-oh-**THAIR**-ah-pee	R/CF R/	**radi/o-** *radiation* **-therapy** *treatment*	Treatment using radiation
radiotherapist	**RAY**-dee-oh-**THAIR**-ah-pist	S/ R/	**-ist** *specialist* **-therap-** *treatment*	Specialist in the use of radiation in the treatment of patients
stereotactic	**STER**-ee-oh-**TAK**-tik	S/ R/CF R/	**-ic** *-pertaining to* **stere/o-** *three-dimensional* **-tact-** *orderly arrangement*	Pertaining to a precise three-dimensional method to locate a lesion or a tumor

Check Point Section 21.2

A. To improve your knowledge of radiology terms, complete the following exercises by selecting the correct answer. LO 21.2, 21.6

1. Which term best describes two-dimensional imaging?

   a. ultrasound

   b. scintigraphy

   c. PET scan

   d. MRI scan

   e. interventional

2. What is a tracer?

   a. a red line that appears on the scan

   b. a radioactive agent

   c. a plastic object you swallow for the test

   d. a record produced by the test

   e. a tiny camera you swallow for the test

3. A tracer is used in which type of imaging?

   a. ultrasound

   b. MRI

   c. scintigraphy

   d. radiation

4. The type of radioactive positron that is used to detect thyroid disorders:

   a. glucose

   b. iodine

   c. thallium

   d. technetium

5. The production of "slice" views of body structures used with scintigraphy:

   a. SPECT

   b. PET

   c. FDG

   d. IR

B. Differentiate between the different types of x-ray therapy for malignant tumors. *Choose the best answer for each question.* **LO 20.7**

1. A brand name for this type of therapy is Gamma Knife:

   a. proton beam therapy

   b. conventional external-beam radiation therapy

   c. intensity-modulated radiation therapy

   d. stereotactic radiation

2. Of all of the types of x-ray therapy, this one has the greatest incidence of radiation being applied to normal, healthy tissue:

   a. proton beam therapy

   b. conventional external-beam radiation therapy

   c. intensity-modulated radiation therapy

   d. stereotactic radiation

3. The next generation of 3DCRT is:

   a. proton beam therapy

   b. conventional external-beam radiation therapy

   c. intensity-modulated radiation therapy

   d. stereotactic radiation

4. This therapy can treat cancer with high doses of radiation without adjacent normal tissue damage:

   a. proton beam therapy

   b. conventional external-beam radiation therapy

   c. intensity-modulated radiation therapy

   d. stereotactic radiation

C. Identify the following elements. *Match the word element in the first column to its correct definition in the second column.* **LO 21.3**

_____ 1. *stere/o*

_____ 2. *hypo-*

_____ 3. *fract*

_____ 4. *mono-*

_____ 5. *clon*

_____ 6. *brachy-*

a. short

b. small amount

c. below

d. three-dimensional

e. cutting

f. one

Table 21.1 Chapter 21 Abbreviations

Abbreviations	Meaning
AP	anteroposterior
CT	computed tomography
DR	digital radiography
EGD	esophagogastroduodenoscopy
FFDM	full-field digital mammography
FDG	fludeoxyglucose
GI	gastrointestinal
IR	interventional radiology
I-131	radioactive iodine
IMRT	intensity-modulated radiation therapy
MLO	mediolateral oblique
MRI	magnetic resonance imaging
PA	posteroanterior
PET	positron emission tomography
RIT	radioimmunotherapy
SBRT	stereotactic body radiation treatment
SRS	stereotactic radiosurgery
SPECT	single-photon emission computed tomography
US	ultrasound
3DCRT	three-dimensional conformal radiation therapy

Challenge Your Knowledge

A. **Review the planes and directional terms because they are very important in diagnostic radiology.** Fill in the blanks. **LO 21.1**

1. front of the body

   _____

2. divides the body into upper and lower portions

   _____

3. side of the body

   _____

4. toward the midline of the body

   _____

5. head of the body

   _____

6. back of the body

   _____

7. divides the body into right and left portions

   _____

8. only horizontal plane in the body

   _____

9. head to foot

   _____

B. **Choose the correct answer. LO 21.1**

1. Which x-ray characteristic is electromagnetic?

   a. speed

   b. velocity

   c. wavelength

   d. ionization

C. **The most basic element in any medical term is its root or combining form.** In each of these terms, identify the root/combining form and define the meaning of the element and the term. **LO 21.3**

Term	Identify Root/ Combining Form	Meaning of Element	Meaning of Term
mammogram	1.	2.	3.
fluoroscopy	4.	5.	6.
sagittal	7.	8.	9.
scintigraphy	10.	11.	12.
monoclonal	13.	14.	15.
radiograph	16.	17.	18.

D. **Each of these medical terms has a function in radiology.** Write the correct term with its correct definition. Fill in the blank. **LO 21.2**

1. Materials placed into the body to enhance the image of an organ or structure in radiographic procedures. _____

2. Internal radiation therapy delivered by placing radiation sources into the tumor. _____

3. Radioactive agent used in nuclear medicine to visualize metabolic processes of cells and organs. _____

4. The use of high-frequency sound waves to visualize structures. _____

5. A computer-generated cross-sectional image. _____

E. Choose the best answer. LO 21.8

1. Which pair of terms could appear in a radiology report?
   a. impacted   cerumen
   b. oblique   opaque
   c. sublingual   subcutaneous
   d. tonometer   otolith
   e. cannula   catheter

F. Read the following paragraph and then choose the correct answers. LO 21.2, 21.6, 21.7, 21.8

In fluoroscopy and angiography, a fluorescent screen and image intensifier tube are connected to a closed-circuit television system. This allows real-time imaging of structures in motion; for example, blood vessels or the GI tract. Radiocontrast agents, such as barium sulfate and iodine, are administered orally, rectally, intravenously, or into an artery and enhance the real-time imaging of dynamic processes such as blood flow in arteries and veins or peristalsis in the GI tract. Iodine contrast also may be concentrated in tumors, cysts, or inflamed areas to make them more opaque and conspicuous.

1. What is *real-time imaging*?
   a. You take pictures during a scan and view them later.
   b. You see images on a screen as the scan is actually happening.
   c. You take pictures before any tracer is administered.
   d. You can only take pictures at night.
   e. You can only take pictures in the morning.

2. What does *angiography* look at specifically?
   a. organs
   b. tissue
   c. blood vessels
   d. muscle
   e. tendons

3. What is the purpose of a radiocontrast agent?
   a. to enhance the image being filmed
   b. to soften the structure being filmed
   c. to block out of the picture any organs not being filmed
   d. to administer chemotherapy to a tumor being filmed
   e. to add more liquid volume to the body

4. What does radiocontrast specifically identify in the GI tract?
   a. outline of organs
   b. tumors or masses
   c. peristalsis
   d. edema
   e. clots

G. Alphabet soup. Use the correct letters to form the abbreviations necessary to match the definitions. Fill in the blanks with the correct abbreviation. **LO 21.9**

A   B   C   D   E   F   G   H   I   J   K   L   M   N   O   P   Q   R   S   T   U   V   W   X   Y   Z

1. This term refers to the stomach and intestines.   _____
2. This replaces film screen radiography.   _____
3. X-rays travel from an anterior source to a posterior receiver.   _____
4. This uses minimally invasive procedures.   _____
5. High-frequency sound waves are used to visualize soft tissue structures.   _____
6. This test gives the best soft tissue contrast of all the imaging modalities.   _____
7. This scan produces a computer-generated cross-sectional image in the axial plane.   _____
8. This scan will produce multiplanar images of the body.   _____

H. **All the following terms are composed of various combinations of elements.** Answer the questions, using your knowledge of the elements of the language of radiology. Fill in the blank. Not all terms will be used. **LO 21.3**

anteroposterior	opaque	fluoroscopy	posteroanterior
claustrophobia	teleradiology	coronal	tomography
ultrasound	radiopharmaceutical	oblique	

1. Which of the above terms means *impervious to light*? _____

2. Which of the above terms means *fear of closed spaces*? _____

3. Which of the above terms has an element meaning *distant*? _____

4. Which of the above terms pertains to a *vertical plane*? _____

5. Which of the above terms has an element meaning *section*? _____

6. Which of the above terms has an element meaning *drugs*? _____

I. **Build the correct medical terms by using elements from the element bank that follows (you will not use all the elements provided) to complete the terms.** **LO 21.5, 21.6, 21.7**

hypo	immune	mono	stereo	ary
brachy	fract	bi	al	mammo

1. therapy of short duration: _____ /therapy

2. larger measures of a dose of radiation given less frequently: _____ / _____ /ionation

3. protein from a single clone of cells: _____ /clon/ _____

4. record of the breast: _____ /gram

J. **Construct medical terms with your knowledge of the language of radiology.** **LO 21.5, 21.6, 21.7, 21.10**

1. Combine the R/CF *mamm/o* with various suffixes to complete the sentences below.

   graphy   **plasty**   **gram**

   The patient underwent _____ at her physician's request. After she read the _____, she recommended that the patient undergo a _____ to repair her breast.

2. Select the correct terms to complete the sentences below.

   radiographer   **radiologist**   **radiographic**   **radiographs**

   The chief _____ ordered various _____ studies to help determine the patient's diagnosis. The _____ performed the requested studies and after viewing the _____, the doctor was able to determine a diagnosis for the patient.

K. Which of the following medical terms are diagnostic, and which are therapeutic? Write D is the term is diagnostic. Write T if the term is therapeutic. **LO 21.6, 21.7**

Medical Term	D (Diagnostic) or T (Therapeutic)
brachytherapy	1.
radiotherapy	2.
hypofractionation	3.
Cyberknife	4.
mammogram	5.
angiography	6.
PET scan	7.
fluoroscopy	8.

L. In the following exercise, which statement is incorrect? Choose T if the statement is true. Choose F if the statement is false. **LO 21.2**

1. A tracer is a radioactive agent.   T   F

2. MRIs use gamma cameras.   T   F

3. Nuclear medicine uses high doses of radiation.   T   F

4. Ionizing radiation works by damaging the DNA of tissues exposed to it.   T   F

5. *Hypofractionation* refers to the dosage of radiation.   T   F

M. Choose the correct answer. **LO 21.8**

1. Which of the following pairs of terms would *not* appear in a radiology report?

    a. anterior   posterior

    b. medial   lateral

    c. coronal   caudal

    d. platelet   capillary

    e. tarsus   malleolus

N. Assign the correct term from the word bank (you will have more choices than you will need) to complete the statements. Fill in the blank. **LO 21.1, 21.2, 21.6, 21.7**

Word Bank:

intravenously	back	teleradiology	CT scan
radiocontrast agents	ultrasonography	tomogram	concurrently
sagittal	interventional	scintigraphy	front

1. Barium sulfate and iodine are _____.

2. Delineation of dynamic structures using sound waves is _____.

3. Radiocontrast agents are administered orally, rectally, and _____.

4. A radiographic image of a selected section or slice of tissue is a(n) _____.

5. Anteroposterior x-ray beams pass through the patient from _____ to _____.

6. Digitized diagnostic images transmitted from a distance are called _____.

7. A _____ produces two-dimensional imaging.

8. The term _____ means *happening together* or *at the same time.*

O. **Pronunciation is important whether you are saying the word or listening to a word from a coworker.** Identify the proper pronunciation of the following medical terms. Correctly spell the term. **LO 21.1, 21.4, 21.5, 21.7**

   1. The correct pronunciation for the process of causing an atom or group of atoms to gain or lose one or more electrons

     a. **EYE**-on-ih-**ZA**-shun   **c.** ray-dee-oh-**PAKE**

     b. **EYE**-nigh-zay-shun   **d.** **RAY**-day-oh-**PAKE**

     Correctly spell the term: _____

   2. The correct pronunciation for the process of taking a radiographic image of a selected section or slice of tissue

     a. toh-**MO**-gra-fee   **c.** **STER**-ee-oh-**TAK**-tik

     b. toh-**MOG**-rah-fee   **d.** steer-ee-oh-**TAK**-tik

     Correctly spell the term: _____

   3. The correct pronunciation for recording of radioactivity with gamma cameras

     a. **HIGH**-pro-frak-**SHUN**-ay-shun

     b. **HIGH**-poh-frak-shun-**AY**-shun

     c. sin-**TI**-gra-fee

     d. sin-**TIG**-rah-fee

     Correctly spell the term: _____

   4. The correct pronunciation for pertaining to x-rays

     a. ray-dee-oh-**GRAF**-ik

     b. **RAY**-dee-oh-graf-ik

     c. **RAY**-dee-oh-graf-ik-al

     d. **RAY**-dee-oh-**GRAY**-ict

     Correctly spell the term: _____

   5. The correct pronunciation for examination of the structures of the body by x-rays

     a. **TELL**-ur-ay-dee-oh-**LO**-jee

     b. **TEL**-eh-ray-dee-**OL**-oh-jee

     c. flow-er-**OS**-koh-pay

     d. flor-**OS**-koh-pee

     Correctly spell the term: _____

Case Reports

A. **After reading the following Case Report, correctly answer the following questions.** The answers to the questions may not be in the Case Report itself but can be found in the chapter content. **LO 21.2, 21.4, 21.6, 21.7, 21.9, 21.10**

 Case Report (CR) 21.2

You are a...

. . .Tyrone Shaw, a nuclear medicine technologist working in the nuclear medicine department at Fulwood Medical Center.

Your patient is

. . .Mr. Rodney Billington, a 59-year-old computer programmer who feels tightness in his chest during his evening walks. Dr. Oren, his cardiologist, suspects that he may have myocardial ischemia (low blood flow to his heart muscle). Because Mr. Billington was unable to complete his cardiac stress test due to ECG abnormalities, Dr. Oren has ordered a **SPECT technetium-99m** cardiac rest-stress study.

You obtain IV (intravenous) and then begin the study by injecting technetium-99m. Mr. Billington does well and does not complain of any discomfort during the study. Dr. Oren reviews the images and determines that Mr. Billington has decreased perfusion (blood flow) to his left ventricle during the stress phase of the study. She will consult Dr. Larsen, a cardiovascular surgeon, for further evaluation.

---

1. Technetium-99m is a:

   a. proton

   b. radiocontrast

   c. brachytherapy

   d. radiopharmaceutical

2. Provide the correct abbreviation for Technetium-99m: _____

3. Provide the words that SPECT stands for (one word per blank): _____

   _____   _____   _____

4. The medical specialist that oversees your department is a:

   a. radiologist.

   b. cardiologist.

   c. cardiovascular surgeon.

   d. pharmacologist.

5. Mr. Billington is concerned about the medication you administered during the study. Which of the follow statements is the best reply to his concern?

   a. "The medication will decay and be eliminated through normal renal mechanisms."

   b. "Thallium-201 is not dangerous to those around you."

   c. "The dose of technetium-99m you were given has a very low risk for causing cancer."

   d. "The study revealed that perfusion of your myocardium is impaired."

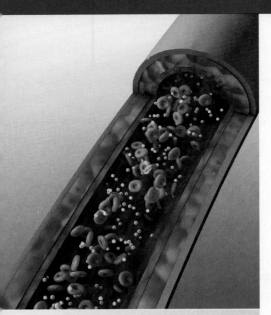

2014 Nucleus Medical Media

Pharmacology
The Language of Pharmacology

Chapter Learning Outcomes

Upon completion of this chapter, you will be able to:

LO 22.1 Recognize the differences between the chemical name, generic name, and brand name of a drug.

LO 22.2 Define the methods used for setting and referencing the standards for the effectiveness and purity of drugs used in the United States.

LO 22.3 Use roots, combining forms, suffixes, and prefixes to construct and analyze medical terms used in pharmacology.

LO 22.4 Spell medical terms related to pharmacology.

LO 22.5 Pronounce medical terms related to pharmacology.

LO 22.6 Explain the methods used to ensure safety and accuracy in drug administration by the different persons administering the drugs.

LO 22.7 Describe the different routes of administration of drugs.

LO 22.8 Apply knowledge of medical terms relating to pharmacology to documentation, medical records, and communication.

LO 22.9 Identify correct abbreviations and abbreviations that should not be used for medical terms used in pharmacology and pharmacy.

LO 22.10 Identify health professionals involved in the preparation and administration of drugs.

No matter in which health profession you are working, the following medical terms will be used frequently:

- **Pharmacology** is the study of drugs (**medications**) and their sources, preparation, chemistry, actions, and uses.
- A **pharmacologist,** usually a medical professional with an additional PhD, is a specialist who develops and tests drugs for medicinal use.
- A **pharmacist** is licensed to prepare and dispense drugs and compounds when given written orders from a physician. Pharmacists are knowledgeable about drugs' properties and are able to advise patients and practitioners about their effects and interactions.
- A **pharmacy** is a facility licensed to prepare and dispense drugs (medications) to the public.
- A **pharmacy technician** is trained to work under the supervision of a pharmacist to provide medications to patients.
- A **medication aide** is licensed by the state to assist competent individuals, caretakers, and licensed health care professionals to administer medications. They work mostly in nursing homes and assisted living facilities.

Section 22.1 Drug Names, Standards, and References

Drug Names

There are more than 3,000 drugs that can be **prescribed** by licensed practitioners. Each drug has three different names:

- The drug's **chemical** name (e.g., 8-chloro-1-methyl-6-phenyl4H-s-triazolo-benzodiazepine), which specifies the chemical makeup of the drug, is often long and complicated.
- The drug's **generic** name (e.g., alprazolam), which identifies the drug legally and scientifically; there is only one generic name for each drug.
- The drug's **brand (trade)** name (e.g., *Xanax*), which each manufacturer gives to the drug. These names are the manufacturer's private property. There can be several brand names of a particular drug, depending on how many different companies are manufacturing the drug. The brand names are always capitalized (e.g., *Xanax*).

When a drug manufacturer receives U.S. **Food and Drug Administration (FDA)** approval to sell a particular drug, it is allowed to have 20 years of protected proprietary manufacture of the drug (patent) from the date of invention, which means that no other company can manufacture and sell the same drug during that period of time. After that period of time, however, the generic name of the drug becomes public property, and any drug manufacturer can manufacture and sell the drug under that generic name.

However, if a specific brand name is ordered on a **prescription** by a physician and is designated "dispense as written," no generic or other brand name may be substituted. Generic drugs are usually cheaper than brand-name drugs because several companies are competing with one another to sell them and the generic companies have not had the initial research and development costs.

Drug Standards

Over-the-Counter (OTC) Drugs

Over-the-counter (OTC) drugs *(Figure 22.1)*, which also are called nonprescription drugs, are used to treat conditions that do not generally require care or a prescription from a health professional. Examples of these drugs include **analgesics,** such as aspirin or acetaminophen; **antihistamines,** such as chlorpheniramine, loratadine, cetirizine, fexofenadine, and some sleeping aids, such as doxylamine or diphenhydramine (Benadryl; antihistamines). In addition, herbal preparations, vitamins, minerals, and supplements are available without a prescription.

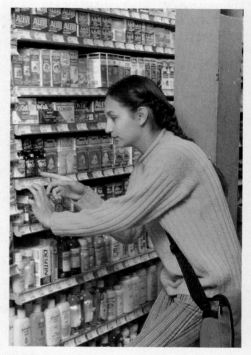

▲ **Figure 22.1** Shopping in a pharmacy for over-the-counter (OTC) medicines.
Ken Karp/McGraw Hill

S = Suffix P = Prefix R = Root R/CF = Combining Form

WORD	PRONUNCIATION	ELEMENTS		DEFINITION
antihistamine	an-tee-**HISS**-tah-meen	P/ R/ R/CF	anti- *against* -hist- *derived from histidine* -amin/e *nitrogen compound*	Drug used to treat allergic symptoms because of its action antagonistic to histamine
histamine	**HISS**-tah-meen			Compound liberated in tissues as a result of injury or an allergic response
drug	DRUG		Old English *drug*	A therapeutic agent or an addictive substance
generic	jeh-**NER**-ik	S/ R/	-ic *pertaining to* gener- *birth*	A nonproprietary name for a drug
pharmacist	**FAR**-mah-sist	S/ R/	-ist *specialist* pharmac- *drug* Greek *to administer drugs*	Person licensed by the state to prepare and dispense drugs
pharmacy	**FAR**-mah-see			Facility licensed to prepare and dispense drugs
pharmacology	far-mah-**KOL**-oh-jee	S/ R/CF	-logy *study* pharmac/o- *drug*	Science of the preparation, uses, and effects of drugs
pharmacologist	far-mah-**KOL**-oh jist	S/	-logist *specialist*	A medical specialist in pharmacology
prescribe	pree-**SKRIBE**	P/ R/	pre- *before* -scribe *write*	To give directions in writing for the preparation and administration of a remedy
prescription	pree-**SKRIP**-shun	S/ R/	-ion *process, action* -script- *writing*	A written direction for the preparation and administration of a remedy

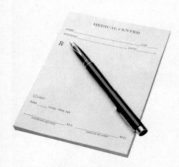

Prescription Drugs

A prescription **medication** is legally regulated, which means that a person needs a medical prescription to receive it *(Figure 22.2)*. Prescriptions can only be written by physicians, licensed medical practitioners, dentists, optometrists, veterinarians, and advanced nurse practitioners. Prescribed drugs must have a package insert detailing the intended effects of the drug and its **side effects.**

Regulating the safety and effectiveness of prescription drugs in the United States is the responsibility of the **FDA.** Another agency, the **United States Pharmacopeia (USP),** sets the standards for the quality, purity, and safety of the medications to be enforced by the FDA to protect the public health.

Controlled Substance Schedules

Certain groups of prescription drugs that are considered to have a potential for abuse are called **controlled drugs.** Regulation of these drugs is the responsibility of the U.S. Department of Justice **Drug Enforcement Administration (DEA).** These controlled substances are divided into five schedules, depending on their currently accepted medical use in treatment, their potential for abuse, and their likelihood of causing dependence.

- **Schedule I** controlled substances have a high potential for abuse and have no accepted medical use in treatment in the United States. Examples include heroin, marijuana, ecstasy, peyote and **LSD.** Drugs listed in Schedule I cannot be prescribed, federally marijuana is Schedule I, but at the time of this writing, at least 36 states have approved medical marijuana for "medically qualified" individuals. In addition, at least 17 states, as well as Washington DC, and Guam, have legalized recreational marijuana, but it is still Schedule I.
- **Schedule II** controlled substances have a high potential for abuse. Abuse of these substances may lead to severe psychological or physical dependence. Examples include some **narcotics,** such as morphine, methadone, meperidine (*Demerol*), fentanyl, hydromorphone (Dilaudid) and oxycodone (*OxyContin*); **stimulants,** such as amphetamine, methamphetamine, dextroamphetamine/amphetamine (Adderall) and methylphenidate (*Ritalin*); cocaine; and barbiturates, such as pentobarbital. Combination products with less than 15 milligrams of hydrocodone per dose (e.g., Vicodin) are now classified as Schedule II narcotics.
- **Schedule III** controlled substances have less potential for abuse than substances in Schedules I and II. Abuse of these substances may lead to moderate or low physical dependence or high psychological dependence. Examples include combination products with less than 90 milligrams of codeine per dose (e.g., acetaminophen [*Tylenol*] with codeine). Other Schedule III nonnarcotics include **anabolic steroids,** such as oxandrolone and testosterone.
- **Schedule IV** controlled substances have a lower potential for abuse than Schedule III drugs. Schedule IV substances include benzodiazepines. Examples are alprazolam (Xanax), diazepam (Valium), chlordiazepoxide (Librium); and sedative hypnotics like zolpidem (Ambien), zaleplon (Sonata), eszopiclone (Lunesta). Miscellanous analgesics such as tramadol (Ultram) and butorphanol (Stadol) are also Schedule IV.

Did you know...

- Drug Facts & Comparisons contains detailed information on individual drugs, including their intended effects, side effects, interactions, dosage, and administration. The information is updated monthly and includes both prescription and OTC products.
- A **hospital formulary** provides similar information about the medications the hospital's physicians can prescribe.
- An insurance company's formulary provides similar information about the medications it will pay for.

- **Schedule V** controlled substances have a lower potential for abuse compared to Schedule IV substances and consist primarily of preparations containing limited quantities of certain narcotics. These are generally used for **antitussive, antidiarrheal,** and **analgesic** purposes. Examples include *Robitussin AC* and *Phenergan* with codeine.

Drugs listed in Schedules II through V have accepted medical uses and therefore may be prescribed, administered, or dispensed for medical use.

Word Analysis and Definition: Prescription Drugs

S = Suffix P = Prefix R = Root R/CF = Combining Form

WORD	PRONUNCIATION	ELEMENTS		DEFINITION
anabolic steroid	an-a-**BOL**-ik **STER**-oyd	S/ R/ S/ R/	**-ic** *pertaining to* **anabol-** *to raise up* **-oid** *resemble* **ster-** *solid*	Prescription drug abused by some athletes to increase muscle mass
analgesic	an-al-**JEE**-zik	S/ P/ R/	**-ic** *pertaining to* **an-** *without* **-alges-** *sensation of pain*	Substance that produces a reduction in the sensation of pain
antitussive	an-tee-**TUS**-iv	S/ P/ R/	**-ive** *nature of, quality of* **anti-** *against* **-tuss-** *cough*	A cough remedy
control	kon-**TROLE**		Latin *to check an account*	To regulate, correct
formulary	**FORM**-you-lair-ee	S/ R/	**-ary** *pertaining to* **formul-** *form*	An official list of drugs approved for use by health-systems, managed care, or group of physicians
medication	med-ih-**KAY**-shun	R/ S/	**medic-** *physician* **-ation** *healing*	A substance having curative properties
narcotic	nar-**KOT**-ik	S/ R/CF	**-tic** *pertaining to* **narc/o-** *sleep, stupor*	Drug derived from opium, or a synthetic drug with similar effects
side effect	SIDE ee-**fekt**		**side** Old English *side* **effect** Old English *result*	An undesirable result of drug or other therapy
stimulant	**STIM**-you-lant	S/ R/	**-ant** *agent* **stimul-** *excite*	Agent that excites or strengthens functional activity

Check Point Section 22.1

A. The differences between the chemical name, generic name, and brand name of a drug. *Match the name in the first column with its correct definition in the second column.* **LO 22.1**

_____ 1. chemical name

_____ 2. brand name

_____ 3. generic name

a. identifies the drug legally and scientifically

b. specifies the chemical makeup of the drug

c. name of the drug given by the manufacturer

B. Identify the different names given to the one drug. *All of the following names are applied to the same drug. Identify its name type by choosing the correct answer.* **LO 22.1**

1. diphenhydramine

   a. chemical name   b. brand name   c. generic name

2. 2-(diphenylmethoxy)-*N,N*-dimethylethanamine

   a. chemical name   b. brand name   c. generic name

3. *Benadryl*

   a. chemical name   b. brand name   c. generic name

C. Use the words of the language of pharmacology in context. *Use the terms from the provided word bank to complete the sentences. Not all terms will be used. Fill in the blanks.* **LO 22.2, 22.3, 22.9**

| USP | FDA | DEA | narcotic | antitussive | analgesic | I | II | IV | V |

Mr. Hatfield arrives to the clinic complaining of a cough that occurs frequently. The physician prescribed a(n) _____ **(1)** to control the coughing episodes. The medication contains a(n) _____ **(2)**. Because of this, the _____ **(3)** regulates the drug. Generally speaking, this type of drug is usually a Schedule _____ **(4)** drug.

D. Create words using the correct root/combining form. *Construct medical terms related to pharmacology using the correct root/combining form.* *Fill in the blank.* **LO 22.2, 22.3**

1. Agent that excites or strengthens functional activity: _____ /ant

2. A cough remedy: anti/ _____ /ive

3. Official list of drugs approved for use in a health-system: _____ /ary

4. Agent that reduces the sensation of pain: an/_____ /ic

5. A medication that treats pain but also induces sleep: _____ /ic

Section 22.2 The Administration of Drugs

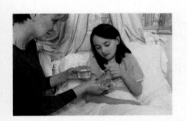

▲ **Figure 22.3 Mother gives medication.** Image Source/Alamy Stock Photo

Routes of Administration

A route of administration in pharmacology and toxicology is the path by which a drug or other substance is taken into the body. Routes of administration are usually classified according to the location on the body to which the drug is applied. The routes of administration distinguish whether a drug's effect is local (as in topical) or systemic (as in enteral or parenteral administration).

The bioavailability of a drug reveals what proportion of the drug reaches the systemic blood circulation and is available to reach the intended site(s) of action. A drug's route of administration (e.g., oral or intravenous [IV]) and its formulation (e.g., tablet, capsule, or liquid) clearly influence its bioavailability.

The path that a drug takes from the point of its application to reach the tissue where its effect is targeted is part of pharmacokinetics—the absorption, distribution, metabolism, and elimination of drugs. A drug's interaction at its target site(s) of action is called pharmacodynamics.

Enteral Administration

Enteral administration is through the gastrointestinal **(GI)** tract. **Oral** is the most frequently used, convenient, and economical method of drug administration *(Figure 22.3)*. However, absorption of a drug by this route is affected by the unpredictable nature of the GI tract. For example, by affecting the gastric motility and emptying time, the presence of food influences the rate and extent of drug absorption. Solid-dose forms such as tablets and capsules have a high degree of drug stability and provide accurate dosage. The use of liquids and soluble preparations is less reliable. Modified-release preparations aim to maintain plasma drug concentrations for extended periods. If they are chewed or crushed, the full dose is released immediately, leading to **toxicity.**

The **sublingual** and **buccal** routes provide a rich supply of blood vessels through which drugs can be directly absorbed into the systemic circulation. Wafer-based versions of drugs, such as glyceryl trinitrate in the treatment of acute angina pectoris *(see Chapter 10),* placed under the tongue give rapid responses to their effects.

Rectal administration in the form of **suppositories** or **enemas** is popular in some European countries but is not easily accepted by patients in America. **Antiemetics** can be administered rectally for nausea and vomiting.

Topical Administration

Topical administration allows a drug to be available directly at the site of action without going through the systemic circulation. For example, topical applications include steroid ointments for treating dermatitis *(Chapter 4)*, beta blocker eye drops for treating glaucoma *(Chapter 16)*, nasal medications instilled via drops or a spray, bronchodilators that are inhaled to treat asthma *(Chapter 13)*, and **pessaries** or creams containing clotrimazole *(Lotrimin, Mycelex)* that are inserted to treat vaginal candidiasis *(Chapter 8)*. Thus, *topical* refers to more than just application on the skin.

Drugs also can be administered into the systemic circulation through the skin. Adhesive **transdermal** patches can contain drugs that migrate across the epidermis into the blood vessel–rich dermis, where they are absorbed into the systemic circulation. Medications for motion sickness, cardiac problems, birth control, and the chemicals testosterone and nicotine are administered by transdermal patches.

WORD	PRONUNCIATION	ELEMENTS		DEFINITION
antiemetic	**AN**-tee-eh-**MET**-ik	S/ P/ R/	**-tic** pertaining to **anti-** against **-eme-** to vomit	A medication that helps to control nausea and vomiting
bioavailability	**BIE**-oh-ah-**VALE**-ah-**BIL**-ih-tee	S/ R/CF R/	**-ity** condition, state **bi/o-** life **-availabil-** to be worth	The amount of a drug that reaches the systemic circulation and is available to reach the intended site of action
buccal	**BUK**-al	S/ R/	**-al** pertaining to **bucc-** cheek	Inside the cheek—a site for the administration of certain medications
enema	**EN**-eh-mah		Greek injection	An injection of fluid into the rectum
enteral	**EN**-ter-al	S/ R/	**-al** pertaining to **enter-** intestine	Administration of medications by way of the GI tract
formulation	**FORM**-you-**LAY**-shun	S/ R/	**-ation** process **formul-** form	The form in which a drug is presented—tablet, capsule, liquid, etc.
oral	**OR**-al	S/ R/	**-al** pertaining to **or-** mouth	Pertaining to the mouth
pessary	**PES**-ah-ree		Greek an oval stone	Appliance inserted into the vagina
pharmacodynamics	**FAR**-mah-coh-die-**NAM**-iks	S/ R/CF R/	**-ics** pertaining to **pharmac/o-** drug **-dynam-** force	The uptake and action of drugs at their tissue site(s) of action
pharmacokinetics	**FAR**-mah-coh-ki-**NET**-iks	S/ R/CF R/	**-ics** pertaining to **pharmac/o-** drug **-kinet-** moving	The movement of drugs within the body affecting absorption, distribution, metabolism, and excretion
rectal	**REK**-tal	S/ R/	**-al** pertaining to **rect-** rectum	Pertaining to the rectum
sublingual	sub-**LING**-wal	S/ P/ R/	**-al** pertaining to **sub-** underneath **-lingu-** tongue	Underneath the tongue
suppository	suh-**PAH**-zih-tor-ee		Latin placed underneath	A small solid body containing medication that is placed in a body orifice other than the mouth to release the medication
topical	**TOP**-ih-kal	S/ R/	**-al** pertaining to **topic-** local	Medication applied to a local area
toxin	**TOK**-sin		Greek poison	Poisonous substance formed by a cell or organism
toxicity	tok-**SIS**-ih-tee	S/ S/ R/	**-ity** state, condition **-ic-** pertaining to **tox-** poison	The state of being poisonous
toxicology	tok-sih-**KOL**-oh-jee	S/ R/CF	**-logy** study of **toxic/o-** poison	The science of poisons, including their source, chemistry, actions, and antidotes
transdermal	trans-**DER**-mal	S/ P/ R/	**-al** pertaining to **trans-** across, through **-derm-** skin	Going across or through the skin

Parenteral Administration

Parenteral administration, which literally means *not through the GI tract,* is the injection of a drug directly into the body that bypasses the skin and mucous membranes.

The common routes of parenteral administration are:

- **intramuscular (IM)** *(Figure 22.4a)*
- **intravenous (IV)** *(Figure 22.4b)*
- **subcutaneous (SC)**

Less common routes include:

- **intradermal (ID)**
- **intrathecal** *(Figure 22.4c)*

Intramuscular and **subcutaneous injections** establish a "depot" for a drug that is released gradually, depending on the drug's formulation, into the systemic circulation. For example, oil-based medications are released more slowly than water based. An IM injection of *Depo-Provera,* a birth control drug, works steadily for a 3-month period. The **intradermal** route for medications is rarely used.

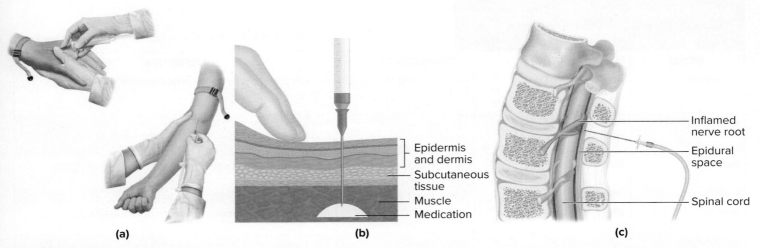

				Epidermis and dermis
				Subcutaneous tissue
				Muscle
				Medication

				Inflamed nerve root
				Epidural space
				Spinal cord

(a) (b) (c)

▲ **Figure 22.4** **Routes for parenteral administration.** (a) Inserting an intravenous (IV) cannula, (b) IM injection, and (c) intrathecal injection.

Intravenous injections enable a drug to reach its sites of action within seconds. An IV **infusion** also can deliver continuous medication—for example, morphine to patients in continuous pain or a saline drip for people needing fluids. The medications also can be given in a small solution through a **port** in intravenous tubing (**bolus**), or attached in smaller infusion containers to a larger infusion (piggyback).

Disadvantages of IV injections or infusions include the fact that patients are not typically able to self-administer them and the fact that, because it bypasses most of the body's natural defenses, IV is the most dangerous route of administration. Also, the preparation and administration of IV drugs require the use of **aseptic** techniques. Careful training is necessary to achieve competence in the administration of IV medications.

Intrathecal injections are given into the subarachnoid space surrounding the spinal cord in the spinal canal *(see Chapter 9)*. An epidural block, which is an injection of a local anesthetic agent into the epidural space *(Figure 22.4c)*, is used often for pain management during labor *(see Chapter 8)* and occasionally for chemotherapy. An intrathecal injection's primary advantage is that the drug avoids the blood–brain barrier (BBB; *see Chapter 9*).

Methods to ensure accuracy and safety in the administration of drugs are described in the next lesson of this chapter.

Word Analysis and Definition: Routes of Administration

S = Suffix P = Prefix R = Root R/CF = Combining Form

WORD	PRONUNCIATION	ELEMENTS		DEFINITION
aseptic (adj) (**Note:** The final "s" of the root is not used to allow the pronunciation to flow)	ay-**SEP**-tik	S/ P/ R/	-tic *pertaining to* a- *without* -seps- *decay*	Pertaining to the absence of living organisms
bolus	**BOH**-lus		Greek *a lump*	Single mass of a substance
infusion	in-**FYU**-zhun	P/ R/	in- *in* -fusion *to pour*	Introduction intravenously of a substance other than blood
injection	in-**JEK**-shun	R/	-jection *to throw*	Introduction of a medical substance parenterally
intradermal (adj)	**IN**-trah-**DER**-mal	S/ P/ R/	-al *pertaining to* intra- *within* -derm- *skin*	Within the dermis
intramuscular (adj)	**IN**-trah-**MUS**-kew-lar	S/ R/	-ar *pertaining to* -muscul- *muscle*	Within the muscle
intrathecal (adj)	**IN**-trah-**THEE**-kal	R/	-thec- *sheath*	Within the subarachnoid or subdural space
intravenous (adj)	**IN**-trah-**VEE**-nus	S/ R/	-ous *pertaining to* -ven- *vein*	Inside a vein
parenteral	pah-**REN**-ter-al	S/ P/ R/	-al *pertaining to* par- *abnormal, beside* -enter- *intestine*	Administering medication by any means other than the GI tract
port	PORT		Latin *gate*	A point of entry into an IV system
subcutaneous (adj)	sub-kew-**TAY**-nee-us	S/ P/ R/	-ous *pertaining to* sub- *below* -cutane- *skin*	Below the skin
hypodermic (syn)	high-poh-**DER**-mik			

A. Differentiate the different routes of administration of drugs. *Match the route of administration in the first column with its correct definition in the second column.* **LO 22.7**

_____ 1. *rectal*	a. applied to a local area
_____ 2. *sublingual*	b. inside the cheek
_____ 3. *oral*	c. medication given via the GI tract
_____ 4. *transdermal*	d. under the tongue
_____ 5. *buccal*	e. pertaining to the mouth
_____ 6. *topical*	f. going across the skin
_____ 7. *enteral*	g. pertaining to the rectum

B. Use the correct abbreviation for the described procedure. *Abbreviations are commonly used when communicating verbally and in writing. Use the correct abbreviation for the words written in italics.* **LO 22.7, 22.8**

1. The injection was *given into the muscles* of the buttocks. _____

2. The nurse practitioner ordered that the medication be given *under the subcutaneous tissue.* _____

3. The allergy test involves placing an allergen *within the skin.* _____

4. Give the patient his medication *via his vein.* _____

C. The definitions of the terms are given to you. *Write the correct terms on the lines.* **LO 22.7**

1. absence of living organisms: _____

2. within the dermis: _____

3. point of entry into an IV system: _____

4. same as hypodermic: _____

5. single mass of a substance: _____

Section 22.3 Accuracy and Safety in Drug Administration

Self-Administration of Medications in the Elderly

The most common route of administration of medications is the self-administered oral route. Eighty-nine percent of adults older than 65 are on at least one prescription medications, with 54% of them taking four or more prescription drugs and 90% of them also taking over-the-counter (OTC) drugs. In a recent study published in early 2021, 95% of adults 65 and older were prescribed a drug with a risk for causing falls. According to the Centers for Disease Control, nearly $50 billion is spent on medical costs related to fall injuries among older adults. Even minor falls are dangerous for older adults. Falls that do not lead to fatalities can still cause severe injuries like hip fractures and head trauma, that can significantly impair a patient's quality of life. A drug-induced fall is considered an **adverse effect (AE).** Adverse effects are harmful and undesired effects secondary to the main or therapeutic effect of the medication. Research also has found that **adverse drug reactions (ADR)** caused by intolerance,

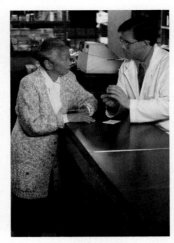

▲ **Figure 22.5** Pharmacist consults with elderly patient.
Keith Brofsky/Getty Images

susceptibility, or interaction with another drug occurred in the hospitalization of some 35% of patients. In addition to hospitalization, severe adverse drug reactions can result in death or permanent **impairment** of physical activities and/or quality of life. ADRs result in four times as many hospitalizations in older, versus younger, adults. Prescribing cascades (using a drug/s to treat another drug/s side effects), drug-drug interactions, and inappropriate drug doses are causes of preventable ADRs. Lists of inappropriate drugs/doses to use in elderly patients have been developed, and are used by clinicians, including geriatric pharmacists (*Figure 22.5*) and geriatric physicians, and other healthcare professionals, when caring for elderly patients. One common tool/list is the Beers criteria.

Opioids such as morphine and codeine are naturally derived from opium poppy plants. Hydrocodone (*Vicodin*) and oxycodone (*Percocet*) are manufactured semi-synthetic opioids. In 2019, nearly 50,000 people in the United States died from opioid-involved overdoses and that same number of people tried heroin for the first time. An additional 1.6 million people misused prescription pain relievers for the first time. Fentanyl is a fully synthetic opioid, 100 times more powerful than morphine. Methadone is another fully synthetic opioid. Heroin is an illegal drug synthesized from morphine and caused 14,996 deaths in 2018. There were five deaths for every 100,000 people. The number of heroin-involved overdoses was seven times greater in 2018 than in 1999. Nearly one-third of all opioid deaths involve heroin.

Naloxone (*Narcan*) blocks the effects of opioids, particularly in overdose. Given IV, it works within 2 minutes, IM within 5 minutes. Sprayed into the nose, the effect is variable. Intranasal naloxone is commonly used outside healthcare facilities (e.g., given to family members for use at home, outdoors, on the street) to reverse opioid/narcotic effects when an emergency department is not nearby. Intranasal naloxone is to be given immediately when a suspected or known opioid overdose has occurred. Emergency assistance (911) should be called immediately after administration of the first dose.

Word Analysis and Definition: Self-Administration of Medications

S = Suffix P = Prefix R = Root R/CF = Combining Form

WORD	PRONUNCIATION	ELEMENTS		DEFINITION
adverse	**AD**-vers	P/ R/	ad- *toward* -verse *turned*	Noxious, unintended, undesired
impairment	im-**PAIR**-ment	S/ R/	-ment *action, state* impair- *worsen*	Diminishing of normal function
interaction	in-ter-**AK**-shun	P/ R/	inter- *between* -action *to do*	The action between two entities to produce or prevent an effect
opioid	**OH**-pee-oyd		Latin *bringing sleep*	A narcotic substance, either natural or synthetic.
reaction	ree-**AK**-shun	P/ R/	re- *again, backward* -action *to do*	The response of a living tissue or organism to a stimulus
synergist	**SIN**-er-jist	S/ P/ R/	-ist *specialist* syn- *together* -erg- *work*	Agent or process that aids the actions of another
synergism	**SIN**-er-jism	S/	-ism *condition, process*	Coordinated action of two or more agents or processes so that the combined action is greater than that of each acting separately
synergistic (adj)	sin-er-**JIS**-tik	S/	-ic *pertaining to*	Pertaining to synergism
tranquilizer	**TRANG**-kwih-lie-zer	S/ R/	-izer *affects in a particular way* tranquil- *calm, serene*	Agent that calms without sedating or depressing

Caregiver Administration of Medications

Five Rights

Before a caregiver administers a drug (medication) to a patient by any route, five factors should be addressed by the caregiver (*Figure 22.6*).

- **Right patient**
  - Identify the patient by a bracelet or name badge. Asking the patient's name can lead to confusion, particularly in the assisted living environment.
- **Right drug**
  - Check the medication record for the name of the drug and compare with the drug in hand at three points:
    1. When taking hold of the package that contains the drug.
    2. When opening the package.
    3. When returning the package to storage.
- **Right route**
  - Check the medication record for how to administer the drug and check the labeling of the drug to make sure it matches the prescribed route.
- **Right dose**
  - Check that the medication record orders the same **dose** as that in hand.
- **Right time**
  - Check that the time ordered or the frequency matches the current time.

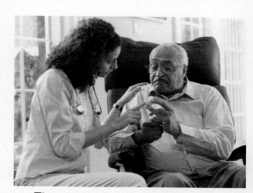

▲ **Figure 22.6** Patient is shown how to check a medication label. Fuse/Getty Images

In addition, the caregiver must actually watch the patient take the medication. Caregivers should not leave medications unattended and should ensure that the medication does not come into contact with any potentially **contaminated** surface or object.

Documentation of having given medication is a vital responsibility of the caregiver. Medication errors must be documented, and should clearly state if it was one or more of the **Five Wrongs**—namely the **wrong patient,** the **wrong drug,** the **wrong route,** the **wrong dose,** or the **wrong time.**

Abbreviations that should not be used

The Institute for Safe Medication Practices (ISMP) is a nonprofit organization devoted entirely to preventing medication errors. Throughout their 25-year existence the ISMP has helped make a difference in the lives of millions of patients and healthcare professionals who care for patients. The ISMP produces a list of "error-prone" abbreviations, symbols, and dose designations that have been misinterpreted and involved in harmful or potentially harmful medication errors. These abbreviations, symbols, and dose designations should NEVER be used when communicating medical information verbally, electronically, and/or in handwritten applications. This list has been adopted by health-systems and is used in the accreditation process of U.S. hospitals. This list is known as the "Do Not Use" list because these abbreviations can be misinterpreted for another meaning. Some of the more common abbreviations on this list are: IU (International Units), U (units), Q.D., QD, q.d., or qd (mistaken as daily or four times daily rather than once a day); Q.O.D., QOD, q.o.d., or qod (mistaken as daily or four times daily rather than every other day); and o.d. or OD (daily mistaken as right eye, leading to oral liquid medications administered in the eye).

Self-Administration of Drugs

For a patient at home administering his/her own medications, usually orally, the Five Rights also apply at the time of administration:

- **Right patient:** The patient should make sure that the container or package holding the medication has his or her name on it.
- **Right drug:** The patient should check his or her own medication record to ensure that the medication has been prescribed and stored correctly.
- **Right route:** The patient should check whether the medication should be swallowed whole as a **capsule** or **tablet,** or taken as directed if a liquid.
- **Right dose:** The patient should check with his or her medication record and the label on the package that the number of tablets or capsules or the amount of liquid is correct.
- **Right time:** The patient should check his or her medication record and the label on the package to ensure that the medication is being taken at the right time.

Documentation of the administration of all drugs as part of the patient's medical record should be encouraged, particularly among the elderly.

Self-Administration of Insulin

Some 34.2 million people in the United States have been diagnosed with **diabetes.** There are 7.4 million diabetics who self-administer insulin into their subcutaneous tissue either by **syringe, pen injection,** high-pressure jet injection, or subcutaneous infusion pumps *(Figure 22.7).* Inhalation of an insulin powder (*Afrezza* inhalation powder) is also available but not yet widely used. It is essential that the right dose of the right drug (i.e., the right type of insulin *[see Chapter 17]*) is given in response to the patient's blood sugar level.

The different drugs used in each body system are described in the appropriate chapter.

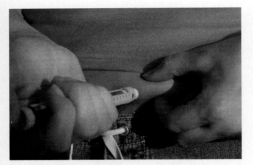

▲ **Figure 22.7** **Injecting insulin using a pen device.** Insulin pens are pen-like devices that allow diabetics to give themselves insulin injections without using vials and syringes. Mark Harmel/ Science Source

Word Analysis and Definition: Self-Administration of Drugs

S = Suffix P = Prefix R = Root R/CF = Combining Form

WORD	PRONUNCIATION	ELEMENTS		DEFINITION
capsule	**KAP**-syul	S/ R/	-ule *little* caps- *box*	A solid dosage form in which a drug is enclosed in a hard or soft shell
document (verb)	**DOK**-you-ment	S/ R/	-ment *resulting state, action* docu- *to teach*	To provide written proof
documentation (noun)	**DOK**-you-men-**TAY**-shun	S/	-ation *process*	The process of providing written proof
dose	DOHS		Greek *a giving*	The quantity of a drug to be taken at one time
syringe	si-**RINJ**		Greek *pipe* or *tube*	An instrument used for injecting or withdrawing fluids
tablet	**TAB**-let		Latin *small table*	A solid, flattish dosage form containing medication

Check Point Section 22.3

A. Table search and find. *The elements are given in the first column. Fill in the answers to the element questions in columns 2 and 3.* **LO 22.3**

Name of Element	Identity of Element (Prefix, Root, Combining Form, Suffix)	Meaning of Element
syn	1.	2.
impair	3.	4.
erg	5.	6.
ic	7.	8.
ist	9.	10.

B. Which of the following statements is true? *Choose T if the statement is true. Choose F if the statement is false.* **LO 22.6**

1. A synergist is a medical professional.   T   F

2. A tranquilizer will make you sleep.   T   F

3. A reaction is a response to a stimulus.   T   F

4. An impairment is the inability to sleep.   T   F

5. An interaction involves at least five entities.   T   F

C. Match the form of the medication with the route by which it is given. *The form of a drug is specific to the route by which it is to be given. Given the medication, choose the correct route by which it is to be given.* **LO 22.6**

1. tablet
   - **a.** rectal
   - **b.** topical
   - **c.** oral
   - **d.** intravenous

2. ointment
   - **a.** rectal
   - **b.** topical
   - **c.** oral
   - **d.** intravenous

3. capsule
   - **a.** rectal
   - **b.** topical
   - **c.** oral
   - **d.** intravenous

4. syringe with attached needle
   - **a.** rectal
   - **b.** topical
   - **c.** oral
   - **d.** intravenous

5. suppository
   - **a.** rectal
   - **b.** topical
   - **c.** oral
   - **d.** intravenous

Table 22.1 "Do not use" list of abbreviations

Do not Use	Issue with use	Use Instead
U, u (unit)	Mistaken for "O" (zero), the number "4" (four) or "cc"	Write "unit"
IU (International Unit)	Mistaken for IV (intravenous) or the number 10 (ten)	Write "International Unit"
Q.D., QD, q.d., qd (daily)	Mistaken for each other	Write "daily"
Q.O.D., QOD, q.o.d, qod (every other day)	Period after the Q mistaken for "I" and the "O" mistaken for "I	Write "every other day"
Trailing Zero (X.0 mg)* Lack of leading zero (.X mg)	Decimal point is missed	Write X mg Write 0.X mg
MS MSO4 and MgSO4	Can mean morphine sulfate or magnesium sulfate Confused for one another	Write "morphine sulfate" or "magnesium sulfate"

*Exception: A "trailing zero" may be used only where required to demonstrate the level of precision of the value being reported, such as for laboratory results, imaging studies that report size of lesions, or catheter/tube sizes. It may not be used in medication orders or other medication-related documentation.

Table 22.2 Chapter 22 Abbreviations

Abbreviations	Meaning
a.c.	before meals
ADR	adverse drug reaction
AE	adverse effect
b.i.d.	twice each day
CDC	Centers for Disease Control and Prevention
CNS	central nervous system
DEA	U.S. Drug Enforcement Agency
FDA	U.S. Food and Drug Administration
GI	gastrointestinal
h.s.	at bedtime
ID	intradermal
IM	intramuscular
IV	intravenous
LSD	lysergic acid diethylamide
OTC	over the counter
p.c.	after meals
PCP	primary care physician
p.o.	by mouth
pr	per rectum
p.r.n.	when necessary
Rx	prescribe
SC	subcutaneous
STAT	immediately
t.i.d	three times each day
USP	United States Pharmacopeia

Challenge Your Knowledge

A.   Abbreviations are an important part of clinical documentation. Make sure you know what they mean. Insert the correct abbreviation in the appropriate space. **LO 22.7, 22.8, 22.9**

a.c.   b.i.d.   t.i.d.   q.i.d.   on   p.o.   p.r.n.   GI   IM   p.c.   q.d.   h.s.

1. Mr. Baker's doctor has told you to administer his medication _____ (before meals).

2. The medicine prescribed by the doctor will help Mr. Baker's _____ (gastrointestinal) problem.

3. This medication is to be given to the patient _____ (at night).

4. The patient needs the medication _____ (three times each day).

5. Because her coughing is improving, the patient only needs the medication _____ (when necessary).

6. This medicine should be given _____ (after meals); otherwise, it will upset the patient's stomach.

7. Administer this medication for the patient by _____ (intramuscular) injection.

8. The prescription was written to be taken _____ (twice a day) _____ (by mouth).

9. Do not confuse _____ (daily) with _____ (four times each day).

B.   What is the purpose of a port? Choose the correct answer. LO 22.7

1. to divert fluids away from the site

2. to provide an entry site for IV fluids

3. to separate veins and arteries

4. to speed the process of blood circulation

5. to help prevent clots

C.   Deconstruction. Deconstruction of medical terms is a tool for analyzing the meaning. In the following chart, you are given a medical term. Deconstruct the term into its prefix, root (or combining form), and suffix. Write the element and its meaning in the appropriate column and the meaning of the term in the last column. If the term does not have a word element, write n/a. *The first one is done for you.* **LO 22.3**

Medical Term	Prefix	Meaning of Prefix	Root/Combining Form	Meaning of Root/Combining Form	Suffix	Meaning of Suffix	Meaning of Term
syngerism	*syn-*	together	*-erg-*	work	*-ism*	process	Coordinated action of two agents so that the combined action is greater than that of each acting separately
subcutaneous	1.	2.	3.	4.	5.	6.	7.
prescription	8.	9.	10.	11.	12.	13.	14.
interaction	15.	16.	17.	18.	19.	20.	21.
tranquilizer	22.	23.	24.	25.	26.	27.	28.
antitussive	29.	30.	31.	32.	33.	34.	35.

D. Who are the only health care personnel currently licensed to write prescriptions in most states? Choose Yes if the particular health care professional can prescribe medications; choose No if they cannot. **LO 22.2, 22.10**

1. dentist

   a. Yes

   b. No

2. pharmacist

   a. Yes

   b. No

3. nurse practitioner

   a. Yes

   b. No

4. optometrist

   a. Yes

   b. No

5. registered nurse

   a. Yes

   b. No

6. physical therapist

   a. Yes

   b. No

7. doctor of osteopathy

   a. Yes

   b. No

8. pediatrician

   a. Yes

   b. No

9. obstetrician

   a. Yes

   b. No

10. physician assistant

    a. Yes

    b. No

E. One element changes the meaning of medical terms. *Many medical terms are similar, with one element making the difference between terms. Given the definition, complete each term with the correct element.* **LO 22.3, 22.7, 22.10**

1. Specialist that is licensed to dispense and prepare medications: pharmac _____

2. The study of the preparation, uses, and effects of drugs: pharmac _____

3. Specialist in the study of the science of the preparation, uses, and effects of drugs: pharmac _____

4. Substance given into the skin: intra _____al

5. Substance given into the subarachnoid space: intra _____al

6. The movement of drugs within the body: pharmaco _____ics

7. The uptake of drugs at the site(s) of action: pharmaco _____ics

F. Fill in the blanks with the correct abbreviations. LO 22.9

1. by mouth _____

2. medication (drug) information in this reference _____

3. federal government agency that sets standards for drug quality, purity, and safety _____

4. when necessary _____

5. medication that does not need a prescription _____

G. Practice the language of pharmacology. Choose the correct answer that answers each question. **LO 22.1–22.10**

1. The path by which a drug or other substance is taken into the body is called:

   a. bioavailability

   b. digestion

   c. absorption

   d. a route of administration

   e. biokinetics

2. The method by which a medication is prepared for administration is called its:

   a. formulation

   b. route

   c. pharmacokinetics

   d. prescription

3. What would an ENT physician prescribe for a patient with a heavy cough?

   a. antiemetic

   b. antihistamine

   c. antitussive

   d. anticoagulant

   e. antidepressant

4. Which of the following does *not* refer to a drug name?

   a. chemical

   b. generic

   c. brand

   d. trade

   e. popular

5. Which U.S. agency sets the standards for the quality, purity, and safety of medications?

   a. USP

   b. USPS

   c. CDC

   d. BATF

   e. AAP

6. The physician wrote for the medication to be placed in the buccal cavity. You would instruct the patient to place it:

   a. under the tongue

   b. in the nose

   c. between the cheek and gum

   d. in the eye

7. You are online researching antibiotics. The following medication is listed as: metronidazole, *Flagyl,* 2-Methyl-5-nitroimidazole-1-ethanol. *Flagyl* is the:

   a. chemical name

   b. brand name

   c. generic name

8. A prescription medication that has a high potential for abuse would be classified as Schedule:

   a. I

   b. II

   c. III

   d. IV

   e. V

9. The federal agency that monitors prescriptions written by physicians:

   a. USP

   b. DEA

   c. FBI

   d. PDR

10. A professional that dispenses medication under the supervision of a pharmacist:

   a. occupational therapist

   b. pharmacologist

   c. medication aide

   d. pharmacy technician

H. **Identify the different routes of drug administration.** Choose from the following terms the correct route of administration. Fill in the blanks. You will not use all the choices. **LO 22.4**

enteral   oral   rectal   buccal   sublingual   transdermal   intravenous

1. You have placed a patch containing pain medicine on the skin of your patient's back. Which route of administration

   is that? _____

2. Mr. Matthews has to put his medicine under his tongue. Which route of administration is that? _____

3. Dr. Philips has ordered a suppository for Mrs. Johnson. Which route of administration is that? _____

4. Dr. Mallard prescribed pain pills for Mr. Cosmos. Which route of administration is that? _____

I. **Identify abbreviations used to describe drugs, their routes of administration, and their timing.** Match the abbreviation to the correct statement. **LO 22.9**

_____ 1. p.r.n.   a. intramuscular

_____ 2. t.i.d.   b. by mouth

_____ 3. b.i.d.   c. when necessary

_____ 4. IM   d. twice each day

_____ 5. p.o.   e. three times each day

Case Reports

A. **After reading the following Case Report, correctly answer the following questions.** The answers to the questions may not be in the Case Report itself but can be found in the chapter content. **LO 22.4, 22.7, 22.8, 22.9**

Case Report (CR) 22.1

You are

. . . a pharmacist in the pharmacy at Fulwood Medical Center. Your patient has been sent to you by Susan Lee, MD, a primary care physician at Fulwood Medical Center.

Your patient is

. . . Mrs. Rebecca Borodin, a frail 80-year-old widow living in an assisted living facility. She has recently begun to complain that she has difficulty recognizing and naming her fellow residents and knowing when to go to the facility's dining room for meals. In addition, it has been hard for her to eat because she suffers from dry mouth and difficulty in swallowing. She also has complained of dizziness and problems with balance; recently, she fell as a result of these problems. Her past medical history includes osteoarthritis, osteopenia, hypertension, congestive heart failure, persistent pain following herpes zoster, and stress incontinence.

Mrs. Borodin has brought in a bag containing all her medications, which include famotidine, acetaminophen with codeine *(Tylenol #3)*, oxybutynin, digoxin, atenolol, alprazolam, zolpidem *(Ambien)*, and naproxen. In addition, she takes an OTC multivitamin and melatonin.

Dr. Lee has asked you to make sure that Mrs. Borodin knows what each of the medications is for and when to take it. She also has asked you to review the drugs themselves to see if any of them could be causing her recent symptoms.

Review her medications, see if they have side effects, make sure that knows what they are what are for.

All the drugs that Mrs. Borodin has brought in for your inspection are administered orally.

Her medications, and their times of administration, include famotidine 200 mg **b.i.d.**; *Tylenol #3* when necessary **p.r.n.** for pain; oxybutinin 5 mg **t.i.d.**; digoxin 0.25 mg twice each day **b.i.d.**; atenolol **100 mg h.s.**; alprazolam 0.5 mg **b.i.d.**; *Ambien* 5 mg **h.s.**; and naproxen 500 mg **b.i.d.** In addition, she takes an OTC multivitamin daily, and melatonin 1 mg **h.s.**

1. Which of the medications is classified as a Schedule IV drug?

   a. naproxen

   b. famotidine

   c. digoxin

   d. alprazolam

2. What condition does zolpidem treat?

   a. insomnia

   b. depression

   c. stress incontinence

   d. osteoarthritis

3. List the medications that do not require a prescription: _____

4. List the medications that are scheduled drugs: _____

5. The route of delivery for these medications is:

   a. parenteral.

   b. enteral.

   c. subcutaneous.

   d. intrathecal.

6. Mrs. Borodin takes acetaminophen with codeine *(Tylenol #3)*. The trade name of this medication is:

   a. acetaminophen only

   b. codeine only

   c. acetaminophen and codeine

   d. *Tylenol #i3* only

7. The purpose of your meeting with Mrs. Borodin is to determine her:

   _____

8. Provide the three words that OTC stands for. _____ _____ _____

9. You talk to Mrs. Borodin to make sure she takes atenolol:

   a. in the morning.

   b. at night.

   c. as needed.

   d. twice a day.

   e. three times a day.

10. How many times a day is she to take famotidine medication?

    f. as needed

    g. once

    h. twice

    i. three

    j. four

11. Which medication is to be taken three times a day?

    k. *Tylenol #3*

    l. naproxen 500

    m. oxybutnin

    n. multivitamin

Appendices

Word Parts

Note: For easy identification, the word parts in this appendix appear in the same colors as they do in the Word Analysis and Definition boxes: suffix, prefix, root, root/combining form. Any term that is used in the text in both root and combining form is shown in this appendix only as a combining form. Sometimes the same element (for example, "ac") can function in different parts of the medical term.

WORD PART	DEFINITION
a-	not, without, into
ab-	away from
abdomin/o	abdomen
ability	competence
ablat	take away
-able	capable of
abort	fail at onset
absorpt	to swallow, take in
ac-	toward
-ac	pertaining to
-acea	condition, remedy
acetyl	acetyl
acid/o	acid, low pH
acin	grape
acous	hearing
acr/o	peak, extremity, highest point
acromi/o	acromion
act	to do, perform, performance
actin	ray
activ/e	movement
acumin	to sharpen
ad-	to, toward, near, into
adapt	to adjust
-ade	process
aden/o	gland
adip	fat
adjust	alter
adjuv	give help
adnex	connected parts
adolesc	beginning of adulthood
adren/o	adrenal gland
aer/o	air, gas
ag-	to
-age	related to

WORD PART	DEFINITION
agglutin	sticking together, clumping
-ago	disease
-agon	contest
agon	contest against, fight against
agor/a	marketplace
-agra	rough
-al	pertaining to
alanine	an amino acid, protein synthesized in muscle
albin/o	white
albumin	albumin
ald/o	organic compound
-ale	pertaining to
alges	sensation of pain
-algia	pain, painful condition
aliment	nourishment
-alis	pertaining to
alkal	base
all/o	strange, other, different
allo-	other, different, strange
alopec	baldness, mange
alpha-	first letter in Greek alphabet
alveol	alveolus, air sac
-aly	condition
ambi-	both, double
ambly-	dull
ambulat	to walk, walking
amin/o	nitrogen compound
-amine	nitrogen-containing
ammon	ammonia
amni/o	amnion, fetal membrane
amoeb	amoeba
amph-	around
ampull	bottle-shaped
amput	to prune, lop off

S = Suffix   P = Prefix   R = Root   R/CF = Combining Form

WORD PART	DEFINITION
amyl	starch
-an	pertaining to
an-	not, lack of, without
an/o	anus
ana-	away from, excessive
anabol	build up
analysis	process to define
analyst	one who defines
anastom	join together
-ance	condition, state of
-ancy	state of
andr/o	male, masculine
aneurysm	dilation
angi/o	blood vessel, lymph vessel
angina	sore throat, chest pain radiating to throat
ankyl	stiff
-ant	forming, pertaining to, agent
ante-	before, forward
anter	before, front part
anthrac	coal
anti-	against
aort	aorta
apo-	different from, separation from, off
append	appendix
apse	clasp
aqu/a	watery
-ar	pertaining to
arachn	cobweb, spider
-arche	beginning
aria	air
-arian	one who is
-aris	pertaining to
aroma	smell, sweet herb
array	place in order
arteri/o	artery
arteriosus	like an artery
arthr/o	joint
articul	joint
-ary	pertaining to

WORD PART	DEFINITION
asbest	asbestos
asc	belly
ascit	fluid in the belly
-ase	enzyme
aspartate	an amino acid
aspirat	remove by suction
assay	evaluate
assist	aid, help
astr/o	star
-ata	action, place, use
-ate	composed of, pertaining to, process
-ated	process, composed of
atel-	incomplete
ather/o	porridge, gruel, fatty substance
athet	without position, uncontrolled
-atic	pertaining to
-ation	process
-ative	pertaining to, quality of
-ator	agent, instrument, person or thing that does something
atri/o	entrance, atrium
-atric	treatment
attent	awareness
attenu	to weaken
audi/o	to hear
audit	hearing
aur	ear
auscult	listen to
auto-	self, same
avail	useful
axill	armpit
ayur-	life
azot	nitrogen
back	back, return
bacter	bacterium
bacteri/o	bacteria
balan	glans penis
bar	pressure, weight
bas/o	base, opposite of acid
basal/e	deepest part

S = Suffix   P = Prefix   R = Root   R/CF = Combining Form

WORD PART	DEFINITION
basil	base, support
be	life
behav	mental activity
beta	second letter of Greek alphabet
bi-	two, twice, double
-bic	life
-bil	able
bil/i	bile
bio	life
biot	life
-blast	embryo, germ cell, immature cell
blast/o	immature cell, germ cell
blephar/o	eyelid
body	body, mass, substance
bov	cattle
brachi/o	arm
brachy-	short
brady-	slow
bride	rubbish, rubble
bronch/i, bronch/o	bronchus
bronchiol	small bronchus
bucc	cheek
buccin	cheek
bulb/o	bulb
burs	bursa
calc/i	calcium
calcan/e	calcaneus
calcul	stone, little stone
callos	thickening
calor	heat
cancer	cancer
candid	*Candida*, a yeast
capill	hairlike structure, capillary
capit	head
capn	carbon dioxide
caps	box, cover, shell
capsul	little box
carb/o	carbon
carboxy	group of organic compounds
carcin/o	cancerous, cancer

WORD PART	DEFINITION
cardi	heart
cardi/o	heart
care	be responsible for
caroten/e	yellow-red pigment
carotid	large neck artery
carp/o	bones of the wrist
cartilag/e	cartilage
cata-	down
catabol	break down
catechol	benzene derivative
cathet	insert, catheter
caud/a	tail
cava	cave
cavern	cave
cec	cecum
-cele	cave, hernia, swelling
celi	abdomen
cellul	small cell
cent-	hundred
cent	hundred
-centesis	to puncture
centr/o	central
cephal/o	head
-cephalus	head
cephalus	head
cephaly	condition of the head
-ceps	head
cept	to receive
cerebell	little brain, cerebellum
cerebr/o	brain
cervic	neck, cervix
cess	going forward
chancr	chancre
chem/o	chemical
chemic	chemical
-chete	hair
-chezia	pass a stool
chir/o	hand
chlor/o	green
chol/e	bile

WORD PART	DEFINITION
cholangi	bile duct
cholecyst	gallbladder
choledoch/o	common bile duct
choline	choline
chondr/o	cartilage, rib
chori/o	chorion, membrane
chorion	chorion
chrom/o	color
chromat	color
chron/o	time
chym/o	chyme
-cidal	pertaining to killing
-cide	to kill
cili	hairlike structure, eyelid
circum-	around
cirrh	yellow
cis	to cut
-clast	break, break down
claudic	limp
claustr/o	confined space
clav	clavicle
clave	lock
clavicul	clavicle
-cle	small
clitor	clitoris
clon	cutting used for propagation
-clonus	violent action
co-	with, together
coagul/o	clotting, clump
coarct	press together, narrow
cobal	cobalt
cocc	spherical bacterium, berry
cochle	cochlea
code	information system
cognit	thinking
coit	sexual intercourse
col-	before
col	colon
coll/a	glue
colon	colony

WORD PART	DEFINITION
colp/o	vagina
com-	with, together
combin	combine
comminut	break into small pieces
commodat	adjust
compat	tolerate
compet	strive together
complete	fill in
complex	woven together
compli	fulfill
compress	press together
compuls	drive, compel
con-	with, together
concav	arched, hollow
concept	become pregnant
concuss	shake violently
condyl	knuckle
confus	bewildered
congest	accumulation of fluid
coni	dust
coniz	cone
conjunctiv	conjunctiva
conscious	aware
constip	press together
constrict	narrow, to narrow
contagi/o	transmissible by contact
contamin	to corrupt, make unclean
contin	hold together
contra-	against
contract	draw together, pull together
contus	bruise
convalesc	recover
cor	heart, pupil
cori	skin
corne	having a horn
corne/o	cornea
coron	crown, coronary
corpor/a	body
corpus	body
cort	cortex

S = Suffix   P = Prefix   R = Root   R/CF = Combining Form

WORD PART	DEFINITION
cortic/o	cortex, cortisone
cortis	cortisone
costo	rib
crani/o	cranium, skull
cre	separation
crease	groove
creat	flesh
creatin	creatine
cret	to separate
cretin	cretin
crimin	distinguish
crin/o	secrete
crista	crest
-crit	to separate
crown	crown
crur	leg
cry/o	icy cold
crypt-	hidden
cub	cube
cubit	elbow
cubitus	lying down
cune/i	wedge
cur	cleanse, cure
curat	to care for
curett	to cleanse
curr	to run
cursor	run
cusp	point
cutane/o	skin
cyan/o	blue
-cyst	cyst, sac, bladder
cyst/o	bladder, sac, cyst
cysteine	an amino acid
cyt/o	cell
-cyte	cell
dacry/o	tears, lacrimal duct
dai	day
de-	from, take away, out of, without
defec	clear out waste
deferens	carry away

WORD PART	DEFINITION
defici	failure, lacking, inadequate
degenerat	deteriorate
deglutit	to swallow
del	visible, manifest
deliri	confusion, disorientation
delt	Greek letter delta
delus	deceive
demi-	half
dendr/o	treelike, branching structure
dent	tooth
depend	relying on
depress	press down
derm/a	skin
dermat/o	skin
dermis	skin
-desis	bind together, fixation of bone or joint
di-	two, complete
dia-	complete, through
diabet	diabetes
diagnost	decision
diaphor	sweat
diaphragm/a	diaphragm
dict	consent, surrender
didym/o	testis
didymis	testis
diet	a way of life
different	not identical
digest	to break down, break up
digit	finger or toe
dilat	open up, expand, open out
dips	thirst
dis-	apart, away from
discipl	understand
disciplin	disciple, instruction
dist	away from the center
-dium	appearance
diverticul	by-road
dorm	sleep
dors/i	back
drome	running

S = Suffix   P = Prefix   R = Root   R/CF = Combining Form

WORD PART	DEFINITION
duce	to lead
ducer	to lead, leader
duct	to lead
ductus	leading
duoden	twelve, duodenum
dur/a	hard, dura mater
dwarf	miniature
dynam	power
-dynia	pain
dys-	bad, difficult, painful
e-	out of, from
-eal	pertaining to
ease	normal function, freedom from pain
ec-	out, outside
ech/o	sound wave
eclamps	shining forth
eco-	environment
-ectasis	dilation
-ectomy	excision, surgical excision
ectop	on the outside, displaced
eczema	eczema
-ed	pertaining to
edema	edema, swelling
efface	wipe out
ejacul	shoot out
electr/o	electric, electricity
elimin	throw away, expel
-elle	small
em-	in, into
-ema	result
emac/i	make thin
embol	plug
embry/o	embryo, fertilized egg
eme	to vomit
-emesis	to vomit, vomiting
-emia	blood, blood condition
-emic	in the blood
emmetr-	measure
emuls	suspend in a liquid
emulsific	to milk out, to drain out

WORD PART	DEFINITION
en-	in
-ence	forming, quality of, state of
encephal/o	brain
encephaly	condition of the brain
-ency	condition, state of, quality, quality of
end-	inside, within
endo-	inner, inside, within
-ent	end result, pertaining to, state of, end, forming
enter/o	intestine
entery	intestine
enur	urinate
environ	surroundings
-eon	one who does
eosin/o	dawn
ependym	lining membrane
epi-	above, upon, over
epilep	seizure
epiphys/e	growth
episi/o	vulva
equi-	equal
equin/a	horse
-er	agent, one who does
erect	straight, to set up
erg/o	work
-ergy	process of working
-ery	condition, process of
erythemat	redness
erythr/o	red
-escent	process
-esis	abnormal condition
eso-	inward
esophag/e	esophagus
esthes	sensation
esthet	sensation, perception
estr/i estr/o	woman
ethm	sieve
eti/o	cause
-etic	pertaining to
-etics	pertaining to
-ette	little

S = Suffix   P = Prefix   R = Root   R/CF = Combining Form

WORD PART	DEFINITION
eu-	good, normal
ex-	away from, out, out of
exacerb	increase, aggravate
examin	test, examine
excret	separate, discharge
exo-	outside, outward
expect	await
expir	breathe out
extra-	out of, outside
fac/i	face
factor	maker
farct	stuff
fasci/o	fascia
febr	fever
fec	feces
feed	to give food, nourish
femor	femur
fer	to bear, carry
ferrit	iron
fertil	able to conceive
fertiliz	to bear, make fruitful
fet/o	fetus
fibr/o	fiber, fibrous
fibril	small fiber
fibrin/o	fibrin
-fication	remove
fida	split
field	definite area
filtr	strain through
fiss	split
fistul	tube, pipe
flatul	excessive gas
flavon	yellow
flex	bend
fluid/o	to flow
fluo-	fluorine
fluor/o	flux, flow, x-ray beam
flux	flow
foc	center, focus
follicul	follicle

WORD PART	DEFINITION
foramin	opening, foramen
fore-	in front
-form	appearance of, resembling
fract	break
free	free
frequ	repeated, often
front	front, forehead
fruct	fruit
funct	perform
fund/o	fundus
fung/i	fungus
fusion	to pour
galact/o	milk
gall	bile
gastr/o	stomach
gastrin	stomach hormone
gastrocnem	calf of leg
gemin	twin, double
-gen	create, produce, form
-gene	producer, give birth
gener	produce
-genesis	creation, origin, formation, source
-genic	creation, producing
genit	bring forth, birth, primary male or female sex organ
genitor	offspring
ger	old age
geront/o	process of aging
gest	gestation, pregnancy, produce
gestat	gestation, pregnancy, to bear
gigant	giant
gingiv	gums
gland	gland
glauc	lens opacity, gray
gli/o	glue, supportive tissue of nervous system
glia	glue, supportive tissue of nervous system
glob	globe
globin/o	protein
globul	globular, protein
glomerul/o	glomerulus

S = Suffix　　P = Prefix　　R = Root　　R/CF = Combining Form

WORD PART	DEFINITION
gloss/o	tongue
glottis	windpipe
gluc/o	glucose, sugar
glut/e	buttocks
glutin	glue, stick together
glyc/o	glycogen, glucose, sugar
glycer	glycerol, sweet
gnath	jaw
gnose	recognize an abnormal condition
gnosis	knowledge
gomph	bolt, nail
gon/o	seed
gonad/o	gonads, testes or ovaries
-grade	going, level
graft	splice, transplant
graine	head pain
-gram	a record, drawing, recording
grand-	big
granul/o	granule, small grain
-graph	to record, write
-grapher	one who records
-graphy	process of recording
gravid	pregnant
gravida	pregnant woman
gravis	serious
green	green
gru	to move
guan	dung
gurgit	flood
gynec/o	woman, female
habilitat	restore
hale	breathe
halit	breath
hallucin	imagination
hallux	big toe
hem/o	blood
hemangi/o	blood vessel
hemat/o	blood
heme	red iron-containing pigment
hemi-	half

WORD PART	DEFINITION
hepar	liver
hepat/o	liver
heredit	inherited through genes
herni/o	hernia, rupture
herp	blister
hetero-	different
hist	derived from histidine
hist/o	tissue
holist	entire, whole
hom/i	man
home/o	the same
homo-	same, alike
hormone	excite, stimulate
humor	fluid
hyal	glass
hydr/o	water
hyp-	below
hyper-	above, beyond, excess, excessive
hypn/o	sleep
hypo-	below, deficient, smaller, low, under
hyster/o	uterus
-ia	condition
-iac	pertaining to
-ial	pertaining to
-ian	one who does, specialist
-ias	condition
-iasis	condition, state of
-iatric	relating to medicine, medical knowledge
-iatrist	practitioner, one who treats
iatro-	medical treatment, treatment
-iatry	treatment, field of medicine
-ible	can do, able to
-ic	pertaining to
-ica	pertaining to
-ical	pertaining to
-ician	expert, specialist
-ics	knowledge of
ict	seizure
icterus	jaundice
ichthy	fish

S = Suffix   P = Prefix   R = Root   R/CF = Combining Form

WORD PART	DEFINITION
-id	having a particular quality, pertaining to
-ide	having a particular quality
idi/o	personal, distinct, unknown
ifer	to bear, carry
-ify	to become
-il	capability
-ile	capable, capability, pertaining to
ile/o	ileum
-ility	having the quality of, state of
im-	not, in
immun/o	immune, immune response, immunity
impair	worsen
imperfecta	unfinished
-imus	most
-in	chemical, chemical compound, substance
in-	not, into, in, without
incis	cut into
incub	sit on, lie on, hatch
index	to declare
-ine	pertaining to, substance
infect/i	tainted, internal invasion
infer	below, beneath
infest	invade, attack
inflammat	set on fire
inflat	blow up
infra-	below, beneath
-ing	quality of, doing
ingest	carry in
inguin	groin
inhal	breathe in
inhibit	repress
inject	force in
ino	sinew
insect/i	insect
insert	put together
inspir	breathe in
insul	island
integument	covering of the body
integr	whole
intellect/u	perception, discernment

WORD PART	DEFINITION
inter-	between
interstit	spaces within tissues
intestin	gut, intestine
intra-	inside, within
intrins	on the inside
intus-	within
iod/o	violet, iodine
-ion	action, condition, process
-ior	pertaining to, suffix for comparatives
-iosum	pertaining to
-ious	pertaining to
irrigat	to water
-is	belonging to, pertaining to, condition
isch	to keep back
-ism	action, condition, process
-ismus	take action
iso-	equal
-isone	cortisone
-ist	agent, specialist
-istic	pertaining to
-istry	specialty
-isy	inflammation
-ite	resembling
-ites	associated with
-itic	pertaining to
-ition	process
-itis	inflammation, infection
-ity	condition, state
-ium	structure
-ius	pertaining to
-ive	nature of, quality of, pertaining to
-ization	process of creating, process of affecting in a specific way
-ize	action, affect in a specific way, policy
-ized	affected in a specific way
-izer	affects in a particular way, line of action
jejun	jejunum
jugul	throat
junct	joining together
juxta-	beside, near, close to

S = Suffix   P = Prefix   R = Root   R/CF = Combining Form

WORD PART	DEFINITION
kal	potassium
kary/o	nucleus
kel/o	tumor
kerat/o	cornea, horny
keratin/o	keratin
kern	nucleus
ket/o	ketone
keton	ketone
ketone	organic compound, ketone
kin	motion
kinase	enzyme
-kine	movement
kines/i	movement
kinet	motion
-kinin	move in
klept/o	to steal
kyph/o	bent
labi	lip
labyrinth	inner ear
lacer	to tear
lacrim	tears, tear duct
lact/e	milk
lactat	secrete milk
lapar/o	abdomen in general
-lapse	fall together, slide
lapse	clasp, fall together
laryng/o	larynx
laser	acronym for light amplification by stimulated emission of radiation
lash	end of whip
lat	to take
later	side, at the side
latiss	wide
-le	small
lei/o	smooth
-lemma	covering
-lepsy	seizure
lept	thin, small
-let	small
leuk/o	white

WORD PART	DEFINITION
lex	word
librium	balance
ligament	ligament
ligat	tie up, tie off
lign	line
line	a mark
-ling	small
lingu	tongue
lip/o	fat, fatty tissue
lipid	fat
lith/o	stone
liv	life
lob	lobe
locat	a place
log	to study, study of
-logist	one who studies, specialist
logous	relation
-logy	to study, study of
longev	long life
lord	curve, swayback
lubric	make slippery
lucid	bright, clear
lumb	lower back, loin
lump	piece
lun	moon
-lus	small
lute	yellow
luxat	dislocate
-ly	going toward, every
ly	break down, separate
lymph/o	lymph
lymphaden/o	lymph node
lymphangi/o	lymphatic vessels
lys/o	decompose, decomposition, dissolve
-lysis	destroy, destruction, dissolve, separate, break down
lyt	dissolve
-lyte	soluble
-lytic	relating to destruction
lyze	destruct, dissolve, destroy

S = Suffix   P = Prefix   R = Root   R/CF = Combining Form

WORD PART	DEFINITION
macro-	large
macul	spot
-maker	one who makes
mal-	bad, inadequate
-malacia	abnormal softness
malign	harmful, bad, cancer
malleol	small hammer, malleolus
mamm/o	breast
man/o	pressure
mandibul	the jaw
-mania	frenzy, madness
manic	affected by frenzy
manipul	handful, use of hands
marker	sign
mast	breast
mastic	chew
mastoid	mastoid process
mater	mother
matern	mother
matur	ripe, ready
mature	ripe, ready, fully developed
medi	middle
media-	middle
medic	medicine
medulla	middle
mega-	enormous
-megaly	enlargement
mei	lessening
mela	black
melanin	black
melan/o	melanin, black pigment, black
mellit	sweetened with honey
membran/o	cover, skin
men/o	menses, monthly, month
mening/o	meninges
meningi/o	membranes
menisc	crescent, meniscus
menstru	menses, occurring monthly
-ment	action, state, resulting state
ment	mind, chin

WORD PART	DEFINITION
mere	part
mero-	partial
mes-	middle
meso-	middle
meta-	after, subsequent to, beyond
metabol	change
metacarp	bones of the hand
metatars	bones of the foot
meter	measure
metr/i metr/o	uterus
mi-	derived from hemi, half
micro-	small
mictur	make urine, pass urine
mid-	middle
mileusis	lathe
milli-	one-thousandth
miner	mines
mineral/o	inorganic materials
miss	send
mit/o	thread, threadlike structure
mitr-	having two points
mitt	to send
mod	nature, form, method
molec	mass
mollusc	soft
mon-	single
mono-	one, single
morbid	disease
morph/o	shape
morphin	morphine
mort	death
mot	move
motiv	move
muc/o	mucous membrane, mucus
mucos/a	lining of a cavity
multi-	many
muscul/o	muscle
mut	silent
muta	genetic change
mutil	to maim

WORD PART	DEFINITION
my/o	muscle
myc/o	fungus
myel/o	spinal cord, bone marrow
myelin	in the spinal cord, myelin
myo-	to blink
myos	muscle
myring/o	tympanic membrane, eardrum
myx-	mucus
narc/o	stupor, sleep
narciss	self-love
nas/o	nose
nat/e	birth, born
natr/i	sodium
nebul	cloud
necr/o	death
neo-	new
nephr/o	kidney
nerv	nerve
-ness	quality, state
neur/o	nerve, nervous tissue, nerve tissue
neutr/o	neutral
-nic	pertaining to
nitr/o	nitrogen
noct-	night
noia	to think
nom	law
non-	no
nor-	normal
norm-	normal
nos/o	disease
nucl	nucleus
nucle/o	nucleus
nucleol	small nucleus
nutri	nourish
nutrit	nourishment
o/o	egg
oblong	elongated
obsess	besieged by thoughts
obstetr	midwifery
occipit	back of head

WORD PART	DEFINITION
occult/a	hidden
occupation	work
ocul/o	eye
ode	way, road, path
odont	tooth
-oid	appearance of, resemble, resembling
-ol	alcohol, chemical substance
-ole	small
olfact	smell
oligo-	too little, scanty
-oma	tumor, mass
-ome	a mass of something
onc/o	tumor
-one	chemical substance, hormone
onych/o	nail
ophthalm/o	eye
opia	sight
opportun	take advantage of
-opsis	vision
-opsy	to view
opt/o	vision
-or	a doer, one who does, that which does something
or/o	mouth
orbit	orbit
orch/o	testicle
ordin	arrange
orex	appetite
organ	organ, tool, instrument, organic
orth/o	straight
orthot	correct
-orum	function of
-ory	having the function of
os	mouth
-osa	like
-ose	full of, condition
-osis	condition
osmo	push
osmol	concentration
oss/i	bone

S = Suffix   P = Prefix   R = Root   R/CF = Combining Form

WORD PART	DEFINITION
oste/o	bone
-osus	condition
ot/o	ear
-otomy	incision
-ous	pertaining to
ov/i	egg
ovari	ovary
ovul	ovum, egg
ox/y	oxygen
-oxia	oxygen condition
oxid	oxidize
oxytoc	swift birth
pace	step, pace
pact	driven in
palat	palate
palliat	reduce suffering
palpat	touch, stroke
palpit	throb
pan-	all
pancreat	pancreas
papill/o	pimple
par-	abnormal, beside
para-	adjacent to, alongside, beside, abnormal
para	to bring forth
parasit	parasite
paresis	weakness
pareun	lying beside, sexual intercourse
pariet	wall
paroxysm	irritation
particul	little piece
partum	childbirth, to bring forth
pat	lie open
patell	patella
patent	lie open
path/o	disease
pathet	suffering
pathic	pertaining to a disease
pathy	emotion, disease
pause	cessation
pector	chest

WORD PART	DEFINITION
ped	child, foot
pedicul	louse
pelv	pelvis
pen	penis
-penia	deficient, deficiency
peps	digestion
pepsin/o	pepsin
pept/i	digest, digestion, amino acid
per-	intense, through
perforat	bore through
perfus/e	to pour
peri-	around
perin/e	perineum
peripher	external boundary, outer part, outer edge
periton/e	stretch over, peritoneum
perium	bringing forth
perm/e	pass through
person	person
personal	individual
pes	foot
pest/i	pest, nuisance
petit-	small
-pexy	fixation, surgical fixation
phac/o	lens
phag/e	to eat
phagia	swallowing, eating
phalang/e	phalanx
pharmac/o	drug
pharyng/e	pharynx
pharynx	throat, pharynx
phen/o	appearance
pheo-	gray
pher-	carrying
-pheresis	removal
phery	outer edge
-phil	attraction
-phile	attraction
-philia	attraction
phim	muzzle
phleb/o	vein

S = Suffix   P = Prefix   R = Root   R/CF = Combining Form

WORD PART	DEFINITION
-phobia	fear
phobia	fear
phon/o	sound, voice
phor/e	bear, carry
phosph	phosphorus
phot/o	light
phren	mind
phylac	protect
phylaxis	protection
phys	nature
physema	blowing
physi/o	body
physic	body
physis	growth
phyt/o	plant
pia	delicate
pituit	pituitary
placed	in an area
plak	plate, plaque
plant	insert, plant
planus	flat surface
plas	molding, formation
-plasia	formation
-plasm	something formed
plasm/o	to form
-plasty	formation, repair, surgical repair
plate	flat
pleg	paralysis
plete	filled
pleur	pleura
plexy	stroke
-pnea	to breathe
pneum/o	air, lung
pneumat	structure filled with air
pneumon	air, lung
pod	foot
-poiesis	to make
-poiet	the making
-poietin	the maker
poikilo-	irregular

WORD PART	DEFINITION
point	to pierce
pol	pole
polio-	gray matter
pollut	to defile
poly-	excessive, many, much
polyp	polyp
poplit/e	ham, back of knee
por/o	opening
post-	after
poster	coming behind
pract	efficient, practical
prand/i	breakfast
pre-	before, in front of
precis	accurate
predn	a derivative of cholesterol
pregn	with child, pregnant
presby	old person
press	press close, press down, squeeze
prevent	prevent
primi-	first
pro-	before, in front, projecting forward
proct/o	anus and rectum
product	lead forth
prol/i	bear offspring
prolifer	bear offspring
pronat	bend down
prost/a	prostate
prot/e	first
protein	protein
proto-	first
proton	first
provis	provide
proxim	nearest
prurit	itch
pseudo-	false
psych/o	mind, soul
pteryg	wing
-ptosis	drooping
ptysis	spit
pub	pubis

S = Suffix   P = Prefix   R = Root   R/CF = Combining Form

WORD PART	DEFINITION
puber	growing up
pubesc	to reach puberty
puer	child
pulmon/o	lung
puls	to drive
pump	pump
punct	puncture
pur	pus
purg	cleanse, evacuate, throw up
purif	make pure
purul	pus
py/o	pus
pyel/o	renal pelvis
pylor	gate, pylorus
pyr/o	fire, heat, fever
pyret	fever
pyrex	fever, heat
quadri-	four
radi/o	x-ray, radiation, radius
radial	radius
radic	root
re-	again, back, backward
recept	receive
rect/o	rectum
reflex/o	to reflect, bend back
regul	to rule
remiss	send back, give up
ren	kidney
replic	reply
rescein	resin
resect/o	cut off
resid/u	left over, what is left over
resist	to withstand
restor	renew
resuscit	revival from apparent death
reticul	fine net, network
retin/o	retina
retinacul	hold back
retro-	backward
rhabd/o	rod-shaped, striated

WORD PART	DEFINITION
-rhaphy	suture, repair
rheumat	a flow, rheumatism
rhin/o	nose
rhythm	rhythm
rib/o	like a rib
rigid	stiff
rotat	rotate
-rrhage	to flow profusely
-rrhagia	excessive flow, discharge
-rrhaphy	suture
-rrhea	flow, discharge
-rrhoid	flow
rrhythm	rhythm
-rubin	rust colored
rumin	throat
-ry	occupation
sacchar	sugar
sacr/o	sacrum
sagitt	arrow
saliv	saliva
salping/o	uterine tube
san	sound, healthy
sarc/o	flesh, sarcoma, muscle
satur	to fill
scapul	scapula
schiz/o	to split, cleave
scinti	spark
scler/o	hard, white of eye, hardness
-scope	instrument for viewing, instrument
scope	instrument for viewing
-scopy	to examine, to view, visual examination
script	writing, thing copied
scrot	scrotum
seb/o	sebum
sebac/e	wax
secret	secrete, produce, separate
sect	cut off
sedat	to calm
sedent	sitting
segment	section

WORD PART	DEFINITION
seiz	to grab, convulse
self	me, own individual
semi-	half
semin	scatter seed
semin/i	semen
sen	old age
senesc	growing old
senil	characteristic of old age
sens	feel
sensitiv	sensitive, feeling, sensitivity
sensor/i	sensation, sensory
separat	move apart
seps	decay, infection
sept/o	septum, partition
septic	infected
ser/o	serum, serous
sib	relative
sigm	Greek letter sigma, "S"
sigmoid/o	sigmoid colon
silic	silicon, glass
simul	imitate
sin/o	sinus
sinus	sinus
sipid	flavor
-sis	abnormal condition, process
sit/u	place
skelet	skeleton
soci/o	partner, ally, community
-sol	solution
soma	body
somat/o	body
-some	body
somn/o	sleep
somy	chromosome
son/o	sound
sorpt	swallow
sound	noise
spad	tear or cut
spasm	spasm, sudden involuntary tightening
spast	tight

WORD PART	DEFINITION
specif	species
sperm/i	sperm
spermat/o	sperm
sphen	wedge
spher/o	sphere
sphygm/o	pulse
spin/o	spine, spinal cord
spir/o	spiral, coil
spirat	breathe
spiro-	spiral, coil
splen/o	spleen
spondyl	vertebra
spong/i	sponge
spongios	sponge
stabil	stand firm
stalsis	to constrict
staphyl/o	bunch of grapes
-stasis	control, stop, stand still
stat	stand still
-static	to make stand, stop
-statin	inhibit
stax	fall in drops
steat	fat
stein	stone
sten/o	narrow, contract
ster	solid, steroid
stere/o	three-dimensional
steril	barren
stern	chest, breastbone
-steroid	steroid
-sterol	steroid
steron	steroid
-sterone	sterol
steth/o	chest
sthen	strength
stick	branch, twig
stigmat	focus
stimul	excite, strengthen
stin	partition
stit/i	space

S = Suffix   P = Prefix   R = Root   R/CF = Combining Form

WORD PART	DEFINITION
stoma	mouth
-stomy	new opening
stone	stone, pebble
storm	crisis
strab	squint
strat	layer
strepto-	curved
su/i	self
sub-	below, under, slightly, underneath
sucr	sucrose, table sugar
suffic/i	enough
sulf	sulfur
sum	pick up
super	above
supinat	bend backward
suppress	pressed under, push under
supra-	above, excessive
surf	surface
surg	operate
suscept	to take up
-sylated	linked
sym-	together
symptomat	symptom
syn-	together
syndesm	bind together
syring/o	tube, pipe
system	body system
systol/e	contraction
tachy-	rapid
tact	orderly arrangement
tali	ankle bone
tamin	touch
tampon	plug
tangent/i	touch
tars/o	ankle
tax	coordination
tect/o	to shelter
tempor/o	time, temple, side of head
ten/o	tendon
tendin	tendon

WORD PART	DEFINITION
tens	pressure
-tensin	tense, taut
terat/o	monster, malformed fetus
term	normal gestation
test/o	testis, testicle
testicul	testicle, testis
tetra-	four
thalam	thalamus
thalass	sea
thec	sheath
thel	breast, nipple
thel/i	lining
thenar	palm
therap/o	healing, treatment
therapeut	healing, treatment
therapy	medical treatment
therm/o	heat
thesis	to arrange, place
thet	place, arrange
thora	chest
thorac/o	chest
-thorax	chest
thromb/o	blood clot, clot
thrombin	clot
thym	thymus gland, the mind
thyr/o	an oblong shield, thyroid
thyroid	an oblong shield, thyroid
-tic	pertaining to
-tion	process, being
-tiz	pertaining to
toc	labor, birth
toler	endure
tom/o	section, incise, cut
-tome	instrument to cut
-tomy	surgical incision
-tory	pertaining to
ton/o	pressure, tension
tonsil	tonsil
tonsill/o	tonsil
tope	part, location

S = Suffix   P = Prefix   R = Root   R/CF = Combining Form

WORD PART	DEFINITION
topic	local
-tous	pertaining to
tox/o	poison
-toxic	able to kill
toxic/o	poison
toxin	poison
trache/o	trachea, windpipe
tract	draw, pull
tranquil	calm
trans-	across, through
trauma	wound, injury
tresia	a hole
tri-	three
trich/o	hair, flagellum
trichin/o	hair
-tripsy	to crush
-tripter	crusher
trochle	pulley
trop	turn, turning
troph	development, nourishment
trophy	development, nourishment
-tropic	stimulator, change
-tropin	nourishing, stimulation
tryps	friction
tub/a	tube
tubercul	swelling, tuberculosis, nodule
tubul	small tube
tuss/i	cough
tussis	cough
-ty	quality, state
tympan/o	eardrum, tympanic membrane
-type	model, particular kind, group
-ula	small thing
ulcer	a sore
-ule	little, small
-ulent	abounding in
uln/a	forearm bone
ultra-	higher, beyond
-um	tissue, structure
umbilic	belly button, navel, umbilicus

WORD PART	DEFINITION
un-	not
un	one
uni-	one
ur/o	urinary system
-ure	process, result of
uresis	to urinate
uret	ureter, urine, urination
ureter/o	ureter
urethr/o	urethra
urin/a	urine
-us	pertaining to
uter/o	uterus
uve	uvea
uvul	uvula
vaccin	vaccine, giving a vaccine
vag	vagus nerve
vagin	sheath, vagina
valgus	turn out
valv	valve
varic/o	varicosity; dilated, tortuous vein
vas/o	blood vessel, duct
vascul	blood vessel
vegetat	growth
ven/o	vein
ventil	wind
ventr	belly
ventricul	ventricle
vers	turned
verse	travel
-version	change
vert	to turn
vertebr/a	vertebra
vesic	sac containing fluid
vestibul/o	vestibule of inner ear
via	the way
violet	bluish purple
vir	virus
viril	masculine
virus	poison
visc/o	sticky

S = Suffix   P = Prefix   R = Root   R/CF = Combining Form

WORD PART	DEFINITION
viscer	an internal organ
visu	sight
vit/a	life
voc	voice
vol	volume
volunt	free will
-volut	rolled up
volut/e	shrink, roll up
vuls	tear, pull

WORD PART	DEFINITION
vulv/o	vulva
whip	to swing
xanth	yellow
xeno-	foreign
-yl	substance
-zoa	animal
zyg	zygote
-zyme	enzyme
zyme	fermenting, enzyme, transform

Abbreviations

ABBREVIATION	DEFINITION
↑	increase/ above
↓	decrease/ below
1°	primary
2°	secondary
99mTc	technetium 99m, a radionuclide
ABG	arterial blood gas
ABI	ankle/brachial index
ABO	a blood group system
AC	acromioclavicular
ACE	angiotensin-converting enzyme
ACEP	American College of Emergency Physicians
ACL	anterior cruciate ligament
ACTH	adrenocorticotropic hormone
AD	Latin, auris dextra right ear
ADD	attention deficit disorder
ADH	antidiuretic hormone
ADHD	attention deficit hyperactivity disorder
ADLs	activities of daily living
AED	automatic external defibrillator
AFP	alpha-fetoprotein
AIDS	acquired immunodeficiency syndrome
ALL	acute lymphoblastic leukemia
ALP	alkaline phosphatase
ALS	amyotrophic lateral sclerosis
ALT	alanine aminotransferase
AMAS	anti-malignin antibody screen
ANS	autonomic nervous system
AOM	acute otitis media
AP	anteroposterior
APP	advanced practice provider
aPTT	activated partial thromboplastin time
ARDS	acute respiratory distress syndrome
ARF	acute respiratory failure
ARF	acute renal failure
AROM	active range of motion
AS	Latin, auris sinistra left ear

ABBREVIATION	DEFINITION
ASD	atrial septal defect
ASD	autism spectrum disorder
ASHD	arteriosclerotic heart disease
AST	aspartate aminotransferase
AU	Latin, aures unitas or auris uterque both ears
AV	atrioventricular
AVM	arteriovenous malformation
BAL	bronchoalveolar lavage
BBB	blood-brain barrier
BD	brain death
BKA	below-the-knee amputation
BM	bowel movement
BMD	bone mineral density
BMR	basal metabolic rate
BNP	B-type natriuretic peptide
BOM	bilateral otitis media
BP	blood pressure
BPD	borderline personality disorder
BPH	benign prostatic hyperplasia
BPPV	benign paroxysmal positional vertigo
BRCA1	a gene that, when mutated, increases risk for breast and ovarian cancer (BReast CAncer 1)
BRCA2	a gene that, when mutated, increases risk for breast cancer (BReast CAncer 2)
BSE	bovine spongiform encephalopathy
BSE	breast self-examination
BUN	blood urea nitrogen
C1–C8	cervical spinal nerves
C5	fifth cervical vertebra or nerve
CA	cancer
CABG	coronary artery bypass graft
CAD	coronary artery disease
CAO	chronic airway obstruction
CAPD	continuous ambulatory peritoneal dialysis
CBC	complete blood count
CBT	cognitive behavioral therapy

ABBREVIATION	DEFINITION
CD	cluster of differentiation; coreceptors of cell membranes to recognize specific antigens
CD	conduct disorder
CD8	helper T cell
CDC	Centers for Disease Control and Prevention
CEA	carcinoembryonic antigen
CF	cystic fibrosis
CHART	continuous hyperfractionated accelerated radiotherapy
CHD	congenital heart disease
CHES	Certified Health Education Specialist
CHF	congestive heart failure
CIS	carcinoma in situ
CJD	Creutzfeldt-Jakob disease
CK	creatine kinase
CKD	chronic kidney disease
CMA	Certified Medical Assistant
CMV	cytomegalovirus
CNA	Certified Nurse Assistant
CNS	central nervous system
c/o	complains of
CO_2	carbon dioxide
COPD	chronic obstructive pulmonary disease
COT	Certified Occupational Therapist
COTA	Certified Occupational Therapist Assistant
CP	cerebral palsy
CPAP	continuous positive airway pressure
CPR	cardiopulmonary resuscitation
CPT	cognitive processing therapy
CRF	chronic renal failure
CRP	C-reactive protein
C-section	cesarean section
CSF	cerebrospinal fluid
CT	computed tomography
CVA	cerebrovascular accident
CVP	central venous pressure
CVS	cardiovascular system
CVT	cardiovascular technician
CXR	chest x-ray
D&C	dilation and curettage
DEXA	dual-energy x-ray absorptiometry
DHEA	dehydroepiandrosterone
DI	diabetes insipidus

ABBREVIATION	DEFINITION
DIC	disseminated intravascular coagulation
DID	dissociative identity disorder
DIFF	differential white blood cell count
DJD	degenerative joint disease
DKA	diabetic ketoacidosis
dL	deciliter; one-tenth of a liter
DM	diabetes mellitus
DMD	Duchenne muscular dystrophy
DNA	deoxyribonucleic acid
DNR	do not resuscitate
DO	doctor of osteopathy
DRE	digital rectal examination
DSM-V	*Diagnostic and Statistical Manual of Mental Disorders*, fifth edition
DUB	dysfunctional uterine bleeding
DVT	deep vein thrombosis
Dx	diagnosis
EBT	electron beam tomography
EBV	Epstein-Barr virus
ECG	electrocardiogram
E. coli	*Escherichia coli*
ECT	electroconvulsive therapy
ED	erectile dysfunction
EEG	electroencephalogram
EKG	electrocardiogram
ELISA	enzyme-linked immunosorbent assay
EMDR	eye movement desensitization and reprocessing
EMG	electromyogram
EMR	emergency medical responder
EMS	emergency medical services
EMT	emergency medical technician
EP	evoked potential
EPA	U.S. Environmental Protection Agency
ER	Emergency Room
ERCP	endoscopic retrograde cholangiopancreatography
ESR	erythrocyte sedimentation rate
ESRD	end-stage renal disease
ESWL	extracorporeal shock wave lithotripsy
ETS	environmental tobacco smoke
FAS	fetal alcohol syndrome
FDA	U.S. Food and Drug Administration
FEV1	forced expiratory volume in 1 second

ABBREVIATION	DEFINITION
fL	femtoliter; one-quadrillionth of a liter
FOBT	fecal occult blood test
FSH	follicle-stimulating hormone
FTT	failure to thrive
FVC	forced vital capacity
Fx	fracture
g	gram
GAD	generalized anxiety disorder
GDM	gestational diabetes mellitus
GERD	gastroesophageal reflux disease
GFR	glomerular filtration rate
GGT	gamma-glutamyl transpeptidase
GH	growth hormone, somatotropin
GI	gastrointestinal
GI	glycemic index
GL	glycemic load
GnRH	gonadotropin-releasing hormone
GSR	galvanic skin response
GTT	glucose tolerance test
GYN	gynecology
H1N1	swine flu virus
H$_2$-blocker	histamine-2 receptor antagonist
H5N1	subtype of avian influenza virus
HAV	hepatitis A virus
Hb	hemoglobin
Hb A1c	glycosylated hemoglobin A1c
HBV	hepatitis B virus
HCG	human chorionic gonadotropin
HCL	hydrochloric acid
Hct	hematocrit
HCV	hepatitis C virus
HDL	high-density lipoprotein
HDN	hemolytic disease of the newborn
Hg	mercury
Hgb	hemoglobin
HIPAA	Health Insurance Portability and Accountability Act
HIV	human immunodeficiency virus
HLA	human leukocyte antigen
HLD	high-level disinfection
HMD	hyaline membrane disease
H/O	history of
HPI	history of present illness

ABBREVIATION	DEFINITION
HPV	human papillomavirus
HRT	hormone replacement therapy
HSV	herpes simplex virus
HSV-1	herpes simplex virus, type 1
HUS	hemolytic uremic syndrome
IADLs	instrumental activities of daily living
IBS	irritable bowel syndrome
ICD	implantable cardioverter/defibrillator
IDDM	insulin-dependent diabetes mellitus
Ig	immunoglobulin
IgA	immunoglobulin A
IgD	immunoglobulin D
IgE	immunoglobulin E
IGF	insulinlike growth factor
IgG	immunoglobulin G
IgM	immunoglobulin M
IM	intramuscular
INR	international normalized ratio
ITP	idiopathic (or immunologic) thrombocytopenic purpura
IU	international unit(s)
IUD	intrauterine device
IV	intravenous
IVC	inferior vena cava
IVF	in vitro fertilization
IVP	intravenous pyelogram
JC	Joint Commission
JRA	juvenile rheumatoid arthritis
KUB	x-ray of abdomen to show kidneys, ureters, and bladder
L	liter
L1–L5	lumbar spinal nerves or vertebrae
LASER	light amplification by stimulated emission of radiation
LCC-ST	Liaison Council on Certification for the Surgical Technologist
LD	learning disability
LDL	low-density lipoprotein
LED	light-emitting diode
LEEP	loop electrosurgical excision procedure
LFT	liver function test
LH	luteinizing hormone
LLQ	left lower quadrant
LOC	loss of consciousness

ABBREVIATION	DEFINITION
LPN	licensed practical nurse
LSD	lysergic acid diethylamide (acid)
LUQ	left upper quadrant
LVN	licensed vocational nurse
MAOI	monoamine oxidase inhibitor
mcg	microgram; one-millionth of a gram
MCH	mean corpuscular hemoglobin (the average amount of hemoglobin in the average red blood cell)
MCHC	mean corpuscular hemoglobin concentration (the average concentration of hemoglobin in a given volume of red blood cells)
MCP	metacarpophalangeal
MCS	minimally conscious state
MCV	mean corpuscular volume (the average volume of a red blood cell)
MD	doctor of medicine
MDMA	methylenedioxymethamphetamine (ecstasy)
mg	milligram
MHC	major histocompatibility complex
MI	myocardial infarction
mL	milliliter
mm³	cubic millimeter
MOAB	monoclonal antibody
MODY	mature-onset diabetes of youth
MPD	multiple personality disorder
MRA	magnetic resonance angiography
MRI	magnetic resonance imaging
mRNA	messenger RNA
MRSA	methicillin-resistant *Staphylococcus aureus*
MS	multiple sclerosis
NCI	National Cancer Institute
NHGRI	National Human Genome Research Institute
NHLBI	National Heart, Lung, and Blood Institute
NIDDM	non-insulin-dependent diabetes mellitus
NIH	National Institutes of Health
NKA	no known allergies
NLM	National Library of Medicine
NMS	neurally mediated syncope
NO	nitric oxide
NPH	neutral protamine Hagedorn insulin
NRDS	neonatal respiratory distress syndrome
NSAID	nonsteroidal anti-inflammatory drug
O₂	oxygen

ABBREVIATION	DEFINITION
OA	osteoarthritis
OB	obstetrics
OCD	obsessive-compulsive disorder
OD	doctor of osteopathy
OD	Latin, oculus dexter right eye
OGTT	oral glucose tolerance test
OME	otitis media with effusion
omega-3	alpha-linolenic acid
OR	operating room
OS	Latin, oculus sinister left eye
OSHA	Occupational Safety and Health Administration
OT	ophthalmic technician
OXT	oxytocin
OT	occupational therapist, occupational therapy
OTC	over-the-counter
OU	Latin, oculus uterque both eyes
P	pulse (rate)
PA	posteroanterior
PaO₂	partial pressure of arterial oxygen
Pap	Papanicolaou (Pap test, Pap smear)
PAT	paroxysmal atrial tachycardia
PCBs	polychlorinated biphenyls
PCD	programmed cell death
PCL	posterior cruciate ligament
PCOS	polycystic ovarian syndrome
PCP	phencyclidine (angel dust), primary care provider
PDA	patent ductus arteriosus
PDT	postural drainage therapy
PE	pressure equalization (tube)
PEEP	positive end-expiratory pressure
PEFR	peak expiratory flow rate
PET	positron emission tomography
PFT	pulmonary function test
pg	picogram; one-trillionth of a gram
PGY	pregnancy
pH	hydrogen ion concentration
PhD	doctor of philosophy
PID	pelvic inflammatory disease
PIP	proximal interphalangeal (joint)
PKD	polycystic kidney disease
PMDD	premenstrual dysphoric disorder
PMNL	polymorphonuclear leukocyte

ABBREVIATION	DEFINITION
PMS	premenstrual syndrome
PNS	peripheral nervous system
p.o.	Latin, per os by mouth
polio	poliomyelitis
PPH	postpartum hemorrhage
PPI	proton pump inhibitor
PPS	postpolio syndrome
PRL	prolactin
p.r.n.	Latin, pro re nata when necessary
PSA	prostate-specific antigen
PsyD	doctor of psychology
PT	physiotherapy
PT	prothrombin time
PT	physical therapy, physical therapist
PTA	physical therapy assistant
PTCA	percutaneous transluminal coronary angioplasty
PTH	parathyroid hormone
PTSD	posttraumatic stress disorder
PVC	premature ventricular contraction
PVD	peripheral vascular disease
PVS	persistent vegetative state
q.4.h.	Latin, quaque quarta hora every 4 hours
q.i.d.	Latin, quater in die four times a day
R	respiration (rate)
RA	rheumatoid arthritis
RBC	red blood cell
RDS	respiratory distress syndrome
RF	radiofrequency
Rh	Rhesus
RhoGAM	Rhesus immune globulin
RLQ	right lower quadrant
RN	registered nurse
RNA	ribonucleic acid
ROM	range of motion
RSV	respiratory syncytial virus
RT	radiology technician
RU-486	mifepristone
RUQ	right upper quadrant
S1–S5	sacral nerves or vertebrae
SA	sinoatrial
SAD	seasonal affective disorder
SBS	shaken baby syndrome

ABBREVIATION	DEFINITION
SC	subcutaneous
SCI	spinal cord injury
SET	self-examination of the testes
SG	specific gravity
SGOT	serum glutamic oxaloacetic acid transaminase (AST)
SGPT	serum glutamic-pyruvic transaminase (ALT)
SI	sacroiliac
SLE	systemic lupus erythematosus
SMI	sustained maximal inspiration
SNRI	serotonin and norepinephrine reuptake inhibitor
SOB	short(ness) of breath
SRS	stereotactic radiosurgery
SSA	Sjögren syndrome antibodies A
SSB	Sjögren syndrome antibodies B
SSRI	selective serotonin reuptake inhibitor
STAT	Latin, statim immediately
STD	sexually transmitted disease
SVC	superior vena cava
T	temperature
T1	first thoracic vertebra or nerve
T1–T12	thoracic spinal nerves or vertebrae
T_3	triiodothyronine
T_4	tetraiodothyronine (thyroxine)
TB	tuberculosis
TBI	traumatic brain injury
TCA	tricyclic antidepressant
TEE	transesophageal echocardiography
TENS	transcutaneous electrical nerve stimulation
THC	tetrahydrocannabinol (marijuana)
THR	total hip replacement
TIA	transient ischemic attack
TIBC	total iron-binding capacity
t.i.d.	(Latin ter in die) three times a day
TMJ	temporomandibular joint
TNM	tumor-node-metastasis (staging system for cancer)
TOF	tetralogy of Fallot
tPA	tissue plasminogen activator
TS	tumor suppressor
TSH	thyroid-stimulating hormone
TTM	trichotillomania

ABBREVIATION	DEFINITION
TTP	thrombotic thrombocytopenic purpura
TURP	transurethral resection of the prostate
U	unit
UA	urinalysis
URI	upper respiratory infection
UTI	urinary tract infection
UV	ultraviolet
VCUG	voiding cystourethrogram
VEP	visual evoked potential

ABBREVIATION	DEFINITION
V-fib	ventricular fibrillation
VS	vital signs
VSD	ventricular septal defect
vWD	von Willebrand disease
vWF	von Willebrand factor
WAD	Word Analysis and Definition (box)
WBC	white blood cell; white blood (cell) count
WNL	within normal limits

A

abdomen (AB-doh-men) Part of the trunk between the thorax and the pelvis.

abdominal (ab-DOM-in-al) Pertaining to the abdomen.

abdominopelvic (ab-DOM-ih-noh-PEL-vik) Pertaining to the abdomen and pelvis.

abducens (ab-DYU-senz) Sixth (VI) cranial nerve; responsible for eye movement.

abduction (ab-DUK-shun) Action of moving away from the midline.

ablation (ab-LAY-shun) Removal of tissue to destroy its function.

abortus (ah-BOR-tus) Product of abortion.

abrasion (ah-BRAY-shun) Area of skin or mucous membrane that has been scraped off.

abruptio (ab-RUP-shee-oh) Placenta abruptio is the premature detachment of the placenta.

absorption (ab-SORP-shun) Uptake of nutrients and water by cells in the GI tract.

accessory (ak-SESS-oh-ree) Eleventh (XI) cranial nerve; supplying neck muscles, pharynx, and larynx.

acetabulum (ass-eh-TAB-you-lum) The cup-shaped cavity of the hip bone that receives the head of the femur to form the hip joint.

acetaminophen (ah-seet-ah-MIN-oh-fen) Medication that is an analgesic and an antipyretic.

acetone (ASS-eh-tone) Ketone that is found in blood, urine, and breath when diabetes mellitus is out of control.

acetylcholine (AS-eh-til-KOH-leen) Parasympathetic neurotransmitter.

Achilles tendon (ah-KIL-eez TEN-dun) A tendon formed from the gastrocnemius and soleus muscles and inserted into the calcaneus. Also called *calcaneal tendon*.

achondroplasia (ay-kon-droh-PLAY-zee-ah) Condition with abnormal conversion of cartilage into bone, leading to dwarfism.

acid (ASS-id) Substance with a pH below 7.0.

acinar cells (ASS-in-ar SELLS) Enzyme-secreting cells of the pancreas.

acne (AK-nee) Inflammatory disease of sebaceous glands and hair follicles.

acquired immunodeficiency syndrome (AIDS) (ah-KWIRED IM-you-noh-dee-FISH-en-see SIN-drome) Infection with the HIV virus.

acromegaly (ak-roh-MEG-ah-lee) Enlargement of the head, face, hands, and feet due to excess growth hormone in an adult.

acromioclavicular (AC) (ah-CROH-mee-oh-klah-VIK-you-lar) The joint between the acromion and the clavicle.

acromion (ah-CROH-mee-on) Lateral end of the scapula, extending over the shoulder joint.

acrophobia (ak-roh-FOH-bee-ah) Pathologic fear of heights.

actinic (ak-TIN-ik) Pertaining to the sun.

activities of daily living (ADLs) (ak-TIV-ih-teez of DAY-lee LIV-ing) Daily routines for mobility and personal care: bathing, dressing, eating, and moving.

acuminata (a-KYU-min-AH-ta) Tapering to a point.

addiction (ah-DIK-shun) Habitual psychological and physiologic dependence on a substance or practice.

addictive (ah-DIK-tiv) Pertaining to or causing addiction.

Addison disease (ADD-ih-son diz-EEZ) An autoimmune disease leading to decreased production of adrenocortical steroids.

adduction (ah-DUK-shun) Action of moving toward the midline.

adenocarcinoma (AD-eh-noh-kar-sih-NOH-mah) A cancer arising from glandular epithelial cells.

adenohypophysis (AD-en-oh-high-POF-ih-sis) Anterior lobe of the pituitary gland.

adenoid (ADD-eh-noyd) Single mass of lymphoid tissue in the midline at the back of the throat.

adenoma (AD-eh-NOH-mah) Benign tumor that originates from glandular tissue.

adherence (ad-HEER-ents) The act of sticking to something.

adipose (ADD-i-pose) Containing fat.

adjuvant (AD-joo-vant) Additional treatment after a primary treatment has been used.

adnexa (ad-NEK-sa) Parts accessory to an organ or structure. Singular *adnexum*.

adrenal gland (ah-DREE-nal GLAND) The suprarenal, or adrenal, gland on the upper pole of each kidney.

adrenalectomy (ah-DREE-nal-EK-toh-mee) Removal of part or all of an adrenal gland.

adrenaline (ah-DREN-ah-lin) One of the catecholamines. Also called *epinephrine*.

adrenocortical (ah-DREE-noh-KOR-tih-kal) Pertaining to the cortex of the adrenal gland.

adrenocorticotropic hormone (ah-DREE-noh-KOR-tih-koh-TROH-pik HOR-mohn) Hormone of the anterior pituitary that stimulates the cortex of the adrenal gland to produce its own hormones.

adrenogenital syndrome (ah-DREE-noh-JEN-it-al SIN-drome) Hypersecretion of androgens from the adrenal gland.

advance medical directive (ad-VANTS MED-ih-kal die-REK-tiv) Legal document signed by the patient dealing with issues of prolonging or ending life in the event of life-threatening illness.

adventitia (ad-ven-TISH-ah) Outer layer of connective tissue covering blood vessels or organs.

affect (AF-fekt) External display of feelings, thoughts, and emotions.

afferent (AF-eh-rent) Conducting impulses inward *toward* the spinal cord or brain.

agglutinate (ah-GLUE-tin-ate) Stick together to form clumps.

agglutination (ah-glue-tih-NAY-shun) Process by which cells or other particles adhere to each other to form clumps.

aging (AY-jing) The process of human maturation and decline.

agonist (AG-on-ist) Agent that combines with receptors to initiate drug actions.

agoraphobia (ah-gor-ah-FOH-bee-ah) Pathologic fear of being trapped in a public place.

agranulocyte (ay-GRAN-you-loh-site) A white blood cell without any granules in its cytoplasm.

alanine aminotransferase (ALT) (AL-ah-neen ah-MEE-noh-TRANS-fer-aze) Enzyme that is found in liver cells and leaks out into the bloodstream when the cells are damaged, enabling liver damage to be diagnosed.

albinism (AL-bih-nizm) Genetic disorder with lack of melanin.

albumin (al-BYU-min) Simple, soluble protein.

aldosterone (al-DOS-ter-ohn) Mineralocorticoid hormone of the adrenal cortex.

aldosteronism (al-DOS-ter-ohn-izm) Condition caused by excessive secretion of aldosterone. Also called *Conn syndrome.*

aldosteronoma (al-DOS-ter-oh-NOH-mah) Benign adenoma of the adrenal cortex.

alimentary (al-ih-MEN-tar-ee) Pertaining to the digestive tract.

alkaline (AL-kah-line) Substance with a pH above 7.0. Also called *basic.*

alkaloid (AL-ka-loyd) Alkaline substances with pharmacologic activity synthesized from plants.

allergen (AL-er-jen) Substance producing a hypersensitivity (allergic) reaction.

allergic (ah-LER-jik) Pertaining to being hypersensitive.

allergy (AL-er-jee) Hypersensitivity to an allergen.

allogen (AL-oh-jen) Antigen from someone else in the same species.

allograft (AL-oh-graft) Tissue graft from another person or cadaver.

alloimmune (AL-oh-im-YUNE) Reaction directed against foreign tissue.

alopecia (al-oh-PEE-shah) Partial or complete loss of hair, naturally or from medication.

alpha-fetoprotein (AL-fah-fee-toh-PROH-teen) Protein normally produced only by the fetus.

alveolus (al-VEE-oh-lus) Small empty hollow or sac. It is a terminal element of the respiratory tract. Plural *alveoli.*

Alzheimer disease (AWLZ-high-mer diz-EEZ) Common form of dementia.

amblyopia (am-blee-OH-pee-ah) Failure or incomplete development of the pathways of vision to the brain.

amenorrhea (a-men-oh-REE-ah) Absence or abnormal cessation of menstrual flow.

amino acid (ah-MEE-noh ASS-id) The basic building block of protein.

ammonia (ah-MOHN-ih-ah) Toxic breakdown product of amino acids.

amnesia (am-NEE-zee-ah) Total or partial inability to remember past experiences.

amniocentesis (AM-nee-oh-sen-TEE-sis) Removal of amniotic fluid for diagnostic purposes.

amnion (AM-nee-on) Membrane around the fetus that contains amniotic fluid.

ampulla (am-PULL-ah) Dilated portion of a canal or duct.

amputation (am-pyu-TAY-shun) Process of removing a limb, a part of a limb, a breast, or some other projecting part.

amylase (AM-il-aze) One of a group of enzymes that break down starch.

amyotrophic (a-my-oh-TROH-fik) Pertaining to muscular atrophy.

anabolism (an-AB-oh-lizm) The buildup of complex substances in the cell from simpler ones as a part of metabolism.

analgesic (an-al-JEE-zik) Substance that reduces the response to pain.

anaphylactic (AN-ah-fih-LAK-tik) Pertaining to anaphylaxis.

anaphylaxis (AN-ah-fih-LAK-sis) Immediate severe allergic response.

anastomosis (ah-NAS-to-MOH-sis) A surgically made union between two tubular structures. Plural *anastomoses.*

anatomic (an-ah-TOM-ik) Pertaining to anatomy.

androgen (AN-droh-jen) Hormone that promotes masculine characteristics.

anemia (ah-NEE-mee-ah) Decreased number of red blood cells.

anencephaly (AN-en-SEF-ah-lee) Born without cerebral hemispheres.

anesthesiologist (AN-es-thee-zee-OL-oh-jist) Medical specialist in anesthesia.

anesthetic (an-es-THET-ik) Substance that takes away feeling and pain.

aneurysm (AN-yur-izm) Circumscribed dilation of an artery or cardiac chamber.

angiogenesis (AN-jee-oh-JEN-eh-sis) Creation of new blood vessels.

angiogram (AN-jee-oh-gram) Radiograph obtained after injection of radiopaque contrast material into blood vessels.

angiography (an-jee-OG-rah-fee) Radiography of vessels after injection of contrast material.

angioplasty (AN-jee-oh-PLAS-tee) Recanalization of a blood vessel by surgery.

anomaly (ah-NOM-ah-lee) A structural abnormality.

anorchism (an-OR-kizm) Absence of testes.

anorexia (an-oh-RECK-see-ah) Severe lack of appetite; *or* an aversion to food.

anoscopy (A-nos-koh-pee) Endoscopic examination of the anus.

anoxia (an-OK-see-ah) Without oxygen.

antacid (ant-ASS-id) Agent that neutralizes acidity.

antagonist (an-TAG-oh-nist) An opposing structure, agent, disease, or process.

antagonistic (an-TAG-oh-nis-tik) Having an opposite function.

anterior (an-TER-ee-or) Front surface of body; situated in front.

anteverted (an-teh-VERT-ed) Tilted forward.

anthracosis (an-thra-KOH-sis) Lung disease caused by the inhalation of coal dust.

anti-inflammatory (AN-tee-in-FLAM-ah-tor-ee) Agent that reduces inflammation by acting on the body's response mechanisms without affecting the causative agent.

antiangiogenesis (AN-tee-AN-jee-oh-JEN-eh-sis) The prevention of growth of new blood vessels.

antibiotic (AN-tih-bye-OT-ik) A substance that has the capacity to destroy bacteria and other microorganisms.

antibody (AN-tih-bodee) Protein produced in response to an antigen. Plural *antibodies.*

anticoagulant (AN-tee-koh-AG-you-lant) Substance that prevents clotting.

antidiuretic hormone (ADH) (AN-tih-die-you-RET-ik HOR-mohn) Posterior pituitary hormone that decreases urine output by acting on the kidney. Also called *vasopressin*.

antiemetic (AN-tee-eh-MEH-tik) Agent that prevents vomiting.

antiepileptic (AN-tee-eh-pih-LEP-tik) A pharmacologic agent capable of preventing or arresting epilepsy.

antigen (AN-tih-jen) Substance capable of triggering an immune response.

antihistamine (an-tee-HISS-tah-meen) Drug used to treat allergic symptoms because of its action antagonistic to histamine. Some can also be effective against vomiting.

antioxidant (an-tee-OKS-ih-dant) Substance that can prevent cell damage by neutralizing free radicals.

antipruritic (AN-tee-pru-RIT-ik) Medication against itching.

antipsychotic (AN-tih-sigh-KOT-ik) An agent helpful in the treatment of psychosis.

antipyretic (AN-tee-pie-RET-ik) Agent that reduces fever.

antisocial personality disorder (AN-tee-SOH-shal per-son-AL-ih-tee dis-OR-der) Disorder of people who lie, cheat, and steal and have no guilt about their behavior.

antithyroid (an-tee-THIGH-royd) A substance that inhibits production of thyroid hormones.

antrum (AN-trum) A nearly closed cavity or chamber.

anuria (an-YOU-ree-ah) Absence of urine production.

anus (AY-nuss) Terminal opening of the digestive tract through which feces are discharged.

anxiety (ang-ZIE-eh-tee) Distress caused by fear.

aorta (ay-OR-tuh) Main trunk of the systemic arterial system.

apex (AY-peks) Tip or end of cone-shaped structure, such as the heart.

aphonia (ay-FOH-nee-ah) Loss of voice.

aphthous ulcer (AF-thus UL-ser) Painful small oral ulcer (canker sore).

aplastic anemia (ay-PLAS-tik ah-NEE-mee-ah) Condition in which the bone marrow is unable to produce sufficient red cells, white cells, and platelets.

apnea (AP-nee-ah) Absence of spontaneous respiration.

apocrine (AP-oh-krin) Apocrine sweat glands that open into the hair follicle.

apoptosis (AP-op-TOH-sis) Programmed normal cell death.

appendicitis (ah-pen-dih-SIGH-tis) Inflammation of the appendix.

appendix (ah-PEN-dicks) Small blind projection from the pouch of the cecum.

aqueous humor (AYK-wee-us HEW-mor) Watery liquid in the anterior and posterior chambers of the eye.

arachnoid mater (ah-RAK-noyd MAY-ter) Weblike middle layer of the three meninges.

areola (ah-REE-oh-luh) Circular reddish area surrounding the nipple.

arrhythmia (ah-RITH-mee-ah) An abnormal heart rhythm.

arteriography (ar-teer-ee-OG-rah-fee) X-ray visualization of an artery after injection of contrast material.

arteriole (ar-TEER-ee-ole) Small terminal artery leading into the capillary network.

arteriosclerosis (ar-TEER-ee-oh-skler-OH-sis) Hardening of the arteries.

arteriosclerotic (ar-TEER-ee-oh-skler-OT-ik) Pertaining to or suffering from arteriosclerosis.

arteriovenous malformation (ar-TEER-ee-oh-VEE-nus mal-for-MAY-shun) An abnormal communication between an artery and a vein.

artery (AR-ter-ee) Thick-walled blood vessel carrying blood away from the heart.

arthrocentesis (AR-throh-sen-TEE-sis) Withdrawal of fluid from a joint through a needle.

arthrodesis (AR-throh-DEE-sis) Fixation or stiffening of a joint by surgery.

arthrography (ar-THROG-rah-fee) X-ray of a joint taken after the injection of a contrast medium into the joint.

arthroplasty (AR-throh-plas-tee) Surgery to restore as far as possible the function of a joint.

arthroscope (AR-throh-skope) Endoscope used to examine the interior of a joint.

arthroscopy (ar-THROS-koh-pee) Visual examination of the interior of a joint.

articulation (ar-tik-you-LAY-shun) Joint formed to allow movement.

asbestosis (as-bes-TOH-sis) Lung disease caused by the inhalation of asbestos particles.

ascites (ah-SIGH-teez) Accumulation of fluid in the abdominal cavity.

aspartate aminotransferase (AST) (as-PAR-tate ah-MEE-noh-TRANS-fer-aze) Enzyme that is found in liver cells and leaks out into the bloodstream when the cells are damaged, enabling liver damage to be diagnosed.

aspiration (AS-pih-RAY-shun) Removal by suction of fluid or gas from a body cavity.

assistive device (ah-SIS-tiv dee-VICE) Tool, software, or hardware to assist in performing daily activities.

asthma (AZ-mah) Episodes of breathing difficulty due to narrowed or obstructed airways.

astigmatism (ah-STIG-mah-tism) Inability to focus light rays that enter the eye in different planes.

astrocyte (ASS-troh-site) Star-shaped connective tissue cell in the nervous system.

asystole (ay-SIS-toh-lee) Absence of contractions of the heart.

ataxia (a-TAK-see-ah) Inability to coordinate muscle activity, leading to jerky movements.

atelectasis (at-el-EK-tah-sis) Collapse of part of a lung.

atherectomy (ath-er-EK-toh-mee) Surgical removal of the atheroma.

atheroma (ath-er-ROH-mah) Lipid deposit in the lining of an artery.

atherosclerosis (ATH-er-oh-skler-OH-sis) Atheroma in arteries.

athetosis (ath-eh-TOH-sis) Slow, writhing involuntary movements.

atom (AT-om) A small unit of matter.

atopy (AY-toh-pee) State of hypersensitivity to an allergen; allergic.

atrioventricular (AV) (AY-tree-oh-ven-TRIK-you-lar) Pertaining to both the atrium and the ventricle.

GLOSSARY

atrium (AY-tree-um) Chamber where blood enters the heart on both right and left sides. Plural *atria*.

atrophy (AT-roh-fee) The wasting away or diminished volume of tissue, an organ, or a body part.

atropine (AT-roh-peen) Pharmacologic agent used to dilate pupils.

attenuated (ah-TEN-you-ay-ted) Weakened.

audiologist (aw-dee-OL-oh-jist) Specialist in evaluation of hearing function.

audiology (aw-dee-OL-oh-jee) Study of hearing disorders.

audiometer (aw-dee-OM-eh-ter) Instrument to measure hearing.

auditory (AW-dih-tor-ee) Pertaining to the sense or the organs of hearing.

aura (AWE-rah) Sensory experience preceding an epileptic seizure or a migraine headache.

auricle (AW-ri-kul) The shell-like external ear.

auscultation (aws-kul-TAY-shun) Diagnostic method of listening to body sounds with a stethoscope.

autoantibody (aw-toh-AN-tee-bod-ee) Antibody produced in response to an antigen from the host's own tissue.

autograft (AWE-toh-graft) A graft using tissue taken from the individual who is receiving the graft.

autoimmune (aw-toh-im-YUNE) Immune reaction directed against a person's own tissue.

autologous (awe-TOL-oh-gus) Blood transfusion with the same person as donor and recipient.

autolysis (awe-TOL-ih-sis) Self-destruction of cells by enzymes within the cells.

autonomic (awe-toh-NOM-ik) Not voluntary; pertaining to the self-governing visceral motor division of the peripheral nervous system.

autopsy (AWE-top-see) Examination of the body and organs of a dead person to determine the cause of death.

avascular (ay-VAS-cue-lar) Without a blood supply.

axilla (ak-SIL-ah) Medical name for the armpit. Plural *axillae*.

axon (AK-son) Single process of a nerve cell carrying nervous impulses away from the cell body.

azotemia (az-oh-TEE-me-ah) Excess nitrogenous waste products in the blood.

B

bacterium (bak-TEER-ee-um) A unicellular, simple, microscopic organism. Plural *bacteria*.

balanitis (bal-ah-NIE-tis) Inflammation of the glans and prepuce of the penis.

bariatric (bar-ee-AT-rik) Treatment of obesity.

basal metabolic rate (BAY-sal met-ah-BOL-ic RATE) Energy the body requires to function at rest.

basilar (BAS-ih-lar) Pertaining to the base of a structure.

basophil (BAY-so-fill) A basophil's granules attract a basic blue stain in the laboratory.

behavior (be-HAYV-yur) Mental or motor activity.

Bell palsy (BELL PAWL-zee) Paresis or paralysis of one side of the face.

benign (bee-NINE) Denoting the nonmalignant character of a neoplasm or illness.

beta (BAY-tah) Second letter in the Greek alphabet.

biceps brachii (BIE-sepz BRAY-kee-eye) A muscle of the upper arm that has two heads or points of origin on the scapula.

biconcave (BIE-kon-KAVE) Having a hollowed surface on both sides of a structure.

bicuspid (by-KUSS-pid) Having two points; a bicuspid heart valve has two flaps, and a bicuspid (premolar) tooth has two points.

bifocal (bi-FOH-cal) Two powers on lens.

bilateral (by-LAT-er-al) On two sides; for example, in both ears.

bile (BILE) Fluid secreted by the liver into the duodenum.

bile acids (BILE ASS-ids) Steroids synthesized from cholesterol.

biliary (BILL-ee-air-ee) Pertaining to bile or the biliary tract.

bilirubin (bill-ee-RU-bin) Bile pigment formed in the liver from hemoglobin.

biofeedback (bie-oh-FEED-bak) Training techniques to achieve voluntary control of responses to stimuli.

biomarker (BIE-oh-MARK-er) A biological marker or product by which a cell can be identified.

biopsy (BIE-op-see) Removing tissue from a living person for laboratory examination.

biopsy removal (BI-op-see re-MUV-al) Used for small tumors when complete removal provides tissue for a biopsy and cures the lesion. Also called *excisional biopsy*.

bipolar disorder (bi-POH-lar dis-OR-der) A mood disorder with alternating episodes of depression and mania.

bladder (BLAD-er) Hollow sac that holds fluid; for example, urine or bile.

blastocyst (BLAS-toh-sist) The developing embryo during the first 2 weeks.

blepharitis (blef-ah-RIE-tis) Inflammation of the eyelid.

blepharoptosis (BLEF-ah-rop-TOH-sis) Drooping of the upper eyelid.

blood-brain barrier (BBB) (BLUD BRAYN BAIR-ee-er) A selective mechanism that protects the brain from toxins and infections.

bolus (BOH-lus) Single mass of a substance.

botulism (BOT-you-lizm) Food poisoning caused by the neurotoxin produced by *Clostridium botulinum*.

bovine spongiform encephalopathy (BOH-vine SPON-jee-form en-sef-ah-LOP-ah-thee) Disease of cattle (mad cow disease) that can be transmitted to humans, causing Creutzfeldt-Jakob disease.

bowel (BOUGH-el) Another name for intestine.

brace (BRAYS) Appliance to support a part of the body in its correct position.

brachial (BRAY-kee-al) Pertaining to the arm.

brachialis (BRAY-kee-al-is) Muscle that lies underneath the biceps and is the strongest flexor of the forearm.

brachiocephalic (BRAY-kee-oh-seh-FAL-ik) Pertaining to the head and arm, as an artery supplying blood to both.

brachioradialis (BRAY-kee-oh-RAY-dee-al-is) Muscle that helps flex the forearm.

brachytherapy (brah-kee-THAIR-ah-pee) Radiation therapy in which the source of irradiation is implanted in the tissue to be treated.

bradycardia (brad-ee-KAR-dee-ah) Slow heart rate (below 60 beats per minute).

bradypnea (brad-ip-NEE-ah) Slow breathing.

brainstem (BRAYN-stem) Region of the brain that includes the thalamus, pineal gland, pons, fourth ventricle, and medulla oblongata.

breech (BREECH) Buttocks-first presentation of the fetus at delivery.

bronchiectasis (brong-kee-EK-tah-sis) Chronic dilation of the bronchi following inflammatory disease and obstruction.

bronchiole (BRONG-key-ole) Increasingly smaller subdivisions of bronchi.

bronchiolitis (brong-kee-oh-LIE-tis) Inflammation of the small bronchioles.

bronchoalveolar (BRONG-koh-al-VEE-oh-lar) Pertaining to the bronchi and alveoli.

bronchoconstriction (BRONG-koh-kon-STRIK-shun) Reduction in diameter of a bronchus.

bronchodilator (BRONG-koh-die-LAY-tor) Agent that increases the diameter of a bronchus.

bronchogenic (brong-koh-JEN-ik) Arising from a bronchus.

bronchopneumonia (BRONG-koh-new-MOH-nee-ah) Acute inflammation of the walls of smaller bronchioles with spread to lung parenchyma.

bronchoscope (BRONG-koh-skope) Endoscope used for bronchoscopy.

bronchoscopy (brong-KOS-koh-pee) Examination of the interior of the tracheobronchial tree with an endoscope.

bronchus (BRONG-kuss) One of two subdivisions of the trachea. Plural *bronchi.*

buffer (BUFF-er) Substance that resists a change in pH.

bulbourethral (BUL-boh-you-REE-thral) Pertaining to the bulbous penis and urethra.

bulla (BULL-ah) Bubblelike dilated structure. Plural *bullae.*

bundle of Hiss (BUN-del of Hiss) Pathway for electrical signals to be transmitted to the ventricles of the heart.

bunion (BUN-yun) A swelling at the base of the big toe.

bursa (BURR-sah) A closed sac containing synovial fluid.

bursitis (burr-SIGH-tis) Inflammation of a bursa.

C

calcaneus (kal-KAY-nee-us) Bone of the tarsus that forms the heel.

calcimimetic (kal-sih-mi-MET-ick) Substance that imitates calcium.

calcitonin (kal-sih-TONE-in) Thyroid hormone that moves calcium from blood to bones.

calculus (KAL-kyu-lus) Small stone. Plural *calculi.*

callus (KAL-us) The mass of fibrous connective tissue that forms at a fracture site and becomes the foundation for the formation of new bone.

calyx (KAY-licks) Funnel-shaped structure. Plural *calyces.*

cancellous (KAN-sell-us) Bone that has a spongy or latticelike structure.

cancer (KAN-ser) General term for a malignant neoplasm.

Candida **(KAN-did-ah)** A yeastlike fungus.

candidiasis (kan-dih-DIE-ah-sis) Infection with the yeastlike fungus *Candida.* Also called *thrush.*

canker; canker sore (KANG-ker SOAR) Nonmedical term for aphthous ulcer. Also called *mouth ulcer.*

canthus (KAN-thus) Corner of the eye where the upper and lower lids meet. Plural *canthi.*

capillary (KAP-ih-lair-ee) Minute blood vessel between the arterial and venous systems.

capsule (KAP-syul) Fibrous tissue layer surrounding a joint or some other structure; or a solid dosage form in which a drug is enclosed in a hard or soft shell.

carbohydrate (kar-boh-HIGH-drate) Group of organic food compounds that includes sugars, starch, glycogen, and cellulose.

carboxypeptidase (kar-box-ee-PEP-tid-ase) Enzyme that breaks down protein.

carbuncle (KAR-bunk-ul) Infection of many furuncles in a small area, often on the back of the neck.

carcinogen (kar-SIN-oh-jen) Cancer-producing agent.

carcinogenesis (KAR-sin-oh-JEN-eh-sis) Origin and development of cancer.

carcinoma (kar-sih-NOH-mah) A cancerous (malignant) and invasive epithelial tumor.

carcinoma in situ (kar-sih-NOH-mah IN SIGH-tyu) Carcinoma that has not invaded surrounding tissues.

cardiac (KAR-dee-ak) Pertaining to the heart.

cardiogenic (KAR-dee-oh-JEN-ik) Of cardiac origin.

cardiologist (kar-dee-OL-oh-jist) A medical specialist in diagnosis and treatment of the heart (cardiology).

cardiology (kar-dee-OL-oh-jee) Medical specialty of diseases of the heart.

cardiomegaly (KAR-dee-oh-MEG-ah-lee) Enlargement of the heart.

cardiomyopathy (KAR-dee-oh-my-OP-ah-thee) Disease of heart muscle, the myocardium.

cardiopulmonary resuscitation (KAR-dee-oh-PUL-moh-nair-ee ree-sus-ih-TAY-shun) The attempt to restore cardiac and pulmonary function.

cardiovascular (KAR-dee-oh-VAS-kyu-lar) Pertaining to the heart and blood vessels.

cardioversion (KAR-dee-oh-VER-shun) Restoration of a normal heart rhythm by electrical shock. Also called *defibrillation.*

cardioverter (KAR-dee-oh-VER-ter) Device used to generate electrical shock for cardioversion.

caries (KARE-eez) Bacterial destruction of teeth.

carotid (kah-ROT-id) Main artery of the neck.

carpal (KAR-pal) Pertaining to the wrist.

cartilage (KAR-tih-lij) Nonvascular, firm connective tissue found mostly in joints.

cast (KAST) A cylindrical mold formed by materials in kidney tubules.

catabolism (kah-TAB-oh-lizm) Breakdown of complex substances into simpler ones as a part of metabolism.

cataplexy (KAT-ah-plek-see) Sudden loss of muscle tone with brief paralysis.

cataract (KAT-ah-rakt) Complete or partial opacity of the lens.

catatonia (kat-ah-TOH-nee-ah) Syndrome characterized by physical immobility and mental stupor.

catecholamine (kat-eh-KOHL-ah-meen) Any major hormones in stress response; includes epinephrine and norepinephrine.

catheter (KATH-eh-ter) Hollow tube that allows passage of fluid into or out of a body cavity, organ, or vessel.

catheterization (KATH-eh-ter-ih-ZAY-shun) Introduction of a catheter.

cauda equina (KAW-dah eh-KWIE-nah) Bundle of spinal nerves in the vertebral canal below the ending of the spinal cord.

caudal (KAW-dal) Pertaining to or nearer to the tail.

cautery (KAW-ter-ee) Agent or device used to burn or scar a tissue.

cavernosa (kav-er-NOH-sah) Resembling a cave.

cavity (KAV-ih-tee) Hollow space or body compartment. Plural *cavities*.

cecum (SEE-kum) Blind pouch that is the first part of the large intestine.

celiac disease (SEE-lee-ak diz-EEZ) Disease caused by sensitivity to gluten.

cell (SELL) The smallest unit capable of independent existence.

cellular (SELL-you-lar) Pertaining to a cell.

cellulitis (sell-you-LIE-tis) Infection of subcutaneous connective tissue.

cephalic (se-FAL-ik) Pertaining to or nearer to the head.

cerebellum (ser-eh-BELL-um) The most posterior area of the brain.

cerebrospinal fluid (CSF) (SER-eh-broh-SPY-nal FLU-id) Fluid formed in the ventricles of the brain; surrounds the brain and spinal cord.

cerebrum (ser-EE-brum) The major portion of the brain divided into two hemispheres (cerebral hemispheres) separated by a fissure.

cerumen (seh-ROO-men) Waxy secretion of the ceruminous glands of the external ear.

cervical (SER-vih-kal) Pertaining to the cervix or to the neck region.

cesarean section (seh-ZAH-ree-an SEK-shun) Extraction of the fetus through an incision in the abdomen and uterine wall. Also called *C-section*.

chalazion (kah-LAY-zee-on) Cyst on the outer edge of an eyelid.

chancre (SHAN-ker) Primary lesion of syphilis.

chancroid (SHAN-kroyd) Infectious, painful, ulcerative STD not related to syphilis.

Charcot joint (SHAR-koh JOYNT) Bone and joint destruction secondary to a neuropathy and loss of sensation.

chemotherapy (KEE-moh-THAIR-ah-pee) Treatment using chemical agents.

chiasm (KIE-asm) X-shaped crossing of the two optic nerves at the base of the brain. Alternative term *chiasma*.

chickenpox (CHICK-en-pocks) Acute, contagious viral disease. Also called *varicella*.

chiropractor (kie-roh-PRAK-tor) Practitioner of chiropractic.

chlamydia (klah-MID-ee-ah) A species of bacteria causing a sexually transmitted disease.

chlorine (KLOR-een) A toxic agent used as a disinfectant and bleaching agent.

cholecystitis (KOH-leh-sis-TIE-tis) Inflammation of the gallbladder.

cholecystokinin (KOH-leh-sis-toh-KIE-nin) Hormone secreted by the lining of the intestine that stimulates secretion of pancreatic enzymes and contraction of the gallbladder.

choledocholithiasis (koh-LED-oh-koh-lih-THIGH-ah-sis) Presence of a gallstone in the common bile duct.

cholelithiasis (KOH-leh-lih-THIGH-ah-sis) Condition of having bile stones (gallstones).

cholelithotomy (KOH-leh-lih-THOT-oh-mee) Surgical removal of a gallstone(s).

cholesteatoma (koh-less-tee-ah-TOH-mah) Yellow, waxy tumor arising in the middle ear.

cholesterol (koh-LESS-ter-ol) Steroid formed in liver cells; it is the most abundant steroid in tissues and circulates in the plasma attached to proteins of different densities.

chondromalacia (KON-droh-mah-LAY-shee-ah) Softening and degeneration of cartilage.

chondrosarcoma (KON-droh-sar-KOH-mah) Cancer arising from cartilage cells.

chordae tendineae (KOR-dee ten-DIN-ee-ee) Tendinous cords attaching the bicuspid and tricuspid valves to the heart wall.

chorea (kor-EE-ah) Involuntary, irregular spasms of limb and facial muscles.

choriocarcinoma (KOH-ree-oh-kar-sih-NOH-mah) Highly malignant cancer in a testis or ovary.

chorion (KOH-ree-on) The fetal membrane that forms the placenta.

chorionic (koh-ree-ON-ik) Pertaining to the chorion.

chorionic villus (koh-ree-ON-ik VILL-us) Vascular process of the embryonic chorion to form the placenta.

choroid (KOR-oid) Region of the retina and uvea.

chromatin (KROH-ma-tin) Substance composed of DNA that forms chromosomes during cell division.

chromosome (KROH-moh-sohm) Body in the nucleus that contains DNA and genes.

chronic (KRON-ik) Describes a persistent, long-term disease.

chronotropic (KRONE-oh-TROH-pik) Affecting the heart rate.

chyle (KILE) A milky fluid that results from the digestion and absorption of fats in the small intestine.

chyme (KIME) Semifluid, partially digested food passed from the stomach into the duodenum.

chymotrypsin (kie-moh-TRIP-sin) Trypsin found in chyme.

ciliary body (SILL-ee-air-ee BOD-ee) Muscles that make the eye lens thicker and thinner.

cilium (SILL-ee-um) Hairlike motile projection from the surface of a cell. Plural *cilia*.

circulation (SER-kyu-LAY-shun) Continuous movement of blood through the heart and blood vessels.

circumcision (ser-kum-SIZH-un) To remove part or all of the prepuce.

circumduction (ser-kum-DUK-shun) Movement of an extremity in a circular motion.

cirrhosis (sir-ROH-sis) Extensive fibrotic liver disease.

claudication (klaw-dih-KAY-shun) Intermittent leg pain and limping.

claustrophobia (klaw-stroh-FOH-bee-ah) Pathologic fear of being trapped in a confined space.

clavicle (KLAV-ih-kul) Curved bone that forms the anterior part of the pectoral girdle.

clitoris (KLIT-oh-ris) Erectile organ of the vulva.

clonic (KLON-ik) State of rapid successions of muscular contractions and relaxations.

closed fracture (KLOHZD FRAK-chur) A bone is broken, but the skin over it is intact.

Clostridium botulinum **(klos-TRID-ee-um bot-you-LIE-num)** Bacterium that causes food poisoning.

clot (KLOT) The mass of fibrin and cells that is produced in a wound.

coagulation (koh-ag-you-LAY-shun) The process of blood clotting.

coagulopathy (koh-ag-you-LOP-ah-thee) Disorder of blood clotting. Plural *coagulopathies.*

coarctation (koh-ark-TAY-shun) Constriction, stenosis, particularly of the aorta.

coccyx (KOK-siks) Small tailbone at the lower end of the vertebral column.

cochlea (KOK-lee-ah) An intricate combination of passages; used to describe the part of the inner ear used in hearing.

cochlear (KOK-lee-ar) Pertaining to the cochlea.

cognition (kog-NIH-shun) Process of acquiring knowledge through thinking, learning, and memory.

cognitive (KOG-nih-tiv) Pertaining to the mental activities of thinking and learning.

cognitive behavioral therapy (CBT) (KOG-nih-tiv be-HAYV-yur-al THAIR-ah-pee) Psychotherapy that emphasizes thoughts and attitudes in one's behavior.

cognitive processing therapy (KOG-nih-tiv PROS-es-ing THAIR-ah-pee) Psychotherapy to build skills to deal with effects of the trauma in other areas of life.

coitus (KOH-it-us) Sexual intercourse.

colic (KOL-ik) Spasmodic, crampy pains in the abdomen; in young infants, persistent crying and irritability thought to be arising from pain in the intestines.

colitis (koh-LIE-tis) Inflammation of the colon.

collagen (KOL-ah-jen) Major protein of connective tissue, cartilage, and bone.

collateral (koh-LAT-er-al) Situated at the side, often to bypass an obstruction.

Colles fracture (KOL-ez FRAK-chur) Fracture of the distal radius at the wrist.

colloid (COLL-oyd) Liquid containing suspended particles.

colon (KOH-lon) The large intestine, extending from the cecum to the rectum.

colonoscopy (koh-lon-OSS-koh-pee) Examination of the inside of the colon by endoscopy.

color Doppler ultrasonography (DOP-ler UL-trah-soh-NOG-rah-fee) Computer-generated color image to show directions of blood flow.

colostomy (ko-LOS-toh-mee) Artificial opening from the colon to the outside of the body.

colostrum (koh-LOSS-trum) The first breast secretion at the end of pregnancy.

colpopexy (KOL-poh-pek-see) Surgical fixation of the vagina.

coma (KOH-mah) State of deep unconsciousness.

comedo (KOM-ee-doh) A whitehead or blackhead caused by too much sebum and too many keratin cells blocking the hair follicle. Plural *comedones.*

comminuted fracture (KOM-ih-nyu-ted FRAK-chur) A fracture in which the bone is broken into pieces.

comorbidity (koh-mor-BID-ih-tee) Presence of two or more diseases at the same time.

complement (KOM-pleh-ment) Group of proteins in serum destroy bacteria and other cells.

complete fracture (kom-PLEET FRAK-chur) A bone is fractured into at least two separate pieces.

compliance (kom-PLY-ance) Measure of the capacity of a chamber or hollow viscus to expand; for example, compliance of the lungs.

compression (kom-PRESH-un) A squeezing together so as to increase density and/or decrease a dimension of a structure.

compression fracture (kom-PRESH-un FRAK-chur) Fracture of a vertebra causing loss of height of the vertebra.

compulsion (kom-PUL-shun) Uncontrollable impulses to perform an act repetitively.

compulsive (kom-PUL-siv) Possessing uncontrollable impulses to perform an act repetitively.

concave (con-CAVE or CON-cave) Curve inward.

conception (kon-SEP-shun) Fertilization of the egg by sperm to form a zygote.

concha (KON-kah) Shell-shaped bone on the medial wall of the nasal cavity. Plural *conchae.*

concussion (kon-KUSH-un) Mild head injury.

condom (KON-dom) A sheath or cover for the penis or vagina to prevent conception and infection.

conduction (kon-DUCK-shun) Process of transmitting energy.

conductive hearing loss (kon-DUK-tiv HEER-ing LOSS) Hearing loss caused by lesions in the outer ear or middle ear.

condyle (KON-dile) Large, smooth, rounded expansion of the end of a bone that forms a joint with another bone.

condyloma (kon-dih-LOH-ma) Warty growth on external genitalia. Plural *condylomata.*

confusion (kon-FEW-zhun) Mental state in which environmental stimuli are not processed appropriately.

congenital (kon-JEN-ih-tal) Present at birth, either inherited or due to an event during gestation up to the moment of birth.

congruent (KON-gru-ent) Coinciding or agreeing with.

conization (koh-nih-ZAY-shun) Surgical excision of a cone-shaped piece of tissue.

conjunctiva (kon-junk-TIE-vah) Inner lining of the eyelids.

conjunctivitis (kon-junk-tih-VIE-tis) Inflammation of the conjunctiva.

Conn syndrome (KON SIN-drohm) Condition caused by excessive secretion of aldosterone. Also called *aldosteronism.*

consciousness (KON-shus-ness) The state of being aware of and responsive to the environment.

constipation (kon-stih-PAY-shun) Hard, infrequent bowel movements.

contagious (kon-TAY-jus) Able to be transmitted, as infections transmitted from person to person or from person to air or surface to person.

contaminate (kon-TAM-in-ate) To cause the presence of an infectious agent to be on any surface.

contraception (kon-trah-SEP-shun) Prevention of conception.

contraceptive (kon-trah-SEP-tiv) An agent that prevents conception.

contract (kon-TRAKT) Draw together or shorten.

contracture (kon-TRAK-chur) Muscle shortening due to spasm or fibrosis.

contrecoup (KON-treh-koo) Injury to the brain at a point directly opposite the point of original contact.

contusion (kon-TOO-zhun) Bruising of a tissue, including the brain.

conversion disorder (kon-VER-shun dis-OR-der) An unconscious emotional conflict is expressed as physical symptoms with no organic basis.

convex (CON-vecks or con-VECKS) Curved outward.

cor pulmonale (KOR pul-moh-NAH-lee) Right-sided heart failure arising from chronic lung disease.

coreceptor (koh-ree-SEP-tor) Cell surface protein that enhances the sensitivity of an antigen receptor.

cornea (KOR-nee-ah) The central, transparent part of the outer coat of the eye covering the iris and pupil.

coronal (KOR-oh-nal) Pertaining to the vertical plane dividing the body into anterior and posterior portions.

coronal plane (KOR-oh-nal PLAIN) Vertical plane dividing the body into anterior and posterior portions.

coronary circulation (KOR-oh-nair-ee SER-kyu-LAY-shun) Blood flow through the vessels supplying the heart.

corpus (KOR-pus) Major part of a structure. Plural *corpora*.

corpus albicans (KOR-pus AL-bih-kanz) An atrophied corpus luteum.

corpus callosum (KOR-pus kah-LOH-sum) Bridge of nerve fibers connecting the two cerebral hemispheres.

corpus luteum (KOR-pus LOO-tee-um) Yellow structure formed at the site of a ruptured ovarian follicle.

cortex (KOR-teks) Outer portion of an organ, such as bone; *or* gray covering of cerebral hemispheres. Plural *cortices*.

corticoid (KOR-tih-koyd) One of the steroid hormones produced by the adrenal cortex. Also called *corticosteroid*.

corticosteroid (KOR-tih-koh-STEHR-oyd) A hormone produced by the adrenal cortex.

corticotropin (KOR-tih-koh-TROH-pin) Pituitary hormone that stimulates the cortex of the adrenal gland to secrete corticosteroids.

cortisol (KOR-tih-sol) One of the glucocorticoids produced by the adrenal cortex; has anti-inflammatory effects. Also called *hydrocortisone*.

coryza (koh-RIE-zah) Viral inflammation of the mucous membrane of the nose. Also called *rhinitis*.

cosmetic (koz-MET-ik) A concern for appearance.

coup (KOO) Injury to the brain occurring directly under the skull at the point of impact.

cranial (KRAY-nee-al) Pertaining to the skull.

cranium (KRAY-nee-um) The upper part of the skull that encloses and protects the brain.

craving (KRAY-ving) Deep longing or desire.

creatine kinase (KREE-ah-teen KIE-naze) Enzyme elevated in plasma following heart muscle damage in myocardial infarction.

creatinine (kree-AT-ih-neen) Breakdown product of the skeletal muscle protein creatine.

cretinism (KREH-tin-ism) Condition of severe congenital hypothyroidism.

Creutzfeldt-Jakob disease (KROITS-felt-YAK-op diz-EEZ) Progressive incurable neurologic disease caused by infectious prions.

cricoid (CRY-koyd) Ring-shaped cartilage in the larynx.

crista ampullaris (KRIS-tah am-pull-AIR-is) Mound of hair cells and gelatinous material in the ampulla of a semicircular canal.

criterion (krie-TEER-ee-on) Standard or rule for judging. Plural *criteria*.

Crohn's disease (KRONES diz-EEZ) Inflammatory bowel disease with narrowing and thickening of the terminal small bowel. Also called *regional enteritis*.

croup (KROOP) Infection of the upper airways in children; characterized by a barking cough. Also called *laryngotracheobronchitis*.

crown (KROWN) Part of tooth above the gum.

crowning (KROWN-ing) During childbirth, when the maximum diameter of the baby's head comes through the vulvar ring.

cruciate (KRU-shee-ate) Shaped like a cross.

cryopexy (CRY-oh-PEK-see) Repair of a detached retina by freezing it to surrounding tissue.

cryosurgery (cry-oh-SUR-jer-ee) Use of liquid nitrogen or argon gas in a probe to freeze and kill abnormal tissue.

cryotherapy (CRY-oh-THAIR-ah-pee) The use of cold in the treatment of injury.

cryptorchism (krip-TOR-kizm) Failure of one or both testes to descend into the scrotum.

culture (KUL-chur) The growth of microorganisms on or in media.

curative (KYUR-ah-tiv) That which heals or cures.

curettage (kyu-reh-TAHZH) Scraping of the interior of a cavity.

curette (kyu-RET) Scoop-shaped instrument for scraping the interior of a cavity or removing new growths.

Cushing syndrome (KUSH-ing SIN-drome) Hypersecretion of cortisol (hydrocortisone) by the adrenal cortex.

cuspid (KUSS-pid) Tooth with one point.

cutaneous (kyu-TAY-nee-us) Pertaining to the skin.

cuticle (KEW-tih-cul) Nonliving epidermis at the base of the fingernails and toenails, and the outer layer of hair.

cyanosis (sigh-ah-NOH-sis) Blue discoloration of the skin, lips, and nail beds due to low levels of oxygen in the blood.

cyst (SIST) An abnormal, fluid-containing sac.

cystic (SIS-tik) Relating to a cyst.

cystic fibrosis (CF) (SIS-tik fie-BROH-sis) Genetic disease in which excessive viscid mucus obstructs passages, including in the pancreas and in the bronchi of the lungs.

cystitis (sis-TIE-tis) Inflammation of the urinary bladder.

cystocele (SIS-toh-seal) Hernia of the bladder into the vagina.

cystopexy (SIS-toh-pek-see) Surgical procedure to support the urinary bladder.

cystoscope (SIS-toh-skope) An endoscope inserted to view the inside of the bladder.

cystoscopy (sis-TOS-koh-pee) The process of using a cystoscope.

cystourethrogram (sis-toh-you-REETH-roh-gram) X-ray image during voiding to show the structure and function of the bladder and urethra.

cytogenetics (SIGH-toh-jeh-NET-iks) Study of chromosomal abnormalities in a cell.

cytokine (SIGH-toh-kine) Proteins produced by different cells that communicate with other cells in the immune system.

cytology (sigh-TOL-oh-jee) Study of the cell.

cytoplasm (SIGH-toh-plazm) Clear, gelatinous substance that forms the substance of a cell except for the nucleus.

cytosol (SIGH-toe-sawl) Liquid portion of the cell between the cell membrane and the nucleus.

cytotoxic (sigh-toh-TOK-sik) Destructive to cells.

D

dacryocystitis (DAK-ree-oh-sis-TIE-tis) Inflammation of the lacrimal sac.

dacryostenosis (DAK-ree-oh-steh-NOH-sis) Narrowing of the nasolacrimal duct.

dandruff (DAN-druff) Seborrheic scales from the scalp.

death (DETH) Total and permanent cessation of all vital functions.

debridement (day-BREED-mon) The removal of injured or necrotic tissue.

decongestant (dee-con-JESS-tant) Agent that reduces the swelling and fluid in the nose and sinuses.

decubitus ulcer (de-KYU-bit-us UL-ser) Sore caused by lying down for long periods of time.

decussate (DEE-kuss-ate) Cross over like the arms of an "X."

defecation (def-eh-KAY-shun) Evacuation of feces from the rectum and anus.

defect (DEE-fect) An absence, malformation, or imperfection.

defibrillation (dee-fib-rih-LAY-shun) Restoration of uncontrolled twitching of cardiac muscle fibers to normal rhythm.

defibrillator (dee-FIB-rih-lay-tor) Instrument for defibrillation.

deformity (dee-FOR-mih-tee) A permanent structural deviation from the normal.

degenerative (dee-JEN-er-a-tiv) Relating to the deterioration of a structure.

deglutition (dee-glue-TISH-un) The act of swallowing.

dehydration (dee-high-DRAY-shun) Process of losing body water.

dehydroepiandrosterone (DHEA) (dee-HIGH-droh-eh-pee-an-DROS-ter-ohn) Precursor to testosterone; produced in the adrenal cortex.

delirium (deh-LIR-ee-um) Acute altered state of consciousness with agitation and disorientation; condition is reversible.

deltoid (DEL-toyd) Large, fan-shaped muscle connecting the scapula and clavicle to the humerus.

delusion (dee-LOO-shun) Fixed, unyielding, false belief or judgment held despite strong evidence to the contrary.

dementia (deh-MEN-shee-ah) Chronic, progressive, irreversible loss of the mind's cognitive and intellectual functions.

demyelination (dee-MY-eh-lin-A-shun) Process of losing the myelin sheath of a nerve fiber.

dendrite (DEN-dright) Branched extension of the nerve cell body that receives nervous stimuli.

dental (DEN-tal) Pertaining to the teeth.

dentin (DEN-tin) Dense, ivorylike substance located under the enamel in a tooth.

deoxyribonucleic acid (DNA) (dee-OCK-see-RYE-boh-noo-KLEE-ik ASS-id) Source of hereditary characteristics found in chromosomes.

dependence (dee-PEN-dense) State of needing someone or something.

depressant (dee-PRESS-ant) Substance that diminishes activity, sensation, or tone.

depression (dee-PRESH-un) Mental disorder with feelings of deep sadness and despair.

dermatitis (der-mah-TYE-tis) Inflammation of the skin.

dermatologist (der-mah-TOL-oh-jist) Medical specialist in diseases of the skin.

dermatology (der-mah-TOL-oh-jee) Medical specialty concerned with disorders of the skin.

dermatome (DER-mah-tome) The area of skin supplied by a single spinal nerve; alternatively, an instrument used for cutting thin slices.

dermatomyositis (DER-mah-toh-MY-oh-SIGH-tis) Inflammation of the skin and muscles.

dermis (DER-miss) Connective tissue layer of the skin beneath the epidermis.

detoxification (dee-TOKS-ih-fih-KAY-shun) Removal of poison from a tissue or substance.

deviation (dee-vee-AY-shun) A turning aside from a normal course.

diabetes insipidus (die-ah-BEE-teez in-SIP-ih-dus) Excretion of large amounts of dilute urine as a result of inadequate ADH production.

diabetes mellitus (die-ah-BEE-teez MEL-ih-tus) Metabolic syndrome caused by absolute or relative insulin deficiency and/or insulin ineffectiveness.

diabetic (die-ah-BET-ik) Pertaining to or suffering from diabetes.

diagnosis (die-ag-NO-sis) The determination of the cause of a disease. Plural *diagnoses.*

diagnostic (die-ag-NOS-tik) Pertaining to or establishing a diagnosis.

dialysis (die-AL-ih-sis) An artificial method of filtration to remove excess waste materials and water from the body.

dialyzer (DIE-ah-lie-zer) Machine for dialysis.

diaphoresis (DIE-ah-foh-REE-sis) Abnormal amount of sweat or perspiration.

diaphoretic (DIE-ah-foh-RET-ic) Pertaining to sweat or perspiration.

diaphragm (DIE-ah-fram) A ring and dome-shaped material inserted in the vagina to prevent pregnancy; *or* the musculomembranous partition separating the abdominal and thoracic cavities.

diaphysis (die-AF-ih-sis) The shaft of a long bone.

diarrhea (die-ah-REE-ah) Abnormally frequent and loose stools.

diascopy (die-AS-koh-pee) Examination of superficial skin lesions with pressure.

diastasis (die-ASS-tah-sis) Separation of normally joined parts.

diastole (die-AS-toh-lee) Dilation of heart cavities, during which they fill with blood.

diffusion (dih-FYU-zhun) The means by which small particles move between tissues.

DiGeorge syndrome (dee-JORJ SIN-drome) Congenital absence of the thymus gland.

digestion (die-JEST-shun) Breakdown of food into elements suitable for cell metabolism.

digestive (die-JEST-iv) Relating to digestion.

digital (DIJ-ih-tal) Pertaining to a finger or toe.

dilation (die-LAY-shun) Stretching or enlarging of an opening.

dioxin (die-OK-sin) Carcinogenic contaminant in pesticides.

diplegia (die-PLEE-jee-ah) Paralysis of all four limbs, with the two legs affected most severely.

disability (dis-ah-BILL-ih-tee) Diminished capacity to perform certain activities or functions.

disaccharide (die-SACK-ah-ride) A combination of two monosaccharides; for example, table sugar.

discrimination (DIS-krim-ih-NAY-shun) Ability to distinguish between different things.

dislocation (dis-loh-KAY-shun) The state of being completely out of joint.

displaced fracture (dis-PLAYSD FRAK-chur) A fracture in which the fragments are separated and are not in alignment.

disseminate (dih-SEM-in-ate) Widely scattered throughout the body or an organ.

dissociative identity disorder (dih-SOH-see-ah-tiv eye-DEN-tih-tee dis-OR-der) Mental disorder in which an individual's personality is separated from the rest, leading to multiple personalities.

distal (DISS-tal) Situated away from the center of the body.

distract (dis-TRAKT) To turn the mind away.

distractibility (dis-TRAK-ti-BILL-ih-tee) Inability to keep the mind on topic.

diuresis (die-you-REE-sis) Excretion of large volumes of urine.

diuretic (die-you-REH-tik) Agent that increases urine output.

diverticulitis (DIE-ver-tick-you-LIE-tis) Inflammation of the diverticula.

diverticulosis (DIE-ver-tick-you-LOH-sis) Presence of a number of small pouches in the wall of the large intestine.

diverticulum (die-ver-TICK-you-lum) A pouchlike opening or sac from a tubular structure (e.g., gut). Plural *diverticula*.

dizygotic (die-zie-GOT-ik) Twins from two separate zygotes.

dopamine (DOH-pah-meen) Neurotransmitter in some specific small areas of the brain.

dormant (DOR-mant) Inactive.

dorsal (DOR-sal) Pertaining to the back or situated behind.

dorsum (DOR-sum) Upper, posterior, or back surface.

Duchenne muscular dystrophy (DOO-shen MUSS-kyu-lar DISS-troh-fee) A condition with symmetrical weakness and wasting of pelvic, shoulder, and proximal limb muscles.

duct (DUKT) A tube to carry gas or fluid.

ductus deferens (DUK-tus DEH-fuh-renz) Tube that receives sperm from the epididymis. Also known as *vas deferens*.

duodenum (du-oh-DEE-num) The first part of the small intestine; approximately 12 finger-breadths (9 to 10 inches) in length.

Dupuytren contracture (du-pweh-TRAHN kon-TRAK-chur) A thickening and shortening of fibrous bands in the palm of the hand.

dura mater (DYU-rah MAY-ter) Hard, fibrous outer layer of the meninges.

dwarfism (DWORF-izm) Short stature due to underproduction of growth hormone.

dysentery (DIS-en-tare-ee) Disease with diarrhea, bowel spasms, fever, and dehydration.

dysfunctional (dis-FUNK-shun-al) Having difficulty in performing.

dysmenorrhea (dis-men-oh-REE-ah) Painful and difficult menstruation.

dysmorphic (dis-MOR-fik) Possessing a developmental structural defect.

dyspareunia (dis-pah-RUE-nee-ah) Pain during sexual intercourse.

dyspepsia (dis-PEP-see-ah) "Upset stomach," epigastric pain, nausea, and gas.

dysphagia (dis-FAY-jee-ah) Difficulty in swallowing.

dysplasia (dis-PLAY-zee-ah) Abnormal tissue formation.

dyspnea (disp-NEE-ah) Difficulty breathing.

dysrhythmia (dis-RITH-mee-ah) An abnormal heart rhythm.

dysuria (dis-YOU-ree-ah) Difficulty or pain with urination.

E

eccrine (EK-rin) Coiled sweat gland that occurs in skin all over the body.

echocardiography (EK-oh-kar-dee-OG-rah-fee) Ultrasound recording of heart function.

echoencephalography (EK-oh-en-sef-ah-LOG-rah-fee) Use of ultrasound in the diagnosis of intracranial lesions.

eclampsia (eh-KLAMP-see-uh) Convulsions in a patient with preeclampsia.

ectopic (ek-TOP-ik) Out of place, not in a normal position.

eczema (EK-zeh-mah) Inflammatory skin disease often with a serous discharge.

edema (ee-DEE-mah) Excessive accumulation of fluid in cells and tissues.

edematous (ee-DEM-ah-tus) Pertaining to or marked by edema.

effacement (ee-FACE-ment) Thinning of the cervix in relation to labor.

efferent (EF-eh-rent) Conducting impulses outward away from the brain or spinal cord.

effusion (eh-FYU-shun) Collection of fluid that has escaped from blood vessels into a cavity or tissues.

ejaculate (ee-JACK-you-late) To expel suddenly; *or* the semen expelled in ejaculation.

ejaculation (ee-JACK-you-LAY-shun) Process of expelling semen suddenly.

electrocardiogram (ECG or EKG) (ee-LEK-troh-KAR-dee-oh-gram) Record of the electrical signals of the heart.

electrocardiograph (ee-LEK-troh-KAR-dee-oh-graf) Machine that makes the electrocardiogram.

electroconvulsive therapy (ee-LEK-troh-kon-VUL-siv THAIR-ah-pee) Passage of electric current through the brain to produce convulsions and treat persistent depression, mania, and other disorders.

electrode (ee-LEK-trode) A device for conducting electricity.

electroencephalogram (EEG) (ee-LEK-troh-en-SEF-ah-loh-gram) Record of the electrical activity of the brain.

electroencephalography (ee-LEK-troh-en-SEF-ah-LOG-rah-fee) The process of recording the electrical activity of the brain.

electrolyte (ee-LEK-troh-lite) Substance that, when dissolved in a suitable medium, forms electrically charged particles.

electromagnetic (ee-LEK-troh-mag-NET-ik) Pertaining to energy propagated through matter and space.

electromyography (ee-LEK-troh-my-OG-rah-fee) Recording of electrical activity in muscle.

electroneurodiagnostic (ee-LEK-troh-NYUR-oh-die-ag-NOS-tik) Pertaining to the use of electricity in the diagnosis of a neurologic disorder.

elimination (e-lim-ih-NAY-shun) Removal of waste material from the digestive tract.

embolus (EM-boh-lus) Detached piece of thrombus, mass of bacteria, quantity of air, or foreign body that blocks a vessel.

embryo (EM-bree-oh) Developing organism from conception until the end of the eighth week.

embryonic (em-bree-ON-ic) Pertaining to the embryo.

emesis (EM-eh-sis) Vomit.

emmetropia (em-eh-TROH-pee-ah) Normal refractive condition of the eye.

empathy (EM-pah-thee) Ability to place yourself into the feelings, emotions, and reactions of another person.

emphysema (em-fih-SEE-mah) Dilation of respiratory bronchioles and alveoli.

empyema (EM-pie-EE-mah) Pus in a body cavity, particularly in the pleural cavity.

emulsify (ee-MUL-sih-fie) Break up into very small droplets to suspend in a solution (emulsion).

enamel (ee-NAM-el) Hard substance covering a tooth.

encephalitis (en-SEF-ah-LIE-tis) Inflammation of brain cells and tissues.

encephalomyelitis (en-SEF-ah-loh-MY-eh-LIE-tis) Inflammation of the brain and spinal cord.

endarterectomy (END-ar-ter-EK-toh-mee) Surgical removal of plaque from an artery.

endocarditis (EN-doh-kar-DIE-tis) Inflammation of the lining of the heart.

endocardium (EN-doh-KAR-dee-um) The inside lining of the heart.

endocrine (EN-doh-krin) Pertaining to a gland that produces an internal or hormonal secretion and secretes it into the bloodstream.

endocrine gland (EN-doh-krin GLAND) A gland that produces an internal or hormonal secretion and secretes it into the bloodstream.

endocrinologist (EN-doh-krih-NOL-oh-jist) A medical specialist in endocrinology.

endocrinology (EN-doh-krih-NOL-oh-jee) Medical specialty concerned with the production and effects of hormones.

endometriosis (EN-doh-mee-tree-OH-sis) Endometrial tissue in the abdomen outside the uterus.

endometrium (EN-doh-MEE-tree-um) Inner lining of the uterus.

endoplasmic reticulum (EN-doh-PLAZ-mik reh-TIC-you-lum) Structure inside a cell that synthesizes steroids, detoxifies drugs, and manufactures cell membranes.

endorphin (en-DOR-fin) Natural substance in the brain that has the same effect as opium.

endoscope (EN-doh-skope) Instrument for examining the inside of a tubular or hollow organ.

endoscopy (en-DOSS-koh-pee) The use of an endoscope.

endosteum (en-DOSS-tee-um) A membrane of tissue lining the inner (medullary) cavity of a long bone.

endothelial (en-doh-THEE-lee-al) A type of epithelial cell that lines the inside of blood vessels, lymphatic vessels, and the heart.

endothelium (en-doh-THEE-lee-um) Tissue found lining the inside of blood vessels and lymphatic vessels.

endotracheal (en-doh-TRAY-kee-al) Pertaining to being inside the trachea.

enema (EN-eh-mah) An injection of fluid into the rectum.

enteroscopy (en-ter-OSS-koh-pee) The examination of the lining of the digestive tract.

environment (en-VIE-ron-ment) All the external conditions affecting the life of an organism.

environmental (en-VIE-ron-MEN-tal) Pertaining to the environment.

enzyme (EN-zime) Protein that induces changes in other substances.

eosinophil (ee-oh-SIN-oh-fill) An eosinophil's granules attract a rosy-red color on staining.

ependyma (ep-EN-dih-mah) Membrane lining the central canal of the spinal cord and the ventricles of the brain.

epicardium (EP-ih-KAR-dee-um) The outer layer of the heart wall.

epicondyle (ep-ih-KON-dile) Projection above the condyle for attachment of a ligament or tendon.

epidermis (ep-ih-DER-miss) Top layer of the skin.

epididymis (EP-ih-DID-ih-miss) Coiled tube attached to the testis.

epididymitis (EP-ih-did-ih-MY-tis) Inflammation of the epididymis.

epididymoorchitis (ep-ih-DID-ih-moh-or-KIE-tis) Inflammation of the epididymis and testicle. Also called *orchitis*.

epidural (ep-ih-DYU-ral) Above the dura.

epidural space (ep-ih-DYU-ral SPASE) Space between the dura mater and the wall of the vertebral canal or skull.

epigastric (ep-ih-GAS-trik) Abdominal region above the stomach.

epigenetics (EP-ih-jeh-NET-iks) The study of disorders produced by the effects of chemical compounds (e.g., pollutants) or environmental influences (such as diet) on genes.

epiglottis (ep-ih-GLOT-is) Leaf-shaped plate of cartilage that shuts off the larynx during swallowing.

epiglottitis (ep-ih-glot-TIE-tis) Inflammation of the epiglottis.

epilepsy (EP-ih-LEP-see) Chronic brain disorder due to paroxysmal excessive neuronal discharges.

epinephrine (ep-ih-NEF-rin) Main catecholamine produced by the adrenal medulla. Also called *adrenaline.*

epiphyseal plate (eh-pih-FIZ-ee-al PLATE) Layer of cartilage between the epiphysis and metaphysis where bone growth occurs.

epiphysis (eh-PIF-ih-sis) Expanded area at the proximal and distal ends of a long bone that provides increased surface area for attachment of ligaments and tendons.

episiotomy (eh-peez-ee-OT-oh-mee) Surgical incision of the vulva.

epispadias (ep-ih-SPAY-dee-as) Condition in which the urethral opening is on the dorsum of the penis.

epistaxis (ep-ih-STAK-sis) Nosebleed.

epithelium (ep-ih-THEE-lee-um) Tissue that covers surfaces or lines cavities.

equilibrium (ee-kwih-LIB-ree-um) Being evenly balanced.

erectile (ee-REK-tile) Capable of erection or being distended with blood.

erection (ee-REK-shun) Distended and rigid state of an organ.

erosion (ee-ROH-shun) A shallow ulcer in the lining of a structure.

erythroblast (eh-RITH-roh-blast) Precursor to a red blood cell.

erythroblastosis fetalis (eh-RITH-roh-blas-TOH-sis fee-TAH-lis) Hemolytic disease of the newborn due to Rh incompatibility.

erythrocyte (eh-RITH-roh-site) Another name for a red blood cell.

erythropoiesis (eh-RITH-roh-poy-EE-sis) The formation of red blood cells.

erythropoietin (eh-RITH-roh-POY-ee-tin) Protein secreted by the kidney that stimulates red blood cell production.

eschar (ESS-kar) The burned, dead tissue lying on top of third-degree burns.

esophagitis (ee-SOF-ah-JIE-tis) Inflammation of the lining of the esophagus.

esophagus (ee-SOF-ah-gus) Tube linking the pharynx and the stomach.

esotropia (es-oh-TROH-pee-ah) A turning of the eye inward toward the nose.

estriol (ESS-tree-ol) One of the three main estrogens.

estrogen (ES-troh-jen) Generic term for hormones that stimulate female secondary sex characteristics.

ethmoid bone (ETH-moyd BOHN) Bone that forms the back of the nose and part of the orbits and encloses numerous air cells, forming the ethmoid sinuses.

eumelanin (YOU-mel-ah-nin) The dark form of the pigment melanin.

euphoria (yoo-FOR-ee-ah) Exaggerated feeling of well-being.

eupnea (yoop-NEE-ah) Normal breathing.

eustachian tube (you-STAY-shun TYUB) Tube that connects the middle ear to the nasopharynx. Also called *auditory tube.*

euthyroid (you-THIGH-royd) Normal thyroid function.

eversion (ee-VER-shun) A turning outward.

exacerbation (ek-zas-er-BAY-shun) Period in which there is an increase in the severity of a disease.

excoriate (eks-KOR-ee-ate) To scratch.

excrete (eks-KREET) To pass out of the body waste products of metabolism.

excretion (eks-KREE-shun) Removal of waste products of metabolism out of the body.

exhale (EKS-hail) Breathe out.

exocrine gland (EK-soh-krin GLAND) A gland that secretes outwardly through excretory ducts.

exophthalmos (ek-sof-THAL-mos) Protrusion of the eyeball.

exotropia (ek-soh-TROH-pee-ah) A turning of the eye outward away from the nose.

expectorate (ek-SPEC-toh-rate) Cough up and spit out mucus from the respiratory tract.

expiration (EKS-pih-RAY-shun) Breathe out.

extension (eks-TEN-shun) Straighten a joint to increase its angle.

extracorporeal (EKS-trah-kor-POH-ree-al) Outside the body.

extravasate (eks-TRAV-ah-sate) To ooze out from a vessel into the tissues.

extrinsic (eks-TRIN-sik) Extrinsic eye muscles are located on the outside of the eye, as opposed to intrinsic muscles, which are located inside the eye.

F

facet (FAS-et) Small smooth area around a pain-producing nerve.

facial (FAY-shal) Seventh (VII) cranial nerve; supplying the forehead, nose, eyes, mouth, and jaws.

facies (FASH-eez) Facial expression and features characteristic of a specific disease.

fallopian tubes (fah-LOH-pee-an TUBES) Uterine tubes connected to the fundus of the uterus.

fascia (FASH-ee-ah) Sheet of fibrous connective tissue.

fascicle (FAS-ih-kull) Bundle of muscle fibers.

fasciectomy (fash-ee-EK-toh-mee) Surgical removal of fascia.

fasciitis (fash-ee-IE-tis) Inflammation of the fascia.

fasciotomy (fash-ee-OT-oh-mee) An incision through a band of fascia, usually to relieve pressure on underlying structures.

fatty acid (FAT-ee ASS-id) An acid obtained from the hydrolysis of fats.

fecal (FEE-kal) Pertaining to feces.

feces (FEE-sees) Undigested waste material discharged from the bowel.

femoral (FEM-oh-ral) Pertaining to the femur.

femur (FEE-mur) The thigh bone.

ferritin (FER-ih-tin) Iron-protein complex that regulates iron storage and transport.

fertilization (FER-til-eye-ZAY-shun) Union of a male sperm and a female egg.

fertilize (FER-til-ize) To penetrate an oocyte with a sperm so as to impregnate.

festinant (FES-tih-nant) Shuffling, falling-forward gait.

fetal (FEE-tal) Pertaining to the fetus.

fetus (FEE-tus) Human organism from the end of the eighth week after conception to birth.

fiber (FIE-ber) Carbohydrate not digested by intestinal enzymes; *or* a strand or filament.

fibrillation (fih-brih-LAY-shun) Uncontrolled quivering or twitching of the heart muscle.

fibrin (FIE-brin) Stringy protein fiber that is a component of a blood clot.

fibrinogen (fie-BRIN-oh-jen) Precursor of fibrin in blood-clotting process.

fibroadenoma (FIE-broh-ad-en-OH-mah) Benign tumor containing much fibrous tissue.

fibroblast (FIE-broh-blast) Cell that forms collagen fibers.

fibrocartilage (fie-broh-KAR-til-ij) Cartilage containing collagen fibers.

fibrocystic disease (fie-broh-SIS-tik diz-EEZ) Benign breast disease with multiple tiny lumps and cysts.

fibroid (FIE-broyd) Uterine tumor resembling fibrous tissue.

fibromyalgia (fie-broh-my-AL-jee-ah) Pain in the muscle fibers.

fibromyoma (FIE-broh-my-OH-mah) Benign neoplasm derived from smooth muscle containing fibrous tissue.

fibrosis (fie-BROH-sis) Repair of dead tissue cells by formation of fibrous tissue.

fibrous (FIE-brus) Tissue containing fibroblasts and fibers.

fibula (FIB-you-lah) The smaller of the two bones of the lower leg.

filter (FIL-ter) A porous substance through which a liquid or gas is passed to separate out contained particles; or to use a filter.

filtrate (FIL-trate) That which has passed through a filter.

fimbria (FIM-bree-ah) A fringelike structure on the surface of a cell or microorganism. Plural *fimbriae.*

fissure (FISH-ur) Deep furrow or cleft. Plural *fissures.*

fistula (FIS-tyu-lah) Abnormal passage.

flagellum (fla-JELL-um) Tail of a sperm. Plural *flagella.*

flatus (FLAY-tus) Gas or air expelled through the anus.

flexion (FLEK-shun) Bend a joint to decrease its angle.

flexor (FLEK-sor) Muscle or tendon that flexes a joint.

flexure (FLEK-shur) A bend in a structure.

fluoresce (flor-ESS) Emit a bright-colored light when irradiated with ultraviolet or violet-blue rays.

fluorescein (flor-ESS-ee-in) Dye that produces a vivid green color under a blue light to diagnose corneal abrasions and foreign bodies.

fluoroscopy (flor-OS-koh-pee) Examination of the structures of the body by x-rays.

folic acid (FOH-lik ASS-id) Synthetic B_9 vitamin.

follicle (FOLL-ih-kull) Spherical mass of cells containing a cavity or a small cul-de-sac, such as a hair follicle.

follicular (fo-LIK-you-lar) Pertaining to a follicle.

foramen (foh-RAY-men) An opening through a structure. Plural *foramina.*

forceps extraction (FOR-seps ek-STRAK-shun) Assisted delivery of the baby by an instrument that grasps the head of the baby.

fornix (FOR-niks) Arch-shaped, blind-ended part of the vagina behind and around the cervix. Plural *fornices.*

fovea centralis (FOH-vee-ah sen-TRAH-lis) Small pit in the center of the macula that has the highest visual acuity.

free radical (FREE RAD-ih-kal) Short-lived product of oxidation in a cell that can be damaging to the cell.

frenulum (FREN-you-lum) Fold of mucous membrane between the glans and the prepuce.

frequency (FREE-kwen-see) The number of times something happens in a given time (e.g., passing urine).

frontal (FRON-tal) Pertaining to the vertical plane dividing the body into anterior and posterior portions.

frontal bone (FRON-tal BOHN) Bone that forms the forehead and the roofs of the orbits and contains a pair of right and left frontal sinuses above the orbits.

frontal lobe (FRON-tal LOBE) Area of brain behind the frontal bone.

fructosamine (FRUK-toe-sah-meen) Organic compound with fructose as its base.

function (FUNK-shun) The ability of an organ or tissue to perform its special work.

fundoscopy (fun-DOS-koh-pee) Examination of the fundus (retina) of the eye.

fundus (FUN-dus) Part farthest from the opening of a hollow organ.

furuncle (FU-rung-kel) An infected hair follicle that spreads into the tissues around the follicle.

G

galactorrhea (gah-LAK-toh-REE-ah) Abnormal flow of milk from the breasts.

gallbladder (GAWL-blad-er) Receptacle on the inferior surface of the liver for storing bile.

gallstone (GAWL-stone) Hard mass of cholesterol, calcium, and bilirubin that can be formed in the gallbladder and bile duct.

ganglion (GANG-lee-on) Collection of nerve cell bodies outside the CNS; *or* a fluid-containing swelling attached to the synovial sheath of a tendon. Plural *ganglia.*

gastric (GAS-trik) Pertaining to the stomach.

gastrin (GAS-trin) Hormone secreted in the stomach that stimulates secretion of HCl and increases gastric motility.

gastritis (gas-TRY-tis) Inflammation of the lining of the stomach.

gastrocnemius (gas-trok-NEE-mee-us) Major muscle in back of the lower leg (the calf).

gastrocolic reflex (gas-troh-KOL-ik REE-fleks) Taking food into the stomach leads to mass movement of feces in the colon and the desire to defecate.

gastroenteritis (GAS-troh-en-ter-EYE-tis) Inflammation of the stomach and intestines.

gastroenterologist (GAS-troh-en-ter-OL-oh-jist) Medical specialist in gastroenterology.

gastroenterology (GAS-troh-en-ter-OL-oh-jee) Medical specialty of the stomach and intestines.

gastroesophageal (GAS-troh-ee-sof-ah-JEE-al) Pertaining to the stomach and esophagus.

gastrointestinal (GI) (GAS-troh-in-TESS-tin-al) Relating to the stomach and intestines.

gastroscopy (gas-TROS-koh-pee) Endoscopic examination of the stomach.

gene (JEEN) Functional segment of the DNA molecule.

genetic (jeh-NET-ik) Pertaining to a gene.

genetics (jeh-NET-iks) Science of the inheritance of characteristics.

genital (JEN-ih-tal) Relating to reproduction or to the male or female sex organs.

genitalia (JEN-ih-TAY-lee-ah) External and internal organs of reproduction.

genome (JEE-nome) Complete set of genes.

geriatrician (jer-ee-ah-TRISH-an) Medical specialist in geriatrics.

geriatrics (jer-ee-AT-riks) Medical specialty that deals with the problems of old age.

gerontologist (jer-on-TOL-oh-jist) Medical specialist in gerontology.

gerontology (jer-on-TOL-oh-jee) Study of the process and problems of aging.

Giardia **(jee-AR-dee-ah)** Parasite in the small intestine.

gigantism (jie-GAN-tizm) Abnormal height and size of the entire body.

gingiva (JIN-jih-vah) Tissue surrounding teeth and covering the jaw.

gingivitis (jin-jih-VIE-tis) Inflammation of the gums.

glans (GLANZ) Head of the penis or clitoris.

glaucoma (glaw-KOH-mah) Increased intraocular pressure.

glia (GLEE-ah) Connective tissue that holds a structure together.

glioblastoma multiforme (GLIE-oh-blas-TOH-mah MULL-tih-FOR-mee) A malignant form of brain cancer.

glioma (glie-OH-mah) Tumor arising in a glial cell.

globulin (GLOB-you-lin) Family of blood proteins.

glomerulonephritis (glo-MER-you-loh-nef-RIE-tis) Infection of the glomeruli of the kidney.

glomerulus (glo-MER-you-lus) Plexus of capillaries; part of a nephron. Plural *glomeruli.*

glossodynia (gloss-oh-DIN-ee-ah) Painful, burning tongue.

glossopharyngeal (GLOSS-oh-fah-RIN-jee-al) Ninth (IX) cranial nerve; supplying the tongue and pharynx.

glottis (GLOT-is) Vocal apparatus of the larynx.

glucagon (GLUE-kah-gon) Pancreatic hormone that supports blood glucose levels.

glucocorticoid (glue-koh-KOR-tih-koyd) Hormone of the adrenal cortex that helps regulate glucose metabolism.

gluconeogenesis (GLUE-koh-nee-oh-JEN-eh-sis) Formation of glucose from noncarbohydrate sources.

glucose (GLU-kose) The final product of carbohydrate digestion and the main sugar in the blood.

gluten (GLU-ten) Insoluble protein found in wheat, rye, and barley.

gluteus (GLUE-tee-us) Term that refers to a muscle in the buttocks.

glycogen (GLIE-koh-jen) The body's principal carbohydrate reserve, stored in the liver and skeletal muscle.

glycogenolysis (GLIE-koh-jeh-NOL-ih-sis) Conversion of glycogen to glucose.

glycosuria (GLIE-koh-SYU-ree-ah) Presence of glucose in urine.

glycosylated hemoglobin (Hb A1c) (GLIE-koh-sih-lay-ted HEE-moh-GLOH-bin) Hemoglobin A fraction linked to glucose; used as an index of glucose control.

goiter (GOY-ter) Enlargement of the thyroid gland.

gomphosis (gom-FOH-sis) Joint formed by a peg and socket. Plural *gomphoses.*

gonad (GOH-nad) Testis or ovary. Plural *gonads.*

gonadotropin (GOH-nad-oh-TROH-pin) Hormone capable of promoting gonad function.

gonorrhea (gon-oh-REE-ah) Specific contagious sexually transmitted infection.

gout (GOWT) Painful arthritis of the big toe and other joints.

grade (GRAYD) In cancer pathology, a classification of the rate of growth of cancer cells.

grand mal (GRAHN MAL) Old name for a generalized tonic-clonic seizure.

granulation (gran-you-LAY-shun) New fibrous tissue formed during wound healing.

granulocyte (GRAN-you-loh-site) A white blood cell that contains multiple small granules in its cytoplasm.

granulosa cell (gran-you-LOH-sah SELL) Cell lining the ovarian follicle.

Graves disease (GRAYVZ diz-EEZ) Hyperthyroidism with toxic goiter.

gravida (GRAV-ih-dah) A pregnant woman.

gravidarum (gra-vih-DAR-um) Relating to pregnant women.

gray matter (GRAY MATT-er) Regions of the brain and spinal cord occupied by cell bodies and dendrites.

greenstick fracture (GREEN-stik FRAK-chur) A fracture in which one side of the bone is partially broken and the other side is bent; occurs mostly in children.

Guillain-Barré syndrome (GEE-yan-bah-RAY SIN-drome) Disorder in which the body makes antibodies against myelin, disrupting nerve conduction.

gynecologist (guy-nih-KOL-oh-jist) Specialist in gynecology.

gynecology (guy-nih-KOL-oh-jee) Medical specialty for the care of the female reproductive system.

gynecomastia (GUY-nih-koh-MAS-tee-ah) Enlargement of the breast.

gyrus (JIE-rus) Rounded elevation on the surface of the cerebral hemispheres. Plural *gyri.*

H

hairline fracture (HAIR-line FRAK-chur) A fracture without separation of the fragments.

halitosis (hal-ih-TOE-sis) Bad odor of the breath.

hallucination (hah-loo-sih-NAY-shun) Perception of an object or event when there is no such thing present.

hallux valgus (HAL-uks VAL-gus) Deviation of the big toe toward the lateral side of the foot.

handicap (HAND-ee-cap) Condition that interferes with a person's ability to function normally.

hapten (HAP-ten) Small molecule that has to bind to a larger molecule to form an antigen.

Hashimoto disease (hah-shee-MOH-toh diz-EEZ) Autoimmune disease of the thyroid gland. Also called *Hashimoto thyroiditis.*

haversian canals (hah-VER-shan ka-NALS) Vascular canals in bone. Also called *central canals.*

head (HED) The rounded extremity of a bone.

Heberden node (HEH-ber-den NOHD) Bony lump on the terminal phalanx of the fingers in osteoarthritis.

helix (HEE-liks) A line in the shape of a coil.

hematemesis (he-mah-TEM-eh-sis) Vomiting of red blood.

hematochezia (he-mat-oh-KEY-zee-ah) The passage of red, bloody stools.

hematocrit (Hct) (hee-MAT-oh-krit) Percentage of red blood cells in blood.

hematology (hee-mah-TOL-oh-jee) Medical specialty of disorders of blood.

hematoma (hee-mah-TOH-mah) Collection of blood that has escaped from the blood vessels into tissue. Also called *bruise*.

hematopoietic (HEE-mah-toh-poy-ET-ik) Pertaining to the making of red blood cells.

hematuria (hee-mah-TYU-ree-ah) Blood in the urine.

heme (HEEM) The iron-based component of hemoglobin that carries oxygen.

hemifacial (hem-ee-FAY-shal) Pertaining to one side of the face.

hemiparesis (HEM-ee-pah-REE-sis) Weakness of one side of the body.

hemiplegia (hem-ee-PLEE-jee-ah) Paralysis of one side of the body.

Hemoccult test (HEEM-oh-kult TEST) Trade name for a fecal occult blood test.

hemochromatosis (HEE-moh-kroh-mah-TOH-sis) Dangerously high levels of iron in the body with deposition of iron pigments in tissues.

hemodialysis (HEE-moh-die-AL-ih-sis) An artificial method of filtration to remove excess waste materials and water directly from the blood.

hemoglobin (HEE-moh-GLOH-bin) Red-pigmented protein that is the main component of red blood cells.

hemoglobinopathy (HEE-moh-GLOH-bih-NOP-ah-thee) Disease caused by the presence of an abnormal hemoglobin in the red blood cells.

hemolysis (hee-MOL-ih-sis) Destruction of red blood cells so that hemoglobin is liberated.

hemolytic (hee-moh-LIT-ik) Pertaining to the process of destruction of red blood cells.

hemophilia (hee-moh-FILL-ee-ah) An inherited disease from a deficiency of clotting factor VIII.

hemoptysis (hee-MOP-tih-sis) Bloody sputum.

hemorrhage (HEM-oh-raj) To bleed profusely.

hemorrhoid (HEM-oh-royd) Dilated rectal vein producing painful anal swelling. Plural *hemorrhoids*.

hemostasis (hee-moh-STAY-sis) Controlling or stopping bleeding.

hemothorax (hee-moh-THOR-aks) Blood in the pleural cavity.

heparin (HEP-ah-rin) An anticoagulant secreted particularly by liver cells.

hepatic (hep-AT-ik) Pertaining to the liver.

hepatitis (hep-ah-TIE-tis) Inflammation of the liver.

hepatocellular (HEP-ah-toh-SELL-you-lar) Pertaining to liver cells.

heredity (heh-RED-ih-tee) Transmission of characteristics from parents to offspring through genes.

hernia (HER-nee-ah) Protrusion of a structure through the tissue that normally contains it.

herniate (HER-nee-ate) To protrude.

herniation (HER-nee-AY-shun) Protrusion of an anatomical structure from its normal location.

herniorrhaphy (HER-nee-OR-ah-fee) Repair of a hernia.

herpes simplex virus (HSV) (HER-peez SIM-pleks VIE-rus) Disease that manifests with painful, watery blisters on the skin and mucous membranes.

herpes zoster (HER-pees ZOS-ter) Painful eruption of vesicles that follows a dermatome or nerve root on one side of the body. Also called *shingles*.

heterograft (HET-er-oh-graft) A graft using tissue taken from another species. Also known as *xenograft*.

hiatus (high-AY-tus) An opening through a structure.

hilum (HIGH-lum) The site where the nerves and blood vessels enter and leave an organ. Plural *hila*.

hirsutism (HER-sue-tizm) Excessive body and facial hair.

histamine (HISS-tah-meen) Compound liberated in tissues as a result of injury or an allergic response.

histology (his-TOL-oh-jee) Structure and function of cells, tissues, and organs.

histone (HIS-tone) A simple protein found in the cell nucleus.

Hodgkin lymphoma (HOJ-kin lim-FOH-muh) Disease marked by chronic enlargement of lymph nodes, spreading to other nodes in an orderly way.

homeostasis (hoh-mee-oh-STAY-sis) Stability or equilibrium of a system or the body's internal environment.

homicidal (hom-ih-SIDE-al) Having a tendency to commit homicide.

homocysteine (hoh-moh-SIS-teen) An amino acid similar to cysteine.

homograft (HOH-moh-graft) Skin graft from another person or a cadaver.

hordeolum (hor-DEE-oh-lum) Abscess in an eyelash follicle. Also called *stye*.

hormone (HOR-mohn) Chemical formed in one tissue or organ and carried by the blood to stimulate or inhibit a function of another tissue or organ.

Horner syndrome (HOR-ner SIN-drome) Disorder of the sympathetic nerves to the face and eye.

hospice (HOS-pis) Facility or program that provides care to the dying and their families.

human immunodeficiency virus (HIV) (HYU-man IM-you-noh-dee-FISH-en-see VIE-rus) Etiologic agent of acquired immunodeficiency syndrome (AIDS).

human papilloma virus (HPV) (HYU-man pap-ih-LOH-mah VIE-rus) Causes warts on the skin and genitalia and can increase the risk for cervical cancer.

humerus (HYU-mer-us) Single bone of the upper arm.

humoral immunity (HYU-mor-al im-YOU-nih-tee) Defense mechanism arising from antibodies in the blood.

Huntington disease (HUN-ting-ton diz-EEZ) Progressive inherited, degenerative, incurable neurologic disease. Also called *Huntington chorea*.

hyaline (HIGH-ah-line) Cartilage that looks like glass and contains fine collagen fibers.

hyaline membrane disease (HIGH-ah-line MEM-brain diz-EEZ) Respiratory distress syndrome of the newborn.

hydrocele (HIGH-droh-seal) Collection of fluid in the space of the tunica vaginalis.

hydrocephalus (HIGH-droh-SEF-ah-lus) Enlarged head due to excess CSF in the cerebral ventricles.

hydrochloric acid (HCl) (high-droh-KLOR-ic ASS-id) The acid of gastric juice.

hydrocortisone (high-droh-KOR-tih-sohn) Potent glucocorticoid with anti-inflammatory properties. Also called *cortisol*.

hydronephrosis (HIGH-droh-neh-FROH-sis) Dilation of the pelvis and calyces of a kidney.

hymen (HIGH-men) Thin membrane partly occluding the vaginal orifice.

hyperactive (HIGH-per-ac-TIV) Excessive restlessness and movement.

hyperactivity (HIGH-per-ac-TIV-ih-tee) Condition of being hyperactive.

hypercalcemia (HIGH-per-kal-SEE-mee-ah) Excessive level of calcium in the blood.

hyperemesis (high-per-EM-eh-sis) Excessive vomiting.

hyperflexion (high-per-FLEK-shun) Flexion of a limb or part beyond the normal limits.

hyperfractionated (high-per-FRAK-shun-ay-ted) Given in smaller amounts and more frequently.

hyperglycemia (HIGH-per-glie-SEE-mee-ah) High level of glucose (sugar) in blood.

hyperglycemic (HIGH-per-glie-SEE-mik) Pertaining to high blood sugar.

hyperinflation (HIGH-per-in-FLAY-shun) Overdistension of pulmonary alveoli with air resulting from airway obstruction.

hyperopia (high-per-OH-pee-ah) Able to see distant objects but unable to see close objects.

hyperosmolar (HIGH-per-os-MOH-lar) Marked hyperglycemia without ketoacidosis.

hyperparathyroidism (HIGH-per-pair-ah-THIGH-royd-ism) Excessive levels of parathyroid hormone.

hyperplasia (high-per-PLAY-zee-ah) Increase in the *number* of the cells in a tissue or organ.

hyperpnea (high-perp-NEE-ah) Deeper and more rapid breathing than normal.

hypersecretion (HIGH-per-seh-KREE-shun) Excessive secretion of mucus (or enzymes or waste products).

hypersensitivity (HIGH-per-sen-sih-TIV-ih-tee) Exaggerated abnormal reaction to an allergen.

hypersplenism (high-per-SPLEN-izm) Condition in which the spleen removes blood components at an excessive rate.

hypertension (HIGH-per-TEN-shun) Persistent high arterial blood pressure.

hyperthyroidism (high-per-THIGH-royd-ism) Excessive production of thyroid hormones.

hypertrophy (high-PER-troh-fee) Increase in size, but not in number, of an individual tissue element.

hypochondriac (high-poh-KON-dree-ack) A person who exaggerates the significance of symptoms; *or* pertaining to below the cartilage below the ribs.

hypochondriasis (HIGH-poh-kon-DRIE-ah-sis) Belief that a minor symptom indicates a severe disease.

hypochromic (high-poh-CROH-mik) Pale in color, as in RBCs when hemoglobin is deficient.

hypodermis (high-poh-DER-miss) Tissue layer below the dermis.

hypogastric (high-poh-GAS-trik) Abdominal region below the stomach.

hypoglossal (high-poh-GLOSS-al) Twelfth (XII) cranial nerve; supplying muscles of the tongue.

hypoglycemia (HIGH-poh-glie-SEE-mee-ah) Low level of glucose (sugar) in the blood.

hypogonadism (HIGH-poh-GOH-nad-izm) Deficient gonad production of sperm or eggs or hormones.

hypokalemia (HIGH-poh-kah-LEE-mee-ah) Low level of potassium in the blood.

hypoparathyroidism (HIGH-poh-pair-ah-THIGH-royd-ism) Deficient levels of parathyroid hormone.

hypophysis (high-POF-ih-sis) Another name for the pituitary gland.

hypopigmentation (HIGH-poh-pig-men-TAY-shun) Below-normal melanin relative to the surrounding skin.

hypopituitarism (HIGH-poh-pih-TYU-ih-tah-rizm) Condition of one or more deficient pituitary hormones.

hypospadias (high-poh-SPAY-dee-as) Urethral opening more proximal than normal on the ventral surface of the penis.

hypotension (HIGH-poh-TEN-shun) Persistent low arterial blood pressure.

hypothalamus (high-poh-THAL-ah-muss) Area of gray matter forming part of the walls and floor of the third ventricle.

hypothenar (high-poh-THEE-nar) Fleshy eminence at the base of the little finger.

hypothyroidism (high-poh-THIGH-royd-ism) Deficient production of thyroid hormones.

hypovolemic (HIGH-poh-voh-LEE-mik) Having decreased blood volume in the body.

hypoxia (high-POK-see-ah) Decrease below normal levels of oxygen in tissues, gases, or blood.

hypoxic (high-POK-sik) Deficient in oxygen.

hysterectomy (his-ter-EK-toh-mee) Surgical removal of the uterus.

hysterosalpingogram (HIS-ter-oh-sal-PING-oh-gram) Radiograph of the uterus and uterine tubes after injection of contrast material.

hysteroscopy (his-ter-OS-koh-pee) Visual inspection of the uterine cavity using an endoscope.

I

ictal (IK-tal) Pertaining to, or condition caused by, a stroke or epilepsy.

icterus (ICK-ter-us) Yellow staining of tissues with bile pigments, including bilirubin.

idiopathic (ID-ih-oh-PATH-ik) Pertaining to a disease of unknown etiology.

ileocecal (ILL-ee-oh-SEE-cal) Pertaining to the junction of the ileum and cecum.

ileocecal sphincter (ILL-ee-oh-SEE-cal SFINK-ter) Band of muscle that encircles the junction of the ileum and cecum.

ileostomy (ill-ee-OS-toh-mee) Artificial opening from the ileum to the outside of the body.

ileum (ILL-ee-um) Third portion of the small intestine.

ilium (ILL-ee-um) Large wing-shaped bone at the upper and posterior part of the pelvis. Plural *ilia.*

immune (im-YUNE) Protected from an infectious disease.

immune serum (im-YUNE SEER-um) Serum taken from another human or animal that has antibodies to a disease. Also called *antiserum.*

immunity (im-YOU-nih-tee) State of being protected.

immunization (im-you-nih-ZAY-shun) Administration of an agent to provide immunity.

immunoassay (IM-you-noh-ASS-ay) Biochemical test to measure the amount of a substance in a liquid, using the reaction of an antibody to its antigen.

immunodeficiency (IM-you-noh-dee-FISH-en-see) Failure of the immune system.

immunoglobulin (IM-you-noh-GLOB-you-lin) Specific protein evoked by an antigen. All antibodies are immunoglobulins.

immunologist (im-you-NOL-oh-jist) Medical specialist in immunology.

immunology (im-you-NOL-oh-jee) The science and practice of immunity and allergy.

immunosuppression (IM-you-noh-suh-PRESH-un) Suppression of the immune response by an outside agent, such as a drug.

impacted (im-PAK-ted) Immovably wedged, as with earwax blocking the external canal.

impacted fracture (im-PAK-ted FRAK-chur) A fracture in which one bone fragment is driven into the other.

impairment (im-PAIR-ment) Diminishing of normal function.

impetigo (im-peh-TIE-go) Infection of the skin producing thick, yellow crusts.

implantable (im-PLAN-tah-bul) Able to be inserted into tissues.

implantation (im-plan-TAY-shun) Attachment of a fertilized egg to the endometrium.

impotence (IM-poh-tence) Inability to achieve an erection.

in situ (IN SIGH-tyu) In the correct place.

in vitro fertilization (IVF) (IN VEE-troh FER-til-eye-ZAY-shun) Process of combining a sperm and egg in a laboratory dish and placing the resulting embryos inside a uterus.

incision (in-SIZH-un) A cut or surgical wound.

incisor (in-SIGH-zor) Chisel-shaped tooth.

incompatible (in-kom-PAT-ih-bul) Substances that interfere with each other physiologically.

incompetence (in-KOM-peh-tense) Failure of valves to close completely.

incomplete fracture (in-kom-PLEET FRAK-chur) A fracture that does not extend across the bone, as in a hairline fracture.

incontinence (in-KON-tin-ens) Inability to prevent discharge of urine or feces.

incubation (in-kyu-BAY-shun) Process of developing an infection.

incus (IN-cuss) Middle one of the three ossicles in the middle ear; shaped like an anvil.

index (IN-deks) A standard indicator of measurement. Plural *indices*.

infarction (in-FARK-shun) Sudden blockage of an artery.

infection (in-FEK-shun) Invasion of the body by disease-producing microorganisms.

infectious (in-FEK-shus) Capable of being transmitted; *or* caused by infection by a microorganism.

inferior (in-FEE-ree-or) Situated below.

infertility (in-fer-TIL-ih-tee) Inability to conceive over a long period of time.

infestation (in-fes-TAY-shun) Act of being invaded on the skin by a troublesome other species, such as a parasite.

infiltration (in-fil-TRAY-shun) The invasion into a tissue or cell.

inflation (in-FLAY-shun) Process of expanding with air.

infundibulum (IN-fun-DIB-you-lum) Funnel-shaped structure. Plural *infundibula*.

infusion (in-FYU-zhun) Introduction intravenously of a substance other than blood.

ingestion (in-JEST-shun) Intake of food, either by mouth or through a nasogastric tube.

inguinal (IN-gwin-al) Pertaining to the groin.

inhale (IN-hail) Breathe in.

inotropic (IN-oh-TROH-pik) Affecting the contractility of cardiac muscle.

insanity (in-SAN-ih-tee) Nonmedical term for a person unable to be responsible for his or her actions.

insecticide (in-SEK-tih-side) Agent for destroying insects.

insemination (in-sem-ih-NAY-shun) Introduction of semen into the vagina.

insertion (in-SIR-shun) The attachment of a muscle to a more movable part of the skeleton, as distinct from the origin.

insomnia (in-SOM-nee-ah) Inability to sleep.

inspiration (in-spih-RAY-shun) Breathe in.

instability (in-stah-BIL-ih-tee) Abnormal tendency of a joint to partially or fully dislocate; *or* difficulty in balance.

insufficiency (in-suh-FISH-en-see) Lack of completeness of function; in the heart, failure of a valve to close properly.

insulin (IN-syu-lin) A hormone secreted by the pancreas.

integumentary (in-TEG-you-MEN-tah-ree) Pertaining to the covering of the body.

interatrial (IN-ter-AY-tree-al) Between the atria of the heart.

intercostal (IN-ter-KOS-tal) The space between two ribs.

intermittent (IN-ter-MIT-ent) Alternately ceasing and beginning again.

internal (IN-tur-nal) Inside a structure or organ.

interphalangeal (IN-ter-fah-LAN-jee-al) Pertaining to the joints between two phalanges.

interstitial (in-ter-STISH-al) Pertaining to spaces between cells in a tissue or organ.

interventricular (IN-ter-ven-TRIK-you-lar) Between the ventricles of the heart.

intervertebral (IN-ter-VER-teh-bral) The space between two vertebrae.

intestine (in-TES-tin) The digestive tube from stomach to anus.

intima (IN-tih-ma) Inner layer of a structure, particularly a blood vessel.

intolerance (in-TOL-er-ance) Inability of the small intestine to digest and dispose of a particular dietary constituent.

intracellular (in-trah-SELL-you-lar) Within the cell.

intracranial (in-trah-KRAY-nee-al) Within the cranium (skull).

intradermal (IN-trah-DER-mal) Within the dermis.

intramuscular (IN-trah-MUS-kew-lar) Within the muscle.

intraocular (in-trah-OK-you-lar) Pertaining to the inside of the eye.

intrathecal (IN-trah-THEE-kal) Within the subarachnoid or subdural space.

intrauterine (IN-trah-YOU-ter-ine) Inside the uterine cavity.

intravenous (IN-trah-VEE-nus) Inside a vein.

intrinsic (in-TRIN-sik) Any muscle whose origin and insertion are entirely within the structure under consideration; for example, muscles inside the vocal cords or the eye.

intrinsic factor (in-TRIN-sik FAK-tor) Substance that makes the absorption of vitamin B_{12} happen.

intubation (IN-tyu-BAY-shun) Insertion of a tube into the trachea.

intussusception (IN-tuss-sus-SEP-shun) The slipping of one part of the bowel inside another to cause obstruction.

inversion (in-VER-shun) A turning inward.

involute (in-voh-LUTE) To return to a former condition; *or* decline associated with advanced age.

involution (in-voh-LOO-shun) A decrease in size or vigor.

iodine (EYE-oh-dine or EYE-oh-deen) Chemical element, the lack of which causes thyroid disease.

iris (EYE-ris) Colored portion of the eye with the pupil in its center.

irrigation (ih-rih-GAY-shun) Use of water to wash out a canal or wound.

ischemia (is-KEE-mee-ah) Lack of blood supply to a tissue.

ischium (ISS-kee-um) Lower and posterior part of the hip bone. Plural *ischia.*

Ishihara color system (ish-ee-HAR-ah KUH-ler SIS-tem) Test for color vision defects.

islet cells (EYE-let SELLS) Hormone-secreting cells of the pancreas.

islets of Langerhans (EYE-lets ov LAHNG-er-hahnz) Areas of pancreatic cells that produce insulin and glucagon.

isotope (EYE-soh-tope) Radioactive element used in diagnostic procedures.

isthmus (IS-mus) Part connecting two larger parts; for example, the uterus to the uterine tube.

J

Jaeger reading card (YAY-ger REED-ing CARD) Type in different sizes of print for testing near vision.

jaundice (JAWN-dis) Yellow staining of tissues with bile pigments, including bilirubin.

jejunum (je-JEW-num) Segment of small intestine between the duodenum and the ileum where most of the nutrients are absorbed.

jugular (JUG-you-lar) Pertaining to the throat.

juvenile (JU-ven-ile) Between the ages of 2 and 17 years.

K

Kaposi sarcoma (ka-POH-see sar-KOH-mah) A malignancy often seen in AIDS patients.

karyotype (KAIR-ee-oh-type) Map of chromosomes of an individual cell.

Kegel exercises (KEE-gal EKS-er-size-ez) Contraction and relaxation of the pelvic floor muscles to improve urethral and rectal sphincter function.

keloid (KEY-loyd) Raised, irregular, lumpy, shiny scar due to excess collagen fiber production during healing of a wound.

keratin (KER-ah-tin) Protein found in the dead outer layer of skin and in nails and hair.

keratinocyte (ke-RAT-in-oh-site) Cell producing a tough, horny protein (keratin) in the process of differentiating into the dead cells of the stratum corneum.

keratomileusis (KER-ah-toh-mie-LOO-sis) A surgical procedure that involves cutting and shaping the cornea.

keratosis (ker-ah-TOH-sis) Epidermal lesion of circumscribed overgrowth of the horny layer.

keratotomy (KER-ah-TOT-oh-mee) Incision in the cornea.

kernicterus (ker-NIK-ter-us) Bilirubin staining of the basal nuclei of the brain.

ketoacidosis (KEY-toh-ass-ih-DOH-sis) Excessive production of ketones, making the blood acid.

ketone (KEY-tone) Chemical formed in uncontrolled diabetes or in starvation.

ketosis (key-TOH-sis) Excess production of ketones.

kidney (KID-nee) Organ of excretion.

kleptomania (klep-toh-MAY-nee-ah) Uncontrollable need to steal.

kyphosis (kie-FOH-sis) A normal posterior curve of the thoracic spine that can be exaggerated in disease.

L

labium (LAY-bee-um) Fold of the vulva. Plural *labia.*

labor (LAY-bore) Process of expulsion of the fetus.

labrum (LAY-brum) Cartilage that forms a rim around the socket of the hip joint.

labyrinth (LAB-ih-rinth) The inner ear.

laceration (lass-eh-RAY-shun) A tear of the skin.

lacrimal (LAK-rim-al) Pertaining to tears.

lactase (LAK-tase) Enzyme that breaks down lactose to glucose and galactose.

lactation (lak-TAY-shun) Production of milk.

lacteal (LAK-tee-al) A lymphatic vessel carrying chyle away from the intestine.

lactiferous (lak-TIF-er-us) Pertaining to or yielding milk.

lactose (LAK-toes) The disaccharide found in cow's milk.

lacuna (la-KOO-nah) Small space or cavity within the matrix of bone. Plural *lacunae.*

lanugo (la-NYU-go) Fine, soft hair on the fetal body.

laparoscope (LAP-ah-roh-skope) Instrument (endoscope) used for viewing the abdominal contents.

laparoscopic (LAP-ah-rah-SKOP-ik) Pertaining to laparoscopy.

laparoscopy (lap-ah-ROS-koh-pee) Examination of the contents of the abdomen using an endoscope.

laryngitis (lair-in-JIE-tis) Inflammation of the larynx.

laryngopharynx (lah-RING-oh-FAIR-inks) Region of the pharynx below the epiglottis that includes the larynx.

laryngoscope (lah-RING-oh-skope) Hollow tube with a light and camera used to visualize or operate on the larynx.

laryngotracheobronchitis (lah-RING-oh-TRAY-kee-oh-brong-KIE-tis) Inflammation of the larynx, trachea, and bronchi. Also called *croup.*

larynx (LAIR-inks) Organ of voice production.

laser (LAY-zer) Intense, narrow beam of monochromatic light.

laser surgery (LAY-zer SUR-jer-ee) Use of a concentrated, intense narrow beam of electromagnetic radiation for surgery.

lateral (LAT-er-al) Situated at the side of a structure.

latex (LAY-tecks) Manufactured from the milky liquid in rubber plants; used for gloves in patient care.

latissimus dorsi (lah-TISS-ih-muss DOR-sigh) The widest (broadest) muscle in the back.

lavage (lah-VAHZH) Washing out of a hollow cavity, tube, or organ.

leiomyoma (LIE-oh-my-OH-mah) Benign neoplasm derived from smooth muscle.

lens (LENZ) Transparent refractive structure behind the iris.

lentigo (len-TIE-goh) Age spot; small, flat, brown-black spot in the skin of older people. Plural *lentigines*.

leptin (LEP-tin) Hormone secreted by adipose tissue.

lesion (LEE-zhun) Pathologic change or injury in a tissue.

leukemia (loo-KEE-mee-ah) Disease in which the blood is taken over by white blood cells and their precursors.

leukocoria (loo-koh-KOH-ree-ah) Reflection in the pupil of a white mass in the eye.

leukocyte (LOO-koh-site) Another term for *white blood cell*. Alternative spelling *leucocyte*.

leukocytosis (LOO-koh-sigh-TOH-sis) An excessive number of white blood cells.

leukopenia (loo-koh-PEE-nee-ah) A deficient number of white blood cells.

leukoplakia (loo-koh-PLAY-kee-ah) White patch on the oral mucous membrane, often precancerous.

libido (li-BEE-doh) Sexual desire.

life expectancy (LIFE ek-SPEK-tan-see) Statistical determination of the number of years an individual is expected to live.

life span (LIFE SPAN) The age that a person reaches.

ligament (LIG-ah-ment) Band of fibrous tissue connecting two structures.

ligate (LIE-gate) Tie off a structure, such as a bleeding blood vessel.

ligation (lie-GAY-shun) Use of a tie to close a tube.

limbic (LIM-bic) Pertaining to the limbic system, an array of nerve fibers surrounding the thalamus.

linear fracture (LIN-ee-ar FRAK-chur) A fracture running parallel to the length of the bone.

lipase (LIE-paze) Enzyme that breaks down fat.

lipectomy (lip-EK-toh-mee) Surgical removal of adipose tissue.

lipid (LIP-id) General term for all types of fatty compounds; for example, cholesterol, triglycerides, and fatty acids.

lipoprotein (LIE-poh-proh-teen) Molecules made of combinations of fat and protein.

lithotripsy (LITH-oh-trip-see) Crushing stones by sound waves.

lithotripter (LITH-oh-trip-ter) Instrument that generates sound waves.

liver (LIV-er) Body's largest internal organ, located in the right upper quadrant of the abdomen.

lobe (LOBE) Subdivision of an organ or some other part.

lobectomy (loh-BEK-toh-mee) Surgical removal of a lobe of the lungs or the thyroid gland.

lochia (LOH-kee-uh) Vaginal discharge following childbirth.

longevity (lon-JEV-ih-tee) Duration of life beyond the normal expectation.

loop of Henle (LOOP of HEN-lee) Part of the renal tubule where reabsorption occurs.

lordosis (lore-DOH-sis) An exaggerated forward curvature of the lumbar spine.

louse (LOWSE) Parasitic insect. Plural *lice*.

lumbar (LUM-bar) Pertaining to the region in the back and sides between the ribs and pelvis.

lumen (LOO-men) The interior space of a tubelike structure.

lumpectomy (lump-EK-toh-mee) Removal of a lesion with preservation of surrounding tissue.

lutein (LOO-tee-in) Yellow pigment.

Lyme disease (LIME diz-EEZ) Disease transmitted by the bite of an infected deer tick.

lymph (LIMF) A clear fluid collected from tissues and transported by lymph vessels to the venous circulation.

lymphadenectomy (lim-FAD-eh-NEK-toh-mee) Surgical excision of a lymph node.

lymphadenitis (lim-FAD-eh-NIE-tis) Inflammation of a lymph node.

lymphadenopathy (lim-FAD-eh-NOP-ah-thee) Any disease process affecting a lymph node.

lymphangiogram (lim-FAN-jee-oh-gram) Radiographic images of lymph vessels and nodes following injection of contrast material.

lymphatic (lim-FAT-ik) Pertaining to lymph or the lymphatic system.

lymphedema (LIMF-eh-DEE-mah) Tissue swelling due to lymphatic obstruction.

lymphocyte (LIM-foh-site) Small white blood cell with a large nucleus.

lymphoid (LIM-foyd) Resembling lymphatic tissue.

lymphoma (lim-FOH-mah) Any neoplasm of lymphatic tissue.

lysosome (LIE-soh-sohm) Enzyme that digests foreign material and worn-out cell components.

lysozyme (LIE-soh-zime) Enzyme that dissolves the cell walls of bacteria.

M

macrocytic (mak-roh-SIT-ik) Pertaining to macrocytes.

macrophage (MAK-roh-fayj) Large white blood cell that removes bacteria, foreign particles, and dead cells.

macula (MAK-you-lah) Small area of special function; in the ear, a sensory receptor. Plural *maculae*.

macula lutea (MAK-you-lah LOO-tee-ah) Yellowish spot on the back of the retina; contains the fovea centralis.

majus (MAY-jus) Bigger or greater; for example, labia majora. Plural *majora*.

malabsorption (mal-ab-SORP-shun) Inadequate gastrointestinal absorption of nutrients.

malfunction (mal-FUNK-shun) Inadequate or abnormal function.

malignant (mah-LIG-nant) Capable of invading surrounding tissues and metastasizing to distant organs.

malleus (MAL-ee-us) Outer (lateral) one of the three ossicles in the middle ear; shaped like a hammer.

malnutrition (mal-nyu-TRISH-un) Inadequate nutrition from poor diet or inadequate absorption of nutrients.

mammary (MAM-ah-ree) Relating to the lactating breast.

mammogram (MAM-oh-gram) The record produced by x-ray imaging of the breast.

mammography (mah-MOG-rah-fee) Process of x-ray examination of the breast.

mandible (MAN-di-bel) Lower jawbone.

mania (MAY-nee-ah) Mood disorder with hyperactivity, irritability, and rapid speech.

manic-depressive disorder (MAN-ik dee-PRESS-iv dis-OR-der) An outdated name for bipolar disorder.

marijuana (mar-ih-HWAN-ah) Dried, flowering leaves of the plant *Cannabis sativa.*

marrow (MAH-roh) Fatty, blood-forming tissue in the cavities of long bones.

mastalgia (mass-TAL-jee-uh) Pain in the breast.

mastectomy (mass-TEK-toh-mee) Surgical excision of the breast.

masticate (MAS-tih-kate) To chew.

mastitis (mass-TIE-tis) Inflammation of the breast.

mastoid (MASS-toyd) Small bony protrusion immediately behind the ear.

maternal (mah-TER-nal) Pertaining to or derived from the mother.

matrix (MAY-triks) Substance that surrounds cells, is manufactured by the cells, and holds them together.

maximus (MAKS-ih-mus) The gluteus maximus muscle is the largest muscle in the body, covering a large part of each buttock.

McBurney point (mack-BUR-nee POYNT) One-third the distance from the anterior superior iliac spine to the umbilicus.

meatus (mee-AY-tus) Passage or channel; also used to denote the external opening of a passage.

meconium (meh-KOH-nee-um) The first bowel movement of the newborn.

media (MEE-dee-ah) Middle layer of a structure, particularly a blood vessel.

medial (MEE-dee-al) Nearer to the middle of the body.

mediastinoscopy (MEE-dee-ass-tih-NOS-koh-pee) Examination of the mediastinum using an endoscope.

mediastinum (MEE-dee-ah-STIE-num) Area between the lungs containing the heart, aorta, venae cavae, esophagus, and trachea.

medius (MEE-dee-us) The gluteus medius muscle is partly covered by the gluteus maximus; it originates on the ilium and is inserted into the femur.

medulla (meh-DULL-ah) Central portion of a structure surrounded by cortex.

medulla oblongata (meh-DULL-ah ob-lon-GAH-tah) Most posterior subdivision of the brainstem; continuation of the spinal cord.

megakaryocyte (MEG-ah-KAIR-ee-oh-site) Large cell with a large nucleus. Parts of the cytoplasm break off to form platelets.

meiosis (my-OH-sis) Two rapid cell divisions, resulting in half the number of chromosomes.

melanin (MEL-ah-nin) Black pigment found in the skin, hair, and retina.

melanocyte (MEL-an-oh-cyte) Cell that synthesizes (produces) melanin.

melanoma (MEL-ah-NOH-mah) Malignant neoplasm formed from cells that produce melanin.

melasma (meh-LAZ-mah) Patchy pigmentation of the skin.

melatonin (mel-ah-TONE-in) Hormone formed by the pineal gland.

melena (mel-EN-ah) The passage of black, tarry stools.

membrane (MEM-brain) Thin layer of tissue covering a structure or cavity.

Ménière disease (men-YEAR diz-EEZ) Disorder of the inner ear with a cluster of symptoms of acute attacks of tinnitus, vertigo, and hearing loss.

meninges (meh-NIN-jeez) Three-layered covering of the brain and spinal cord.

meningioma (meh-NIN-jee-OH-mah) Tumor arising from the arachnoid layer of the meninges.

meningitis (men-in-JIE-tis) Acute infectious disease of children and young adults.

meningocele (meh-NING-oh-seal) Protrusion of the meninges from the spinal cord or brain through a defect in the vertebral column or cranium.

meningococcal (meh-nin-goh-KOK-al) Pertaining to the *meningo-coccus* bacterium.

meningomyelocele (meh-NING-oh-MY-el-oh-seal) Protrusion of the spinal cord and meninges through a defect in the vertebral arch of one or more vertebrae.

meniscectomy (men-ih-SEK-toh-mee) Excision (cutting out) of all or part of a meniscus.

meniscus (meh-NISS-kuss) Disc of connective tissue cartilage between the bones of a joint; for example, in the knee joint. Plural *menisci.*

menopause (MEN-oh-paws) Permanent ending of menstrual periods.

menorrhagia (men-oh-RAY-jee-ah) Excessive menstrual bleeding.

menstruation (men-stru-AY-shun) Synonym of *menses.*

mental (MENT-tal) Pertaining to the mind.

merocrine (MARE-oh-krin) Another name for *eccrine.*

mesentery (MESS-en-ter-ree) A double layer of peritoneum enclosing the abdominal viscera.

mesothelioma (MEEZ-oh-thee-lee-OH-mah) Cancer arising from the cells lining the pleura or peritoneum.

metabolic acidosis (met-ah-BOL-ik ass-ih-DOH-sis) Decreased pH in the blood and body tissues as a result of an upset in metabolism.

metabolism (meh-TAB-oh-lizm) The constantly changing physical and chemical processes occurring in the cell.

metacarpal (MET-ah-KAR-pal) The five bones between the carpus and the fingers.

metacarpophalangeal (MET-ah-KAR-poh-fah-LAN-jee-al) Pertaining to the joints between the metacarpal bones and the phalanges.

metaphysis (meh-TAF-ih-sis) Region between the diaphysis and the epiphysis where bone growth occurs.

metastasis (meh-TAS-tah-sis) Spread of a disease from one part of the body to another. Plural *metastases.*

metastasize (meh-TAS-tah-size) To spread to distant parts.

metrorrhagia (MEH-troh-RAY-jee-ah) Irregular uterine bleeding between menses.

microalbuminuria (MY-kroh-al-byu-min-YOU-ree-ah) Presence of very small quantities of albumin in urine that cannot be detected by conventional urine testing.

microaneurysm (my-kroh-AN-yu-rizm) Focal dilation of retinal capillaries.

microangiopathy (MY-kroh-an-jee-OP-ah-thee) Disease of the very small blood vessels (capillaries).

microarray (MY-kroh-ah-RAY) Technique for studying one gene in one experiment. Also called *gene chips.*

microcephaly (MY-kroh-SEF-ah-lee) An abnormally small head.

microcytic (my-kroh-SIT-ik) Pertaining to a small cell.

microglia (my-KROH-glee-ah) Small nervous tissue cells that are phagocytes.

microscope (MY-kroh-skope) Instrument for viewing something small that cannot be seen in detail by the naked eye.

micturition (mik-choo-RISH-un) Act of passing urine.

migraine (MY-grain) Paroxysmal severe headache confined to one side of the head.

mimetic (mi-MET-ick) A substance that imitates another substance.

mineral (MIN-er-al) Inorganic compound usually found in earth's crust.

mineralocorticoid (MIN-er-al-oh-KOR-tih-koyd) Hormone of the adrenal cortex that influences sodium and potassium metabolism.

minimus (MIN-ih-mus) The gluteus minimus is the smallest of the gluteal muscles and lies under the gluteus medius.

minus (MY-nus) Smaller or lesser; for example, labia minora. Plural *minora.*

mitochondrion (my-toe-KON-dree-on) Organelle that generates, stores, and releases energy for cell activities. Plural *mitochondria.*

mitosis (my-TOH-sis) Cell division to create two identical cells, each with 46 chromosomes.

mitral (MY-tral) Shaped like the headdress of a Catholic bishop.

molar (MOH-lar) One of six teeth in each jaw that grind food.

mole (MOLE) Benign localized area of melanin-producing cells.

molecule (MOLL-eh-kyul) Very small particle consisting of two or more atoms held tightly together.

molluscum contagiosum (moh-LUS-kum kon-TAY-jee-oh-sum) An STD caused by a virus.

monoclonal (MON-oh-KLOH-nal) Derived from a protein from a single clone of cells, all molecules of which are the same.

monocyte (MON-oh-site) Large white blood cell with a single nucleus.

monoglyceride (mon-oh-GLISS-eh-ride) A fatty substance with a single fatty acid.

mononeuropathy (MON-oh-nyu-ROP-ah-thee) Disorder affecting a single nerve.

mononucleosis (MON-oh-nyu-klee-OH-sis) Presence of large numbers of mononuclear leukocytes.

monoplegia (MON-oh-PLEE-jee-ah) Paralysis of one limb.

monosaccharide (MON-oh-SACK-ah-ride) Simplest form of sugar; for example, glucose.

Monospot test (MON-oh-spot TEST) Detects heterophile antibodies in infectious mononucleosis.

monozygotic (MON-oh-zie-GOT-ik) Twins from a single zygote.

mons pubis (MONZ PYU-bis) Fleshy pad with pubic hair, overlying the pubic bone.

morphine (MOR-feen) Derivative of opium used as an analgesic or sedative.

mortality (mor-TAL-ih-tee) Fatal outcome or death rate.

morula (MOR-you-lah) Ball of cells formed from divisions of a zygote.

motile (MOH-til) Capable of spontaneous movement.

motility (moh-TILL-ih-tee) The ability for spontaneous movement.

motor (MOH-tor) Pertaining to nerves that send impulses out to cause muscles to contract or glands to secrete.

mouth (MOWTH) External opening of a cavity or canal.

mucin (MYU-sin) Protein element of mucus.

mucolytic (MYU-koh-LIT-ik) Agent capable of dissolving or liquefying mucus.

mucopurulent (myu-koh-PYUR-you-lent) Mixture of pus and mucus.

mucosa (myu-KOH-sah) Lining of a tubular structure. Another name for *mucous membrane.*

mucus (MYU-kus) Sticky secretion of cells in mucous membranes.

multimodal (mul-tee-MOH-dal) Using many methods.

multipara (mul-TIP-ah-ruh) Woman who has given birth to two or more children.

murmur (MUR-mur) Abnormal sound heard on auscultation of the heart or blood vessels.

Murphy sign (MUR-fee SINE) Tenderness in the right subcostal area on inspiration, associated with acute cholecystitis.

muscle (MUSS-el) Tissue consisting of contractile cells.

muscular (MUSS-kyu-lar) Pertaining to muscle or muscles.

muscularis (muss-kyu-LAR-is) The muscular layer of a hollow organ or tube.

mutagen (MYU-tah-jen) Agent that produces a mutation in a gene.

mutation (myu-TAY-shun) Change in the chemistry of a gene.

mutism (MYU-tizm) Absence of speech.

myasthenia gravis (my-as-THEE-nee-ah GRAH-vis) Disorder of fluctuating muscle weakness.

myelin (MY-eh-lin) Material of the sheath around the axon of a nerve.

myelitis (MY-eh-LIE-tis) Inflammation of the spinal cord.

myelography (my-eh-LOG-rah-fee) Radiography of the spinal cord and nerve roots after injection of a contrast medium into the subarachnoid space.

myeloid (MY-eh-loyd) Resembling cells derived from bone marrow.

myocarditis (MY-oh-kar-DIE-tis) Inflammation of the heart muscle.

myocardium (MY-oh-KAR-dee-um) All the heart muscle.

myoglobin (MY-oh-GLOH-bin) Protein of muscle that stores and transports oxygen.

myoma (my-OH-mah) Benign tumor of muscle.

myomectomy (my-oh-MEK-toh-mee) Surgical removal of a myoma (fibroid).

myometrium (my-oh-MEE-tree-um) Muscle wall of the uterus.

myopia (my-OH-pee-ah) Able to see close objects but unable to see distant objects.

myringotomy (mir-in-GOT-oh-mee) Incision in the tympanic membrane.

myxedema (mik-seh-DEE-mah) Severe hypothyroidism.

N

narcissistic (NAR-sih-SIS-tik) Relating everything to oneself.

narcolepsy (NAR-coh-lep-see) Condition with frequent incidents of sudden, involuntary deep sleep.

narcotic (nar-KOT-ik) Drug derived from opium, or a synthetic drug with similar effects.

naris (NAH-ris) Nostril. Plural *nares.*

nasal (NAY-zal) Pertaining to the nose.

nasolacrimal duct (NAY-zoh-LAK-rim-al DUKT) Passage from the lacrimal sac to the nose.

nasopharynx (NAY-zoh-FAIR-inks) Region of the pharynx at the back of the nose and above the soft palate.

natriuretic peptide (NAH-tree-you-RET-ik PEP-tide) Protein that increases the excretion of sodium.

nebulizer (NEB-you-lize-er) Device used to deliver liquid medicine in a fine mist.

necrosis (neh-KROH-sis) Pathologic death of cells or tissue.

necrotic (neh-KROT-ik) Affected by necrosis.

necrotizing fasciitis (neh-kroh-TIZE-ing fash-eh-EYE-tis) Inflammation of fascia, producing death of the tissue.

neonate (NEE-oh-nate) A newborn infant.

neoplasm (NEE-oh-plazm) A new growth, either a benign or malignant tumor.

nephritis (neh-FRIE-tis) Inflammation of the kidney.

nephroblastoma (NEF-roh-blas-TOH-mah) Cancerous kidney tumor of childhood. Also known as *Wilms tumor.*

nephrolithiasis (NEF-roh-lih-THIGH-ah-sis) Presence of a kidney stone.

nephrolithotomy (NEF-roh-lih-THOT-oh-mee) Incision for removal of a stone.

nephrologist (neh-FROL-oh-jist) Medical specialist in disorders of the kidney.

nephron (NEF-ron) Filtration unit of the kidney; glomerulus + renal tubule.

nephropathy (neh-FROP-ah-thee) Any disease of the kidney.

nephroscope (NEF-roh-skope) Endoscope used to view the inside of the kidney.

nephrotic syndrome (neh-FROT-ik SIN-drome) Glomerular disease with marked loss of protein. Also known as *nephrosis.*

nerve (NERV) A cord of fibers in connective tissue that conduct impulses.

nerve conduction study (NERV kon-DUK-shun STUD-ee) Procedure for measuring the speed at which an electrical impulse travels along a nerve.

nervous (NER-vus) Pertaining to a nerve.

neural tube (NYU-ral TYUB) Embryologic tubelike structure that forms the brain and spinal cord.

neuralgia (nyu-RAL-jee-ah) Pain in the distribution of a nerve.

neurilemma (nyu-ri-LEM-ah) Covering of a nerve around the myelin sheath.

neuroglia (nyu-ROH-glee-ah) Connective tissue holding nervous tissue together.

neurohypophysis (NYUR-oh-high-POF-ih-sis) Posterior lobe of the pituitary gland.

neurologist (nyu-ROL-oh-jist) Medical specialist in disorders of the nervous system.

neurology (nyu-ROL-oh-jee) Medical specialty of disorders of the nervous system.

neuromuscular (NYUR-oh-MUSS-kyu-lar) Pertaining to both nerves and muscles.

neuron (NYUR-on) Technical term for a nerve cell; consists of the cell body with its dendrites and axons.

neuropathy (nyu-ROP-ah-thee) Any disease of the nervous system.

neurosurgeon (NYU-roh-SUR-jun) Specialist in operating on the nervous system.

neurosurgery (NYU-roh-SUR-jer-ee) Medical specialty in surgery of the nervous system.

neurotoxin (NYUR-oh-tock-sin) Agent that poisons the nervous system.

neurotransmitter (NYUR-oh-trans-MIT-er) Chemical agent that relays messages from one nerve cell to the next.

neutropenia (NEW-troh-PEE-nee-ah) A deficiency of neutrophils.

neutrophil (NEW-troh-fill) A neutrophil's granules take up (purple) stain equally, whether the stain is acid or alkaline.

neutrophilia (NEW-troh-FILL-ee-ah) An increase in neutrophils.

nevus (NEE-vus) Congenital or acquired lesion of the skin. Plural *nevi.*

nipple (NIP-el) Projection from the breast into which the lactiferous ducts open.

nitrite (NIE-trite) Chemical formed in urine by *E. coli* and other microorganisms.

nitrogenous (ni-TROJ-en-us) Containing or generating nitrogen.

nocturia (nok-TYU-ree-ah) Excessive urination at night.

node (NOHD) A circumscribed mass of tissue.

nodule (NOD-yule) Small node or knotlike swelling.

norepinephrine (NOR-ep-ih-NEF-rin) Parasympathetic neurotransmitter that is a catecholamine hormone of the adrenal gland. Also called *noradrenaline.*

nuchal cord (NYU-kul KORD) Loop of umbilical cord around the fetal neck.

nucleolus (nyu-KLEE-oh-lus) Small mass within the nucleus.

nucleotide (NYU-klee-oh-tide) Combination of a DNA base, a sugar molecule, and a phosphate molecule.

nucleus (NYU-klee-us) Functional center of a cell or structure.

null cells (NULL SELLS) Lymphocytes with no surface markers, unlike T cells or B cells.

nutrient (NYU-tree-ent) A substance in food required for normal physiologic function.

nutrition (nyu-TRISH-un) The study of food and liquid requirements for normal function of the human body.

O

obesity (oh-BEE-sih-tee) Excessive amount of fat in the body.

oblique fracture (ob-LEEK FRAK-chur) A diagonal fracture across the long axis of the bone.

obsession (ob-SESH-un) Persistent, recurrent, uncontrollable thoughts or impulses.

obsessive (ob-SES-iv) Possessing persistent, recurrent, uncontrollable thoughts or impulses.

obstetrician (ob-steh-TRISH-un) Medical specialist in obstetrics.

obstetrics (OB) (ob-STET-riks) Medical specialty for the care of women during pregnancy and the postpartum period.

occipital bone (ok-SIP-it-al BOHN) Bone that forms the back and part of the base of the cranium.

occipital lobe (ok-SIP-it-al LOBE) Posterior area of the cerebral hemispheres.

occlude (ok-KLUDE) To close, plug, or completely obstruct.

occult (oh-KULT) Not visible on the surface.

occupational therapy (OK-you-PAY-shun-al THAIR-ah-pee) Use of work and recreational activities to increase independent function.

oculomotor (OK-you-loh-MOH-tor) Third (III) cranial nerve; moves the eye.

olfaction (ol-FAK-shun) Sense of smell.

olfactory (ol-FAK-toh-ree) First (I) cranial nerve; carries information related to the sense of smell.

oligodendrocyte (OL-ih-goh-DEN-droh-site) Connective tissue cell of the central nervous system that forms a myelin sheath.

oligohydramnios (OL-ih-goh-high-DRAM-nee-os) Too little amniotic fluid.

oliguria (ol-ih-GYUR-ee-ah) Scanty production of urine.

omentum (oh-MEN-tum) Membrane that encloses the bowels.

oncogene (ONG-koh-jeen) One of a family of genes involved in cell growth that work in concert to cause cancer.

oncologist (on-KOL-oh-jist) Medical specialist in oncology.

oncology (on-KOL-oh-jee) The science dealing with cancer.

onychomycosis (oh-ni-koh-my-KOH-sis) Condition of a fungus infection in a nail.

oocyte (OH-oh-site) Female egg cell.

oogenesis (oh-oh-JEN-eh-sis) Development of a female egg cell.

open fracture (OH-pen FRAK-chur) The skin over the fracture is broken.

ophthalmia neonatorum (off-THAL-mee-ah nee-oh-nay-TOR-um) Conjunctivitis of the newborn.

ophthalmologist (off-thal-MALL-oh-jist) Medical specialist in ophthalmology.

ophthalmoscope (off-THAL-moh-skope) Instrument for viewing the retina.

ophthalmoscopic (OFF-thal-moh-SKOP-ik) Pertaining to the use of an ophthalmoscope.

opiate (OH-pee-ate) A drug derived from opium.

opportunistic (OP-or-tyu-NIS-tik) An organism or a disease in a host with lowered resistance.

opportunistic infection (OP-or-tyu-NIS-tik in-FEK-shun) An infection that causes disease when the immune system is compromised for other reasons.

optic (OP-tik) Pertaining to the eye; *or* second (II) cranial nerve, which carries visual information.

optometrist (op-TOM-eh-trist) Someone who is skilled in the measurement of vision but cannot treat eye diseases or prescribe medication.

oral (OR-al) Pertaining to the mouth.

orbit (OR-bit) The bony socket that holds the eyeball.

orchiectomy (or-kee-ECK-toh-mee) Removal of one or both testes.

orchiopexy (OR-kee-oh-PEK-see) Surgical fixation of a testis in the scrotum.

orchitis (or-KIE-tis) Inflammation of the testis. Also called *epididymoorchitis.*

organ (OR-gan) Structure with specific functions in a body system.

organelle (OR-gah-nell) Part of a cell having a specialized function(s).

organophosphate (OR-ga-no-FOS-fate) Organic phosphorus compound used as an insecticide.

origin (OR-ih-gin) Fixed source of a muscle at its attachment to bone.

oropharynx (OR-oh-FAIR-inks) Region at the back of the mouth between the soft palate and the tip of the epiglottis.

orthopedic (or-thoh-PEE-dik) Pertaining to the correction and cure of deformities and diseases of the musculoskeletal system; originally, most of the deformities treated were in children. Also spelled *orthopaedic.*

orthopedist (or-thoh-PEE-dist) Specialist in orthopedics.

orthopnea (or-THOP-nee-ah) Difficulty in breathing when lying flat.

orthotic (or-THOT-ik) Orthopedic appliance used to correct an abnormality.

orthotist (or-THOT-ist) Maker and fitter of orthopedic appliances.

os (OS) Opening into a canal; for example, the cervix.

osmosis (oz-MOH-sis) The passage of water across a cell membrane.

ossicle (OS-ih-kel) A small bone, particularly relating to the three bones in the middle ear.

osteoarthritis (OS-tee-oh-ar-THRIE-tis) Chronic inflammatory disease of the joints with pain and loss of function.

osteoblast (OS-tee-oh-blast) Bone-forming cell.

osteoclast (OS-tee-oh-klast) Bone-removing cell.

osteocyte (OS-tee-oh-site) Bone-maintaining cell.

osteogenesis (OS-tee-oh-JEN-eh-sis) Creation of new bone.

osteogenesis imperfecta (OS-tee-oh-JEN-eh-sis im-per-FEK-tah) Inherited condition in which bone formation is incomplete, leading to fragile, easily broken bones.

osteogenic sarcoma (OS-tee-oh-JEN-ik sar-KOH-mah) Malignant tumor originating in bone-producing cells.

osteomalacia (OS-tee-oh-mah-LAY-shee-ah) Soft, flexible bones lacking in calcium (rickets).

osteomyelitis (OS-tee-oh-my-eh-LIE-tis) Inflammation of bone tissue.

osteopathy (OS-tee-OP-ah-thee) Medical practice based on maintaining the structural integrity of the musculoskeletal system.

osteopenia (OS-tee-oh-PEE-nee-ah) Decreased calcification of bone.

osteoporosis (OS-tee-oh-poh-ROH-sis) Condition in which the bones become more porous, brittle, and fragile and are more likely to fracture.

osteosarcoma (OS-tee-oh-sar-KOH-mah) Cancer arising in bone-forming cells.

ostomy (OS-toh-mee) Surgery to create an artificial opening into a tubular structure.

otitis media (oh-TIE-tis MEE-dee-ah) Inflammation of the middle ear.

otolith (OH-toh-lith) A calcium particle in the vestibule of the inner ear.

otologist (oh-TOL-oh-jist) Medical specialist in diseases of the ear.

otomycosis (OH-toh-my-KOH-sis) Fungal infection of the external ear.

otorhinolaryngologist (OH-toh-RIE-noh-LAH-rin-GOL-oh-jist) Ear, nose, and throat medical specialist.

otosclerosis (oh-toh-skler-OH-sis) Hardening at the junction of the stapes and oval window that causes loss of hearing.

otoscope (OH-toh-skope) Instrument for examining the ear.

otoscopic (oh-toh-SKOP-ik) Pertaining to examination with an otoscope.

otoscopy (oh-TOS-koh-pee) Examination of the ear.

ovarian (oh-VAIR-ee-an) Pertaining to the ovary.

ovary (OH-va-ree) One of the paired female egg-producing glands.

ovulation (OV-you-LAY-shun) Release of an oocyte from a follicle.

oxyhemoglobin (OK-see-HEE-moh-GLOH-bin) Hemoglobin in combination with oxygen.

oxytocin (OK-see-TOH-sin) Pituitary hormone that stimulates the uterus to contract.

P

pacemaker (PACE-may-ker) Device that regulates cardiac electrical activity.

palate (PAL-uht) Roof of the mouth.

palatine (PAL-ah-tine) Bone that forms the hard palate and parts of the nose and orbits.

palliative care (PAL-ee-ah-tiv KAIR) Care that relieves symptoms and pain without curing.

pallor (PAL-or) Paleness of the skin.

palm (PAHLM) The flat anterior surface of the hand.

palpate (PAL-pate) To examine with the fingers and hands.

palpation (pal-PAY-shun) An examination with the fingers and hands.

palpitation (pal-pih-TAY-shun) Forcible, rapid beat of the heart felt by the patient.

palsy (PAWL-zee) Paralysis or paresis from brain damage.

pancreas (PAN-kree-as) Lobulated gland, the head of which is tucked into the curve of the duodenum.

pancreatic (pan-kree-AT-ik) Pertaining to the pancreas.

pancreatitis (PAN-kree-ah-TIE-tis) Inflammation of the pancreas.

pancytopenia (PAN-sigh-toh-PEE-nee-ah) Deficiency of all types of blood cells.

panendoscopy (pan-en-DOS-koh-pee) Examination of the inside of the esophagus, stomach, and upper duodenum using a flexible fiber-optic endoscope.

panhypopituitarism (pan-HIGH-poh-pih-TYU-ih-tah-rizm) Deficiency of all the pituitary hormones.

Pap test (PAP TEST) Examination of cells taken from the cervix.

papilla (pah-PILL-ah) Any small projection. Plural *papillae*.

papilledema (pah-pill-eh-DEE-mah) Swelling of the optic disc in the retina.

papilloma (pap-ih-LOH-mah) Benign projection of epithelial cells.

papule (PAP-yul) Small, circumscribed elevation on the skin.

para (PAH-rah) Abbreviation for number of deliveries.

paralysis (pah-RAL-ih-sis) Loss of voluntary movement.

paralyze (PAR-ah-lize) To make incapable of movement.

paranasal (PAIR-ah-NAY-zal) Adjacent to the nose.

paranoid (PAIR-ah-noyd) Having delusions of persecution.

paraphimosis (PAR-ah-fi-MOH-sis) Condition in which a retracted prepuce cannot be pulled forward to cover the glans.

paraplegia (par-ah-PLEE-jee-ah) Paralysis of both lower extremities.

parasite (PAR-ah-site) An organism that attaches itself to, lives on or in, and derives its nutrition from another species.

parasympathetic (par-ah-sim-pah-THET-ik) Pertaining to division of the autonomic nervous system; has opposite effects of the sympathetic division.

parathyroid (pair-ah-THIGH-royd) Endocrine glands embedded in the back of the thyroid gland.

paraurethral (PAR-ah-you-REE-thral) Situated around the urethra.

parenchyma (pah-RENG-kih-mah) Characteristic functional cells of a gland or organ that are supported by the connective tissue framework.

parenteral (pah-REN-ter-al) Giving medication by any means other than the gastrointestinal tract.

paresis (par-EE-sis) Partial paralysis.

paresthesia (par-es-THEE-zee-ah) An abnormal sensation; for example, tingling, burning, pricking. Plural *paresthesias*.

parietal (pah-RYE-eh-tal) Pertaining to the wall of an organ or a body cavity.

parietal bones (pah-RYE-eh-tal BOHNZ) Bones that form the bulging sides and roof of the cranium.

parietal lobe (pah-RYE-eh-tal LOBE) Area of the brain under the parietal bone.

parity (PAIR-ih-tee) Number of deliveries.

Parkinson disease (PAR-kin-son diz-EEZ) Disease of muscular rigidity, tremors, and a masklike facial expression.

paronychia (pair-oh-NICK-ee-ah) Infection alongside the nail.

parotid (pah-ROT-id) Parotid gland is the salivary gland beside the ear.

paroxysmal (par-ok-SIZ-mal) Occurring in sharp, spasmodic episodes.

particle (PAR-tih-kul) A small piece of matter.

particulate (par-TIK-you-let) Relating to a fine particle.

patella (pah-TELL-ah) Thin, circular bone in front of the knee joint and embedded in the patellar tendon. Also called the *kneecap*.

patent (PAY-tent) Open.

patent ductus arteriosus (PAY-tent DUK-tus ar-TEER-ee-oh-sus) An open, direct channel between the aorta and the pulmonary artery.

pathogen (PATH-oh-jen) A disease-causing microorganism.

pathologic fracture (path-oh-LOJ-ik FRAK-chur) Fracture occurring at a site already weakened by a disease process, such as cancer.

pathologist (pah-THOL-oh-jist) A specialist in pathology (study of disease or characteristics of a particular disease).

pathology (pah-THOL-oh-jee) Medical specialty dealing with the structural and functional changes of a disease process; *or* the cause, development, and structural changes in disease.

pectoral (PEK-tor-al) Pertaining to the chest.

pectoral girdle (PEK-tor-al GIR-del) Incomplete bony ring that attaches the upper limb to the axial skeleton.

pedal (PEED-al) Pertaining to the foot.

pediatrician (PEE-dee-ah-TRISH-an) Medical specialist in pediatrics.

pediculosis (peh-dick-you-LOH-sis) An infestation with lice.

pelvic (PEL-vic) Pertaining to the pubic bone.

pelvis (PEL-vis) A cup-shaped cavity, as in the pelvis of the kidney; *or* a cup-shaped ring of bone.

penis (PEE-nis) Conveys urine and semen to the outside.

pepsin (PEP-sin) Enzyme produced by the stomach that breaks down protein.

pepsinogen (pep-SIN-oh-jen) Converted by HCl in stomach to pepsin.

peptic (PEP-tik) Relating to the stomach and duodenum.

perforated (PER-foh-ray-ted) Punctured with one or more holes.

perforation (per-foh-RAY-shun) Erosion that progresses to become a hole through the wall of a structure.

perfuse (per-FYUSE) To force blood to flow through a lumen or a vascular bed.

pericarditis (PER-ih-kar-DIE-tis) Inflammation of the pericardium, the covering of the heart.

pericardium (per-ih-KAR-dee-um) Structure around the heart.

perimeter (peh-RIM-eh-ter) An edge or border.

perimetrium (per-ih-MEE-tree-um) The covering of the uterus; part of the peritoneum.

perinatal (per-ih-NAY-tal) Around the time of birth.

perineum (PER-ih-NEE-um) Area between the thighs, extending from the coccyx to the pubis.

periodontal (PER-ee-oh-DON-tal) Around a tooth.

periodontitis (PER-ee-oh-don-TIE-tis) Inflammation of tissues around a tooth.

periorbital (per-ee-OR-bit-al) Pertaining to tissues around the orbit.

periosteum (PER-ee-OSS-tee-um) Fibrous membrane covering a bone.

peripheral (peh-RIF-er-al) Pertaining to the periphery or external boundary.

peripheral vision (peh-RIF-er-al VIZH-un) Ability to see objects as they come into the outer edges of the visual field.

periphery (peh-RIF-eh-ree) Outer part of a structure away from the center.

peristalsis (per-ih-STAL-sis) Waves of alternate contraction and relaxation of the intestinal wall to move food along the digestive tract.

peritoneum (per-ih-toh-NEE-um) Membrane that lines the abdominal cavity.

peritonitis (PER-ih-toh-NIE-tis) Inflammation of the peritoneum.

peritubular (PER-ih-TOO-byu-lar) Surrounding the small renal tubules.

permeable (PER-mee-ah-bull) Allows passage of substances through a membrane.

pernicious anemia (per-NISH-us ah-NEE-mee-ah) Chronic anemia due to lack of vitamin B_{12}.

peroneal (pair-uh-NEE-al) Pertaining to the lateral part (fibula) of the lower leg, or the nerve named after it.

pertussis (per-TUSS-is) Infectious disease with a spasmodic, intense cough ending on a whoop (stridor). Also known as *whooping cough*.

pes planus (PES PLAY-nuss) A flat foot with no plantar arch.

pessary (PES-ah-ree) Appliance inserted into the vagina to support the uterus.

pesticide (PES-tih-side) Agent for destroying flies, mosquitoes, and other pests.

petechia (peh-TEE-kee-ah) Pinpoint capillary hemorrhagic spot in the skin. Plural *petechiae*.

petit mal (peh-TEE MAL) Old name for an absence seizure.

Peyronie disease (pay-ROH-nee diz-EEZ) Penile bending and pain on erection.

phacoemulsification (FAK-oh-ee-mul-sih-fih-KAY-shun) Technique used to fragment the center of the lens into very tiny pieces and suck them out of the eye.

phagocytize (FAG-oh-site-ize) Ingest foreign particles and cells.

phagocytosis (FAG-oh-sigh-TOH-sis) Process of ingestion and destruction.

phalanx (FAY-lanks) A bone of a finger or toe. Plural *phalanges*.

pharmacist (FAR-mah-sist) Person licensed by the state to prepare and dispense drugs.

pharmacology (far-mah-KOL-oh-jee) Science of the preparation, uses, and effects of drugs.

pharmacy (FAR-mah-see) Facility licensed to prepare and dispense drugs.

pharyngitis (fair-in-JIE-tis) Inflammation of the pharynx.

pharynx (FAIR-inks) Air tube from the back of the nose to the larynx.

phenotype (FEE-noh-type) A visible trait.

pheochromocytoma (fee-oh-KROH-moh-sigh-TOH-mah) Adenoma of the adrenal medulla secreting excessive catecholamines.

pheomelanin (FEE-oh-mel-ah-nin) The lighter form of melanin.

pheromone (FAIR-oh-moan) Substance that carries and generates a physical attraction for other people.

phimosis (fi-MOH-sis) Condition in which the prepuce cannot be retracted.

phlebitis (fleh-BIE-tis) Inflammation of a vein.

phlegm (FLEM) Abnormal amounts of mucus expectorated from the respiratory tract.

phobia (FOH-bee-ah) Pathologic fear or dread.

phosphatase (FOS-fah-tase) Enzyme that liberates phosphorus.

photocoagulation (foh-toh-koh-ag-you-LAY-shun) The use of light (laser beam) to form a clot.

photophobia (foh-toh-FOH-bee-ah) Fear of the light because it hurts the eyes.

photoreceptor (foh-toh-ree-SEP-tor) A photoreceptor cell receives light and converts it into electrical impulses.

photosensitivity (foh-toh-sen-sih-TIV-ih-tee) Condition in which light produces pain in the eye.

physiatrist (fih-ZIE-ah-trist) Specialist in physical medicine.

physiatry (fih-ZIE-ah-tree) Physical medicine.

physical medicine (FIZ-ih-cal MED-ih-sin) Diagnosis and treatment by means of remedial agents, such as exercises, manipulation, and heat.

physical therapy (FIZ-ih-cal THAIR-ah-pee) Use of remedial processes to overcome a physical defect. Also known as *physiotherapy*.

pia mater (PEE-ah MAY-ter) Delicate inner layer of the meninges.

pineal (PIN-ee-al) Pertaining to the pineal gland.

pink eye (PINK EYE) Conjunctivitis.

pinna (PIN-ah) Another name for *auricle*. Plural *pinnae*.

pituitary (pih-TOO-ih-tair-ee) Pertaining to the pituitary gland.

placenta (plah-SEN-tah) Organ that allows metabolic interchange between the mother and the fetus.

plaque (PLAK) Patch of abnormal tissue.

plasma (PLAZ-mah) Fluid, noncellular component of blood.

plasma cell (PLAZ-mah SELL) Cell derived from B lymphocytes and active in formation of antibodies.

platelet (PLAYT-let) Cell fragment involved in the clotting process. Also called *thrombocyte*.

pleura (PLOOR-ah) Membrane covering the lungs and lining the ribs in the thoracic cavity. Plural *pleurae*.

pleurisy (PLOOR-ih-see) Inflammation of the pleura.

plexus (PLEK-sus) A weblike network of joined nerves. Plural *plexuses*.

plica (PLEE-cah) Fold in a mucous membrane. Plural *plicae*.

pneumatic (new-MAT-ik) Pertaining to a structure filled with air.

pneumoconiosis (new-moh-koh-nee-OH-sis) Fibrotic lung disease caused by the inhalation of different dusts.

pneumonectomy (NEW-moh-NEK-toh-mee) Surgical removal of a whole lung.

pneumonia (new-MOH-nee-ah) Inflammation of the lung parenchyma.

pneumothorax (new-moh-THOR-aks) Air in the pleural cavity.

podiatrist (poh-DIE-ah-trist) Practitioner of podiatry.

podiatry (poh-DIE-ah-tree) Specialty concerned with the diagnosis and treatment of disorders and injuries of the foot.

poikilocytic (POY-kee-loh-SIT-ik) Pertaining to an irregular-shaped RBC.

poliomyelitis (POH-lee-oh-MY-eh-LIE-tis) Inflammation of the gray matter of the spinal cord, leading to paralysis of the limbs and muscles of respiration.

pollutant (poh-LOO-tant) Substance that makes an environment unclean or impure.

pollution (poh-LOO-shun) Condition that is unclean, impure, and a danger to health.

polycystic (pol-ee-SIS-tik) Composed of many cysts.

polycythemia vera (POL-ee-sigh-THEE-me-ah VEH-rah) Chronic disease with bone marrow hyperplasia and an increase in the number of RBCs and blood volume.

polydipsia (pol-ee-DIP-see-ah) Excessive thirst.

polyhydramnios (POL-ee-high-DRAM-nee-os) Too much amniotic fluid.

polymenorrhea (POL-ee-men-oh-REE-ah) More than normal frequency of menses.

polymorphonuclear (POL-ee-more-foh-NEW-klee-ar) White blood cell with a multilobed nucleus.

polyneuropathy (POL-ee-nyu-ROP-ah-thee) Disorder affecting many nerves.

polyp (POL-ip) Mass of tissue that projects into the lumen of the bowel.

polyphagia (pol-ee-FAY-jee-ah) Excessive eating.

polysaccharide (pol-ee-SACK-ah-ride) A combination of many saccharides; for example, starch.

polysomnography (pol-ee-som-NOG-rah-fee) Test to monitor brain waves, muscle tension, eye movement, and oxygen levels in the blood as the patient sleeps.

polyuria (pol-ee-YOU-ree-ah) Excessive production of urine.

pons (PONZ) Part of the brainstem.

popliteal (pop-LIT-ee-al) Pertaining to the back of the knee.

popliteal fossa (pop-LIT-ee-al FOSS-ah) The hollow at the back of the knee.

portal; portal vein (POR-tal VANE) The vein that carries blood from the intestines to the liver.

postcoital (post-KOH-ih-tal) After sexual intercourse.

posterior (pos-TEER-ee-or) Pertaining to the back surface of the body; situated behind.

postictal (post-IK-tal) Occurring after a seizure.

postmature (post-mah-TYUR) Infant born after 42 weeks of gestation.

postmaturity (post-mah-TYUR-ih-tee) Condition of being postmature.

postpartum (post-PAR-tum) After childbirth.

postpolio syndrome (PPS) (post-POH-lee-oh SIN-drome) Progressive muscle weakness in a person previously affected by polio.

postprandial (post-PRAN-dee-al) Following a meal.

postpubescent (post-pyu-BESS-ent) After the period of puberty.

posttraumatic (post-traw-MAT-ik) Occurring after and caused by trauma.

posture (POSS-chur) The carriage of the body as a whole and the position of the limbs.

Pott fracture (POT FRAK-chur) Fracture of the lower end of the fibula, often with fracture of the tibial malleolus.

precancerous (pree-KAN-sir-us) Lesion from which a cancer can develop.

precursor (pree-KUR-sir) Cell or substance formed earlier in the development of the cell or substance.

preeclampsia (pree-eh-KLAMP-see-uh) Hypertension, edema, and proteinuria during pregnancy.

pregnancy (PREG-nan-see) State of being pregnant.

prehypertension (pree-HIGH-per-TEN-shun) Precursor to hypertension.

premature (pree-mah-TYUR) Occurring before the expected time; for example, an infant born before 37 weeks of gestation.

prematurity (pree-mah-TYUR-ih-tee) Condition of being premature.

prenatal (pree-NAY-tal) Before birth.

prepatellar (pree-pah-TELL-ar) In front of the patella.

prepuce (PREE-puce) Fold of skin that covers the glans penis.

presbyopia (prez-bee-OH-pee-ah) Difficulty in nearsighted vision occurring in middle and old age.

preterm (PREE-term) Baby delivered before 37 weeks of gestation. Also called *premature.*

prevention (pree-VEN-shun) Process undertaken to prevent occurrence of a disease or health problem.

previa (PREE-vee-ah) Anything blocking the fetus during its birth; for example, an abnormally situated placenta, *placenta previa.*

priapism (PRY-ah-pizm) Persistent erection of the penis.

primary care (PRY-mah-ree KAIR) Comprehensive and preventive health care services that are the first point of care for a patient.

primigravida (pree-mih-GRAV-ih-dah) First pregnancy.

primipara (pree-MIP-ah-ruh) Woman who has given birth for the first time.

prion (PREE-on) Small infectious protein particle.

proctitis (prok-TIE-tis) Inflammation of the lining of the rectum.

proctoscopy (prok-TOSS-koh-pee) Examination of the inside of the anus by endoscopy.

progesterone (proh-JESS-ter-ohn) Hormone that prepares the uterus for pregnancy.

progestin (pro-JESS-tin) A synthetic form of progesterone.

prognathism (PROG-nah-thizm) Condition of a forward-projecting jaw.

prognosis (prog-NO-sis) Forecasting of the probable course of a disease.

prolactin (proh-LAK-tin) Pituitary hormone that stimulates the production of milk.

prolactinoma (proh-lak-tih-NOH-mah) Prolactin-producing tumor.

prolapse (proh-LAPS) The falling or slipping of a body part from its normal position.

proliferate (proh-LIF-eh-rate) To increase in number through reproduction.

pronate (PROH-nate) Rotate the forearm so that the surface of the palm faces posteriorly in the anatomical position.

pronation (proh-NAY-shun) Process of lying facedown or of turning a hand or foot with the volar (palm or sole) surface down.

prone (PRONE) Lying facedown, flat on your belly.

prophylaxis (pro-fih-LAX-is) Prevention of disease.

prostaglandin (PROS-tah-GLAN-din) Hormone present in many tissues, but first isolated from the prostate gland.

prostate (PROS-tate) Organ surrounding the beginning of the urethra.

prostatectomy (pross-tah-TEK-toh-mee) Surgical removal of the prostate.

prostatitis (pross-tah-TIE-tis) Inflammation of the prostate.

prosthesis (pros-THEE-sis) A manufactured substitute for a missing or diseased part of the body.

protease (PROH-tee-aze) Group of enzymes that break down protein.

protection (proh-TEK-shun) Defense against attack or invasion.

protein (PRO-teen) Class of food substances based on amino acids.

proteinuria (pro-tee-NYU-ree-ah) Presence of protein in urine.

prothrombin (proh-THROM-bin) Protein formed by the liver and converted to thrombin in the blood-clotting mechanism.

proton pump inhibitor (PPI) (PROH-ton PUMP in-HIB-ih-tor) Agent that blocks production of gastric acid.

protooncogene (pro-toh-ONG-koh-jeen) A normal gene involved in normal cell growth.

provisional diagnosis (proh-VISH-un-al die-ag-NOH-sis) A temporary diagnosis pending further examination or testing. Also called *preliminary diagnosis.*

proximal (PROK-sih-mal) Situated nearest to the center of the body.

pruritus (proo-RYE-tus) Itching.

psoriasis (so-RYE-ah-sis) Rash characterized by reddish, silver-scaled patches.

psychedelic (sigh-keh-DEL-ik) Agent that intensifies sensory perception.

psychiatric (sigh-kee-AH-trik) Pertaining to psychiatry.

psychiatrist (sigh-KIE-ah-trist) Licensed medical specialist in psychiatry.

psychiatry (sigh-KIE-ah-tree) Diagnosis and treatment of mental disorders.

psychoactive (sigh-koh-AK-tiv) Able to alter mood, behavior, and/or cognition.

psychoanalysis (sigh-koh-ah-NAL-ih-sis) Method of psychotherapy.

psychoanalyst (sigh-koh-AN-ah-list) Practitioner of psychoanalysis.

psychological (sigh-koh-LOJ-ik-al) Pertaining to psychology.

psychologist (sigh-KOL-oh-jist) Licensed specialist in psychology.

psychology (sigh-KOL-oh-jee) Scientific study of the human mind and behavior.

psychopath (SIGH-koh-path) Person with antisocial personality disorder.

psychosis (sigh-KOH-sis) Disorder causing mental disruption and loss of contact with reality.

psychosomatic (sigh-koh-soh-MAT-ik) Pertaining to disorders of the body usually resulting from disturbances of the mind.

psychotherapist (sigh-koh-THAIR-ah-pist) Practitioner of psychotherapy.

psychotherapy (sigh-koh-THAIR-ah-pee) Treatment of mental disorders through communication.

ptosis (TOH-sis) Sinking down of an eyelid or an organ.

puberty (PYU-ber-tee) Process of maturing from child to young adult capable of reproducing.

pubic (PYU-bik) Pertaining to the pubis.

pubis (PYU-bis) Bony front arch of the pelvis of the hip. Also called *pubic bone.*

puerperium (pyu-er-PEE-ree-um) Six-week period after birth in which the uterus involutes.

pulmonary (PULL-moh-NAIR-ee) Pertaining to the lungs and their blood supply.

pulmonologist (PULL-moh-NOL-oh-jist) Medical specialist in pulmonary disorders.

pulp (PULP) Dental pulp is the connective tissue in the cavity in the center of the tooth.

pupil (PYU-pill) The opening in the center of the iris that allows light to reach the lens. Plural *pupillae.*

Purkinje fibers (per-KIN-jee FIE-bers) Network of nerve fibers in the myocardium.

purpura (PUR-pyu-rah) Skin hemorrhages that are red initially and then turn purple.

purulent (PURE-you-lent) Showing or containing a lot of pus.

pustule (PUS-tyul) Small protuberance on the skin that contains pus.

pyelitis (pie-eh-LIE-tis) Inflammation of the renal pelvis.

pyelogram (PIE-el-oh-gram) X-ray image of renal pelvis and ureters.

pyelonephritis (PIE-eh-loh-neh-FRIE-tis) Inflammation of the kidney and renal pelvis.

pyloric (pie-LOR-ik) Pertaining to the pylorus.

pylorus (pie-LOR-us) Exit area of the stomach.

pyorrhea (pie-oh-REE-ah) Purulent discharge.

pyrexia (pie-REK-see-ah) An abnormally high body temperature or fever.

pyromania (pie-roh-MAY-nee-ah) Morbid impulse to set fires.

Q

quadrant (KWAD-rant) One-quarter of a circle.

quadrantectomy (kwad-ran-TEK-toh-mee) Surgical excision of a quadrant of the breast.

quadriceps femoris (KWAD-rih-seps FEM-or-is) An anterior thigh muscle with four heads.

quadriplegia (kwad-rih-PLEE-jee-ah) Paralysis of all four limbs.

R

radial (RAY-dee-al) Pertaining to the forearm.

radiation (ray-dee-AY-shun) A spreading out, as of anatomical parts.

radical (RAD-ih-kal) Extensive, as in complete removal of a diseased part.

radioactive (RAY-dee-oh-AK-tiv) Spontaneously emitting alpha, beta, or gamma rays.

radioactive iodine (RAY-dee-oh-AK-tiv EYE-oh-dine) Any of the various tracers that emit alpha, beta, or gamma rays.

radiologist (ray-dee-OL-oh-jist) Medical specialist in the use of x-rays and other imaging techniques.

radiology (ray-dee-OL-oh-jee) The study of medical imaging.

radionuclide (RAY-dee-oh-NYU-klide) Radioactive agent used in diagnostic imaging.

radiotherapy (RAY-dee-oh-THAIR-ah-pee) Treatment using radiation.

radius (RAY-dee-us) The forearm bone on the thumb side.

rale (RAHL) Crackle heard through a stethoscope when air bubbles through liquid in the lungs. Plural *rales.*

raphe (RAY-fee) Line separating two symmetrical structures.

reabsorption (ree-ab-SORP-shun) The taking back into the blood of substances that had previously been filtered out from it.

recombinant DNA (ree-KOM-bin-ant DEE-en-a) DNA (deoxyribonucleic acid) altered by inserting a new sequence of DNA into the chain.

rectocele (REK-toh-seal) Hernia of the rectum into the vagina.

rectum (RECK-tum) Terminal part of the colon from the sigmoid to the anal canal.

recurrent (ree-KUR-ent) Symptoms or lesions returning after an intermission.

reflex (REE-fleks) An involuntary response to a stimulus.

reflux (REE-fluks) Backward flow.

regenerate (ree-JEN-eh-rate) Reconstitution of a lost part.

regimen (REJ-ih-men) Program of treatment.

regulate (REG-you-late) To control the way in which a process progresses.

regurgitate (ree-GUR-jih-tate) To flow backward; for example, through a heart valve.

regurgitation (ree-gur-jih-TAY-shun) The flow of material in backward direction. In the digestive system, it means to expel contents of the stomach into the mouth, short of vomiting.

rehabilitation (REE-hah-bil-ih-TAY-shun) Therapeutic restoration of an ability to function as before.

remission (ree-MISH-un) Period in which there is a lessening or absence of the symptoms of a disease.

renal (REE-nal) Pertaining to the kidney.

renin (REE-nin) Enzyme secreted by the kidney that causes vasoconstriction.

replicate (REP-lih-kate) To produce an exact copy.

replication (rep-lih-KAY-shun) Reproduction to produce an exact copy.

reproductive (ree-pro-DUC-tiv) Relating to the process by which organisms produce offspring.

resection (ree-SEK-shun) Removal of a specific part of an organ or structure.

residual (ree-ZID-you-al) Pertaining to anything left over.

resistance (ree-ZIS-tants) Ability of an organism to withstand the effects of an antagonistic agent.

resorption (ree-SORP-shun) Loss of substance, such as bone.

respiration (RES-pih-RAY-shun) Fundamental process of life used to exchange oxygen and carbon dioxide.

respiratory (RES-pir-ah-TOR-ee) Relating to the process of exchanging oxygen and carbon dioxide.

restorative rehabilitation (ree-STOR-ah-tiv REE-hah-bil-ih-TAY-shun) Promote renewal of health and strength.

rete testis (REE-teh TES-tis) Network of tubules between the seminiferous tubules and the epididymis.

retention (ree-TEN-shun) Holding back in the body what should normally be discharged (e.g., urine).

reticulum (reh-TIK-you-lum) Fine network of cells in the medulla oblongata.

retina (RET-ih-nah) Light-sensitive innermost layer of the eyeball.

retinaculum (ret-ih-NAK-you-lum) Fibrous ligament that keeps the tendons in place on the wrist so that they do not "bowstring" when the forearm muscles contract.

retinoblastoma (RET-in-oh-blas-TOH-mah) Malignant neoplasm of primitive retinal cells.

retinoid (RET-ih-noyd) A class of keratolytic agents.

retinopathy (ret-ih-NOP-ah-thee) Degenerative disease of the retina.

retraction (ree-TRAK-shun) A pulling back, as a pulling back of the intercostal spaces and the neck above the clavicle.

retrograde (RET-roh-grade) Reversal of a normal flow; for example, back from the bladder into the ureters.

retroverted (REH-troh-vert-ed) Tilted backward.

retrovirus (REH-troh-VIE-rus) Virus that replicates in a host cell by converting its RNA core into DNA.

Reye syndrome (RAY SIN-drome) Encephalopathy and liver damage in children following an acute viral illness; linked to aspirin use.

rhabdomyolysis (RAB-doh-my-OL-ih-sis) Destruction of muscle to produce myoglobin.

rhabdomyosarcoma (RAB-doh-MY-oh-sar-KOH-mah) Cancer derived from skeletal muscle.

rheumatoid arthritis (RA) (RHU-mah-toyd ar-THRIE-tis) Disease of connective tissue, with arthritis as a major manifestation.

rhinitis (rye-NIE-tis) Inflammation of the nasal mucosa. Also called *coryza*.

rhinoplasty (RYE-noh-plas-tee) Surgical procedure to change the size or shape of the nose.

rhonchus (RONG-kuss) Wheezing sound heard on auscultation of the lungs; made by air passing through a constricted lumen. Plural *rhonchi*.

ribosome (RYE-bo-sohm) Structure in the cell that assembles amino acids into protein.

rickets (RIK-ets) Disease due to vitamin D deficiency, producing soft, flexible bones.

Rinne test (RIN-eh TEST) Test for conductive hearing loss.

root (ROOT) Fundamental or beginning part of a structure.

rosacea (roh-ZAY-she-ah) Persistent erythematous rash of the central face.

rotator cuff (roh-TAY-tor CUFF) Part of the capsule of the shoulder joint.

Roux-en-Y (ROO-on-Y) Surgical procedure to reduce the size of the stomach.

ruga (ROO-gah) A fold, ridge, or crease. Plural *rugae*.

rupture (RUP-tyur) Break or tear of any organ or body part.

S

sacral (SAY-kral) In the neighborhood of the sacrum.

sacroiliac joint (SAY-kroh-ILL-ih-ak JOYNT) The joint between the sacrum and the ilium.

sacrum (SAY-krum) Segment of the vertebral column that forms part of the pelvis.

sagittal (SAJ-ih-tal) Pertaining to the vertical plane through the body, dividing it into right and left portions.

saliva (sa-LIE-vah) Secretion in the mouth from salivary glands.

salpingectomy (sal-pin-JEK-toh-mee) Surgical removal of fallopian tube(s).

salpingitis (sal-pin-JIE-tis) Inflammation of the uterine tube.

saphenous (SAF-ih-nus) Relating to the saphenous vein in the thigh.

sarcoidosis (sar-koy-DOH-sis) Granulomatous lesions of the lungs and other organs; cause is unknown.

sarcoma (sar-KOH-mah) A malignant tumor originating in connective tissue.

sarcopenia (sar-koh-PEE-nee-ah) Progressive loss of muscle mass and strength in aging.

scab (SKAB) Crust that forms over a wound or sore during healing.

scabies (SKAY-bees) Skin disease produced by mites.

scapula (SKAP-you-lah) Shoulder blade. Plural *scapulae*.

scar (SKAR) Fibrotic seam that forms when a wound heals.

schizoid (SKITZ-oyd) Withdrawn, socially isolated.

schizophrenia (skitz-oh-FREE-nee-ah) Disorder of perception, thought, emotion, and behavior.

Schwann cell (SHWANN SELL) Connective tissue cell of the peripheral nervous system that forms a myelin sheath.

sciatic (sigh-AT-ik) Pertaining to the sciatic nerve or sciatica.

sciatica (sigh-AT-ih-kah) Pain from compression of L5 or S1 nerve roots.

scintigraphy (sin-TIG-rah-fee) Recording of radioactivity with a special camera.

sclera (SKLAIR-ah) Fibrous outer covering of the eyeball and the white of the eye.

scleritis (sklair-RIE-tis) Inflammation of the sclera.

scleroderma (sklair-oh-DERM-ah) Thickening and hardening of the skin due to new collagen formation.

sclerose (skleh-ROZE) To harden or thicken.

sclerotherapy (SKLAIR-oh-THAIR-ah-pee) To collapse a vein by injecting a solution into it to harden it.

scoliosis (skoh-lee-OH-sis) An abnormal lateral curvature of the vertebral column.

scrotum (SKROH-tum) Sac containing the testes.

seasonal affective disorder (SEE-zon-al af-FEK-tiv dis-OR-der) Depression that occurs at the same time every year, often in winter.

sebaceous glands (se-BAY-shus GLANDZ) Glands in the dermis that open into hair follicles and secrete an oily fluid called sebum.

seborrhea (seb-oh-REE-ah) Excessive amount of sebum.

sebum (SEE-bum) Waxy secretion of the sebaceous glands.

secrete (seh-KREET) To release or give off, as substances produced by cells.

secretin (se-KREE-tin) Hormone produced by the duodenum to stimulate pancreatic juice.

sedative (SED-ah-tiv) Agent that calms nervous excitement.

sedentary (sed-en-TAIR-ee) Accustomed to little exercise or movement.

segment (SEG-ment) A section of an organ or structure.

segmentectomy (seg-men-TEK-toh-mee) Surgical excision of a segment of a tissue or organ.

seizure (SEE-zhur) Event due to excessive electrical activity in the brain.

self-examination (SELF-ek-zam-ih-NAY-shun) The examination of part of one's own body.

self-mutilation (self-myu-tih-LAY-shun) Injury or disfigurement made to one's own body.

semen (SEE-men) Penile ejaculate containing sperm and seminal fluid.

semilunar (sem-ee-LOO-nar) Appears like a half moon.

seminal vesicle (SEM-in-al VES-ih-kull) Sac of the ductus deferens that produces seminal fluid.

seminiferous tubule (sem-ih-NIF-er-us TU-byul) Coiled tubes in the testes that produce sperm.

seminoma (sem-ih-NOH-mah) Neoplasm of germ cells of a testis.

senescence (seh-NES-ens) The state of being old.

senile (SEE-nile) Characteristic of old age.

senility (seh-NIL-ih-tee) Old age.

sensorineural hearing loss (SEN-sor-ih-NYUR-al HEER-ing LOSS) Hearing loss caused by lesions of the inner ear or the auditory nerve.

sensory (SEN-soh-ree) Having the function of sensation; relating to structures of the nervous system that carry impulses to the brain.

septum (SEP-tum) A wall dividing two cavities. Plural *septa*.

serosa (seh-ROH-sa) Outermost covering of the alimentary tract.

serotonin (ser-oh-TOH-nin) A neurotransmitter in the central and peripheral nervous systems.

serous (SEER-us) Thicker and less transparent than water.

serum (SEER-um) Fluid remaining after removal of cells and fibrin clot.

shock (SHOCK) Sudden physical or mental collapse or circulatory collapse.

shunt (SHUNT) A bypass or diversion of fluid, such as blood.

sibling (SIB-ling) Brother or sister.

sigmoid (SIG-moyd) Sigmoid colon is shaped like an "S."

sigmoidoscopy (sig-moi-DOS-koh-pee) Endoscopic examination of the sigmoid colon.

sign (SINE) Physical evidence of a disease process.

silicosis (sil-ih-KOH-sis) Fibrotic lung disease from inhaling silica particles.

sinoatrial (SA) node (sigh-noh-AY-tree-al NODE) The center of modified cardiac muscle fibers in the wall of the right atrium that acts as the pacemaker for the heart rhythm.

sinus (SIGH-nus) Cavity or hollow space in a bone or other tissue.

sinus rhythm (SIGH-nus RITH-um) The normal (optimal) heart rhythm arising from the sinoatrial node.

sinusitis (sigh-nuh-SIGH-tis) Inflammation of the lining of a sinus.

skeletal (SKEL-eh-tal) Pertaining to the bones.

smegma (SMEG-mah) Oily material produced by the glans and prepuce.

Snellen letter chart (SNEL-en LET-er CHART) Test for acuity of distance vision.

snore (SNOR) Noise produced by vibrations in the structures of the nasopharynx.

sociopath (SOH-see-oh-path) Person with antisocial personality disorder.

soleus (SOH-lee-us) Large muscle of the calf.

somatic (soh-MAT-ik) Relating to the body in general; *or* pertaining to a division of the peripheral nervous system serving the skeletal muscles.

somatoform (soh-MAT-oh-form) Physical symptoms occurring without identifiable physical cause.

somatostatin (SOH-mah-toh-STAT-in) Hormone that inhibits release of growth hormone and insulin.

somatotropin (SOH-mah-toh-TROH-pin) Hormone of the anterior pituitary that stimulates growth of body tissues. Also called *growth hormone.*

sonographer (so-NOG-rah-fer) The technician who performs a sonogram.

spasmodic (spaz-MOD-ik) Having intermittent spasms or contractions.

spastic (SPAS-tik) Increased muscle tone on movement.

specificity (spes-ih-FIS-ih-tee) State of having a fixed relation to a particular entity.

sperm (SPERM) Mature male sex cell. Also called *spermatozoon.*

spermatic (SPER-mat-ik) Pertaining to sperm.

spermatid (SPER-mah-tid) A cell late in the development process of sperm.

spermatocele (SPER-mat-oh-seal) Cyst of the epididymis that contains sperm.

spermatogenesis (SPER-mat-oh-JEN-eh-sis) The process by which male germ cells differentiate into sperm.

spermatozoa (SPER-mat-oh-ZOH-ah) Sperm (plural of *spermatozoon*).

spermicidal (SPER-mih-SIDE-al) Pertaining to sperm.

spermicide (SPER-mih-side) Agent that destroys sperm.

sphenoid bone (SFEE-noyd BONE) Wedge-shaped bone that forms part of the base of the cranium and the orbits.

spherocyte (SFEER-oh-site) A spherical cell.

spherocytosis (SFEER-oh-sigh-TOH-sis) Presence of spherocytes in the blood.

sphincter (SFINK-ter) Band of muscle that encircles an opening; when it contracts, the opening squeezes closed.

sphygmomanometer (SFIG-moh-mah-NOM-ih-ter) Instrument for measuring arterial blood pressure.

spina bifida (SPY-nah BIH-fih-dah) Failure of one or more vertebral arches to close during fetal development.

spina bifida cystica (SPY-nah BIH-fih-dah SIS-tik-ah) Meninges and spinal cord protrude through the absent vertebral arch and have the appearance of a cyst.

spina bifida occulta (SPY-nah BIH-fi-dah oh-KUL-tah) The deformity of the vertebral arch is not apparent from the skin surface.

spiral fracture (SPY-ral FRAK-chur) A fracture in the shape of a coil.

spirochete (SPY-roh-keet) Spiral-shaped bacterium causing a sexually transmitted disease (syphilis).

spirometer (spy-ROM-eh-ter) An instrument used to measure respiratory volumes.

spirometry (spy-ROM-eh-tree) Use of a spirometer.

spleen (SPLEEN) Vascular, lymphatic organ in the left upper quadrant of the abdomen.

splenectomy (spleh-NEK-toh-mee) Surgical removal of the spleen.

splenomegaly (spleh-noh-MEG-ah-lee) Enlarged spleen.

spondylosis (spon-dih-LOH-sis) Degenerative osteoarthritis of the spine.

spongiosum (spun-jee-OH-sum) Spongelike tissue.

sputum (SPYU-tum) Matter coughed up and spat out by individuals with respiratory disorders.

squamous cell (SKWAY-mus SELL) Flat, scalelike epithelial cell.

stage (STAYJ) Definition of the extent and dissemination of a malignant neoplasm.

staging (STAY-jing) Process of determining the extent of the distribution of a neoplasm.

stapes (STAY-pees) Inner (medial) one of the three ossicles of the middle ear; shaped like a stirrup.

status epilepticus (STAT-us ep-ih-LEP-tik-us) A recurrent state of seizure activity lasting longer than a specific time frame (usually 30 minutes).

stem cell (STEM SELL) Undifferentiated cell found in a differentiated tissue that can divide to yield the specialized cells in that tissue.

stenosis (steh-NOH-sis) Narrowing of a canal or passage, as in the narrowing of a heart valve.

stent (STENT) Wire mesh tube used to keep arteries open.

stereopsis (ster-ee-OP-sis) Three-dimensional vision.

stereotactic (STER-ee-oh-TAK-tik) Pertaining to a precise three-dimensional method to locate a lesion.

sterile (STER-ill) Free from all living organisms and their spores; *or* unable to fertilize or reproduce.

sternum (STIR-num) Long, flat bone forming the center of the anterior wall of the chest.

steroid (STER-oyd) Large family of chemical substances found in many drugs, hormones, and body components.

stethoscope (STETH-oh-skope) Instrument for listening to cardiac and respiratory sounds.

stimulant (STIM-you-lant) Agent that excites or strengthens functional activity.

stimulation (stim-you-LAY-shun) Arousal to increased functional activity.

stoma (STOH-mah) Artificial opening.

strabismus (strah-BIZ-mus) A turning of an eye away from its normal position.

strain (STRAIN) Overstretch or tear in a muscle or tendon.

stratum basale (STRAH-tum ba-SAL-eh) Deepest layer of the epidermis, from which the other cells originate and migrate.

streptokinase (strep-toh-KIE-nase) An enzyme that dissolves clots.

striated muscle (STRIE-ay-ted MUSS-el) Another term for *skeletal muscle.*

striation (strie-AY-shun) Stripes.

stricture (STRICK-shur) Narrowing of a tube.

stridor (STRIE-door) High-pitched noise made when there is a respiratory obstruction in the larynx or trachea.

stroke (STROHK) Acute clinical event caused by an impaired cerebral circulation.

stroma (STROH-mah) Connective tissue framework that supports the parenchyma of an organ or gland.

subarachnoid space (sub-ah-RAK-noyd SPASE) Space between the pia mater and the arachnoid membrane.

subclavian (sub-CLAY-vee-an) Underneath the clavicle.

subcutaneous (sub-kew-TAY-nee-us) Below the skin. Also known as *hypodermic.*

subdural (sub-DUR-al) Located in the space between the dura mater and the arachnoid membrane.

sublingual (sub-LING-wal) Underneath the tongue.

subluxation (sub-luk-SAY-shun) An incomplete dislocation in which some contact between the joint surfaces remains.

submandibular (sub-man-DIB-you-lar) Underneath the mandible.

submucosa (sub-mew-KOH-sa) Tissue layer underneath the mucosa.

suicidal (SOO-ih-SIGH-dal) Wanting to kill oneself.

sulcus (SUL-cuss) Groove on the surface of the cerebral hemispheres that separates gyri. Plural *sulci.*

superior (soo-PEE-ree-or) Situated above.

supinate (SOO-pih-nate) Rotate the forearm so that the surface of the palm faces anteriorly in the anatomical position.

supination (soo-pih-NAY-shun) Process of lying face upward or turning an arm or foot so that the palm or sole is facing up.

supine (soo-PINE) Lying face up, flat on your spine.

suprapubic (SOO-prah-PYU-bik) Above the symphysis pubis.

surfactant (ser-FAK-tant) A protein and fat compound that creates surface tension to hold lung alveolar walls apart.

susceptible (suh-SEP-tih-bull) Capable of being affected by.

suture (SOO-chur) Place where two bones are joined together by a fibrous band continuous with their periosteum, as in the skull; *or* a stitch to hold the edges of a wound together. Plural *sutures.*

sympathetic (sim-pah-THET-ik) Pertaining to the part of the autonomic nervous system operating at the unconscious level.

sympathy (SIM-pa-thee) Appreciation and concern for another person's mental and emotional state.

symphysis (SIM-feh-sis) Two bones joined by fibrocartilage. Plural *symphyses.*

symptom (SIMP-tum) Departure from normal health experienced by the patient.

symptomatic (simp-toh-MAT-ik) Pertaining to the symptoms of a disease.

synapse (SIN-aps) Junction between two nerve cells, or a nerve fiber and its target cell, where electrical impulses are transmitted between the cells.

synchondrosis (sin-kon-DROH-sis) A rigid articulation (joint) formed by cartilage. Plural *synchondroses.*

syncope (SIN-koh-pee) Temporary loss of consciousness and postural tone due to diminished cerebral blood flow.

syndesmosis (sin-dez-MOH-sis) A rigid articulation (joint) formed by ligaments. Plural *syndesmoses*.

syndrome (SIN-drohm) Combination of signs and symptoms associated with a particular disease process.

synovial (sih-NOH-vee-al) Pertaining to synovial fluid and synovial membrane.

synthesis (SIN-the-sis) The process of building a compound from different elements.

synthetic (sin-THET-ik) Built up or put together from simpler compounds.

syphilis (SIF-ih-lis) Sexually transmitted disease caused by a spirochete.

syringomyelia (sih-RING-oh-my-EE-lee-ah) Abnormal longitudinal cavities in the spinal cord that cause paresthesias and muscle weakness.

systemic (sis-TEM-ik) Relating to the entire organism.

systemic lupus erythematosus (sis-TEM-ik LOO-pus er-ih-THEE-mah-toh-sus) Inflammatory connective tissue disease affecting the whole body.

systole (SIS-toh-lee) Contraction of the heart muscle.

T

tachycardia (tak-ih-KAR-dee-ah) Rapid heart rate (above 100 beats per minute).

tachypnea (tak-ip-NEE-ah) Rapid breathing.

tactile (TAK-tile) Relating to touch.

talipes (TAL-ip-eez) Deformity of the foot involving the talus.

talus (TAY-luss) The tarsal bone that articulates with the tibia to form the ankle joint.

tampon (TAM-pon) Plug or pack in a cavity to absorb or stop bleeding.

tamponade (tam-poh-NAID) Pathologic compression of an organ such as the heart.

tangent (TAN-jent) Sudden change of course.

tangentiality (tan-jen-shee-AL-ih-tee) Disturbance in thought processes, which move rapidly from one topic to another.

tarsus (TAR-sus) The collection of seven bones in the foot that form the ankle and instep; *or* the flat fibrous plate that gives shape to the outer edges of the eyelids.

tartar (TAR-tar) Calcified deposit at the gingival margin of the teeth. Also called *dental calculus*.

taste (TAYST) Sensation from chemicals on the taste buds.

Tay-Sachs disease (TAY-SAKS diz-EEZ) Congenital fatal disorder of fat metabolism.

temporal bones (TEM-por-al BONES) Bones that form the sides and part of the base of the cranium.

temporal lobe (TEM-por-al LOBE) Posterior two-thirds of the cerebral hemispheres.

temporomandibular joint (TMJ) (TEM-por-oh-man-DIB-you-lar JOYNT) The joint between the temporal bone and the mandible.

tendinitis (ten-dih-NIE-tis) Inflammation of a tendon. Also spelled *tendonitis*.

tendon (TEN-dun) Fibrous band that connects muscle to bone.

tenosynovitis (TEN-oh-sine-oh-VIE-tis) Inflammation of a tendon and its surrounding synovial sheath.

teratogen (TER-ah-toh-jen) Agent that produces fetal deformities.

teratogenesis (TER-ah-toh-JEN-eh-sis) Process involved in producing fetal deformities.

teratoma (ter-ah-TOH-mah) Neoplasm of a testis or ovary containing multiple tissues from other sites in the body.

testicle (TES-tih-kul) One of the male reproductive glands. Also called *testis*.

testis (TES-tis) A synonym for testicle. Plural *testes*.

testosterone (tes-TOSS-ter-ohn) Powerful androgen produced by the testes.

tetanus (TET-ah-nuss) A disease with painful, tonic, muscular contractions caused by the toxin produced by *Clostridium tetani*.

tetany (TET-ah-nee) Severe muscle twitches, cramps, and spasms.

tetralogy of Fallot (TOF) (teh-TRAL-oh-jee OV fah-LOH) Set of four congenital heart defects occurring together.

thalamus (THAL-ah-mus) Mass of gray matter underneath the ventricle in each cerebral hemisphere.

thalassemia (thal-ah-SEE-mee-ah) Group of inherited blood disorders that produce a hemolytic anemia.

thenar (THEE-nar) The fleshy mass at the base of the thumb.

therapeutic (THAIR-ah-PYU-tik) Relating to the treatment of a disease or disorder.

therapist (THAIR-ah-pist) Professional trained in the practice of a particular therapy.

therapy (THAIR-ah-pee) Systematic treatment of a disease, dysfunction, or disorder.

thoracentesis (THOR-ah-sen-TEE-sis) Insertion of a needle into the pleural cavity to withdraw fluid or air. Also called *pleural tap*.

thoracic (thor-ASS-ik) Pertaining to the chest (thorax).

thoracoscopy (thor-ah-KOS-koh-pee) Examination of the pleural cavity with an endoscope.

thoracotomy (thor-ah-KOT-oh-mee) Incision through the chest wall.

thrombin (THROM-bin) Enzyme that forms fibrin.

thrombocyte (THROM-boh-site) Another name for *platelet*.

thrombocytopenia (THROM-boh-sigh-toh-PEE-nee-ah) Deficiency of platelets in circulating blood.

thromboembolism (THROM-boh-EM-boh-lizm) A piece of detached blood clot (embolus) blocking a distant blood vessel.

thrombolysis (throm-BOL-ih-sis) Dissolving a thrombus (clot).

thrombophlebitis (THROM-boh-fleh-BIE-tis) Inflammation of a vein with clot formation.

thrombosis (throm-BOH-sis) Formation of a thrombus.

thrombus (THROM-bus) A clot attached to a diseased blood vessel or heart lining.

thrush (THRUSH) Infection with *Candida albicans*.

thymectomy (thigh-MEK-toh-mee) Surgical removal of the thymus gland.

thymoma (thigh-MOH-mah) Benign tumor of the thymus gland.

thymus (THIGH-mus) Endocrine gland located in the mediastinum.

thyroid (THIGH-royd) Endocrine gland in the neck; *or* a cartilage of the larynx.

thyroid hormone (THIGH-royd HOR-mohn) Collective term for the two thyroid hormones, T_3 and T_4.

thyroid storm (THIGH-royd STORM) Medical crisis and emergency due to excess thyroid hormones.

thyroidectomy (thigh-roy-DEK-toh-mee) Surgical removal of the thyroid gland.

thyroiditis (thigh-roy-DIE-tis) Inflammation of the thyroid gland.

thyrotoxicosis (THIGH-roh-tok-sih-KOH-sis) Disorder caused by excessive thyroid hormone production.

thyrotropin (thigh-roh-TROH-pin) Hormone from the anterior pituitary gland that stimulates function of the thyroid gland.

thyroxine (thigh-ROK-seen) Thyroid hormone T_4, tetraiodothyronine.

tibia (TIB-ee-ah) The larger bone of the lower leg.

tic (TIK) Sudden, involuntary, repeated contraction of muscles.

tic douloureux (TIK duh-luh-RUE) Painful, sudden, spasmodic involuntary contractions of the facial muscles supplied by the trigeminal nerve. Also called *trigeminal neuralgia.*

tinea (TIN-ee-ah) General term for a group of related skin infections caused by different species of fungi.

tinnitus (TIN-ih-tus) Persistent ringing, whistling, clicking, or booming noise in the ears.

tissue (TISH-you) Collection of similar cells.

tolerance (TOL-er-ants) The capacity to become accustomed to a stimulus or drug.

tomography (toh-MOG-rah-fee) Radiographic image of a selected slice of tissue.

tone (TONE) Tension present in resting muscles.

tongue (TUNG) Mobile muscle mass in the mouth; bears the taste buds.

tonic-clonic seizure (TON-ik-KLON-ik SEE-zhur) Generalized seizure due to epileptic activity in all or most of the brain.

tonometer (toh-NOM-eh-ter) Instrument for determining intraocular pressure.

tonometry (toh-NOM-eh-tree) The measurement of intraocular pressure.

tonsil (TON-sill) Mass of lymphoid tissue on either side of the throat at the back of the tongue.

tonsillectomy (ton-sih-LEK-toh-mee) Surgical removal of the tonsils.

tonsillitis (ton-sih-LIE-tis) Inflammation of the tonsils.

topical (TOP-ih-kal) Medication applied to the skin to obtain a local effect.

torsion (TOR-shun) The act or result of twisting.

Tourette syndrome (tur-ET SIN-drome) Disorder of multiple motor and vocal tics.

toxic (TOK-sick) Pertaining to a toxin.

toxicity (tok-SIS-ih-tee) The state of being poisonous.

toxin (TOK-sin) Poisonous substance formed by a cell or organism.

trachea (TRAY-kee-ah) Air tube from the larynx to the bronchi.

trachealis (tray-kee-AY-lis) Pertaining to the trachea.

tracheostomy (tray-kee-OST-oh-mee) Surgical opening into the windpipe, usually so that a tube can be inserted to assist breathing.

tracheotomy (tray-kee-OT-oh-mee) Incision made into the trachea to create a tracheostomy.

tract (TRAKT) Bundle of nerve fibers with a common origin and destination.

tranquilizer (TRANG-kwih-lie-zer) Agent that calms without sedating or depressing.

transcriptionist (tran-SCRIP-shun-ist) One who makes the copy of dictated material.

transdermal (trans-DER-mal) Going across or through the skin.

transducer (trans-DYU-sir) Device that converts energy from one form to another.

transfusion (trans-FYU-zhun) Transfer of blood or a blood component from donor to recipient.

transplant (TRANZ-plant) The tissue or organ used; *or* the act of transferring tissue from one person to another.

transplantation (TRANZ-plan-TAY-shun) The moving of tissue or an organ from one person or place to another.

transverse (trans-VERS) Pertaining to the horizontal plane dividing the body into upper and lower portions.

transverse fracture (trans-VERS FRAK-chur) A fracture perpendicular to the long axis of the bone.

tremor (TREM-or) Small, shaking, involuntary, repetitive movements of hands, extremities, neck, or jaw.

triceps brachii (TRY-sepz BRAY-kee-eye) Muscle of the arm that has three heads or points of origin.

Trichomonas **(trik-oh-MOH-nas)** A parasite causing a sexually transmitted disease.

trichomoniasis (TRIK-oh-moh-NIE-ah-sis) Infection with *Trichomonas vaginalis.*

tricuspid (try-KUSS-pid) Having three points; a tricuspid heart valve has three flaps.

trigeminal (try-GEM-in-al) Fifth (V) cranial nerve, with its three different branches supplying the face.

triglyceride (trie-GLISS-eh-ride) Any of a group of fats containing three fatty acids.

triiodothyronine (trie-EYE-oh-doh-THIE-roh-neen) Thyroid hormone T_3.

trimester (TRY-mes-ter) One-third of the length of a full-term pregnancy.

triplegia (try-PLEE-jee-ah) Paralysis of three limbs.

trochlear (TROHK-lee-ar) Fourth (IV) cranial nerve; supplies one muscle of the eye.

tropic (TROH-pik) Tropic hormones stimulate other endocrine glands to produce hormones.

trypsin (TRIP-sin) Enzyme that breaks down protein.

tuberculosis (too-BER-kyu-LOH-sis) Infectious disease that can infect any organ or tissue.

tumor (TOO-mer) Any abnormal swelling.

tunica (TYU-nih-kah) A layer in the wall of a blood vessel or other tubular structure.

tunica vaginalis (TYU-nih-kah vaj-ih-NAHL-iss) Covering, particularly of a tubular structure. The tunica vaginalis is the sheath of the testis and epididymis.

turbinate (TUR-bin-ate) Another name for the nasal conchae on the lateral walls of the nasal cavity.

tympanic (tim-PAN-ik) Pertaining to the tympanic membrane or tympanic cavity.

tympanostomy (tim-pan-OS-toh-mee) Surgically created new opening in the tympanic membrane to allow fluid to drain from the middle ear.

U

ulcer (ULL-sir) Erosion of an area of skin or mucosa.

ulcerative (UL-sir-ah-tiv) Marked by an ulcer or ulcers.

ulna (UL-nah) The medial and larger bone of the forearm.

ulnar (UL-nar) Pertaining to the ulna or any of the structures (artery, vein, nerve) named after it.

ultrasonography (UL-trah-soh-NOG-rah-fee) Delineation of deep structures using sound waves.

ultrasound (UL-trah-sownd) Use of very-high-frequency sound waves.

umbilical (um-BIL-ih-kal) Pertaining to the umbilicus or the center of the abdomen.

umbilicus (um-BIL-ih-kus) Pit in the abdomen where the umbilical cord entered the fetus.

unipolar disorder (you-nih-POLE-ar dis-OR-der) Depression.

uranium (you-RAY-nee-um) Radioactive metallic element.

urea (you-REE-ah) End product of nitrogen metabolism.

uremia (you-REE-mee-ah) The complex of symptoms arising from renal failure.

ureter (you-REET-er) Tube that connects the kidney to the urinary bladder.

ureteroscope (you-REE-ter-oh-skope) Endoscope to view the inside of the ureter.

ureteroscopy (you-REE-ter-OS-koh-pee) Examination of the ureter.

urethra (you-REE-thra) Canal leading from the bladder to outside.

urethritis (you-ree-THRIE-tis) Inflammation of the urethra.

urethrotomy (you-ree-THROT-oh-mee) Incision of a stricture of the urethra.

urinalysis (you-rih-NAL-ih-sis) Examination of urine to separate it into its elements and define their kind and/or quantity.

urinary (YUR-in-air-ee) Pertaining to urine.

urination (yur-ih-NAY-shun) The act of passing urine.

urine (YUR-in) Fluid and dissolved substances excreted by the kidney.

urologist (you-ROL-oh-jist) Medical specialist in disorders of the urinary system.

urology (you-ROL-oh-jee) Medical specialty of disorders of the urinary system.

urticaria (ur-tih-KARE-ee-ah) Rash of itchy wheals (hives).

uterus (YOU-ter-us) Organ in which an egg develops into a fetus.

uvea (YOU-vee-ah) Middle coat of the eyeball—includes the iris, ciliary body, and choroid.

uveitis (you-vee-IE-tis) Inflammation of the uvea.

uvula (YOU-vyu-lah) Fleshy projection of the soft palate.

V

vaccination (vak-sih-NAY-shun) Administration of a vaccine.

vaccine (vak-SEEN) Preparation to generate active immunity.

vagina (vah-JIE-nah) Female genital canal extending from the uterus to the vulva.

vaginal (VAJ-in-al) Pertaining to the vagina.

vaginitis (vah-jih-NIE-tis) Inflammation of the vagina.

vaginosis (vah-jih-NOH-sis) Any disease of the vagina.

vagus (VAY-gus) Tenth (X) cranial nerve; supplies many different organs throughout the body.

varicocele (VAIR-ih-koh-seal) Varicose veins of the spermatic cord.

varicose (VAIR-ih-kos) Characterized by or affected with varices.

varix (VAIR-iks) Dilated, tortuous vein. Plural *varices*.

vasectomy (vah-SEK-toh-mee) Excision of a segment of the ductus deferens.

vasoconstriction (VAY-soh-con-STRIK-shun) Reduction in diameter of a blood vessel.

vasodilation (VAY-soh-die-LAY-shun) Increase in diameter of a blood vessel.

vasopressin (vay-soh-PRESS-in) Pituitary hormone that constricts blood vessels and decreases urine output. Also called *antidiuretic hormone (ADH)*.

vasovasostomy (VAY-soh-vay-SOS-toh-mee) Reanastomosis of the ductus deferens to restore the flow of sperm. Also called *vasectomy reversal*.

vegetative (VEJ-eh-tay-tiv) Functioning unconsciously as plant life is assumed to do.

vein (VANE) Blood vessel carrying blood toward the heart.

vena cava (VEE-nah KAY-vah) One of the two largest veins in the body. Plural *venae cavae*.

venogram (VEE-noh-gram) Radiograph of veins after injection of radiopaque contrast material.

venous (VEE-nus) Pertaining to venous blood or the venous circulation.

ventilation (ven-tih-LAY-shun) Movement of gases into and out of the lungs.

ventral (VEN-tral) Pertaining to the belly or situated nearer to the surface of the belly.

ventricle (VEN-trih-kel) A cavity of the heart or brain.

venule (VEN-yule) Small vein leading from the capillary network.

vermiform (VER-mih-form) Worm shaped; used as a descriptor for the appendix.

vernix caseosa (VER-niks kay-see-OH-sah) Cheesy substance covering the skin of the fetus.

verruca (ver-ROO-cah) Wart caused by a virus.

vertex (VER-teks) Topmost point of the vault of the skull.

vertigo (VER-tih-goh) Sensation of spinning or whirling.

vesicle (VES-ih-kull) Small sac containing liquid; for example, a blister or semen.

vestibule (VES-tih-byul) Space at the entrance to a canal.

vestibulectomy (ves-tib-you-LEK-toh-mee) Surgical excision of the vulva.

vestibulocochlear (ves-TIB-you-loh-KOK-lee-ar) Eighth (VIII) cranial nerve; carrying information for the senses of hearing and balance.

villus (VILL-us) Thin, hairlike projection, particularly of a mucous membrane lining a cavity. Plural *villi*.

virilism (VIR-ih-lizm) Development of masculine characteristics by a woman or girl.

virulent (VIR-you-lent) Extremely toxic or pathogenic.

virus (VIE-rus) Group of infectious agents that require living cells for growth and reproduction.

visceral (VISS-er-al) Pertaining to the internal organs.

viscosity (vis-KOS-ih-tee) The resistance of a fluid to flowing.

viscous (VISS-kus) Sticky; resistant to flow.

visual acuity (VIH-zhoo-wal ah-KYU-ih-tee) Sharpness and clearness of vision.

vital signs (VIE-tal SIGNS) A procedure during a physical examination in which temperature (T), pulse (P), respirations (R), and blood pressure (BP) are measured to assess general health and cardiorespiratory function.

vitamin (VIE-tah-min) Essential organic substance necessary in small amounts for normal cell function.

vitiligo (vit-ill-EYE-go) Nonpigmented white patches on otherwise normal skin.

vitreous humor (VIT-ree-us HEW-mor) A gelatinous liquid in the posterior cavity of the eyeball with the appearance of glass.

vocal (VOH-kal) Pertaining to the voice.

void (VOYD) To evacuate urine or feces.

voluntary muscle (VOL-un-tare-ee MUSS-el) Muscle that is under the control of the will.

vomer (VOH-mer) Lower nasal septum.

vulva (VUL-vah) Female external genitalia.

vulvodynia (vul-voh-DIN-ee-uh) Chronic vulvar pain.

vulvovaginitis (VUL-voh-vaj-ih-NIE-tis) Inflammation of the vagina and vulva.

W

Weber test (VAY-ber TEST) Test for sensorineural hearing loss.

whiplash (WHIP-lash) Symptoms caused by sudden, uncontrolled extension and flexion of the neck, often in an automobile accident.

white matter (WITE MATT-er) Regions of the brain and spinal cord occupied by bundles of axons.

whooping cough (WHO-ping KAWF) Infectious disease with spasmodic, intense cough ending on a whoop (stridor). Also called *pertussis*.

Wilms tumor (WILMZ TOO-mor) Cancerous kidney tumor of childhood. Also known as *nephroblastoma*.

wound (WOOND) Any injury that interrupts the continuity of skin or a mucous membrane.

X

xenograft (ZEN-oh-graft) A graft from another species. Also known as *heterograft*.

Y

yolk sac (YOKE SACK) Source of blood cells and future sex cells for the fetus.

Z

zygote (ZIE-goht) Cell resulting from the union of the sperm and egg.

Reflux, 115, 116, 151
Refract, 531
Refraction, 530, 531
Refractive error, 542
Refractive surgery, 545
Refractometer, 542, 544
Refractory, 194, 195
Regenerate, 76
Regeneration, 76
Regimens, 668, 669
Regional enteritis, 118, 119
Regional lymphadenectomy, 413
Regions, abdominal, 45–46
Registered nurse (RN), 221, 574
Registered respiratory therapists (RRTs),
    424, 444
Regulate, 147
Regurgitate, 331, 332
Regurgitation, 115, 116
Rehabilitation, 517
Rehabilitation medicine, 517
Reminiscence therapy (RT), 647
Remissions, 291
Renal, 147, 325
Renal adenoma, 152
Renal angiogram, 159
Renal arteries, 324
Renal cell carcinoma, 152, 162, 173
Renal drugs, 162
Renal pelvis, 148
Renal stones, 160
Renal transplant, 162
Renal tubule, 148
Renin, 147, 149
Renin-angiotensin, 346
Repetitive transcranial magnetic
    stimulation, 626
Replicate, 40, 41
Reproduction, 185
Reproductive, 37, 38, 184, 185
Reproductive system. *See* Female
    reproductive system; Male
    reproductive system
Resect, 130, 447
Resection, 130, 195, 447
Resectoscope, 194, 195
Reservoir, 399, 400
Resistance, 402, 589
Resistant, 402
Resorption, 481, 482, 491
Respiration, 425, 426, 433, 503
Respirator, 426
Respiratory, 37, 38, 426

Respiratory care practitioners, 424
Respiratory center, 270
Respiratory distress syndrome (RDS), 239
Respiratory drugs, 447–448
Respiratory membrane, 433
Respiratory system, 424–447
    lower, 431–433
        diagnostic and therapeutic procedures
            for, 446
        disorders of, 437–439, 441
        lungs of, 431–433
        pharmacology for, 444–445
        pulmonary function tests for, 433,
            444–445
        respiration in, 433
        trachea of, 431
    organs and functions of, 37, 425l
    senescence of, 643
    symptoms and signs of disorders of,
        437–438
    upper, 427–428
        disorders of, 435–437
        larynx of, 428
        nose of, 427
        pharynx of, 427
Respiratory therapist, 15
Respiratory therapy technician (RT), 424
Restorative rehabilitation, 517, 519
Retained placenta, 234, 239
Rete testis, 184, 185
Retention, 156
Reticular, 271
Reticular formation, 270
Reticulocytes, 365, 366
Reticulum, 271
Retina, 530–532
    diseases of, 538–539
    examination of, 545
Retinal, 531
Retinal cryopexy, 545
Retinal detachment, 538
Retinoblastoma, 538, 539, 543
Retinoids, 81, 82
Retinopathy, 538, 539, 545
Retraction, 439, 440
Retrograde, 130, 160
Retrograde pyelogram, 159
Retroversion, 219
Retrovert, 8
Retroverted, 218, 219
Retrovirus, 164, 408, 409
Reye syndrome, 285, 286
Rh, 370

Rhabdomyolysis, 510, 511
Rhabdomyosarcoma, 659, 660
Rhesus (Rh) blood group, 370–371
Rhesus factor, 370, 371
Rheumatic, 484
Rheumatic fever, 331
Rheumatic nodules, 484
Rheumatism, 484
Rheumatoid arthritis (RA), 484, 491, 493
Rhinitis, 435, 437
Rhinoplasty, 446, 447
Rhonchi, 445
Rhonchus, 445, 446
Rhythm method, 242
Ribosomes, 34, 35
Rickets, 481, 482
Right common carotid artery, 324
Right lower quadrant (RLQ), 45
Right lymphatic duct, 396
Right subclavian artery, 324
Right subclavian vein, 396
Right upper quadrant (RUQ), 45
Rinne test, 557, 558
RIT, 689
Rivaroxaban, 382
RLQ, 45
RN, 221, 574
Robot-assisted laparoscopic
    surgery, 227
Rods, 531
Root canals, 97
Roots, 2, 3, 97, 98
    word, 2, 3
Rosacea, 70, 71
Rotation, 467
Rotation tests, 558
Rotational atherectomy, 344
Rotator cuff, 505, 510
Rotator cuff muscles, 505
Rotator cuff tears, 510
Routes of administration, 702–704
Routine urinalysis (UA), 158
Roux-en-Y, 129, 130
RRT, 424
RT, 424
Ruga, 97, 207
Rugae, 96, 97, 206, 207
Rule of Nines, 76
Runner's knee, 486
Rupture, 71, 72
Ruptured spleen, 405
RUQ, 45
Rx, 710